Immunology of Human Infection

Part I: Bacteria, Mycoplasmae, Chlamydiae, and Fungi

Comprehensive Immunology

Series Editors: ROBERT A. GOOD and STACEY B. DAY
Memorial Sloan-Kettering Cancer Center
New York, New York

Immunology of Human Infection

Part I: Bacteria, Mycoplasmae, Chlamydiae, and Fungi

Edited by
ANDRÉ J. NAHMIAS
Emory University
Atlanta, Georgia

and
RICHARD J. O'REILLY
Memorial Sloan-Kettering Cancer Center
New York, New York

PLENUM MEDICAL BOOK COMPANY
New York and London

Library of Congress Cataloging in Publication Data

Main entry under title:

Bacteria, mycoplasmae, chlamydiae, and fungi.

(Immunology of human infection; pt. 1) (Comprehensive immunology; v. 8)
Bibliography: p.
Includes index.
1. Bacterial diseases — Immunological aspects. 2. Chlamydia infections — Immunological
aspects. 3. Mycoplasma diseases — Immunological aspects. 4. Mycoses — Immunological
aspects. I. Nahmias, André J. II. O'Reilly, Richard J. III. Series. IV. Series: Comprehensive
immunology; v. 8. [DNLM: 1. Communicable diseases — Immunology. 2. Infection —
Immunology. QW700 I335]
RC110.I45 pt. 1 [RC115]   616.9s [616.9'2]   79-9162
ISBN 0-306-40257-2

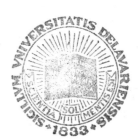

© 1981 Plenum Publishing Corporation
233 Spring Street, New York, N. Y. 10013

Plenum Medical Book Company is an imprint of Plenum Publishing Corporation

Printed in the United States of America

Contributors

Arthur J. Ammann   Division of Pediatric Immunology, Pediatric Clinical Research Center, and Department of Pediatrics, University of California, San Francisco, California

Lane Barksdale   Department of Microbiology, New York University School of Medicine and Medical Center, New York, New York

Ward E. Bullock   Department of Medicine, University of Kentucky Medical Center, Lexington, Kentucky

Wallace A. Clyde, Jr.   Department of Pediatrics, University of North Carolina School of Medicine, Chapel Hill, North Carolina

Dan Danielsson   Department of Clinical Bacteriology and Immunology, Central County Hospital, Orebro, Sweden

Floyd W. Denny   Department of Pediatrics, University of North Carolina School of Medicine, Chapel Hill, North Carolina

Richard D. Diamond   Infectious Disease Division, Department of Medicine, University Hospital, and Boston University School of Medicine, Boston, Massachusetts

Gerald W. Fernald   Department of Pediatrics, University of North Carolina School of Medicine, Chapel Hill, North Carolina

Richard A. Finkelstein   Department of Microbiology, University of Missouri School of Medicine, Columbia, Missouri

Alan A. Glynn   Bacteriology Department, Wright–Fleming Institute, St. Mary's Hospital Medical School, London, England

Ronald Gold   Hospital for Sick Children, Toronto, Canada

Sarah F. Grappel   Skin and Cancer Hospital, Temple University Health Sciences Center, Philadelphia, Pennsylvania. *Present address:* Smith Kline & French Laboratories, Philadelphia, Pennsylvania

W. Lee Hand   V.A. Medical Center (Atlanta), Decatur, Georgia, and Department of Medicine, Emory University School of Medicine, Atlanta, Georgia

Richard B. Hornick   Division of Infectious Diseases, University of Maryland School of Medicine, Baltimore, Maryland

Dexter H. Howard   Department of Microbiology and Immunology, School of Medicine, University of California, Los Angeles, California

Dwight W. Lambe, Jr.   Department of Microbiology, College of Medicine, East Tennessee State University, Johnson City, Tennessee

Hayes C. Lamont   Department of Microbiology, Harvard School of Public Health, Boston, Massachusetts. *Present address:* Department of Biology, Suffolk University, Boston, Massachusetts

Maurice J. Lefford   Department of Immunology and Microbiology, Wayne State University of Medicine, Detroit, Michigan

T. Lehner   Guy's Hospital Medical and Dental Schools, London Bridge, London, England

Martha L. Lepow   Department of Pediatrics, Albany Medical College, Albany, New York

Myron M. Levine   Division of Infectious Diseases, University of Maryland School of Medicine, Baltimore, Maryland

Stephen I. Morse   State University of New York, Downstate Medical Center, Brooklyn, New York

E. Richard Moxon   Eudowood Division of Infectious Diseases, Department of Pediatrics, The Johns Hopkins University School of Medicine, Baltimore, Maryland

Roger L. Nichols   Department of Microbiology, Harvard School of Public Health, Boston, Massachusetts

Robert J. North   Trudeau Institute, Inc., Saranac Lake, New York

J. Pepys   Clinical Immunology, Cardiothoracic Institute, University of London, Brompton, London, England

Peter L. Perine   Center for Disease Control, Venereal Disease Control Division, Atlanta, Georgia

Phillip K. Peterson   Departments of Pediatrics and Medicine, University of Minnesota School of Medicine, Minneapolis, Minnesota

Paul G. Quie   Departments of Pediatrics and Medicine, University of Minnesota School of Medicine, Minneapolis, Minnesota

James W. Smith   V.A. Medical Center and Department of Medicine, University of Texas (Southwestern) Medical School at Dallas, Dallas, Texas

Jan Verhoef   Departments of Pediatrics and Medicine, University of Minnesota School of Medicine, Minneapolis, Minnesota

Lewis W. Wannamaker   Departments of Pediatrics and Microbiology, University of Minnesota, Minneapolis, Minnesota

J. M. A. Wilton   Guy's Hospital Medical and Dental Schools, London Bridge, London, England

Preface

When we were first approached by the senior editors of this series to edit a book on interactions between the host and infectious agents, we accepted this offer as an exciting challenge. The only condition, readily agreed upon, was that such a book should focus on the immunology of infections in humans. Our reasons, if not biases, were severalfold. We sensed that the fields of microbiology and immunology, which had diverged as each was focusing on its individual search, were coming together. In agreement with the opinions expressed by Dr. Richard Krause in the Introduction, we strongly believed that the development of the immune system evolved in response to infectious agents and that the evolution of these agents was influenced in turn by the character of the host's responses. An intensive examination of the multitude of primitive or more recently developed host defense mechanisms to determine their relative contribution to man's resistance to a given infectious agent appeared to us to be of crucial basic and practical interest. Many immune mechanisms studied in animals were being explored in humans and it appeared timely to focus particularly on what was known about man's resistance to infectious agents, correlating this information with lessons learned from relevant experiments in animal models.

Having been involved ourselves in investigations of several different infectious agents, we immediately realized that general chapters on host interactions with one group of agents, such as bacteria, or even with agents within a family, such as herpesviruses, would not be sufficient. We thus had to come to grips with the need for selecting for review specific agents pathogenic for man. In general, we concentrated on agents of particular clinical importance. We included, however, opportunistic pathogens such as the anaerobic bacteria and *Pneumocystis carinii*, which have emerged to frustrate modern medicine's complex and intensive assault on malignant diseases, as well as the parasitic diseases that continue to ravage populations in countries where public health measures are inadequate to abort or contain the spread of infection. We included a chapter on the poxviruses, which have provided both a classical model for studying the immune response and a clear testimony to the potential of immunoprevention for eradicating a human disease. We also tried to anticipate future developments by incorporating, for example, a chapter on the immunology of oncornaviruses, a class of agents that, to date, has only been studied in animals.

In order to provide the reader with a broad yet comprehensive view of the variety and complexity of host–parasite interactions, we planned a series of chapters describing the systems contributing to the human host's resistance against exogenous pathogens, the biological processes that lead to infection, eradication of invading pathogens, and secondary immunopathology, and the factors intrinsic or extrinsic to the host, such as the host's genetic background, the endogenous microflora, concurrent infections, and modes of therapeutic intervention, which may modulate susceptibility or resistance. We also included chapters and discussions detailing the spectra of infections seen in hosts with known abnormalities of one or more of these defense systems, to provide the reader with some measures for assessing their relative contribution to resistance to a given pathogen. We also thought it would be valuable to include chapters on immunodiagnosis and on immunoprevention, to provide critical reviews of current and emerging techniques for serodiagnosis and to assess the impact of both established and recently developed vaccines on public health. What started out then to be one volume ultimately required three to achieve the necessary comprehensiveness.

The selections made may not satisfy some of our readers, who may find that their favorite "bug" was left out. This may not be entirely our fault, as we could no longer wait for two "promised" chapters. We apologize for the delay to some of our contributors. To all, however, we are most grateful for their enthusiastic response to our request to review current knowledge on the general or specific aspects of host interactions with infectious agents. We are also thankful to Ms. Hilary Evans and Mr. Peter Strupp of Plenum Publishing Corporation for all their assistance.

André J. Nahmias
Richard J. O'Reilly

Atlanta and New York

Introduction

A comprehensive series on the Immunology of Human Infection is long overdue. While books on the principles of immunology and those on infectious diseases serve important specialized purposes, in the end neither type of book adequately covers the complex interrelationships that underlie the immunology of infection. In the last analysis, the study of infection cannot proceed without the study of immunity. Indeed, infection and immunity are so intertwined that they are inseparable; they cannot be pulled apart. While this has always been the case, this reality has not necessarily been the guiding principle for those who are interested in either infection or immunity. For a variety of reasons, all too frequently there has been a polarization, with students of infection working outside the discipline of immunology and, contrariwise, those immersed in immunology working outside the discipline of microbiology. It is for these reasons that I welcome the opportunity to comment on this intimate relationship in the Introduction to this treatise edited by Drs. Nahmias and O'Reilly.

My theme then will be the interrelationships between microbiology and immunology. I would like to underscore three aspects of this relationship:

1. The dependence of the immune system upon the microbial world. The point of emphasis here is that persistent exposure to a variety of microbes is a propelling force behind the development and maturation of the immune system.
2. The occurrence of certain immunologic disorders that appear to be a strange amalgam of both infection and immunity.
3. The new opportunities for immunization, recognizing that we must remain alert because the risk of infection still prevails.

The development of the immune system occurs through the constant exposure throughout life to the ubiquitous microbes and viruses that inhabit the respiratory tract, the gastrointestinal tract, and other body surfaces. The immune system is relatively immature at birth, and its development depends upon this continuous bombardment by bacteria, viruses, and other antigens. At birth, the immune system in man is still incompletely prepared to perform its protective role. Many functions need to be primed by exposure to microorganisms in the environment. The usually harmless indigenous microbes are the antigenic stimuli that drive the immune system to maturation. It is this concept, it seems to me, that highlights the intimate relationship between microbes and the immune system.

The influence of immunity on the microbial world is as important as the influence of microbes on immunity. For example, the occurrence of widespread immunity to prevalent current serotypes of bacteria and viruses functions as a relentless selective pressure on the emergence of new serotypes.

We cannot escape these evolutionary considerations. We will shore up, to be sure, the defensive posture of immunity through new immunizations and new opportunities for manipulation of the immune system. But this will have countereffects on the microbial world to which we must remain alert. These countereffects have genetic, biochemical, and medical aspects. At the practical level we are all too aware, for example, of the emergence of antibiotic resistance among bacteria and parasites. So we must remain dedicated to understanding the basic biology and the medical microbiology of bacteria, viruses, parasites, and fungi. Knowledge from such research is needed to counter the persistent challenge that stems from microbial mutability.

My second point concerns those special immunologic disorders that appear to be a consequence of both infectious and immunologic processes. Still obscured in mystery are the pathways that lead from microbial infection through the immune system to a variety of diseases, such as rheumatoid arthritis, lupus erythematosus, acute nephritis, and acute rheumatic fever. The most celebrated examples, of course, are acute rheumatic fever and acute glomerulonephritis. Yet we remain largely in the dark about the pathogenic processes involved and the mechanisms whereby disease is initiated by prior infection.

We have been aware of the relationship between Group A streptococcal infections and acute rheumatic fever for at least 50 years. Most investigators argue that some sort of immune mechanism is involved in pathogenesis. Yet there is no absolute proof for a particular immunologic process. Indeed, the facts that bear on pathogenesis are precious few, despite all the work that has been done. I only hope that investigators interested in the new associations between infection and immunologic diseases will have greater success than did those of us who harvested disappointment from our effort to solve the rheumatic fever riddle.

What then are the new opportunities in immunization? Infectious diseases still remain the fifth most common cause of death in the United States. But beyond this issue of mortality, we all know the influence that an infectious disease has on the quality of life and the burden that infectious diseases place upon the health care delivery system. (The etymological origins of the word *influenza* are not accidental.) Several studies have called attention to the fact that at least one-fifth of patient visits to doctors' offices are for the treatment of infectious diseases.

Faced with the burden of infectious diseases, what is our plan of attack? First, I think we must recognize that there is no simple solution. There are many different infections, each with a distinctive biology and epidemiology. Given the rising tide of antibiotic resistance in many different bacteria and given the fact that infections spread from index cases to susceptible subjects prior to successful antibiotic treatment, we must remain alert to the new opportunities for immunization.

I cannot review here all of the new opportunities in immunization that stem from the application of recombinant DNA technology and hybridoma cell fusion. "Live" virus vaccines, perhaps new and resourceful uses of specially devised adjuvants—these and other developments may influence control of hepatitis, influenza, diarrhea, and other viral infections. We will capitalize also on the successful use of purified bacterial polysaccharides as vaccines. But overall, and for the work ahead, I doubt if we can break significant new ground by reapplying the conventional principles of immunochemical prophylaxis. We will need a new dimension, which will be the legacy of the future.

This legacy will draw on the new immunology, which is focused on the regulatory processes of the immune system. Revelation of these internal processes should illuminate new opportunities to manipulate the immune system. Equally important in this legacy of the future are studies of the genetics and biochemistry of microbes. Advances in molecular biology are penetrating the mysteries of antibiotic resistance, genetic and regulatory mechanisms, and biochemical determinants of infectious diseases.

In summary, I have emphasized the intimate and close association between the microbial world and the immune system. Without the microbial world, there would be no development of the immune system. Without the immune system, there would be no defense against the invasion of infection. But as immunity strikes back against infection, counterforces are erected that apply evolutionary pressures for the selection of new variants of pathogens. And when, for reasons that are still obscure to us, microbes induce distortions in the natural biological rhythms of the immune system, a whole series of immunologic disorders can occur.

I have stressed the importance of improving our immunization resources, if for no other reason than the fact that the drift toward antibiotic resistance will continue. We cannot escape these evolutionary events.

Finally, we must be alert to new opportunities if we are to develop novel or alternative approaches to immunologic manipulation and intervention for the prevention of infectious diseases and for the prevention and/or treatment of immunologic disorders. There may also emerge new opportunities for treatment, if not prevention, of those chronic diseases that now appear to be a strange amalgam of both infection and immunity, such as rheumatoid arthritis, chronic nephritis, multiple sclerosis, and lupus erythematosus.

Richard M. Krause

Director, National Institute of
Allergy and Infectious Diseases
National Institutes of Health
Bethesda, Maryland 20205

Contents

Bacteria

Chapter 8

Immunobiology of Diphtheria   171

Lane Barksdale

Chapter 15

Immunobiology of Leprosy   369

Ward E. Bullock

Chapter 16

Immunology of Syphilis   391

Peter L. Perine

Mycoplasmas

Chapter 17

Immunology of Mycoplasma Infection   **415**

Gerald W. Fernald, Wallace A. Clyde, Jr., and Floyd W. Denny

Chlamydiae

Fungi

Chapter 22

Fungi in Pulmonary Allergic Diseases   **561**

   J. Pepys

1

Bacterial Immunity

ALAN A. GLYNN

1. Introduction

1.1. Outline

This chapter outlines the major features of bacterial immunity and provides a framework in which to place the more detailed analyses presented later. The remarkable specificity of some host–parasite relations is illustrated by some clinical examples. A detailed description of the methods of bacterial attack is followed by a discussion of the ways in which they are contained by host defense mechanisms.

It is not possible in a single chapter to deal comprehensively with all the interactions between pathogenic bacteria and host defenses. Some of the most important will be discussed, arranged by site, since the site of an infection, surface, local tissue, or general systemic, is perhaps the major factor in determining which group of defense reactions is most effective.

1.2. Immune Responses to Bacteria

1.2.1. Specificity and Interactions

Immunity to infection has been studied with increasing intensity since Jenner and Pasteur. During the salad days of antibiotic optimism there was a transient neglect of immunity, but it was soon clear that, when host defenses are impaired, antibiotics provide only temporary and uncertain support. Knowledge of immune

responses is based partly on infection but owes much to fundamental work in transplant and tumor immunology and to experiments with red cells and proteins. Nevertheless, infections are more frequent than transplants or tumors, and more complex than a simple collection of antigenic stimuli.

The action and significance of host defenses can be properly analyzed only in relation to the sort of attack they may have to withstand. One result of recent preoccupation with immune deficiencies, congenital or iatrogenic, is the realization that the failure of any one defense mechanism usually gives rise not to a general increased risk of infection but to characteristic infections with specific organisms. For example, children with hypogammaglobulinemia get infected with pyogenic cocci or *Haemophilus influenzae,* which need opsonic antibodies. Patients with deficient cell-mediated immunity are more likely to suffer from chronic intracellular infections. More specific relationships occur as in chronic granulomatous disease, where the failure of the myeloperoxidase system results in infection by catalase-positive staphylococci (Klebanoff, 1971).

Each of the "experiments of nature" just described illustrates the action of a particular defense mechanism. A more frequent clinical situation is where a particular infection characteristically complicates some general disorder. The pathogenesis of such infections is not always clear.

It is easy to see why, in cirrhosis of the liver, the failure of the Kuppfer cells to sequestrate bacteria coming from the intestine, so that

ALAN A. GLYNN ● Bacteriology Department, Wright-Fleming Institute, St. Mary's Hospital Medical School, London W2 1PG, England.

1

more reach the spleen, gives rise to gram-negative bacteremias and high serum antibody levels to gut organisms (Bjorneboe *et al.*, 1972). Where impaired clearance of particles from the blood is combined with impaired production of antibody, as after splenectomy, there is a risk of fulminating bacteremias due to pneumococci and *H. influenzae* (Editorial, 1976b).

It is more difficult to understand why salmonellae, which normally do not cause osteomyelitis, should do so not infrequently in patients with sickle cell anemia (Hook *et al.*, 1957). The localization is probably the result of local ischemia due to intravascular sickling and obstruction. In addition, comparison of experimental hemolytic and hemorrhagic anemias (Kaye *et al.*, 1967; Kaye and Hook, 1963) suggests that in the former saturation of macrophages by damaged red cells impairs their bactericidal activities.

Even such general poisons as alcohol may be associated with specific susceptibilities such as to pneumococcal and *H. influenzae* infection (Capps and Coleman, 1923; Johnson *et al.*, 1968). An unknown metabolite decreases serum complement activity (Marr and Spilberg, 1975). In chronic alcoholics, polymorph chemotaxis but not phagocytosis and intracellular killing were impaired (Brayton *et al.*, 1970). Experimentally, alcohol decreased the bactericidal activity of lung macrophages (Green, 1968). Less specifically, acute alcoholism increases the risk of inhaling food or vomit, and at the same time depresses ciliary activity of the respiratory mucosa.

In contrast, severe chronic malnutrition is associated with a wide variety of infections depending largely on local epidemiological conditions (Gontzea, 1974).

1.2.2. Protective and Harmful Responses

The immune responses set in motion by an infection may promote resistance, produce tissue damage, or do both. The two phenomena are frequently, although not inevitably, inseparable, as the old arguments on the protective value of the Koch phenomenon (Rich, 1951) show. Moreover, since the system is mechanistic rather than teleological, the responses may well be irrelevant to resistance, although some pick up a secondary value if they become diagnostically useful. Responses

which increase resistance are not simply directed to killing the infecting organisms. Some prevent their attachment or penetration at the site of what Miles *et al.* (1957) have called the primary lodgement. At such sites, particularly on mucosal surfaces, Besredka's long-neglected local immunity is significant. Some infections may be neither prevented nor overcome but may continue, with or without progressive tissue damage. They may be accompanied by immunity of infection or premunition, a characteristic feature of chronic and intracellular infections such as those due to syphilis, protozoa, and, above all, viruses.

1.3. Routes and Sites of Infection

1.3.1. Routes of Clinical Infections

The route of arrival determines the primary and often the major site of a bacterial infection. A flea bite causes bubonic, and inhalation of infected droplets pneumonic, plague. Butcher's warts follow skin inoculation of anthrax spores from an animal carcass, while woolsorter's disease follows their inhalation from hides. Bovine tubercle bacilli ingested in milk reach the cervical or mesenteric glands, while inhaled human bacilli reach the lungs. The site of infection and hence route of toxin absorption markedly affect the clinical picture in diphtheria and tetanus.

1.3.2. Routes of Experimental Infections

In experimental infections inconclusive arguments as to which route is the most natural and hence the most significant are less important than the light each route throws on the workings of the defense mechanisms involved.

Even with enterobacteria, infection by mouth has been little used because of the large inocula required and the unpredictable variations resulting from the hazards of bacterial survival in the alimentary tract. However, variability can be reduced by using specific pathogen-free mice, and smaller inocula are effective if the mice are first starved and fed bicarbonate (Collins, 1972) or streptomycin (Miller and Bohnhoff, 1963).

The intraperitoneal route is widely used, although when both immunization and challenge are given in this way nonspecific inflammatory effects may contribute to any increased resistance which develops. However, no such protection against *Salmonella typhimurium* was given by a prior injection of starch (Kenny and Herzberg, 1968). Blanden *et al.* (1966) and Collins (1969) suggest that opsonizing antibodies are most effective in salmonella infections started intraperitoneally; they prefer the intravenous route for experiments. The early and intimate contact of the bacteria with the central reticuloendothelial system so produced may be the reason for the predominant role of cell-mediated immunity in this form of infection. Subcutaneous infection provides a less abrupt challenge to the liver and spleen and allows some local multiplication before spread.

Intracerebral, like intraperitoneal, injection introduces bacteria to a relatively defenseless site. Its most widespread use is in challenging young mice with *Bordetella pertussis* for testing pertussis vaccine. Surprisingly, this route gives results more in line with field trials of the vaccine than does nasal challenge (Standfast, 1967).

The injection of *Neisseria gonorrhoeae* into subcutaneous chambers prepared by the implantation of springs or plastic tubes (Arko, 1972) gives a more convenient model of gonococcal infection than using chimpanzees. However, although very useful, it does not copy the mucosal infection of the natural disease.

Locally administered extraneous agents such as cotton dust (Noble, 1965) enhance infection but complicate interpretation. The clinical inspiration for the cotton dust was the stitch abscess (Elek and Conen, 1957), itself but one example of infection complicating an implanted foreign body.

1.4. Measurement of Resistance to Infection

Whether one is judging the virulence of a microorganism or the resistance of the host, what has to be measured is the frequency of an infection and its severity. The epidemiological and clinical problems of such measurements are well known. In experimental animal infection lesion size has been used frequently where appropriate (Miles *et al.*, 1957; Noble, 1965), but for systemic infection mortality is still easier to measure than morbidity. However, mortality, whether expressed as time to death, death rate, or LD_{50} of the infecting

agent, remains a crude index. Finer discrimination can be obtained by following the numbers of viable bacteria in blood or organs at suitable times (Mackaness *et al.*, 1966). Where such a system is well established, a single viable count at a critical time can be used to determine the resistance of individual animals from a population known to be genetically heterogeneous (Plant and Glynn, 1976).

However, the method must not be taken to extremes. Whatever viable counts or secondary phenomena such as antibodies or cell-mediated immune responses may suggest, survival and death must be the final arbiters.

2. Bacterial Attack

2.1. Bacterial Growth

In many biochemical and structural investigations bacteria are examined in the logarithmic growth phase. Such organisms are healthy and vigorous, with a full complement of enzymes and substrates, but are not necessarily best adapted for growth *in vivo*.

Logarithm-phase *Escherichia coli* organisms are less resistant than those in stationary phase to killing by complement (Davis and Wedgwood, 1965). On the other hand, the staphylococcal cell wall impedin, which suppresses inflammation, can be extracted only from young cultures (Hill, 1968). Under optimal conditions *in vitro*, *S. typhimurium* may have a generation time as short as 20 min, yet in the infected mouse spleen it is 6–8 hr (Maw and Meynell, 1968). It seems unlikely that the augmentation of virulence which follows animal passage depends on the slowing of growth.

2.2. Bacterial Structure and Components

Any discussion of the interactions between immunological defense mechanisms and bacteria must take into account the microanatomical and chemical structure of the latter. Most significance attaches to the cell wall, although soluble toxins and enzymes and cytoplasmic components such as ribosomes are obviously important.

2.2.1. Cytoplasmic Membrane

In all bacteria the cytoplasm is bounded by a trilaminar lipoprotein membrane, forming a permeability barrier no different in principle from the cytoplasmic membrane of cells in general. Mycoplasma have no other cell wall. In protoplasts and L forms derived from "complete" bacteria, biochemical traces of outer wall layers may remain but have little or no functional structure.

2.2.2. The Rigid Layer

Immediately outside the cytoplasmic membrane in all the remaining forms of bacteria is a characteristic mucopeptide or peptidoglycan layer found only in bacteria and blue-green algae. The peptidoglycan forms one giant molecule, enclosing the whole cell in a sort of chain mail, imposing its geometric form and giving mechanical strength. Peptidoglycans are heteropolymers composed of long polysaccharide chains cross-linked to form a three-dimensional lattice by short peptide chains. The polysaccharide chains consist of alternating *N*-acetylglucosamine and *N*-acetylmuramic acid units joined by β-1,4-glycoside links. Muramic acid is simply *N*-acetylglucosamine joined by an ether link to D-lactic acid. The peptidoglycan backbone therefore resembles a substituted chitin. The carboxyl groups of most of the muramic acid units are substituted by a short peptide chain or four or five alternating D- and L-amino acids. Their variety is restricted, a very typical example being (muramic acid)–L-alanine–D-glutamine–*m*-diaminopimelic acid–D-alanine–D-alanine. Position 3 is always occupied by a diamino acid, although diaminopimelic may be replaced by L-lysine. The peptide subunits of different chains are cross-linked between the second amino group of the diamino acid in one and the carboxyl group of the D-alanine in position 4 of another. The link may be direct or via a short pentapeptide bridge. Although the general structures just described are common to all peptidoglycans, there is scope for many variations in detail between species; these have been described and classified by Schleifer and Kandler (1972). Gram-positive species vary more than gram-negative ones.

Unlike the inner and outer layers of the wall, peptidoglycans do not form a permeability barrier. Their porosity is large, the experimental estimates varying from 2.5-nm-diameter pores allowing the passage of molecules up to 70,000

daltons (Hughes *et al.*, 1975) to 10-nm pores allowing molecules of 3×10^6 daltons to pass (Hurst and Stubbs, 1969).

Apart from its general structure, the features which distinguish peptidoglycan from all other biological compounds are muramic acid and the presence of D-amino acids. It is not surprising, therefore, that many metabolic inhibitors of peptidoglycan synthesis find a use as antibiotics, the outstanding one being penicillin.

Many of the biological properties of peptidoglycan depend on the size of the polymer and decrease with its degradation. The key enzyme involved is lysozyme, which splits the *N*-acetylglucosamine–*N*-acetylmuramic acid link (Strominger and Tipper, 1974).

Provided that osmotic and mechanical stresses are not too great, most bacteria can survive damage to their rigid layer. Lysozyme and other hydrolytic enzymes in the lysosomes and granules of phagocytes are more likely to have a digestive than a bactericidal function. However, the relatively simple walled *Micrococcus lysodeikticus* is killed after phagocytosis by polymorphs or macrophages, while its lysozyme-resistant mutant strain is not (Brumfitt and Glynn, 1961). Persistence and transport of bacterial degradation products in phagocytes have been implicated in the pathogenesis of chronic inflammatory processes (Ginsburg and Sela, 1976).

The biological effects of peptidoglycan are incompletely worked out. Since methods of preparation are not standard, it is not always clear whether an effect is due to peptidoglycan itself or to traces of attached polysaccharides or proteins. Nor need all peptidoglycans behave similarly.

Direct inflammatory effects on injection of streptococcal peptidoglycans have been described (Abdulla and Schwab, 1966; Heymer *et al.*, 1971). In contrast, preparations from virulent *Staphylococcus aureus* suppressed inflammation (Hill, 1968). Both effects were reduced by treating the peptidoglycan with lysozyme. Inhibition of macrophage and polymorph motility and chemotaxis reported by many workers is probably a direct toxic effect (Heymer *et al.*, 1973; Weksler and Hill, 1969).

In view of the wide distribution of peptidoglycans, it is surprising that antibodies to them are not better known, although they have recently been detected in one-third of a normal population (Schachenmayr *et al.*, 1975). There is much cross-reaction between peptidoglycans of different bacteria, and three principal antigenic determinants have been recognized. In the glycan backbone *N*-acetylglucosamine is the immunodominant sugar. In the non-cross-linked pentapeptide side chains the immunodominant site is the two terminal D-alanines. The third determinant is the interpeptide bridge (Heymer *et al.*, 1975; Schleifer and Krause, 1971; Seidl and Schleifer, 1975).

What part these antibodies play in the pathogenesis of infectious disease remains to be determined. One, at least, against staphylococcal peptidoglycan, is protective (Hill, 1969; Easmon and Glynn, 1975a). Whether the antibodies to streptococcal peptidoglycan reported to be frequent in patients with rheumatoid arthritis (Braun and Holm, 1970) are protective, are involved in noxious autoimmune processes, or are artifacts due to cross-reactions with rheumatoid factor is also uncertain (Krause, 1975).

Peptidoglycans can produce a surprising number of effects usually attributed to endotoxin. As reviewed by Rotta (1975), they include fever, leukopenia, nonspecific resistance to infection, and local but not general Shwartzman reactions. Preparations from gram-positive organisms, which never make lipopolysaccharide, are effective, so there is no question of contamination. Since the two classes of compound are quite different chemically, any similarity of their actions may be due to their both triggering the same mechanisms in the mammalian host. The suggestion that many endotoxin effects are the result of delayed hypersensitivity was put forward many years ago by Stetson (1964).

Not much is known in general about delayed hypersensitivity to peptidoglycans. It is certainly important in local staphylococcal infections, where it contributes to tissue damage (Easmon and Glynn, 1975b; Taubler, 1968). However, Misaki *et al.* (1966) could not detect delayed hypersensitivity to the peptidoglycan of BCG.

Like lipopolysaccharide, peptidoglycan can activate complement by both the classical and alternative pathways. Activation of the classical pathway is not necessarily via antibody and may involve a direct effect on Clq (Bokisch, 1975).

The extremely interesting adjuvant properties of peptidoglycans are discussed more fully later.

2.2.3. Outer Membrane Layer of the Bacterial Cell Wall

Two main types of outer membranes are known. Those of gram-negative bacteria characteristically contain lipopolysaccharide, probably anchored to the peptidoglycan by a structural lipoprotein (Braun, 1973), and phospholipid. The outer membranes of gram-positive bacteria contain protein, teichoic or teichuronic acid, and other polysaccharides. Although otherwise gram positive, *Mycobacteria* are a special case, with walls containing complex waxes and lipids.

Still farther outside, many bacteria possess a capsule, usually of some highly polymerized carbohydrate as in the pneumococci, although some polypeptide capsules are known, e.g., in *Bacillus anthracis*. The acid polysaccharide K antigens of *E. coli* and the corresponding Vi antigen of some salmonellae are sometimes classed as microcapsules. Many although not all capsules act as impedins.

a. Teichoic Acids. The teichoic acids are polymers of either glycerol or ribitol held together by phosphate diester links (Dziarski, 1976). Antigenic and presumably functional variety is provided by substitution of OH groups with D-alanine, sugars, or amino sugars. Teichoic acids are covalently linked to the peptidoglycan and may be partly within its meshes. Some lie deeper, attached to the cytoplasmic membrane.

Toxic effects of teichoic acid have been reported but have not always been distinguished from those of peptidoglycan. Antibodies to teichoic acids have been used to detect staphylococcal endocarditis (Crowder and White, 1972) but, as is the case with delayed hypersensitivity to these bacterial constituents, a general account of their role in pathogenesis and immunity is difficult.

b. Lipopolysaccharides. Impure preparations of endotoxin contain protein, but all the characteristic biological effects have been reproduced with lipopolysaccharide alone prepared by the phenol water extraction method (Westphal and Jann, 1965). The significance of the protein fraction, however, may well have been underestimated, and the role of outer membrane proteins in general is only now being explored.

Lipopolysaccharides consist of three regions. Region I is made of chains of repeating oligosaccharides forming the specific O antigens characterizing many gram-negative bacteria. The chains are linked to region II, an oligosaccharide core containing heptose. The core in turn is linked via a ketodeoxyoctonate trisaccharide to region III, or lipid A. The lipid A structure includes long-chain fatty acids and amino sugars (Lüderitz et al., 1973).

Westphal and his colleagues have long held that the toxic properties of lipopolysaccharides reside in the lipid A part but are made manifest by the increased water solubility of the complete molecule. The polysaccharide fraction by itself is nontoxic. These views are confirmed by recent work (Galanos et al., 1972) in which lipid A, made soluble by complexing it with albumin, showed the toxic properties of lipopolysaccharide.

Defective lipopolysaccharide from Re mutants contains only lipid A and ketodeoxyoctonate but is fully toxic (Kim and Watson, 1967; Kasai and Nowotny, 1967).

To what degree cross-resistance to different Salmonellae and other gram-negative bacteria may be due to common antibodies to lipid A (Galanos et al., 1971) or to lipid A and core polysaccharide (McCabe et al., 1973) remains to be seen.

The relationship of lipopolysaccharide to virulence has been particularly studied in the salmonellae.

Loss of O side chains is paralleled by loss of virulence (Roantree, 1967; Nakano and Saito, 1969). However, not all smooth strains are virulent, and it is difficult to explain the difference between typhoid and food poisoning in man by the small difference in O antigens between Salmonella typhi (0, 1, 9, 12) and Salmonella typhimurium (0, 1, 4, 12), a difference based on the substitution of one dideoxy sugar for another. Moreover, in the mouse S. typhimurium produces a typhoidlike illness, while S. typhi does not establish a systemic infection.

These differences have been ingeniously tested by Makela et al. (1973), who by transduction or conjugation modified the lipopolysaccharide of S. typhimurium, converting it from the original 0, 1, 4, 12 antigenic pattern to 0, 1, 9, 12 or to 0, 6, 7 by transfer of genes from S. enteritidis or S. montevideo, so reducing its virulence on intraperitoneal injection tenfold or a hundredfold. However, wild-type strains of S. typhimurium and S. enteritidis can vary over this range. Since the differences between the natural and transduced strains persist even in thymectomized irradiated mice, specific immunity does not explain the strain differences (Valtonen et al., 1971). According to Makela et al. (1973), only a small number of other genes would have been transferred, and the chance that they too would be concerned with virulence is small. However, closely associated genes may control quite different products with related general functions.

Innumerable biological effects of lipopolysaccharide have been described. Lipopolysaccharides are highly immunogenic in very small doses, and, although generally said to induce only IgM antibodies, IgG and IgA responses have been described (Turner and Rowe, 1964; Rossen et al., 1967). Delayed hypersensitivity to lipopolysaccharides also occurs, although it is less well characterized (Kawakami et al., 1971).

With or without antibody, lipopolysaccharides can activate the classical and alternative complement pathways (Gewurz et al., 1971), as well as Hageman factor, and hence directly or indirectly the kinin and clotting systems (Cochrane et al., 1972). In turn, complement may detoxify lipopolysaccharide since animals deficient in C5 and C6 are unduly susceptible (Johnson and Ward, 1971, 1972).

Lipopolysaccharides bind to the surface of many cells, including platelets and polymorphs. Activation of macrophages (Allison et al., 1973) and mitogenicity for B lymphocytes (Oppenheim and Rosenstreich, 1976) have been suggested as the basis of their adjuvant action and ability to induce antibody formation without the help of T cells.

Animals become extremely sensitive to lipopolysaccharide after X irradiation or administration of cortisone or BCG. Chedid (1973) points out that, although detailed mechanisms may differ, these and other sensitizing agents either stimulate or suppress immune responses. Susceptibility to endotoxin may therefore be an important factor in clinical problems of immunological manipulation.

On repeated injection of lipopolysaccharide, both animals and man become transiently resistant to its effects. Such resistance, originally attributed by Beeson (1947) to increased activity of the reticuloendothelial system, is also due in part to antibody production and can be transferred passively by serum (Greisman and Hornick, 1973).

The precise role of lipopolysaccharide and resistance to its toxic effects in the pathogenesis of signs and symptoms of febrile disease such as typhoid (Greisman et al., 1964), pyelonephritis (McCabe, 1963), or gram-negative bacteremia with shock (Kass et al., 1973) is still not clearly defined in spite of the introduction of the rapid and sensitive if not very precise limulus assay for measuring blood endotoxin levels.

2.3. Impedins

2.3.1. Definition

In some species of bacteria pathogenicity is determined predominantly by one factor, e.g., toxin production by *Clostridium tetani* or *Corynebacterium diphtheriae*; more commonly, it depends on several factors. Toxins, although the most obvious, are not the only agents of bacterial virulence. Bail (1900) introduced the term "aggressin" to indicate a new class of bacterial products which, although themselves nontoxic, were able to enhance infection while they did not stimulate bacterial growth *in vitro*. Bail thought that aggressins impeded host defense mechanisms and were not produced to any extent *in vitro*. Since then, the term "aggressin" has often been loosely applied to many sorts of virulence factors, including toxins. Aggressin gives the impression of something which actively damages the host. A more appropriate collective term for compounds not overtly toxic but able to inhibit a variety of host defenses would be "impedin" (Torikata, 1917). "Impedin" could be used for a bacterial factor capable of inhibiting any defense mechanism of multicellular organisms against infection. A pragmatic approach based on func-tion is preferable to a formal definition which would eventually need to be modified.

Many impedins have been described (Glynn, 1972), ranging from the antiphagocytic capsules of pneumococci to ill-defined factors suppressing antibody formation (Malakian and Schwab, 1967), lymphocyte transformation (Copperman and Morton, 1966), or cell-mediated immunity (Schwab, 1975).

2.3.2. Types of Impedin

An impedin may be necessary for virulence but not adequate by itself to determine it. A good example is the inflammation-suppressing factor described by Agarwal (1967a) in strains of *Staphylococcus aureus*. Important though this cell wall impedin is in skin lesions, it is less so in intraperitoneal infections, where capsulated strains are more virulent (Easmon and Glynn, 1976). As discussed in Section 4, other factors such as toxin production and hypersensitivity are also involved in virulence.

Most human strains of *S. aureus* also produce protein A (Kronvall et al., 1971), which reacts in some specific way with the Fc portion of human IgG subgroups 1, 2, and 4 but not IgG3 (Kronvall and Williams, 1969). In so doing it may activate complement and set off many immune reactions. How far this and its antiphagocytic activity (Dossett et al., 1969) further virulence is not known.

Virulent strains of *Neisseria gonorrhoeae* grow as characteristic colonies, types I and II of Kellogg et al. (1963, 1968), and produce pili (Jephcott et al., 1971; Swanson et al., 1971). Pili enable gonococci to adhere to surface mucosal cells (Ward and Watt, 1972) but not to polymorphs, and may even have an antiphagocytic effect (Ofek et al., 1974; Punsalang and Sawyer, 1973; Thongthai and Sawyer, 1973).

Freshly isolated strains of gonococci are resistant to killing by complement (Ward et al., 1970). The factor responsible for such resistance is distinct from the pili and is rapidly lost on subculture except on media rich in prostatic extract (Watt et al., 1972). The importance of this factor to bacterial survival in acute inflammatory exudates containing complement has not been established. Gonococci adapted for growth in guinea pigs are more resistant to killing by complement (Penn et al., 1976) and by polymorphs (Veale et al., 1976). Such animal-adapted gonococci develop more pili and peptidoglycan and are more resistant to complement (Arko et al., 1976).

The waxy nature of the cell wall of mycobacteria protects them against noxious agents in vitro. It may act similarly in vivo, although it is hard to be sure since the nature of the antimycobacterial mechanisms is not known. Virulent strains of Mycobacterium tuberculosis H37RV when taken up by macrophages inhibit the fusion of lysosomes, with phagosomes so evading exposure to lysosomal enzymes (Armstrong and Hart, 1971). With Mycobacterium leprae and M. lepraemurium, however, normal fusion occurs (Hart et al., 1972). Some chlamydiae (Lawn et al., 1973) and Toxoplasma gondii (Jones and Hirsch, 1972) may also prevent fusion. The inhibition was overcome when the mycobacteriae were first treated with antibody, but, although phagolysosomes were then readily produced, the bacteria still survived. The possibility that lysosomes of immune macrophages would be more lethal remains (Armstrong and Hart, 1975). Incidentally, this illustrates an unusual example of antibody functioning intracellularly.

Their surface K antigens may make Escherichia coli inagglutinable by O sera (Kauffmann, 1943) and resistant to killing by complement and to phagocytosis (Glynn and Howard, 1970; Howard and Glynn, 1971a). Specific anti-K sera improve phagocytosis but do not affect complement killing.

The K antigens, which are acid polysaccharides, act by inhibiting the attachment of antibody, IgG or IgM, to neighboring determinants and also reduce the activation of complement by antibody (Glynn and Howard, 1970). The inhibitory activity of K antigens depends more on their degree of polymerization than on their surface charge (Howard and Glynn, 1971b). Their effect is nonspecific. Thus group A red cells treated with a K antigen are no longer agglutinable by anti-A.

K-rich strains of E. coli are more lethal than K-poor strains on intracerebral injection in mice (Howard and Glynn, 1971a). A pathogenic role for K antigens in urinary infection was suggested by Sjostedt (1946), although he did not quantitate them. K-rich strains are no better than K-poor strains at producing bladder infections but are more likely to be asso-

ciated with infection of the kidney both experimentally in mice (Nicholson and Glynn, 1975) and naturally in women (Glynn et al., 1971). The relation of K antigens to human kidney infection has been confirmed by Kaijser (1973) and McCabe et al. (1975). In Kaijser's series the specific K1 antigen was particularly noticeable. Since K-rich strains were not isolated particularly from patients with bacteremia, McCabe et al. suggested that they may have a nephrogenic rather than a general pathogenic action.

Unfortunately, through the idiosyncrasies of historical nomenclature, the adhesion-promoting surface protein antigens of enteropathogenic E. coli are also termed K, e.g., K88 (Ørskov and Ørskov, 1970).

Quite another group of impedins are the complex chelating agents by which bacteria obtain adequate supplies of iron otherwise tightly bound to host transferrin (Glynn, 1972; Weinberg, 1966).

Additional iron can enable bacteria to overcome serum bactericidal or bacteriostatic mechanisms in vitro as shown for M. tuberculosis (Kochan, 1969), Clostridium welchii (Rogers, 1967), and E. coli (Bullen and Rogers, 1969), among others. Iron can also exacerbate experimental infections, such as with Klebsiella (Martin et al., 1963), Listeria (Sword, 1966), and C. welchii (Bullen et al., 1967). Clinical evidence of the role of iron in infections is suggestive rather than conclusive, but, given therapeutically for anemia, it may exacerbate infection in children with kwashiokor and low serum transferrin levels (Macfarlane et al., 1970).

Lipopolysaccharide may suppress antibody formation (Finger et al., 1971). The transient reduction in nonspecific resistance induced by endotoxin (Rowley, 1956) may correspond to the negative phase of Almroth Wright (Shaw, 1911), during which immunization was thought to do more harm than good.

2.4. Bacterial Adjuvants

The mycobacteria in Freund's complete adjuvant are the best-known and the most effective example of the adjuvant action of bacteria. Similar activity has been found in many other bacterial species. Indeed, one function of the Bordetella pertussis used in the triple antigen given to children is to act as an adjuvant for the other two. *Corynebacterium parvum* and other anaerobic coryneform bacteria also stimulate antibody production, even to thymus-independent antigens, but not usually cell-mediated immunity, which they may depress. They are more often used for a variety of effects on the immune system, e.g., in efforts to induce tumor immunity, than as straightforward adjuvants (White, 1976).

Lipopolysaccharides given at the right time strongly enhance antibody responses (Johnson *et al.*, 1956). The effect is not due to the lipid A component since various derivatives are equally effective (Chedid *et al.*, 1975). Similarly, derivatives, some water soluble, of mycobacterial cell walls and of the peptidoglycans of many bacteria are good adjuvants, although some are better when incorporated in oil-in-water emulsions (Audibert and Chedid, 1976).

The minimal structure required for adjuvant action by these cell wall derivatives has turned out to be a relatively simple muramyl dipeptide, *N*-acetyl-muramyl-1-alanyl-*d*-isoglutamine (Ellouz *et al.*, 1974). Nauciel *et al.* (1974) suggested a very similar structure.

Many bacterial products are mitogens (Ling, 1968), particularly for B cells, but, although compounds may be both mitogens and adjuvants, the two properties can sometimes be dissociated (Rook and Stewart-Tull, 1976). A peptidoglycan polymer from *E. coli* was both a mitogen and an adjuvant, but the monomer was an adjuvant only, the suggestion being that mitogens required a repetitive structure (Damais *et al.*, 1975).

Many mitogenic and adjuvant properties of bacterial products given in large amounts are mainly of pharmacological significance. A role in pathogenesis and immunity cannot be entirely ruled out. For example, Campbell *et al.* (1976) have tried to link the B-cell mitogen and adjuvant factor isolated from the cell walls of *Listeria monocytogenes* with resistance to infection.

Mycobacterium tuberculosis in Freund's adjuvant is needed to produce delayed hypersensitivity to soluble antigens (Nelson and Boyden, 1964). Peptidoglycans from gram-negative bacteria have similar properties, and an active tetrapeptide has been isolated by Fleck *et al.* (1974).

2.5. Cross-Reacting Antigens

2.5.1. Bacterial Antigens Cross-Reacting with Tissue Antigens

The earliest examples of cross-reactions between some bacterial antigens and antigens of other bacterial or mammalian species were exploited for diagnostic purposes, as in the Wassermann and Weil-Felix reactions. Later, interest developed in the pathogenic significance of such relationships. Bacteria mimicking their hosts' antigens could conceivably gain some selective advantage by not provoking protective immune responses. Where mimicry was incomplete, the responses could break the normal tolerance for self antigens and result in autoimmune disease.

The suggestion (Rowley and Jenkin, 1962) that *S. typhimurium* bearing the 05 antigen was virulent for mice because the latter possess a similar antigen is unlikely because strains of mice differing a thousandfold in susceptibility both possess the antigen, as do resistant rats (Boyle, 1967).

Many cross-reactions between bacteria and blood group substances have been described (Springer, 1971), but suggestions that the world distribution of ABO groups is the result of past epidemics of plague and smallpox said to contain antigens reacting with O and A blood group substances (Pettenkofer *et al.*, 1962) are only speculative. Cross-reactions between *Strep. pyogenes* group A and heart muscle and kidney basement membrane form the basis of autoimmune theories of rheumatic fever and acute nephritis (Zabriskie, 1967). Cross-reaction works both ways; *E. coli* 086 which carries blood group B specificity can be killed by complement or phagocytosed by polymorphs if first treated with anti-B serum (Muschel and Osawa, 1959; Check *et al.*, 1972).

2.5.2. Cross-Reactions between Bacteria

Many antigenic relationships have been described between the polysaccharide capsules of *Streptococci pneumoniae* and *Klebsiella* strains (Heidelberger and Nimmich, 1972), between cell wall mucopeptides of staphylococci and streptococci (Karakawa *et al.*, 1968), and between cell wall proteins (Rittenhouse *et al.*, 1973).

Many lipopolysaccharides vary little in their

core specificity (Lüderitz *et al.*, 1966). Mc-Cabe (1972) produced good heterologous immunity to experimental salmonella infection by means of Re mutants of *S. minnesota*, i.e., which had only core lipopolysaccharides. In patients with gram-negative bacteremias the severity and mortality of the disease were less when anti-Re titers were high (McCabe *et al.*, 1972). It could be argued that such antibodies would be more likely to occur after infection with rough and hence less virulent strains.

The gradual development with age of antibodies protective against *Haemophilus influenzae* and *Neisseria meningitidis*, although partly due to subclinical infections, is also the result of stimulation by antigens of the normal body flora. Strains of *E. coli* bear antigens similar to the b type capsule of *H. influenzae*, to the A and C group polysaccharides of *N. meningitidis*, or to some pneumococcal serotypes (Robbins *et al.*, 1972). Schneerson and Robbins (1975) stimulated bactericidal antibody to *H. influenzae* b in men using *E. coli* of serotype 075:K100:H5.

The K1 antigen of *E. coli* is serologically identical with group B meningococcal antigen, both being sialic acid polymers. Unfortunately, *E. coli* K1 does not appear to be a useful substitute for the poorly immunogenic B antigen (Kasper *et al.*, 1973). *E. coli* bearing K1 is also common in renal infections (Kaijser, 1973).

3. Surface Infections

3.1. Introduction

The ability of a bacterial strain to adhere to the cells of mucous membranes may be critical in the establishment of an infection whether this is confined to the mucosal surface or is followed by penetration and spread. The causative organisms of whooping cough, cholera, and gonorrhea all have to cope with mechanical forces trying to dislodge them. Different immune defenses are appropriate according to how much a bacterium's pathogenicity depends on adhesion, penetration or toxin production. *E. coli*, *Vibrio cholerae*, salmonellae, and shigellae form a most instructive series of examples. Most enteropathogenic *E. coli*, like the completely noninvasive cholera vibrios,

act on the mucosa of the small intestine. A few strains of *E. coli*, however, act like dysentery bacilli in the colon and penetrate the mucous membrane (DuPont *et al.*, 1971). Salmonellae involve either the small or large intestine and may penetrate still farther.

3.2. Toxigenic Bacteria

Cholera is noninvasive, and the intestinal mucosa of patients with the acute disease is intact (Gangarosa *et al.*, 1960). All the manifestations of cholera can be produced by purified toxin given by mouth (Finkelstein, 1975). Ligated intestinal loops can be used to demonstrate cholera toxin and the toxins of enteropathogenic *E. coli* (Smith and Halls, 1968). The heat-labile enterotoxin of *E. coli* is antigenically very similar to cholera toxin (Gyles, 1974); both are proteins and have the same ganglioside receptor sites in the cell membrane (Holmgren, 1973). Both stimulate adenyl cyclase in the intestinal epithelial cells, thus increasing the concentration of cyclic adenosine monophosphate (cAMP) and provoking excessive though otherwise normal fluid secretion (Field, 1971).

An enterotoxin from *Shigella dysenteriae* type 1 provoked secretion in ileal loops (Keutsch *et al.*, 1972) but did not act via cAMP (Donowitz *et al.*, 1975). No toxins have yet been described for other species of shigellae, but antitoxin was found in patients infected by them, suggesting that toxin may be produced *in vivo*. However, experimental infection has been produced by nontoxigenic mutants (Formal *et al.*, 1972).

There is only preliminary evidence of enterotoxin production by salmonellae (Koupal and Deibel, 1975). Even with strains producing choleralike diarrhea, the mechanism of secretion is different and invasion of the mucosa by the salmonella is essential (Giannella *et al.*, 1971, 1973).

Even where toxin is responsible for all symptoms, as in cholera, antitoxin or immunization with toxoid is of little help clinically, whatever they do in experimental models. This may be because, unlike diseases such as diphtheria or tetanus, in cholera the toxin is produced at the surface of the cells it affects and may never be adequately exposed to antibody.

3.3. Bacterial Adhesion

3.3.1. *Vibrio Cholerae*

Attachment of the vibrios to the intestinal mucous membrane is an important feature of experimental and perhaps of natural cholera. Experimentally, attachment can be reduced by antibody (Freter, 1972a). Some but not all of the antibody is locally formed IgA (Fubara and Freter, 1973). A surface killing mechanism requiring antibody and live cells but not complement may be more important (Freter, 1972b).

Agglutination by producing aggregates of a hundred to a thousand bacteria reduced attachment and protected infant mice (Bellamy et al., 1975). Antibody to H antigens was effective, acting presumably by agglutination or inhibition of motility or both.

The anti-H serum had no bactericidal or antitoxic activity, and its protective value was reduced by adsorption with flagella antigen. Since dogma has long held that H antibodies are of no protective value, this is a most striking finding. Much of the evidence on which H antigens have been dismissed is based on experiments involving parenteral routes of infection. Flagellae may be of significance only at mucosal surfaces, and a reappraisal of salmonella infection, including typhoid, from this point of view would be useful.

Bivalent F(ab')$_2$ fragments of antibody protected infant mice, as well as whole IgG molecules did, again suggesting that cross-linking of vibrios by antibody rather than any opsonic or complement-dependent bactericidal mechanism was involved (Steele et al., 1975).

Fab' monomeric fragments had only 10% of the original protective capacity and presumably blocked receptors for adhesion on the bacterial surface.

3.3.2. *Escherichia coli*

The anterior small intestine is normally sterile in infants and young animals, although small numbers of E. coli have been recorded (Smith and Jones, 1963). The proliferation and adhesion of E. coli in this area occur in pigs and calves with diarrhea (Smith and Halls, 1968). Adhesion of enteropathogenic E. coli to mucosa was demonstrated by fluorescent microscopy in piglets (Arbuckle, 1970). To induce diarrhea, the bacteria must be not only toxigenic but also able to multiply in the an-terior intestine; adhesion enables them to maintain themselves *in situ*. The protein K88 antigen is important for E. coli adhesion in piglets, and antibody to it protects against diarrhea (Jones and Rutter, 1972). Some piglets are genetically resistant to K88 adhesion. The presumptive corresponding antigen in human E. coli remains undiscovered.

Adhesion by some strains of E. coli to the lining of the urinary tract also occurs and may be inhibited by antibody (Eden et al., 1976).

3.3.3. Streptococci

Some species of streptococci adhere to oral epithelium, others to teeth (Gibbons and van Houte, 1971). S. mutans, implicated in the production of dental caries, attaches to teeth if sucrose is available, because only with sucrose and not glucose can it synthesize sticky glucans. IgA antibodies can prevent adhesion (Williams and Gibbons, 1972) and inhibit enzymes (Fukui et al., 1973).

3.4. Bacterial Invasion

3.4.1. Salmonellae

All salmonellae invade the intestinal mucosa, but most go no farther, although, for example, *Salmonella typhi* in man and *S. typhimurium* in mice give rise to bacteremia and general infection. Salmonellae traverse the epithelium unharmed in lysosomal vacuoles and are released in the submucosa, where they cause inflammation (Takeuchi, 1971). Intestinal hypersecretion in ileal loops occurred only with invasive strains, not with all strains, and was not related to the degree of inflammation, the number of bacteria present, or their ability to invade more generally (Gianella et al., 1973). Lipopolysaccharide-deficient mutants could invade; pili and flagellae were irrelevant (Tannock et al., 1975). Protection by antibody has not been reported. Macromolecular antigens can penetrate the intestinal mucosa intact, but local antibodies can inhibit this process (Walker et al., 1972).

3.4.2. Shigellae

Shigellae characteristically penetrate colonic epithelium and multiply in the submucosa but do not spread further (LaBrec and Formal, 1961). Noninvasive mutants of *Sh. flexneri* 2a no longer caused diarrhea in monkeys or starved guinea pigs (LaBrec et al., 1964).

In contrast, some avirulent hybrids of Sh. flexneri and E. coli, although they penetrated the intestinal mucosa, failed to survive and produced only transient inflammatory changes (Formal et al., 1965).

4. Local Infections

4.1. Inflammation

The characteristic feature of a range of conditions from a minor boil to infection of a major organ as in pneumonia, meningitis, or pyelonephritis is inflammation. Not only are polymorphs and serum factors focused at the site of an acute infection, but also the T lymphocytes responsible for the macrophage activation accumulate in inflamed areas (Koster et al., 1971). The anaphylactoid, chemotactic, and opsonizing effects of complement are all involved. Local inflammatory responses were found to be reduced in mice depleted of complement (Willoughby et al., 1969) or in genetically deficient mice (Medhurst et al., 1969).

Some of the rare experiments in which the significance of a defense mechanism has been expressed in quantitative terms have been reported by Miles et al. (1957). From the change in dose–response relationships in skin lesions due to Pseudomonas aeruginosa in guinea pigs, when inflammation was prevented early by local injection of minute doses of epinephrine, they were able to calculate that the early defenses so suppressed were worth a 99% kill of the bacteria. The first few hours were critical, and suppression of inflammation later had no effect.

The lessened inflammatory response to staphylococcal skin infection in C5-deficient mice compared with normal mice could be reduced even further by cobra venom factor, suggesting that C3 also normally played a part (Easmon and Glynn, 1976). Comparison of early exudation in response to infection in immunized, unimmunized, normal, and C5-deficient mice with and without cobra venom factor, suggested that in immune mice most of the exudate was due to C3.

Similarly, with some strains of S. aureus given intraperitoneally, treatment of the mice with cobra venom factor, i.e., removal of both

C3 and C5 at least, reduced the lethal dose tenfold. Deficiency of C5 alone reduced the lethal dose 2–5 times (Easmon and Glynn, 1976).

Agarwal (1967a,b) related virulence of strains of S. aureus in skin lesions in mice to their ability to suppress the early inflammatory response. The factor involved was isolated only from young, actively growing cultures and was part of or intimately linked to the mucopeptide (Hill, 1968). The factor had no action on complement but prevented the synthesis or release of kinins and histamine (Easmon et al., 1973). It also inhibited chemotaxis in vitro, probably by a direct effect on the polymorphs (Weksler and Hill, 1969). In the local staphylococcal lesion model used by Agarwal, an early inflammatory response, however provoked, was the major protective factor. Although specific neutralizing antibodies, e.g., anti-α-toxin, helped, the most important result of antigen–antibody reactions was to cause local inflammation by some kind of immediate hypersensitivity reaction (Easmon and Glynn, 1975a).

Conversely, delayed hypersensitivity reaction to the staphylococcal antigens exacerbated the lesions, a result quite unlike the protective role of cell-mediated immunity in, say, listeria infections, but similar to the local necrosis found in tuberculosis (Easmon and Glynn, 1975b).

4.2. Opsonins

4.2.1. Antibody

Opsonization and phagocytosis are of great importance in local infections, although not, of course, confined to them. Resistance to phagocytosis is generally taken as a mark of virulence and is associated with surface impedins. Current investigations are particularly concerned with the opsonic activities of the different classes of antibody and with the role of heat-labile opsonin, i.e., complement, whether activated by the classical or the alternative pathways.

IgM antibodies were said to be more active as opsonins than were IgG molecules (Robbins et al., 1965), but the converse has been reported (Smith et al., 1967). Opsonic activity of IgA has been described (Knop et al., 1971;

Kaplan *et al.*, 1972) and also denied (Eddie *et al.*, 1971; Wilson, 1972). The kind of antibody required and how much help gained from complement vary with the species of bacterium.

4.2.2. Complement

Only the first four components of complement are needed for good opsonization (Gigli and Nelson, 1968), and phagocytosis of salmonellae and *E. coli* in C5-deficient mice is normal (Stiffel *et al.*, 1964). There is a possible supplementary role for C5 in opsonizing pneumococci (Shin *et al.*, 1969) and yeasts (Miller and Nilsson, 1970). The LD_{50} of a strain of pneumococci for the C5-deficient mice B10D2 old line was one-tenth that for the normal B10D2 new line (Shin *et al.*, 1969), but *in vivo* chemotaxis, where C5 has a clear part, may have contributed to the difference.

Since antibody takes time to appear, Wood (1960) suggested that surface phagocytosis might be important in the early stages of an infection such as pneumonia. A more efficient mechanism is the activation of the alternative complement path by pneumococci (Winkelstein *et al.*, 1972; Alper *et al.*, 1970). The activating factor responsible is not yet known. Although many capsulated serotypes of pneumococci could activate the alternative pathway, not all the polysaccharides were able to when purified. Moreover, a noncapsulated mutant of pneumococcus type 2 was as effective as the capsulated wild strain (Winkelstein *et al.*, 1975). That such activation may occur *in vivo* is suggested by the low levels of factor B and C3 in the blood in patients with early pneumococci (Reed *et al.*, 1976). Evidence for opsonization via the alternative complement pathway is increasing. *Staph. albus*, *Serratia marscens*, *Strep. viridans*, and *Strep. faecalis* could all be phagocytosed in this way (Forsgren and Quie, 1974), as could *E. coli*, but probably not *Staph. aureus* (Forsgren and Quie, 1974). Opsonization of *Staph. aureus* by complement did occur and was not necessarily due to activation of the classical pathway by protein A, since strains low in this were also phagocytosed. C2-deficient human serum opsonized *E. coli*, *Proteus mirabilis*, pneumococci, and *Staph. aureus* (Johnston *et al.*, 1972). C1q-deficient serum was also opsonic for *E. coli* but less so for *Staph. aureus* (Jasin, 1972).

5. Systemic Infections

5.1. Introduction

In systemic infections where intracellular bacterial survival is short—in meningitis, for example—the main conflict with host defenses is in the events leading to phagocytosis and involves largely complement and antibody, although cell-mediated immune responses may occur. The principles involved, therefore, are similar to those discussed in Section 4. Direct bactericidal effects of complement can occur locally but are more easily considered in relation to bacteremia.

Although much is known about phagocytic clearance of bacteria from the circulation, there is little information about their entry from the tissues. In rats given *Haemophilus influenzae* b intraperitoneally, 93% of the bacteria present were extravascular. If 1% of these entered the circulation each hour, they would have balanced the observed clearance rate (Shaw *et al.*, 1976).

In general, in infections with facultative or obligate intracellular parasites, e.g., tuberculosis, syphilis, salmonellosis, and brucellosis, cell-mediated immunity is of major importance, not least, in augmenting intracellular bactericidal mechanisms.

5.2. Bactericidal Action of Complement

5.2.1. Mechanisms

The fundamental processes of the system have been worked out by the study of hemolysis. Although convenient, it is risky to transfer the results uncritically to bacteria, which grow, multiply, and die and in general vary more than red cells.

Complement can damage the outer lipopolysaccharide-containing membrane of gram-negative bacteria (Humphrey and Dourmashkin, 1969; Bladen *et al.*, 1967; Glynn and Milne, 1967) as well as the inner cytoplasmic membrane (Muschel and Jackson, 1966). Since complement acts before lysozyme, which breaks up the rigid middle layer, the probable sequence of complement attack is from without inward (Glynn, 1969). Damage to the inner, cytoplasmic membrane may also be mechanical, secondary to fracture and disintegration of the rigid mucopeptide (Wilson and Spitznagel, 1968). Further evidence of a primary attack on the lipopolysaccharide region is the complete resistance of gram-positive bacteria, although their cytoplasmic membrane is susceptible and their outer walls can activate complement to opsonization.

The actual lesion is presumably formed, as in red cells, by a trimolecular complex C567 bound to the wall and carrying one molecule of C8 and six of C9, forming, so to speak, a ten-molecule drilling rig (Kolb *et al.*, 1972).

The key lethal event is uncertain, although changes described include release of phospholipids (Wilson and Spitznagel, 1971) and neutral lipids (Wilson and Glynn, 1975), and inhibition of RNA synthesis (Melching and Vas, 1971).

5.2.2. Bacterial Resistance

Within gram-negative species, resistance has been attributed to complete lipopolysaccharides (Nelson and Roantree, 1967), acid polysaccharide K antigens (Glynn and Howard, 1970), and surface proteins (Taylor, 1975).

Complement needs to be activated close to its site of action or some components decay before reaching it. Hence activation by antibodies to very peripheral structures such as long strands of lipopolysaccharide (Shands, 1965), flagellae (Felix and Olitzki, 1926), and large, passively attached antigens (Rowley and Turner, 1968) may not be lethal.

5.2.3. Initiation

Killing via the classical pathway is better initiated by IgM than by IgG antibodies (Robbins *et al.*, 1965), although both are effective. Killing by complement and lysozyme initiated by secretory IgA (Adinolfi *et al.*, 1966; Hill and Porter, 1974) is presumably via the alternative path. So is killing initiated by IgG1 guinea pig antibodies (Sirotak *et al.*, 1976). Activation of the alternative pathway by lipopolysaccharide or of either by lipid A (Bitter-Suerman *et al.*, 1975) may explain the wide bactericidal spectrum of normal serum, including antibody-free neonatal piglet serum (Sterzl *et al.*, 1962).

The alternative pathway in C4-deficient guinea pigs kills *E. coli* relatively slowly (Root *et al.*, 1972). It is also somewhat slower tested in human serum *in vitro* and appears to require antibody (Wilson and Glynn, 1977).

5.2.4. Significance

Although it is currently fashionable to attribute greater importance to the inflammatory chemotactic and opsonic functions of complement than to its bactericidal effects, much depends not only on the pathogen but also on the route and site of infection.

There is an inverse relationship between the level of bactericidal antibodies in a population and the incidence of meningitis due to either *Haemophilus influenzae* (Fothergill and Wright, 1933) or *Neisseria meningitidis* (Goldschneider *et al.*, 1969). Although bactericidal antibodies have usually been measured in these diseases, opsonic antibodies are present and may be equally important. The antibodies produced in response to immunization with capsular polysaccharide of *H. influenzae* b gave both bactericidal and opsonic antibodies, and both reactions required complement (Johnston *et al.*, 1973; Newman *et al.*, 1973). Useful protection against meningococcal meningitis is induced by vaccines containing the surface polysaccharides of types A and C, but not so far B (Editorial, 1976a). Interestingly, complement sensitivity of type B strains is not related to their surface polysaccharide (Frasch and Chapman; 1972, Frisch, 1968).

Bacteremic strains of *E. coli* are more complement resistant than are fecal strains. Roantree and Rantz (1960). Vosti and Randall (1970), and McCabe *et al.* (1975) did not find a significant predominance of such strains in patients with bacteremia, but they did not measure complement sensitivity directly.

Bacteremic strains of *Pseudomonas aeruginosa* resisted killing by complement but not by polymorphs (Young and Armstrong, 1972). Bacteremic strains of *Bacteroides fragilis* were resistant to complement (Casciato *et al.*, 1975).

In the examples so far given, resistance to killing is paralleled by resistance to opsonization, and either or both could be important. The first unequivocal evidence for the value of the bactericidal effect *in vivo* is the description of one certain and two more probable attacks of disseminated gonococcal infection in a girl genetically deficient in C8 and hence with normal serum chemotactic and opsonic function (Petersen *et al.*, 1976).

Unlike organisms isolated from local lesions, gonococci from the blood of patients with disseminated gonococcal infection are resistant to complement and may be of a particular auxotype (Schoolnik *et al.*, 1976).

This now increases the potential significance of the complement resistance of gonococci grown *in vivo* (Watt *et al.*, 1972) and of the meningitis data. The evolutionary selective value of a mechanism coping with a sterilizing disease like gonorrhea and a lethal one like meningitis would be great.

The role of complement in gram-negative bacteremia is complex and not entirely beneficial. Complement activation may contribute to clinical shock. In patients in whom shock develops, the alternate pathway is activated, as shown by low levels of properdin factor B and the late complement components C3, C5, C6, and C9, while C1, C4, and C2 levels remain normal (Fearon *et al.*, 1975). Whatever the role of complement, McCabe *et al.* (1972) suggest on the basis of extensive clinical data that while IgM antibodies acting via the bactericidal action of complement may help prevent gram-negative bacteremia, they are of no use in controlling it once it is established. In contrast, IgG antibodies, perhaps by virtue of their greater opsonic efficiency, are protective (Zinner and McCabe, 1976).

5.3. Cell-Mediated Immunity

5.3.1. Activated Macrophages

The field of cell-mediated immunity has been dominated for the last 15 years or so by the theory of activated macrophages developed by Mackaness and his colleagues (Mackaness and Blanden, 1967). Briefly, this postulates that, in infections due to facultative or obligate intracellular parasites, specific T lymphocytes are stimulated to release a variety of soluble factors which act on macrophages. As a result, macrophages accumulate at the site of infection and become activated; that is, their phagocytic and bactericidal capacities increase. The crucial point is that while stimulation of the lymphocytes is specific, the increased macrophage activity is not, and can be directed against organisms other than those initiating the process. However, maintenance or augmentation of the immune response requires the original specific stimulus. A good illustration is given by some transfer experiments of Mackaness (1964, 1969). Mice given lymphoid cells from BCG-immunized mice were not resistant to *Listeria*, although the donors were. However, resistance developed if the cell recipients were themselves given BCG before challenge with *Listeria*. The donated lymphocytes could respond specifically to BCG-releasing factors which then activated the recipients' macrophages.

5.3.2. Protective Value of Cell-Mediated Immunity

Formal proofs of the activated macrophage theory and detailed analysis of the number and nature of all the cells involved, and the kinetics of their changes on infection, have been presented in numerous papers. Indeed, the model presented by Mackaness is so attractive that its widespread acceptance threatens to lead to undue neglect of other defense systems. Several systems can occur in parallel, and the significance as distinct from the presence of any one needs to be assessed for each infection separately. For example, Coppel and Youmans (1969a–c) have tried to assess the relative importance of the specific and nonspecific components of immunity in listeria and tuberculous infections. Mice were immunized with either *L. monocytogenes* or *M. tuberculosis*. A few weeks later, when immunity was waning, the mice were given a second injection of the homologous organisms and the next day were challenged intravenously with *L. monocytogenes*. Progress was followed by serial viable counts of bacteria in the livers and spleens. Mice immunized and boosted with *Listeria* were far more resistant to challenge with *L. monocytogenes* than were mice immunized and boosted with *M. tuberculosis*, although in both groups of animals the macrophages should have been at their most active.

Although cell-mediated immunity of the type discussed has been demonstrated for *salmonella*, *brucella*, *listeria*, and *mycobacteria* infections, among others, remarkably little is known in chemical terms about why these organisms should stimulate it so strongly. Intracellular survival is perhaps the key, but needs explaining in its turn. Further help may come from studies of cell wall fractions in relation to adjuvance and to tolerance, and perhaps especially from a study of the relative stimulation by bacteria of effector or suppressor cells (Asherson and Zembala, 1976).

5.4. Spectrum of Responses to Infection

An important concept in chronic infections is that variations in their clinical manifestations depend more on the form of the host's immunological response than on changes in the infecting microorganism. The best example is leprosy, where the spectrum ranges from the tuberculoid form through several intermediates to the lepromatous form. In tuberculoid leprosy the main clinical feature is nerve damage and its consequences. The lesions contain few bacteria but many lymphocytes, there is delayed hypersensitivity to lepromin, and there are few antibodies. In lepromatous leprosy there are large, nodular lesions packed with bacteria. Plasma cells and antibodies are prominent; lymphocytes and delayed hypersensitivity are not. How and how far environmental, host genetic, and bacterial factors determine these differences remains to be analyzed. Similar spectra, although less clear, can be detected in tuberculosis, syphilis, and the protozoan infection leishmaniasis (Turk and Bryceson, 1971).

5.5. Ribosomal Immunity

Ribosomal preparations came into prominence following the work of Youmans and his colleagues, who were looking for an effective nonliving vaccine against tuberculosis and found what turned out to be mycobacterial RNA. This not only induced resistance to an intracellular parasite as good as that given by live attenuated bacteria but also did so without any accompanying delayed hypersensitivity (Youmans and Youmans, 1969). The problem has not been made easier by the extension of ribosomally induced immunity to bacteria such as streptococci, pneumococci, meningococci, staphylococci, pseudomonas, and cholera bacilli, in which cell-mediated responses are not usually thought to contribute to protection.

A second odd feature of ribosomal vaccines is that, unlike most protective antigens, they

come from the bacterial cytoplasm and not from the bacterial surface or extracellular products which form the significant interface with the host. However, this peculiarity may be more apparent than real since in some preparations traces of lipopolysaccharide are necessary for activity (Hoops *et al.*, 1976). There is still considerable argument, too, between workers using different species of bacteria, or even the same species, as to the relative importance of the RNA and protein fractions of active preparation.

6. Conclusion

This survey of the interactions between bacteria and immune responses is necessarily incomplete. In particular, although phagocytosis has been referred to repeatedly in connection with inflammation, chemotaxis, and opsonization, little has been said about intracellular killing mechanisms or the factors governing intracellular survival. These aspects of phagocytosis and a general assessment of the role of the great phagocytic systems of the body are dealt with in Part III of this treatise. Bacterial virulence and host defense mechanisms can properly be assessed only in relation to each other. While many aggressive and defensive mechanisms have been analyzed, often in great detail, more needs to be known of their quantitative significance *in vivo* in natural infections.

References

Abdulla, E. M., and Schwab, J. H., 1966, Biological properties of streptococcal cell wall particles. III. Dermonecrotic reaction to cell wall mucopeptides, *J. Bacteriol.* **91:**374–383.

Adinolfi, M., Glynn, A. A., Lindsay, M., and Milne, C. M., 1966, Serological properties of γ A antibodies to *Escherichia coli* present in human colostrum, Immunology **10:**517–526.

Agarwal, D. S., 1967a, Subcutaneous staphylococcal infection in mice. I. The role of cotton dust in enhancing infection, *Br. J. Exp. Pathol.* **48:**436–439.

Agarwal, D. S., 1967b, Subcutaneous staphylococcal infection in mice. II. The inflammatory response to different strains of staphylococci and micrococci, *Br. J. Exp. Pathol.* **48:**468–482.

Allison, A. C., Davies, J. D., and Page, R. C., 1973, Effect of endotoxin on macrophages and other lymphoreticular cells, *J. Infect. Dis.* **128**:S213–219.

Alper, C. A., Abramson, N., Johnston, R. B., Jandl, J. H., and Rosen, F. S., 1970, Increased susceptibility to infection associated with abnormalities of complement mediated functions and of the third component of complement (C3), *N. Engl. J. Med.* **282**:349–354.

Arbuckle, J. B. R., 1970, The location of *Escherichia coli* in the pig intestine, *J. Med. Microbiol.* **3**:333–340.

Arko, R. J., 1972, *Neisseria gonorrhoeae* experimental infection of laboratory animals, *Science* **177**:1200–1201.

Arko, R. J., Bullard, J. C., and Duncan, W. P., 1976, Effects of laboratory maintenance on the nature of surface reactive anigens of *Neisseria gonorrhoeae*, *Br. J. Vener. Dis.* **52**:316–325.

Armstrong, J. A., and Hart, P. D'Arcy, 1971, Response of cultured macrophages to *Mycobacterium tuberculosis* with observations on fusion of lysosomes with phagosomes, *J. Exp. Med.* **134**:713–740.

Armstrong, J. A., and Hart, P. D'Arcy, 1975, Phagosome and lysosome interaction in cultured macrophages infected with virulent tubercle bacilli, *J. Exp. Med.* **142**:1–16.

Asherson, G. L., and Zembala, M., 1976, Suppressor T cells in cell-mediated immunity, *Br. Med. Bull.* **32**:158–164.

Audibert, F., and Chedid, L., 1976, Activity in saline of phthalylated or succinylated derivatives of mycobacterial water-soluble adjuvant, *Infect. Immun.* **14**:1263–1268.

Bail, 1900, cited by Wilson, G. S., and Miles, A. A., 1975, in: *Principles of Bacteriology and Immunity* (Topley and Wilson, eds.), 6th ed., p. 1556, Edward Arnold, London.

Bellamy, J. E. C., Knop, J., Steele, E. J., Chaicumpa, W., and Rowley, D., 1975, Antibody cross-linking as a factor in immunity to cholera in infant mice, *J. Infect. Dis.* **132**:181–188.

Beeson, P. B., 1947, Tolerance to bacterial pyrogens. II. Role of the reticuloendothelia system, *J. Exp. Med.* **86**:39–44.

Bitter-Suerman, D., Hadding, V., Schorlemmer, H. V., Limbert, M., Dierich, M., and Dukor, P., 1975, Activation by some T-independent antigens and B cell mitogens of the alternative pathway of the complement system, *J. Immunol.* **115**:425–430.

Bjorneboe, M., Prytz, H., and Orskov, F., 1972, Antibodies to intestinal microbes in serum of patients with cirrhosis of the liver, *Lancet* **1**:58–60.

Bladen, H. A., Gewurz, H., and Mergenhagen, S., 1967, Interaction of the complement system with the surface and endotoxin lipopolysaccharide of *Veillonella alkalescens*, *J. Exp. Med.* **125**:767–786.

Blanden, R. V., Mackaness, G. B., and Collins, F. M., 1966, Mechanisms of acquired resistance in mouse typhoid, *J. Exp. Med.* **124**:585–600.

Bokisch, V. A., 1975, Interaction of peptidoglycans with anti-IgGs and with complement, *Z. Immunitaetsforsch.* **149**:320–330.

Boyle, W., 1967, An antigen common to mouse cells and *Salmonella typhimurium*, *J. Immunol.* **98**:256–259.

Braun, D. G., and Holm, S. E., 1970, Streptococcal antigroup A precipitin in sera from patients with rheumatoid arthritis and acute glomerulonephritis, *Int. Arch. Allergy Appl. Immunol.* **37**:216–224.

Braun, V., 1973, Molecular organization of the rigid layer and the cell wall of *Escherichia coli*, *J. Infect. Dis.* **128**:S9–S29.

Brayton, R. G., Stokes, P. F., Schwartz, M. S., and Louria, D. B., 1970, Effect of alcohol and various diseases on leukocyte mobilization, phagocytosis and intracellular bacterial killing, *N. Engl. J. Med.* **282**:123–128.

Brumfitt, W., and Glynn, A. A., 1961, Intracellular killing of *Micrococcus lysodeikticus* by macrophages and polymorphonuclear leucocytes: A comparative study, *Br. J. Exp. Pathol.* **62**:408–423.

Bullen, J. J., and Rogers, H. J., 1969, Bacterial iron metabolism and immunity to *Pasteurella septica* and *Escherichia coli*, *Nature (London)* **224**:380–382.

Bullen, J. J., Cushnie, G. H., and Rogers, H. J., 1967, The abolition of the protective effect of *Clostridium welchii* type A antiserum by ferric iron, *Immunology* **12**:303–312.

Campbell, P. A., Schuffler, C., and Rodriguez, G. E., 1976, *Listeria* cell wall fraction: A B cell adjuvant, *J. Immunol.* **116**:590–594.

Capps, J. A., and Coleman, G. H., 1923, Influence of alcohol on prognosis of pneumonia in Cook County Hospital. A statistical report. *J. Am. Med. Assoc.* **30**:750–752.

Casciato, D. A., Rosenblatt, J. E., Goldberg, L. S., and Bluestone, R., 1975, *In vitro* interaction of *Bacteroides fragilis* with polymorphonuclear leucocytes and serum factors, *Infect. Immun.* **11**:337–342.

Check, J. H., O'Neill, E. A., O'Neill, K. E., and Fuscaldo, K. E., 1972, Effect of anti-B serum on the phagocytosis of *Escherichia coli*, *Infect. Immun.* **6**:95–96.

Chedid, L., 1973, Possible role of endotoxemia during immunologic imbalance, *J. Infect. Dis.* **128**:S112–S117.

Chedid, L., Audibert, F., and Bona, C., 1975, Activités adjuvantes et mitogenes de lipopolysaccharides détoxifiés, *C.R. Acad. Sci. Ser. D* **280**:1197–1200.

Cochrane, C. G., Revak, S., Atkin, B. S., and Wuepper, K. D., 1972, The structural characteristics and activation of Hageman factor, in: *Inflammation* (I. H. Lepow and P. A. Ward, eds.), pp. 119–138, Academic Press, New York.

Collins, F. M., 1969, Effect of specific immune mouse serum on the growth of *Salmonella enteritidis* in non-vaccinated mice challenged by varous routes, *J. Bacteriol.* **97**:667–675.

Collins, F. M., 1972, Salmonellosis in orally infected specific pathogen free C57B1 mice, *Infect. Immun.* **5**:191–198.

Coppel, S., and Youmans, G. P., 1969a, Specificity of acquired resistance to immunization with mycobacterial cells and mycobacterial fractions, *J. Bacteriol.* **97:**114–120.

Coppel, S., and Youmans, G. P., 1969b, Specificity of acquired resistance to immunization with *Listeria monocytogenes* and *Listeria* fractions, *J. Bacteriol.* **97:**121–126.

Coppel, S., and Youmans, G. P., 1969c, Specificity of the anamnestic response produced by *Listeria monocytogenes* or *Mycobacterium tuberculosis* to challenge with *Listeria monocytogenes*, *J. Bacteriol.* **97:**127–133.

Copperman, R., and Morton, H. E., 1966, Reversible inhibition of mitosis in lymphocyte cultures by non-viable mycoplasma, *Proc. Soc. Exp. Biol. Med.* **123:**790–795.

Crowder, J. G., and White, A., 1972, Teichoic acid antibodies in staphylococcal and non-staphylococcal endocarditis, *Ann. Int. Med.* **77:**87–90.

Damais, C., Bona, C., and Chedid, L., 1975, Mitogenic effect of bacterial peptidoglycans possessing adjuvant activity, *J. Immunol.* **115:**268–271.

Davis, S. D., and Wedgwood, R. J., 1965, Kinetics of the bactericidal action of normal serum on gram negative bacteria, *J. Immunol.* **95:**75–79.

Donowitz, M., Keusch, G. T., and Bindes, H. J., 1975, Effect of *Shigella* enterotoxin on electrolytic transport in rabbit ileum, *Gastroenterology* **69:**1230–1237.

Dossett, J. H., Kronvall, G., Williams, R. C., Jr., and Quie, P. G., 1969, Antiphagocytic effects of staphylococcal protein A, *J. Immunol.* **103:**1405–1410.

DuPont, H. L., Formal, S. B., Hornick, R. B., Snyder, M. J., Libonati, J. P., Sheahan, D. G., LaBrec, E. H., and Kalas, J. P., 1971, Pathogenesis of *Escherichia coli* diarrhea, *N. Engl. J. Med.* **285:**1–9.

Dziarski, R., 1976, Teichoic acids, *Curr. Top. Microbiol. Immunobiol.* **74:**113–135.

Easmon, C. S. F., and Glynn, A. A., 1975a, The role of humoral immunity and acute inflammation in protection against staphylococcal dermonecrosis, *Immunology* **29:**67–74.

Easmon, C. S. F., and Glynn, A. A., 1975b, Cell-mediated immune responses in *Staphylococcus aureus* infections in mice, *Immunology* **29:**75–85.

Easmon, C. S. F., and Glynn, A. A., 1976, Comparison of subcutaneous and intraperitoneal staphylococcal infections in normal and complement deficient mice, *Infect. Immun.* **13:**399–406.

Easmon, C. S. F., Hamilton, I., and Glynn, A. A., 1973, Mode of action of a staphylococcal anti-inflammatory factor, *Br. J. Exp. Pathol.* **54:**638–645.

Eddie, D. S., Schulkind, M. L., and Robbins, J. B., 1971, The isolation and biologic activities of purified secretory IgA and IgG anti-*Salmonella typhimurium* "O" antibodies from rabbit intestinal fluid and colostrum, *J. Immunol.* **106:**181–190.

Eden, C. S., Hanson, L. A., Jodal, V., Lindberg, U., and Akerlund, A. S., 1976, Variable adherence to normal human urinary tract epithelial cells of *Escherichia coli* strains associated with various forms of urinary tract infection, *Lancet* **2:**490–492.

Editorial, 1976a, Vaccination against meningitis, *Br. Med. J.* **1:**919–920.

Editorial, 1976b, Infective hazards of splenectomy, *Lancet* **1:**1167–1168.

Elek, S. D., and Conen, P. E., 1957, The virulence of *Staphylococcus pyogenes* for man. A study of the problems of wound infection, *Br. J. Exp. Pathol.* **38:**573–586.

Ellouz, F., Adam, A., Ciorbaru, R., and Lederer, E., 1974, Minimal structural requirements for adjuvant activity of bacterial peptidoglycan derivatives, *Biochem. Biophys. Res. Commun.* **59:**1317–1325.

Fearon, D. T., Ruddy, S., Schur, P. H., and McCabe, W. R., 1975, Activation of the properdin pathway of complement in patients with gram-negative bacteremia, *N. Engl. J. Med.* **292:**937–940.

Felix, A., and Olitzki, A. L., 1926, The qualitative receptor analysis. II. Bactericidal serum action and qualitative receptor analysis, *J. Immunol.* **11:**31–80.

Field, M., 1971, Intestinal secretion: Effect of cyclic AMP and its role in cholera, *N. Engl. J. Med.* **284:**1137–1144.

Finger, H., Fresenius, H., and Angerer, M., 1971, Bacterial endotoxins as immunosuppressive agents, *Experientia* **27:**456–458.

Finkelstein, R. A., 1975, Cholera enterotoxin, in: *Microbiology 1975* (D. Schlesinger, ed.), pp. 236–241, ASM, Washington D.C.

Fleck, J., Mock, M., Tytgat, F., Nauciel, C., and Mink, R., 1974, Adjuvant activity in delayed hypersensitivity of the peptidic part of bacterial peptidoglycans, *Nature (London)* **250:**517–518.

Formal, S. B., LaBrec, E. H., Kent, T. H., and Falkow, S., 1965, Abortive intestinal infection with an *Escherichia coli–Shigella flexneri* hybrid strain, *J. Bacteriol.* **89:**1374–1382.

Formal, S. B., Gemski, P., Giannella, R. A., and Austin, S., 1972, Mechanisms of *Shigella* pathogenesis, *Am. J. Clin. Nutrition* **25:**1427–1432.

Forsgren, A., and Quie, P. G., 1974, Influence of the alternate complement pathway on opsonization of several bacterial species, *Infect. Immun.* **10:**402–404.

Fothergill, L. D., and Wright, J., 1933, Influenzal meningitis: The relation of age incidence to the bactericidal power of the blood against the causal organism *J. Immunol.* **24:**273–284.

Frasch, C. E., and Chapman, S. S., 1972, Classification of *Neisseria meningitidis* group B into distinct serotypes. I. Serological typing by a microbactericidal method, *Infect. Immun.* **5:**98–102.

Freter, R., 1972a, Parameters affecting the association of vibrios with the intestinal surface in experimental cholera, *Infect. Immun.* **6:**134–141.

Freter, R., 1972b, Mechanism of action of intestinal antibody in experimental cholera. II. Antibody-mediated antibacterial reaction at the mucosal surface, *Infect. Immun.* **2:**556–562.

Frisch, A. W., 1968, The meningococcidal power of heparinised blood for group B organisms, *Am. J. Clin. Pathol.* **50**:221–228.

Fubara, E. S., and Freter, R., 1973, Protection against enteric bacterial infection by secretory IgA antibodies, *J. Immunol.* **111**:395–403.

Fukui, Y., Fukui, K., and Moriyama, T., 1973, Inhibition of enzymes by human salivary immunoglobulin A, *Infect. Immun.* **8**:335–340.

Galanos, C., Lüderitz, O., and Westphal, O., 1971, Preparation and properties of antisera against the lipid A component of bacterial lipopolysaccharides, *Eur. J. Biochem.* **24**:116–122.

Galanos, C., Rietschel, E. T., Lüderitz, O., Westphal, O., Kim, Y. B., and Watson, D. W., 1972, Biological activities of lipid A complexed to bovine serum albumin, *Eur. J. Biochem.* **31**:230–233.

Gangarosa, E. F., Beisel, W. R., Benyajati, C., Sprinz, H., and Piyaratn, P., 1960, The nature of the gastrointestinal lesion in Asiatic cholera and its relation to pathogenesis: A biopsy study. *Am. J. Trop. Med. Hyg.* **9**:125–135.

Gewurz, H., Snyderman, R., Mergenhagen, S. E., and Shin, H. S., 1971, Effect of endotoxic lipopolysaccharide on the complement system, in: *Microbial Toxins*, Vol. 5 (S. Kadis, G. Weinbaum, and S. J. Ajl, eds.), pp. 127–150, Academic Press, New York.

Giannella, R. A., Broitman, S. A., and Zamcheck, N., 1971, Salmonella enteritis. II. Fulminant diarrhea in and effects on the small intestine, *Am. J. Dig. Dis.* **16**:1007–1013.

Giannella, R. A., Formal, S. B., Dammin, G. J., and Collins, H., 1973, Pathogenesis of salmonellosis: Studies of fluid secretion, mucosal invasion and morphologic reaction in the rabbit ileum, *J. Clin. Invest.* **52**:441–453.

Gibbons, R. J., and van Houte, J., 1971, Selective bacterial adherence to oral epithelial surfaces and its role as an ecological determinant, *Infect. Immun.* **3**:567–573.

Gigli, I., and Nelson, R. A., 1968, Complement dependent immune phagocytosis. I. Requirements for C'1, C'4, C'2, C'3, *Exp. Cell Res.* **51**:45–67.

Ginsburg, I., and Sela, M. N., 1976, The role of leukocytes and their hydrolases in the persistence, degradation and transport of bacterial constituents in tissues: Relation to chronic inflammatory processes in staphylococcal, streptococcal and mycobacterial infections and in chronic periodontal disease, *Crit. Rev. Microbiol.* **4**:249–332.

Glynn, A. A., 1969, The complement lysozyme sequence in immune bacteriolysis, *Immunology* **16**:463–471.

Glynn, A. A., 1972, Bacterial factors inhibiting host defence mechanisms *Symp. Soc. Gen. Microbiol.* **22**:75–112.

Glynn, A. A., and Howard, C. J., 1970, The sensitivity to complement of strains of *Escherichia coli* related to their K antigens, *Immunology* **18**:331–346.

Glynn, A. A., and Milne, C. M., 1967, A kinetic study of the bacteriolytic action of human serum, *Immunology* **12**:639–653.

Glynn, A. A., Brumfitt, W., and Howard, J. C., 1971, K

antigens of *Escherichia coli* and renal involvement in urinary tract infections, *Lancet* **1**:514–516.

Goldschneider, I., Gottschlich, E. C., and Artenstein, M. S., 1969, Human immunity to the meningococcus. I. The role of humoral antibodies, *J. Exp. Med.* **129**:1307–1326.

Gontzea, I., 1974, *Nutrition and Anti-infectious Defense*, Karger, Basel.

Green, G. M., 1968, Pulmonary clearance of infectious agents, *Annu. Rev. Med.* **19**:315–336.

Greisman, S. E., and Hornick, R. B., 1973, Mechanisms of endotoxin tolerance with special reference to man, *J. Infect. Dis.* **128**:S265–S276.

Greisman, S. E., Hornick, R. B., and Woodward, T. D., 1964, The role of endotoxin during typhoid fever and tularemia in man. III. Hyperreactivity to endotoxin during infection, *J. Clin. Invest.* **43**:1747–1757.

Gyles, C. L., 1974, Relationships among heat-labile enterotoxins of *Escherichia coli* and *Vibrio cholerae*, *J. Infect. Dis.* **129**:277–283.

Hart, P. D'Arcy, Armstrong, J. A., Brown, C. A., and Draper, P., 1972, Ultrastructural study of the behaviour of macrophages toward parasitic mycobacteria, *Infect. Immun.* **5**:803–807.

Heidelberger, M., and Nimmich, W., 1972, Additional immunochemical relationships of capsular polysaccharides of *Klebsiella* and pneumococci, *J. Immunol.* **109**:1337–1344.

Heymer, B., Bültmann, B., and Haferkamp, D., 1971, Toxicity of streptococcal mucopeptides *in vivo* and *in vitro*, *J. Immunol.* **106**:858–861.

Heymer, B., Bültmann, B., Schachenmayr, W., Spanel, R., Haferkamp, O., and Schmidt, W. C., 1973, Migration inhibition of rat peritoneal cells induced by streptococcal mucopeptides. Characteristics of the reaction and properties of the mucopeptide preparations, *J. Immunol.* **116**:1743–1754.

Heymer, B., Bernstein, D., Schleifer, K. H., and Krause, R. M., 1975, Measurement of peptidoglycan antibodies by a radioimmunoassay, *Z. Immunitaets Forsch.* **149**:168–178.

Hill, M. J., 1968, A staphylococcal aggressin, *J. Med. Microbiol.* **1**:33–43.

Hill, M. J., 1969, Protection of mice against infection by *Staphylococcus aureus*, *J. Med. Microbiol.* **2**:1–7.

Hill, I. R., and Porter, P., 1974, Studies of bactericidal activity to *Escherichia coli* of porcine serum and colostral immunoglobulins and the role of lysozyme with secretory IgA, *Immunology* **26**:1239–1250.

Holmgren, J., 1973, Comparison of the tissue receptors for *Vibrio cholerae* and *Escherichia coli* enterotoxins by means of gangliosides and natural cholera toxoid, *Infect. Immun.* **8**:851–859.

Hook, E. W., Campbell, G. C., Weens, H. S., and Cooper, G. R., 1957, *Salmonella osteomyelitis* in patients with sickle cell anaemia, *N. Engl. J. Med.* **257**:403–407.

Hoops, P. Prather, N. E., Berry, L. J., and Ravel, J. M., 1976, Evidence for an extrinsic immunogen in effective ribosomal vaccines from *Salmonella typhimurium*, *Infect. Immun.* 13:1184–1192.

Howard, C. J., and Glynn, A. A., 1971a, The virulence for mice of strains of *Escherichia coli* related to the effect of K antigens on their resistance to phagocytosis and killing by complement, *Immunology* 20:767–777.

Howard, C. J., and Glynn, A. A., 1971b, Some physical properties of K antigens of *Escherichia coli* related to their biological activity, *Infect. Immun.* 4:6–11.

Hughes, R. C., Thurman, P. F., and Stokes, E., 1975, Estimates of the porosity of *Bacillus licheniformis* and *Bacillus subtilis* cell walls, *Z. Immunitaets forsch.* 149:126–135.

Humphrey, J. H., and Dourmashkin, R. R., 1969, The lesion in cell membranes caused by complement, *Adv. Immunol.* 11:75–115.

Hurst, A., and Stubbs, J. M., 1969, Electron microscopy of membranes and walls of bacteria and changes occurring during growth initiation, *J. Bacteriol.* 97:1466–1479.

Jasin, H. E., 1972, Human heat labile opsonins: Evidence for their mediation via the alternate pathway of complement activation, *J. Immunol.* 109:26–31.

Jephcott, A. E., Reyn, A., and Birch-Andersen, A., 1971, *Neisseria gonorrhoeae*. III. Demonstration of presumed appendages to cells from different colony types, *Acta Pathol. Microbiol. Scand. Sec. B* 79:437–439.

Johnson, A. G., Gaines, S., and Landy, M., 1956, Studies on the O antigen of *Salmonella typhosa*. V. Enhancement of antibody response to protein antigens by the purified lipopolysaccharide, *J. Exp. Med.* 103:225–246.

Johnson, K. J., and Ward, P. A., 1971, Protective function of C6 in rabbits treated with bacterial endotoxin, *J. Immunol.* 106:1125–1127.

Johnson, K. J., and Ward, P. A., 1972, The requirement for serum complement in the detoxification of bacterial endotoxin, *J. Immunol.* 108:611–616.

Johnson, W. E., Kaye, D., and Hook, E. W., 1968, *Haemophilus influenzae* in adults: Report of five cases and review of the literature, *Am. Rev. Resp. Dis.* 97:1112–1117.

Johnston, F. R., Agnello, V., and Williams, R. C., 1972, Opsonic activity in human serum deficient in C2, *J. Immunol.* 109:141–145.

Johnston, R. B., Anderson, P., Rosen, F. S., and Smith, D. H., 1973, Characterisation of human antibody to polyribophosphate, the capsular antigen of *Hemophilus influenzae*, Type B, *Clin. Immunol. Immunopathol.* 1:234–240.

Jones, G. W., and Rutter, J. M., 1972, Role of the K88 antigen in the pathogenesis of neonatal diarrhea caused by *Escherichia coli* in piglets, *Infect. Immun.* 6:918–927.

Jones, T. C., and Hirsch, J. G., 1972, The interaction between *Toxoplasma gondii* and mammalian cells, *J. Exp. Med.* 136:1173–1194.

Kaijser, B., 1973, Immunology of *Escherichia coli* K antigen and its relation to urinary tract infection, *J. Infect. Dis.* 127:670–677.

Kaplan, M. E., Dalmasso, A. P., and Woodson, M., 1972, Complement-dependent opsonization of incompatible erythrocytes by human secretory IgA, *J. Immunol.* 108:275–278.

Karakawa, W. W., Braun, D. G., Lackland, H., and Krause, R. M., 1968, Immunochemical studies on the cross-reactivity between streptococcal and staphylococcal mucopeptide, *J. Exp. Med.* 128:325–340.

Kasai, N., and Nowotny, A., 1967, Endotoxic glycolipid from a heptoseless mutant of *Salmonella minnesota*, *J. Bacteriol.* 94:1824–1836.

Kasper, D. L., Winkchaker, J. L., Zollinger, W. D., Brandt, B. L., and Artenstein, M. S., 1973, Immunochemical similarity between polysaccharide antigens of *Escherichia coli* 07:K1(L):NM and group B *Neisseria meningitidis*, *J. Immunol.* 110:262–268.

Kass, E. H., Porter, P. J., McGill, M. W., and Vivaldi, E., 1973, Clinical and experimental observations on the significance of endotoxemia, *J. Infect. Dis.* 128:S299–S302.

Kauffmann, F., 1943, Über neue thermolabile Körperentigene der Coli-bakterien. *Acta Pathol. Microbiol. Scand.* 20:21–44.

Kawakami, M., Hara, Y., and Osawa, N., 1971, Experimental salmonellosis: Hypersensitivity to cell wall lipopolysaccharide and anti infectious resistance of mice infected with *Salmonella*, *Infect. Immun.* 4:519–524.

Kaye, D., and Hook, E. W., 1963, The influence of hemolysis or blood loss on susceptibility to infection, *J. Immunol.* 91:65–75.

Kaye, D., Gill, F. A., and Hook, E. W., 1967, Factors influencing host resistance to *Salmonella* infections: The effects of hemolysis and erythrophagocytosis, *Am. J. Med. Sci.* 254:205–215.

Kellogg, D. S., Peacock, W. L., Deacon, W. E., Brown, L., and Pirkle, C. I., 1963, *Neisseria gonorrhoeae*. I. Virulence genetically linked to clonal variation. *J. Bacteriol.* 85:1274–1279.

Kellogg, D. S., Cohen, I. R., Norins, L. C., Schroeter, A. L., and Reising, G., 1968, *Neisseria gonorrhoeae*. II. Colonia variation and pathogenicity during 35 months *in vitro*, *J. Bacteriol.* 96:596–605.

Kenny, K., and Herzberg, M., 1968, Antibody response and protection induced by immunization with smooth and rough strains in experimental salmonellosis, *J. Bacteriol.* 95:406–417.

Keutsch, G. J., Grady, G. F., Maya, L. J., and McIver, J., 1972, The pathogenesis of *Shigella diarrhea*. I. Enterotoxin production by *Shigella dysenteriae* 1, *J. Clin. Invest.* 51:1212–1218.

Kim, Y. G., and Watson, D. W., 1967, Biologically active endotoxins from *Salmonella* mutants deficient in O- and R-polysaccharides and heptose, *J. Bacteriol.* 94:1320–1326.

Klebanoff, S. J., 1971, Intraleucocytic microbicidal defects, *Annu. Rev. Med.* 22:39–62.

Knop, J., Breu, H., Wernet, P., and Rowley, D., 1971, The relative antibacterial efficiency of IgM, IgG and IgA from pig colostrum, *Aust. J. Exp. Biol. Med. Sci.* **49**:405–413.

Kochan, I., 1969, Mechanism of tuberculostasis in mammalian serum. I. Role of transferrin in human serum tuberculostasis, *J. Infect. Dis.* **119**:11–18.

Kolb, W. P., Haxby, J. A., Arroyave, C. M., and Muller-Eberhard, H. J., 1972, Molecular analysis of the molecular attack mechanism of complement, *J. Exp. Med.* **135**:549–566.

Koster, F. T., McGregor, D. D., and Mackaness, G. B., 1971, Migration of immunologically committed lymphocytes into inflammatory exudates, *J. Exp. Med.* **133**:389–399.

Koupal, L. R., and Deibel, R. H., 1975, Assay, characterisation and localization of an enterotoxin produced by *Salmonella, Infect. Immun.* **11**:14–22.

Krause, R. M., 1975, Immunological activity of the peptidoglycan, *Z. Immunitaets forsch.* **149**:136–150.

Kronvall, G., and Williams, R. C., 1969, Differences in anti-Protein A activity among IgG subgroups, *J. Immunol.* **103**:828–833.

Kronvall, G., Dossett, J. H., Quie, P. Q., and Williams, R. C., 1971, Occurrence of protein A in staphylococcal strains: Quantitative aspects and correlation to antigenic and bacteriophage types, *Infect. Immun.* **3**:10–15.

LaBrec, E. H., and Formal, S. B., 1961, Experimental *Shigella* infections. IV. Fluorescent antibody studies of an infection in guineapigs, *J. Immunol.* **87**:562–572.

LaBrec, E. H., Schneider, H., Magnani, T. J., and Formal, S. B., 1964, Epithelial cell penetration as an essential step in the pathogenesis of bacillary dysentery, *J. Bacteriol.* **88**:1503–1518.

Lawn, A. M., Blyth, W. A., and Taverne, J., 1973, Interactions of TRIC agents with macrophages and BHK-21 cells observed by electron microscopy, *J. Hyg.* **71**:515–528.

Ling, N. R., 1968, in: *Lymphocyte Stimulation*, pp. 152, 154, North-Holland, Amsterdam.

Lüderitz, O., Staub, A. M., and Westphal, O., 1966, Immunochemistry of O and R antigens of *Salmonella* and related Enterobacteriaceae, *Bacteriol. Rev.* **30**:192–255.

Lüderitz, O., Galanos, C., Lehmann, V., Nurminen, M., Rietschel, E. T., Rosenfelder, G., Simon, M., and Westphal, O., 1973, Lipid A: Chemical structure and biological activity, *J. Infect. Dis.* **128**:S17–S29.

McCabe, W. R., 1963, Endotoxin tolerance. II. Its occurrence in patients with pyelonephritis, *J. Clin. Invest.* **42**:618–625.

McCabe, W. F., 1972, Immunization with R. mutants of *S. minnesota.* I. Protection against challenge with heterologous gram-negative bacteria, *J. Immunol.* **108**:601–610.

McCabe, W. R., Kreger, B. E., and Johns, M., 1972, Type specific and cross-reactive antibodies in gram negative bacteremia, *N. Engl. J. Med.* **287**:261–267.

McCabe, W. R., Greely, A., Di Genio, T., and Johns, M. A., 1973, Humoral immunity to type specific and cross reactive antigens of gram negative bacilli, *J. Infect. Dis.* **128**:S284–S294.

McCabe, W. R., Carling, P. C., Bruins, S., and Greely, A., 1975, The relation of K-antigen to virulence of *Escherichia coli, J. Infect. Dis.* **131**:6–10.

Macfarlane, H., Reddy, S., Adcock, K. J., Adeshina, H., Cooke, A. R., and Akene, J., 1970, Immunity and survival in kwashiorkor, *Br. Med. J.* **4**:268–270.

Mackaness, G. B., 1964, The immunological basis of acquired cellular resistance, *J. Exp. Med.* **120**:105–120.

Mackaness, G. B., 1969, The influence of immunologically committed lymphoid cells on macrophage activity *in vivo, J. Exp. Med.* **129**:973–992.

Mackaness, G. B., and Blanden, R. V., 1967, Cellular immunity, *Progr. Allergy* **11**:89–140.

Mackaness, G. B., Blanden, R. V., and Collins, F. M., 1966, Host–parasite relations in mouse typhoid, *J. Exp. Med.* **124**:573–584.

Makela, P. H., Valtonen, V. V., and Valtonen, M., 1973, Role of O-antigen lipopolysaccharide factors in the virulence of *Salmonella, J. Infect. Dis.* **128**:S81–S85.

Malakian, A., and Schwab, J., 1967, Immunosuppressant from group A streptococci, *Science* **159**:880–881.

Marr, J. J., and Spilberg, I., 1975, A mechanism for decreased resistance to infection by gram-negative organisms during acute alcoholic intoxication, *J. Lab. Clin. Med.* **86**:253–258.

Martin, C. M., Jandl, J. H., and Finland, M., 1963, Enhancement of acute bacterial infections in rats and mice by iron and their inhibition by human transferrin, *J. Infect. Dis.* **112**:158–163.

Maw, J., and Meynell, G. G., 1968, The true division and death rates of *Salmonella typhimurium* in the mouse spleen determined with superinfecting phage P22, *Br. J. Exp. Pathol.* **49**:597–613.

Medhurst, F. A., Hill, M. J., and Glynn, A. A., 1969, The effect of antilymphocyte serum on subcutaneous staphylococcal infections in normal immune and complement deficient mice, *J. Med. Microbiol.* **2**:147–159.

Melching, L., and Vas, S. I., 1971, Effects of serum components on gram-negative bacteria during bactericidal reactions, *Infect. Immun.* **3**:107–115.

Miles, A. A., Miles, E. M., and Burke, J., 1957, The value and duration of defence reactions of the skin to the primary lodgement of bacteria, *Br. J. Exp. Pathol.* **38**:79–96.

Miller, C. P., and Bohnhoff, M., 1963, Changes in the mouse's enteric microflora associated with enhanced susceptibility to *Salmonella* infection following streptomycin treatment, *J. Infect. Dis.* **113**:59–66.

Miller, M. E., and Nilsson, U. R., 1970, A familial deficiency of the phagocytosis enhancing activity of serum related to a dysfunction of the fifth component of complement (C5), *N. Engl. J. Med.* **282**:354–358.

Misaki, A., Yukawa, S., Tsuchiya, K., and Yamasaki, T., 1966, Studies on the cell walls of *Mycobacteria.* I. Chemical and biological properties of the cell walls and the mucopeptide of BCG, *J. Biochem.* **59**:388–396.

Muschel, L. H., and Jackson, J. E., 1966, The reactivity

of serum against protoplasts and spheroplasts, *J. Immun.* **97:**46–51.

Muschel, L. H., and Osawa, E., 1959, Human blood group substance B and *Escherichia coli* 086, *Proc. Soc. Exp. Biol. Med.* **101:**614–617.

Nakano, M., and Saito, K., 1969, Chemical components in the cell wall of *Salmonella typhimurium* affecting its virulence and immunogenicity in mice, *Nature (London)* **222:**1085–1086.

Nauciel, C., Fleck, J., Martin, J. P., Mock, M., and Nguyen-Huy, H., 1974, Adjuvant activity of bacterial peptidoglycans on the production of delayed hypersensitivity and on antibody response, *Eur. J. Immunol.* **4:**352–356.

Nelson, D. S., and Boyden, S. V., 1964, The cutaneous reactivity of guinea pigs to pure protein antigens, *Int. Arch. Allergy* **25:**279–303.

Nelson, B. W., and Roantree, R. J., 1967, Analyses of lipopolysaccharides extracted from penicillin-resistant, serum-sensitive *Salmonella* mutants, *J. Gen. Microbiol.* **48:**179–188.

Newman, S. L., Waldo, B., and Johnston, R. B., 1973, Separation of serum bactericidal and opsonizing activities for *Haemophilus influenzae*, *Infect. Immun.* **8:**488–490.

Nicholson, A. M., and Glynn, A. A., 1975, Investigation of the effect of K antigen in *Escherichia coli* urinary tract infections by use of a mouse model, *Br. J. Exp. Pathol.* **56:**549–553.

Noble, W. C., 1965, The production of subcutaneous staphylococcal skin lesions in mice, *Br. J. Exp. Pathol.* **46:**254–262.

Ofek, I., Beachey, E. H., and Bisno, A. L., 1974, Resistance of *Neisseria gonorrhoeae* to phagocytosis: Relationship to colonial morphology and surface pili, *J. Infect. Dis.* **129:**310–316.

Oppenheim, J. J., and Rosenstreich, D. L., 1976, Signals regulating *in vitro* activation of lymphocytes, *Progr. Allergy* **20:**65–194.

Ørskov, I., and Ørskov, F., 1970, The K antigens of *Escherichia coli*. Re-examination and re-evaluation of the nature of L antigens, *Acta Pathol. Microbiol. Scand. Ser.* B **78:**593–604.

Penn, C. W., Sen, D., Veale, D. R., Parsons, N. J., and Smith, H., 1976, Morphological biological and antigenic properties of *Neisseria gonorrhoeae* adopted to growth in guinea pig subcutaneous chambers, *J. Gen. Microbiol.* **97:**35–43.

Petersen, B. H., Graham, J. A., and Brooks, G. F., 1976, Human deficiency of the eighth component of complement. The requirement of C8 for serum *Neisseria gonorrhoeae* bactericidal activity, *J. Clin. Invest.* **57:**283–290.

Pettenkofer, H. J., Stors, B., Helmbold, W., and Vogel, F., 1962, Alleged causes of the present day world distribution of blood groups, *Nature (London)* **193:**445–446.

Plant, J., and Glynn, A. A., 1976, Genetics of resistance to infection with *Salmonella typhimurium* in mice, *J. Infect. Dis.* **133:**72–78.

Punsalang, A. P., and Sawyer, W. D., 1973, Role of pili

in the virulence of *Neisseria gonorrhoeae*, *Infect. Immun.* **8:**255–263.

Reed, W. P., Davidson, M. S., and Williams, R. C., 1976, Complement system in pneumococcal infections, *Infect. Immun.* **13:**1120–1125.

Rich, A. R., 1951, *The Pathogenesis of Tuberculosis*, 2nd ed., p. 509, Blackwells, Oxford.

Rittenhouse, H. G., Roda, J. B., and McFadden, B. A., 1973, Immunologically cross reacting proteins in cell walls of many bacteria, *J. Bacteriol.* **113:**1400–1403.

Roantree, R. J., 1967, *Salmonella* O antigens and virulence, *Annu. Rev. Microbiol.* **21:**443–446.

Roantree, R. J., and Rantz, L. A., 1960, A study of the relationship of the normal bactericidal activity of human serum to bacterial infection, *J. Clin. Invest.* **39:**72–81.

Robbins, J. B., Kenny, K., and Suter, E., 1965, The isolation and biological activities of rabbit M and G anti-*Salmonella typhimurium* antibodies, *J. Exp. Med.* **122:**385–402.

Robbins, J. B., Myerowitz, R. L., Whisnant, J. K., Argaman, M., Schneerson, R., Handzel, Z. T., and Gotschlich, E. C., 1972, Enteric bacteria cross reactive with *Neisseria meningitidis* groups A and C and *Diplococcus pneumoniae* types I and III, *Infect. Immun.* **6:**651–656.

Rogers, H. J., 1967, Bacteriostatic effects of horse sera and serum fractions on *Clostridium welchii* type A, and the abolition of bacteriostasis by iron salts, *Immunology* **12:**285–301.

Rook, G. A. W., and Stewart-Tull, D. E. S., 1976, The dissociation of adjuvant properties of mycobacterial components from mitogenicity, and from the ability to induce the release of mediators from macrophages, *Immunology* **31:**389–396.

Root, R. K., Ellman, L., and Frank, M. M., 1972, Bactericidal and opsonic properties of C4 deficient guinea pig serum, *J. Immunol.* **109:**477–486.

Rossen, R. G., Wolff, S. M., and Butler, W. T., 1967, The antibody response in nasal washings and serum to *S. typhosa* endotoxin administered intravenously, *J. Immunol.* **99:**246–254.

Rotta, J., 1975, Endotoxin-like properties of the peptidoglycan, *J. Immunitaets forsch.* **149:**230–244.

Rowley, D., 1956, Rapidly induced changes in the level of non-specific immunity in laboratory animals, *Br. J. Exp. Pathol.* **37:**223–234.

Rowley, D., and Jenkin, C. R., 1962, Antigenic cross-reaction between host and parasite as a possible cause of pathogenicity, *Nature (London)* **193:**151–154.

Rowley, D., and Turner, K. J., 1968, Passive sensitization of *Salmonella adelaide* to the bactericidal action of antibody and complement, *Nature (London)* **217:**657–658.

Schachenmayr, W., Heymer, B., and Haferkamp, O., 1975, Antibodies to peptidoglycan in the sera from population surveys, *Z. Immunitaetsforsch.* **149:**179–186.

Schleifer, K. H., and Kandler, O., 1972, Peptidoglycan types of bacterial cell walls and their taxonomic implications, *Bacteriol. Rev.* **36:**407–477.

Schleifer, K. H., and Krause, R. M., 1971, The immunochemistry of peptidoglycan. Separation and characterisation of antibodies to the glycan and to the peptide sabunit, *Eur. J. Biochem.* **19**:471–478.

Schneerson, R., and Robbins, J. B., 1975, Induction of serum *Haemophilus influenzae* type B capsular antibodies in adult volunteers fed cross-reacting *Escherichia coli* 075:K100:H5, *N. Engl. J. Med.* **292**:1093–1096.

Schoolnik, G. K., Buchanan, T. M., and Holmes, K. K., 1976, Gonococci causing disseminated gonococcal infection are resistant to the bactericidal action of normal human sera, *J. Clin. Invest.* **58**:1163–1173.

Schwab, J. H., 1975, Suppression of the immune response by microorganisms, *Bacteriol. Rev.* **39**:121–143.

Seidl, P. H., and Schleifer, K. H., 1975, Immunochemical studies with synthetic immunogens chemically related to peptidoglycan, *Z. Immunitaetsforsch.* **149**:157–164.

Shands, J. W., 1965, Localisation of somatic antigen on gram-negative bacteria by electron microscopy, *J. Bacteriol.* **90**:266–270.

Shaw, G. B., 1911, *The Doctor's Dilemma*, Constable, London.

Shaw, S., Smith, A. L., Anderson, P., and Smith, D. H., 1976, The paradox of *Haemophilus influenzae* type B bacteremia in the presence of serum bactericidal activity, *J. Clin. Invest.* **58**:1019–1029.

Shin, H. S., Smith, M. R., and Wood, W. B., 1969, Heat labile opsonins to pneumococcus. II. Involvement of C3 and C5, *J. Exp. Med.* **130**:1229–1241.

Siroták, L., Inoue, K., Okada, M., and Amano, T., 1976, Immune bactericidal reactions by guinea pig γ 1 and γ 2 antibodies, *Immunology* **30**:435–441.

Sjostedt, S., 1946, Pathogenicity of certain serological types of *B. coli*, *Acta Pathol. Microbiol. Scand. Suppl.* **63**:1–148.

Smith, H. W., and Halls, S., 1968, The production of oedema disease and diarrhoea in weaned pigs by the oral administration of *Escherichia coli*: Factors that influence the course of the experimental disease, *J. Med. Microbiol.* **1**:45–60.

Smith, H. W., and Jones, J. E. T., 1963, Observations on the alimentary tract and its bacterial flora in healthy and diseased pigs, *J. Pathol. Bacteriol.* **86**:387–412.

Smith, J. W., Barnett, J. A., May, R. P., and Sanford, J. P., 1967, Comparison of the opsonic activity of γ G and γ M anti-*Proteus* globulins, *J. Immunol.* **98**:336–343.

Springer, G. F., 1971, Blood-group and Forssman antigenic determinants shared between microbes and mammalian cells, *Progr. Allergy* **15**:9–77.

Standfast, A. F. B., 1967, Bacterial antigens, in: *Modern Trends in Immunology*, 2nd ed. (R. Cruickshank and D. Weir, eds.), pp. 1–27, Butterworths, London.

Steele, E. J., Chaicumpa, W., and Rowley, D., 1975, Further evidence for cross-linking as a protective factor in experimental cholera: Properties of antibody fragments, *J. Infect. Dis.* **132**:175–180.

Sterzl, J., Kostka, J., and Lanc, A., 1962, Development of bactericidal properties against gram-negative organisms in the serum of young animals, *Folia Microbiol. (Prague)* **7**:162–174.

Stetson, C. A., 1964, Role of hypersensitivity in reactions to endotoxin, in: *Bacterial Endotoxins* (M. Landy and W. Braun, eds.), pp. 658–662, Rutgers University Press, New Brunswick, N.J.

Stiffel, C., Biozzi, G., Mouton, D., Bouthillier, Y., and Decreusefond, C., 1964, Studies on phagocytosis of bacteria by the reticuloendothelial system in a strain of mice lacking hemolytic complement, *J. Immunol.* **93**:246–249.

Strominger, J. L., and Tipper, D. J., 1974, Structure of bacterial cell walls: The lysozyme substrate, in: *Lysozyme* (E. F. Osserman, R. E. Canfield, and S. Beychok, eds.), pp. 169–184, Academic Press, New York and London.

Swanson, J., Kraus, S. J., and Gotschlich, E. C., 1971, Studies on gonococcus infection. I. Pili and zones of adhesion: Their relation to gonococcal growth patterns, *J. Exp. Med.* **134**:886–906.

Sword, C. P., 1966, Mechanisms of pathogenesis in *Listeria monocytogenes* infection. I. Influence of iron, *J. Bacteriol.* **92**:536–542.

Takeuchi, A., 1971, Penetration of the intestinal epithelium by various microorganisms, *Curr. Top. Pathol.* **54**:1–27.

Tannock, G. W., Blumershine, R. V. H., and Savage, D. C., 1975, Association of *Salmonella typhimurium* with, and its invasion of, the ileal mucosa in mice, *Infect. Immun.* **11**:365–370.

Taubler, J. H., 1968, Staphylococcal delayed hypersensitivity in mice. I. Induction and *in vivo* demonstration of delayed hypersensitivity, *J. Immunol.* **101**:546–549.

Taylor, P. W., 1975, Genetical studies of serum resistance in *Escherichia coli*, *J. Gen. Microbiol.* **89**:57–66.

Thongthai, C., and Sawyer, W. D., 1973, Studies on the virulence of *Neisseria gonorrhoeae*. I. Relation of colonial morphology and resistance to phagocytosis by polymorphonuclear leucocytes, *Infect. Immun.* **7**:373–379.

Torikata, R., 1917, in: J. P. Scott, 1931, Aggressins. An outline of the development of the theory and notes on the use of these products, *J. Bacteriol.* **22**:323–337.

Turk, J. L., and Bryceson, A. D. M., 1971, Immunological phenomena in leprosy and related diseases, *Adv. Immunol.* **13**:209–266.

Turner, M. W., and Rowe, D. S., 1964, Characterization of human antibodies to *Salmonella typhi* by gel-filtration and antigenic analysis, *Immunology* **7**:639–656.

Valtonen, V. V. Aird, J., Valtonen, M., Makela, O., and Makela, P. H., 1971, Mouse virulence of *Salmonella*: Antigen-dependent differences are demonstrable also after immunosuppression, *Acta Pathol. Scan. Ser. B* **79**:715–718.

Veale, D. R., Finch, H., Penn, C. W., Sen, D., and Smith, H., 1976, Resistance of *Neisseria gonorrhoeae* grown *in vivo* to ingestion and digestion by phagocytes of human blood, *J. Gen. Microbiol.* **96**:341–350.

Vosti, K. L., and Randall, E., 1970, Sensitivity of serologically classified strains of *Escherichia coli* of human origin to the serum bactericidal system. *Am. J. Med. Sci.* **259:**114–119.

Walker, W. A., Isselbacher, K. J., and Bloch, K. J., 1972, Intestinal uptake of macromolecules: Effect of oral immunization, *Science* **177:**608–610.

Ward, M. E., and Watt, P. J., 1972, Adherence of *Neisseria gonorrhoeae* to urethral mucosal cells: An electron microscopic study of human gonorrhoea, *J. Infect. Dis.* **126:**601–605.

Ward, M. E., Watt, P. J., and Glynn, A. A., 1970, Gonococci in urethral exudates possess a virulence factor lost on subculture, *Nature (London)* **227:**382–384.

Watt, P. J., Glynn, A. A., and Ward, M. E., 1972, Maintenance of virulent gonococci in laboratory culture, *Nature (London) New Biol.* **236:**186–187.

Weinberg, E. D., 1966, Roles of metallic ions in host-parasite interactions, *Bacteriol. Rev.* **30:**136–151.

Weksler, B. B., and Hill, M. J., 1969, Inhibition of leukocyte migration by a staphylococcal factor, *J. Bacteriol.* **98:**1030–1035.

Westphal, O., and Jann, K., 1965, in: *Methods of Carbohydrate Chemistry*, Vol. 5 (R. L. Whistler and M. L. Wolfrom, eds.), pp. 83–91, Academic Press, New York.

White, R. G., 1976, The adjuvant effect of microbial products on the immune response, *Annu. Rev. Microbiol.* **30:**579–600.

Williams, R. C., and Gibbons, R. J., 1972, Inhibition of bacterial adherence by secretory immunoglobulin A: A mechanism of antigen disposal, *Science* **177:**697–699.

Willoughby, D. A., Coote, E., and Turk, J. L., 1969, Complement in acute inflammation, *J. Pathol.* **97:**295–305.

Wilson, B. M., and Glynn, A. A., 1975, Release of ^{14}C label and complement killing of *Escherichia coli*, *Immunology* **28:**391–400.

Wilson, B. M., and Glynn, A. A., 1977, Comparison of the bactericidal effects of the classical and alternative pathways of human complement on *Escherichia coli*, *Proc. Soc. Gen. Microbiol.* **4:**118–119.

Wilson, I. D., 1972, Studies on the opsonic activity of human secretory IgA using an *in vitro* phagocytosis system, *J. Immunol.* **108:**726–730.

Wilson, L. A., and Spitznagel, J. K., 1968, Molecular and structural damage to *Escherichia coli* produced by antibody complement and lysozyme systems, *J. Bacteriol.* **96:**1339–1348.

Wilson, L. A., and Spitznagel, J. K., 1971, Characteristics of complement-dependent release of phospholipid from *Escherichia coli*, *Infect. Immun.* **4:**23–28.

Winkelstein, J. A., Shin, H. S., and Wood, W. B., 1972, Heat labile opsonins to pneumococcus. III. The participation of immunoglobulin and of the alternate pathway of C3 activation, *J. Immunol.* **108:**1681–1689.

Winkelstein, J. A., Smith, M. R., and Shin, H. S., 1975, The role of C3 as an opsonin in the early stages of infection, *Proc. Soc. Exp. Biol. Med.* **149:**397–401.

Winkelstein, J. A., Bocchini, J. A., and Schiffman, G., 1976, The role of the capsular polysaccharide in the activation of the alternative pathway by the pneumococcus, *J. Immunol.* **116:**367–378.

Wood, B. W., 1960, Phagocytosis, with particular reference to encapsulated bacteria, *Bacteriol. Rev.* **24:**41–49.

Youmans, G. P., and Youmans, A. S., 1969, Recent studies on acquired immunity in tuberculosis, *Curr. Top. Microbiol. Immunol.* **48:**129–178.

Young, L. S., and Armstrong, D., 1972, Human immunity to *Pseudomonas aeruginosa*. I. *In-vitro* interaction of bacteria, polymorphonuclear leukocytes, and serum factors, *J. Infect. Dis.* **126:**257–276.

Zabriskie, J. B., 1967, Mimetic relationships between group A streptococci and mammalian tissues, *Adv. Immunol.* **7:**147–188.

Zinner, S. H., and McCabe, W. F., 1976, Effects of IgM and IgG antibody in patients with bacteremia due to gram-negative bacilli, *J. Infect. Dis.* **133:**37–45.

2

Immunology of *Streptococcus pneumoniae*

ARTHUR J. AMMANN

1. Introduction

In 1909, Sir William Osler termed pneumonia "captain of the men of death" (Osler, 1909). Today, pneumonia ranks as the only infectious illness among the ten leading causes of death in the United States (Austrian, 1976). From 1900 to 1968, the annual mortality fell from approximately 200 per 100,000 population to 35 per 100,000. In a report by the Respiratory Disease Task Force (1972), it was noted that there were 2,700,000 hospitalizations for infectious pneumonia in 1975 and that these hospitalizations accounted for 8.5% of admissions that year. The early treatment of pneumococcal pneumonia required the isolation and typing of the causative organism with subsequent administration of type-specific antiserum. Typing and the use of antiserum became unnecessary with the introduction of antibiotics, initially in the form of sulfonamides and subsequently penicillin.

In spite of the striking decrease in mortality from pneumococcal infections, several observations indicate that significant problems remain: (1) the mortality for uncomplicated bacteremic pneumococcal pneumonia treated with penicillin or other antibiotics is 17–18%, and in patients over 50 years of age, or with underlying systemic illness, greater than 25%

(Austrian, 1976); (2) pneumococcal infections remain among the primary causes of bacterial otitis media, pneumonia, and meningitis in infants and children (Loda *et al.*, 1975).

2. Immunochemistry

2.1. Basic Chemistry

A significant number of bacteria, including *Streptococcus pneumoniae,* develop a thick envelope termed a capsule. Numerous methods have been used to demonstrate this capsule including india ink (Bott *et al.*, 1936) and the Neufeld Quellung reaction utilizing specific antibody. The majority of bacterial capsules consist of polysaccharides with a high proportion of acidic constituents, including neuraminic acid, hexuronic acids, or pyruvate (Luderitz *et al.*, 1968). Microorganisms frequently are found to have a capsule when they are obtained from pathogenic material, but this capsule may be lost on prolonged cultivation. Encapsulation may be a measure of the pathogenicity of the organism, as evidenced by the observation that the capsule may result in bacterial resistance to phagocytosis and to the reaction of antibody or complement (Schwarzmann and Boring, 1971; Glynn, 1969).

A variety of methods have been utilized to isolate capsular polysaccharides, including block electrophoresis and gels (Holmgren *et al.*, 1971), ion-exchange chromatography (Yurewicz *et al.*, 1971), precipitation with cetav-

ARTHUR J. AMMANN • Division of Pediatric Immunology, Pediatric Clinical Research Center, and Department of Pediatrics, University of California, San Francisco, California 94143.

lon (Jann and Westphal, 1975). These purification methods usually are utilized following extraction with saline or buffer at temperatures between 20°C and 50°C or with a 5% aqueous phenol (Jann and Westphal, 1975).

The capsular polysaccharide serves to distinguish more than 75 serologically distinct types of pneumococci which are designated by individual numbers. Table 1 lists the composition of pneumococcal polysaccharides 3, 4, 8, and 18. Many of the polysaccharides are charged either through the hexuronic acid constituents or through the phosphate or pyruvic substitution. Pneumococcal polysaccharides contain three different neutral sugars with a high incidence of L-rhamnose. The complete structure of the pneumococcal polysaccharides is known in some cases. Structures of some of the type-specific capsular polysaccharides are listed in Table 2.

A species-specific C polysaccharide is produced by many strains of pneumococci. It has some features in common with certain type-specific polysaccharides (types 6 and 24), in that it contains ribitol phosphate. In addition, N-acetylgalactosamine, glucose, 2-acetamido-4-amino-2,4,6-trideoxyhexose, and phosphorylcholine are found (Jann and Westphal, 1975).

2.2. Immunochemical Analysis of Polysaccharide Antigens

A variety of serological methods have been utilized to study the immunochemistry of polysaccharide antigens and include precipitation (Heidelberger and Kendall, 1929), agglutination (Neter, 1956), complement fixation (Wasserman and Levine, 1961), precipitation in gels (Ouchterlony, 1958; Hanson, 1959), and coating of specific polysaccharides onto red cells by the indirect hemagglutination technique (Baker *et al.*, 1969; Ammann and Pelger, 1972). Antigen-binding studies have been performed utilizing equilibrium dialysis (Pinckard

and Weir, 1973) or binding of the intrinsically or extrinsically labeled polysaccharide to an antigen–antibody and precipitation of the antibody–antigen complex with ammonium sulfate (Minden and Farr, 1967).

Several investigators (Kabat, 1966; Mage and Kabat, 1966; Gelzer and Kabat, 1964) have studied the inhibitory capacity of oligosaccharides in antibody–polysaccharide precipitating systems. The conclusions reached are that the antigenic specificity of polysaccharides centers around single hexose units and the sequential groupings and conformational relationships of these units along the polysaccharide chain over regions of different lengths.

Because many polysaccharides are branched, the question has been raised as to whether it is the oligosaccharide sequences within the branch or the branch itself which represents the antigenic determinants (Jann and Westphal, 1975). Although some workers have reported that the side chains are usually the immunodeterminant in branched polysaccharides (Ballou, 1970; Suzuki *et al.*, 1968), the serological specificity of the branched pneumococcal polysaccharide is not necessarily restricted to the side chains and substituent monosaccharide units alone (Heidelberger and Elliot, 1966). The role of conformational changes in antigenicity has been well studied with proteins. However, information on the influence of conformation on the antigenicity of polysaccharides has not been evaluated. It may be that conformational determinants, as opposed to structural determinants, also may play a role in polysaccharides (Kabat, 1966).

The elaboration of the immunogenic determinants of a polysaccharide may be critical in a study of protection against infection. When the immunogenic determinant was used to produce antibodies, such as cellobiuronic acid, the repeating unit of pneumococcal polysaccharide 3, animals were protected against fatal

TABLE 1. Composition of Certain Pneumococcal Capsular Polysaccharides

Polysaccharide	Amino sugar (N-acetylated)	Neutral sugar	Hexuronic acid	Noncarbohydrate
3	—	Glc	GlcUA	—
4	GalN ManN FucN	Gal	—	Pyruvate
8	—	GalGlc	GlcUA	—
18	—	GalGlc Rha		Glycerolphosphate

TABLE 2. Structure of Certain Pneumococcal Capsular
Polysaccharides

Polysaccharide	Repeating unit
3	$\xrightarrow{\ 3\ }$ GlcUA $\xrightarrow{\beta1,4}$ Glc $\xrightarrow{\ 1\ }$
6	$\xrightarrow{\ 2\ }$ Gal $\xrightarrow{\alpha1,3}$ Glc $\xrightarrow{1,3}$ L-Rha $\xrightarrow{1,3}$ Ribitol $\longrightarrow$ P $\longrightarrow$
7	$\xrightarrow{\ 4\ }$ GlcUA $\xrightarrow{\beta1,4}$ Glc $\xrightarrow{\beta1,4}$ Glc $\xrightarrow{\alpha1,4}$ Gal $\xrightarrow{\alpha1}$

infection with highly pathogenic type 3 organisms (Goebel, 1940).

The immunogenicity of pure polysaccharide may vary with the animal utilized for immunization (Jann and Westphal, 1975). For example, some pneumococcal polysaccharides are relatively nonimmunogenic in rabbits but excellent immunogens for man. Polysaccharide may be transformed into an immunogen by several means, including diazotization and coupling of the polysaccharide to protein (Goebel, 1940; Himmelspach *et al.,* 1971), coupling to polypeptides (Sela, 1966), and tyrosylation (Sorg *et al.,* 1970).

In addition to the cell wall (C) polysaccharide of the pneumococcus, a C-like capsular polysaccharide or soluble polysaccharide (Cs) has been isolated (Schiffman *et al.,* 1971). Immunochemical analysis has shown heterogeneity of both the C and C-like polysaccharides from a variety of pneumococcal strains. The dissimilarities reside in the mucopeptide portion of the molecule or the region of its attachment to the teichoic acid moiety. It is of interest that vaccines made from the Cs mutants are highly antigenic in rabbits, in contrast to other polysaccharides.

2.3. Cross-Reactions between Microbial Polysaccharides

Antibody directed against capsular polysaccharide has been utilized to determine cross-reactivity between various microbial agents. In a heterologous system, such as pneumococcal polysaccharides 3, 8, anti-3, and anti-8, the antigen–antibody binding may be inhibited completely by low concentrations of tetrasaccharides (Sela, 1966). Cellobiuronic acid, which is common to both polysaccharides, will also completely inhibit the antigen–antibody reaction. Cellobiuronic acid is therefore the

cause of the cross-reactivity detected in this heterologous system. Cross-reactivity also causes difficulty in serological classifications. In early investigations, atypical forms of pneumococci were reported, e.g., types 2A and 3A. Subsequently, it was discovered that these strains represented independent types and were designated type 5 and type 8, respectively. The analysis of a variety of cross-reactions between the polysaccharides of pneumococci and of other microbial agents allowed for characterization of the antibodies reacting with partial structures of these polysaccharides. The phenomenon of cross-reactivity has become a useful tool in the structural elucidation of polysaccharides. Usually, antibody directed against a known structure is used to identify similar structures in an unknown polysaccharide. Alternatively, oligosaccharides of known structure may be used to inhibit an antigen–antibody reaction with polysaccharides for partial identification.

Comparative immunochemistry has shown cross-reactivity between pneumococcal polysaccharide antigens, *Escherichia coli* polysaccharide and plant polysaccharides. Specifically, pneumococcal polysaccharides 3 and 8, oat glucan, and the K87 antigen of *E. coli* have common antigenic determinants (Jann and Westphal, 1975). Antigenic similarities have been detected between the teichoic acid of streptococcus group N and acetylphosphogalactan from *Sporobloyces* and the capsular polysaccharides from pneumococcus types 6, 16, 18, and 22 (Heidelberger and Elliot, 1966). Klebsiella polysaccharides also cross-react with pneumococcal polysaccharides (Heidelberger and Nimmich, 1972). The Klebsiella polysaccharide K1 reacts with antibody to pneumococcal polysaccharide 10. K2, K4, K8, and K9 react strongly with antibody to pneumococcal polysaccharide 2. Other cross-reactions exist between K32, K47, and K48 and various pneumococcal polysaccharide types.

Certain cross-reactivities may have important implications regarding the development of natural immunity. Previously, it was believed that virtually all antibody directed against specific bacterial antigens developed as a result of exposure to a specific bacteria. Thus the demonstration of antibody directed against pneumococcal polysaccharide type 3, in an individual without a history of clinical infection, was interpreted as indicating a subclinical infection. An understanding of the phenomenon of cross-reactivity between microbial species resulted in an alternative explanation, i.e., colonization by nonpathogenic bacteria resulting in antibody production with cross-reactivity against pathogenic bacteria. Several investigators have shown cross-reactivity between pathogenic strains of *Neisseria, Hemophilus,* and *Diplococcus.* The capsular polysaccharides of pneumococcus type 1 and type 3 cross-react with several strains of *E. coli* (WHO 11, WHO 42, WHO 30, WHO 252, WHO 165, BOS Y2, ISB 353, and LH) (Robbins *et al.,* 1972). *B. cereus* shares antigenic determinants with pneumococcal polysaccharide type 3; *B. alvei* cross-reacts with pneumococcal polysaccharide 3, as well as with *H. influenzae* type B (Myerowitz *et al.,* 1974).

2.4. Immunogenicity of Pneumococcal Polysaccharides

Proteins and natural polysaccharides have similar molecular weights. However, in contrast to proteins, polysaccharides have a simple composition and conformation. The molecular weight is one of the major determinants in the immunogenicity of a polysaccharide. Extensive studies on comparative immunogenicity of dextrans indicate that those dextrans with a mean molecular weight of 90,000 and above are good immunogens, while dextrans with an average molecular weight of below 50,000 are poor immunogens (Kabat and Bezer, 1958). Studies on the imunogenicity of degraded products of the native polysaccharide type 3 have been performed utilizing plaque-forming cells as an indication of antibody formation (Howard *et al.,* 1971). The studies, conducted in mice, indicated that immunogenicity was related to molecular weight. Native polysaccharide type 3, wth a molecular weight of 220,000, elicited a hundred fold greater response than degradation products with a molecular weight of 4000. Degradation products with molecular weights of 30,000 and 120,000 resulted in intermediate antibody responses.

Dose–response studies indicate that the immunogenicity of polysaccharide is related to a more narrow dose range than that of protein antigens. Large amounts of polysaccharide (about 500 μg) render mice unresponsive, whereas small amounts (0.5–1 μg) protected mice against subsequent challenge with specific bacteria (Felton and Ottinger, 1942). Further, it was shown that a single injection of 500 μg of polysaccharide abbrogated the subsequent immune response to immunizing doses. This form of "immunological paralysis" persisted for at least 15 months. It was postulated that this effect was achieved by persistence of polysaccharide antigen which could not be degraded by enzymes of the animal. Polysaccharide thus would persist in cells, be excreted intact from such cells, and continue to recirculate, resulting in continuous neutralization of antibody and inability to detect the antibody response. This phenomenon also may exist in humans who have undergone infection with polysaccharide containing organisms. Significant numbers of individuals who have experienced infection with polysaccharide containing organisms such as *H. influenzae* fail to form antibody during the convalescent phase (O'Reilly *et al.,* 1975). We have studied the immune response in an infant with a pneumococcal polysaccharide type 14 meningitis. The infant failed to respond with antibody formation following immunization with pneumococcal polysaccharide type 14, given 4 weeks after recovery from the meningitis. As long as 18 weeks following immunization, no antibody to type 14 polysaccharide could be detected. Immunization with an unrelated pneumococcal polysaccharide (type 4) resulted in a 512-fold increase in antibody titer.

3. Antibody-Mediated Immunity to *Streptococcus pneumoniae*

3.1. Basic Antibody Response

The majority of studies on antibody-mediated immunity to pneumococcal antigens have been performed in mice utilizing pneumococcal polysaccharide. Several of these studies indicate that the antibody response following immunization occurs quite rapidly. Utilizing a bentonite-adherence method, the interval between the intravenous injection of an optimal dose (1 μg) and the appearance of antibody-forming cells was between 4 and 8 hr (Baker and Landy, 1967). Utilizing a rosette technique, circulating antibody has been detected 12 hr following immunization (Howard, 1969; Howard *et al.,* 1969). Use of the hemolytic plaque technique has shown detectable antibody forming cells at 12–48 hr following immunization (Kearney and Halliday, 1970; Baker and Stashak, 1969). Assay methods utilizing single-cell techniques, such as the hemolytic plaque or bentonite-adherence method, may not be so restricted in the determination of antibody as more classical antibody methods. The problems of detecting antibody in the presence of excess polysaccharide antigen will be discussed later in greater detail.

Calculations, utilizing the hemolytic plaque assay, suggest that the doubling time of cells is in the range of 6–7 hr. Since this is less than the generation time for immunocompetent cells by most methods, it has been suggested that new potential antibody-forming cells are activated continuously rather than formed by cell division (Baker and Stashak, 1969).

The duration of antibody response has been studied primarily in humans immunized with pneumococcal polysaccharide (Heidelberger, 1953). In these studies, antibody was found to persist for periods up to 8 years following initial immunization. Few additional studies are available.

Although the majority of studies in animals indicate that the antibody class formed following immunization with polysaccharide antigens is primarily IgM, recent studies suggest that IgG and IgA also may be produced (Barthold *et al.,* 1974). Some species of mice undergoing an allogeneic effect (an enhanced immunoreactive state associated with graft-vs.-host reaction) when immunized with pneumococcal polysaccharide type 3 produce IgG antibody (Braley-Mullen, 1974). Mice also may produce IgG antibody when the polysaccharide is coupled to a thymic-dependent antigen, e.g., type 3 coupled to sheep erythrocytes.

In studies performed in man to determine the degree of antibody responsiveness following immunization with 25–100 μg of purified pneumococcal polysaccharides (Austrian, 1976), the antigenicity of each individal polysaccharide varied considerably. Of the types used (types 1, 2, 3, 4, 6, 7, 8, 9, 12, 14, 18, 19, and 23), type 3 was consistently highly immunogenic, whereas types 1, 19, and 23 do not result in so significant an antibody increase. Mean antibody titers, expressed as micrograms of antibody nitrogen per milliliter, varied from 0.03 to 0.95 before immunization and from 0.48 to 13.50 after immunization (Austrian, 1976).

Detailed studies of the class of antibody formed following immunization with pneumococcal polysaccharide in man have not been reported previously. Following immunization with 50 μg of polysaccharide type 3 in three normal individuals, we determined antibody titers 3 weeks later by the indirect hemagglutination method. Titers were 1:128, 1:132, and 1:512. Following inactivation with 2-mercaptoethanol, the hemagglutinating titers were 1:2, 1:8, and 1:512, respectively. These studies suggest that the early antibody response is composed primarily of IgM but in some instances may consist of a 7 S response. Additional studies were performed following ultracentrifugation and sucrose density separation of serum samples obtained 5 and 7 days following immunization with type 2 and type 3 polysaccharide in three individuals. Antibody activity was found in both the IgG and IgM fractions at 5 and 7 days following immunization, indicating that the early antibody response consists of both IgG and IgM. These studies did not determine if IgA antibody is formed.

Studies on paired maternal and fetal samples indicated that significant amounts of antibody to pneumococcal polysaccharide exist in the IgG class. Maternal titers to four pneumococcal polysaccharide types (1, 2, 8, 23) were compared to paired cord serum titers. A significant titer of antibody was found in the cord blood samples which contained only IgG.

The protective function of antibody produced following immunization or natural infection has not been studied in detail in animals or man. It is generally accepted that IgM antibody may be more protective in animal studies. Horse IgM directed against polysaccharide was found to be 100 times as active as IgG in the mouse protection assay (Hill and Robbins, 1966).

Some of the difficulties encountered in the determination of antibody following immunization and/or natural infection result from persistence of polysaccharide antigens in the circulation. This is one of the most remarkable properties of these antigens, and studies in mice indicate that the antigen may persist for weeks to months in the circulation (Howard and Siskind, 1969). Other investigations indicate that the antigen may remain in the spleen and other tissues for at least a year and that these antigens can be extracted in a form which can be precipitated by rabbit antibody or used to immunize other animals (Felton, 1949; Felton et al., 1955). As a result of these studies, it has been postulated that antibody formed in animals following immunological paralysis by pneumococcal polysaccharides continuously unite with the antigen present in the circulation and tissues and may be interpreted as a lack of immunological response.

Immunological paralysis in animals can be produced by a variety of antigenic pneumococcal polysaccharide types. The route of administration of the antigens does not appear to be as important as the dose of antigen administered. Two forms of immunological paralysis have been produced, "low zone" and "high zone" (Halliday, 1971). Low-zone tolerance, however, has been observed only with pneumococcal polysaccharide type 3 (Baker et al., 1971b). In these studies, prior immunization, irrespective of the doses employed, resulted in transient low-dose paralysis demonstrable upon reimmunization with optimal doses of antigen. This effect persisted for several weeks.

High-zone tolerance is produced in mice utilizing 100 to 500 mcgm doses of polysaccharide for immunization. As previously indicated, this phenomenon may be a result of continuous binding of antibody by persistent antigen. It is probable that polysaccharides are phagocytized but are resistant to degradation, and that the antigen which is detectable in the blood has been released chronically by a process of exocytosis (Halliday, 1971). Such antigen is excreted slowly as partially degraded polymer in the urine (Coonrad and Rytel, 1973). Paralyzed mice eventually may become immune months after the initial antigen administration, indicating either a persistence or a renewed synthesis of antibody (Siskind, 1962; Siskind et al., 1963).

A secondary or anamnestic response following immunization with purified polysaccharide antigens does not exist under normal circumstances. This has been true in both animals (Halliday, 1971) and man (Heidelberger, 1953). The two exceptions relate to a longer time interval between doses (10 months or more) and a small first dose with a larger second dose and a shortened time interval (Halliday, 1971).

3.2. Genetic Control of Antibody Response

Several studies have indicated that the antibody response to polysaccharides and lipopolysaccharides is under genetic control (Coutinho et al., 1975; Amsbaugh et al., 1972; Amsbaugh et al., 1974; Braley-Mullen et al., 1974). In the case of lipopolysaccharide, it has been postulated that the responsiveness of mice, either high or low responders, is determined by one single, codominantly expressed, autosomal gene (Coutinho et al., 1975). Studies on the response to pneumococcal polysaccharide type 3, in high- and low-responder mice, indicate that a major component of the control of IgM antibody response is X linked (Amsbaugh et al., 1972). These studies also suggest that other factors, probably autosomal genes, regulate the magnitude of the antibody response produced in mice possessing the X-linked gene. Responsiveness was not associated with the ability to synthesize normal quantitative levels of IgM (Amsbaugh et al., 1974). Other investigators have shown that the genetic control of the immune response in mice to pneumococcal polysaccharide type 3 is located at a single autosomal locus, rather than an X-linked locus (Braley-Mullen et al., 1974).

3.3. Tolerance to Polysaccharide Antigens

Young offspring of immunologically paralyzed mice are more susceptible to the induction of paralysis and immunity following immunization with purified polysaccharide than normal mice of the same age (Kerman et al., 1970). The administration of purified specific antipneumococcal antibody or normal IgG has the ability of restoring the offspring of paralyzed mice to the same level of susceptibility to the induction of paralysis and immunity as normal mice. These investigators concluded that a relative deficiency of naturally occurring specific antipneumococcal antibodies was responsible for an altered immunological response in paralyzed mice. They postulated that the results were compatible with a role of preformed antibody in the regulation of antibody formation. These results may be important in immunization studies of infants with purified pneumococcal polysaccharides.

Although it is not certain whether the phenomena of high- and low-zone tolerance to polysaccharides exist in man, several pieces of evidence suggest that they might. Following infection with pneumococcal and *H. influenzae* organisms, large amounts of polysaccharide can be detected in the circulation (Dochez and Avery, 1917; Alexander, 1943). Detailed studies of antigen clearance in *H. influenzae* infection have been performed utilizing a radioimmunoassay to detect the persistence of the capsular polysaccharide, polyribophosphate (O'Reilly *et al.*, 1975). The antigen could be detected in an unbound form in the cerebrospinal fluid and serum for 1–30 days after initiation of effective therapy. Antigen–antibody complexes could be detected as long as 145 days after initial infection. Antibody responses were detected during the first 100 days of convalescence by a radioimmunoassay technique in approximately 80% of the children. However, the intensity of antibody responses was of low magnitude in patients with prolonged antigenemia. Patients who failed to develop antibody also exhibited impaired antigen clearance.

In a study of two patients who developed pneumococcal meningitis, we were able to demonstrate specific immunological unresponsiveness to the polysaccharide as a cause of infection. In the first instance, a normal infant, who was part of a study to determine the effect of immunization with purified polysaccharide in normal infants and children, developed pneumococcal meningitis 8 weeks following a booster immunization with an octavalent pneumococcal polysaccharide vaccine. The initial immunization had been given 22 weeks prior to the development of meningitis. The infant had demonstrated a significant antibody response only to pneumococcal polysaccharide type 1 contained in the vaccine. The meningitis was due to a type 23 pneumococcal infection. No antibody response had been demonstrated to pneumococcal polysaccharide type 23 following 2 immunizations prior to the meningitis, nor was an antibody response detected 4 weeks following the meningitis.

In a second infant, no antibody could be detected to pneumococcal polysaccharide type 14, which was the cause of meningitis. Antibody titers were determined up to 18 weeks following recovery from infection and none could be detected. Immunization with the polysaccharide of the type responsible for infection did not result in an antibody response, whereas immunization with unrelated polysaccharides resulted in a 512-fold increase in antibody response.

4. Cell-Mediated Immunity to *Streptococcus pneumoniae*

4.1. Morphological Alterations following Antigenic Challenge

Conflicting reports are available concerning the effect of pneumococcal antigens on histological changes in various tissues. The reaction of lymph nodes to small intradermal doses of polysaccharide appears to be directed primarily toward antibody formation, with the development of prominent germinal centers in the cortex of lymph nodes and increased numbers of plasma cells in the medulla. No development of pyroninophilic cells or proliferation of lymphocytes in the paracortical, thymic-dependent areas was reported (Turk and Heather, 1965). No lymph node reactivity following immunization has been reported in another study (Davies *et al.*, 1970). Comparison between salmonella flagellar and pneumococcal polysaccharide antigen was recently investigated in normal mice and thymectomized, irradiated, bone-marrow-injected mice with and without a thymus graft (Davies *et al.*, 1970). A chromosome marker was used to differentiate between the response of cells derived from the bone marrow and the thymus graft. Cells of thymic origin were not stimulated into mitosis by pneumococcal polysaccharide.

4.2. Delayed Hypersensitivity

Initial results in animals indicated that delayed hypersensitivity did not develop following immunization with pneumococcal polysaccharide (Turk and Heather, 1965). Subsequently, it was found that administration of polysaccharide subcutaneously in complete Freund's adjuvant resulted in a typical delayed hypersensitivity reaction (Gerety et al., 1970). Cellular reactivity induced by polysaccharide in the absence of adjuvant had the characteristics of a "Jones–Mote" reactivity. This type of delayed reactivity may be related to the early phase of antibody synthesis.

In humans with pneumococcal pneumonia, the intradermal injection of pneumococcal polysaccharide derived from the infecting organism gave rise to immediate-type reactions (Tillett and Francis, 1929). Similar results have been observed with blood group substances where antibodies are produced against the sugar components, while delayed reactivity is a result of the peptide moiety of the substances (Holborow and Loewi, 1962).

4.3. Stimulation of T Cells by Pneumococcal Antigens

No studies have been reported which indicate that purified polysaccharide is capable of inducing blastogenesis of T cells in immunized individuals. Lipopolysaccharides, in contrast, are very effective in this respect as a result of both specific recognition and of the mitogenic properties of purified lipopolysaccharides (Coutinho et al., 1975).

Although the majority of studies indicate that polysaccharides are thymic-independent antigens, recent investigations have shown that T cells may express both a suppressor and an amplifier effect on the antibody response to pneumococcal polysaccharides (Barthold et al., 1974; Baker et al., 1971a,b, 1973; Morse et al., 1976). Initial studies were performed in mice utilizing pneumococcal polysaccharide type 3 (Baker et al., 1973). Under normal conditions, two types of antibody-producing or plaque-forming cells were detected (direct and indirect). The administration of antilymphocyte serum produced a significant increase in the magnitude of direct plaque-forming cells. Treatment of nude mice with antilymphocyte serum did not influence the degree of antibody

formation (Baker et al., 1973). Subsequent studies indicated that the magnitude of the IgG and IgA plaque-forming cells as well as the IgM plaque-forming cells could be increased with antilymphocyte serum treatment (Barthold et al., 1974).

Additional studies performed in mice at different ages suggested that the ontogeny of suppressor and amplifier T cells varies with age. Amplifier T-cell activity was shown to be minimal at 2–4 weeks of age and did not reach a maximum until 8–10 weeks of age. By contrast, suppressor T-cell activity was fully developed as early as 2 weeks of age. In these studies, suppressor T-cell activity could be abrogated by depletion of T cells (Morse et al., 1976). Studies conducted with adult thymectomized mice showed that both amplifier and suppressor T cells, once seeded to the periphery, were stable and did not depend on the presence of an intact thymus for continued activity (Baker et al., 1973).

5. Phagocytosis of Streptococcus pneumoniae

The role of the macrophage in the antibody response to pneumococcal polysaccharide is not clear. The rapid appearance of antibody-forming cells following immunization has led some investigators to suggest that macrophages are not required for normal antibody synthesis following immunization with pneumococcal polysaccharides. It has been shown, however, that two populations of cells are required for the formation of normal numbers of specific plaque forming cells. The two populations consist of a "lymphocyte-rich" and a "macrophage-rich" population. Neither population alone results in a normal antibody response (Mosier, 1967). Certain investigators have suggested that macrophages handle pneumococcal polysaccharides differently from other antigens (Morgan et al., 1953), a view supported by the observed association of slow intracellular degradation and high paralytogenic potency of polysaccharides. Indirect evidence for a difference in the processing of polysaccharide vs. protein antigen is obtained from studies of patients with Wiskott-Aldrich syndrome. These patients are unable to form antibody to polysaccharide antigens but are capable of forming a normal antibody response to protein antigen. The defect is believed to reside in the macrophage (Cooper *et al.*, 1964).

The clearance of pneumococci from the blood of normal and immunized animals indicates that phagocytosis plays an important role. Immunity is easily transferred utilizing immune serum, suggesting that antibody is capable of enhancing phagocytosis.

It has been found that the polysaccharide capsule increases bacterial virulence (Howard and Glynn, 1971; Howard and Siskind, 1969). In contrast, antibodies directed against capsular polysaccharides have the ability to enhance phagocytosis. Capsular polysaccharides have an antiphagocytic effect which probably is not specific but rather is related to charge and thickness of capsular material (Jann and Westphal, 1975).

The nude mouse model, an animal deficient in T-cell function, was utilized to determine the requirement of T cells for resistance to pneumococcal infection. Studies revealed normal serum opsonizing activity and *in vivo* phagocytosis of pneumococci. The mean lethal dose for pneumococcus was equivalent to normal control mice These studies suggested that T cells are not necessary for a normal host defense against pneumococcal infection (Winkelstein and Swift, 1975).

6. Complement and *Streptococcus pneumoniae*

Encapsulated pneumococci are resistant to ingestion by phagocytic cells unless certain serum factors, termed opsonins, are available. Although the majority of opsonins are related to specific antibodies, it has been shown that certain pneumococcal serotypes can be opsonized efficiently by complement components. Specific antibody may behave as an opsonin by attaching directly to immunoglobulin receptors on phagocytic cell membranes. Antibody may participate indirectly in opsonization by the activation of the first component of complement, C1q, with subsequent activation via the classical complement pathway. This results in activation of the third complement component, C3, and in deposition of a cleavage fragment, C3b, on the antigen. A receptor for C3b is present on the cell membrane of phagocytic cells. Activation of the alternate complement pathway does not require antibody. Both the classical and the alternate pathway have been implicated in opsonization of pneumococci.

Pneumococcal organisms activate the terminal complement components (C3–C9) by means of the classical pathway or the alternative pathway (Winkelstein *et al.*, 1976). The cleavage of C3 and the fixation of C3b to the bacterial surface result from activation of either pathway. Activation of the classical pathway is accomplished through immune complexes consisting of type-specific antipneumococcal antibody combined with specific capsular polysaccharide. Opsonization via the classical pathway plays an essential role in acquired immunity.

Complement activation by means of the alternative pathway may be an important factor in natural immunity (Winkelstein *et al.*, 1976). It has been shown that some capsular polysaccharides are capable of activating the alternative pathway (polysaccharide types 1, 4, and 25), whereas other types (2, 3, 14, and 19) are unable to activate the alternate pathway. The differences observed in the activation of the alternative complement pathway by purified pneumococcal polysaccharides are not observed with intact encapsulated pneumococci, all of which are capable of activating the alternate pathway. It also has been found that certain nonencapsulated pneumococci, derived from homologous organisms, are capable of activating the alternate pathway as well as fully encapsulated pneumococci. Other investigators have found that pneumococcal types 7, 12, 14, and 25 activate readily the alternate pathway in the presence or absence of antibody. In contrast, types 1, 3, 4, and 8 lack intrinsic ability to activate the alternate pathway, while types 3, 4, and 8 can do so in conjunction with specific antibody. Pneumococcal type 1 lacked the ability to activate the complement system. (Fine, 1975).

The complement system has been studied in pneumococcal infections in man (Reed *et al.*, 1976). Twenty-two patients with pneumococcal infection were studied acutely and during convalescence for levels of C1q, C4, properdin factor B, C3, and hemolytic complement. Acute and recovery values were nearly identical for C1q and C4, two early components of the classical pathway. The mean level of properdin factor B was depressed significantly but was associated with a normal value in the recovery phase. During the acute phase, the level of C3 was depressed and was subsequently found to be normal during the recovery period. Total hemolytic complement was not significantly different during the acute phase when compared to the recovery phase. The authors concluded that factor B was turned over rapidly, or consumed early, in the course of pneumococcal infections, or that persons with low values of factor B may be susceptible to pneumococcal infection.

Certain polysaccharide-containing bacteria are considered to be relatively complement resistant. It has been found that charged capsular polysaccharides inhibit red cell agglutination and hemolysis by hemolysin and complement (Glynn and Howard, 1970). Antibodies directed against the capsular polysaccharide cannot overcome complement resistance. The thickness of the capsule, as well as the surface charge, may play a role in complement resistance. These same properties are important in the antiphagocytic effect of capsular polysaccharides.

7. Increased Susceptibility to Pneumococcal Infection

7.1. Increased Susceptibility to Pneumococcal Infection in Infants

Streptococcus pneumoniae is the most frequent cause of pneumonia, otitis media, and septicemia in infants more than 1 month old (Loda *et al.*, 1975). The susceptibility to infection of infants under 6 months of age is unlikely to be due to an intrinsic defect of phagocytic function. Rather, a deficiency of opsonins in the form of antibody and/or complement most likely is responsible. Studies of complement function in the newborn infant have revealed a deficiency of C3, C4, and factor B (Johnston and Stroud, 1977; Norman *et al.*, 1975). We performed studies comparing maternal and newborn cord serum sample levels of antibody to a variety of type-specific pneumococcal polysaccharides. The amount of antibody passively transferred varied with the pneumococcal polysaccharide type analyzed by the indirect hemagglutination technique.

The antibody class which is passively transferred consists of IgG and significant antibody levels are detected, even with a hemagglutination technique. As the infant matures and approaches childhood, the levels of antibody directed against a variety of pneumococcal polysaccharides begin to increase and continue to increase until late adulthood. It was previously believed that "natural antibody" was derived from subclinical or unrecognized exposure to bacterial organisms. Recently, it has been appreciated that colonization by nonpathogenic bacteria may result in a significant antibody response to antigens which cross-react with pathogenic bacteria (Robbins *et al.*, 1972).

It appears that the susceptibility of infants and young children to pneumococcal infection resides in three major aberrations. One abnormality consists of a deficiency in complement function which is self-corrective with advancing age. The second abnormality consists of a deficiency of specific antibody directed against pneumococcal polysaccharides. This deficiency varies with the amount of antibody which has been transferred from the maternal circulation. This in turn may vary with maternal exposure to specific pneumococcal polysaccharides or may be related to specific transfer of immunoglobulin across the placenta. The third aberration consists of a deficiency in "naturally occurring antibodies" which is most likely related to the acquisition of nonpathogenic microbial species with the capability of inducing cross-reacting antibody.

7.2. Increased Susceptibility to Pneumococcal Infection in Old Age

The incidence and mortality of pneumococcal infection are significantly greater in persons 50 years of age or older (Austrian, 1976; Shapera and Matsen, 1972). Many older patients have underlying diseases, including heart failure, malignancy, chronic liver disease, chronic renal disease, and chronic pulmonary disease. Adults and elderly individuals are more susceptible to pneumococcal infection with the lower types, e.g., types 1–8. Young infants and children have infections caused by *S. pneumoniae* of the higher types, e.g., types 14, 18, and 23. The reason for this dissociation is not known. There also is a discrepancy between the incidence of bacteremia in adults with pneumococcal infection and children with pneumococcal infection—33% v. 5% respectively (Shapera and Matsen, 1972).

A variety of immunological abnormalities have been described in elderly individuals, including decreased delayed hypersensitivity, decreased numbers of T cells, diminished reactivity of lymphocytes to phytohemagglutinin and allogeneic cells (Weksler and Hutteroth, 1974; Heidrick and Makinodan, 1973). None of these appears to explain adequately the increased susceptibility to pneumococcal infection. Detailed studies of complement function and phagocytic function have not been performed in the aged population. Studies on quantitative immunoglobulin levels in the aged population have revealed increased values for serum IgG and IgA (Hallgren *et al.*, 1973).

We performed immunological evaluations in 66 elderly individuals (age range 57–100 years, mean age 78 years) prior to immunization. Lymphocyte transformation and response to phytohemagglutinin, as a measure of T-cell immunity, and a semiquantitative nitroblue tetrazolium dye test, as a measure of phagocytic function, were normal in all individuals tested (Table 3). Analysis of IgG and IgM serum levels revealed no significant difference between adult controls and elderly patients. However, serum IgA values were significantly higher in elderly individuals (Table 3).

To analyze possible relationships between the ability to respond with antibody formation following immunization with type-specific pneumococcal polysaccharide, the elderly patients were divided into individuals who did not show an antibody titer change and those who showed a greater than twofold increase in antibody titer following immunization with pneumococcal polysaccharide type 3 and type 8 (Tables 4 and 5). The mean IgM values in each group were calculated and compared statistically. A significant difference was demonstrated between the IgM values of those individuals who did not respond following immunization to pneumococcal polysaccharide type 3 and type 8, serum IgM values being considerably lower in the nonresponder group. A similar analysis was performed between responders and nonresponders comparing the mean serum IgA value. Again, a statistically significant difference was shown between the responders and nonresponders, responders having a significantly lower serum IgA value. These studies suggest that the inability of elderly individuals to respond to pneumococcal polysaccharide may be related to the ability to form IgM and/or IgA antibody.

7.3. Increased Susceptibility to Pneumococcal Infection in Immunodeficiency Disorders

7.3.1. Hypogammaglobulinemia

A variety of primary and acquired immunodeficiency disorders demonstrate enhanced susceptibility to infection with polysaccharide-containing organisms. The majority of these disorders have in common an inability to form antibody against such organisms.

Infants and children with congenital hypogammaglobulinemia, and children and adults with acquired hypogammaglobulinemia, have repeated sinopulmonary infections with *S. pneumoniae* as well as pyogenic organisms. The susceptibility to infection in these patients

TABLE 3.   Immunological Studies in Aged Individuals

Lymphocyte transformation (PHA): Normal in all

Nitroblue tetrazolium test: Normal

Immunoglobulins:

	IgG	IgM	IgA
Controls (adults)[a]	1158 ± 305	99 ± 27	200 ± 61
Patients (old age)[b]	1394 ± 356	111 ± 88	301 ± 134
Significance	N.S.	N.S.	$p = < 0.0005$

[a] Age range 23–42 years, mean 28 years.
[b] Sixty-six elderly individuals, range 57–100 years, mean 78 years.

TABLE 4.   Comparison of IgM Values in Aged Patients
with and without Titer Change following Immunization
with Pneumococcal Polysaccharide

	Number	IgM	
PPS 8			
No titer change	14	71 ± 57	$p < 0.05$
Titer change > twofold	52	118 ± 110	
PPS 3			
No titer change	6	45 ± 33	$p < 0.05$
Titer change > twofold	60	104 ± 88	

is due to a deficiency of antibody, as the majority of these individuals have been found to
have intact phagocytic function, complement
function, and T-cell immunity (Davis, 1973).
These patients have excellent control of recurrent infections with regular administration
of antibody, provided as γ-globulin injections
or fresh frozen plasma. γ-Globulin injections
usually are administered on a 3- to 4-week
basis, and in the majority of patients provide
adequate passive protection. As the γ-globulin
contains primarily IgG and virtually no IgM
or IgA, it is apparent that passive protection
is provided by IgG, which has a half-life of
25–30 days. In studies to determine the level
of pneumococcal antibody associated with
protection in patients receiving γ-globulin injections, the amount has been calculated to be
approximately 1–2 μg of antibody nitrogen/ml.

7.3.2. Wiskott–Aldrich Syndrome

Patients with the Wiskott–Aldrich syndrome
(immunodeficiency with eczema and thrombocytopenia) are uniquely susceptible to infection with polysaccharide-containing organisms. The susceptibility to infection appears
in early infancy with an increased incidence
of otitis media, pneumonia, and meningitis.
Characteristically, the patients are unable to
form antibody following immunization with
polysaccharide antigens, while the antibody
response following immunization with protein
antigens is entirely normal (Cooper et al.,
1964). Patients have low isohemagglutinin titers, believed to be due to an inability to form
cross-reacting antibody against blood group
substances following colonization by nonpathogenic polysaccharide-containing organisms.
Immunoglobulin patterns in patients demonstrate a typical pattern of normal IgG, depressed IgM, and increased IgA and IgE. The
decreased IgM is likely to be secondary to the
inability to form antibody to polysaccharides
in the IgM class. When splenectomy has been
performed to correct the thrombocytopenia,
fatal infection has been the usual outcome,
regardless of the age at which the splenectomy
is performed (Huntley and Dees, 1957). Although no adequate basic defect has been described to explain the multisystem abnormalities, it is believed that all patients are unable
to form antibody to polysaccharide antigens.

TABLE 5.   Comparison of IgA Values in Aged Patients with
and without Titer Change following Immunization with
Pneumococcal Polysaccharide

	Number	IgA	
PPS 8			
No titer change	14	256 ± 127	$p < 0.0005$
Titer change > twofold	52	313 ± 129	
PPS 3			
No titer change	6	235 ± 121	$p < 0.0005$
Titer change > twofold	60	306 ± 133	

Some authors have postulated that this defect resides in macrophage processing rather than in a primary B-cell defect (Cooper *et al.*, 1964).

7.3.3. Selective IgM Deficiency

The rare immunodeficiency disorder of selective IgM deficiency is associated with normal values of other immunoglobulins, and a selective deficiency of serum IgM. Some but not all patients are capable of a normal antibody response in other immunoglobulin classes. Detailed studies of T-cell immunity have not been performed. These patients are susceptible to autoimmune diseases, as well as to overwhelming infection with polysaccharide-containing organisms such as *S. pneumoniae* and *H. influenzae* (Hobbs *et al.*, 1967). The mortality rate is extremely high. It appears that the extreme susceptibility to infection is directly related to the deficiency of serum IgM and perhaps to the inability to form antibody against polysaccharide antigen.

7.3.4. Complement Deficiencies

Certain complement deficiencies are associated with increased susceptibility to microbial infection. As complement factors are necessary for normal opsonization, bacterial killing, and neutrophil chemotaxis, it is not surprising to find an association of complement deficiency and enhanced susceptibility to bacteria including pneumococcal infection. The types of complement deficiency which have been described in association with increased susceptibility to infection are C1q (Wara *et al.*, 1975), C1r, C1s, C2 (Day *et al.*, 1972), C3 (Alper *et al.*, 1976), C4 (Lim *et al.*, 1976), and C5 (Rosenfeld *et al.*, 1976). These deficiencies can be detected by the hemolytic complement screening assay or, in the case of C3 deficiency, by a direct quantitation of C3. Patients with C3 deficiency who have been treated with plasma have shown a decreased susceptibility to infection. Frozen plasma infusions should be used with caution, however, in patients with C1r, C1s, and C2 deficiency, as these disorders also are associated with autoimmune diseases, e.g., systemic lupus erythematosus. Provision of complement components may improve the susceptibility to infection but may alter the course of the autoimmune disease.

7.4. Increased Susceptibility to Pneumococcal Infection in Patients with Nephrotic Syndrome and Cirrhosis

The etiology of the occurrence of pneumococcal peritonitis in patients with the nephrotic syndrome is unclear. The original observations date back to a time when adequate treatment with steroids and immunosuppressive agents was not available (Pahmer, 1940). More recent studies suggest that a decreased incidence in such patients is perhaps due to more adequate treatment of the underlying disease (Burke *et al.*, 1971). Pneumococcal peritonitis has also been found in patients with ascites secondary to liver cirrhosis (Shapera and Matsen, 1972). In the case of ascites, it has been postulated that pneumococci, which commonly are present in the respiratory tract of all individuals, may cause transient bacteremia. The ascitic fluid would provide an optimal environment for growth of organisms which might seed the peritoneal cavity. An additional factor might be related to secondary hypogammaglobulinemia. Although high molecular weight immunoglobulins, such as IgM, may be normal in the serum of patients with the nephrotic syndrome, the low molecular weight immunoglobulins may be severely reduced secondary to renal protein loss. Frequently, the serum levels of IgG are comparable to those found in congenital hypogammaglobulinemia. A deficiency of serum antibody thus might predispose these patients to pneumococcal bacteremia with subsequent growth of the organism in the ascitic fluid.

7.5. Increased Susceptibility to Pneumococcal Infection in Anatomical and Functional Asplenia

It is well recognized that splenectomy in infants markedly increases the susceptibility to overwhelming pneumococcal infection (King and Shumacker, 1952; Eraklis *et al.*, 1967; Robinson and Watson, 1966). Although it is not known which immunological defects predispose young infants to overwhelming infection following splenectomy, it is possible that the lack of "natural" antibody in the absence of the spleen permits rapid multiplication of pneumococcal organisms. Thus young infants have in common with immunodeficient patients a lack of preformed antibody directed against pneumococcal polysaccharide. The additional removal of a major phagocytic organ might therefore be expected to markedly enhance susceptibility to infection. Overwhelming pneumococcal infection following splenectomy may not be confined to young infants. Numerous reports of overwhelming pneumococcal sepsis have been described in older patients who have had traumatic splenectomies performed (Maron and Maloney, 1972; Grinblat and Gilboa, 1975).

We have performed a study on the antibody response in 19 infants and children who had splenectomies performed for a variety of reasons, including two with congenital asplenia, four with hereditary spherocytosis, 12 with idiopathic thrombocytopenic purpura, and one with trauma. The patients were immunized with octavalent pneumococcal polysaccharide vaccine. Results were compared to normal age-matched populations. There was no significant difference between the antibody response, as measured by indirect hemagglutination in the postsplenectomy group, and in the normals. This would indicate that, at least in this group of patients a susceptibility to pneumococcal infection is not a result of an inability to form antibody to purified polysaccharide.

Patients with sickle cell disease also are susceptible to overwhelming pneumococcal infection. This susceptibility begins at approximately 1 year of age and continues until the patients reach 8–10 years of age. After 10 years of age, the susceptibility decreases markedly (Powars, 1975). The spectrum of *S. pneumoniae* types is similar to that observed in the normal population (Seeler and Jacobs, 1977). A number of abnormalities have been described following splenectomy, including decreased properdin levels (Carlisle and Saslaw, 1959), increased transferrin levels (Schumacker, 1970), and decreased tuftsin levels (Constantopoulos and Najjar, 1973). In patients with sickle cell disease who undergo autosplenectomy, additional aberrations of immune function have been described, including decreased opsonizing activity (Winkelstein and Drachman, 1968) and abnormalities in the alternate complement pathway (Johnston *et al.*, 1973). A decrease in the splenic clearance of ^{99m}Tc-sulfa colloid has been described by Falter *et al.* (1973). Other investigators have

reported an impaired antibody response to particulate antigenic material, such as red blood cells (Schwartz and Pearson, 1972). However, the ability of patients with splenectomy and sickle cell disease to respond normally following parenteral immunization with a variety of antigens has been well documented (Robbins and Parson, 1965).

We have studied 77 patients with sickle cell disease following immunization with octavalent pneumococcal polysaccharide vaccine. Our results indicate that patients with sickle cell disease are able to respond in a manner comparable to that of a normal control population. The response to each individual pneumococcal polysaccharide may vary considerably but is comparable in the sickle cell and control group. The mean fold increase 3 weeks following immunization varied from 1.65 to 12.55, and the percent responders varied from 47% to 82%.

An additional defect in patients with sickle cell disease may be the inability to form adequate amounts of serum IgM antibody. Gavrilis *et al.* (1974) have reported low concentrations of serum IgM in patients with sickle cell disease and decreased splenic function. We were unable to confirm these results in a study of our own patients. The discrepancy in results may be related to the wide range of values obtained in patients with sickle cell disease at various ages. To further analyze whether there might be a relationship between serum IgM values and antibody response to individual polysaccharides, we compared the mean fold increase in a group of sickle cell patients with serum IgM values less than 2 standard deviations below normal to the response in sickle cell patients with a normal serum IgM. No significant difference was found between the two groups.

In summary, it is likely that multiple immunological abnormalities explain the increased susceptibility to infection in patients with asplenia and functional asplenia. Lack of preformed antibody, as found in infants and immunodeficient patients, likely is a predisposing cause. Removal of the spleen, or decreased splenic function, results in a significant loss of phagocytic mass. Additional defects, such as aberrations in the alternate complement pathway and other opsonizing components, contribute to the susceptibility to overwhelming infection. Impaired ability to form antibody to whole organisms exists in many patients, although the ability to respond to purified polysaccharides is normal in the majority of patients.

8. Immunodiagnosis of Pneumococcal Infection

8.1. Identification of Type-Specific Pneumococci

Classically, the type of *S. pneumoniae* has been identified utilizing antisera directed against purified polysaccharides. Currently, commercially available rabbit antipneumococcal sera are used for screening with pools containing antibodies to several types. Antibody reactive with a single pneumococcal polysaccharide then is used to identify specifically the organism isolated. The methodology used is the Quellung reaction, whereby capsular swelling occurs when the specific antibody reacts with the organism being tested.

8.2. Detection of Pneumococcal Antigens in Body Fluids

Fluorescein-conjugated antipneumococcal sera can be used to detect pneumococci in the cerebrospinal fluid and other body fluids (Sloyer *et al.,* 1974) while type-specific antipneumococcal polysaccharide antigen present in blood, pleural fluid, cerebrospinal fluid, and urine (Coonrod and Rytel, 1973; Anhalt and Yu, 1975; Coonrod and Leach, 1976) can be detected utilizing a method of counterimmunoelectrophoresis. Commercially available pneumococcal antisera and test solutions are placed in wells cut in agarose slides and subjected to electrophoresis. Precipitin lines form in the presence of antibody plus specific polysaccharide. As little as 0.05 µg/ml of polysaccharide can be detected by this method. In urine, following twentyfold concentration, as little as 0.0025 µg/ml of antigen can be detected.

Recent methods of determining antibody responses following immunization with pneumococcal polysaccharide have utilized sensitive radioimmunoassay techniques. These methods also have been useful for detecting the amount of circulating antigen in serum and body fluids. These sensitive methods have confirmed and extended previous observations that circulating polysaccharide may be present following infection for periods of months or longer.

8.3. Determination of Antibody Response

A variety of methods are available for the detection of antibody in serum and body fluids in man and animals. Previously, precipitation, agglutination, capsular swelling activity of serum, mouse protection tests, and intradermal injection of polysaccharides have been utilized. These tests suffer from lack of sensitivity and may be time consuming for large studies.

More recently, the indirect hemagglutination technique has been used for studies in animals (Baker *et al.,* 1969) and man (Ammann and Pelger, 1972). In the indirect hemagglutination technique, highly purified pneumococcal polysaccharides are coated onto sheep red blood cells or human O Rh-negative red blood cells. The use of human O Rh-negative red blood cells for studies has reduced nonspecific agglutination of red cells due to heterophil antibodies. In most methods, the polysaccharides are coated onto the red cells by a chromic chloride technique. Although the method may favor the determination of IgM antibody to polysaccharide, it is also capable of determining a significant amount of IgG antibody (Ammann and Pelger, 1972). In this method, results usually are expressed as the reciprocal of the titer, e.g., $1:32 = 32$. Serial twofold dilutions are used to titer the antibody response. Results may be expressed as fold increase, that is, the postimmunization titer divided by the preimmunization titer. In order to standardize results, pre- and postimmunization or pre- and postinfection sera usually are run in the same microtiter plates.

The indirect hemagglutination method has several advantages. Results are rapid, with coating of cells and titering of the serum performed on a single day. The method is relatively inexpensive, requiring only human red cells, buffers, disposable microtiter plates, purified polysaccharide, and hand-diluting equipment. Semiautomatic equipment is available which permits the determination of antibody titers in large numbers of samples (Ammann and Pelger, 1972). The method is reproducible and is accurate to within a two-fold dilution. Disadvantages of the method relate to the absence of an absolute standard. Indirect hemagglutination titers usually are compared to those of control samples and may vary with the degree of coating.

The radioimmunoassay technique was developed to overcome some of the problems encountered with indirect hemagglutination techniques (Schiffman and Austrian, 1971). Antigens, utilized for the determination of antibody, are obtained by growing individual strains of *S. pneumoniae* in the presence of [^{14}C]glucose. Specific pneumococcal polysaccharides subsequently are isolated and utilized for the radioimmunoassay. Sera or body fluids containing antibody are incubated with the radiolabeled polysaccharide. Antigen–antibody complexes are precipitated in the presence of amonium sulfate and the counts precipitated and measured in a scintillation counter. The method is standardized by comparison with the quantitative precipitin test and is applicable to all but a few pneumococcal polysaccharide types. The assay has the capability of being modified to permit the measurement of capsular polysaccharide in the serum and other body fluids. The most effective utilization of the method has been in the determination of antibody response following immunization with purified capsular polysaccharides. The method also has been modified to determine circulating immune complexes in the serum of patients following natural infection (Schiffman *et al.*, 1974).

The radioimmunoassay technique has the advantage of expressing results in absolute terms such as nanograms of antibody nitrogen. This method also has increased sensitivity when utilized to determine the antibody response in low responders. It has an additional advantage in determining the total amount of antibody precipitated without distinguishing between antibody subclasses. Variants of this assay utilizing class-specific antiglobulins also may be used to differentiate class specificity. Disadvantages of the method lie primarily in increased expense of supplies as a result of utilization of radioactive material and the necessity for expensive equipment to count the radioactivity. In addition, the pneumococci

must be radiolabeled individually and the polysaccharides subsequently purified.

9. Immunoprevention and Treatment

9.1. Passive Antibody

Before the introduction of antibiotics, pneumococcal infection was treated with type-specific antisera which required the isolation of causative organisms. Large amounts of antisera were necessary, and side reactions were frequent. Following the introduction of sulfonamides and, subsequently, penicillin, antibody therapy no longer was of use. However, with the discovery of hypogammaglobulinemia and other immunodeficiency disorders, γ-globulin therapy became the mainstay of passive protection in patients unable to form antibody against microbial agents. It has been estimated that the amount of antibody which is necessary to prevent infection by *S. pneumoniae* or *H. influenzae* is 1–2 μg of antibody nitrogen/ml. This amount of antibody usually is present 4 weeks following the administration of adequate amounts of γ-globulin. It is apparent that very small amounts of passive antibody in the IgG class are capable of protecting an individual who is unable to form antibody against certain microbial agents.

9.2. Active Immunization

In 1891, Klemperer and Klemperer showed that rabbits could be immunized intravenously with whole pneumococci, resulting in the animal's becoming immune to subsequent challenge with homologous organisms. Studies in man were first performed in 1911 by Wright *et al.* Initial attempts at immunization utilized bacterial vaccines at a time when the diversity of pneumococcal capsular polysaccharides was not appreciated. Francis and Tillett (1930) discovered the immunogenicity of pneumococcal capsular polysaccharides following attempts to evaluate intradermal injections of polysaccharides. Large-scale trials were reported by Ekwurzel *et al.* (1938) utilizing a bivalent vaccine containing pneumococcal polysaccharide types 1 and 2. A quadravalent vaccine containing 50 μg of the pneumococcal polysaccharide types 1, 2, 5, and 7 was evaluated by MacLeod *et al.* (1945) and demonstrated significant type-specific protection in a pneumococcal pneumonia epidemic involving 16,000 individuals. Heidelberger *et al.* (1948) demonstrated the antigenicity of six individual pneumococcal polysaccharides when combined as a single immunization. They also were able to show that antibody persisted for 5–8 years following the initial immunization (Heidelberger *et al.*, 1953). In spite of the studies which had demonstrated the safety, antigenicity, and efficacy of immunization with type-specific pneumococcal polysaccharides, the advent of antibiotic therapy resulted in a marked decline in demand for such vaccines. Renewed interest in pneumococcal polysaccharide vaccines has been brought about by recent studies indicating that the mortality from pneumococcal infection in infants and elderly individuals remains significant. In addition, *S. pneumoniae* infections continue to be a primary cause of bacterial otitis media, pneumonia, and meningitis in infants. The marked susceptibility of patients with splenectomy and functional asplenia to pneumococcal infection also has prompted renewed interest in immunization. Recently, the report of pneumococci resistant to penicillin has provided an additional impetus toward the development of an effective polyvalent pneumococcal vaccine.

In 1967, studies were instituted to determine the incidence of pneumococcal infections and the types of *S. pneumoniae* responsible for infection (Austrian, 1976). Highly purified pneumococcal polysaccharides were then developed and tested, first in a monovalent form and subsequently in a polyvalent form. Immunization trials were performed on infants, children, adults, and patients with increased susceptibility to pneumococcal infection, such as functional asplenia.

In all of the groups tested, immunization with the polysaccharides was associated with a low rate of complication. Local pain, redness, and swelling at the site of injection were seen in some individuals. Febrile reactions were unusual, and no systemic reactions were observed (Austrian, 1976). In adults, the response to individual pneumococcal polysaccharides was determined utilizing a radioimmunoassay technique. Ten to 100 μg of each individual polysaccharide was utilized for immunization and found to be immunogenic in the majority of patients. Fifty micrograms of polysaccharide appeared to be an optimal immunizing dose. Serum antibody was measured 3 weeks following immunization and expressed as micrograms of antibody nitrogen/ per milliliter. The response varied with each pneumococcal polysaccharide and ranged from 0.48 to 13.50 μg antibody nitrogen/ml. The fold increase (postimmunization divided by preimmunization) varied from 3.2 to 30.6. It also was shown that when monovalent vaccines of heterologous types were injected sequentially the administration of a second or third polysaccharide had no effect on the levels of antibody of the initial type given. In addition, the titer of antibody to the second polysaccharide was not influenced by the preexisting antibody to the first polysaccharide administered. We also have found that the preexisting antibody titer does not appear to influence whether patients will or will not respond to polysaccharide immunization.

Immunization studies in infants and children indicate a definite relationship of age to antibody response. It is known that, following immunization with both meningococcal polysaccharide and *H. influenzae* polysaccharide, antibody responsiveness is poor prior to 2 years of age (Smith *et al.*, 1973; Gotschlich *et al.*, 1972). The response to pneumococcal polysaccharide immunization varies with each individual polysaccharide type. In studies performed by us, 69% of infants less than 3 months of age responded following immunization with pneumococcal polysaccharide type 3 with greater than a twofold increase in antibody titer. On the other hand, only 8% of infants responded following immunization with pneumococcal polysaccharide type 23. The response to the majority of pneumococcal polysaccharides under 3 months of age is poor. In the 4- to 6-month age range, the number of infants responding to most pneumococcal polysaccharides increases. Between 7 and 13 months of age, the response rate varies from 18% to 88%. Over 24 months of age, the response rate is comparable to that of adults. The diminished response in infants under 24 months of age does not appear to be due to the presence of passive antibody, as evidenced by the high response rate to pneumococcal polysaccharide type 3. As it is thought that the response to pneumococcal polysaccharides does not require the presence of T-helper cells, it is unlikely that the low response rate in young infants is due to a maturational defect in T cells. It is possible that maturation of B cells is required. Alternatively, macrophage maturation may play a role in determining the response to polysaccharide antigens as suggested by poor clearance in young infants.

Parenteral immunization with polysaccharides does not result in an increase in antibody in secretions. We immunized five individuals with pneumococcal polysaccharide 2 and determined the antibody response 3 weeks later in serum and saliva. Significant increases in antibody titer were observed in the serum, without any antibody detected in concentrated saliva samples.

Immunization of individuals with impaired splenic function has resulted in similar antibody responses as matched controls. Thus patients with anatomical asplenia and functional asplenia are capable of forming normal antibody responses following immunization with purified pneumococcal polysaccharide, although having impaired responses following immunization with particulate polysaccharide-containing material, such as red blood cells or whole organisms.

The efficacy of pneumococcal polysaccharide immunization in preventing pneumococcal infection has been well documented. The most recent studies of Austrian (1976) indicate that the use of a polyvalent pneumococcal polysaccharide vaccine is capable of preventing pneumococcal pneumonia, sepsis, and meningitis in populations at high risk. The duration of protection has not been determined from recent studies. The effectiveness of pneumococcal polysaccharide immunization in infants and children in preventing otitis media, pneumonia, meningitis, and sepsis has not been determined. In a recent study, however, we have immunized 77 patients with sickle cell disease with an octavalent pneumococcal polysaccharide vaccine. These patients responded in a manner comparable to that of normal age-matched controls. In a 2-year follow-up study, no episodes of pneumococcal infection were observed in the immunized group. On the other hand, nine episodes of pneumococcal infection, with two deaths, were observed in the unimmunized group of 106 patients with sickle cell disease. All of these infections were with *S. pneumoniae* of the type found in the vaccine. These studies strongly suggest that immunization with polyvalent pneumococcal polysaccharide vaccines may be useful in high-risk populations such as infants, elderly individuals, and individuals with impaired immunological function.

References

Alexander, H. E., 1943, Experimental basis for treatment of *Haemophilus influenzae* infections, *Am. J. Dis. Child.* **66**:160–171.

Alper, C. A., Colten, H. R., Gear, J. S. S., Rabson, A. R., and Rosen, F. S., 1976, Homozygous human C3 deficiency: The role of C3 in antibody production, C1s-induced vasopermeability, and cobra venom-induced passive hemolysis, *J. Clin. Invest.* **57**:222–229.

Ammann, A. J., and Pelger, R. J., 1972, Determination of antibody to pneumococcal polysaccharides following immunization using chromic chloride treated red blood cells and indirect hemagglutination, *Appl. Microbiol.* **24**:679–683.

Amsbaugh, D. F., Hansen, C. T., Prescott, B., Stashak, P. W., Barthold, D. R., and Baker, P. J., 1972, Genetic control of the antibody response to type III pneumococcal polysaccharide in mice. I. Evidence that an X-linked gene plays a decisive role in determining responsiveness, *J. Exp. Med.* **136**:931–949.

Amsbaugh, D. F., Hansen, C. T., Prescott, B., Stashak, P. W., Asofsky, R., and Baker, P. J., 1974, Genetic control of the antibody response to type III pneumococcal polysaccharide in mice. II. Relationship between IgM immunoglobulin levels and the ability to give an IgM antibody response, *J. Exp. Med.* **139**:1499–1512.

Anhalt, J. P., and Yu, P. K. W., 1975, Counterimmunoelectrophoresis of pneumococcal antigens: Improved sensitivity for the detection of types VII and XIV, *J. Clin. Microbiol.* **2**:510–515.

Austrian, R., 1976, Vaccines of the pneumococcal capsular polysaccharide and the prevention of pneumococcal pneumonia, in: *The Role of Immunologic Factors in Infectious, Allergic and Autoimmune Processes* (R. F. Beers and E. G. Bassett, eds.), pp. 79–89, Raven Press, New York.

Baker, P. J., and Landy, M., 1967, Brevity of the inductive phase in the immune response of mice to capsular polysaccharide antigens, *J. Immunol.* **99**:687–694.

Baker, P. J., and Stashak, P. W., 1969, Quantitative and qualitative studies on the primary antibody response to pneumococcal polysaccharides at the cellular level, *J. Immunol.* **103**:1342–1348.

Baker, P. J., Stashak, P. W., and Prescott, B., 1969, Use of erythrocytes sensitized with purified pneumococcal polysaccharides for the assay of antibody and antibody-producing cells, *Appl. Microbiol.* **17**:422–426.

Baker, P. J., Prescott, B., Stashak, P. W., and Amsbaugh, D. F., 1971a, Characterization of the antibody response to type III pneumococcal polysaccharide at the cellular level. III. Studies on the average avidity of the antibody produced by specific plaque-forming cells. *J. Immunol.* **107**:719–724.

Baker, P. J., Stashak, P. W., Amsbaugh, D. F., and Prescott, B., 1971b, Characterization of the antibody response to type III pneumococcal polysaccharide at the cellular level. I. Dose–response studies and the effect of prior immunization on the magnitude of the antibody response, *Immunology* **20**:469–480.

Baker, P. J., Reed, N. D., Stashak, P. W., Amsbaugh, D. F., and Prescott, B., 1973, Regulation of the antibody response to type III pneumococcal polysaccharide. I. Nature of regulatory cells, *J. Exp. Med.* **137**:1431–1441.

Ballou, C. E., 1970, A study of the immunochemistry of three yeast mannans, *J. Biol. Chem.* **245**:1197–1203.

Barthold, D. R., Prescott, B., Stashak, P. W., Amsbaugh, D. F., and Baker, P. J., 1974, Regulation of the antibody response to type III pneumococcal polysaccharide. III. Role of regulatory T cells in the development of an IgG and IgA antibody response, *J. Immunol.* **112**:1042–1050.

Bott, E. M., Bonynge, C. W., and Joyce, R. L., 1936, The demonstration of capsules about hemolytic streptococci with india ink or azo blue, *J. Infect. Dis.* **58**:5–9.

Braley-Mullen, H., 1974, Regulatory role of T cells in IgG antibody formation and immune memory to type III pneumococcal polysaccharide, *J. Immunol.* **113**:1909–1920.

Braley-Mullen, H., Chase, G. R., Sharp, G. C., and Freeman, M. J., 1974, Genetic control of the immune response of mice to type III pneumococcal polysaccharide, *Cell. Immunol.* **10**:280–286.

Burke, J. P., Klein, J. O., Gezon, H. M., and Finland, M., 1971, Pneumococcal bacteremia: Review of 111 cases, 1957–1969, with special reference to cases with undetermined focus, *Am. J. Dis. Child.* **121**:353–359.

Carlisle, H. N., and Saslaw, S., 1959, Properidin levels in splenectomized persons, *Proc. Soc. Exp. Biol. Med.* **102**:150–154.

Constantopoulos, A., and Najjar, V. A., 1973, Tuftsin deficiency syndrome. A report of two cases, *Acta Paediatr. Scand.* **62**:645–648.

Coonrod, J. D., and Leach, R. P., 1976, Antigenemia in fulminant pneumococcemia, *Ann. Intern. Med.* **84**:561–563.

Coonrod, J. D., and Rytel, M. W., 1973, Detection of type-specific pneumococcal antigens by counterimmunoelectrophoresis. I. Methodology and immunologic properties of pneumococcal antigens, *J. Lab. Clin. Med.* **81**:770–777.

Cooper, M. D., Krivit, W., Peterson, R. D. A., and Good, R. A., 1964, An immunological defect in Wiskott-Ald-

rich patients, in: *Transactions American Pediatric Society 74th Annual Meeting,* Seattle, Wash., June 16–18

Coutinho, A., Moller, G., and Gronowicz, E., 1975, Genetic control of B cell responses. IV. Inheritance of the unresponsiveness to lipopolysaccharides, *J. Exp. Med.* **142**:253–258.

Davies, A. J. S., Carter, R. L., Leuchars, E., Wallis, V., and Dietrich, F. M., 1970, The morphology of immune reactions in normal, thymectomized and reconstituted mice. III. Response to bacterial antigens: salmonellar, flagellar antigen and pneumococcal polysaccharide, *Immunology* **19**:945–957.

Davis, S. D., 1973, Antibody deficiency diseases, in: *Immunologic Disorders in Infants and Children* (E. R. Stiehm and V. Fulginiti, eds.), pp. 184–198, Saunders Co., Philadelphia.

Day, N. K., Geiger, H., Stroud, R., deBracco, M., Mancado, B., Windhorst, D., and Good, R. A., 1972, C1r deficiency: An inborn error associated with cutaneous and renal disease, *J. Clin. Invest.* **51**:1102–1108.

Dochez, A. R., and Avery, O. T., 1917, The elaboration of specific soluble substance by pneumococcus during growth, *J. Exp. Med.* **26**:477–493.

Ekwurzel, G. M., Simmons, J. S., Dublin, L. I., and Felton, L. D., 1938, Studies on immunizing substances in penumococci. VIII. Report on field tests to determine the prophylactic value of a pneumococcus antigen, *Public Health Rep.* **53**:1877–1893.

Eraklis, A. J., Kevy, S. V., Diamond, L. K., and Gross, R. E., 1967, Hazard of overwhelming infection after splenectomy in childhood, *N. Engl. J. Med.* **276**:1225–1229.

Falter, M. L., Robinson, M. G., Kim, O. S., Go, S. C., and Taubkin, S. P., 1973, Splenic function and infection in sickle cells anemia, *Acta Haematol.* **50**:154–161.

Felton, F. D., 1949, The significance of antigen in animal tissues, *J. Immunol.* **61**:107–117.

Felton, L. D., and Ottinger, B., 1942, Pneumococcus polysaccharide as a paralyzing agent on the mechanism on immunity in white mice, *J. Bacteriol.* **43**:94–95.

Felton, L. D., Prescott, B., Kauffman, G., and Ottinger, B., 1955, Pneumococcal antigenic polysaccharide substances from animal tissues, *J. Immunol.* **74**:205–213.

Fine, D. P., 1975, Pneumococcal type-associated variability in alternate complement pathway activation, *Infect. Immun.* **12**:772–778.

Francis, T., and Tillett, W. S., 1930, Cutaneous reactions in pneumonia. The development of antibodies following the intradermal injection of type specific polysaccharide, *J. Exp. Med.* **52**:573–585.

Gavrilis, P., Rothenberg, S. P., and Guy, R., 1974, Correlation of low serum IgM levels with absence of functional splenic tissue in sickle cell disease syndromes, *Am. J. Med.* **57**:542–545.

Gelzer, J., and Kabat, E. A., 1964, Specific fractionation of human anti-dextran antibodies. III. Fractionation of anti-dextran by sequential extraction with oligosaccharides of increasing chain length and attempts at subfractionation, *Immunochemistry* 1:303–316.

Gerety, R. J., Ferraresi, R. W., and Raffel, S., 1970, Polysaccharide in delayed hypersensitivity. I. Pneumococcal polysaccharide as inducer and elicitor of delayed reactivity in guinea pigs, *J. Exp. Med.* 131:189–206.

Glynn, A. A., 1969, The complement lysozyme sequence in immune bacteriolysis, *Immunology* 16:463–471.

Glynn, A. A., and Howard, C. J., 1970, The sensitivity to complement of strains of *Escherichia coli* related to their K antigens, *Immunology* 18:331–346.

Goebel, W. F., 1940, Studies on antibacterial immunity induced by artificial antigens. II. Immunity to experimental pneumococcal infection with antigens containing saccharides of synthetic origin, *J. Exp. Med.* 72:33–48.

Gotschlich, E. C., Rey, M., Triau, R., and Sparks, K. J., 1972, Quantitative determination of the human immune response to immunization meningococcal vaccines, *J. Clin. Invest.* 51:89–96.

Grinblat, J., and Gilboa, Y., 1975, Overwhelming pneumococcal sepsis 25 years after splenectomy, *Am. J. Med. Sci.* 270:523–524.

Hallgren, H. M., Buckley, C. E., III, Gilbertsen, V. A., and Yunis, E. J., 1973, Lymphocyte phytohemagglutinin, responsiveness, immunoglobulins and autoantibodies in aging humans, J. Immunol. 111:1101–1107.

Halliday, W. J., 1971, Immunological paralysis of mice with pneumococcal polysaccharide antigens, *Bacteriol. Rev.* 35:267–289.

Hanson, L. A., 1959, Immunological analysis of streptococcal antigens and human sera by means of diffusion-in-gel methods, Int. Arch. Allergy Appl. Immunol. 14:279–291.

Heidelberger, M., 1953, Persistence of antibodies in man after immunization, in: *The Nature and Significance of the Immune Response* (A. M. Pappenheimer, Jr., ed.), pp.90–101, Columbia University Press, New York.

Heidelberger, M., and Elliot, S., 1966, Cross reactions of streptococcal group N teichoic acid antipneumococcal horse sera of types VI, XIV, XVI and XXVII, *J. Bacteriol.* 92:281–283.

Heidelberger, M., and Kendall, F. G., 1929, A quantitative study of the precipitin reaction between type III pneumococcus polysaccharide and purified homologous antibody, *J. Exp. Med.* 50:809–823.

Heidelberger, M., and Nimmich, W., 1972, Additional immunochemical relationships of capsular polysaccharides of Klebsiella and Pneumococci, *J. Immunol.* 109:1337–1344.

Heidelberger, M., MacLeod, C. M., and Dilapi, M. M., 1948, The human antibody response to simultaneous injection of six specific polysaccharides of pneumococcus, *J. Exp. Med.* 88:369–372.

Heidrick, M. L., and Makinodan, T., 1972, Nature of cellular deficiencies in age-related decline of the immune system, *Gerontologia* 18:305–320.

Hill, W. C., and Robbins, J. B., 1966, Horse anti-pneu-

mococcal immunoglobulins. II. Specific mouse protective activity, *Proc. Soc. Exp. Biol. Med.* 123:105–108.

Himmelspach, K., Westphal, O., and Teichman, B., 1971, Use of 1-(m-aminophenyl) flavazoles for the preparation of immunogens with oligosaccharide determinant groups, *Eur. J. Immunol.* 1:106–112.

Hobbs, J. R., Milner, R. D. G., and Watt, P. J., 1967, Gamma-M deficiency predisposing to meningococcal septicemia, *Br. Med. J.* 4:583–586.

Holborow, E. J., and Loewi, G., 1962, The immune response to blood group substances, *Immunology* 5:278–286.

Holmgren, J., Hanson, L. A., Holm, S. E., and Kaijser, B., 1971, An antigenic relationship between kidney and certain Escherichia coli strains, *Int. Arch. Allergy Appl. Immunol.* 41:463–474.

Howard, C. J., and Glynn, A. A., 1971, The virulence for mice of strains of Escherichia coli related to the effects of K antigens on their resistance to phagocytosis and killing by complement, *Immunology* 20:767–777.

Howard, J. G., 1969, Discussion, in: *Immunologic Tolerance* (M. Landy and W. Braun, eds.), pp. 28–31, Academic Press, New York.

Howard, J. G., and Siskind, G. W., 1969, Studies on immunological paralysis. I. A consideration of macrophage involvement in the induction of immunity and paralysis by type II pneumococcal polysaccharide, *Clin. Exp. Immunol.* 4:29–39.

Howard, J. G., Elson, J., Christie, G. H., and Kinsky, R. G., 1969, Studies on immunological paralysis. II. The detection and significance of antibody-forming cells in the spleen during immunologic paralysis with type III pneumococcal polysaccharide, *Clin. Exp. Immunol.* 4:29–37.

Howard, J. G., Zola, H., Christie, G. H., and Courtenay, B. M., 1971, Studies on immunological paralysis. V. The influence of molecular weight on the immunogenicity, tolerogenicity and antibody-neutralizing activity of type III pneumococcal polysaccharide, *Immunology* 21:535–546.

Huntley, C. C., and Dees, S. C., 1957, Eczena associated with thrombcytopenic purpura and purulent otitis media. Report of five fatal cases, *Pediatrics* 19:351–361.

Jann, K., and Westphal, O., 1975, Microbial polysaccharides, in: *The Antigens* (M. Sela, ed.), pp. 1–125, Academic Press, New York.

Johnston, R. B., and Stroud, R. M., 1977, Complement and host defense against infection, *J. Pediatr.* 90:169–170.

Johnston, R. B., Newman, S. L., and Struth, A. G., 1973, An abnormality of the alternate pathway of complement activation in sickle-cell disease, *N. Engl. J. Med.* 288:803–808.

Kabat, E. A., 1966, The nature of an antigenic determinant, *J. Immunol.* 97:1–11.

Kabat, E. A., and Bezer, A. E., 1958, The effect of variation in molecular weight on the antigenicity of dextran in man, *Arch. Biochem. Biophys.* 78:306–318.

Kearney, R., and Halliday, W. J., 1970, Humoral and cellular responses of mice to a pneumococcal polysaccharide antigen. Plaques and paralysis, *in vivo* and *in vitro*, *Aust. J. Exp. Biol. Med. Sci.* **48:**227–235.

Kerman, R., Segre, D., and Myers, W. L., 1970, The role of immune and natural specific antibodies in immunologic paralysis and immunity of mice to pneumococcal polysaccharide type III, *J. Immunol.* **104:**656–664.

King, H., and Shumacker, H. B., Jr., 1952, Splenic studies I. Susceptibility to infection after splenectomy performed in infancy, *Ann. Surg.* **136:**239–242.

Klemperer, G., and Klemperer, F., 1891, Versuche über Immunisirung und Heilung bei der Pneumokokeninfection, *Berl. Klin. Wochenschr.* **28:**833–869.

Lim, D., Gewurz, A., Lint, T. F., Ghaze, M., Sepheri, B., and Gewurz, H., 1976, Absence of the sixth component of complement in a patient with repeated episodes of meningococcal meningitis, *J. Pediatr.* **89:**42–47.

Loda, F. A., Collier, A. M., Glezen, W. P., Strangert, K., Clyde, W. A., Jr., and Denny, F. W., 1975, Occurrence of *Diplococcus pneumoniae* in the upper respiratory tract of children, *J. Pediatr.* **87:**1087–1093.

Luderitz, O., Gmeiner, J., Kickhofen, B., Mayer, H., Westphal, O., and Wheat, R. W., 1968, Identification of D-mannosamine and Quinovosamine in salmonella and related bacteria, *J. Bacteriol.* **95:**490–493.

MacLeod, C. M., Hodges, R. G., Heidelberger, M., and Bernhard, W. B., 1945, Prevention of pneumococcal pneumonia by immunization with specific polysaccharides, *J. Exp. Med.* **82:**445–465.

Mage, R. G., and Kabat, E. A., 1963, The combining regions of the type III pneumococcus polysaccharide and homologous antibody, *Biochemistry* **2:**1278–1288.

Maron, B. J., and Maloney, J. R., 1972, Septicemia following traumatic or incidental splenectomy, *Johns Hopkins Med. J.* **130:**266–268.

Minden, P., and Farr, S. R., 1967, The ammonium sulfate method to measure antigen-binding, in: *The Handbook of Experimental Immunology* (D. W. Weir, ed.), pp. 463–492, Blackwell Scientific Publications, England.

Morgan, P., Watson, D. W., and Cromartie, W. J., 1953, Type-specificity of "immunological paralysis" induced in mice with pneumococcal polysaccharide, *J. Bacteriol.* **65:**224–225.

Morse, H. C., III, Prescott, B., Cross, S. S., Stashak, P. W., and Baker, P. J., 1976, Regulation of the antibody response to type III pneumococcal polysaccharide. V. Ontogeny of factors influencing the magnitude of the plaque-forming cell response, *J. Immunol.* **116:**279–287.

Mosier, D. E., 1967, A requirement for two cell types for antibody formation *in vitro*, *Science* **158:**1573–1575.

Myerowitz, R. L., Gordon, R. E., and Robbins, J. B., 1974, Polysaccharides of the genus *Bacillus* cross-reactive with the capsular polysaccharides of *Diplococcus pneumoniae* type III, *Haemophilus influenzae* type b and *Neisseria meningitis* group A, *Infect. Immun.* **8:**896–900.

Neter, E., 1956, Bacterial hemagglutination and hemolysis, *Bacteriol. Rev.* **20:**166–188.

Norman, M. E., Gall, E. P., Taylor, A., Laster, L., and Nilsson, U. R., 1975, Serum complement profiles in infants and children, *J. Pediatr.* **87:**912–916.

O'Reilly, R. J., Anderson, P., Ingram, D. L., Peter, G., and Smith, D. H., 1975, Circulating polyribophosphate in *Hemophilus influenzae* type b meningitis: Correlation with clinical course and antibody response, *J. Clin. Invest.* **56:**1012–1022.

Osler, W., 1909, *The Principles and Practice of Medicine,* p. 165, Appleton, New York.

Ouchterlony, O., 1958, Diffusion-in-gel methods for immunological analysis, *Progr. Allergy* **5:**1–78.

Pahmer, M., 1940, Pneumococcus peritonitis in nephrotic and nonnephrotic children, *J. Pediatr.* **17:**90–105.

Pinckard, R. N., and Weir, D. M., 1973, Equilibrium dialysis and preparation of hapten-conjugates, in: *Handbook of Experimental Immunology* (D. W. Weir, ed.), pp. 16.1–16.21, Blackwell, Oxford.

Powars, D. R., 1975, Natural history of sickle cell disease: The first ten years. *Semin. Hematol.* **12:**267–285.

Reed, W. P., Davidson, M. S., and Williams, R. C., Jr., 1976, Complement systemic in pneumococcal infections, *Infect. Immun.* **13:**1120–1125.

Respiratory Disease Task Force Report on Problems, Research, Approaches, Needs, 1972, National Heart and Lung Institute, DHEW Publication No. 73432, p. 118, U.S. Government Printing Office, Washington, D.C.

Robbins, J. B., and Parson, H. A., 1965, Normal response of sickle cell patients to immunization with Salmonella vaccines, *J. Pediatr.* **66:**877.

Robbins, J. B., Myerowitz, R. L., Whisnant, J. K., Argaman, M., Schneerson, R., Handzel, Z. T., and Gotschlich, E. C., 1972, Enteric bacteria cross-reactive with Nesissera meningitidis groups A and C and Diplococcus pneumoniae types I and III, *Infect. Immun.* **6:**651–656.

Robinson, M. G., and Watson, R. J., 1966, Pneumococcal meningitis in sickle-cell anemia, *N. Engl. J. Med.* **274:**1006–1008.

Rosenfeld, S. I., Kelly, M. E., and Leddy, J. P., 1976, Hereditary deficiency of the fifth component of complement in man. I. Clinical immunochemical and family studies, *J. Clin. Invest.* **57:**1626–1634.

Schiffman, G., and Austrian, R., 1971, A radioimmunoassay for the measurement of pneumococcal capsular antigens and of antibodies thereto, *Fed. Proc.* **30**(2):651.

Schiffman, G., Bornstein, D. L., and Austrian, R., 1971, Capsulation of pneumococcus with soluble cell wall-like polysaccharide. II. Nonidentity of cell wall and soluble cell wall-like polysaccharides derived from the same and from different pneumococcal strains, *J. Exp. Med.* **134:**600–617.

Schiffman, G., Summerville, J. E., Costagna, R., Douglas, R., Bonner, M. J., and Austrian, R., 1974, Quantitation of antibody, antigen, and antigen-antibody complexes in sera of patients with pneumococcal pneumonia, *Fed. Proc.* **33**(3):758.

Schumacker, M. J., 1970, Serum immunoglobulin and transferrin levels after childhood splenectomy, *Arch. Dis. Child.* **45**:114–117.

Schwartz, A. D., and Pearson, H. A., 1972, Impaired antibody response to intravenous immunization in sickle cell anemia, *Pediatr. Res.* **6**:145–149.

Schwarzmann, S., and Boring, J. R., III., 1971, Antiphagocytic effect of slime from a mucoid strain of pseudomonas aeruginosa, *Infect. Immun.* **3**:762–767.

Seeler, R. A., and Jacobs, N. M., 1977, Pyogenic infections in children with sickle hemoglobinopathy, *J. Pediatr.* **90**:161–162.

Sela, M., 1966, Immunological studies with synthetic polypeptides, *Adv. Immunol.* **5**:29–129.

Shapera, R. M., and Matsen, J. M., 1972, Host factors and capsular typing of body fluid isolates in fulminant pneumococcal infections, *Infect. Immun.* **5**:132–136.

Siskind, G. W., 1962, Immunological response of newborn and adult mice to pneumococcal polysaccharide, *Fed. Proc.* **21**:34.

Siskind, G. W., Paterson, P. Y., and Thomas, L., 1963, Induction of unresponsiveness and immunity in newborn and adult mice with pneumococcal polysaccharide, *J. Immunol.* **90**:929–934.

Sloyer, J. L., Howie, V. M., Ploussard, J. H., Ammann, A. J., Austrian, R., and Johnston, R. B., 1974, Immune response to acute otitis media, *Infect. Immun.* **9**:1028–1032.

Smith, D. H., Peter, G., Ingram, D. L., Harding, A. L., and Anderson, P., 1973, Responses of children immunized with the capsular polysaccharide of Hemophilus influenzae, type b, *Pediatrics* **52**:637–644.

Sorg, C., Rude, E., and Westphal, O., 1970, Immunological properties of amylose, dextran and polyvinylalcohol conjugated with polytyrosylpeptides, *Eur. J. Biochem.* **17**:85–90.

Suzuki, S., Sunayama, H., and Saito, T., 1968, Studies on the antigenic activity of yeasts. I. Analysis of the determinant groups of the mannam of *Saccharamyces cerevisae*, *Jpn. J. Microbiol.* **12**:19–24.

Tillett, W. S., and Francis, T., 1929, Cutaneous reactions to the polysaccharides and proteins of pneunococcus in lobar pneumonia, *J. Exp. Med.* **52**:687–691.

Turk, J. L., and Heather, C. J., 1965, A histological study of lymph nodes during the development of delayed hypersensitivity to soluble antigens, *Int. Arch. Allergy Appl. Immunol.* **27**:199–212.

Wara, D. W., Reiter, E. O, Doyle, N. E., Gewurz, H., and Ammann, A. J., 1975, Persistent C1q deficiency in a patient with a systemic lupus erythematosus-like syndrome, *J. Pediatr.* **86**:743–745.

Wasserman, E., and Levine, L., 1961, Quantitative microcomplement fixation and its use in the study of antigenic structure by specific antigen-antibody inhibition, *J. Immunol.* **87**:290–295.

Weksler, M. E., and Hutteroth, T. H., 1974, Impaired lymphocyte function in aged humans, *J. Clin. Invest.* **53**:99–104.

Winkelstein, J. A., and Drachman, R. H., 1968, Deficiency of pneumococcal serum opsonizing activity in sickle-cell disease, *N. Engl. J. Med.* **279**:459–466.

Winkelstein, J. A., and Swift, A. J., 1975, Host defense against the pneumococcus in T-lymphocyte deficient, nude mice, *Infect. Immun.* **12**:1222–1223.

Winkelstein, J. A., Bocchinit, J. A., Jr., and Schiffman, G., 1976, The role of the capsular polysaccharide in the activation of the alternative pathway by the pneumococcus, *J. Immunol.* **116**:367–370.

Yurewicz, E. G., Ghalambor, M. A., and Heath, E. C., 1971, The structure of aerobacter aerogenes capsular polysaccharide, *J. Biol. Chem.* **246**:5596–5606.

3

Immunology of Streptococci

LEWIS W. WANNAMAKER

1. Introduction

The wealth of antigens and of immune responses associated with streptococci has provided a wide choice of antibodies for clinical diagnosis of streptococcal infections, abundant materials and models for experimental immunologists and immunogeneticists, and a diversity of hypotheses about the pathogenesis of the nonsuppurative complications of streptococcal infections, acute nephritis and acute rheumatic fever.

Although group A streptococci (*Streptococcus pyogenes*) account for most streptococcal infections in humans, groups B, C, G, and D streptococci and "viridans" streptococci are also important pathogens in man. The pneumococci (*Streptococcus pneumoniae*) are discussed in Chapter 2. Those obligately anaerobic streptococci that do not produce lactic acid as a major metabolic product, now classified as a separate genus, *Peptostreptococcus* will not be considered here.

2. Evolution, Genetics, and Taxonomic Relationships of Streptococci

Little is known about the evolution of streptococci. Many approaches have been used in exploring possible relationships among streptococcal species and between streptococci and other bacteria. The problem here, as with other bacteria, is in distinguishing true phylogenetic relationships from convergent evolutionary trends.

Studies of the immunological relationships of fructose diphosphate aldolases have suggested that streptococci can be placed into antigenic groups, correlating roughly with the Lancefield grouping antigens (see below), and that a tentative phylogenetic map reflecting interrelationships among the Lactobacillaceae can be drawn (London and Kline, 1973). Some evidence of partial correlation between fatty acid profiles and Lancefield groups has also been reported (Drucker and Holmes, 1974)

Of the many extracellular products of streptococci produced by strains of different serological groups of streptococci, some appear to be immunologically identical. For example, nuclease A, produced by group C strains, is also produced by some group A strains. A more striking example is streptolysin O, which is produced by groups C and G as well as group A streptococcal strains and indeed cross-reacts immunologically with the hemolysins of other gram-positive bacteria, e.g., the pneumococcus and the tetanus bacillus (Discussion in Wannamaker and Matsen, 1972a). The existence of such similar hemolysins suggests a possible link among these various bacteria.

The spectra of activity of bacteriocins of streptococci and of other gram-positive cocci (Tagg *et al.*, 1976a) are much broader than those of gram-negative bacteria, with reactivity against strains of many gram-positive species and, in the case of the bacteriocins of "viridans" streptococci, apparently also including some gram-negative bacteria (Dajani *et al.*, 1976). This indicates a widespread relationship among the many bacterial species

LEWIS W. WANNAMAKER • Departments of Pediatrics and Microbiology, University of Minnesota, Minneapolis, Minnesota 55455.

susceptible to these bacteriocins, the basis of which is not understood but which is perhaps attributable to a common receptor.

The host ranges of bacteriophages may also provide some clues about the relationships of streptococci, although interpretation of results is difficult since they may depend on a number of factors including receptors, other (interfering) surface components, lysogeny, bacteriophage interference, and restriction nucleases. Studies of phages indicate some crossover of host ranges of virulent and temperate phages of groups A, C, and G streptococci (Colón *et al.*, 1971; Wannamaker *et al.*, 1973; Wannamaker and Skjold, unpublished observations). It is of interest that the receptor in group A streptococci for the virulent streptococcal phage A25 appears to be peptidoglycan, which is identical or closely related to that of groups C and G streptococci (Cleary *et al.*, 1977).

Streptococci from a large number of different serological groups contain a peptidoglycan that is cross-linked by interpeptide bridges consisting of L-alanyl oligopeptides. The bridges vary in amino acid composition and sequence, permitting division of the peptidoglycans into 12 different types. With the exception of groups D and K, most of the strains from a serological group exhibit only one type of peptidoglycan. Those of groups A and C are identical and are similar to those of some group G strains. Thus the peptidoglycans which serve as the backbone for streptococci and may act as attachment sites for bacteriocins and bacteriophages with broad spectra and host ranges may be good indicators of phylogenetic relationships. The majority of the gram-positive, non-spore-forming, fermenting bacteria such as the streptococci appear to represent a primitive stage exhibiting great variability in peptidoglycan structure which is probably still in the process of evolving (Schleifer and Kandler, 1972).

The teichoic acids (polyglycerophosphates), which appear to be immunologically related in a wide range of streptococci (of different serological groups) and of certain other gram-positive species (McCarty, 1959; Matsuno and Slade, 1970), also suggest a possible genetic or evolutionary relationship.

The carbohydrates of the cell wall, which (except for groups D and N) are responsible for the group designation of streptococci, are related in structure but exhibit terminal *N*-acetyl amino sugars that are largely responsible for their immunological specificity (Krause, 1963). The specificity of A-variant strains resides in the rhamnose moiety of the carbohydrate (McCarty, 1956). It has been suggested that this variant like antigen exists, either masked or overt, in all streptococci and may be the counterpart of the R core of the lipopolysaccharides of the Enterobacteriaceae (Elliott *et al.*, 1971). This postulated variant-like antigen is another possible link among the serological groups of streptococci.

Immunological cross-reactions among capsular polysaccharides of pneumococci and of α and nonhemolytic streptococci have been identified by a number of investigators. Cross-reactions between the cell wall polysaccharides of streptococci and the somatic polysaccharide of pneumococcus have also been demonstrated (Austrian *et al.*, 1972). These and other findings (see following discussion) indicate a close relationship between pneumococci and "viridans" streptococci.

Transformation has been successfully carried out between pneumococci and "viridans" streptococci (Bracco *et al.*, 1957; Ravin and De Sa, 1964; Biswas and Ravin, 1971; Deddish and Ravin, 1974), as well as among a number of other members of the *Streptococcus* genus (see review by Dobrzański, 1972). Intergeneric transformation between *Staphylococcus aureus* and group H streptococci has also been reported by one investigator (Dobrzański *et al.*, 1968). Reciprocal transformation experiments have been useful in confirming the relationships among human viridans streptococci which have proved difficult to classify on the basis of serological reactions (Colman, 1969; Colman and Williams, 1972).

Transduction has been demonstrated not only between strains of homologous group, e.g., strains of group A streptococci (Leonard *et al.*, 1968; Malke, 1969; Malke and Köhler, 1973; Tagg *et al.*, 1976b), but also among strains of different groups, e.g., groups A, C, and G streptococci (Colón *et al.*, 1972; Wannamaker *et al.*, 1973; Malke *et al.*, 1975). Transductional analysis has helped to elucidate the genetic relationships of resistance to various antibiotics in streptococci (Malke, 1972; Malke *et al.*, 1975; Ubukata *et al.*, 1975).

Conjugal transfer of bacteriogenicity and of

antibiotic resistance has been demonstrated in group D streptococci (Tomura *et al.,* 1973; Jacob and Hobbs, 1974; Dunny and Clewell, 1975). Although transfer of antibiotic resistance has been demonstrated in mixed cultures of group A streptococci, the exchange appears to be phage mediated (Malke, 1975).

It is of interest that the mechanisms available for genetic exchange among group A streptococci may be limited to those involving bacteriophages (Wannamaker *et al.,* 1973) and conjugal transfer (Engel *et al.,* 1979). Attempts at transformation with group A streptococci as recipients have never been successful, perhaps because of the large amounts of DNases of diverse kinds produced by group A streptococci (Wannamaker, 1964). In addition to the role of virulent and temperate phages in transduction of group A streptococci (see preceeding discussion), a role for temperate phage in directing the production or release of scarlatinal toxin has been reported, most likely by a mechanism of phage conversion (Zabriskie, 1964; Barksdale, 1964; Zabriskie *et al.,* 1972).

Studies of base composition of diverse strains of streptococci have yielded values ranging from 27 to 40 mol % guanosine plus cytosine (Laskin and Lechevalier, 1973). Like the pathogenic staphylococci, the streptococci show a DNA of predominantly AT type (Belozersky and Spirin, 1960; Marmur *et al.,* 1963). The values reported for the GC content of group A streptococci have varied from 34% to 40% (Laskin and Lechevalier, 1973; Jones and Walker, 1968; Stuart and Ferretti, 1975). Analysis of GC compositions and base sequence homologies has been a valuable tool in examining differences in *Streptococcus sanguis* and *Streptococcus mutans* (Coykendall, 1970, 1974; Coykendall and Specht, 1975).

DNA-RNA homology techniques have been used to examine the relationships among Lancefield groups and M types of streptococci, with good general agreement between serological data and homology findings (Weissman *et al.,* 1966). Organisms in different Lancefield groups were related but could be differentiated from each other, as could serotypes within group A. Strains of Lancefield groups A, C, H, and F exhibited a closer relationship to each other than to strains of group D streptococci. DNA-DNA hybridization techniques have been employed in ex-

amining the relationship of atypical enterococci and of streptococci from plants which exhibit characteristics of both group D and group N streptococci (Roop *et al.,* 1974). DNA-DNA reassociation studies have also been useful in confirming genetic differences among serological types of *S. mutans* (Coykendall, 1974).

Plasmids appear to play an important role in genetic changes of streptococci, as determinants not only of antibiotic resistance but also of bacteriocin production (Tagg and Wannamaker, 1976) and perhaps of virulence (see following discussion). Of possible clinical interest are recent studies in group A streptococci indicating that determinants of resistance to erythromycin and lincomycin are plasmid mediated (Clewell and Franke, 1974; Malke, 1974; Malke *et al.,* 1976) and are transducible with high efficiency by a temperate phage obtained by ultraviolet light induction of a naturally resistant strain (Malke, 1974). Studies in recent years have indicated that erythromycin resistance in group A streptococci, although still uncommon, may be on the increase and may be found in other serological groups of streptococci as well as in several different types of group A streptococci (Dixon and Lipinski, 1974). In addition to the macrolide antibiotics, resistance to chloramphenicol and to tetracycline may be plasmid determined (Nakae *et al.,* 1975). Multiple antibiotic resistance to *Streptococcus faecalis* is also plasmid borne (Jacob and Hobbs, 1974). Plasmid-determined tetracycline resistance in this species, with evidence of gene amplification during growth in the presence of tetracycline, has also been reported (Clewell *et al.,* 1975; Yagi and Clewell, 1976). Similar molecular weights of and demonstration of a high degree of homology between some of the plasmids isolated from groups A and D streptococci suggest the possibility of a common phylogenetic origin (Malke *et al.,* 1976).

The genetics and evolution of streptococci as they relate to virulence, to the appearance and disappearance of the organism (in individual human hosts and in populations), to interactions with normal flora, to immune reactions in the host, and to the development of suppurative and nonsuppurative complications are important areas for careful studies in the future.

Virulence in group A streptococci is primarily related to the type-specific M proteins, antibodies to which confer type-specific immunity (see Section 6). The T antigen is another antigen occurring in multiple serological forms in streptococci. Studies of strains over many years have indicated a frequent but by no means absolute correlation between the occurrence of certain M and T antigens (Maxted and Widdowson, 1972), indicating the possibility of a genetic linkage of varying distance between these two antigens. A much closer linkage appears to exist between certain M proteins and another series of serologically diverse substances, the serum opacity reaction (SOR) factors, produced by some strains of group A streptococci (Krumwiede, 1954; Top and Wannamaker, 1968; Widdowson et al., 1971b; Maxted et al., 1973b). Although recent evidence suggests that M protein and SOR factors are separable epidemiologically and genetically (Cleary, Johnson, and Wannamaker, unpublished observations), the linkage has proved close enough to be useful in screening for M protein changes by the opacity reaction around streptococcal colonies on serum agar plates.

Recent studies, using the SOR detection system, have suggested that the production of M protein may be under extrachromosomal (plasmid or prophage DNA) control (Cleary et al., 1975). This finding is in line with earlier laboratory (Lancefield and Todd, 1928) and epidemiological observations of the genetic instability of M protein. The documented progressive loss of M protein in strains isolated during the chronic carrier state after infection (Rothbard and Watson, 1948; Krause et al., 1962) could result from loss of plasmid(s) or prophage(s), perhaps under selective pressure from the development of M antibody or from "curing" of the lysogenic state by the development of phage antibody. Of interest also are serial observations suggesting that a strain of group A streptococcus persisting in a population for a long period of time may change from one M type to another (Maxted and Valkenburg, 1969). It has long been known that new M types of streptococci may appear in populations (Wannamaker, 1954; Parker, 1969; Anthony et al., 1976), perhaps most often because of introduction from outside sources,

but a change in M type with time among strains with another persisting marker (the T antigen) is highly suggestive of a genetic basis. The explanation for the modification in M type of a persisting strain is not clear, but it is possible that point mutations or genetic exchanges mediated by bacteriophages may play a role. The development of "herd immunity" in the form of either type-specific antibody to the M protein of the parent strain or antibody to the temperate phage carried by the parent strain may result in the emergence of the new M variant as the predominant strain in the population. Of interest in this regard, and supportive of a possible role of bacteriophage, is the observation (Kjems, 1958; Wannamaker et al., 1970) that in naturally lysogenized group A strains the serological specificity of the M type parallels the serological specificity of the harbored phage. This finding, the explanation for which is unknown, requires confirmation by examining a wider range of strains.

Although the production of M proteins was long considered the exclusive province of group A streptococci, recent studies have indicated that group G, and also possibly group C, streptococci may harbor an M protein serologically identical with the M protein of type 12 streptococci (Maxted and Potter, 1967; Cole, 1968). Whether this was acquired by genetic exchange processes is uncertain, but the existence of bacteriophages that cross group lines makes this a possibility. Other studies have indicated that group C streptococci can produce type-specific proteins that may be analogous to the M proteins of group A streptococci, but their role in immunity is not entirely clear (Moore and Bryans, 1969; Woolcock, 1974; Woods and Ross, 1975).

3. Host Ranges of Streptococcal Infection

Since the early studies of Lancefield (1940–1941), it has been recognized that the host ranges of streptococci vary with different serological groups. In some instances these appear to be restrictive and in others quite broad.

The most common streptococci producing infections in man are those belonging to group A. Except for acute mastitis in cattle (Brown,

1946), group A streptococci are rarely associated with natural infection in other animals. The few exceptions have been discussed in recent reviews (Lancefield, 1972; Ginsburg, 1972). Mice have been traditionally used for passage of group A streptococci to enhance virulence and for assays of type-specific protection. However, freshly isolated strains from human epidemics rarely show natural virulence for mice and have to be adapted by serial passage (Dochez *et al.*, 1919). Rabbits and monkeys have also been used in experimental infections, notably in experimental attempts to produce rheumatic fever (Murphy, 1960; Morse *et al.*, 1955; Watson *et al.*, 1946; Vanace, 1960). Hamsters have been used in an experimental model of impetigo (Cushing and Mortimer, 1970; Dajani and Wannamaker, 1970; Cushing, 1975).

A-variant strains have been identified only after serial passage of group A strains in mice (McCarty and Lancefield, 1955) and have not been found in human infections except in one case of a laboratory worker (Lancefield, 1972).

Group B streptococci are a common cause of chronic mastitis in cattle. They may be found in the vagina of normal women and may cause puerperal infection in the mother and sepsis, with or without meningitis, in newborn human infants (see Section 11).

Streptococci exhibiting the group C antigen fall into several different species. Of these, *Streptococcus equi* is of special interest because of its sharp species specificity for horses, in which it causes strangles (Bryans and Moore, 1972). In contrast, *Streptococcus zooepidermicus* and *Streptococcus equisimilis* have been found in a variety of animals; the latter is the most common species of group C streptococci found in humans (Wilson and Miles, 1975).

Group G streptococci of the large colony forms are found chiefly in dogs (Laughton, 1948) and in man, where they can cause sore throat, endocarditis, and urinary tract infections (Hill *et al.*, 1969; MacDonald, 1939; Rantz, 1942).

Group D streptococci are a heterogeneous collection of species found in human, animal, and bird feces and in some plants. They are found in urinary tract infections, endocarditis, and abdominal infections in man (Krause,

1972a; Wannamaker and Ferrieri, 1975) and may also cause infections in swine and sheep (Ross, 1972; Jamieson, 1950; Elliott *et al.*, 1966).

The "viridans" streptococci are found on the body surfaces and in the oropharynx of animals and man and are a common cause of endocarditis in man.

The bacterial and host factors that determine the host ranges of streptococci are not understood. However, it is provocative that the blood of animal species other than man is generally not satisfactory for the performance of bactericidal tests with group A streptococci (see below). Of interest also is the observation that the resistance of guinea pigs to infection with group A streptococci seems to be due to the capacity of guinea pig serum to destroy asparagine, which appears to be a nutritional requirement of most group A streptococci (Bassett, 1972).

4. Host Genetics of Streptococcal Infection

The discovery that rabbits immunized with streptococcal vaccines may produce large amounts of antibody of restricted heterogeneity and that this response may be genetically determined has opened up new horizons and new approaches in immunogenetics. The details of this rapidly proliferating area of research are beyond the scope of this chapter. The reader is referred to other reviews (Krause, 1970; Krause and Kindt, 1977) and to Part III of this treatise. In brief, early studies of Krause and his associates indicated that after immunization with streptococcal vaccines an occasional rabbit develops antibodies with several of the properties of myeloma proteins. The unusual uniformity of these antibodies (directed toward the group-specific carbohydrate) is suggested by their monodisperse distribution on zone electrophoresis (Osterland *et al.*, 1966) and by their individual antigenic specificity (Braun and Krause, 1968). Like myeloma proteins, these rabbit antibodies to streptococcal polysaccharide also show selectivity of expression of the allotypic specificities on both the heavy and light chains (Kindt *et al.*, 1970). With repeated immunization, antibodies with either identical or distinct individual antigenic specificities may occur in the same animal (Eichmann *et al.,* 1970). In some of these rabbits, antibody concentrations exceed 50 mg/ml antisera (Osterland *et al.,* 1966), thereby comprising a large fraction of the total serum protein. The magnitude and the heterogeneity of the antibody response are determined by independent genetic factors (Eichmann *et al.,* 1971; Braun *et al.,* 1973). In addition to antibodies to the streptococcal carbohydrates, some animals develop 19 S and 19 S and 7 S anti-IgG exhibit a specificity for the Fc piece of IgG of their species (Bokisch *et al.,* 1973; Chiao *et al.,* 1974). The production of antibodies of limited heterogeneity in response to streptococcal carbohydrates has now been observed in a number of species—notably the mouse, where studies of inbred strains have identified the streptococcal group A polysaccharide as a thymus-dependent antigen (Braun *et al.,* 1972). They have also facilitated studies of the idiotypic specificity of these antibodies (Eichmann, 1972; Capra *et al.,* 1976) and have resulted in identification of a new immune response gene (Cramer and Braun, 1975). The immunogenetic studies of responses to group A streptococcal carbohydrates are now being extended to man, in whom there is evidence of restriction in class, subclass, and type of antibody produced and in the number of clonotypes of antibody-producing cells stimulated (Riesen *et al.,* 1976).

Animal experiments demonstrating skin graft sensitization after immunization with heat-killed group A streptococci of a variety of serological types have raised the question of a possible cross-reaction between mammalian transplantation antigens and streptococcal antigens (Chase and Rapaport, 1965; Rapaport and Chase, 1964). Among a variety of other bacteria tested, including streptococci of other groups, only staphylococci produced similar results. The responsible antigen in group A streptococci was shown to be a component of the cell membrane. Antisera produced by immunization with group A streptococcal membranes have been shown to mediate skin allograft rejection in guinea pigs (Rapaport *et al.,* 1966). In man, the existence of a relationship between streptococcal antigens and human histocompatibility (HLA) antigens has been postulated from HLA cytotoxicity inhibition

studies. Preparations of type 1 M protein were found to inhibit allogenic antisera against human lymphocytes of all seven HLA specificities tested (Hirata and Terasaki, 1970). M protein preparations of other types, group A polysaccharide, and other bacterial antigens were ineffective. Subsequent studies have indicated that HLA allo- and heteroantisera, without correlation to specificity, are also effective in inhibiting the lymphocyte transformation-inducing activity of type 1 M protein preparations (Pellegrino *et al.,* 1972). In similar studies, the capacity of a type 12 cell membrane preparation to protect human lymphocytes from the cytotoxic effects of isospecific HLA sera was interpreted to result from steric hindrance by binding of the streptococcal antigen to the lymphocyte surface (Rapaport *et al.,* 1973). More recent investigations, using a cell membrane preparation of type 1 streptococci, have demonstrated the same effect but have indicated that the inhibition is due to activation and consumption of components of the alternate complement pathway (Tauber *et al.,* 1976a). The complement-activating factor in streptococcal membranes appears to be protein in nature and to have a molecular weight greater than 40,000–60,000 (Tauber *et al.,* 1976b). In none of these studies has a specificity for any particular HLA type or types been demonstrated, and in none of them have antisera to M protein or to cell membranes been found to be cytotoxic for human lymphocytes. From these latest studies (Tauber *et al.,* 1976a,b) it has been concluded that the accelerated rejection of skin homografts in animals sensitized to streptococcal antigens (Rapaport and Chase, 1964) results from organ-related, rather than HLA, antigens. The authors speculate that the HLA markers characterized by high genetic polymorphism may have evolved as an escape from microbial mimicry (Tauber, 1977). Since the alternate complement pathway has been shown to be inactivated by preparations from many different bacterial species in addition to streptococci, it has been postulated that it represents a nonspecific defense system which appeared early in evolution and persists to fill gaps in specific immunity resulting from microbial mimicry as exhibited by a number of streptococcal antigens (see Section 8).

The possibility that HLA antigens of a specific type or types may be correlated with streptococcal immune responses or with susceptibility to complications (see Section 8) has also been entertained by a number of workers. *In vitro* studies of human lymphocyte blastogenesis by a streptokinase–streptodornase (SK-SD) preparation indicated a statistically significant increase in frequency of HLA-5 antigen among high responders (Greenberg *et al.*, 1975b). The blastogenesis-inducing activity, originally considered to be associated with streptococcal nuclease A, has subsequently been shown to be distinguishable (Gray and Greenberg, personal communication; Chopyk *et al.*, 1976). Preliminary family studies suggesting that the response is HLA haplotype associated support the view that the trait is transmitted by the same chromosome (Greenberg *et al.*, 1975a).

These studies seem to open up new approaches to an understanding of the genetics of immune responses in man, not only to the various streptococcal antigens but to other bacterial antigens as well. Studies of the distribution of HLA types in patients with complications of streptococcal infections will be discussed in Section 8.

5. Pathogenesis of Streptococcal Infection

Group A streptococci can and do infect almost any organ of the human body, but they most commonly produce a localized infection of the upper respiratory tract or of the skin. The many intriguing differences between streptococcal infections at these two sites have been reviewed in detail elsewhere (Wannamaker, 1970a) and are outlined in Table 1.

When group A streptococci are found in the throat, they may reflect a variety of microbe–host interactions, including transitory acquisition, clinical or subclinical infection, or a chronic carrier state. Some of the factors that determine the outcome of contact between group A streptococci and their human hosts are discussed in this and other sections.

Striking differences in streptococcal infections of the respiratory tract as related to age have been noted (Powers and Boisvert, 1944). Thus the infant under 6 months of age presents with a mild (sometimes almost subclinical) illness, the cardinal signs of which are an insidious onset, a low-grade, irregular fever, and a thin, persistent mucoserous nasal discharge resulting in excoriation and crusting around the external nares. Some infection of the throat may be present, but pharyngeal signs are usually minimal. Older infants are often more severely ill with early signs of coryza and a diffusely reddened pharynx but without exudate. An irregular fever and enlarged cervical lymph nodes, which tend to suppurate, may continue in untreated infants for periods up to 2 months. The more generalized and more protracted illness of infants, frequently accompanied by otitis media and sometimes by bacteremia, contrasts sharply with the focalized, short, and stormy course of scarlet fever or acute streptococcal pharyngitis characteristically seen in older children and adults.

The reasons for the differences between infants and older individuals in appearance of streptococcal infections are not well understood. It seems unlikely that they are due to age *per se* since the protracted febrile form is common up to 3 years of age, by which time there should be no residual immaturity in the ability of the human host to respond to streptococcal infection. The more localized and more acute response seen in older children and adults is most probably due to previous experience with the streptococcus and modification of the response by the development of hypersensitivity and of humoral antibodies to streptococcal toxins and enzymes. The infrequency of scarlet fever and of acute rheumatic fever in infants has been attributed to absence of hypersensitivity, which may require repeated or prolonged exposure to streptococcal antigens (see Section 8). Because of the differences in appearance of streptococcal infections with age, an analogy has been drawn with tuberculosis, and the term "streptococcosis" has been introduced to emphasize the variations in clinical manifestations associated with age (Powers and Boisvert, 1943). Some confusion has resulted in the literature, however, by the subsequent use of the term to apply specifically to the infant form of streptococcal infection. Although the analogy is perhaps useful, group A streptococci differ from the human tubercle bacillus in the many serological types, which after untreated infections result in the development of type-specific immunity. Thus the multiple infections which

TABLE 1.   Differences in Streptococcal Infections at Different Sites[a]

Feature	Streptococcal pharyngitis and tonsillitis	Streptococcal impetigo and pyoderma
Epidemiology		
Seasonal occurrence	Winter and spring	Late summer
Geographic distribution	More common in temperate or cold climates	More common in hot or tropical climates
Age	Young school-age children	Preschool children
"Carrier" state	Common in pharynx of many populations	Infecting strain found on skin before lesions develop, appears in throat late in infection
Preceding trauma	Not necessary	May be essential for natural as well as experimental infection
Local factors	Some strains of viridans streptococci may be protective	Local flora and skin lipids may be protective
Mode of transmission and environmental factors	Spread by direct contact with human reservoirs, particularly acutely infected persons and nasal carriers; environmental contamination does not play a role	Hygiene appears to be a factor; contaminated environment and insects may play a role in transmission
Clinical aspects		
Appearance	Generalized erythema usually present; no vesicles; no crusting	Erythema usually minimal; transient vesicular stage; characteristic crusts
Local pain	Common, may be intense	Absent
Systemic reaction	Fever, headache, malaise common	Absent
Bacteremia	Rare, except in infants	May be more frequent
Course	Typically acute, except in infants	May be chronic and recurrent in certain environments
Laboratory findings		
Leukocytosis	Usually present	Often absent
Group A streptococci	Classical serotypes	New types (recently described, with higher numbers); few types are able to cause clinical infection of both respiratory and skin sites
Immune response		
Antistreptolysin O	Good response	Absent or poor response, apparently inhibited by cholesterol in skin
Anti-DNase B and anti-hyaluronidase	Good response	Good response
Type-specific M antibody	Develops in untreated patients; protective against reinfection	Develops less regularly and may not be protective
Nonsuppurative sequelae		
Acute nephritis	Occurs; may be partially preventable by penicillin treatment	Occurs; may develop despite penicillin treatment
Acute rheumatic fever	Occurs; preventable by penicillin treatment	Does not occur

[a] Modified and with additions from Wannamaker (1970a). (See original for more complete listing and description.)

may occur throughout life and particularly during childhood are usually due to different serological types of streptococci. Following untreated infection and sometimes despite treatment, group A streptococci may be identified in throat cultures for weeks or months and probably persist in tonsillar tissue for years, but, except for the rare patient who may show clinical relapse due to treatment failure, there is no convincing evidence that these latent streptococci are responsible for repeated infections.

In order to initiate infection in the upper respiratory tract, group A streptococci must compete with resident flora, must possess a mechanism of adhering to the pharynx or tonsils, and must escape or overcome host defenses.

Clinical and epidemiological studies have indicated that α-hemolytic streptococci, the most abundant flora of the human throat, can interfere with establishment of group A streptococci at this site (Sanders, 1969; Crowe *et al.*, 1973). This mechanism of bacterial interference is not understood but may include competition for nutrients or for sites of adherence (see following discussion), changes in pH, and hydrogen peroxide or bacteriocin production (Tagg *et al.*, 1976a). Recent studies have indicated that some strains of α-hemolytic streptococci may contain intracellular bacteriocinlike substances, called viridins, which have an unusually wide spectrum of bacteriostatic or bactericidal activity, including the inhibition of group A streptococci (Dajani *et al.*, 1976). Other members of the throat flora, e.g., staphylococci (Fredericq, 1946; Tagg *et al.*, 1976a), may produce bacteriocins. Bacteriocins are also produced by some strains of group A streptococci (Tagg *et al.*, 1973); if such strains are currently being "carried" in the throat, they may theoretically prevent the establishment of new strains of group A streptococci.

A mechanism of adherence is an important first step in initiating infection. The anatomical structures in group A streptococci responsible for adherence are the abundant "pili" or "fimbriae" on their surface (Ellen and Gibbons, 1972). Two components have been identified in the fimbriae of group A streptococci, M protein and lipoteichoic acid (Swanson *et al.*, 1969; Beachey and Ofek, 1976). Although the original studies suggested that M protein is involved in attachment, current evidence indicates that the lipoteichoic acid component of the fimbriae is responsible for binding of group A streptococci to epithelial cells (Beachey and Ofek, 1976). It has been shown that secretory immunoglobulin in saliva will inhibit the adherence to epithelial cells of some streptococcal species indigenous to human oral mucous surfaces (Williams and Gibbons, 1972). It is possible that secretory immunoglobulins to some surface component could act in a similar fashion to prevent the adherence of group A streptococci to epithelial cells or that viridans streptococci could compete with group A streptococci for the binding sites on epithelial cells. Although there is no clear evidence that nasal or pharyngeal secretions contain IgA directed against streptococcal surface antigens, it is of interest in this regard that local immunization may prevent colonization by group A streptococci (see Section 12).

The factors that influence localization of streptococci at certain sites are not understood. Some studies have indicated that streptococci of different species have specific preferences for adherence to different parts of the oral cavity, e.g., *Streptococcus salivarius* to buccal epithelial cells and *Streptococcus mutans* to the teeth (Gibbons and van Houte, 1971), the latter preference perhaps relating to the role of this species in the pathogenesis of dental caries. However, no information is available to explain the localization of infection with group A streptococci on the posterior pharynx and tonsils, and indeed buccal and nasal rather than pharyngeal epithelial cells have been used in most studies of adherence of group A streptococci. Factors that may relate to localization of streptococcal infection in the skin are discussed below.

After attachment to the epithelial cells of the upper respiratory tract, the streptococcal products and components responsible for invasion of the tissues probably include (1) the specific toxins (streptolysins S and O and the erythrogenic or pyrogenic toxins) which may damage or kill fixed tissue or circulating cells, including leukocytes, by lysis or other mechanisms, (2) specific enzymes such as hyaluronidase and streptokinase which may promote spread of infection, and (3) surface components of the streptococcal cell (M protein and hyaluronic acid).

The host factors responsible for defense against and limitation of primary (preimmune) invasion by streptococci are not well defined and indeed may be feeble, perhaps accounting for the more prolonged course and the tendency toward bacteremia in infections acquired in infancy (see above). In contrast to gram-negative bacteria, the bactericidal and bacteriolytic systems present in normal and immune sera and mediated by immunoglobulins and complement are ineffective in killing or lysing most gram-positive bacteria including group A streptococci (Davis *et al.*, 1972). Moreover, the serum β lysins, which are heat-stable cationic proteins released from platelets during blood coagulation (Weksler and Nachman, 1971) and which are bactericidal for some gram-positive species, do not kill most strains of streptococci (Donaldson, 1973). Although C-reactive protein can be readily demonstrated in the serum of most patients during the acute phase of streptococcal pharyngitis (Kaplan and Wannamaker, 1977) and has been associated with a variety of biological functions (Mortensen *et al.*, 1975; Croft *et al.*, 1976), some of which may have a role in nonspecific resistance to infection or regulation of host responses, no specific information is available concerning the possible role that C-reactive protein or other acute phase reactants may play in host defense against streptococcal infection.

An increase in circulating polymorphonuclear leukocytes is characteristic of acute streptococcal infections. The local appearance of leukocytes is reflected in the formation of pharyngeal exudate, presumably due to increased leukotactic activity as has been demonstrated in patients with streptococcal infections of the skin (see following discussion). However, no increase in the percent of circulating neutrophils with spontaneous reduction of nitroblue tetrazolium (NBT) dye occurs in patients with streptococcal pharyngitis (Shapera and Matsen, 1973; Poretz, 1974).

Some phagocytosis of virulent group A streptococci may occur in the absence of serum or type-specific antibody, particularly on surfaces. Therefore, surface phagocytosis may play an important role in the early stages of defense against streptococcal infection (Foley *et al.*, 1959; Foley and Wood, 1959). Experimental infections suggest that earliest defense is provided by monocytes followed by polymorphonuclear leukocytes, both acting by surface phagocytosis (Sawyer *et al.*, 1954).

Two superficial components of the streptococcal cell, the hyaluronic acid capsule and the M protein (located on the fimbriae), are responsible for the resistance of virulent group A streptococci to phagocytosis (Lancefield, 1962). In man, the M protein appears to play the more important role in resistance to phagocytosis, since human sera contain a factor that neutralizes the retarding effect of the hyaluronic acid capsule on engulfment. The nature of this thermolabile factor in human serum is uncertain, but it appears to be neither an antibody, an enzyme, nor a component of complement (Hirsch and Church, 1960; Stollerman *et al.*, 1967). Most humans, except for rare individuals, have this factor in their blood, whereas most animals, except for monkeys, lack this "streptococcal coopsonin" (Stollerman *et al.*, 1963, 1967). The role of complement (C′) as a possible cofactor for opsonization of group A streptococci is not clear. The coopsonin is removed from fresh human plasma by absorption with bentonite without apparent change of C′ components.

Recently, surface components of group A streptococci have been shown to combine with the Fc portion of γ-globulin (P. Christensen, *et al.*, 1976). The factors, which are analogous in their action to protein A of staphylococci, seem to be heterogeneous and protein in nature but distinct from M protein (Christensen and Holm, 1976; Myhre and Kronvall, 1977). There is no evidence that these factors play a role in resistance to phagocytosis.

The mechanism by which M protein results in resistance to phagocytosis is not clear. Resistance to ingestion does not depend on the cocci being in an active metabolic state since it persists even in killed streptococci (Wiley and Wilson, 1956).

The enhancement of phagocytosis and the consequent protection provided by type-specific antibody are discussed in subsequent sections. Since this antibody is so slow in appearing, it is not likely to play a role in the limitation or termination of acute streptococcal infection.

After phagocytosis, streptococci are enclosed in a digestive vacuole. They may be killed within a period of about 30 min, or they may be egested in a viable or nonviable state, depending on the length of stay in the vacuole (Wilson, 1953). Sometimes the tables will be turned and the ingested group A streptococci will kill the leukocyte (Wilson, 1957). This leukotoxicity has been ascribed to the production of streptococcal nicotinamide-adenine dinucleotidase (NADase) (Bernheimer *et al.*, 1957) and more recently to streptolysin S (Ofek *et al.*, 1970).

It is curious that polymorphonuclear leukocytes from patients with chronic granulomatous disease of childhood retain the ability to kill group A and other streptococci (Kaplan *et al.*, 1968). As a result these patients have no special problem with streptococcal infections as they do with infections due to staphylococci and other catalase-producing organisms (Quie, 1972; Quie and Hill, 1973). The neutrophils of patients with chronic granulomatous disease lack the capacity to generate reactive oxygen radicals such as superoxide and hydrogen peroxide during phagocytosis. These products of oxidative metabolism are produced during phagocytosis by normal leukocytes and together with myeloperoxidase and halide constitute a potent microbicidal system (Klebanoff, 1975). Streptococci, which are catalase negative, generate their own hydrogen peroxide, resulting in self-destruction (Stossel, 1974).

Degradation of streptococci or of streptococcal components (e.g., cell wall) within phatocytes or other tissues may require hours or weeks (Ayoub and Wannamaker, 1967; Spector et al., 1970; Schwab and Ohanian, 1967; Schwab and Brown, 1968; Glick et al., 1971). This raises the question of whether human or other mammalian tissues possess enzymes that can deal efficiently with streptococcal components, particularly the cell wall (Ayoub and McCarty, 1968; Ginsburg, 1974; Ginsburg et al., 1976). The morphological changes and degradation of streptococci by polymorphonuclear leukocytes and by macrophages have been recently reviewed in detail (Ginsburg and Sela, 1976).

Although poorly understood, the factors responsible for localization of streptococcal infection must be relatively efficient, except in infants (see preceding discussions). In experimental infections in adults, in which infectious exudate from a patient with active streptococcal infection is implanted into the throat of a normal volunteer lacking type-specific antibody for that type, throat cultures are negative for the first 32 hr after inoculation and the transferred organism is recovered only a few hours before symptoms appear (Rammelkamp, 1957).

Strict containment of the streptococci to the tissues of the pharynx may not be achieved. Indeed, involvement of the regional (anterior cervical) lymph nodes is common in patients with group A streptococcal infection of the upper respiratory tract, in older individuals and adults as well as in infants (Kaplan et al., 1971). By needle aspiration the infecting organism can often be obtained from tender enlarged cervical nodes, sometimes even when the throat culture is negative (Dajani et al., 1963). Postmortem studies of the cervical lymph nodes of children have also indicated a relatively high frequency of isolation of group A streptococci (Adamson, 1949).

In older children and adults, bacteremia is uncommon with streptococcal infections of the upper respiratory tract. In experimental infections in animals, group A streptococci injected intravenously completely disappear from the bloodstream, apparently through clearance by the reticuloendothelial system, but may persist in the tissues at various sites and, as long as 100 days later, may reappear in the bloodstream after administration of cortisone (Denny and Thomas, 1955).

The ability of group A streptococci to persist in the throat for months after infection is well known, and it is likely that these organisms may persist for longer periods in the tonsils and other lymphoid tissues of the pharynx and also in the regional lymph nodes. Localization and persistence at more distant sites have been postulated to play a role in the pathogenesis of rheumatic fever, but no conclusive evidence is available (see Section 8).

Because tonsils are often the site of streptococcal infection, the role that they may play in immunological responses and in defense is of special interest with respect to streptococcal diseases, but little definitive information is available. Tonsils differ from lymph nodes in that they have no afferent lymph vessels. Presumably, microorganisms and antigens can gain direct access. Experimental work in rabbits suggests that tonsils do take up antigen applied to their epithelial surface and that tonsils function as regional as well as nonregional lymph nodes (Surján and Surján, 1971; Surján et al., 1972; Merler and Silberschmidt, 1972; Godrick and Patt, 1971). Direct lymphatic connections have been demonstrated between tonsils and the heart (Andriushin, 1969), a finding of possible importance in the pathogenesis of rheumatic heart disease (Wannamaker, 1973).

Studies of human tonsils by electron microscopy have verified that they are composed primarily of lymphoid cells (Zucker-Franklin and Berney, 1972). The ratio of B lymphocytes to T lymphocytes varies from one report to another and also apparently from one individual to another. Some reports suggest that B and T cells are almost equally represented in the tonsillar lymphocytes (Delespesse *et al.*, 1976). Lymphocyte forming rosettes with erythrocytes sensitized with IgG are apparently rare or absent in tonsils (Frøland and Natvig, 1973; Delespesse *et al.*, 1976). These reports are difficult to interpret in view of the conflicting claims in the literature about the ability of such complexes to bind to lymphocytes.

All classes of immunoglobulins appear to be represented in tonsils. In comparison with other lymphoid tissues, they are particularly rich in IgE-producing cells (Tada and Ishizaka, 1970). Tonsils are able to synthesize various types of immunoglobulins and specific antibodies (Hoffmann *et al.*, 1973; Surján and Surján, 1971; Godrick and Patt, 1971; Sloyer *et al.*, 1973). From studies in rabbits, tonsils appear to be most immunologically reactive in the early weeks of life at a time when other future antibody-producing cells are not competent or less competent (Godrick and Patt, 1971).

A possible compartmentalization of cellular immune responses to preparations of streptolysin O has been suggested by studies of blastogenic responses, which have been reported to be absent in tonsillar lymphocytes (Oettgen *et al.*, 1966), whereas a number of other studies indicate that lymphocytes from peripheral blood are stimulated by preparations of this antigen (Hirschhorn *et al.*, 1964; Francis and Oppenheim, 1970; Gotoff *et al.*, 1973). Other studies of lymphocytes from peripheral blood suggest that hemolytically active streptolysin O fails to stimulate *in vitro* blast transformation but streptolysin O inactivated by heat or cholesterol does stimulate thymidine uptake by lymphocytes from this same source. Interpretation of these reports is difficult because of problems in determining whether streptolysin O is present in an active or inactive state and whether it may influence cell responses by its action on cell membranes or receptor sites (Bernheimer, 1972).

Although tonsillectomy has often been performed in patients with repeated throat infections and in patients with rheumatic fever, its value in protection against streptococcal infections and recurrences of rheumatic fever is not clear (Wannamaker, 1970b). There is evidence that clinically recognized streptococcal infections may be reduced in tonsillectomized patients (Dingle *et al.*, 1964; Holmes *et al.*, 1958). Other studies indicate that tonsillectomy results in streptococcal infections that are no less frequent but more likely to be subclinical and that tonsillectomy does not reduce the recurrence rate of rheumatic fever (Chamovitz *et al.*, 1960). Still other studies have suggested that large tonsils may be associated with an increased frequency of rheumatic recurrences (Feinstein and Levitt, 1970).

Streptococcal infections of the skin may take the form of erysipelas, impetigo, or pyoderma, the last sometimes superimposed on other skin diseases such as eczema or scabies. Certain serological types of group A streptococci have been associated with impetigo or pyoderma and others with pharyngitis (Wannamaker, 1970a). "Pyoderma" strains are often found in the throat, arriving there after the skin infection is well established, but only a few serological types of streptococci appear to have the capacity to produce clinical infection at either site (Anthony *et al.*, 1976).

In contrast to throat infections in which epidemiological studies and experimental inoculation of human volunteers have indicated that group A streptococci can initiate infection without trauma (Rammelkamp, 1957), initiation of infection of the skin apparently requires local trauma (Duncan *et al.*, 1970; Wannamaker, 1970a). Indeed, group A streptococci of the serological type which will subsequently cause infection are often found on the normal skin for several weeks before impetigo or pyoderma develops (Dudding *et al.*, 1970; Ferrieri *et al.*, 1972), perhaps waiting for access by some local minor trauma, e.g., a scratch or an insect bite.

As in throat infections, bacterial interference and adherence may be important determinants of the success or failure of group A streptococci in initiating infection of the skin. Removal of the resident flora from the skin prolongs the period of survival of applied group A streptococci (Aly *et al.*, 1972). In addition, skin lipids (Ricketts *et al.*, 1951) are bactericidal for group A streptococci *in vitro* and may play a role in protection against the establishment of infection.

Increased leukotactic activity of circulating

polymorphonuclear leukocytes has been demonstrated in streptococcal infection of the skin (Hill *et al.*, 1974) and may be responsible for the prompt infiltration of neutrophils and thus contribute to the localization of infection. Although streptolysin O is capable of inhibiting leukotaxis and random migration of neutrophils (Andersen and Van Epps, 1972), it does not do so, perhaps as a result of the neutralizing effect of free cholesterol, which is found in abundance in the skin and which is apparently also responsible for suppressing the antibody response to this antigen (see Section 6). As in streptococcal infections of the throat (see preceding discussion) and other localized infections, the leukocytes of most patients with well-established streptococcal impetigo do not show increased reduction of nitroblue tetrazolium (NBT) dye (Hill *et al.*, 1974), although an early transitory increase has been demonstrated in experimental streptococcal skin infections in hamsters (Dajani and Wannamaker, 1972).

Involvement of the regional lymph nodes is a less prominent feature of impetigo as compared with throat infections but may occur with extensive pyoderma or with wound infections. Lymphangitis is common with wounds infected with streptococci and in patients with filariasis with secondary streptococcal infection (Yü-K'un *et al.*, 1964). These findings, together with the common involvement in streptococcal upper respiratory infections of the tonsils, the other lymphatic tissues of the throat, and the regional lymph nodes, suggest that streptococci may have a special affinity for lymphatic tissues.

It seems unlikely that secretory immunoglobulins contribute to the defense against skin infection, and indeed it is uncertain whether type-specific immunity plays a protective role in impetigo or other forms of pyoderma as it undoubtedly does in throat infections. Development of type-specific M antibody may occur less regularly after impetigo and may depend on parasitism of the throat by the skin strain (Bisno and Nelson, 1974), which when it occurs is usually a late development (Ferrieri *et al.*, 1972).

Except for the rash of scarlet fever, it is impossible to associate with any degree of confidence the clinical manifestations of streptococcal infection with any specific component or extracellular product of group A streptococci (Dingle, 1954). This unsatisfactory state of affairs is a result of difficulties in obtaining pure preparations and the problems in finding suitable *in vitro* or *in vivo* experimental models. Moreover, it is often difficult to distinguish between direct toxic effects and effects mediated by immunological reactions. Some, perhaps many, streptococcal products appear to have both kinds of effects. For example, the erythrogenic toxins or "streptococcal pyrogenic exotoxins" possess both a primary toxicity and a secondary toxicity mediated by hypersensitivity (Kim and Watson, 1972). Thus human infants do not develop scarlet fever when infected with an erythrogenic toxin-producing strain (Dingle, 1954). This failure of young infants to develop scarlet fever occurs even in infants who apparently have no transplacental antitoxin, suggesting that they have not had an opportunity to become sensitized to the erythrogenic toxin. The streptococcal pyrogenic toxins resemble the gram-negative endotoxins in many of their effects and in exhibiting both primary and secondary toxicity. Other well-defined streptococcal extracellular products and cellular components that exhibit toxicity or enhance cell damage include streptolysin O, streptolysin S, proteinase, streptokinase, and peptidoglycan. A detailed discussion of these and the many other streptococcal substances is beyond the scope of this chapter. The reader is referred to a recent review by Ginsburg (1972) and particularly to its comprehensive list of references. Some of the streptococcal substances that produce immunological responses of use in diagnosis or that may possibly relate to the development of nonsuppurative complications are discussed in the sections below.

6. Humoral Immune Responses

The number and variety of immune responses that occur in humans after group A streptococcal infection are quite large and the techniques used for identifying them are diverse. This and other sections of this chapter emphasize those that have been found to be most useful clinically and epidemiologically and those that are of special interest with respect to the role they may play in the modification or expression of streptococcal infections and their sequelae. A detailed description of the methods for some of the commonly used antibody tests will be found elsewhere (Bisno and Stollerman, 1975).

An indication of the number of circulating antibodies to streptococcal substances found in human blood can be gained from precipitin analysis of pooled human γ-globulin (Halbert, 1958) and from immunoelectrophoretic studies of cellular extracts (Wilson and Wiley, 1963) which have revealed at least 12 distinct extracellular antigens and seven cellular antigens.

Apart from antibody to M protein and to the streptococcal pyrogenic exotoxins (erythrogenic toxins), little specific information is available to indicate how humoral antibody might modify the host response on reexposure to group A streptococci. Evidence in experimental animals (Lancefield, 1962) and epidemiological studies in man (Wannamaker, 1954) indicate that antibody directed toward the type-specific M protein protects against reinfection with the same serological type of streptococcus (see following discussion). Curiously, however, the development of this antibody does not result in eradication of the carrier state, and the role of type-specific antibody in protection against reinfection of the skin is uncertain (see Section 5). The pyrogenic exotoxins (erythrogenic toxins) seem to be rather poor antigens, but antibody to one of these toxins appears to provide protection against that toxin but not against the other two toxins of different serological specificities (Kim and Watson, 1972). The presence or absence of circulating antitoxin determines whether a sensitized individual infected with a strain producing toxin of that serological type will develop a scarlatiniform rash (see Section 5). The role of humoral antibodies to the many other extracellular products and cellular components of the group A streptococci in altering the host response to reinfection is uncertain, but it is possible that by neutralizing the toxic or enzymatic properties of these substances, humoral antibody may exert some influence on the pathological process and the clinical picture, which shows a wide range of severity in the acute stage as well as diversity in suppurative and nonsuppurative sequelae.

Humoral antibodies to streptococcal substances (e.g., antistreptolysin O and probably also type-specific antibodies) can be transmitted through the placenta to the newborn child (Zimmerman and Hill, 1969), in whom they may persist for some months. They may also be found in the mother's milk (Köhler and Dietel, 1968). During late infancy, they may be low or absent if the infant has not acquired a streptococcal infection.

An understanding of the dynamics of streptococcal antibodies is essential for interpretation of titers in clinical situations. Since group A streptococcal infections are common and a series of infections occur during life, one usually finds for common streptococcal antigens a baseline antibody titer, which will vary from person to person and from time to time in a single individual. Population groups will also vary in the distribution of streptococcal antibody titers and in mean titer or "upper limits of normal" (arbitrarily defined as the titer exceeded by only 20% of sera from a normal population). Any factor which correlates with the frequency of streptococcal infection will influence the titers in a normal population and therefore must be considered in interpreting an antibody titer. These include age, sex, season, geographical location, socioeconomic status, size of family, and probably a number of other variables (Wannamaker and Ayoub, 1960; Rantz et al., 1948; Saslaw and Streitfeld, 1959; Markowitz and Gordis, 1972). Ideally, one obtains appropriately timed acute and convalescent serum specimens so that a rise in one or more streptococcal antibodies can be demonstrated. Since variations may occur in titers from one laboratory to another and from day to day in the same laboratory, it is recommended that all sera from the same patient be examined in one laboratory on the same test run. In many clinical situations only a single late bleeding is available, and one must often deduce the likelihood of recent streptococcal infection on the basis of comparison between the titer on this specimen and those in the "normal" population.

Precipitin tests have not been generally useful for measuring the humoral immune response to streptococcal infections in man since highly purified antigens are not readily available and reactions are difficult to quantitate. Most of the streptococcal antibody tests in clinical use measure neutralizing antibody for a specific extracellular biological or enzymatic activity of streptococci (Table 2).

Anti-streptolysin O (ASO) and anti-streptococcal deoxyribonuclease B (anti-DNase B) are the two most valuable and reliable streptococcal antibody tests for clinical use. The ASO test has been widely used and advocated, although it does have some limitations and nonspecific inhibitors may occassionally result in clinical misinterpretation (Table 2). It can be standardized to give reproducible results in a single laboratory, but significant differences in titers on the same serum may occur between laboratories. Streptolysin O is oxygen labile and is active only in the presence of a reducing agent (Bernheimer, 1972). Free cholesterol is a natural inhibitor of streptolysin O, but as usually found in human sera (esterified and bound) cholesterol does not significantly affect the ASO titer. Extremely high titers of ASO have been reported in patients with monoclonal hypergammaglobulinemia (Waldenstrom et al., 1964). Although streptolysin O is closely related to the hemolysins of a number of other gram-positive organisms (e.g., pneumococci, clostridia) and appears to cross-react with these when examined with antisera prepared in horses, this cross-reaction does not seem to occur in human sera (Discussion in Wannamaker and Matsen, 1972a). Whether this is due to some difference in prior exposure to these cross-reacting antigens on the part of horses and man is not certain, but it is of interest and a boon to clinical medicine that humans can apparently distinguish between these closely related antigens in their immunological response.

Anti-DNase B is a reliable streptococcal antibody test for both skin and throat infections and therefore in nephritis after infection at either site. The test is well standardized and reproducible within narrow limits (Table 2). Reagents for the anti-DNase B test are commercially available. It is probably more specific for group A streptococcal infection than the ASO, although the data on the identification of specific nucleases produced by streptococci of other groups and on antibody responses in man after infection with other groups are limited. Most group C strains appear to produce streptococcal DNase A (Wan-

namaker, 1964), and the nucleases of group B streptococci are immunologically distinct from those of group A streptococci (see Section 11). No serum inhibitors (other than specific antibody) for streptococcal DNase B are known. Since group A streptococci can produce at least four different desoxyribonucleases of different serological specificities (Wannamaker, 1964), it is essential to use purified DNase B preparations, which can be obtained by a number of separation techniques, the most simple of which is batch adsorption (Slechta and Gray, 1976).

Both ASO and anti-DNase B can be performed as microtiter tests (Edwards, 1964; Klein et al., 1968; Nelson et al., 1968), and reagents are available commercially for performing both of these antibody tests. The microtiter tests correlate well with the corresponding macroprocedures. Both of these antibodies can be reproducibly titered at close intervals (0.1 log) with either the macro- or the microprocedures. Although some of the dilution schemes in use are at wider and irregular intervals, there is an advantage in using regular, closely spaced dilution increments, particularly for demonstrating antibody changes (Wannamaker and Ayoub, 1960). An international standard serum for ASO is available through WHO (Spaun et al., 1961), and it is hoped that one will soon also be available for streptococcal anti-DNase B.

Other streptococcal antibody tests may be useful but have the disadvantage of being less reproducible at close intervals, less regularly elevated after streptococcal infection, or less specific, or the reagents may not be available commercially (Table 2).

From time to time attempts have been made to introduce agglutination tests, with extracellular antigens such as streptolysin O coated on latex or barium sulfate particles (Klein et al., 1970; Ingram and Hughes, 1972; Mosley and Pickett, 1965), as a substitute for tests measuring neutralizing antibody for specific hemolysins or enzymes. The specificity of such tests is usually doubtful, since it is difficult or impossible to prepare antigens in a sufficiently purified state for such sensitive tests. Recently, an "all-purpose" hemagglutination test for streptococcal antibodies has been introduced which has achieved rather

TABLE 2. Tests for Antibody to Streptococcal Extracellular Products

Antibody test	Basis	Sensitivity	Reproducibility	Clinical usefulness and limitations	References
Antistreptolysin O (ASO)	Neutralization of oxygen-labile hemolytic activity of groups A, C, and G streptococci	Highly sensitive	Reproducible at closely spaced titers	Generally good in throat infections but will not distinguish among infections with groups A, C, and G streptococci; generally poor in impetigo and pyoderma; falsely elevated titers may occur in contaminated sera or in jaundiced patients with liver disease	Bernheimer (1972), El Kholy et al. (1973), Winblad (1966), Killander et al. (1965), Halbert (1970), Watson and Kerr (1975), Kaplan et al. (1970), Bisno et al. (1973), Dillon and Avery-Reeves (1974), Widdowson et al. (1974a)
Antistreptococcal deoxyribonuclease B (anti-DNase B)	Neutralization of most commonly produced nuclease of group A streptococci	Highly sensitive	Reproducible at closely spaced titers	Good in skin as well as throat infections; may be specific for group A infection; use of preparation free of other streptococcal nucleases is essential	Wannamaker (1959), Wannamaker (1964), Ayoub and Wannamaker (1962), Wannamaker (1970a), Kaplan et al. (1970), Bisno et al. (1973), Dillon and Avery-Reeves (1974), Widdowson et al. (1974a)
Antistreptococcal hyaluronidase (ASH)	Neutralization of specific hyaluronidase of group A streptococci	Highly sensitive	Reproducible at widely spaced titers	Good in skin as well as throat infections; apparently specific for group A infections; an acute phase nonspecific inhibitor may result in falsely elevated titers if unheated sera are tested	Harris and Harris (1949), Friou (1949), Good (1952), Wannamaker and Ayoub (1960), Bisno and Stollerman (1975)

(Continued)

wide popularity because of its ease of performance and its reflection of a wide variety of antibody responses in a single simple test. Reagents for the test are available commercially, and it is known as the "streptozyme test," a misnomer since it does not measure enzyme activity but rather antibodies to what appears to be a crude mixture of streptococcal hemolysin(s), enzymes, and possibly other extracellular products coated on red cells. Indeed, there is some evidence that it may contain at least three antigens that have not been

TABLE 2. (*Continued*)

Antibody test	Basis	Sensitivity	Reproducibility	Clinical usefulness and limitations	References
Antistreptococcal nicotinamide adenine dinucleotidase (anti-NADase)	Neutralization of specific enzyme of group A streptococci	Good sensitivity	Reproducible at closely spaced intervals	May be variable depending on the production of this enzyme by infecting strain; generally good in patients with nephritis after throat infection; enzyme reagent not commercially available; requires spectrophotometer	Bernheimer *et al.* (1957), Bernhard and Stollerman (1959), Ayoub and Wannamaker (1962), Wannamaker (1970a), Ofek *et al.* (1971), Lütticken *et al.* (1976a)
Antistreptokinase (ASK)	Neutralization of several streptokinases of group A streptococci	Moderate sensitivity	Reproducible at widely spaced titers	May be variable depending on the kinds of kinases present in the test mixture and produced by the infecting strain	M. Kaplan (1946), Wannamaker and Ayoub (1960), Dillon and Wannamaker (1965), Bisno and Stollerman (1975)
Anti-"streptozyme"	Agglutination of erythrocytes coated with crude mixture of extracellular products	Generally high sensitivity	Reproducible at widely spaced titers	Variation occurs with some lots of reagent; correlates generally well with ASO but less well with other antibodies, especially anti-DNase B	Janeff *et al.* (1971), Klein and Jones (1971), Ofek *et al.* (1973), El Kholy *et al.* (1974), Bisno and Ofek (1974), Bergner-Rabinowitz *et al.* (1975), Kaplan and Wannamaker (1975), Bisno *et al.* (1976), Lütticken *et al.* (1976b)

previously identified (Bisno *et al.,* 1976). In addition to the advantages already mentioned, on the basis of limited data with this test, a response can apparently be demonstrated much earlier (as early as 6–9 days) after a streptococcal infection in man than with conventional antibody tests (Ofek *et al.,* 1973). Animal studies suggest that the early response is due to the appearance of IgM, which is known to be a good agglutinating antibody (Kaplan and Wannamaker, 1975; Bisno *et al.,* 1976). The test seems to correlate generally well with the ASO test, against which it has apparently been standardized (Janeff *et al.,* 1971), but less well

with other streptococcal antibodies, notably anti-DNase B (Klein and Jones, 1971; Lütticken *et al.,* 1976b). Theoretically, this test should identify individuals with elevated titers for one or more of the following—ASO, anti-DNase B, antihyaluronidase, anti-NADase, and antistreptokinase (Janeff *et al.,* 1971)—and should be as good as or better than a combination of these tests. Some, but not all, investigators have found this to be so (Bisno and Ofek, 1974; Ofek *et al.,* 1973; Bergner-Rabinowitz *et al.,* 1975; Lütticken *et al.,* 1976b). One group has found that false-positive and false-negative tests are likely to occur when one or more of the conventional neutralizing antibody titers are at or near the threshold; this group concluded that the test can be used as an adjunct in serodiagnosis of streptococcal infections but is less useful for assessing the level of streptococcal humoral antibody in the general population (El Kholy *et al.*, 1974). Of more concern is the finding of an occasional patient with a high neutralizing titer for one of the conventional specific antibodies (most often anti-DNase B) and a negative "streptozyme test" and the observation that certain lots vary markedly in the reactions obtained (Lütticken *et al.*, 1976b; Kaplan, Ferrieri, and Wannamaker, unpublished observations). A basic problem with this test is that it is probably difficult, if not impossible, to reproduce consistently a reagent containing the same proportions of a complex mixture of antigens, some of which have not been identified. Unless or until this problem can be resolved, this test may continue to give variable results with different lots of the reagent.

The relatively slow response of the ASO and the other conventional neutralizing antibody tests is of interest in view of the fact that most patients have had contact with these antigens before. No change in ASO titer is usually detectable before about the 10th day, and generally 3 weeks, sometimes more, is required before titers reach their maximal level. This seems slow for a secondary immune response. The retarded secondary antibody response to streptolysin O and other streptococcal antigens may be due to the immunosuppressant effect of certain streptococcal substances (see end of this section).

Few studies have examined the class of the neutralizing antibodies formed against extracellular antigens. Some observers have found ASO only in the 7 S γ-globulin fraction (Killander and Philipson, 1964). Others have detected ASO in the IgM (19 S) fraction in children showing an initial response to this antigen (Sonozaki *et al.*, 1970). It is apparent that the timing of the collection of sera was not always ideal in these studies and that examination of sera soon after infection might result in more frequent detection of ASO in the IgM fraction.

The ASO response and probably the response of other streptococcal antibodies can be modified by the administration of penicillin, which may reduce the number of responders

and the magnitude of the response (Kilbourne and Loge, 1948; Wannamaker *et al.*, 1951). Early treatment is likely to result in greater inhibition (Brock and Siegel, 1953). The dosage and duration of penicillin treatment may also influence the frequency or degree of inhibition.

In the absence of a new streptococcal infection, the ASO titer usually begins to decline slowly after 6–8 weeks, reaching its original level within a varying period of 3–12 months.

With any single antibody test, about 20–30% of patients with group A streptococcal infection will fail to show a response. By using several different tests it is possible to show a rise in almost all patients with streptococcal infection and an elevated titer to at least one antibody test in almost all patients with acute rheumatic fever or poststreptococcal acute glomerulonephritis (Stollerman *et al.*, 1956; Ayoub and Wannamaker, 1962). Since chorea often has a long latent period (2–6 months) antibody titers may have begun to decline, but the performance of multiple antibody tests may reveal an elevated titer of at least one streptococcal antibody (Ayoub and Wannamaker, 1966). In patients presenting early in the course of acute nephritis or acute rheumatic fever, the ASO or other antibody titers may not have reached maximal titer. In such patients a repeat antibody determination 1–2 weeks after admission may demonstrate an increase over the admission titer.

Streptococcal antibody tests for the various cellular antigens have been used less frequently in immunodiagnosis of streptococcal infection, in part because they are less often available and usually more difficult to perform and also because they are generally less likely to be helpful. They are nevertheless of interest and may be useful in certain clinical or epidemiological situations.

Antibody to the group A polysaccharide has been demonstrated in human sera by a number of different kinds of tests: hemagglutination of antigen adsorbed directly to tanned, or indirectly to untanned, red cells (Schmidt and Moore, 1965; Goldstein and Caravano, 1967), agglutination of antigen adsorbed on latex particles (Erwa *et al.*, 1969), agglutination by the indirect Coombs test using purified cell walls (Karakawa *et al.*, 1965), and radioimmunoassay using single- or double-labeled antigen

(Dudding and Ayoub, 1968; Krause, personal communication). Although one might expect antibody tests for group A carbohydrate to be highly specific for infection with group A streptococci, in fact some patients also develop antibodies that react with group C polysaccharide (Krause, 1977). From 25% to 42% of patients with group A streptococcal infection have developed a rise in antibody titer or level to the group A polysaccharide (Kaplan et al., 1974; Goedvolk-De Groot et al., 1974). A most interesting observation with respect to the group A carbohydrate antibody is that patients with rheumatic valvular disease have elevated antibody levels which tend to persist for a long period of time (Dudding and Ayoub, 1968), perhaps because of the antigens in heart valves which cross-react with the group A carbohydrate antigen (see below). Patients with congenital heart disease show normal group A carbohydrate antibody levels and patients with endocarditis superimposed on rheumatic or congenital valvular lesions exhibit levels similar to patients without superimposed endocarditis (Ayoub and Dudding, 1970; Shulman et al., 1974). This suggests that valvular damage per se does not contribute to the elevated levels of this antibody found in patients with chronic rheumatic valvular disease. It has also been shown that a significant decrease in the group A carbohydrate antibody occurs in rheumatic patients who have had surgical excision and replacement of an affected valve but not in those who have had a simple commissurotomy (Ayoub et al., 1974). Although the group A carbohydrate antibody test may be useful in differentiating between patients with rheumatic and nonrheumatic valvular disease (when there is an elevated group A carbohydrate antibody level and low titers for other streptococcal antibodies), the frequency of streptococcal infections in children which may result in generally high levels of this and other antibodies makes it less useful in the pediatric age group (Kaplan et al., 1975). Recent studies of the qualitative aspects of the group A carbohydrate antibody response have revealed that acute rheumatic fever patients show low-affinity antibody in hapten-binding studies as compared with patients convalescent from streptococcal infection who do not develop this complication (Shulman and Ayoub, 1974).

It is not known whether this phenomenon is unique for this antigen–antibody system or one that might be found in other streptococcal antigen–antibody systems as well.

In man, type-specific antibody against the M protein of group A streptococci can be measured by the bactericidal test (Rothbard et al., 1948), the long-chain test (Stollerman et al., 1959), and the opsonocytophagic test (Bergner-Rabinowitz et al., 1971). With other kinds of tests such as passive hemagglutination (Vosti and Rantz, 1964) and complement fixation tests (Wittner and Fox, 1971; Beachey et al., 1974a), specificity is often difficult to achieve even with highly purified preparations of M antigens, apparently because of the frequent presence of cross-reacting non-type-specific antibody (see following discussion).

Peptic digestion of rabbit IgG type-specific antibody produces $F(ab')_2$ and Fab' fragments which, according to unconfirmed reports, retain their ability to enhance phagocytosis (Perkins and Hahn, 1968). Evidence from a number of sources suggests that the antigenic determinants for the precipitating and the antiphagocytic properties of M protein and the corresponding antibodies formed against them are distinct (Beachey and Cunningham, 1973; Ofek et al., 1969; Noble and Penny, 1975; El Kholy et al., unpublished observations). Recent studies of M protein extracted with a nonionic detergent indicate that molecular species of M protein in the 28,000–35,000 dalton range exhibit both antiphagocytic and type-specific precipitating properties whereas smaller species (down to 6000 daltons) show only precipitating properties (Fischetti et al., 1976). Both kinds of species are found in living streptococci, and the evidence suggests that the smaller type-specific, precipitating species are used to assemble the larger, antiphagocytic proteins.

After a streptococcal infection, antibodies to M protein are very slow in appearing, sometimes requiring several months before they can be detected (Rothbard et al., 1948; Denny et al., 1957). The slow appearance of type-specific antibody may be explained by the fact that this is a primary immune response rather than a secondary response. Type-specific antibody develops more frequently in patients with prolonged convalescent carriage. In some patients it may persist for many years (Lancefield, 1959), whereas in others it may disappear 6 months to several years after infection (Siegel *et al.,* 1961; Bergner-Rabinowitz *et al.,* 1971). Recall may occur after vaccination (Potter *et al.,* 1962) and perhaps after natural reexposure to strains of the same M type. Some workers have emphasized the importance of subclinical infections or carrier states in the maintenance of type-specific immunity in populations (Dunlap and Harvey, 1967). Penicillin treatment completely inhibits the development of type-specific M antibody (Daikos and Weinstein, 1951; Denny *et al.,* 1957; Siegel *et al.,* 1961). Evidence of placental transfer of M antibody from mother to infant has been obtained (Zimmerman and Hill, 1969).

Epidemiological studies (Anthony *et al.,* 1969) and animal experiments (Dajani and Wannamaker, 1970) indicate that type-specific immunity may develop less frequently after skin infections (impetigo or pyoderma) than after throat infections. The development of type-specific M antibody after streptococcal skin infections (impetigo or pyoderma) appears to be variable and to occur less regularly than after throat infections (Potter *et al.,* 1971; Bergner-Rabinowitz *et al.,* 1971; Bisno and Nelson, 1974; Widdowson *et al.,* 1974a). Type-specific antibody seems to develop more often in patients with skin infections who develop pharyngeal carriage (Bisno and Nelson, 1974). Since the M protein is very sensitive to proteases, it is possible that proteases present in skin may destroy the M protein of streptococci infecting this site.

Another factor which appears to influence the frequency of development of type-specific M antibody, after natural infection in man as well as in immunized animals, is the serological type of the strain. The anti-M response is poor in patients with throat infections caused by strains of M types which produce serum opacity (see following discussion) whereas the anti-M response in patients with throat infections from strains which do not produce serum opacity is generally good (Widdowson *et al.,* 1974a). In this study the anti-M response was poor after skin infections with both serum-opacity-positive and -negative strains.

The serum opacity reaction is associated with group A streptococci of certain serological types (Maxted and Widdowson, 1972).

The factor responsible for this reaction (probably a lipoproteinase) exists in a number of serologically distinct forms which parallel those of the type-specific M proteins (Top and Wannamaker, 1968). Measurement of antibody to the streptococcal opacity factor has been particularly useful as a means of demonstrating a type-specific response in patients infected with streptococci that do not produce a good antigenic response to M protein (Maxted *et al.,* 1973a; Iontova and Totolian, 1975).

The "M-associated" protein is a streptococcal antigen closely associated with the M antigen but not type specific. It can be detected by means of a complement fixation test, and antibody to it can be demonstrated in the sera of patients who have had streptococcal infection (Widdowson *et al.,* 1971a, 1974a,b; Beachey *et al.,* 1974a). Antibody to the non-type-specific M-associated determinant may have pathological significance since it appears to mediate cytotoxicity for platelets and leukocytes in the presence of M proteins (Beachey and Stollerman, 1973).

Methods for measuring antibodies to streptococcal peptidoglycans (Heymer *et al.,* 1976) and to streptococcal teichoic acid (Klesius *et al.,* 1974) have been described but have not been widely used. In view of the extensive cross-reactions of these two streptococcal antigens with similar cellular constituents of other gram-positive bacteria, they may not be specific for streptococcal infection.

Antibodies to cell membranes of streptococci, which are heart reactive and may be useful diagnostically, will be discussed in Section 8.

Before closing this section on humoral immune responses, mention should be made that certain streptococcal substances can have an effect on the immune response to nonstreptococcal antigens (Schwab, 1975). Thus the peptidoglycan component of the streptococcal cell wall has been shown to have an adjuvant effect in rabbits (Holton and Schwab, 1966; Heymer, 1975). In contrast, a potent immunosuppressant has been associated with streptococcal membranes, resulting in suppression of both IgM and IgG plaque-forming cells in the spleens of mice after primary or secondary immunization with sheep erythrocytes (Malakian and Schwab, 1971; Schwab, 1975).

Erythrogenic toxin (streptococcal pyrogenic exotoxin) exerts a biphasic response, with an early immunosuppressive effect on the antibody response to sheep erythrocytes (Hanna and Watson, 1968) frequently followed by elevated antibody and plaque-forming cell levels (Hanna and Watson, 1973). It has been suggested that the early transient immunosuppression produced by the pyrogenic exotoxin(s) may create a favorable environment for the streptococcus and that the deregulation of the antibody response results from a preferential inhibition of a regulatory cell, most likely a suppressor T cell (Hanna and Hale, 1975). It has also been reported that preparations of glycerol teichoic acid from group A streptococci have the capacity to suppress antibody formation to sheep red blood cells in mice (Miller and Jackson, 1973), perhaps acting as a tolerogen (Schwab, 1975). The individual and combined actions and interrelationships of the various streptococcal factors that may influence immune responses in the course of and following streptococcal infection have not been studied but have been the subject of speculation as to the effect on the streptococcal infection itself or its sequelae, on infection with other organisms, and on the host response to tumor cells (Hanna and Hale, 1975; Schwab, 1975).

7. Cellular Immune Responses

Streptococcal antigens have long been employed in studies of cellular immune responses both *in vivo* and *in vitro* (Lawrence, 1952), but the interpretation of results has been hampered by the lack of highly purified and well-defined preparations. For example, the commercial streptokinase–streptodornase (SK-SD) preparation used clinically for skin testing as an indication of T-cell function is a crude mixture of antigens produced by a group C streptococcus. Hypersensitivity as exhibited by skin reactions to streptococcal antigens, both cellular and extracellular, can be easily demonstrated in virtually all human adults, but interpretation of these skin reactions is often perplexing (Stollerman, 1972). There is conflicting information as to whether the cellular response(s) to streptococcal substances is "specific" or "nonspecific" in nature (Francis

et al., 1969; Keiser *et al.*, 1971; Read *et al.*, 1974; Barsumian, 1977); the available evidence suggests that both may occur (see following discussion).

Extracellular preparations of streptococci have been known for some time to induce lymphocyte transformation in sensitized individuals. Transformation-inducing antigens are produced by a variety of group A strains in amounts generally larger than those produced by non-group A streptococci (Taylor, 1972). Moreover, the supernatants of human lymphocytes incubated with extracellular products of group A streptococci, then washed and reincubated, stimulate blastogenesis of homologous lymphocytes. This activity appears to be physically and functionally different from that of extracellular products (Seravalli, 1976). Transformation-inducing activity has been found in several fractions of streptococcal culture supernates (Seravalli and Taranta, 1974; Gray and Greenberg, personal communication). Streptococcal extracellular antigens that stimulate transformation and that have been identified and partially purified include a glycopeptide (Plate and Amos, 1971a,b) and a β-globulin-like component of streptokinase–streptodornase preparations (Tomar *et al.*, 1972). Although some studies originally suggested that transformation-inducing activity is associated with well-defined streptococcal products, such as streptolysin S (Hirschhorn *et al.*, 1964), erythrogenic toxin (Nauciel, 1973) and streptococcal nuclease A (Greenberg *et al.*, 1975b), more recent investigations have indicated that this activity can be dissociated from streptolysin S and from streptococcal nuclease A (Taranta *et al.*, 1969; Plate and Amos, 1969; Taylor, 1969; Hryniewicz *et al.*, personal communication; Gray and Greenberg, personal communication). At present, the association of lymphocyte transformation responses (specific or nonspecific) with well-defined streptococcal products is not clear. Possible exceptions are the pyrogenic exotoxins (erythrogenic toxins) which in highly purified form have shown evidence of a nonspecific blastogenic response (mitogenicity), as suggested by stimulation of lymphocytes in the cord blood of human infants (Barsumian, 1977). Nonspecific stimulation of lymphocyte transformation has also been reported in cellular fractions and acid extracts of group A streptococci on the basis of the uniformity of response in adult subjects, the high percentage of cells transformed, the magnitude of thymidine uptake, and the enhancement of blastogenic transformation in cord blood lymphocytes (Keiser *et al.*, 1971). The nature of this streptococcal factor has not been defined, although it has some properties similar to those described for the lymphocyte-transforming factor present in preparations of streptolysin S, which, on the basis of limited evidence, is apparently also a nonspecific mitogen (Hirschhorn *et al.*, 1964).

The relationship of streptolysin O to blastogenic responses has been intriguing but is rather confusing. Most studies have indicated that streptolysin O stimulates transformation of lymphocytes from peripheral blood (Hirschhorn *et al.*, 1964; Francis and Oppenheim, 1970; Gotoff *et al.*, 1973). Of particular interest is a report indicating that streptolysin O fails to stimulate tonsillar lymphocytes (Oettgen *et al.*, 1966). This raises the possibility of a difference in response of tonsillar and peripheral blood lymphocytes to streptolysin O. Siegel *et al.* (1976) have recently shown profound differences in representatives of T-cell subsets in tonsils and peripheral blood lymphocytes, which may explain this difference. Other studies have suggested that hemolytically active streptolysin O fails to stimulate *in vitro* blast transformation of peripheral blood lymphocytes, whereas streptolysin O inactivated by heat or by cholesterol does stimulate thymidine uptake by lymphocytes (Andersen and Cone, 1974). This latter report also suggests that hemolytically active streptolysin O is an effective inhibitor of phytohemagglutinin-induced stimulation. Additional studies suggest that streptolysin O markedly suppresses chemotaxis and random mobility of human neutrophils, probably on a nonimmune basis (Van Epps and Andersen, 1974). These reports are difficult to interpret because of problems in determining whether streptolysin O is present in an active or inactive state and whether it may influence cellular responses by its action on cell membranes or receptor sites (Bernheimer, 1972).

Macrophage migration inhibition has been associated with fractions of streptococcal culture supernates (Seravalli and Taranta, 1974).

Among the cellular components of streptococci, cell membrane and cell wall fractions have been shown to result in migration inhibition of human peripheral blood leukocytes (Read *et al.*, 1974; Zabriskie *et al.*, 1970b), presumably by stimulation of sensitized lymphocytes to produce migration inhibitory factors. On the other hand, peptidoglycan from group A streptococcal cell walls apparently has the ability to inhibit macrophage migration directly without induction of a detectable migration inhibitory factor by lymphocytes (Heymer *et al.*, 1973).

M protein was one of the first antigens to be used in studies of transfer of delayed-type hypersensitivity in man (Lawrence, 1952). Purified preparations of M protein of different serological types often show cross-reactions in skin testing (Stollerman, 1972). Immunization of guinea pigs with partially purified M protein preparations produced delayed hypersensitivity (by skin tests and macrophage inhibition tests) which was relatively type specific but did show cross reactions (Beachey *et al.*, 1969; Pachman and Fox, 1970).

Further studies on the cellular immune response to streptococci are discussed in the section below on the pathogenesis of nonsuppurative complications.

8. Pathogenesis of Nonsuppurative Complications of Streptococcal Infection (Acute Rheumatic Fever and Acute Glomerulonephritis)

Since almost every group A streptococcal substance (antigenic or nonantigenic) and every kind of streptococcal immune response have at some time been considered important in the pathogenesis of nonsuppurative complications, a comprehensive coverage of this subject is impossible in this chapter.

For a more thorough treatment the reader is referred to several recent reviews (McCarty, 1972; Michael *et al.*, 1972; Stollerman, 1975b; Wannamaker and Kaplan, 1977; Read and Zabriskie, 1976). This section will mention only a few of the observations and hypotheses that have been made, with emphasis on theories that are currently popular and may involve immunological mechanisms.

Although there has been speculation about genetic factors in rheumatic fever for many years, no clear-cut genetic pattern has been detected (Taranta *et al.*, 1959; Stollerman, 1975a; Read and Zabriskie, 1976). Also, studies of HLA antigens in rheumatic subjects have so far failed to reveal any consistent association with a specific antigen or antigens, yet some of the findings in individual studies are intriguing (Falk *et al.*, 1973; Rean and Zabriskie, 1976). For example, the decreased frequency of HLA-B5 reported in one study (Read *et al.*, 1977) is attractive *vis à vis* the report that the absence of HLA-B5 is associated with a poor blastogenic response to a streptococcal antigen (Greenberg *et al.*, 1975a; see Section 7), suggesting a genetic disequilibrium between HLA-B5 and the immune response to this streptococcal antigen. Another study indicates that rheumatic patients may have fewer histocompatibility antigens than normal controls (Falk *et al.*, 1973), which as a result of possible linkage to *Ir* genes might be manifested as a decreased responsiveness to certain streptococcal antigens. A depressed immune response to a streptococcal antigen or blastogen could confer a survival advantage on streptococci (Taranta *et al.*, 1969), resulting in an increased exposure to streptococcal antigens with an ultimate break in tolerance manifested as rheumatic fever (Read and Zabriskie, 1976). Alternatively, it can be hypothesized that rheumatics have a double *Ir* gene dose, resulting in an exaggerated humoral or cellular response to streptococcal antigens (Read and Zabriskie, 1976). Studies of the *HLA-D* locus in rheumatics may help to clarify some of these possibilities since this locus is believed to be more closely linked to the *Ir* genes in man (Read *et al.*, 1977). The recent demonstration that a novel B-cell alloantigen is found at a significantly increased frequency among patients with rheumatic fever (Patarroyo *et al.*, 1979) gives new impetus to the concept that an immunogenetic factor is important in the pathogenesis of rheumatic fever.

In order for acute rheumatic fever to develop, the infecting agent must be a group A streptococcus, there must be an antibody response (probably as an indication of infection rather than a carrier state), and the infection must occur in the upper respiratory tract (Wannamaker, 1973). Moreover, clinical studies of the factors essential for the prevention of rheumatic fever by antibiotic treatment indicate that unless the living streptococcus is present in the throat for more than 10 days, rheumatic fever is not likely to occur (Catanzaro *et al.*, 1954). However, there are no convincing data of the occurrence of living group A streptococci at distant sites (e.g., hearts or joints) in rheumatic patients during life or at carefully performed postmortem examinations (Watson *et al.*, 1961). L forms of group A streptococci have been observed in experimental animals and in human impetigo (Mortimer *et al.*, 1972), but they have not been identified with certainty in throat cultures or in the tissues of rheumatic patients.

Streptococcal components or products with toxic properties that might initiate tissue damage include the two streptolysins, streptococcal proteinase, the pyrogenic exotoxins (erythrogenic toxins), and peptidoglycan. Streptolysin S has attracted attention because it is apparently nonantigenic and therefore would continue to be active during repeated streptococcal infections and in recurrences of rheumatic fever (MacLeod, 1959). Streptolysin O is a potent cardiotoxin (Halbert, 1970). The poor anti-streptolysin O response in patients with streptococcal impetigo, which apparently results from the binding of this toxin by cholesterol or related lipids in the skin, has been postulated to be linked with the failure of rheumatic fever to develop after infections at this site (Kaplan and Wannamaker, 1976). The pyrogenic exotoxins and streptococcal peptidoglycans exhibit many of the properties of endotoxins (Kim and Watson, 1972; Krause, 1972b). Both of these toxic substances, and also streptococcal proteinase, will produce myocardial necrosis in experimental animals. Cell wall complexes containing peptidoglycan and group A carbohydrate produce a chronic relapsing nodular lesion when injected into the skin of rabbits; the phenomenon is related to the persistence of cell wall material and does not appear to be immunological in nature (Ohanian and Schwab, 1967). After phagocytosis group A streptococcal cell walls persist in macrophages; such activated macrophages become cytotoxic (Smialowicz and Schwab, 1977a,b). It has been suggested that the persistence of such indigestible residues of group A streptococci in mononuclear phagocytes results in chronic selective release of acid hydrolases and thereby leads to inflammation and tissue damage (Morrison *et al.*, 1976). Evidence of selective release of lysosomal enzymes by macrophages exposed to group A streptococcal cell walls (containing peptidoglycan and group-specific carbohydrate) has been demonstrated *in vitro* (Page *et al.*, 1974; Davies *et al.*, 1974).

Increased levels of γ-globulin and of humoral antibodies to specific streptococcal antigens have been demonstrated in patients with streptococcal infection who develop rheumatic fever, as compared with those who do not (Anderson *et al.*, 1948). In rheumatics, higher antibody titers have been shown to a variety of streptococcal antigens including streptolysin O and streptokinase (Anderson *et al.*, 1948), hyaluronidase (Harris and Harris, 1949), M-associated protein (Widdowson *et al.*, 1971a,b), and streptococcal membrane-absorbable heart-reactive antibody (Zabriskie *et al.*, 1970a). However, the most extensive data relate to the anti-streptolysin O response, where the risk of both initial and recurrent attacks has been related to the magnitude of the antibody rise (Stetson, 1954; Taranta *et al.*, 1964). This exaggerated immune response to streptococcal antigens in rheumatic patients is not seen with nonstreptococcal antigens (Rammelkamp, 1957). There is also some recent evidence that a significantly higher humoral antibody response to streptococcal antigens may occur in patients who develop acute nephritis (Dillon and Avery Reeves, 1974).

Autoimmunity has been considered as a mechanism of possible importance in both rheumatic fever and acute nephritis. The possibility that autoimmunity involving humoral cross-reacting antibodies may play a role in the pathogenesis of rheumatic fever was suggested by studies of biopsies of auricular appendages from rheumatic patients revealing γ-globulin deposits in these tissues (Kaplan, 1960) and by subsequent studies demonstrating cross-reacting antigens in components of the group A streptococcal cell and various mammalian tissues, including heart and kidney.

A variety of cross-reactive antigens have been described (Ayoub, 1972). These include cross-reactivity (1) between streptococcal hyaluronate and human synovial fluid tissue (Sandson *et al.*, 1968), (2) between group A carbohydrate and the glycoprotein of heart valves (Goldstein *et al.*, 1967), (3) between a protein of the cell wall and the sarcolemma of cardiac and skeletal muscle (Kaplan, 1963), (4) between a protein of the cell membrane and the sarcolemma of cardiac and skeletal muscle (Zabriskie and Freimer, 1966), (5) between a component of the streptococcal cell membrane and human brain (Husby *et al.*, 1976; see following discussion), (6) between a glycoprotein of the streptococcal cell membrane and a glycoprotein of the glomerular basement membrane (Markowitz and Lange, 1964), and (7) between an antigen of the streptococcal cell membrane and skin (Rapaport *et al.*, 1966). The last cross-reaction is demonstrated by accelerated skin graft rejection in the guinea pig (see Section 4). It is of interest that all of these cross reactions show organ specificity.

The heart-reactive antibody that is absorbable with streptococcal membranes appears to be useful diagnostically. The level of this antibody tends to be sustained in rheumatic patients and can be correlated with the development of recurrences (Zabriskie *et al.*, 1970a). A possible relationship between the non-type-specific "M-associated" antibody and heart-reactive antibody has been postulated (Beachey and Stollerman, 1973).

The pathogenesis of Sydenham's chorea has long been obscure. Of interest are recent fluorescent microscopy studies indicating that IgG antibody from sera of patients with rheumatic chorea will react with neuronal cytoplasm of human caudate and subthalamic nuclei and that this antibody is removed by absorption with group A streptococcal membranes (Husby *et al.*, 1976).

The relationship of these multiple cross-reactive systems to the pathogenesis of rheumatic fever, although widely accepted, is still uncertain (Kaplan, 1976; Read and Zabriskie, 1976). There is no evidence that these antibodies damage cells, and there is no consumption of complement as would be expected for antibody-mediated cell lysis. It has been suggested that these antibodies complexed to cell antigens may stimulate sensitized lymphocytes to cytotoxic activity (Read and Zabriskie, 1976).

The possibility that cell-mediated responses

may play a role in nonsuppurative complications of streptococcal infections, particularly rheumatic fever, has been entertained, and there is some information available that tends to support such a hypothesis. Skin reactions as an index of delayed hypersensitivity to streptococcal products are generally more intense in rheumatic than in nonrheumatic subjects (Gibson *et al.*, 1933; Green, 1942). Some early studies also showed that streptococcal antigens produce specific cytotoxic and cellular inhibition effects on explanted host cells from rheumatic patients, as compared with nonrheumatic subjects (Möen, 1936). More recent studies of peripheral blood leukocytes have indicated that patients with acute rheumatic fever exhibit an exaggerated cellular reactivity (migration inhibition) to streptococcal antigens, especially the antigens of group A streptococcal membranes (Read *et al.*, 1974). Other studies have shown that peripheral blood leukocytes from patients with progressive glomerulonephritis of unknown etiology exhibit significant migration inhibition in the presence of streptococcal particulate antigens (including relatively clean preparations of streptococcal membranes) and also that lymphocytes from these patients exhibit enhanced thymidine incorporation after exposure to these particulate antigens (Zabriskie *et al.*, 1970b; Zabriskie, 1971). Patients in the early acute stages of rheumatic fever have demonstrated an increase in proportions and absolute numbers of peripheral blood lymphocytes bearing surface immunoglobulin, which has been interpreted as being compatible with a loss of suppressor T-cell function (Lueker *et al.*, 1975), a possibility also suggested by studies of the effects of the pyrogenic exotoxins on the immune response of experimental animals (see Section 6). Further recent studies (Williams *et al.*, 1977) indicate that, compared with normals, (1) patients with acute rheumatic carditis or chorea showed elevated proportions and numbers of active T-cell rosettes; (2) patients with acute glomerulonephritis showed elevation in cells bearing surface Ig and Fc receptors with diminished proportions of cells producing EAC rosettes; (3) patients in the acute phase of either rheumatic fever or nephritis showed elevation of streptococcal antigen-binding cells (apparently B cells) capable of forming rosettes with autologous cells

coated with group A streptococcal membranes. Careful comparative studies including patients with other disease states and patients in the acute and convalescent phases of uncomplicated streptococcal infections are needed to interpret the possible significance of these findings.

Cell-mediated autoimmunity is a possibility of current interest among students of the pathogenesis of rheumatic fever. Evidence against this hypothesis comes from a study indicating that the peripheral blood leukocytes from patients with acute rheumatic carditis do not exhibit an enhanced cellular immune response to allogeneic heart homogenates (McLaughlin *et al.*, 1972), but the absence of any response in healthy control persons, as would be expected from current concepts of histocompatibility (Hirschhorn *et al.*, 1963), makes this report difficult to interpret. A recently introduced animal model of cytotoxicity (Yang *et al.*, 1977) may facilitate further studies of this possibility. In this model, T lymphocytes from spleens of adult guinea pigs sensitized to group A streptococcal antigens were found to be cytotoxic for cultured fetal guinea pig heart cells. Immunofluorescent studies indicated the presence of antigenic determinants on the membranes of cultured myofibers that cross-reacted with group A streptococcal cellular antigens. Thus a cell-mediated autoimmune mechanism, involving cross-reacting antigens of the streptococcus and the host, appeared to be responsible for the cytotoxicity observed in this model.

Cellular and humoral tolerance to streptococcal membrane antigen has been induced in mice, which then show prolonged survival of heart tissue allografts (Ellis *et al.*, 1975). It has been postulated that rheumatic fever may result from a break in tolerance to cross-reactive antigens or to an enhanced humoral and cellular responsiveness to streptococcal antigens on the basis of a double *Ir* gene dose (see preceding discussion).

No altogether satisfactory model for acute rheumatic fever or rheumatic heart disease has been developed in experimental animals (Thomas, 1972). A rabbit model (Murphy and Swift, 1950; Murphy, 1960) involving repeated intradermal infections with different serological types of group A streptococci and resulting in focal inflammatory aggregates and sometimes myofiber necrosis comes closest to reproducing the cardiac lesions of the human disease, but pathologists have generally been concerned about the question of the resemblance of these lesions to those of rheumatic heart disease.

Current opinion and a good deal of evidence favor the concept that poststreptococcal acute glomerulonephritis is an antigen–antibody complex disease (Michael *et al.,* 1972). However, other possibilities (perhaps acting in conjunction with this mechanism) that need to be considered include a direct effect of a streptococcal toxin (Holm *et al.,* 1967), cross-reacting antigens (Markowitz *et al.,* 1960; Lange, 1969), and autoantibodies (Schwentker and Comploier, 1939; Cavelti and Cavelti, 1945; Humphrey, 1948; Middleton *et al.,* 1953).

Although a good experimental model for acute nephritis using live streptococci has been reported (Becker and Murphy, 1968), and some possible candidates for the responsible streptococcal factor have been described (Markowitz, 1969; Treser *et al.,* 1970), no evidence has emerged clearly relating the streptococcal aspects of human glomerulonephritis to the experimental model of immune complex glomerulonephritis, which is produced by the injection of a nonstreptococcal product, bovine serum albumin (Dixon, 1968). Although it now appears that a variety of infectious agents can result in a similar pathological picture in the kidney, the association of group A streptococci of a limited number of serological types with a high risk of developing this complication is impressive (Rammelkamp and Weaver, 1953; Dillon, 1972). It is of interest that the types producing nephritis after infection of the skin are different from those producing nephritis after infection of the throat (Wannamaker, 1970a). It is probably not the M protein *per se* that is implicated in the development of nephritis, but rather this antigen serves as a generally good marker for these strains. It has been proposed that "rheumatogenic" as well as "nephritogenic" strains exist (Stollerman, 1975a), but the evidence to date is less convincing for the existence of "rheumatogenic" strains. It seems likely that group A streptococci of many, probably most, serological types that produce clinical infection of the throat can be associated with the development of rheumatic fever.

9. Pathogenesis of Bacterial Endocarditis

Streptococci (commonly "viridans" species, less often enterococci) are frequent pathogens in patients with bacterial endocarditis. Recent studies have emphasized the role of adherence ("stickiness") in the initiation of infection and the possibility that the dextran often produced by endocarditis-associated species of streptococci may contribute to this phenomenon (leading article in *Lancet,* 1974; Elliott, 1973; Parker and Ball, 1976). In patients with endocarditis, the infected intravascular surfaces provide constant direct access of antigens to the bloodstream and ultimately to the immune system (Williams, 1977). This heavy antigenic load may produce immunological phenomena such as immune complex nephritis (Gutman *et al.,* 1972; Levy and Hong, 1973; Keslin *et al.,* 1973), rhematoid factors (Williams and Kunkel, 1962; Gutman *et al.,* 1972), and occasionally other autoantibodies, e.g., antinuclear antibodies (Bacon *et al.,* 1974).

10. Special Hosts

A person who has a well-documented history of rheumatic fever or Sydenham's chorea or who has rheumatic heart disease is a special host since he may have a high risk of developing a recurrence if he develops another streptococcal infection (Markowitz and Gordis, 1972; Stollerman, 1975a). Such patients should receive continuous antimicrobial prophylaxis for a period of years after their attack and perhaps indefinitely (Committee on Prevention of Rheumatic Fever and Bacterial Endocarditis of the American Heart Association, 1977a).

Patients with rheumatic valvular disease are prone to the development of bacterial endocarditis and may benefit from antibiotics given at the time of dental or surgical procedures (Committee on Prevention of Rheumatic Fever and Bacterial Endocarditis of the American Heart Association, 1977b).

Some reports indicate that patients with rubella and rubeola are susceptible to secondary streptococcal infection. Patients who develop streptococcal pneumonia usually have evidence of preceding influenza. A rare patient with varicella may develop gangrenous lesions in association with secondary streptococcal infection (Smith *et al.*, 1976).

Patients with classic agammaglobulinemia may be susceptible to streptococcal infection, whereas those with chronic granulomatous disease handle streptococcal infections well (see Section 5).

Group A streptococci can act as opportunistic organisms in compromised hosts, including patients with leukemia (Dudding *et al.*, 1969), solid tumors (Henkel *et al.*, 1970), or other malignancies or collagen diseases (Hable *et al.*, 1973), as well as in postsurgical patients and in patients with burns. In patients with burns who have received skin grafts, infections with this agent often lead to autograft rejection. Recently it has been recognized that infection with group B streptococci can also result in graft rejection (Smith *et al.*, 1973).

The newborn infant is peculiarly susceptible to infection with group B streptococci (see Section 11).

11. Group B Streptococcal Infections

Since group B streptococci have emerged, for reasons unknown, as prominent pathogens in neonatal sepsis (Howard and McCracken, 1974; Eickhoff, 1972; Anthony and Okada, 1977; Baker, 1977), interest has grown in the clinical presentation, epidemiology, and pathogenesis as well as the immunology of infections with these organisms.

Two different clinical entities have been recognized in human neonates and infants: (1) an early-onset, pulmonic and septicemic form, fulminating and often fatal, with an acute onset, most often within the first 48 hr of life, occasionally as late as 5–10 days, and (2) a late- or delayed-onset form, usually with a slower and more insidious beginning, in infants older than 10 days of age, with meningitis as a common feature and less often fatal in outcome (Franciosi *et al.*, 1973; Baker *et al.*, 1973). The early acute-onset form of infection is often associated with obstetrical complications, such as premature labor and prolonged rupture of membranes. Unusual clinical presentations during infancy include "asymptomatic" bacteremia and focal infections at other sites (Howard and McCracken, 1974;

Ferrieri *et al.*, 1977). Curiously, group B streptococcal infections are rare in children beyond infancy (Bayer *et al.*, 1976). Adult infections with group B streptococci may occur in young females in association with obstetrical or gynecological manipulations or in older adults with underlying disease, notably diabetes mellitus and genitourinary problems (Reinarz and Sanford, 1965; Duma *et al.*, 1969; Bayer *et al.*, 1976).

The epidemiology of group B streptococcal infections appears to be closely allied to its presence in the female genital tract (Anthony and Okada, 1977; Baker, 1977). This seems to be the primary reservoir of these organisms, although they can be found in throat cultures (Ferrieri and Blair, 1977), in rectal swabs (Badri *et al.*, 1977), and in uretheral cultures of adult males (Franciosi *et al.*, 1973; K. K. Christensen *et al.*, 1976), the last suggesting the possibility of venereal transmission, for which, however, there is no clear epidemiological support (Wallin and Forsgren, 1975; Baker *et al.*, 1977b). Both pregnant and nonpregnant women commonly harbor group B streptococci in their genital tract, usually without clinical evidence of infection. The frequency of carriage in the female genital tract varies widely in different reports, ranging from less than 5% to 25% as determined by a single culture taken during pregnancy or at delivery (Anthony and Okada, 1977). These differences may be due to variables in culture methods (e.g., use of selective or nonselective media) or to intrinsic differences in population groups (K. K. Christensen *et al.*, 1976). Conversion of culture status, from negative to positive or *vice versa*, is commonly observed on serial bacteriological studies, suggesting that carriage may be intermittent, that the culture sampling error may be great, or that new acquisitions may occur late in pregnancy (Ferrieri *et al.*, 1977). The risk of acquisition of group B streptococci is high (50% or greater) in infants born of colonized mothers (Baker and Barrett, 1973; Anthony and Okada, 1977; Ferrieri *et al.*, 1977), but despite the frequency of heavy contamination of infants, often at multiple sites (Ferrieri *et al.*, 1977), the risk of clinical disease in the contaminated or colonized infant is low, estimated at only one out of every 100 infants with group B streptococci isolated from surface or mucous membrane sites. The overall risk of serious infection at birth has been estimated at two or three per 1000 live births and the mortality rate at one per 1000 live births (Baker and Barrett, 1973; Franciosi et al., 1973). These rates may not be applicable to all population groups. The virtual concordance in the serological types of group B streptococci isolated from the maternal genital tract and from infants with early-onset disease strongly suggests that this form of infection is acquired in utero or during birth (Baker and Barrett, 1973; Aber et al., 1976). The mode of transmission in the delayed form is not certain; nosocomial spread is suggested by some studies (Aber et al., 1976; Paredes et al., 1977; Anthony and Okada, 1977).

Almost no information is available about the pathogenesis of group B streptococcal infections. In the contaminated or colonized infant, the isolation of the organism from various and often multiple orifices and skin sites, including the nares, ear canal, and umbilicus, makes determination of the portal of entry difficult. However, the frequency of respiratory distress and pneumonia in early-onset neonatal infections suggests that in this form of infection the organisms may gain entry through the respiratory tract (Wannamaker and Ferrieri, 1975). The occurrence of infection in newborns, in adult females in association with obstetrical or gynecological procedures or complications, and in older adults with disorders of the genitourinary tract or underlying disease indicates the importance of ill-defined host factors and of trauma in the development of clinical disease. The factors responsible for virulence in group B streptococci are not known, but immunological studies suggest that they may be related to the capsular antigens (see following discussion). It has been suggested that sialic acid, a major constituent of the polysaccharide capsules of group B streptococci, may be a virulence factor for invasion of neonatal meninges, but the presence of sialic acid in all types of group B streptococci does not explain the special propensity of type III organisms for invasion of this site (Baker and Kasper, 1976a,b).

Relatively few studies are available in animals or man on antibodies to specific extracellular products or cellular constituents of group B streptococci, despite the obvious contribution that such studies may make to understanding the epidemiology, pathogenesis, and resistance to infection. Antibodies have been demonstrated to CAMP factor (a factor released by group B streptococci that greatly enhances the hemolytic activity of a staphylococcal β-toxin) in sera from experimentally infected cows and in a few human sera (Brown et al., 1974). Antibodies to hippuricase, a characteristic enzyme of group B streptococci, located intracellularly (Ferrieri et al., 1973), have been occasionally found in adult patients with group B streptococcal infection (Ferrieri, personal communication). Studies currently in progress indicate that the extracellular nucleases of group B streptococci, which are multiple and immunologically distinct from those of group A streptococci, may produce neutralizing antibody in some mothers and infants (Ferrieri et al., 1975).

Present evidence supports the view that immunity against clinical disease due to group B streptococci is mediated by humoral antibody directed toward the carbohydrate and protein components of the capsule. Five serotypes of group B streptococci have been identified (Ia, Ib, Ic, II, and III), based on these components, some of which are shared by two serotypes (Wilkinson and Eagon, 1971; Lancefield et al., 1975; Baker, 1977). Antibody to the capsular antigens have been demonstrated in mouse protection tests, in opsonophagocytic tests, and by radioimmunoassay. A recent preliminary report suggests that the long-chain reaction, used for determination of type-specific antibody for group A streptococci (see above), can be adapted for assaying type-specific antibody for group B streptococci in rabbit and human sera (Stewardson-Krieger et al., 1977a).

Mouse protection studies indicate the occurrence of multiple protective antibodies developed in response to immunization of rabbits with a single strain of group B streptococcus. Specific rabbit antibodies directed toward either the polysaccharide or the protein antigens can be protective against infection of mice with strains containing these antigens (Lancefield et al., 1975). A summary of these protective antibodies in relationship to specific antigens and serological types of group B streptococci is presented in Table 3, reproduced with permission from the paper by Lancefield et al. (1975). The lack of a mouse-

TABLE 3.   Summary of the Occurrence of Multiple Mouse-Protective Antibodies against Group B Streptococci[a]

| Type designation | Mouse-protective antibodies against | | |
| | Polysaccharides[b] | | Antigenic protein determinants (Ibc) (cross-reactive) |
	Major antigens (specific)	Common polysaccharide determinant (Iabc) (cross-reactive)	
Type Ia	Ia	Present	Absent
Type Ib	Ib	Present	Present
Type Ic	Ia	Present	Present
Type II	II	Absent	—[c]
Type III	III[c]	Absent	—[c]

[a] Reproduced, with permission, from Lancefield et al. (1975).
[b] The group-specific cell wall polysaccharide does not give rise to protective antibodies.
[c] Mouse protection for these antigens not yet studied.

virulent type III strain has prevented studies of protective antibody against this type. Antibodies in rabbits directed against the group-specific carbohydrate of group B streptococci do not protect mice.

Opsonophagocytic studies with rabbit antisera have been performed by several investigators. In a system measuring radioactive uptake of killed streptococci by rabbit alveolar macrophages, heat-stable opsonins to various antigens of types Ia, Ib, and Ic (either type-specific or shared, carbohydrate or protein antigens) have been shown to be required for significant phagocytosis to occur (Anthony, 1976). Complement was not required in this assay system. To the contrary, in a different test system employing human polymorphonuclear leukocytes and rabbit immune serum, complement was required for optimal killing of group B streptococci (Baltimore et al., 1977). In this latter system, immune rabbit sera for all five serotypes of group B streptococci were opsonic in high titer for strains of homologous types. In concurrence with the mouse protective studies, cross-opsonization was found in strains of types with known shared antigens, but some crosses could not be explained by currently recognized shared antigens. Of special interest was the finding that one of ten type III strains examined was killed by polymorphonuclear leukocytes in the absence of either complement or antibody.

Some studies employing human sera in opsonophagocytic assays and mouse protection tests have been reported. In a pioneer report of killing of one strain of group B streptococcus by polymorphonuclear leukocytes, opsonic titers were reduced by heating of the serum, and titers in paired sera from mother and infant were similar (Dossett et al., 1969). Other early studies demonstrated that specific opsonins were required for phagocytosis of type Ia organisms and suggested that nonspecific opsonic factors for all of the other serotypes were present in most human and baboon sera (Klesius et al., 1973; Mathews et al., 1974). The existence of nonspecific opsonic factors in human sera was not confirmed in a subsequent study (Baltimore et al., 1977). The role of heat-labile and heat-stable factors in the phagocytosis of group B streptococci is not entirely clear. Some studies indicate the prevalence of heat-labile opsonins for certain serotypes, including type III, in human sera (Anthony et al., 1974; Ferrieri, personal communication). In another study employing type Ia organisms, opsonic activity was found to be partially dependent on heat-labile serum factors (Stewardson-Krieger et al., 1977b). This study compared the mouse protection test with the opsonophagocytic assay and found no discrepancies. Protective antibody was absent in four of seven cord sera in which the corresponding maternal sera all showed protective antibody, indicating that the presence of maternal antibody cannot always be relied on to provide protection to the human newborn. In this same study, pooled human γ-globulin protected mice from bacterial challenge with type Ia group B streptococci, suggesting that passive immunization of newborn infants might be effective in preventing neonatal infection. In another recent report (Hemming *et al.,* 1976), in which a chemiluminescence assay for phagocytosis was used, it was shown that maternal sera frequently contained type-specific opsonins in the IgG fraction, which crossed the placenta to appear in paired cord sera. In this study, the sera of septic newborns were found to lack opsonic activity against the infecting serotype, suggesting that infants at increased risk of developing infection can be identified by immunological studies (see following discussion).

The feasibility of employing a sensitive radioimmunoassay (by a double-label technique) for measuring antibodies specific for the five group B serotypes has been demonstrated with type-specific immune rabbit sera (Wilkinson and Jones, 1976). However, reported studies of human sera have so far used a single-label radioimmunoassay with a broadly reactive antigenic preparation from type III organisms, containing both type-specific and group-specific determinants (Baker and Kasper, 1976a; Baker *et al.,* 1977a). These studies have suggested the following: (1) low concentrations of antibody are present in the acute sera of patients who develop clinical disease; (2) infants with infections of the bones or joints and adult females with puerperal sepsis show striking rises in antibody concentration; (3) infants convalescent from sepsis or meningitis develop much lower levels of antibody; (4) paired maternal and cord sera show a good correlation in antibody concentration; (5) antibody concentrations in the sera of mothers harboring type III strains and whose newborn infants remain healthy are greater than those in sera from mothers whose babies develop serious disease with group B type III streptococci. Because of the nature of the antigenic preparation used, the significance of these last studies is uncertain, particularly with respect to their type specificity. The good correlation of antibody concentration in paired maternal–cord sera found in these studies is at variance with the studies of placental transfer of protective antibody against serotype Ia organisms (see preceding discussion). These intri-

guing observations made with a radioimmunoassay technique need to be confirmed by similar studies using purified type III antigens and purified antigens of other types.

No studies of cellular immune responses to group B streptococci have been reported in humans. Lymphocytes from hyperimmunized cows have shown a lack of response to cellular antigens of group B streptococci (Kelly, 1968).

12. Immunotherapy and Immunoprevention

Since the scarlet fever that is currently prevalent is quite mild and can be adequately treated with penicillin, antitoxin is no longer used. However, the control of group A and group B streptococcal infections by the use of antibiotics has not been completely satisfactory, so other approaches must be sought (Markowitz, 1970; Wannamaker, 1973; Anthony and Okada, 1977; Baker, 1977). For both group A and group B infections, there seems to be a need for a vaccine (discussion in Wannamaker and Matsen, 1972b; Stollerman, 1975c; Baker, 1977), and some progress toward this end has been made. Highly purified preparations of M protein have been prepared from a limited number of serological types of group A streptococci. On injection into skin-test-negative individuals these preparations may elicit both primary and secondary immune responses (Fox *et al.,* 1966, 1969). Protection against a challenge of streptococci of the same serological type has been demonstrated in adult volunteers immunized subcutaneously and also by aerosol spray (Fox *et al.,* 1973; Polly *et al.,* 1975). Local immunization seemed to prevent colonization as well as illness. Attempts to demonstrate type-specific antibody in nasal washings of immunized subjects produced equivocal results. Other current efforts are being directed toward obtaining an M protein preparation free of the non-type-specific moiety, by pepsin digestion or extraction (Cunningham and Beachey, 1974; Beachey *et al.,* 1974b).

Although these results are encouraging, many problems remain not only because of the multiplicity of serotypes but also because some M types are not very antigenic. Attempts to prepare purified M protein that is antigenic have also proved to be difficult. No serious toxic effects have been encountered so far with highly purified preparations, but careful screening has been carried out to eliminate those with a positive skin test reaction or a personal or family history or rheumatic fever or other evidence of clinical abnormalities. Another vaccination study, using a less highly purified preparation of M protein, reported the development of rheumatic fever in several immunized siblings of rheumatic fever patients when they developed a streptococcal infection at a later date (Massell *et al.,* 1969). Although heart-reactive antigens have not been identified in highly purified preparations (Fox and Grossman, 1969), there is still some concern about the possibility of such antigens in vaccine preparations. A new concern has stemmed from the recent observation that *S. mutans* also contains an antigen cross-reactive with heart tissue (Van de Rijn and Zabriskie, 1976), particularly disturbing at a time when there is growing interest in producing a vaccine for dental caries.

With respect to group B streptococcal infections, future studies might be directed toward the possible passive immunization of infants deficient in protective antibody by the use of human pooled or immune γ-globulin (Stewardson-Krieger *et al.,* 1977b). It has also been suggested that active immunization of mothers with antibody deficiency (see Section 11) might result in protection of their infants (Baker, 1977). Further studies are needed to determine whether immunization of adults with purified type-specific carbohydrate antigens will result in the development of protective antibody and whether this antibody will cross the placenta in sufficient amount to protect both premature anf full-term infants.

ACKNOWLEDGMENTS

The author is indebted to Dr. Roger Cole for identifying references pertinent to the evolution of streptococci and to Drs. Paul P. Cleary, Patricia Ferrieri, Tom Kindt, Horst Malke, and Paul G. Quie for reviewing parts of the manuscript. The author is a Career Investigator of the American Heart Association.

References

Aasted, B., 1974, Characterization of the antibody production in rabbits induced by streptococcal group A and C carbohydrate antigens. II. evidence that the appearance of an antibody response of restricted heterogeneity is accompanied by an anti-antibody production, *Scand. J. Immunol.* 3(5):553–558.

Aber, R. C., Allen, N., Howell, J. T., Wilkinson, H. W., and Facklam, R. R., 1976, Nosocomial transmission of group B streptococci, *Pediatrics* 58(3):346–353.

Adamson, C.-A., 1949, A bacteriological study of lymph nodes: Analysis of postmortem specimens with particular reference to clinical, serological and histo-pathological findings, *Acta Medica Scand. Suppl.* 227:27–52, 67–71, 83–90, 94–95.

Aly, R., Maibach, H. I., Shinefield, H. R., and Strauss, W. G., 1972, Survival of pathogenic microorganisms on human skin, *J. Invest. Dermatol.* 58(4):205–210.

Andersen, B. R., and Cone, R., 1974, Inhibition of human lymphocyte blast transformation by streptolysin O, *J. Lab. Clin. Med.* 84:241–248.

Andersen, B. R., and Van Epps, D. E., 1972, Suppression of chemotactic activity of human neutrophils by streptolysin O, *J. Infect. Dis.* 125(4):353–359.

Anderson, H. C., Kunkel, H. G., and McCarty, M., 1948, Quantitative antistreptokinase studies in patients infected with group A hemolytic streptococci: A comparison with serum antistreptolysin and gamma globulin levels with special reference to the occurrence of rheumatic fever, *J. Clin. Invest.* 27(4):425–434.

Andriushin, Y. N., 1969, Some investigations of the anatomical substantiation of the spread of infections from the tonsils and the pharynx to the heart, *Arkh. Anat.* 56:45–48.

Anthony, B. F., 1976, Immunity to the group B streptococci: Interaction of serum and macrophages with types Ia, Ib, and Ic, *J. Exp. Med.* 143:1186–1198.

Anthony, B. F., and Okada, D. M., 1977, The emergence of group B streptococci in infections of the newborn infant, *Annu. Rev. Med.* 28:355–369.

Anthony, B. F., Kaplan, E. L., Wannamaker, L. W., Briese, F. W., and Chapman, S. S., 1969, Attack rates of acute nephritis following type 49 streptococcal infection of the skin and of the respiratory tract, *J. Clin. Invest.* 48:1697–1704.

Anthony, B. F., Concepcion, N. F., Okada, D., and Hobel, C. J., 1974, Serum opsonins to group B streptococci, *Abstracts of the Interscience Conference on Antimicrobial Agents and Chemotherapy,* No. 253.

Anthony, B. F., Kaplan, E. L., Wannamaker, L. W., and Chapman, S. S., 1976, The dynamics of streptococcal infections in a defined population of children: Serotypes associated with skin and respiratory infections, *Am. J. Epidemiol.* 104:652–666.

Austrian, R., Buettger, C., and Dole, M., 1972, Problems in the classification and pathogenic role of alpha and nonhemolytic streptococci of the human respiratory tract, in: *Streptococci and Streptococcal Diseases: Recognition, Understanding, and Management* (L. W. Wannamaker and J. M. Matsen, eds.), pp. 355–370, Academic Press, New York.

Ayoub, E. M., 1972, Cross-reacting antibodies in the pathogenesis of rheumatic myocardial and valvular disease, in: *Streptococci and Streptococcal Diseases: Recognition, Understanding, and Management* (L. W. Wannamaker and J. M. Matsen, eds.), pp. 451–464, Academic Press, New York.

Ayoub, E. M., and Dudding, B. A., 1970, Streptococcal group A carbohydrate antibody in rheumatic and nonrheumatic bacterial endocarditis, *J. Lab. Clin. Med.* 76(2):322–332.

Ayoub, E. M., and McCarty, M., 1968, Intraphagocytic beta-*N*-acetylglucosaminidase: Properties of the enzyme and its activity on group A streptococcal carbohydrate in comparison with a soil bacillus enzyme, *J. Exp. Med.* 127:833–851.

Ayoub, E. M., and Wannamaker, L. W., 1962, Evaluation of the streptococcal desoxyribonuclease B and diphosphopyridine nucleotidase antibody tests in acute rheumatic fever and acute glomerulonephritis, *Pediatrics* 29(4):527–538.

Ayoub, E. M., and Wannamaker, L. W., 1966, Streptococcal antibody titers in Sydenham's chorea, *Pediatrics* 38:946–956.

Ayoub, E. M., and Wannamaker, L. W., 1967, The fate of group A streptococci following phagocytosis: *In vitro* phagocytic studies of isotope-labeled streptococci, *J. Immunol.* 99(6):1099–1105.

Ayoub, E. M., Taranta, A., and Bartley, T. D., 1974, Effect of valvular surgery on antibody to the group A streptococcal carbohydrate, *Circulation* 50:144–150.

Bacon, P. A., Davidson, C., and Smith, B., 1974, Antibodies to candida and autoantibodies in sub-acute bacterial endocarditis, *Q. J. Med.* 43:537–550.

Badri, M. S., Zawaneh, S., Cruz, A. C., Mantilla, G., Baer, H., Spellacy, W. N., and Ayoub, E. M., 1977, Rectal colonization with group B *Streptococcus*: Relation to vaginal colonization of pregnant women, *J. Infect. Dis.* 135(2):308–312.

Baker, C. J., 1977, Summary of the workshop on perinatal infections due to group B *Streptococcus, J. Infect. Dis.* 136(1):137–152.

Baker, C. J., and Barrett, F. F., 1973, Transmission of group B streptococci among parturient women and their neonates, *J. Pediatr.* 83(6):919–925.

Baker, C. J., and Kasper, D. L., 1976a, Correlation of maternal antibody deficiency with susceptibility to neonatal group B streptococcal infection, *N. Engl. J. Med.* 294:753–756.

Baker, C. J., and Kasper, D. L., 1976b, Microcapsule of type III strains of group B *Streptococcus*: Production and morphology, *Infect. Immun.* 13(1):189–194.

Baker, C. J., Barrett, F. F., Gordon, R. C., and Yow, M. D., 1973, Suppurative meningitis due to streptococci of

Lancefield group B: A study of 33 infants, *J. Pediatr.* 82(4):724–729.

Baker, C. J., Kasper, D. L., Tager, I. B., Paredes, A., Alpert, S., McCormack, W. M., and Goroff, D., 1977a, Quantitative determination of antibody to capsular polysaccharide in infection with type III strains of group B *Streptococcus, J. Clin. Invest.* 59:810–818.

Baker, C. J., Goroff, D. K., Alpert, S., Crockett, V. A., Zinner, S. H., Evrard, J. R., Rosner, B., and McCormack, W. M., 1977b, Vaginal colonization with group B *Streptococcus*: A study in college women, *J. Infect. Dis.* 135(3):392–397.

Baltimore, R. S., Kasper, D. L., Baker, C. J., and Goroff, D. K., 1977, Antigenic specificity of opsonophagocytic antibodies in rabbit antisera to group B streptococci, *J. Immunol.* 118(2):673–678.

Barksdale, L., 1964, Discussion of Dr. Zabriskie's paper, in: *The Streptococcus, Rheumatic Fever and Glomerulonephritis* (J. W. Uhr, ed.), pp. 70–82, Williams and Wilkins, Baltimore.

Barsumian, E. L., 1977, The role of hypersensitivity on the toxicity of streptococcal pyrogenic exotoxins, Ph. D. thesis, University of Minnesota (December).

Bassett, D. C. J., 1972, As quoted by Maxted, in: *Streptococci and Streptococcal Diseases: Recognition, Understanding, and Management* (L. W. Wannamaker and J. M. Matsen, eds.), pp. 349–351, Academic Press, New York.

Bayer, A. S., Chow, A. W., Anthony, B. F., and Guze, L. B., 1976, Serious infections in adults due to group B streptococci: Clinical and serotypic characterization, *Am. J. Med.* 61:498–503.

Beachey, E. H., and Cunningham, M., 1973, Type-specific inhibition of preopsonization versus immunoprecipitation by streptococcal M proteins, *Infect. Immun.* 8(1):19–24.

Beachey, E. H., and Ofek, I., 1976, Epithelial cell binding of group A streptococci by lipoteichoic acid on fimbriae denuded of M protein, *J. Exp. Med.* 143:759–771.

Beachey, E. H., and Stollerman, G. H., 1973, Mediation of cytotoxic effects of streptococcal M protein by non-type-specific antibody in human sera, *J. Clin. Invest.* 52(10):2563–2570.

Beachey, E. H., Alberti, H., and Stollerman, G. H., 1969, Delayed hypersensitivity to purified streptococcal M protein in guinea pigs and man, *J. Immunol.* 102:42–52.

Beachey, E. H., Ofek, I., Cunningham, M., and Bisno, A., 1974a, Evaluation of micro complement fixation tests for antibodies against group A streptococcal M and M-associated antigens in rabbit and human sera, *Appl. Microbiol.* 27(1):1–4.

Beachey, E. H., Campbell, G. L., and Ofek, I., 1974b, Peptic digestion of streptococcal M protein. II. Extraction of M antigen from group A streptococci with pepsin, *Infect. Immun.* 9(5):891–896.

Becker, C. G., and Murphy, G. F., 1968, The experimental induction of glomerulonephritis like that in man by infection with group A streptococci, *J. Exp. Med.* 127:1–23.

Belozersky, A. N., and Spirin, A. S., 1960, Chemistry of the nucleic acids of microorganisms, in: *The Nucleic Acids,* Vol. 3 (E. Chargaff and J. N. Davidson, eds.), pp. 147–185, Academic Press, New York.

Bergner-Rabinowitz, S., Ofek, I., Davies, M. A., and Rabinowitz, K., 1971, Type-specific streptococcal antibodies in pyodermal nephritis, *J. Infect. Dis.* 124(5):488–493.

Bergner-Rabinowitz, S., Fleiderman, S., Ferne, M., Rabinowitz, K., and Ginsburg, I., 1975, The new streptozyme test for streptococcal antibodies, *Clin. Pediatr.* 14(9):804–809.

Bernhard, G. C., and Stollerman, G. H., 1959, Serum inhibition of streptococcal diphosphopyridine nucleotidase in uncomplicated streptococcal pharyngitis and in rheumatic fever, *J. Clin. Invest.* 38:1942–1949.

Bernheimer, A. W., 1972, Hemolysins of streptococci: Characterization and effects on biological membranes, in: *Streptococci and Streptococcal Diseases: Recognition, Understanding, and Management* (L. W. Wannamaker and J. M. Matsen, eds.), pp. 19–31, Academic Press, New York.

Bernheimer, A. W., Lazarides, P. D., and Wilson, A. T., 1957, Diphosphopyridine nucleotidase as an extracellular product of streptococcal growth and its possible relation to leukotoxicity, *J. Exp. Med.* 106(1):27–37.

Bisno, A. L., and Nelson, K. E., 1974, Type-specific opsonic antibodies in streptococcal pyoderma, *Infect. Immun.* 10(6):1356–1361.

Bisno, A. L., and Ofek, I., 1974, Serologic diagnosis of streptococcal infection: Comparison of a rapid hemagglutination technique with conventional antibody tests, *Am. J. Dis. Child.* 127:676–681.

Bisno, A. L., and Stollerman, G. H., 1975, Streptococcal antibodies in the diagnosis of rheumatic fever, in: *Laboratory Diagnostic Procedures in the Rheumatic Diseases,* 2nd ed. (A. S. Cohen, ed.), pp. 207–263, Little, Brown, Boston.

Bisno, A. L., Nelson, K. E., Waytz, P., and Brunt, J., 1973, Factors influencing serum antibody responses in streptococcal pyoderma, *J. Lab. Clin. Med.* 81:410–420.

Bisno, A. L., Ofek, I., and Beachey, E. H., 1976, Antigens of group A streptococci involved in passive hemagglutination reactions, *Infect. Immun.* 13(2):407–412.

Biswas, G. D., and Ravin, A. W., 1971, Heterospecific transformation of pneumococcus and streptococcus. IV. Variations in hybrid DNA produced by recombination, *Mol. Gen. Genet.* 110:1–22.

Bokisch, V. A., Bernstein, D., and Krause, R. M., 1972, Occurrence of 19 S and 7 S anti-IgGs during hyperimmunization of rabbits with streptococci, *J. Exp. Med.* 36(1):799–815.

Bokisch, V. A., Chiao, J. W., and Bernstein, D., 1973, Isolation and immunochemical characterization of rabbit 7 S anti-IgG with restricted heterogeneity, *J. Exp. Med.* 137:1354–1368.

Bracco, R. M., Krauss, M. R., Roe, A. S., and MacLeod, C. M., 1957, Transformation reactions between pneumococcus and three strains of streptococci, *J. Exp. Med.* 106:247–258.

Braun, D. G., and Krause, R. M., 1968, The individual antigenic specificity of antibodies to streptococcal carbohydrates, *J. Exp. Med.* 128(2):969–989.

Braun, D. G., Kindred, B., and Jacobson, E. B., 1972, Streptococcal group A carbohydrate antibodies in mice: Evidence for strain differences in magnitude and restriction of the response, and for thymus dependence, *Eur. J. Immunol.* 2:138–143.

Braun, D. G., Kjems, E., and Cramer, M., 1973, A rabbit family of restricted high responders to the streptococcal group A-variant polysaccharide: Selective breeding narrows the isoelectric focusing spectra of dominant clones, *J. Exp. Med.* 138(3):645–658.

Brock, L. L., and Siegel, A. C., 1953, Studies on the prevention of rheumatic fever: The effect of time of initiation of treatment of streptococcal infections on the immune response of the host, *J. Clin. Invest.* 32(7):630–632.

Brown, J. H., 1946, in: *Bovine Mastitis* (R. B. Little and W. N. Plastridge, eds.), p. 417, McGraw-Hill, New York.

Brown, J., Farnsworth, R., Wannamaker, L. W., and Johnson, D. W., 1974, CAMP factor of group B streptococci: Production, assay, and neutralization by sera from immunized rabbits and experimentally infected cows, *Infect. Immun.* 9(2):377–383.

Bryans, J. T., and Moore, B. O., 1972, Group C streptococcal infections of the horse, in: *Streptococci and Streptococcal Diseases: Recognition, Understanding, and Management* (L. W. Wannamaker and J. M. Matsen, eds.), pp. 327–338, Academic Press, New York.

Capra, J. D., Berek, C., and Eichmann, K., 1976, Structural studies on induced antibodies with defined idiotypic specificities. III. *N*-terminal amino acid sequence of the heavy and light chains of mouse anti-streptococcal antibodies—A5A, S8, and S117, *J. Immunol.* 117(1):7–10.

Catanzaro, F. J., Stetson, C. A., Morris, A. J., Chamovitz, R., Rammelkamp, C. H., Jr., Stolzer, B. L., and Perry, W. D., 1954, The role of the streptococcus in the pathogenesis of rheumatic fever, *Am. J. Med.* 17(6):749–756.

Cavelti, P. A., and Cavelti, E. S., 1945, Studies on the pathogenesis of glomerulonephritis. III. Clinical and pathogenic aspects of the experimental glomerulonephritis produced in rats by means of autoantibodies to kidney, *Arch. Pathol.* 40:163–172.

Chamovitz, R., Rammelkamp, C. H., Jr., Wannamaker, L. W., and Denny, F. W., Jr., 1960, The effect of tonsillectomy on the incidence of streptococcal respiratory disease and its complications, *Pediatrics* 26(3):355–367.

Chase, R. M., Jr., and Rapaport, F. T., 1965, The bacterial induction of homograft sensitivity. I. Effects of sensitization with group A streptococci, *J. Exp. Med.* 122(4):721–732.

Chiao, J. W., Bokisch, V. A., Christian, C. L., and Krause, R. M., 1974, A rabbit IgG antigenic marker detected by 19S anti-IgG present in streptococcal antisera, *J. Immunol.* **112**(2):627–632.

Chopyk, R. L., Slechta, T., Gray, E. D., and Greenberg, L. J., 1976, Characterization of blastogenic factors isolated from streptococci for use as genetic probes, *Fed. Proc.* **35**:813.

Christensen, K. K., Ripa, T., Agrup, G., and Christensen, P., 1976, Group B streptococci in human urethral and cervical specimens, *Scand. J. Infect. Dis.* **8**:75–78.

Christensen, P., and Holm, S. E., 1976, Purification of immunoglobulin G Fc-reactive factor from *Streptococcus azgazardah, Acta Pathol. Microbiol. Scand. (Sect. C)* **84**:196–202.

Christensen, P., Johansson, B. G., and Kronvall, G., 1976, Interaction of streptococci with the Fc fragment of IgG, *Acta Pathol. Microbiol. Scand. (Sect. C)* **84**:73–76.

Cleary, P. P., Johnson, Z., and Wannamaker, L., 1975, Genetic instability of M protein and serum opacity factor of group A streptococci: Evidence suggesting extrachromosomal control, *Infect. Immun.* **12**(1):109–118.

Cleary, P. P., Wannamaker, L. W., Fisher, M., and Laible, N., 1977, Studies of the receptor for phage A25 in group A streptococci: The role of peptidoglycan in reversible adsorption, *J. Exp. Med.* **145**:578–593.

Clewell, D. B., and Franke, A. E., 1974, Characterization of a plasmid determining resistance to erythromycin, lincomycin and vernamycin B$_\alpha$ in a strain of *Streptococcus pyogenes, Antimicrob. Agents Chemother.* **5**(5):534–537.

Clewell, D. B., Yagi, Y., and Bauer, B., 1975, Plasmid-determined tetracycline resistance in *Streptococcus faecalis*: Evidence of gene amplification during growth in presence of tetracycline, *Proc. Natl. Acad. Sci. USA* **72**(5):1720–1724.

Cole, R. M., 1968, Informal discussion, in: *Current Research on Group A Streptococcus* (R. Caravano, ed.), pp. 78–79, Excerpta Medica, Paris.

Colman, G., 1969, Transformation of viridans-like streptococci, *J. Gen. Microbiol.* **57**:247–255.

Colman, G., and Williams, R. E. O., 1972, Taxonomy of some human viridans streptococci, in: *Streptococci and Streptococcal Diseases: Recognition, Understanding, and Management* (L. W. Wannamaker and J. M. Matsen, eds.), pp. 281–299, Academic Press, New York.

Colón, A. E., Cole, R. M., and Leonard, C. G., 1971, Lysis and lysogenization of groups A, C, and G streptococci by a transducing bacteriophage induced from a group G *Streptococcus, J. Virol.* **8**:103–110.

Colón, A. E., Cole, R. M., and Leonard, C. G., 1972, Intergroup lysis and transduction by streptococcal bacteriophages, *J. Virol.* **9**:551–553.

Committee on Prevention of Rheumatic Fever and Bacterial Endocarditis, American Heart Association, 1977a, Prevention of rheumatic fever, *Circulation* **55**:1.

Committee on Prevention of Rheumatic Fever and Bacterial Endocarditis, American Heart Association, 1977b, Prevention of bacterial endocarditis, *Circulation* **56**:139a.

Coykendall, A. L., 1970, Base composition of deoxyribonucleic acid isolated from cariogenic streptococci, *Arch. Oral Biol.* **15**:365–368.

Coykendall, A. L., 1974, Four types of *Streptococcus mutans* based on their genetic, antigenic and biochemical characteristics, *J. Gen. Microbiol.* **83**:327–338.

Coykendall, A. L., and Specht, P. A., 1975, DNA base sequence homologies among strains of *Streptococcus sanguis, J. Gen. Microbiol.* **91**:92–98.

Cramer, M., and Braun, D. G., 1975, Genetics of restricted antibodies to streptococcal group polysaccharides in mice. II. The *Ir-A-CHO* gene determines antibody levels, and regulatory genes influence the restriction of the response, *Eur. J. Immunol.* **5**(12):823–830.

Croft, S. M., Mortensen, R. F., and Gewurz, H., 1976, Binding of C-reactive protein to antigen-induced but not mitogen-induced T lymphoblasts, *Science* **193**:685–687.

Crowe, C. C., Sanders, W. E., Jr., and Longley, S., 1973, Bacterial interference. II. Role of the normal throat flora in prevention of colonization by group A *Streptococcus, J. Infect. Dis.* **128**:527–532.

Cunningham, M. W., and Beachey, E. H., 1974, Peptic digestion of streptococcal M protein. I. Effect of digestion at suboptimal pH upon the biological and immunochemical properties of purified M protein extracts, *Infect. Immun.* **9**(2):244–248.

Cushing, A. H., 1975, Relevance of hamster impetigo model to human impetigo, in: *Animal Models in Dermatology* (Maibach, ed.), pp. 273–278, Churchville Livingstone, New York.

Cushing, A. H., and Mortimer, E. A., Jr., 1970, A hamster model for streptococcal impetigo, *J. Infect. Dis.* **122**(3):224–226.

Daikos, G., and Weinstein, L., 1951, Streptococci bacteriostatic antibody in patients treated with penicillin, *Proc. Soc. Exp. Biol. Med.* **78**:160–163.

Dajani, A. S., and Wannamaker, L. W., 1970, Experimental infection of the skin in the hamster simulating human impetigo. I. Natural history of the infection, *J. Infect. Dis.* **122**:196–204.

Dajani, A. S., and Wannamaker, L. W., 1972, Experimental infection of the skin in the hamster simulating human impetigo. IV. Cellular responses after streptococcal and staphylococcal infections, *Infect. Immun.* **5**(6):942–946.

Dajani, A. S., Garcia, R. E., and Wolinsky, E., 1963, Etiology of cervical lymphadenitis in children. *N. Engl. J. Med.* **268**(24):1329–1333.

Dajani, A. S., Tom, M. C., and Law, D. J., 1976, Viridins, bacteriocins of alpha-hemolytic streptococci: Isolation, characterization and partial purification, *Antimicrob. Agents Chemother.* **9**(1):81–88.

Davies, P., Page, R. C., and Allison, A. C., 1974, Changes in cellular enzyme levels and extracellular release of lysosomal acid hydrolases in macrophages exposed to group A streptococcal cell wall substance, *J. Exp. Med.* **139**:1262–1282.

Davis, S. D., Iannetta, A., and Wedgwood, R. J., 1972, Bactericidal reactions of serum, in: *Biological Activities of Complement* (D. G. Ingram, ed.), pp. 43–55, Karger, Basel.

Deddish, P. A., and Ravin, A. W., 1974, Relation of macromolecular synthesis in streptococci to efficiency of transformation by markers of homospecific and heterospecific origin, *J. Bacteriol.* **117**(3):1158–1170.

Delespesse, G., Duchateau, J., Gaussett, Ph., and Govaerts, A., 1976, In vitro response of subpopulations of human tonsil lymphocytes. I. Cellular collaboration in the proliferative response to PHA and Con A, *J. Immunol.* **116**(2):437–445.

Denny, F. W., Jr., and Thomas, L., 1955, Persistence of group A streptococci in tissues of rabbits after infection, *Proc. Soc. Exp. Biol. Med.* **88**:260–263.

Denny, F. W., Jr., Perry, W. D., and Wannamaker, L. W., 1957, Type specific streptococcal antibody, *J. Clin. Invest.* **36**:1092–1100.

Dillon, H. C., 1972, Streptococcal infections of the skin and their complications: Impetigo and nephritis, in: *Streptococci and Streptococcal Diseases: Recognition, Understanding, and Management* (L. W. Wannamaker and J. M. Matsen, eds.), pp. 571–587, Academic Press, New York.

Dillon, H. C., Jr., and Avery-Reeves, M. S., 1974, Streptococcal immune responses in nephritis after skin infection, *Am. J. Med.* **56**:333–346.

Dillon, H. C., and Wannamaker, L. W., 1965, Physical and immunological differences among streptokinases, *J. Exp. Med.* **121**:351–371.

Dingle, J. H., 1954, The clinical pattern of streptococcal infection in man, in: *Streptococcal Infections* (M. McCarty, ed.), pp. 120–129, Columbia University Press, New York.

Dingle, J. H., Badger, G. F., and Jordan, W. S., Jr., 1964, Relation of tonsillectomy to incidence of certain illnesses in children, in: *Illness in the Home* (J. H. Dingle, G. F. Badger, and W. S. Jordan, Jr., eds.), pp. 118–128, The Press of Western Reserve University, Cleveland.

Dixon, F. J., 1968, Editorial: The pathogenesis of glomerulonephritis, *Am. J. Med.* **44**:493–498.

Dixon, J. M. S., and Lipinski, A. E., 1974, Infections with β-hemolytic *Streptococcus* resistant to lincomycin and erythromycin and observations on zonal-pattern resistance to lincomycin, *J. Infect. Dis.* **130**(4):351–356.

Dobrzański, W. T., 1972, Transformation among streptococci: Mechanisms and implications, in: *Streptococci and Streptococcal Diseases: Recognition, Understanding, and Management* (L. W. Wannamaker and J. M. Matsen, eds.), pp. 81–98, Academic Press, New York.

Dobrzański, W. T., Osowiecki, H., and Jagielski, M. A., 1968, Observations on intergeneric transformation between staphylococci and streptococci, *J. Gen. Microbiol.* **53**:187–196.

Dochez, A. R., Avery, O. T., and Lancefield, R. C., 1919, Studies on the biology of streptococcus. I. Antigenic relationships between strains of *Streptococcus haemolyticus*, *J. Exp. Med.* **30**(3):179–213.

Donaldson, D. M., 1973, β-Lysin and host resistance, in:

Non-specific Factors Influencing Host Resistance (W. Braun and J. Ungar, eds.), pp. 316–322, Karger, Basel.

Dossett, J. H., Williams, R. C., Jr., and Quie, P. G., 1969, Studies on interaction of bacteria, serum factors and polymorphonuclear leukocytes in mothers and newborns, *Pediatrics* **44**(1):49–57.

Drucker, D. B., and Holmes, C., 1974, Fatty acid profiles of streptococci of Lancefield groups A, B, C, D, E, F, G, H, K, O, P and Q, *Proc. Soc. Gen. Microbiol.* **2**(1):19–20.

Dudding, B. A., and Ayoub, E. M., 1968, Persistence of streptococcal group A antibody in patients with rheumatic valvular disease, *J. Exp. Med.* **128**(5):1081–1098.

Dudding, B., Humphrey, G. B., and Nesbit, M. E., 1969, Beta-hemolytic streptococcal septicemias in childhood leukemia, *Pediatrics* **43**:359–364.

Dudding, B. A., Burnett, J. W., Chapman, S. S., and Wannamaker, L. W., 1970, The role of normal skin in the spread of streptococcal pyoderma, *J. Hyg.* **68**:19–28.

Duma, R. J., Weinberg, A. N., Medrek, T. F., and Kunz, L. J., 1969, Streptococcal infections: A bacteriologic and clinical study of streptococcal bacteremia, *Medicine* **48**(2):87–127.

Duncan, W. C., McBride, M. E., and Knox, J. M., 1970, Experimental production of infections in humans, *J. Invest. Dermatol.* **54**:319–323.

Dunlap, M. B., and Harvey, H. S., 1967, The carrier state and type-specific immunity in streptococcal disease, *Am. J. Dis. Child.* **114**:229–243.

Dunny, G. M., and Clewell, D. B., 1975, Transmissible toxin (hemolysin) plasmid in *Streptococcus faecalis* and its mobilization of a non-infectious drug resistance plasmid, *J. Bacteriol.* **124**(2):784–790.

Edwards, E. A., 1964, Protocol for micro antistreptolysin O determinations, *J. Bacteriol.* **87**(5):1254–1255.

Eichmann, K., 1972, Idiotypic identity of antibodies to streptococcal carbohydrate in inbred mice, *Eur. J. Immunol.* **2**:301–307.

Eichmann, K., Braun, D. G., Feizi, T., and Krause, R. M., 1970, The emergence of antibodies with either identical or unrelated individual antigenic specificity during repeated immunizations with streptococcal vaccines, *J. Exp. Med.* **131**(2):1169–1188.

Eichmann, K., Braun, D. G., and Krause, R. M., 1971, Influence of genetic factors on the magnitude and the heterogeneity of the immune response in the rabbit, *J. Exp. Med.* **134**:48–65.

Eickhoff, T. C., 1972, Group B streptococci in human infection, in: *Streptococci and Streptococcal Diseases: Recognition, Understanding, and Management* (L. W. Wannamaker and J. M. Matsen, eds.), pp. 533–543, Academic Press, New York.

El Kholy, A., Sorour, A. H., Houser, H. B., Wannamaker, L. W., Robins, M., Poitras, J.-M., and Krause, R. M., 1973, A three-year prospective study of streptococcal infections in a population of rural Egyptian school children, *J. Med. Microbiol.* **6**:101–110.

El Kholy, A., Hafez, K., and Krause, R. M., 1974, Specificity and sensitivity of the streptozyme test for the detection of streptococcal antibodies, *Appl. Microbiol.* **27**(4):748–752.

Ellen, R. P., and Gibbons, R. J., 1972, M protein-associated adherence of *Streptococcus pyogenes* to epithelial surfaces: Prerequisite for virulence, *Infect. Immun.* **5**(5):826–830.

Elliott, S. D., 1973, The incidence of group-H streptococci in blood cultures from patients with subacute bacterial endocarditis (SBE), *J. Med. Microbiol.* **6**:Pxiv.

Elliott, S. D., Alexander, T. J. L., and Thomas, J. H., 1966, Streptococcal infection in young pigs. II. Epidemiology and experimental production of the disease, *J. Hyg.* **64**:213–220.

Elliott, S. D., Hayward, J., and Liu, T. Y., 1971, The presence of a group A variant-like antigen in streptococci of other groups with special reference to group N, *J. Exp. Med.* **133**(3):479–493.

Ellis, R. J., Ebert, P. A., McCarty, M., and Zabriskie, J. B., 1975, Prolongation of myocardial tissue allografts by pretreatment with streptococcal membrane, *Transplant. Proc.* **7**(1):355–359 (Suppl. 1).

Engel, H. W. B., van Embden, J. D. A., van Klingeren, B., and Soedirman, N., 1979, Transferable drug resistance in group-A, -B, and -D, streptococci, in: *Pathogenic Streptococci* (M. T. Parker, ed.), pps. 282–283, Reedbooks, Ltd., Chertsey, Surrey.

Erwa, H. H., Maxted, W. R., and Brighton, W. D., 1969, A latex agglutination test for the measurement of antibodies to group-specific streptococcal polysaccharides, *Clin. Exp. Immunol.* **4**:311–321.

Falk, J. A., Fleischman, J. L., Zabriskie, J. B., and Falk, R. E., 1973, A study of HL-A antigen phenotype in rheumatic fever and rheumatic heart disease patients, *Tissue Antigens* **3**:173–178.

Feinstein, A. R., and Levitt, M., 1970, The role of tonsils in predisposing to streptococcal infections and recurrences of rheumatic fever, *N. Engl. J. Med.* **282**(6):285–291.

Ferrieri, P., and Blair, L. L., 1977, Pharyngeal carriage of group B streptococci: Detection by three methods, *J. Clin. Microbiol.* **6**(2):136–139.

Ferrieri, P., Danjani, A. S., Wannamaker, L. W., and Chapman, S. S., 1972, Natural history of impetigo. I. Site sequence of acquisition and familial patterns of spread of cutaneous streptococci, *J. Clin. Invest.* **51**:2851–2862.

Ferrieri, P., Wannamaker, L. W., and Nelson, J., 1973, Localization and characterization of the hippuricase activity of group B streptococci, *Infect. Immun.* **7**:747–752.

Ferrieri, P., Gray, E. D., and Wannamaker, L. W., 1975, Group B streptococcal nucleases: Further biochemical and immunological characterization, *Abstracts of the Annual Meeting of the American Society for Microbiology*, p. 19.

Ferrieri, P., Cleary, P. P., and Seeds, A. E., 1977, Epidemiology of group-B streptococcal carriage of pregnant women and newborn infants, *J. Med. Microbiol.* **10**:103–114.

Fischetti, V. A., Gotschlich, E. C., Siviglia, G., and Zabriskie, J. B., 1976, Streptococcal M protein extracted by nonionic detergent. I. Properties of the antiphagocytic and type-specific molecules, *J. Exp. Med.* **144**:32–53.

Foley, S. M. J., and Wood, W. B., Jr., 1959, Studies on the pathogenicity of group A streptococci. II. The antiphagocytic effects of the M protein and the capsular gel, *J. Exp. Med.* **110**(4):617–628.

Foley, S. M. J., Smith, M. R., and Wood, W. B., Jr., 1959, Studies on the pathogenicity of group A streptococci. I. Its relation to surface phagocytosis, *J. Exp. Med.* **110**(4):603–616.

Fox, E. N., and Grossman, B. J., 1969, Antigenicity of the M proteins of group A hemolytic streptococci. V. The absence of antigenic determinants common to mammalian heart muscle, *J. Immunol.* **102**(4):970–974.

Fox, E. N., Wittner, M. K., and Dorfman, A., 1966, Antigenicity of the M proteins of group A hemolytic streptococci. III. Antibody responses and cutaneous hypersensitivity in humans, *J. Exp. Med.* **124**(6):1135–1151.

Fox, E. N., Pachman, L. M., Wittner, M. K., and Dorfman, A., 1969, Primary immunization of infants and children with group A streptococcal M protein, *J. Infect. Dis.* **120**(5):598–604.

Fox, E. N., Waldman, R. H., Wittner, M. K., Mauceri, A. A., and Dorfman, A., 1973, Protective study with a group A streptococcal M protein vaccine: Infectivity challenge of human volunteers, *J. Clin. Invest.* **52**:1885–1892.

Franciosi, R. A., Knostman, J. D., and Zimmerman, R. A., 1973, Group B streptococcal neonatal and infant infections, *J. Pediatr.* **82**(4):707–718.

Francis, T. C., and Oppenheim, J. J., 1970, Impaired lymphocyte stimulation by some streptococcal antigens in patients with recurrent aphthous stomatitis and rheumatic heart disease, *Clin. Exp. Immunol.* **6**:573–586.

Francis, T. C., Oppenheim, J. J., and Barile, M. F., 1969, Lymphocyte transformation by streptococcal antigens in guinea pigs and man, in: *Proceedings of the Third Annual Leucocyte Conference* (W. O. Rieke, ed.), pp. 501–518, Appleton-Century-Crofts, New York.

Fredericq, P., 1946, Sur la sensibilité et l'activité antibiotiques des staphylocoques, *C. R. Soc. Biol. Ses Fil.* **140**:1167–1170.

Friou, G. J., 1949, Further observations of an inhibitor in human serums of the hyaluronidase produced by a strain of hemolytic streptococcus, *J. Infect. Dis.* **84**:240–251.

Frøland, S. S., and Natvig, J. B., 1973, Identification of three different human lymphocyte populations by surface markers, *Transplant. Rev.* **16**:114–162.

Gibbons, R. J., and van Houte, J., 1971, Selective bacterial adherence to oral epithelial surfaces and its role as an ecological determinant, *Infect. Immun.* **3**(4):567–573.

Gibson, H. J., Thomson, W. A. R., and Stewart, D., 1933,

The haemolytic streptococcus as a factor in the causation of acute rheumatism, *Arch. Dis. Child.* **8**:57–72.

Ginsburg, I., 1972, Mechanisms of cell and tissue injury induced by group A streptococci: Relation to poststreptococcal sequelae, *J. Infect. Dis.* **126**(3):294–456.

Ginsburg, I., 1974, The localization, translocation, persistence and degradation of group A streptococci in tissues: Relation to poststreptococcal sequelae, in: *Streptococcal Disease and the Community* (M. J. Haverkorn and H. Valkenburg, eds.), pp. 73–83, Excerpta Medica, Amsterdam.

Ginsburg, I., and Sela, M. N., 1976, The role of leukocytes and their hydrolases in the persistence, degradation, and transport of bacterial constituents in tissues: Relation to chronic inflammatory processes in staphylococcal, streptococcal, and mycobacterial infections and in chronic periodontal disease, *CRC Crit. Rev. Microbiol.*, pp. 249–332.

Ginsburg, I., Neeman, N., Gallily, R., and Lahav, M., 1976, Degradation and survival of bacteria in sites of allergic inflammation, in: *Infection and Immunology in the Rheumatic Diseases* (D. C. Dumonde, ed.), pp. 43–59, Blackwell Scientific, Oxford.

Glick, A. D., Getnick, R. A., and Cole, R. M., 1971, Electron microscopy of group A streptococci after phagocytosis by human monocytes, *Infect. Immun.* **4**(6):772–779.

Godrick, E. A., and Patt, G. R., 1971, A comparison of the immune response of tonsils with the appendix and spleen in neonatal rabbits, *Acta Otolaryngol.* **71**:357–364.

Goedvolk-De Groot, L. E., Michel-Bensink, N., Van Es-Boon, M. M., Van Vonno, A. H., and Michel, M. F., 1974, Comparison of the titres of ASO, anti-DNase B, and antibodies against the group polysaccharide of group A streptococci in children with streptococcal infections, *J. Clin. Pathol.* **27**:891–896.

Goldstein, I., and Caravano, R., 1967, Determination of anti-group A streptococcal polysaccharide antibodies in human sera by an hemagglutination technique, *Proc. Soc. Exp. Biol. Med.* **124**:1209–1212.

Goldstein, I., Halpern, B., and Robert, L., 1967, Immunological relationship between streptococcus A polysaccharide and the structural glycoproteins of heart valve, *Nature (London)* **213**:44–47.

Good, R. A., 1952, Acute-phase reactions in rheumatic fever, in: *Rheumatic Fever* (L. Thomas, ed.), pp. 115–135, University of Minnesota Press, Minneapolis.

Gotoff, S. P., Lolekha, S., Lopata, M. Kopp, J., Kopp, R. L., and Malecki, T. J., 1973, A macrophage aggregation assay for cell-mediated immunity in man: Studies of patients with Hodgkin's disease and sarcoidosis, *J. Lab. Clin. Med.* **82**:682–691.

Green, C. A., 1942, Haemolytic streptococcal infections and acute rheumatism, *Ann. Rheum. Dis.* **3**:4–41.

Greenberg, L. J., Gray, E. D., and Yunis, E. J., 1975a, Association between immune responsiveness *in vitro* to streptococcal antigens and histocompatibility determinants, *Fed. Proc.* **34**:980.

Greenberg, L. J., Gray, E. D., and Yunis, E. J., 1975b, Association of HL-A 5 and immune responsiveness *in vitro* to streptococcal antigens, *J. Exp. Med.* **141**(5):935–943.

Gutman, R. A., Striker, G. E., Gilliland, B. C., and Cutler, R. E., 1972, The immune complex glomerulonephritis of bacterial endocarditis, *Medicine* **51**:1–25.

Hable, K. A., Horstmeier, C., Wold, A. D., and Washington, J. A., 1973, Group A β-hemolytic streptococcemia: Bacteriologic and clinical study of 44 cases, *Mayo Clinic Proc.* **48**:336–339.

Halbert, S. P., 1958, The use of precipitin analysis in agar for the study of human streptococcal infections. III. The purification of some of the antigens detected by these methods, *J. Exp. Med.* **108**(3):385–410.

Halbert, S. P., 1970, Streptolysin O, in: *Microbial Toxins,* Vol. III, (T. C. Montie, S. Kadis, and S. J. Ajl, eds.), pp. 69–98, Academic Press, New York.

Hanna, E. E., and Hale, M., 1975, Deregulation of mouse antibody-forming cells *in vivo* and in cell culture by streptococcal pyrogenic exotoxin, *Infect. Immun.* **11**(2):265–272.

Hanna, E. E., and Watson, D. W., 1968, Host–parasite relationships among group A streptococci. IV. Suppression of antibody response by streptococcal pyrogenic exotoxin, *J. Bacteriol.* **95**(1):14–21.

Hanna, E. E., and Watson, D. W., 1973, Enhanced immune response after immunosuppression by streptococcal pyrogenic exotoxin, *Infect. Immun.* **7**(6):1009–1011.

Harris, T. N., and Harris, S., 1949, Studies in the relation of the hemolytic streptococcus to rheumatic fever. V. Streptococcal antihyaluronidase (mucin-clot-prevention) titers in the sera of patients with rheumatic fever, streptococcal infection and others, *Am. J. Med. Sci.* **217**:174–186.

Hemming, V. G., Hall, R. T., Rhodes, P. G., Shigeoka, A. O., and Hill, H. R., 1976, Assessment of group B streptococcal opsonins in human and rabbit serum by neutrophil chemiluminescence, *J. Clin. Invest.* **58**:1379–1387.

Henkel, J. S., Armstrong, D., Blevins, A., and Moody, M. D., 1970, Group A β-hemolytic *Streptococcus* bacteremia in a cancer hospital, *J. Am. Med. Assoc.* **211**:983–986.

Heymer, B., 1975, Biological properties of the peptidoglycan, *Z. Immun. Forsch. Bd.* **149**:245–257.

Heymer, B., Bültmann, B., Schachenmayr, W., Spanel, R., Haferkamp, O., and Schmidt, W. C., 1973, Migration inhibition of rat peritoneal cells induced by streptococcal mucopeptides: Characteristics of the reaction and properties of the mucopeptide preparations, *J. Immunol.* **116**(6):1743–1754.

Heymer, B., Schleifer, K.-H., Read, S., Zabriskie, J. B., and Krause, R. M., 1976, Detection of antibodies to bacterial cell wall peptidoglycan in human sera, *J. Immunol.* **117**(1):23–26.

Hill, H. R., Caldwell, G. G., Wilson, E., Hager, D., and

Zimmerman, R. A., 1969, Epidemic of pharyngitis due to streptococci of Lancefield group G, *Lancet* **2**:371–374.

Hill, H. R., Kaplan, E. L., Dajani, A. S., Wannamaker, L. W., and Quie, P. G., 1974, Leukotactic activity and reduction of nitroblue tetrazolium by neutrophil granulocytes from patients with streptococcal skin infection, *J. Infect. Dis.* **129**(3):322–326.

Hirata, A. A., and Terasaki, P. I., 1970, Cross-reactions between streptococcal M proteins and human transplantation antigens, *Science* **168**:1095–1096.

Hirsch, J. G., and Church, A. B., 1960, Studies of phagocytosis of group A streptococci by polymorphonuclear leucocytes *in vitro, J. Exp. Med.* **111**(3):309–322.

Hirschhorn, K., Bach, F., Kolodny, R. L., Firschein, I. L., and Hashem, N., 1963, Immune response and mitosis of human peripheral blood lymphocytes *in vitro, Science* **142**:1185–1187.

Hirschhorn, K., Schreibman, R. R., Verbo, S., and Gruskin, R. H., 1964, The action of streptolysin S on peripheral lymphocytes of normal subjects and patients with acute rheumatic fever, *Proc. Natl. Acad. Sci. USA* **52**:1151–1157.

Hoffmann, M. K., Schmidt, D., and Oettgen, H. F., 1973, Production of antibody to sheep red blood cells by human tonsil cells *in vitro, Nature (London)* **243**:408–410.

Holm, S. E., Jönsson, J., and Zettergren, L., 1967, Experimental streptococcal nephritis in rabbits, *Acta Pathol. Microbiol. Scand.* **69**:417–430.

Holmes, M. C., Williams, R. E. O., Bloom, C. V., Hirsch, A., Lermit, A., and Woods, E., 1958, Streptococcal infections among children in a residential home. III. Some factors influencing susceptibility to infection, *J. Hyg.* **56**(2):197–210.

Holton, J. B., and Schwab, J. H., 1966, Adjuvant properties of bacterial cell wall mucopeptides, *J. Immunol.* **96**(1):134–138.

Howard, J. B., and McCracken, G. H., Jr., 1974, The spectrum of group B streptococcal infections in infancy, *Am. J. Dis. Child.* **128**:815–818.

Humphrey, J. H., 1948, The pathogenesis of glomerulonephritis: A reinvestigation of the auto-immunization hypothesis. *J. Pathol. Bacteriol.* **60**:211–218.

Husby, G., Van de Rijn, I., Zabriskie, J. B., Abdin, Z. H., and Williams, R. C., Jr., 1976, Antibodies reacting with cytoplasm of subthalamic and caudate nuclei neurons in chorea and acute rheumatic fever, *J. Exp. Med.* **144**:1094–1110.

Ingram, G. B. P., and Hughes, J. E. P., 1972, A modified rapid slide test for anti-streptolysin O, *J. Clin. Pathol.* **25**:543–544.

Iontova, I. M., and Totolian, A. A., 1975, Lipoproteinase of group A streptococci and the antibodies in human sera, *Zentralbl. Bakteriol. Parasitenk. Infektionshr. Hyg. Abt. 1:Orig. Reihe A* **233**:452–463.

Jacob, A. E., and Hobbs, S. J., 1974, Conjugal transfer of plasmid-borne multiple antibiotic resistance in *Streptococcus faecalis* var. *zymogenes, J. Bacteriol.* **117**(2):360–372.

Jamieson, S., 1950, Recent investigations into certain diseases of sheep, *Vet. Rec.* **62**:772–774.

Janeff, J., Janeff, D., Taranta, A., and Cohen, H., 1971, A screening test for streptococcal antibodies, *Lab. Med.* **2**:38–40.

Jones, A. S., and Walker, R. T., 1968, The isolation of nucleic acids from gram-positive bacteria, *Arch. Biochem. Biophys.* **128**:579–582.

Kaplan, E. L., and Wannamaker, L. W., 1975, Dynamics of the immune response in rabbits immunized with streptococcal extracellular antigens: Comparison of the streptozyme agglutination test with three specific neutralization tests, *J. Lab. Clin. Med.* **86**(1):91–99.

Kaplan, E. L., and Wannamaker, L. W., 1976, Suppression of the antistreptolysin O response by cholesterol and by lipid extracts of rabbit skin, *J. Exp. Med.* **144**:754–767.

Kaplan, E. L., and Wannamaker, L. W., 1977, C-reactive protein in streptococcal pharyngitis, *Pediatrics* **60**:28–32.

Kaplan, E. L., Laxdal, T., and Quie, P. G., 1968, Studies of polymorphonuclear leukocytes from patients with chronic granulomatous disease of childhood: Bactericidal capacity for streptococci, *Pediatrics* **41**(3):591–599.

Kaplan, E. L., Anthony, B. F., Chapman, S. S., Ayoub, E. M., and Wannamaker, L. W., 1970, The influence of the site of infection on the immune response to group A streptococci, *J. Clin. Invest.* **49**:1405–1414.

Kaplan, E. L., Top, F. H., Jr., Dudding, B. A., and Wannamaker, L. W., 1971, Diagnosis of streptococcal pharyngitis: Differentiation of active infection from the carrier state in the symptomatic child, *J. Infect. Dis.* **123**(5):490–501.

Kaplan, E. L., Ferrieri, P., and Wannamaker, L. W., 1974, Comparison of the antibody response to streptococcal cellular and extracellular antigens in acute pharyngitis, *J. Pediatr.* **84**(1):21–28.

Kaplan, E. L., Ferrieri, P., and Wannamaker, L. W., 1975, Streptococcal cellular and extracellular antibodies in rheumatic fever (RF) and rheumatic heart disease (RHD), *Circulation* **52**(4):II–45.

Kaplan, M. H., 1946 (with The Commission on Acute Respiratory Diseases), Studies of streptococcal fibrinolysis. III. A quantitative method for the estimation of serum antifibrinolysin, *J. Clin. Invest.* **25**:347–351.

Kaplan, M. H., 1960, The concept of autoantibodies in rheumatic fever and in the postcommissurotomy state, *Ann. N.Y. Acad. Sci.* **86**:974–990.

Kaplan, M. H., 1963, Immunologic relation of streptococci and tissue antigen. I. Properties of an antigen in certain strains of group A streptococci exhibiting an immunologic cross-reaction with human heart tissue, *J. Immunol.* **90**:595–606.

Kaplan, M. H., 1976, Cross reactions of group A streptococci with heart tissue antigens: Implications for pathogenetic mechanisms in rheumatic fever, in: *Immunologic Aspects of Dental Caries* (W. H. Bowen, R. J. Genco, and T. C. O'Brien, eds.), pp. 171–176, Information Retrieval, Inc., Washington, D.C.

Karakawa, W. W., Osterland, C. K., and Krause, R. M., 1965, Detection of streptococcal group-specific antibodies in human sera, *J. Exp. Med.* **122**(2):195–205.

Keiser, H., Kushner, I., and Kaplan, M. H., 1971, "Nonspecific" stimulation of lymphocyte transformation by cellular fractions and acid extracts of group A streptococci, *J. Immunol.* **106**:1593–1601.

Kelly, R. H., 1968, *In vitro* response of the bovine peripheral lymphocyte to simulation with cellular antigens of group B streptococcus and phytohaemagglutinin, *Immunology* **14**:175–180.

Keslin, M. H., Messner, R. P., and Williams, R. C., Jr., 1973, Glomerulonephritis with subacute bacterial endocarditis, *Arch. Intern. Med.* **132**:578–581.

Kilbourne, E. D., and Loge, J. P., 1948, The comparative effects of continuous and intermittent penicillin therapy on the formation of antistreptolysin in hemolytic streptococcal pharyngitis, *J. Clin. Invest.* **27**(4):418–424.

Killander, J., and Philipson, L., 1964, Separation of rheumatoid factors and antistreptolysins by gel filtration and preparative electrophoresis, *Acta Pathol. Microbiol. Scand.* **61**:127–140.

Killander, J., Philipson, L., and Winblad, S., 1965, Studies on non-specific antistreptolysin O titre. 2. Comparison of specific and non-specific antistreptolysins by gel filtration and dextran sulphate precipitation, *Acta Pathol. Microbiol. Scand.* **65**:587–596.

Kim, Y. B., and Watson, D. W., 1972, Streptococcal exotoxins: Biological and pathological properties, in: *Streptococci and Streptococcal Diseases: Recognition, Understanding, and Management* (L. W. Wannamaker and J. M. Matsen, eds.), pp. 33–50, Academic Press, New York.

Kindt, T. J., Todd, C. W. Eichmann, K., and Krause, R. M., 1970, Allotype exclusion in uniform rabbit antibody to streptococcal carbohydrate, *J. Exp. Med.* **131**(1):343–354.

Kjems, E., 1958, Studies on streptococcal bacteriophages. 3. Hyaluronidase produced by the streptococcal phage–host cell system, *Acta Pathol. Microbiol. Scand.* **44**:429–439.

Klebanoff, S. J., 1975, Antimicrobial mechanisms in neutrophilic polymorphonuclear leukocytes, *Semin. Hematol.* **12**(2):117–142.

Klein, G. C., and Jones, W. L., 1971, Comparison of the streptozyme test with the antistreptolysin O, antideoxyribonuclease B, and antihyaluronidase tests, *Appl. Microbiol.* **21**(2):257–259.

Klein, G. C., Moody, M. D., Baker, C. N., and Addison, B. V., 1968, Micro antistreptolysin O test, *Appl. Microbiol.* **16**(1):184.

Klein, G. C., Baker, C. N., and Moody, M. D., 1970, Comparison of antistreptolysin O latex screening test with the antistreptolysin O hemolytic test, *Appl. Microbiol.* **19**(1):60–61.

Klesius, P. H., Zimmerman, R. A., Mathews, J. H., and Krushak, D. H., 1973, Cellular and humoral immune response to group B streptococci, *J. Pediatr.* **83**(6):926–932.

Klesius, P. H., Zimmerman, R. A., Mathews, J. H., and Auernheimer, A. H., 1974, Human antibody response to group A streptococcal teichoic acid, *Can. J. Microbiol.* **20**(6):853–859.

Köhler, W., and Dietel, K., 1968, Antistreptolysin O in Muttermilch, *Z. Immunitaetsforsch.* **136**:347–350.

Krause, R. M., 1963, Symposium on relationship of structure of microorganisms to their immunological properties. IV. Antigenic and biochemical composition of hemolytic streptococcal cell walls, *Bacteriol. Rev.* **27**(4):369–380.

Krause, R. M., 1970, The search for antibodies with molecular uniformity, in: *Advances in Immunology*, Vol. 12 (F. J. Dixon, Jr., and H. G. Kunkel, eds.), pp. 1–56, Academic Press, New York.

Krause, R. M., 1972a, The antigens of group D streptococci, in: *Streptococci and Streptococcal Diseases: Recognition, Understanding, and Management* (L. W. Wannamaker and J. M. Matsen, eds.), pp. 67–74, Academic Press, New York.

Krause, R. M., 1972b, The streptococcal cell: Relationship of structure to function and pathogenesis, in: *Streptococci and Streptococcal Diseases: Recognition, Understanding, and Management* (L. W. Wannamaker and J. M. Matsen, eds.), pp. 3–18, Academic Press, New York.

Krause, R. M., 1977, Symposium on the current status and prospects for improved and new bacterial vaccines: Welcome and introduction, *J. Infect. Dis. Suppl.* **136**:S8–S12.

Krause, R. M., and Kindt, T. J., 1977, Antibodies with molecular uniformity, in: *Plasma Proteins*, 2nd ed., Vol. 3 (F. W. Putnam, ed.), pp. 285–332, Academic Press, New York.

Krause, R. M., Rammelkamp, C. H., Jr., Denny, F. W., Jr., and Wannamaker L. W., 1962, Studies of the carrier state following infection with group A streptococci. I. Effect of climate, *J. Clin. Invest.* **41**(3):568–574.

Krumwiede, E., 1954, Studies on a lipoproteinase of group A streptococci, *J. Exp. Med.* **100**(6):629–639.

Lancefield, R. C., 1940/1941, Specific relationship of cell composition to biological activity of hemolytic streptococci, *Harvey Lect.* **36**:251–290.

Lancefield, R. C., 1959, Persistence of type-specific antibodies in man following infection with group A streptococci, *J. Exp. Med.* **110**:271–292.

Lancefield, R. C., 1962, Current knowledge of type-specific M antigens of group A streptococci, *J. Immunol.* **89**(3):307–313.

Lancefield, R. C., 1972, Group A streptococcal infections in animals—natural and experimental, in: *Streptococci and Streptococcal Diseases: Recognition, Understanding, and Management* (L. W. Wannamaker and J. M. Matsen, eds.), pp. 313–326, Academic Press, New York.

Lancefield, R. C., and Todd, E. W., 1928, Antigenic differences between matt hemolytic streptococci and their glossy variants, *J. Exp. Med.* **48:**769–790.

Lancefield, R. C., McCarty, M., and Everly, W. N., 1975, Multiple mouse-protective antibodies directed against group B streptococci: Special reference to antibodies effective against protein antigens, *J. Exp. Med.* **142**(1):165–179.

Lange, C. F., 1969, Chemistry of cross-reactive fragments of streptococcal cell membrane and human glomerular basement membrane, *Transplant. Proc.* **1:**959–963.

Laskin, A. I., and Lechevalier, H. A., eds., 1973, *Handbook of Microbiology,* Vol. II. p. 638, CRC Press, Cleveland.

Laughton, N., 1948, Canine beta hemolytic streptococci, *J. Pathol. Bacteriol.* **60:**471–476.

Lawrence, H. S., 1952, The cellular transfer in humans of delayed cutaneous reactivity to hemolytic streptococci, *J. Immunol.* **68:**159–178.

Leading article, 1974, Bacterial stickiness, *Lancet* **1:**716–717.

Leonard, C. G., Colón, A. E., and Cole, R. M., 1968, Transduction in group A streptococcus, Biochem. Biophys. Res. Commun. **30:**130–135.

Levy, R. L., and Hong, R., 1973, The immune nature of subacute bacterial endocarditis (SBE) nephritis, *Am. J. Med.* **54:**645–652.

London, J., and Kline, K., 1973, Aldolase of lactic acid bacteria: A case history in the use of an enzyme as an evolutionary marker, *Bacteriol. Rev.* **37:**453–478.

Lueker, R. D., Abdin, Z. H., and Williams, R. C., Jr., 1975, Peripheral blood T and B lymphocytes during acute rheumatic fever, *J. Clin. Invest.* **55:**975–985.

Lütticken, R., Lütticken, D., Johnson, D. R., and Wannamaker, L. W., 1976a, Application of a new method for detecting streptococcal nicotinamide adenine dinucleotide glycohydrolase to various M types of *Streptococcus pyogenes, J. Clin. Microbiol.* **3**(5):533–536.

Lütticken, R., Wannamaker, L. W., Kluitmann, G., Neugebauer, M., and Pulverer, G., 1976b, Antikörper gegen Streptococcus-pyogenes-Exoenzyme: Antistreptolysin O, anti-DNase B und streptozyme-test, *Deutsch. Med. Wochenschr.* **101:**958–963.

McCarty, M., 1956, Variation in the group-specific carbohydrate of group A streptococci. II. Studies on the chemical basis for serological specificity of the carbohydrates, *J. Exp. Med.* **104:**629–643.

McCarty, M., 1959, The occurrence of polyglycerophosphate as an antigenic component of various gram-positive bacterial species. *J. Exp. Med.* **109**(4):361–378.

McCarty, M., 1972, Theories of pathogenesis of streptococcal complications, in: *Streptococci and Streptococcal Diseases: Recognition, Understanding, and Management* (L. W. Wannamaker and J. M. Matsen, eds.), pp. 517–526, Academic Press, New York.

McCarty, M., and Lancefield, R. C., 1955, Variations in the group-specific carbohydrate of group A streptococci. I. Immunochemical studies on the carbohydrates of variant strains, *J. Exp. Med.* **102:**11–28.

MacDonald, I., 1939, Fatal and severe human infections

with haemolytic streptococci group G (Lancefield), *Med. J. Aust.* **1939:**471–474.

McLaughlin, J. F., Paterson, P. Y., Hartz, R. S., and Embury, S. H., 1972, Rheumatic carditis: *In vitro* responses of peripheral blood leukocytes to heart and streptococcal antigens, *Arthritis Rheum.* **15**(6):600–608.

MacLeod, C. M., 1959, Hypersensitivity and disease, in: *New York Academy of Medicine Symposium Volume, Section on Microbiology* (H. S. Lawrence, ed.), pp. 615–627, Chap. 17.

Malakian, A. H., and Schwab, J. H., 1971, Biological characterization of an immunosuppressant from group A streptococci, *J. Exp. Med.* **134**(5):1253–1265.

Malke, H., 1969, Transduction of *Streptococcus pyogenes* K56 by temperature-sensitive mutants of the transducing phage A25, *Z. Naturforsch.* **24b:**1556–1561.

Malke, H., 1972, Transduction in group A streptococci, in: *Streptococci and Streptococcal Diseases: Recognition, Understanding, and Management* (L. W. Wannamaker and J. M. Matsen, eds.)., pp. 119–133, Academic Press, New York.

Malke, H., 1974, Genetics of resistance to macrolide antibiotics and lincomycin in natural isolates of *Streptococcus pyogenes, Mol. Gen. Genet.* **135:**349–367.

Malke, H., 1975, Transfer of a plasmid mediating antibiotic resistance between strains of *Streptococcus pyogenes* in mixed cultures, *Z. Allg. Mikrobiol.* **15:**645–649.

Malke, H., and Köhler, W., 1973, Transduction among group A streptococci: Transducibility of strains representative of thirty different M types, *Zentralbl. Bakteriol. Parasitenk. Infektionskr. Hyg. Abt. 1:Orig. Reihe A* **224:**194–201.

Malke, H., Starke, R., Köhler, W., Kolesnichenko, T. G., and Totolian, A. A., 1975, Bacteriophage P13234mo-mediated intra- and intergroup transduction of antibiotic resistance among streptococci, *Zentralbl. Bakteriol. Parasitenk. Infektionskr. Hyg. Abt. 1:Orig. Reihe A* **233:**24–34.

Malke, H., Jacob, H. E., and Störl, K., 1976, Characterization of the antibiotic resistance plasmid ERL1 from *Streptococcus pyogenes, Mol. Gen. Genet.* **144:**333–338.

Markowitz, A. S., 1969, Streptococcal related glomerulonephritis in the rhesus monkey, *Transplant. Proc.* **1:**985–991.

Markowitz, A. S., and Lange, C. F., Jr., 1964, Streptococcal related glomerulonephritis. I. Isolation, immunochemistry and comparative chemistry of soluble fractions from type 12 nephritogenic streptococci and human glomeruli, *J. Immunol.* **92:**565–575.

Markowitz, A. S., Armstrong, S. H., and Kushner, D. S., 1960, Immunological relationships between the rat glomerulus and nephritogenic streptococci, *Nature (London)* **187:**1095–1097.

Markowitz, M., 1970, Eradication of rheumatic fever: An unfulfilled hope, *Circulation* **41:**1077–1084.

Markowitz, M., and Gordis, L., eds., 1972, Laboratory findings, in: *Rheumatic Fever,* Vol. 2, 2nd ed., pp. 80–89, Saunders, Philadelphia.

Marmur, J., Falkow, S., and Mandel, M., 1963, New approaches to bacterial taxonomy, *Annu. Rev. Microbiol.* **17**:329–372.

Massell, B. F., Honikman, L. H., and Amezcua, J., 1969, Rheumatic fever following streptococcal vaccination: Report of three cases, *J. Am. Med. Assoc.* **207**(6):1115–1119.

Mathews, J. H., Klesius, P. H., and Zimmerman, R. A., 1974, Opsonin system of the group B streptococcus, *Infect. Immun.* **10**(6):1315–1320.

Matsuno, T., and Slade, H. D., 1970, Composition and properties of a group A streptococcal teichoic acid, *J. Bacteriol.* **102**(3):747–752.

Maxted, W. R., and Potter, E. V., 1967, The presence of type 12 M-protein antigen in group G streptococci, *J. Gen. Microbiol.* **49**:119–125.

Maxted, W. R., and Valkenburg, H. A., 1969, Variation in the M-antigen of group-A streptococci, *J. Med. Microbiol.* **2**:199–210.

Maxted, W. R., and Widdowson, J. P., 1972, The protein antigens of group A streptococci, in: *Streptococci and Streptococcal Diseases: Recognition, Understanding, and Management* (L. W. Wannamaker and J. M. Matsen, eds.), pp. 251–266. Academic Press, New York.

Maxted, W. R., Widdowson, J. P., and Fraser, C. A. M., 1973a, Antibody to streptococci opacity factor in human sera, *J. Hyg.* **71**:35–42.

Maxted, W. R., Widdowson, J. P., Fraser, C. A. M., Ball, L. C., and Bassett, D. C. J., 1973b, The use of the serum opacity reaction in the typing of group-A streptococci, *J. Med. Microbiol.* **6**:83–90.

Merler, E., and Silberschmidt, M., 1972, Uptake of antigen by human lymphocytes, *Immunology* **22**:821–831.

Michael, A. F., Hoyer, J. R., Westberg, N. G., and Fish, A. J., 1972, Experimental models for the pathogenesis of acute poststreptococcal glomerulonephritis, in: *Streptococci and Streptococcal Diseases: Recognition, Understanding, and Management* (L. W. Wannamaker and J. M. Matsen, eds.), pp. 481–500, Academic Press, New York.

Middleton, E., Jr., Middleton, E. B., and Seegal, B. C., 1953, Effect of injecting rats with homologous renal tissue mixed with adjuvants or streptococci, *Arch. Pathol.* **56**:125–134.

Miller, G. A., and Jackson, R. W., 1973, The effect of a *Streptococcus pyogenes* teichoic acid on the immune response of mice, *J. Immunol.* **110**(1):148–156.

Möen, J. K., 1936, Tissue culture studies on bacterial hypersensitivity. II. Reactions of tissues from guinea pigs infected with group C hemolytic streptococci, *J. Exp. Med.* **64**:355–367.

Moore, B. O., and Bryans, J. T., 1969, Antigenic classification of group C animal streptococci, *J. Am. Vet. Med. Assoc.* **155**(2):416–421.

Morrison, D. C., Henson, P. M., and Cochrane, C. G., 1976, The activation of inflammatory cells in immunological disease, in: *Infection and Immunology in the Rheumatic Diseases* (D. C. Dumonde, ed.), pp. 355–363, Blackwell Scientific Publications, Oxford.

Morse, S. I., Darnell, J. E., Jr., Thomas, W. A., and

Glaser, R. J., 1955, Cardiac lesions in rabbits after pharyngeal infections with group A streptococci (21892), *Proc. Soc. Exp. Biol. Med.* **89**:613–616.

Mortensen, R. F., Osmand, A. P., and Gewurz, H., 1975, Effects of C-reactive protein on the lymphoid system. I. Binding to thymus-dependent lymphocytes and alteration of their functions, *J. Exp. Med.* **141**:821–839.

Mortimer, E. A., Jr., Cushing, A. H., Jayanetra, P., and Bunch, G. P., 1972, Studies of streptococcal and staphylococcal L forms *in vivo*, in: *Streptococci and Streptococcal Diseases: Recognition, Understanding, and Management* (L. W. Wannamaker and J. M. Matsen, eds.), pp. 433–450, Academic Press, New York.

Mosley, J. B., and Pickett, M. J., 1965, BSSA: An agglutinogen for quantitation of antistreptolysin O, *Am. J. Clin. Pathol.* **44**(5):525–529.

Murphy, G. E., ed., 1960, *Nature of Rheumatic Heart Disease with Special Reference to Myocardial Disease and Heart Failure*, pp. 289–343, Williams and Wilkins, Baltimore.

Murphy, G. E., and Swift, H. F., 1950, The induction of rheumatic-like cardiac lesions in rabbits by repeated focal infections with group A streptococci: Comparison with the cardiac lesions of serum disease, *J. Exp. Med.* **91**:485–498.

Myhre, E. B., and Kronvall, G., 1977, Heterogeneity of nonimmune immunoglobulin Fc reactivity among gram-positive cocci: Description of three major types of receptors for human immunoglobulin G, *Infect. Immun.* **17**(3):475–482.

Nakae, M., Inoue, M., and Mitsuhashi, S., 1975, Artificial elimination of drug resistance from group A beta-hemolytic streptococci, *Antimicrob. Agents Chemother.* **7**(5):719–720.

Nauciel, C., 1973, Mitogenic activity of purified streptococcal erythrogenic toxin of lymphocytes, *Ann. Immunol. (Inst. Pasteur)* **124**(C):383–390.

Nelson, J., Ayoub, E. M., and Wannamaker, L. W., 1968, Streptococcal antidesoxyribonuclease B: Microtechnique determination, *J. Lab. Clin. Med.* **71**:867–873.

Noble, R. C., and Penny, B. B., 1975, Characterization of the antibody response to type 12 M protein of group A streptococcus, *J. Lab. Clin. Med.* **86**(5):713–721.

Oettgen, H. F., Silber, R., Miescher, P. A., and Hirschhorn, K., 1966, Stimulation of human tonsillar lymphocytes *in vitro*, *Clin. Exp. Immunol.* **1**:77–84.

Ofek, I., Bergner-Rabinowitz, S., and Davies, A. M., 1969, Opsonic capacity of type specific streptococcal antibodies, *Israel J. Med. Sci.* **5**(3):293–296.

Ofek, I., Bergner-Rabinowitz, S., and Ginsburg, I., 1970, Oxygen-stable hemolysins of group A streptococcus. VII. The relation of the leukotoxic factor to streptolysin S, *J. Infect. Dis.* **122**:517–522.

Ofek, I., Fleiderman, S., Bergner-Rabinowitz, S., and Ginsburg, I., 1971, Application of enzyme production properties in subtyping of group A streptococci according to T type, *Appl. Microbiol.* **22**:748–751.

Ofek, I., Kaplan, O., Bergner-Rabinowitz, S., Hornstein, L., Lapid, A., and Davies, A. M., 1973, Antibody tests in streptococcal pharyngitis: Streptozyme versus conventional methods, *Clin. Pediatr.* **12**(6):341–344.

Ohanian, S. H., and Schwab, J. H., 1967, Persistence of group A streptococcal cell walls related to chronic inflammation of rabbit dermal connective tissue, *J. Exp. Med.* **125**:1137–1148.

Osterland, C. K., Miller, E. J., Karakawa, W. W., and Krause, R. M., 1966, Characteristics of streptococcal group-specific antibody isolated from hyperimmune rabbits, *J. Exp. Med.* **123**:599–614.

Pachman, L. M., and Fox, E. N., 1970, Cellular and antibody reactions to streptococcal M protein types 1, 3, 6, and 12, *J. Immunol.* **105**:898–907.

Page, R. C., Davies, P., and Allison, A. C., 1974, Pathogenesis of the chronic inflammatory lesion induced by group A streptococcal cell walls, *Lab. Invest.* **30**(5):568–581.

Paredes, A., Wong, P., Mason, E. O., Jr., Taber, L. H., and Barrett, F. F., 1977, Nosocomial transmission of group B streptococci in a newborn nursery, *Pediatrics* **59**(5):679–682.

Parker, M. T., 1969, Streptococcal skin infection and acute glomerulonephritis, *Br. J. Dermatol.* **81**:37–46 (Suppl. 1).

Parker, M. T., and Ball, L. C., 1976, Streptococci and aerococci associated with systemic infection in man, *J. Med. Microbiol.* **9**:275–302.

Patarroyo, M. E., Winchester, R. J., Vejerano, A., Gibofsky, A., Chalem, F., Zabriskie, J. B., Kunkel, H. G., 1979, Association of a B-cell alloantigen with susceptibility to rheumatic fever, *Nature* **278**(5700):173–174.

Pellegrino, M. A., Ferrone, S., Safford, J. W., Jr., Hirata, A. A., Terasaki, P. I., and Reisfeld, R. A., 1972, Stimulation of lymphocyte transformation by streptococcal type Ml protein: Relationship to HL-A antigens, *J. Immunol.* **109**(1):97–102.

Perkins, J. C., and Hahn, J. J., 1968, Enhancement of phagocytosis of group A streptococci by antibody fragments derived from rabbit immunoglobulin by pepsin digestion, *J. Immunol.* **100**(4):898–901.

Plate, J. M., and Amos, D. B., 1969, Studies on a lymphocyte activating factor from group A streptococci, in: *Proceedings of the Third Annual Leucocyte Culture Conference* (W. O. Rieke, ed.), pp. 485–499, Appleton-Century-Crofts, New York.

Plate, J. M., and Amos, B., 1971a, Lymphocyte stimulation by a glycopeptide isolated from *Streptococcus pyogenes* C203S. I. Isolation and partial purification, *Cell. Immunol.* **1**:476–487.

Plate, J. M., and Amos, B., 1971b, Lymphocyte stimulation by a glycopeptide isolated from *Streptococcus pyogenes* C203S. II. Kinetics of the response, *Cell. Immunol.* **1**:488–499.

Polly, S. M., Waldman, R. H., High, P., Wittner, M. K., Dorfman, A., and Fox, E. N., 1975, Protective studies with a group A streptococcal M protein vaccine. II. Challenge of volunteers after local immunization in the upper respiratory tract, *J. Infect. Dis.* **131**(3):217–224.

Poretz, D. M., 1974, The NBT test in bacterial and nonbacterial pharyngitis, *Virg. Med. Month.* **101**:653–656.

Potter, E. V., Stollerman, G. H., and Siegel, A. C., 1962, Recall of type specific antibodies in man by injections of streptococcal cell walls, *J. Clin. Invest.* **41**(2):301–310.

Potter, E. V., Ortiz, J. S., Sharrett, A. R., Burt, E. G., Bray, J. P., Finklea, J. F., Poon-King, T., and Earle, D. P., 1971, Changing types of nephritogenic streptococci in Trinidad, *J. Clin. Invest.* **50**(6):1197–1205.

Powers, G. F., and Boisvert, P. L., 1943, Tuberculosis and streptococcosis, *Yale J. Biol. Med.* **15**:517–530.

Powers, G. F., and Boisvert, P. L., 1944, Age as a factor in streptococcosis, *J. Pediatr.* **25**:481–504.

Quie, P. G., 1972, Bactericidal function of human polymorphonuclear leukocytes: E. Mead Johnson Award Address, *Pediatrics* **50**(2):264–270.

Quie, P. G., and Hill, H. R., 1973, Granulocytopathies, in: *Disease-A-Month*, August, Year Book Medical Publishers, Chicago.

Rammelkamp, C. H., Jr., 1957, Epidemiology of streptococcal infections, in: *The Harvey Lectures, Series LI*, pp. 113–142, Academic Press, New York.

Rammelkamp, C. H., Jr., and Weaver, R. S., 1953, Acute glomerulonephritis: The significance of the variations in the incidence of the disease, *J. Clin. Invest.* **32**(4):345–358.

Rantz, L. A., 1942, The serological and biological classification of hemolytic and nonhemolytic streptococci from human sources, *J. Infect. Dis.* **71**:61–68.

Rantz, L. A., Randall, E., and Rantz, H. H., 1948, Antistreptolysin "O": A study of this antibody in health and in hemolytic streptococcus respiratory disease in man, *Am. J. Med.* **5**(1):3–23.

Rapaport, F. T., and Chase, R. M., Jr., 1964, Homograft sensitivity induction by group A streptococci, *Science* **145**:407–408.

Rapaport, F. T., Chase, R. M., Jr., and Solowey, A. C., 1966, Transplantation antigen activity of bacterial cells in different animal species and intracellular localization, *Ann. N.Y. Acad. Sci.* **129**(1):102–114.

Rapaport, F. T., Bachvaroff, R., and Markowitz, A. S., 1973, Lymphocyte surface effects of soluble extracts of streptococcal membranes (TGCM). I. Relationships between HL-A and species-specific antigenic sites and TGCM binding sites, *J. Immunol.* **110**(4):1058–1066.

Ravin, A. W., and De Sa, J. D. H., 1964, Genetic linkage of mutational sites affecting similar characters in pneumococcus and streptococcus, *J. Bacteriol.* **87**(1):86–96.

Read, S. E., and Zabriskie, J. B., 1976, Immunological concepts in rheumatic fever pathogenesis, in: *Textbook of Immunopathology*, Vol. 1, 2nd ed. (P. A. Miescher and H. J. Müller-Eberhard, eds.), pp. 471–487, Grune and Stratton, New York.

Read, S. E., Fischetti, V. A., Utermohlen, V., Falk, R. E., and Zabriskie, J. B., 1974, Cellular reactivity studies to streptococcal antigens: Migration inhibition studies in patients with streptococcal infections and rheumatic fever, *J. Clin. Invest.* **54**(2):439–450.

Read, S. E., Reid, H., Poon-King, T., Fischetti, V. A., Zabriskie, J. B., and Rapaport, F. T., 1977, HLA and predisposition to the nonsuppurative sequelae of group A streptococcal infections, *Transplant. Proc.* **9**(1):543–546.

Reinarz, J. A., and Sanford, J. P., 1965, Human infections caused by non-group A or D streptococci, *Medicine* **44**:81–95.

Ricketts, C. R., Squire, J. R., and Topley, E., 1951, Human skin lipids with particular reference to the self-sterilising power of the skin, *Clin. Sci.* **10**:89–111.

Riesen, W. F., Skvaril, F., and Braun, D. G., 1976, Natural infection of man with group A streptococci: Levels; restriction in class, subclass and type; and clonal appearance of polysaccharide-group-specific antibodies, *Scand. J. Immunol.* **5**:383–390.

Roop, D. R., Mundt, J. O., and Riggsby, W. S., 1974, Deoxyribonucleic acid hybridization studies among some strains of group D and group N streptococci, *Int. J. Syst. Bacteriol.* **24**:330–337.

Ross, R. F., 1972, Streptococcal infections in swine, in: *Streptococci and Streptococcal Diseases: Recognition, Understanding, and Management* (L. W. Wannamaker and J. M. Matsen, eds.), pp. 339–348, Academic Press, New York.

Rothbard, S., and Watson, R. F., 1948, Variation occurring in group A streptococci during human infection: Progressive loss of M substance correlated with increasing susceptibility to bacteriostatis, *J. Exp. Med.* **87**(6):521–533.

Rothbard, S., Watson, R. F., Swift, H. F., and Wilson, A. T., 1948, Bacteriologic and immunologic studies on patients with hemolytic streptococcic infections as related to rheumatic fever, *Arch. Intern. Med.* **82**:229–250.

Sanders, E., 1969, Bacterial interference. I. Its occurrence among the respiratory tract flora and characterization of inhibition of group A streptococci by viridans *Streptococci, J. Infect. Dis.* **120**:698–707.

Sandson, J., Hamerman, D., Janis, R., and Rojkind, M., 1968, Immunologic and chemical similarities between the streptococcus and human connective tissue, *Tr. Assoc. Am. Physicians* **81**:249–257.

Saslaw, M. S., and Streitfeld, M. M., 1959, Group A beta hemolytic streptococci and rheumatic fever in Miami, Florida. I. Bacteriologic observations from October 1954 through May 1955, *Dis. Chest* **35**:175–193.

Sawyer, W. D., Smith, M. R., and Wood, W. B., Jr., 1954, The mechanisms by which macrophages phagocyte encapsulated bacteria in the absence of antibody, *J. Exp. Med.* **100**:417–424.

Schleifer, K. H., and Kandler, O., 1972, Peptidoglycan types of bacterial cell walls and their taxonomic implications, *Bacteriol. Rev.* **36**:407–477.

Schmidt, W. C., and Moore, D. J., 1965, The determination of antibody to group A streptococcal polysaccharide in human sera by hemagglutination, *J. Exp. Med.* **121**:793–806.

Schwab, J. H., 1975, Suppression of the immune response by microorganisms, *Bacteriol. Rev.* **39**(2):121–143.

Schwab, J. H., and Brown, R. R., 1968, Modification of antigenic structure *in vivo:* Quantitative studies on the processing of streptococcal cell wall antigens in mice, *J. Immunol.* **101**:930–938.

Schwab, J. H., and Ohanian, S. H., 1967, Degradation of streptococcal cell wall antigens *in vivo, J. Bacteriol.* **94**(5):1346–1352.

Schwentker, F. F., and Comploier, F. C., 1939, The production of kidney antibodies by injection of homologous kidney plus bacterial toxins, *J. Exp. Med.* **70**:223–230.

Seravalli, E., 1976, Isolation of isoelectric focusing of a mitogenic substance released by stimulated human lymphocytes, *Cell. Immunol.* **21**:70–78.

Seravalli, E., and Taranta, A., 1974, Lymphocyte transformation and macrophage migration inhibition by electrofocused and gel-filtered fractions of group A streptococcal filtrate, *Cell. Immunol.* **14**:366–375.

Shapera, R. M., and Matsen, J. M., 1973, Nitroblue tetrazolium dye reduction by neutrophils from patients with streptococcal pharyngitis, *Pediatrics* **51**(2):284–287.

Shulman, S. T., and Ayoub, E. M., 1974, Qualitative and quantitative aspects of the human antibody response to streptococcal group A carbohydrate, *J. Clin. Invest.* **54**(4):990–996.

Shulman, S. T., Ayoub, E. M., Victorica, B. E., Gessner, I. H., Tamer, D. T., and Hernandez, F. A., 1974, Differences in antibody response to streptococcal antigens in children with rheumatic and non-rheumatic mitral valve disease, *Circulation* **50**(2):1244–1251.

Siegel, A. C., Johnson, E. E., and Stollerman, G. H., 1961, Controlled studies of streptococcal pharyngitis in a pediatric population. 2. Behavior of the type-specific immune response, *N. Engl. J. Med.* **265**:566–571.

Siegel, I., Grieco, M. H., and Gupta, S., 1976, Fc- and complement-receptor rosette-forming cell ratios in human tonsils and peripheral blood, *Int. Arch. Allergy Appl. Immunol.* **50**:488–496.

Slechta, T., and Gray, E. D., 1976, Isolation of streptococcal nuclease B by batch adsorption, *J. Clin. Microbiol.* **2**:528–530.

Sloyer, J. L., Veltri, R. W., and Sprinkle, P. M., 1973, *In vitro* IgM antibody synthesis by human tonsil-derived lymphocytes, *J. Immunol.* **111**(1):183–188.

Smialowicz, R. J., and Schwab, J. H., 1977a, Cytotoxicity of rat macrophages activated by persistent or biodegradable bacterial cell walls, *Infect. Immun.* **17**(3):599–606.

Smialowicz, R. J., and Schwab, J. H., 1977b, Processing of streptococcal cell walls by rat macrophages and human monocytes *in vitro, Infect. Immun.* **17**(3):591–598.

Smith, E. W. P., Garson, A., Jr., Boyleston, J. A., Katz, S. L., and Wilfert, C. M., 1976, Varicella gangrenosa due to group A β hemolytic streptococcus, *Pediatrics* **57**:306–310.

Smith, R. F., Dayton, S. L., and Chipps, D. D., 1973, Autograft rejection in acutely burned patients: Relation to colonization by *Streptococcus agalactiae, Appl. Microbiol.* **25**(3):493–495.

Sonozaki, H., Takizawa, S., and Torisu, M., 1970, Immunoglobulin analysis of anti-streptolysin-O antibody, *Clin. Exp. Immunol.* **7**:519–531.

Spaun, J., Bentzon, M. W., Olsen Larsen, S., and Hewitt, L. F., 1961, International standard for antistreptolysin-O, *Bull. WHO* **24**:271–279.

Spector, W. G., Reichold, N., and Ryan, G. B., 1970, Degradation of granuloma-inducing micro-organisms by macrophages, *J. Pathol.* **101**:339–354.

Stetson, C. A., Jr., 1954, The relation of antibody response to rheumatic fever, in: *Streptococcal Infections* (M. McCarty, ed.), pp. 208–218, Columbia University Press, New York.

Stewardson-Krieger, P., Albrandt, K., Kretschmer, R. R., and Gotoff, S. P., 1977a, Group B streptococcal long-chain reaction, *Infect. Immun.* **18**(3):666–672.

Stewardson-Krieger, P. B., Albrandt, K., Nevin, T., Kretschmer, R. R., and Gotoff, S. P., 1977b, Perinatal immunity to group B β-hemolytic *Streptococcus* type Ia, *J. Infect. Dis.* **136**(5):649–654.

Stollerman, G. H., 1972, Hypersensitivity and antibody responses in streptococcal disease, in: *Streptococci and Streptococcal Diseases: Recognition, Understanding, and Management* (L. W. Wannamaker and J. M. Matsen, eds.), pp. 501–513, Academic Press, New York.

Stollerman, G. H., ed., 1975a, *Rheumatic Fever and Streptococcal Infection,* Grune and Stratton, New York.

Stollerman, G. H., ed., 1975b, Etiology and pathogenesis, in: *Rheumatic Fever and Streptococcal Infection,* pp. 101–122, Grune and Stratton, New York.

Stollerman, G. H., ed., 1975c, Immunization against group A streptococcal infection: The immunology of M protein, in: *Rheumatic Fever and Streptococcal Infection,* pp. 277–303, Grune and Stratton, New York.

Stollerman, G. H., Lewis, A. J., Schultz, I., and Taranta, A., 1956, Relationship of immune response to group A streptococci to the course of acute, chronic and recurrent rheumatic fever, *Am. J. Med.* **20**:163–169.

Stollerman, G. H., Siegel, A. C., and Johnson, E. E., 1959, Evaluation of the "long chain reaction" as a means for detecting type-specific antibody to group A streptococci in human sera, *J. Exp. Med.* **110**:887–897.

Stollerman, G. H., Rytel, M., and Ortiz, J., 1963, Accessory plasma factors involved in the bactericidal test for type-specific antibody to group A streptococci. II. Human plasma cofactor(s) enhancing opsonization of encapsulated organisms, *J. Exp. Med.* **117**:1–17.

Stollerman, G. H., Alberti, H., and Plemmons, J. A., 1967, Opsonization of group A streptococci by complement deficient blood from a patient with hereditary angioneurotic edema, *J. Immunol.* **99**(1):92–97.

Stossel, T. P., 1974, Phagocytosis (second of three parts), *New Engl. J. Med.* **290**:774–780.

Stuart, J. G., and Ferretti, J. J., 1975, Determination of

guanine plus cytosine content in *Streptococcus pyogenes, Can. J. Microbiol.* **21**:722–724.

Surján, L., and Surján, M., 1971, Immunological role of human tonsils, *Acta Otolaryngol.* **71**:190–193.

Surján, L., Surján, L., Jr., and Surján, M., 1972, Further investigations into the immunological role of tonsils, *Acta Otolaryngol.* **73**:222–226.

Swanson, J., Hsu, K. C., and Gotschlich, E. C., 1969, Electron microscopic studies on streptococci. I. M antigen, *J. Exp. Med.* **130**:1063–1091.

Tada, T., and Ishizaka, K., 1970, Distribution of γE-forming cells in lymphoid tissues of the human and monkey, *J. Immunol.* **104**(2):377–387.

Tagg, J. R., and Wannamaker, L. W., 1976, Genetic basis of streptococcin A-FF22 production, *Antimicrob. Agents Chemother.* **10**:299–306.

Tagg, J. R., Dajani, A. S., Wannamaker, L. W., and Gray, E. D., 1973, Group A streptococcal bacteriocin: Production, purification and mode of action, *J. Exp. Med.* **138**:1168–1183.

Tagg, J. R., Dajani, A. S., and Wannamaker, L. W., 1976a, Bacteriocins of gram-positive bacteria, *Bacteriol. Rev.* **40**(3):722–756.

Tagg, J. R., Skjold, S., and Wannamaker, L. W., 1976b, Transduction of bacteriocin determinants in group A streptococci, *J. Exp. Med.* **143**:1540–1544.

Taranta, A., Torosdag, S., Metrakos, J. D., Jegier, W., and Uchida, I., 1959, Rheumatic fever in monozygotic and dizygotic twins, *Circulation* **20**:778.

Taranta, A., Wood, H. F., Feinstein, A. R., Simpson, R., and Kleinberg, E., 1964, Rheumatic fever in children and adolescents: A long-term epidemiologic study of subsequent prophylaxis, streptococcal infections, and clinical sequelae. IV. Relation of the rheumatic fever recurrence rate per streptococcal infection to the titers of streptococcal antibodies, *Ann. Intern. Med.* **60**:47–57.

Taranta, A., Cuppari, G., and Qualgliata, F., 1969, Dissociation of hemolytic and lymphocyte-transforming activities of streptolysin S preparations, *J. Exp. Med.* **129**(4):605–622.

Tauber, J., 1977, Discussion in Milgram, F., and Zabriskie, J. B., Workshop on cross-reacting antigens, *Transplant. Proc.* **9**:1281–1285.

Tauber, J. W., Falk, J. A., Falk, R. E., and Zabriskie, J. B., 1976a, Nonspecific complement activation by streptococcal structures. I. Re-evaluation of HLA cytotoxicity inhibition, *J. Exp. Med.* **143**:1341–1351.

Tauber, J. W., Polley, M. J., and Zabriskie, J. B., 1976b, Nonspecific complement activation by streptococcal structures. II. Properdin-independent initiation of the alternate pathway, *J. Exp. Med.* **143**:1352–1366.

Taylor, A. G., 1969, The nature of the lymphocyte mitogen in streptolysin S, *Life Sci.* **8**(2):1281–1297.

Taylor, A. G., 1972, Lymphocyte-transforming activity of streptococci belonging to various Lancefield groups, *J. Med. Microbiol.* **5**:61–65.

Thomas, L., 1972, Experimental models for the pathogenesis of rheumatic heart disease, in: *Streptococci and Streptococcal Diseases: Recognition, Understanding, and Management* (L. W. Wannamaker and J. M. Matsen, eds.), pp. 465–471, Academic Press, New York.

Tomar, R. H., Taylor, F. B., Jr., and Green, G. R., 1972, Delayed hypersensitivity to SK-SD: *In vitro* lymphocyte study with an active component, *J. Immunol.* **108**(1):231–235.

Tomura, T., Hirano, T., Ito, T., and Yoshioka, M., 1973, Transmission of bacteriocinogenicity by conjugation in group D streptococci, *Jpn. J. Microbiol.* **17**(6):445–452.

Top, F. H., Jr., and Wannamaker, L. W., 1968, The serum opacity reaction of *Streptococcus pyogenes:* The demonstration of multiple, strain specific lipoproteinase antigens, *J. Exp. Med.* **127**:1013–1034.

Treser, G., Semar, M., Ty, A., Sagel, I., Franklin, M. A., and Lange, K., 1970, Partial characterization of antigenic streptococcal plasma membrane components in acute glomerulonephritis, *J. Clin. Invest.* **49**:762–768.

Ubukata, K., Konno, M., and Fujii, R., 1975, Transduction of drug resistance to tetracycline, chloramphenicol, macrolides, lincomycin and clindamycin with phages induced from *Streptococcus pyogenes, J. Antibiot.* **28**(9):681–688.

Vanace, P. W., 1960, Experimental streptococcal infection in the rhesus monkey, *Ann. N.Y. Acad. Sci.* **85**(3):910–930.

Van de Rijn, I., and Zabriskie, J. B., 1976, Immunological relationship between *Streptococcus mutans* and human myocardium, in: *Immunology Abstracts* (W. J. Bowen, R. J. Genco, and T. C. O'Brien, eds.), pp. 187–194.

Van Epps, D. E., and Andersen, B. R., 1974, Streptolysin O inhibition of neutrophil chemotaxis and mobility: Nonimmune phenomenon with species specificity, *Infect. Immun.* **9**:27–33.

Vosti, K. L., and Rantz, L. A., 1964, The measurement of type- and nontype-specific group A hemolytic streptococcal antibody with an hemagglutination technique, *J. Immunol.* **92**:185–191.

Waldenstrom, J., Winblad, S., Hällén, J., and Liungman, S., 1964, The occurrence of serological "antibody" reagins or similar γ-globulins in conditions with monoclonal hypergammaglobulinemia, such as myeloma, macroglobulinemia, etc. *Acta Med. Scand.* **176**:619–631.

Wallin, J., and Forsgren, A., 1975, Group B streptococci in venereal disease clinic patients, *Br. J. Venereal Dis.* **51**(6):401–404.

Wannamaker, L. W., 1954, The epidemiology of streptococcal infections, in: *Streptococcal Infections* (M. McCarty, ed.), pp. 157–175, Columbia University Press, New York.

Wannamaker, L. W., 1959, The paradox of the antibody response to streptodornase: The usefulness of antidesoxyribonuclease B as an indication of streptococcal infection in patients with acute rheumatic fever, *Am. J. Med.* **27**(4):567–574.

Wannamaker, L. W., 1964, Streptococcal desoxyribonu-

cleases, in: *The Streptococcus, Rheumatic Fever and Glomerulonephritis* (J. W. Uhr, ed.), pp. 140–165, Williams and Wilkins, Baltimore.

Wannamaker, L. W., 1970a, Medical progress: Differences between streptococcal infections of the throat and of the skin, *N. Engl. J. Med.* **282**:23–31, 78–85.

Wannamaker, L. W., 1970b, Tonsils, rheumatic fever and health delivery, *N. Engl. J. Med.* **282**:336–337.

Wannamaker, L. W., 1973, The chain that links the heart to the throat, *Circulation* **48**:9–18.

Wannamaker, L. W., and Ayoub, E. M., 1960, Antibody titers in acute rheumatic fever, *Circulation* **21**(4):598–614.

Wannamaker, L. W., and Ferrieri, P., 1975, Streptococcal infections—updated, in: *Disease-A-Month* (H. F. Dowling, ed.)., pp. 1–40, Year Book Medical Publishers, Chicago.

Wannamaker, L. W., and Kaplan, E. L., 1977, Acute rheumatic fever, in: *Heart Disease in Infants, Children and Adolescents*, 2nd ed. (A. J. Moss, F. H. Adams, and G. C. Emmanouilides, eds.), p. 515, Williams and Wilkins, Baltimore.

Wannamaker, L. W., and Matsen, J. M., eds., 1972a, Discussion of Chapters 1–3, in: *Streptococci and Streptococcal Diseases: Recognition, Understanding, and Management*, pp. 52–53, Academic Press, New York.

Wannamaker, L. W., and Matsen, J. M., eds., 1972b, Roundtable discussion on prospects for a streptococcal vaccine, in: *Streptococci and Streptococcal Diseases: Recognition, Understanding, and Management*, pp. 411–429, Academic Press, New York.

Wannamaker, L. W., Rammelkamp, C. H., Jr., Denny, F. W., Brink, W. R., Houser, H. B., Hahn, E. O., and Dingle, J. H., 1951, Prophylaxis of acute rheumatic fever by treatment of the preceding streptococcal infection with various amounts of depot penicillin, *Am. J. Med.* **10**:673–695.

Wannamaker, L. W., Skjold, S., and Maxted, W. R., 1970, Characterization of bacteriophages from nephritogenic group A streptococci, *J. Infect. Dis.* **121**:407–418.

Wannamaker, L. W., Almquist, S., and Skjold, S., 1973, Inter-group phage reactions and transduction between group C and group A streptococci, *J. Exp. Med.* **137**:1338–1353.

Watson, K. C., and Kerr, E. J. C., 1975, Partial characterization of an inhibitor of streptolysin O produced by bacterial growth in serum, *J. Med. Microbiol.* **8**:465–475.

Watson, R. F., Rothbard, S., and Swift, H. F., 1946, Type-specific protection and immunity following intranasal inoculation of monkeys with group A hemolytic streptococci, *J. Exp. Med.* **84**:127–142.

Watson, R. F., Hirst, G. K., and Lancefield, R. C., 1961, Bacteriological studies of cardiac tissues obtained at autopsy from eleven patients dying with rheumatic fever, *Arth. Rheum.* **4**(1):74–85.

Weissman, S. M., Reich, P. R., Somerson, N. L., and Cole, R. M., 1966, Genetic differentiation by nucleic acid homology. IV. Relationships among Lancefield groups and serotypes of streptococci, *J. Bacteriol.* **92**(5):1372–1377.

Weksler, B. B., and Nachman, R. L., 1971, Rabbit platelet bactericidal protein, *J. Exp. Med.* **134**:1114–1130.

Widdowson, J. P., Maxted, W. R., and Pinney, A. M., 1971a, An M-associated protein antigen (MAP) of group A streptococci, *J. Hyg.* **69**:553–564.

Widdowson, J. P., Maxted, W. R., Grant, D. L., and Pinney, A. M., 1971b, The relationship between M-antigen and opacity factor in group A streptococci, *J. Gen. Microbiol.* **65**:69–80.

Widdowson, J. P., Maxted, W. R., Notley, C. M., and Pinney, A. M., 1974a, The antibody responses in man to infection with different serotypes of group-A streptococci, *J. Med. Microbiol.* **7**:483–496.

Widdowson, J. P., Maxted, W. R., Newrick, C. W., and Parkin, D., 1974b, An outbreak of streptococcal sore throat and rheumatic fever in a Royal Air Force Training camp; significance of serum antibody to M-associated protein, *J. Hyg.* **72**:1–12.

Wiley, G. G., and Wilson, A. T., 1956, The ability of group A streptococci killed by heat or mercury arc irradiation to resist ingestion by phagocytes, *J. Exp. Med.* **103**(1):15–36.

Wilkinson, H. W., and Eagon, R. G., 1971, Type-specific antigens of group B type Ic streptococci, *Infect. Immun.* **4**(5):596–604.

Wilkinson, H. W., and Jones, W. L., 1976, Radioimmunoassay for measuring antibodies specific for group B streptococcal types Ia, Ib, Ic, II, and III, *J. Clin. Microbiol.* **3**(5):480–485.

Williams, R. C., and Gibbons, R. J., 1972, Inhibition of bacterial adherence by secretory immunoglobulin A: A mechanism of antigen disposal, *Science* **177**:697–699.

Williams, R. C., Jr., 1977, Bacterial endocarditis—An analysis of immunopathology, in: *Proceedings of the American Heart Association Symposium on Infective Endocarditis* (E. L. Kaplan and A. V. Taranta, eds.), pp. 20–23, American Heart Association, Dallas.

Williams, R. C., Jr., and Kunkel, H. G., 1962, Rheumatoid factor complement and conglutinin aberrations in patients with subacute bacterial endocarditis, *J. Clin. Invest.* **41**(3):666–674.

Williams, R. C., Jr., Zabriskie, J. B., Mahros, F., Hassaballa, F., and Abdin, Z. H., 1977, Lymphocyte surface markers in acute rheumatic fever and post-streptococcal acute glomerulonephritis, *Clin. Exp. Immunol.* **27**:135–142.

Wilson, A. T., 1953, The egestion of phagocytized particles by leukocytes, *J. Exp. Med.* **98**(4):305–310.

Wilson, A. T., 1957, The leukotoxic action of streptococci, *J. Exp. Med.* **105**(5):463–484.

Wilson, A. T., and Wiley, G. G., 1963, The cellular antigens of group A streptococci: Immunoelectrophoretic studies of the C, M, T, PGP, E$_4$, F, and E antigens of serotype 17 streptococci, *J. Exp. Med.* **118**(4):527–556.

Wilson, G. S., and Miles, A., eds., 1975, in: *Topley and Wilson's Principles of Bacteriology, Virology and Immunity,* p. 737, Williams and Wilkins, Baltimore.

Winblad, S., 1966, Studies on non-specific antistreptolysin O titre. 1. The influence of serum β-lipoproteins on the non-specific antistreptolysin O titre, *Acta Pathol. Microbiol. Scand.* **66**:93–104.

Wittner, M. K., and Fox, E. N., 1971, Micro complement fixation assay for type-specific group A streptococcal antibody, *Infect. Immun.* **4**(4):441–445.

Woods, R. D., and Ross, R. F., 1975, Purification and serological characterization of a type-specific antigen of *Streptococcus equisimilis, Infect. Immun.* **12**(4):881–887.

Woolcock, J. B., 1974, Purification and antigenicity of an M-like protein of *Streptococcus equi, Infect. Immun.* **10**:116–122.

Yagi, Y., and Clewell, D. B., 1976, Plasmid-determined tetracycline resistance in *Streptococcus faecalis:* Tandemly repeated resistance determinants in amplified forms of pAMα1 DNA, *J. Med. Biol.* **102**:583–600.

Yang, L. C., Soprey, P. R., Wittner, M. K., and Fox, E. N., 1977, Streptococcal-induced cell-mediated-immune destruction of cardiac myofibers *in vitro, J. Exp. Med.* **146**:344–360.

Yü-K'un, L., Shu-Chen, H., and Tze-Ying, T., 1964, The role of streptococcal infections in filariasis, *Chinese Med. J.* **83**:17–22.

Zabriskie, J. B., 1964, The role of temperate bacteriophage in the production of erythrogenic toxin by group A streptococci, *J. Exp. Med.* **119**(5):761–779.

Zabriskie, J. B., 1971, The role of streptococci in human glomerulonephritis, *J. Exp. Med.* **134**(3):180s–192s.

Zabriskie, J. B., and Freimer, E. H., 1966, An immunological relationship between the group A streptococcus and mammalian muscle, *J. Exp. Med.* **124**(4):661–678.

Zabriskie, J. B., Hsu, K. C., and Seegal, B. C., 1970a, Heart-reactive antibody associated with rheumatic fever: Characterization and diagnostic significance, *Clin. Exp. Immunol.* **7**(2):147–159.

Zabriskie, J. B., Lewshenia, R., Möller, G., Wehle, B., and Falk, R. E., 1970b, Lymphocytic responses to streptococcal antigens in glomerulonephritic patients, *Science* **168**:1105–1108.

Zabriskie, J. B., Read, S. E., and Fischetti, V. A., 1972, Lysogeny in streptococci, in: *Streptococci and Streptococcal Diseases: Recognition, Understanding, and Management* (L. W. Wannamaker and J. M. Matsen, eds.), pp. 99–118, Academic Press, New York.

Zimmerman, R. A., and Hill, H. R., 1969, Placental transfer of group A type-specific streptococcal antibody, *Pediatrics* **43**(5):809–814.

Zucker-Franklin, D., and Berney, S., 1972, Electron microscope study of surface immunoglobulin-bearing human tonsil cells, *J. Exp. Med.* **135**(3):533–548.

4

Immunology of Staphylococci

JAN VERHOEF, PHILLIP K. PETERSON, and PAUL G. QUIE

1. Introduction

Staphylocci are constant residents of the skin and mucous membranes. The integument is indeed the most crucial organ system for host defense against staphylococcal disease. Once through the anatomical barrier of the skin, *Staphylococcus aureus* has a complex array of toxins and other mechanisms for attacking the host, so that it is a highly pathogenic invader. *Staphylococcus epidermidis* is much less capable of injuring the invaded host. Invasion by this organism is dangerous only in special clinical circumstances. This chapter will review the antigenic structure of staphylococci, the nature of the armament of these organisms, and the response of the human host when invaded.

S. *aureus* is found as a commensal microbe on moist areas of skin and in the anterior nares of approximately 40% of healthy persons (Williams *et al.*, 1966). These healthy carriers serve as a human reservoir of S. *aureus*, and the skin is often a vehicle for spread of these organisms from person to person (Lidwell *et al.*, 1974). The hospital environment is especially favorable for transmission of S. *aureus* because of intimate care of patients by the same attendants. In some surgical units 10% of operative wounds are infected with staphylococci (Williams *et al.*, 1966). Patients with lesions discharging staphylococci are especially serious sources of such infections. Since many patients are carriers of staphylococci of a wide variety of phage types, it is interesting that only a relatively few phage types of S. *aureus* are implicated in the majority of hospital-acquired infections (see Williams *et al.*, 1966).

The staphylococci have a remarkable capacity for adapting to an unfavorable environment. These organisms can change antigenically (Ekstedt, 1974), can develop resistance to antimicrobial agents (Finland, 1972), or can change metabolically and become "indifferent" to antibiotics (McDermott, 1969). All of these properties have assured S. *aureus* of a continuing prominent role as a cause of infectious diseases. Table 1 summarizes a number of the potential virulence factors of S. *aureus* to be discussed in this chapter. S. *epidermidis* can also gain access to the blood and tissues when the skin is broken. Once established in damaged or prosthetic heart valves (Keys and Hewitt, 1973) or atrioventricular shunts (Shurtleff *et al.*, 1974; Morrice and Young, 1974; Schoenbaum *et al.*, 1975), it is difficult to eradicate, and systemic symptoms develop which can be related to immune complex disease (Dobrin *et al.*, 1975).

2. Armament of *Staphylococcus aureus*

2.1. Cell Wall

The cell wall of S. *aureus* plays a major role in host response to this bacterium. Peptidoglycan gives the cell wall rigidity and elicits numerous effects in the host. Teichoic acids are at least in part responsible for the antigenic specificity of staphylococci (Oeding and Grov,

JAN VERHOEF, PHILLIP K. PETERSON, and PAUL G. QUIE • Departments of Pediatrics and Medicine, University of Minnesota School of Medicine, Minneapolis, Minnesota 55455.

TABLE 1. Potential Virulence Factors of
Staphylococcus aureus

Virulence factors	Proposed effect or mechanism of action
Cell surface components	
Peptidoglycan	Inhibition of leukocyte migration; complement activation (endotoxinlike properties); dermonecrosis (induction of delayed-type hypersensitivity)
Protein A	Interference with opsonization
Capsular material	Interference with opsonization
Extracellular products	
Coagulase	Inhibition of phagocytosis (?)
Catalase	Inhibition of intraleukocytic killing
Enterotoxin	Gastrointestinal disturbance
Epidermolytic toxin	Exfoliative skin lesions
Leukocidin	Cytotoxic, leukotoxic
α-Hemolysin	Leukotoxic, induces dermonecrosis
Genotypic changes	Antimicrobial resistance, change in antigenic structure
Phenotypic variability	Bacterial persistence (L forms)
Ability to survive within phagocytic cells	

1972; Oeding, 1974). Protein A, present in the cell walls of most *S. aureus* strains, combines with immunoglobulins in a unique fashion (Forsgren and Sjöquist, 1966) and may have important biological significance (Forsgren and Nordstrom, 1974). Other cell wall components which influence the immune response include agglutinogens, precipitinogens, and capsular antigens.

The basic structure of the cell wall of staphylococci is provided by its peptidoglycan component, which consists of glycan strands of alternating β-1,4-glycosidically linked *N*-acetylglucosamine and *N*-acetylmuramic acid residues attached to a tetrapeptide of alternating L- and D-amino acids through the carboxyl group of muramic acids, the peptide units being connected to pentaglycine bridges (Sal-

ton, 1964). There is evidence to suggest that the peptide component is not exposed to the cell surface and thereby has no antigenic activity (Morse, 1965). Many strains of *S. aureus* have a cell wall peptidoglycan which has been associated with pathogenicity (Hill, 1968; van der Vijver *et al.*, 1975). When injected intradermally in animals, this cell wall "aggressin" inhibits both edema production and migration of leukocytes, allowing bacteria to multiply freely and to produce necropurulent lesions. *S. aureus* peptidoglycan has also been demonstrated to possess endotoxinlike properties (Rotta, 1975), to activate both the classical and alternative pathways of the serum complement system (Pryjma *et al.*, 1976), and to elicit a cell-mediated immune response (Targowski and Berman, 1975).

Teichoic acids are charged polymers composed of repeating units containing either ribitol or glycerol phosphate linked through phosphodiester groups (Baddiley *et al.*, 1961; Archibald, 1972; Schleifer, 1973). Most teichoic acids also contain glycosyl and D-alanyl groups covalently linked to the peptidoglycan through muramic acid phosphate (Liu and Gotschlich, 1967). Most *S. aureus* strains contain glucosaminyl ribitol teichoic acid (Archibald, 1972), which is part of the phage receptor and is decisive for phage inactivation (Coyette and Ghuysen, 1968; Chatterjee, 1969). *S. epidermidis* strains usually have glycerol teichoic acids with glucosyl residues in their cell walls (Morse, 1963; Davison and Baddiley, 1963; Johnsen *et al.*, 1975).

The teichoic acids are responsible in large measure for the serological specificity of staphylococci (Oeding, 1974). Teichoic acid antibodies are highly specific, and high titers of antibodies have been found in patients with recent staphylococcal infections (Crowder and White, 1972). This antibody assay is being explored as a serological diagnostic tool. The teichoic acid preparations used in these assays are not pure and contain at least traces of peptidoglycan. It is therefore possible that antibodies found in this assay are directed toward both peptidoglycan and teichoic acid.

Agglutination of staphylococci by specific antiserum has been studied in an attempt to differentiate pathogenic from nonpathogenic staphylococci. Staphylococci have group agglutinogens shared by all or by the majority of strains and type-specific antigens present in only a limited number of strains (Oeding, 1967; Haukenes, 1967). All of the agglutinogens present in *S. aureus* have been demonstrated in isolated cell walls (Grov and Rude, 1967), but little is known of their exact chemical nature.

Forty-five years ago, Gilbert (1931) isolated an encapsulated strain of *S. aureus* from patients; subsequently many *S. aureus* strains were found to produce a capsule or capsular antigens when cultured under special conditions (Cohn and Morse, 1959; Sall *et al.*, 1960; Wiley, 1972). Wiley and Maverakis (1974) found that 43% of 109 blood donors carried *S. aureus* in their anterior nares, and 44.7% of these naturally occurring strains were encapsulated. Yoshida *et al.* (1974) reported that a large majority of *S. aureus* strains (82 out of 91 tested) were able to produce capsular material at some point during their growth and that *S. aureus* may have a life cycle *in vivo* which includes encapsulated and pseudoencapsulated forms.

At least five different serological types of staphylococcal capsular antigens have been identified (Yoshida, 1971; Yoshida *et al.*, 1974). This material consists of aminoglucuronic acid and *N*-acetyl-L-alanine, which is the immunodeterminant group (Hanessian and Haskell, 1964; Karakawa and Kane, 1975). Conjugates of *N*-acetyl-L-alanine coupled to bovine serum albumin result in a significant precipitin reaction when added to serum containing IgG antibodies against staphylococci.

Although there has been no definite correlation between encapsulation and pathogenicity, several indirect lines of evidence support this possibility. Most adult human sera contain heat-stable opsonins directed against encapsulated staphylococci, suggesting prior exposure to the capsular antigens (Wiley, 1963). Encapsulated strains isolated from infected patients are highly virulent to mice, and when capsules are lost on subculture the strains lose their virulence for mice (Koenig, 1962; Koenig *et al.*, 1962; Wiley and Maverakis, 1968; Yoshida and Takeuchi, 1970; Melly *et al.*, 1974). Staphylococcal capsules are antiphagocytic; opsonization of encapsulated strains requires both heat-stable and heat-labile serum factors (Morse, 1960; Melly *et al.*, 1974). Recent work in our laboratory has demonstrated that encapsulation of *S. aureus* interferes with phagocytosis by inhibiting opsonization both by heat-stable serum factors and by heat-labile factors of the serum complement system (unpublished data).

In 1958, Jensen reported the presence of an *S. aureus* antigen which reacted with sera from 400 individuals in a gel double diffusion test. This antigen was subsequently shown to be a protein (Löfkvist and Sjöquist, 1962) and was called protein A. In addition to human sera, activity against this protein has been found in the sera of a wide variety of animal species (Lind *et al.*, 1970).

Protein A is present in over 90% of *S. aureus* strains but in only 2% of *S. epidermidis* strains (Forsgren, 1970). Kronvall *et al.* (1971) were unable to find a correlation between the staphylococcal phage type or serological type and the presence or absence of protein A. Lind (1972) reported that strains resistant to neomycin also produced large amounts of protein A, whereas those resistant to methicillin produced little or no protein A. Within phage groups I and II the ability to produce large amounts of protein A was found to correlate with a deficiency in hemolysin production.

Forsgren (1969) found that protein A composed 0.9% of the dry weight of *S. aureus*. Approximately 30% of the protein A produced by the *S. aureus* Cowan I strain was released into the medium during the logarithmic phase of growth. Physiochemical studies have recently revealed its molecular weight to be 42,000 (Bjork *et al.*, 1972). Protein A is covalently linked to the peptidoglycan component of the cell wall (Sjöquist, 1973). The syntheses of protein A and the peptidoglycan appear to take place independently of each other (Movitz, 1974). According to Kronvall *et al.* (1970), the Cowan I strain, which is known to be rich in protein A, has an estimated 80,000 protein A residues per bacterium.

A number of methods for the extraction (Forsgren and Sjöquist, 1966; Sjöquist *et al.*, 1972; Sjöquist, 1973) and identification (Lind *et al.*, 1970; Lind, 1973; Winblad and Ericson, 1973) of protein A have been developed.

In 1966 Forsgren and Sjöquist reported that protein A appeared to react with IgG at its Fc fragment and not through the Fab combining site, which is the case for more classical antigen–antibody reactions. This was termed a "pseudoimmune reaction." They found that protein A was capable of precipitating 45% of a pooled γ-globulin preparation. It seemed unlikely that such a large percentage of pooled immunoglobulin contained antibodies specific for this protein. Furthermore, it was found that seven out of ten IgG preparations from patients with multiple myeloma showed precipitation lines in gel diffusion against protein A. Again, it seemed reasonable to assume that these myeloma immunoglobulins did not contain antibodies directed specifically against protein A and that the reaction of protein A with IgG was not a true antigen–antibody reaction. In further experiments using papain-induced fragments of IgG, protein A was found to be more strongly bound to the Fc and F'c fragments than to the Fab fragments.

Kronvall and Williams (1969) found that the anti-protein A reactivity of serum is confined to the IgG1, IgG2, and IgG4 subclasses. The IgG3 subclass lacks this reactivity. Recently a reactive site for protein A has been demonstrated in the Fc region of immunoglobulins of the IgM class (Grov, 1975).

Recent work indicates that a combining site for protein A also exists on $F(ab')_2$ fragments of IgG obtained from rabbits immunized with protein A (Kronvall and Williams, 1971; Lind and Mansa, 1974). Therefore, protein A can combine with IgG with immunological specificity, as well as in an "immunologically nonspecific" fashion.

Sjöquist and Stålenheim (1969) showed that protein A had anticomplementary properties as a result of the formation of protein A–IgG complexes. Protein A–IgG aggregates resembled antigen–antibody complexes in that complement components were depleted on addition of these aggregates to human serum (Stålenheim et al., 1973). Both the classical and alternate pathways were found to be activated. Somewhat paradoxically, protein A was also found to be capable of inhibiting the Cl binding activity of heat-aggregated IgG and immune complexes of guinea pig IgG2. Protein A in this context presumably occupied a site on the Fc region of IgG sufficiently close to the C1 binding site to prevent C1 fixation. It was suggested that in order for complement activation to occur, very large, conformationally different complexes of protein A are necessary which leave Fc sites available for complement fixation.

Dossett et al. (1969) and Forsgren and Quie (1974a) have reported that protein A is antiphagocytic in vitro. These results were obtained when both isolated IgG and fresh serum served as the opsonic source. Their results were consistent with the binding of the Fc portion of opsonic antibody by protein A and of the anticomplementary action of protein A.

Forsgren and Quie (1974a) reported that protein A was not toxic for phagocytic cells but rather inhibited phagocytosis through its effect on opsonins. At high concentrations of protein A (500 μg/ml), however, there was little complement inactivation and likewise there was little inhibition of serum opsonic activity. This finding was compatible with the observations of Stålenheim et al. (1973) that when excess protein A was present the Fc part of IgG molecules was not available for C1 fixation, but at lower concentrations large conformationally different complexes were formed and complement fixation occurred. Considerations with respect to protein A concentration might explain the results of Shayegani et al. (1970), who failed to demonstrate any antiphagocytic effect of protein A. Recently, it has been reported that protein-A-containing staphylococcal strains are efficiently opsonized in agammaglobulinemic serum and that purified protein A reduces the opsonic capacity of this serum (Peterson et al., 1977a). On the basis of these findings it has been hypothesized that when IgG is not present in the opsonic medium, cell wall protein A is capable of activating complement at the bacterial surface and thereby opsonization is promoted.

In the presence of human serum, protein A has been found to be highly chemotactic for human polymorphonuclear leukocytes (Harvey et al., 1970). Laudable pus in staphylococcal infections might thus be the result of activation of chemotactic complement components generated by the reaction between protein A and immunoglobulins.

Nonimmunized guinea pigs develop local reactions and systemic anaphylaxis after the injection of protein A. When protein A is injected into the skin after intravenous administration of human IgG (Gustafson et al., 1968), an Arthus reaction develops. Preformed protein A human IgG aggregates also elicit an Arthus-type reaction in nonimmunized rabbits. These *in vivo* effects of protein A are not of a toxic nature but result from the reaction between protein A and IgG. Certain reactions appear to be mediated in part through histamine or a similar substance, since they may be blocked by antihistamine drugs.

Mouse LD_{50} studies using protein-A-deficient mutants have indicated that protein A does not by itself account for the virulence of staphylococci (Forsgren, 1973). Virulence undoubtedly depends on several potential pathogenicity factors, including protein A, coagulase, nuclease, fibrinolysin, and α-hemolysin.

Protein A has become an important immunological and diagnostic tool because of its unique capacity to bind the Fc fragment of IgG. This agent has been used to identify surface IgG determinants of lymphocytes (Ghetie *et al.*, 1974; Dorval *et al.*, 1974) as a specific B-lymphocyte mitogen (Forsgren *et al.*, 1976), for the serotyping of streptococci (Christensen *et al.*, 1973), in a serological test for rubella infection (Ankerst *et al.*, 1974), and as an aid in the diagnosis of meningococcal meningitis (Olcen *et al.*, 1975) and gonococcal infection (Christensen *et al.*, 1976).

2.2. Extracellular Products of *Staphylococcus aureus*

Many *S. aureus* strains produce a large number of extracellular, enzymatically active factors believed to have biological effects with significant consequences for the host (Anderson, 1974; van der Vijver *et al.*, 1975; Wadstrom *et al.*, 1974). One of these factors, coagulase, is used as a major means of separating the genus *Staphylococcus* into the species *S. aureus*, which is coagulase positive, and the species *S. epidermidis*, which is coagulase negative. However, the role of coagulase *per se* as a virulence factor has not been established. Hale and Smith (1945) suggested that coagulase production protected staphylococci from phagocytosis. Coagulase-positive staphylococci were poorly phagocytosed when suspended in citrated blood containing fibrinogen but were rapidly phagocytosed in defibrinated blood. Coagulase-negative staphylococci were phagocytosed by polymorphonuclear leuko-

cytes with equal avidity whether suspended in defibrinated or in citrated blood. It was believed that coagulase formed a shield of fibrin around the bacteria which inhibited phagocytosis. These results have been disputed (Cawdery *et al.*, 1969).

At least seven antigenically distinct coagulases have been demonstrated, and antibodies specific for these antigens have been shown to exist (Zen-Yoji *et al.*, 1961). However, antibodies against coagulase apparently do not play a role in host defense against staphylococcal disease (Cybulska and Jeljaszewicz, 1966).

Almost all *S. aureus* strains produce hyaluronidase (Abramson and Friedman, 1967). The importance of this enzyme in terms of pathogenicity is unknown. Schmidt (1966) demonstrated that whereas no antihyaluronidase was present in healthy individuals, 22.4% of patients with mastitis had this antibody. Abramson (1974) has been able to distinguish three molecular forms of this enzyme which correlate with the type of staphylococcal infection. Strains isolated from respiratory tract infections produce hyaluronidase isoenzyme group I, strains from furuncles, abscesses, and wound infections produce isoenzyme group II, and bacteremic and endocarditis isolates produce isoenzyme group III.

Catalase, which converts hydrogen peroxide into water and oxygen, is another enzyme produced by all *S. aureus* strains. Mandell (1975) has suggested that this enzyme might protect ingested staphylococci from the lethal effects of hydrogen peroxide produced by phagocytes. There was good correlation between catalase production and lethality of *S. aureus* for mice.

Approximately one-third of clinical isolates of *S. aureus* strains produce a toxin capable of causing food poisoning (Casman, 1965), characterized by vomiting and diarrhea developing 1–6 hr after ingestion of food containing staphylococcal enterotoxin (Dack, 1956). Five different enterotoxins have been identified (Bergdoll, 1972). These toxins consist of single polypeptide chains containing relatively large amounts of lysine, tyrosine, and aspartic and glutamic acids.

It is believed that enterotoxin enters the circulation via the digestive tract in an unchanged state. Since antibodies to the enterotoxins develop after systemic staphylococcal infection (Jozefczyk, 1974), it might be assumed that the development of resistance to their effects would follow the formation of significant antibody levels. Indeed, animals have been shown to become resistant to the effects of the toxin after repeated oral doses (Bergdoll, 1972).

Recently, enterotoxin B has been found to be mitogenic for thymus-dependent lymphocytes in *in vitro* cultures of human spleen cells (Paevy *et al.*, 1970). The significance of this observation in terms of pathogenesis is not known.

A disease caused by an epidermolytic toxin produced by staphylococci was originally described by Ritter Von Rittershain in 1878 as a bullous exfoliative disease occurring in newborn infants. Twenty years later, Winternitz linked Ritter's disease to infections with *S. aureus* (see Melish *et al.*, 1974). Following the advent of staphylococcal phage typing, it was discovered that only strains belonging to phage group II were associated with Ritter's disease (Gillespie *et al.*, 1957; Benson *et al.*, 1962). In 1967, Lyell described a similar syndrome in adults. It has since been established that two types of toxic epidermal necrolysis exist: (1) a syndrome associated with staphylococcal epidermolytic toxin which occurs primarily in infants and (2) a syndrome with similar clinical manifestation but related to multiple etiologies (drugs, viral infection, etc.) which occurs in older children and adults.

The staphylococcal epidermolytic toxin has been separated from γ- and β-hemolysins by isoelectric focusing and has been shown to have a molecular weight of 30,000. Warren *et al.* (1975) have shown that staphylococci no longer produce exfoliative toxin after treatment with ethidium bromide, suggesting that an extrachromosomal gene is responsible for its production.

Melish *et al.* (1974), Kapral and Miller (1971), and Arbuthnott *et al.* (1971, 1972) have developed animal models for studying the epidermolytic toxin of staphylococci. When neonatal mice less than 6 days old were injected with a tenfold dilution of the lethal dose of toxin, exfoliation of the skin developed 16–20 hr later. All the strains isolated from patients with the staphylococcal "scaled skin

syndrome" were able to produce epidermolysis in neonatal mice.

Host factors which contribute to the clinical manifestations of epidermolytic toxin include intrinsic characteristics of the skin and general antistaphylococcal and antitoxic immunity (Lyell, 1967). Easmon and Glynn (1975) showed that repeated staphylococcal infections in mice protected against dermonecrosis by virulent strains. This protection was antibody mediated. Also, the third and fifth components of complement appear to play an important role. Mice deficient in C5 are more susceptible to *S. aureus* skin infection, and C3 depletion enhances staphylococcal virulence. A 54-year-old patient with chronic renal failure and staphylococcal toxic epidermal necrosis has been described (Reid *et al.*, 1974). It is possible that an immunological defect contributed to this adult's development of the syndrome since the patient had a deficiency in cell-mediated immunity. Wiley *et al.* (1974) were able to produce staphylococcal scalded skin syndrome in adult mice by immunosuppression. Of the ten adult patients with staphylococcal scalded skin syndrome reported in the literature, the majority have had underlying conditions known to adversely affect host defense against staphylococcal infections (Peterson *et al.*, 1977b).

Another extracellular product produced by *S. aureus* that might have a role in pathogenicity is leukocidin, which has been shown to be cytotoxic for human and rabbit polymorphonuclear leukocytes (Woodin, 1972). Treatment of leukocytes with leukocidin results in permeability of the cell membrane to cations. However, the role of staphylococcal leukocidin in staphylococcal virulence remains unclear (Jeljaszewicz *et al.*, 1976). Also, α-hemolysin (Jeljaszewicz, 1972) and β-hemolysin (Jeljaszewicz, 1972) have been proposed as staphylococcal virulence factors. α-Hemolysin may play a role in the dermonecrosis of skin after intradermal injection of staphylococci (Easmon and Glynn, 1976). α-Hemolysin decreases ATP synthesis in mitochondria of leukocytes, resulting in a loss of lysozyme and acid phosphatase activity. This toxin also appears to damage lysosomes, an effect that is much less pronounced with β-hemolysin. Deoxyribonuclease (Abramson, 1972), exolipases (Abramson, 1972), lysozyme (Abramson, 1972), and staphylokinase (Quie and Wannamaker, 1962) may also play roles as staphylococcal virulence factors.

2.3. Genotypic and Phenotypic Variability

The staphylococcus is a tremendously adaptable microbe capable of rapidly changing its phenotypic and genotypic characteristics (see Mudd, 1970). The development of staphylococcal resistance to many major antimicrobial agents is an example of this adaptability. The staphylococcus can present a different "face" to the host by changing its antigenic structure and opsonic requirements; subsequently, phagocytosis is less efficient and the healing process is consequently delayed (see Ekstedt, 1974).

Genotypic variability of *S. aureus* has been shown to occur through mutation, transduction, or transformation (see Hayes, 1968). Genotypic change is especially important in the development of resistance to antibiotics (Novick, 1969; Lacey and Richmond, 1974). Many of the genes responsible for the resistance of staphylococci to antimicrobial agents are carried by plasmids (extrachromosomal circular DNA molecules). When a mutation occurs *in vivo* or the genotype of the bacterium changes by the acceptance of a new plasmid, growth under the prevailing conditions of the host may be improved, e.g., by inactivation of a therapeutic agent or by change in antigenic structure or both (Jagicza, 1973). The mutant can thereby escape the effects of therapeutic agents and evade the host's existing immunological defenses. Such mutants eventually become the predominant bacterial population. Mutation inhibitors such as atabrine have been demonstrated to reduce emergence of antibiotic resistance (Sevag, 1964).

During transformation, exogenous DNA is taken up directly and integrated into chromosomal structures (Rudin *et al.*, 1974). During the process of transduction, genetic material (e.g., a plasmid) is transported to a new bacterial cell by a bacteriophage. Winkler *et al.* (1965) showed that lysogenization with serological group F phages resulted in the loss of β-hemolysin production, suggesting that staphylococcal toxin production may be phage related. In spite of the fact that most staphylococci are equipped with specific endonucleases—enzymes which can degrade foreign DNA (Verhoef *et al.*, 1972)—transduction and subsequent selection of resistant organisms play an important role in the emergence of resistant strains (Lacey and Richmond, 1974).

Genetic changes in the staphylococcus have been shown to alter the bacterial growth rate and bacterial cell surfaces (Lacy and Chopra, 1975). Such altered staphylococcal strains were found to be significantly less virulent for 10-day chick embryos than for the corresponding parent cultures.

Staphylococci also have variable phenotypic characteristics. Cell wall structure and virulence may vary according to the environment in which the bacteria are grown (Archibald, 1972; Gladstone *et al.*, 1974). Staphylococci cultured in hypertonic media, or in media containing penicillin, a cell-wall-inhibiting drug, grow as small protoplasmic bodies without cell walls and are called L forms (Kagan, 1972). L forms may revert to parent bacterial morphology when the inhibiting conditions are withdrawn, or they may persist as stable L forms. It has been suggested that L forms may play a role in bacterial persistence during antibiotic therapy, or they may be responsible for relapse after therapy. However, the clinical importance of L forms has not been established. In several studies the virulence of L forms was found to be greatly reduced compared to that of the parent strain (Linnemann *et al.*, 1973; Watanakunakorn and Bakie, 1974).

Under certain growth conditions, dwarf colony forms (G variants) of staphylococci can be isolated. These variants are occasionally recovered from infected patients (Quie, 1969). The basis for this phenotypic change and the role of such bacterial forms in pathogenesis are unclear.

3. Armament of the Host

As stated previously, the skin and mucous membrane barriers are of primary importance in host defense against staphylococcal disease. But this exterior does not function as a simple armor, for it is, in fact, colonized with bacteria. By allowing a normal skin flora to prosper, a phenomenon called "bacterial interference'' ensues which can contribute indirectly but significantly toward host defense.

The phenomenon of bacterial interference based on the ability of one strain to interfere with the growth of a second strain has been applied clinically. A relatively benign commensal strain was established on the skin to prevent colonization by virulent or antibiotic-resistant strains. An *S. aureus* strain of relatively low pathogenicity (502A) was found capable of establishing itself in the anterior nares and umbilicus of babies (see Shinefield *et al.,* 1972, 1974). This artificial colonization with strain 502A offered a high degree of protection against subsequent acquisition and infection by other staphylococcal strains in nurseries with outbreaks of *S. aureus* infection.

The mechanisms of interaction between bacterial species are complex and are incompletely understood. Some investigators suggest that interference is mediated through nutrient exhaustion by the interfering strain and subsequent inhibition of growth of the challenging strain (Ribble and Shinefield, 1967). Many strains belonging to the family of Micrococcaceae possess strong antagonistic properties against *S. aureus in vitro* (Pulverer and Jeljaszewicz, 1976). It is conceivable that these micrococcins play an important role in the ecology of the skin. Many individuals produce skin surface lipids that are antimicrobial to *S. aureus* (Aly *et al.,* 1976). The indigenous skin flora are also influenced by the pH of the skin and mucous membranes and by antibodies, tissue macrophages, and neutrophils (McCabe, 1968). McCabe (1968) has proposed that host defense mechanisms may also play an important role in the phenomenon of interference.

3.1. Phagocytic Defense against Staphylococci

Once the outer barriers have been breached, phagocytosis and intracellular killing of the staphylococcus represent the major line of host defense. Both a sufficient number and adequate function of phagocytes are essential for the eradication of invading organisms. The monocyte and fixed tissue phagocytes, as well as the polymorphonuclear leukocytes, play significant roles in this regard.

In 1904, Wright and Douglas observed that serum was essential for effective phagocytosis

by human polymorphonculear leukocytes. They introduced the concept that both heat-stable and heat-labile humoral factors in serum were essential for efficient phagocytosis of staphylococci. Many years later these findings were confirmed when Cohn and Morse (1959) and Rogers and Melly (1960) described the opsonic requirements for the encapsulated Smith strains of staphylococci. A thermostable phagocytosis-promoting factor was found to be present in all of the eight normal adult sera tested. Sera from rabbits immunized with the Smith strain greatly enhanced phagocytosis of this strain.

Studies by Laxdal *et al.* (1968) and Messner *et al.* (1968) indicated that patients with subacute bacterial endocarditis have high titers of heat-stable opsonins, which belong to the IgG class of immunoglobulins. The addition of factors which block the Fc fragments of IgG, such as anti-γ-globulin factors (rheumatoid factor) and staphylococcal protein A, significantly diminished the opsonic properties of these immunoglobulins. In addition, using several methods which degrade or alter the Fc fragment of IgG, they abolished opsonic activity (Quie *et al.,* 1968). These findings suggest that antibody molecules act as ligands binding bacteria and phagocytic cells. The Fab part of the antibody molecule attaches with immunological specificity to the antigenic surface of the bacterium and the Fc portion attaches to receptors on the phagocyte surface.

The heat-labile opsonic factors for staphylococci have received considerable attention. Li and Mudd (1965) demonstrated that guinea pig complement restored effective phagocytosis of *S. aureus* in heated serum. Furthermore, if serum was treated in a manner that inactivated C3 or C4, *S. aureus* phagocytosis was greatly reduced. The heat-labile opsonic factors in human serum were also found to be components of the hemolytic complement system.

Although opsonization with heat-labile factors is primarily mediated through activation of complement via IgG at the bacterial cell surface, thermolabile components may become fixed to microorganisms without the participation of antibody (Hirsch, 1964). Laxdal *et al.* (1968) showed that heat-labile opsonic factors, prepared by adsorbing human serum with *S. aureus* to remove IgG from the serum, continued to promote phagocytosis of the homologous staphylococcal strain. Normal opsonic activity has also been reported in serum from patients with agammaglobulinemia (Williams and Quie, 1971; Verhoef et al., 1977a). In conflict with these studies, however, is the finding of Humphreys et al. (1974) that adsorption of normal human serum with S. aureus at 4°C resulted in a significant decrease in IgG levels and completely eliminated opsonic activity. Complement levels (C3 and C4) were not significantly changed by the adsorption procedure.

In order to determine which complement pathway(s) is important for opsonization of S. aureus, Forsgren and Quie (1974b) blocked the classical complement pathway by chelating calcium ions with ethylene glycol tetraacetic acid. Under these conditions, the alternate pathway of complement activation remains intact, and such chelated serum is an excellent opsonin for several bacterial species. Two S. aureus strains, however, were not opsonized by chelated serum, which suggested that the classical pathway was essential for effective opsonization of this bacterial species. In earlier studies Jasin (1972) noted that complement activation by a protein-A-deficient S. aureus strain was mediated via the alternate pathway. Johnson et al. (1972) also found normal opsonic activity for staphylococci in serum from a patient with a deficiency in the second complement component, suggesting that the classical complement pathway may not be essential for opsonization of S. aureus. It is possible that these discrepant findings reflect a heterogeneity of opsonic requirements among different strains of S. aureus. Indeed, strains of S. aureus capable of activating the alternate pathway have been identified in this laboratory (Verhoef et al., 1977a). Polymorphonuclear leukocyte receptors with specificity for C3b have been described (Lay and Nussenzweig, 1968; Scribner and Fahrney, 1976), and recent evidence suggests that these receptors play a major role in phagocytosis of staphylococci opsonized in normal serum (Verhoef et al., 1977b).

The opsonic requirements of S. epidermidis are not clearly established. Although a report by Miller and Beck (1975) suggested that neither antibody nor complement is needed for opsonization of S. epidermidis, other investigators have reported that both heat-stable and heat-labile serum factors promote phagocytosis of this bacterium (Laxdal et al., 1968; Williams and Quie, 1971; Forsgren and Quie, 1974a; Verhoef et al., 1977a). Of interest, S. epidermidis shunt nephritis, due to chronic colonization of ventriculoatrial shunts or infection of damaged heart valves by S. epidermidis, has been reported to involve the deposition of early complement components, immunoglobulin, and S. epidermidis antigens in the form of immune complexes within the renal glomeruli (Dobrin et al., 1975).

After being phagocytosed, most intracellular staphylococci are rapidly killed and degraded within phagocytic vacuoles. Staphylococci are not facultative intracellular organisms, such as Mycobacterium tuberculosis; however, a small percentage of phagocytosed S. aureus survive within leukocytes for prolonged periods of time (Kapral and Shayegani, 1959; Melly et al., 1960). This incomplete killing of S. aureus contrasts with the rapid complete killing of other pyogenic organisms, such as pneumococci and streptococci (Mudd, 1970). Staphylococci may outlive the cells which have ingested them, and later multiply extracellularly. This may in part explain the chronicity of staphylococcal infections (Mudd, 1970).

Although the data are conflicting, opsonins may influence the intracellular fate of staphylococci, as well as aiding phagocytosis per se. Li et al. (1963) found increased intracellular killing in the presence of heat-labile factors; inactivation of serum complement by several means led to enhanced intracellular survival (Li and Mudd, 1965). Other investigators have not been able to confirm an enhancement of intraleukocytic staphylococcal killing by serum opsonins (Downey and Kejima, 1967; Hawiger et al., 1969).

3.2. Defects in Phagocytic Defense

Abnormal phagocytosis resulting from a deficiency in heat-labile opsonic activity of serum has been described in several clinical situations. Alper et al. (1970) reported two patients with C3 deficiency who suffered recurrent episodes of sepsis and cutaneous infections. S. aureus was a frequent cause of infection in these patients. Two infants with C5 deficiency and staphylococcal infection have been described by Miller *et al.* (1969). Immunochemical evaluation revealed normal levels of C5; however, C5 was found to be biologically inactive. Although reports of patients with recurrent episodes of respiratory tract infections and C2 deficiency have appeared (Friend *et al.*, 1975) and serum opsonizing activity for *S. aureus* 502A was demonstrated to be deficient, significant staphylococcal infection has not been reported in patients with C2 deficiency.

Heat-stable opsonins are diminished in patients with primary agammaglobulinemia and immune deficiency associated with certain lymphoreticular malignancies, disorders in which recurrrent infection is a serious problem. As noted previously, Williams and Quie (1971) found that serum from patients with agammaglobulinemia somewhat surprisingly had opsonic activity for staphylococci.

A number of clinical entities have been described in which a defective staphylocidal function of leukocytes has been found (see Table 2). The first clinical syndrome in which the pathogenesis of disease was clearly shown to be associated with defective bactericidal function of polymorphonuclear leukocytes was chronic granulomatous disease (Quie *et al.*, 1967). Chronic granulomatous disease is a phagocytic cell defect inherited primarily as an X-linked recessive trait; autosomal recessive inheritance has also been described (Quie *et al.*, 1974). In patients with this disease the staphylococcus is the most frequent pathogen (Lazarus and Neu, 1975); staphylococcal infections are both frequent and severe.

Leukocytes from patients with chronic granulomatous disease do not respond normally to phagocytosis with an increase in oxygen uptake. There is therefore little shift in metabolism to the hexose monophosphate shunt, and hydrogen peroxide does not accumulate in the phagocytic vacuoles. Organisms which pro-

**TABLE 2. Conditions with Defective
Leukocyte Staphylocidal Activity**

1. Chronic granulomatous disease
2. Myeloperoxidase deficiency
3. Chediak–Higashi syndrome
4. Lipochrome histiocytosis
5. Ataxia telangiectasia
6. Cryoglobulinemia
7. Extremely severe bacterial infections

**TABLE 3. Conditions with Defective
Leukotaxis**

1. Diabetes mellitus
2. Lazy leukocyte syndrome
3. Chediak–Higashi syndrome
4. Rheumatoid arthritis
5. Extremely severe bacterial infection
6. Elevated IgE immunoglobulins
7. Job's syndrome
8. Wiskott–Aldrich syndrome
9. Down's syndrome
10. Measles

duce their own hydrogen peroxide, however, do not survive within this intraleukocyte environment. *S. aureus* produces catalase, an enzyme that breaks down hydrogen peroxide, and it is thus well equipped for prolonged survival in such leukocytes with defective hydrogen-peroxide-producing capacity.

Patients with leukemia and patients on cytotoxic chemotherapy may have both qualitative and quantitative leukocyte defects, and staphylococcal infections are serious and recurrent in such patients. Diminished intracellular killing capacity of ingested *S. aureus* has been reported in leukocytes from patients with lymphoblastic leukemia (Thompson and Williams, 1974), and defects in both phagocytosis and killing of *S. aureus* were found in leukocytes from patients with acute and chronic myelocytic leukemia (Goldman and Th'ng, 1973; Koch, 1975).

The role of leukotaxis (directional locomotion of leukocytes toward an inflammatory site) in host defense against staphylococci is not clearly understood. A number of conditions with defective leukotaxis have been reported (see Table 3), and recurrent staphylococcal infections have been associated with such defects. One such association has been found in patients with elevated serum IgE levels. Buckley *et al.* (1972) reported two adolescent males with IgE levels greater than 5000 ng/ml and recurrent severe abscesses due to *S. aureus*. Clark *et al.* (1973), have described an 11-year-old female with a similar condition. More recently, Hill and Quie (1974) reported three such patients with severe eczema early in life followed by recurrent, severe infections. Hill *et al.* (1974) have also demonstrated defective neutrophil chemotaxis in a group of female patients with recurrent cold staphylococcal abscesses and chronic eczema (Job's syndrome). The decreased leukotactic responsiveness of these patients was not related to a direct effect of the high concentrations of IgE, since the serum from these patients did not impair the chemotactic activity of control leukocytes. It is postulated that histamine and histamine-induced cyclic adenosine monophosphate may accumulate within the neutrophils of these patients and depress chemotactic responsiveness.

3.3. Acquired Immunity to Staphylococci

Koenig *et al.* (1962) were able to demonstrate a clear distinction between antibacterial and antitoxic immunity to *S. aureus*. Mice which had been immunized by repeated subcutaneous injections of crude α toxoid were completely resistant to challenge with α toxin, but there was no protective effect against infection after challenge with whole organisms. In contrast, animals immunized by repeated intravenous injection of a heat-killed whole cell vaccine were highly resistant to challenge with viable organisms but were as susceptible as normal mice to challenge with α toxin. Although a considerable literature dealing with various aspects of antitoxic immunity has emerged (see Ekstedt, 1972), the importance of specific antibodies directed against any of the extracellular products of *S. aureus* for protection against staphylococcal infection has not been established.

The serum of rabbits immunized with live staphylococci has enhanced opsonic activity, and such vaccination provides complete protection against reinfection (Brodie *et al.*, 1958). This protection was found to be type specific, i.e., *S. aureus* Cowan I vaccinated animals were not protected against Cowan III. Greenberg and Cooper (1960) and Greenberg *et al.* (1961) developed a vaccine using a mixture of bacterial lysates obtained from four different phage groups of *S. aureus*. These lysates gave a high degree of protection in rabbits, and a good correlation was found between serum agglutinin titers and protection.

Similarly, capsular antigens appear to provide a protective effect when used as a vaccine against infection with encapsulated strains of *S. aureus*. Fisher (1960) and Morse (1962) iso-

lated antigens from supernatants of cultures of the encapsulated Smith strain, which were termed "Smith surface antigen" and "Smith polysaccharide antigen." When antisera against whole cells were adsorbed with Smith surface antigen or Smith polysaccharide antigen, the agglutinating and opsonizing titers were significantly reduced, suggesting that opsonic antibodies to these bacterial antigens may be protective. However, the purity of these antigen preparations has been questioned. Ekstedt (1963a,b; 1972) has found that supernatants of cultures from encapsulated *S. aureus* Smith contained teichoic acid and protein A, as well as a polysaccharide and other antigens, so the precise target of protective antibody is uncertain.

A primary role of teichoic acid antibodies in the development of humoral immunity to *S. aureus* has been suggested. From the results of their experiments, Mudd *et al.* (1963) concluded that sera adsorbed with teichoic acid had decreased heat-stable opsonic activity. Wysokinska (1973) reported that when teichoic acid was used as a vaccine there was protection against heterologous strains of *S. aureus*. Immune sera prepared from animals vaccinated with teichoic acid protected nonvaccinated animals when challenged with *S. aureus*. However, Shayegani *et al.* (1970) found that heat-stable opsonic activity of serum for *S. aureus* could not be adsorbed with *S. aureus* teichoic acid; rather, serum opsonic titers were significantly lowered after adsorption by purified peptidoglycan from the *S. aureus* cell wall. Humphreys *et al.* (1974) demonstrated that heat-stable opsonins in sera of patients infected with *S. aureus* were directed against the pentaglycine bridge of the cell wall peptidgolycan. Recent work in our laboratory measuring neutrophil uptake of [^{3}H]glycine-labeled purified cell wall components has supported the view that the peptidoglycan is the key cell wall constituent involved in opsonization by both IgG and the classical and alternative pathways of the serum complement system (unpublished data).

It must be remembered that the great adaptibility of *S. aureus* and its ability to change its antigenic structure may allow these organisms to escape opsonization by specific antibodies and thereby efficient phagocytosis by neutrophils. Although the theoretical basis for antistaphylococcal vaccination has been provided and there has been some limited application of its principles (Greenberg and Cooper, 1960; Eisenstein *et al.*, 1968), the value of immunization and serotherapy of humans has never passed the rigors of a controlled study. The complexity of the *S. aureus* antigenic structure and its amazing versatility may account for some of the difficulties encountered with attempts to induce active immunity to staphylococci.

Some reports suggest that cell-mediated immune mechanisms may play an important role in host defense against staphylococcal infections. There is an enhanced inflammatory response in animals vaccinated with heat-killed staphylococci. This enhancement was observed in animals passively sensitized by transfer of peritoneal exudate cells but not in animals given immune serum (Kowalski and Berman, 1971; Mudd, 1971). Several investigators have described patients with recurrent staphylococcal abscesses and a severe delayed-type hypersensitivity reaction to the injection of staphylococcal antigens (Ekstedt, 1974; Mudd *et al.*, 1970; Shayegani *et al.*, 1973). The role of cellular immunity in host defense against *S. aureus* is a promising field for laboratory and clinical investigators. At present, it is difficult to judge the relative importance and the exact mechanisms by which cellular immunity is involved in staphylococcal infection.

3.4. Other Factors Influencing Host Resistance to Staphylococcus

Staphylococcal infections are in general more severe in patients at either end of the age spectrum and in patients with nutritional deficiency. Certain endocrine disorders such as hypothyroidism, adrenal insufficiency, and diabetes mellitus are associated with increased susceptibility to infection. Yotis and Fitzgerald (1974) found that the synthetic estrogen diethylstilbesterol administered in therapeutic concentrations had a significant antistaphylococcal effect *in vivo* and *in vitro*. A similar effect was produced by other gonadal hormones, and it was suggested that staphylococci have hormone receptors on their cell surface.

Antibiotic therapy may have several effects on microbes as well as on host defense mechanisms. Friedman and Warren (1974) reported that nafcillin, in subinhibitory concentrations, enhanced phagocytosis of *S. aureus* by mouse peritoneal exudate cells. Tetracyclines, on the other hand, have been shown to inhibit phagocytosis of *Escherichia coli* and yeast particles but not phagocytosis of *S. aureus* (Forsgren *et al.*, 1974). Johnston *et al.* (1975) reported that sulfisoxazole may enhance intracellular staphylococcal killing in patients with chronic granulomatous disease.

Levamisole, an antihelminthic drug, has been suggested to be an immunostimulatory agent (Editorial, *Lancet,* 1975). Fischer *et al.* (1975) have found a marked enhancement of staphylococcal killing in suckling rats treated with levamisole for 24 hr prior to bacterial challenge. Their results suggest that levamisole treatment stimulated neutrophil chemotaxis and phagocytosis. The mechanisms of action of levamisole are not known; however, it has been suggested that this drug activates phosphodiesterase, thereby leading to a reduction in intracellular cyclic AMP. Levamisole has been demonstrated to stimulate phagocytic cells by increasing cellular cyclic guanosine monophosphate.

Constantopoulos *et al.* (1972) have described two families with recurrent *S. aureus* infections. The serum of these patients had low levels of a specific leukophilic γ-globulin fraction which has been reported to stimulate phagocytosis and has been named tuftsin. The role of this serum factor is uncertain.

Larson and Blades (1976) have shown that influenza virus incubated with human neutrophils *in vitro* inhibited the phagocytosis of staphylococcus by neutrophils. They suggested that the inhibitory effect of the virus on phagocytes might be related to the high incidence and severity of staphylococcal pneumonia in patients with influenza virus infection.

The presence of a foreign body may have a profound influence on the host's ability to clear staphylococci from such an infected site. Indeed, for *S. epidermidis,* which is usually a harmless commensal, a foreign body is often essential in the pathogenesis of infection by this organism. Complete eradication is usually not possible unless the foreign body is removed.

4. Immunodiagnosis

Although the detection of antitoxin antibodies against leukocidin (Towers and Gladstone, 1958; Lack and Towers, 1962; Bänffer and Franken, 1967), hemolysin (Taylor and Plommet, 1973), and staphylokinase (Queneau *et al.*, 1972) has been used as a tool in the diagnosis of staphylococcal infection, false-positive and false-negative reactions have limited the value of some of these tests.

Using a gel diffusion method, Martin *et al.* (1966) found a significantly higher titer of teichoic acid antibodies in patients with *S. aureus* infections than in the control group. Crowder and White (1972) found that all the sera from 15 patients with *S. aureus* endocarditis showed precipitation lines after 4 or more days of infection, while none of the sera from 75 control patients showed detectable precipitins. Using the gel diffusion method, Nagel *et al.* (1975) found that 85% of patients with *S. aureus* endocarditis had positive serum precipitins against teichoic acid. A counterimmunoelectrophoresis method was found to be more sensitive (96% positive reaction) but was less specific (10% false-negative reactions). A combination of the two methods may provide the most sensitive and accurate serodiagnostic results. The value of these tests in the diagnosis of staphylococcal infections other than endocarditis has not been shown.

5. Conclusion

Considering the incredible arsenal of the staphylococcus, i.e., its plethora of toxins and other damaging extracellular products, the antiphagocytic components of its cell wall, its ability to alter its genotypic and phenotypic structure, and its capacity to survive the intraphagocytic environment, it is not surprising that this bacterial species remains a serious cause of human infection. Although marked by major triumphs, chemotherapy alone has not solved the clinical problems of serious staphylococcal infections.

The pathogenesis of staphylococcal infections remains poorly understood in spite of decades of effort. Pathogenesis, as is evident in this chapter, cannot be separated from the immunology of infection. Investigations of normal cellular and humoral response to staphylococci have provided some insight into the significant microbial and host factors in staphylococcal disease, and the study of these responses in patients with defective immunological mechanisms has been especially valuable in increasing our knowledge of host response to this bacteria. At the same time, our appreciation of staphylococcal response to the host has also grown. We have begun to understand how this organism evades host defense mechanisms and antimicrobial therapy by adaptation. Future advances in the prevention and therapy of staphylococcal disease will depend on simultaneous advances in our knowledge of the molecular biology of the microbe and the mechanisms of host defense.

ACKNOWLEDGMENTS

J. V. is supported by the Netherlands Organization for the Advancement of Pure Research (ZWO). P. K. P. is the recipient of a Bristol Research Fellowship in Infectious Diseases. P. G. Q. is American Legion Memorial Heart Research Professor of Pediatrics and Microbiology.

References

Abramson, C., 1972, Staphylococcal enzymes, in: *The Staphylococci* (J. Cohen, ed.), pp. 187–248, Wiley-Interscience, New York.

Abramson, C., 1974, Staphylococcal hyaluronidase isoenzyme profiles related to staphylococcal disease, *Ann. N.Y. Acad. Sci.* **236**:495–507.

Abramson, C., and Friedman, H., 1967, Enzymatic activity of primary isolates of staphylococci in relation to antibiotic resistance and phage type, *J. Infect. Dis.* **117**:242–248.

Alper, C. A., Abramson, N., Johnston, R. B., Jandl, J. H., and Rosen, F. S., 1970, Studies *in vivo* and *in vitro* on an abnormality in the metabolism of C3 in a patient with increased susceptibility to infection, *J. Clin. Invest.* **49**:1975–1985.

Aly, R., Maibach, H. I., Mandel, A., and Shinefield, H. R., 1976, Factors controlling the survival of *Staphylococcus aureus* on human skin, in: *Staphylococci and Staphylococcal Disease* (J. Jeljaszewicz, ed.), pp. 941–946, Fischer-Verlag, New York.

Anderson, J. C., 1974, Experimental staphylococcal mastitis in the mouse: Effects of extracellular products and whole bacterial cells from a high-virulence and a low-virulence strain of *Staphylococcus aureus, J. Med. Microbial.* **7**:205–212.

Ankerst, J., Christensen, P., Kjellen, L., and Kronvall, G., 1974. A routine diagnostic test for IgA and IgM antibodies to rubella virus: Absorption of IgG with *Staphylococcus aureus, J. Infect. Dis.* **130**:268–273.

Arbuthnott, J. P., Kent, J., Lyell, A., and Gemmell, C. G., 1971, Toxic epidermal necrolysis produced by an extracellular product of *Staphylococcus aureus, Br. J. Dermatol.* **85**:145–149.

Arbuthnott, J. P., Kent, J., Lyell, A., and Gemmell, C. G., 1972, Studies of staphylococcal toxins in relation to toxic epidermal necrolysis (the scalded skin syndrome), *Br. J. Dermatol.* **86**:35–39.

Archibald, A. R., 1972, The chemistry of staphylococcal cell walls, in: *The Staphylococci* (J. Cohen, ed.), pp. 75–110, Wiley-Interscience, New York.

Baddiley, J., Buchanan, J. G., Hardy, F. E., Martin, R. O., RajBhandary, U. L., and Sanderson, A. R., 1961, The structure of the ribitol teichoic acid of *Staphylococcus aureus* H, *Biochim. Biophys. Acta* **52**:406–407.

Bänffer, J. R. J., and Franken, J. F., 1967, Immunization with leucocidan toxoid against staphylococcal infection, *Pathol. Microbiol.* **30**:166–174.

Benson, P. F., Raulein, G. L. S., and Rippey, J. J., 1962, An outbreak of exfoliative dermatitis of the newborn (Ritter's disease) due to *Staphylococcus aureus* phagetype 55/71, *Lancet* **1**:999–1002.

Bergdoll, M. S., 1972, The entertoxins, in: *The Staphylococci* (J. Cohen, ed.), pp. 301–332, Wiley-Interscience, New York.

Bjork, I., Peterson, B. A., and Sjöquist, J., 1972, Some physicochemical properties of protein A from *Staphylococcus aureus, Eur. J. Biochem.* **29**:579–584.

Brodie, J., Guthrie, W., and Sommerville, T., 1958, An attenuated variant of *Staphylococcus aureus* with specific immunizing properties, *Br. J. Exp. Pathol.* **39**:199–202.

Buckley, R. H., Wray, R. B., and Belmaker, E. Z., 1972, Extreme hyperimmunoglobulinemia E and undue susceptibility to infection, *Pediatrics* **49**:59–70.

Casman, E. P., 1965, Staphylococcal enterotoxin, *Ann. N.Y. Acad. Sci.* **128**:124–131.

Cawdery, M., Foster, W. D., Hawgood, B. C., and Taylor, C., 1969, The role of coagulase in the defense of *Staphylococcus aureus* against pahgocytosis, *Br. J. Exp. Pathol.* **50**:408–412.

Chatterjee, A. N., 1969, Use of bacteriophage-resistant mutants to study the nature of the bacteriophage receptor site of *Staphylococcus aureus, J. Bacteriol.* **98**:519–527.

Christensen, K. K., Christensen, P., Mardh, P., and Weström, L., 1976, Quantitation of serum antibodies to surface antigens of *Neisseria gonorrhoeae* with radiolabeled protein A of *Staphylococcus aureus, J. Infect, Dis.* **134**:317–323.

Christensen, P., Kahlmeter, G., Jonsson, S., and Kronvall, G., 1973, New method for the serological grouping of streptococci with specific antibodies absorbed to protein A-containing staphylococci, *Infect. Immun.* **7**:881–885.

Clark, R. A., Root, R. K., Kimball, H. R., and Kirkpatrick, C. H., 1973, Defective neutrophil chemotaxis and cellular immunity to a child with recurrent infections, *Ann. Intern. Med.* **78**:515–519.

Cohn, Z. A., and Morse, S. I., 1959, Interactions between rabbit polymorphonuclear leukocytes and staphylococci, *J. Exp. Med.* **110**:419–443.

Constantopoulos, A., Najjas, V. A., and Smith, J. W., 1972, Tuftsin deficiency: A new syndrome with defective phagocytosis, *J. Pediatr.* **80**:564–572.

Coyette, J., and Ghuysen, J. M., 1968, Structure of the cell wall of *Staphylococcus aureus* strain Copenhagen. IX. Teichoic acid and phage absorption, *Biochemistry* **7**:2385–2389.

Crowder, J. G., and White, A., 1972, Teichoic acid antibodies in staphylococcal and nonstaphylococcal endocarditis, *Ann. Intern. Med.* **77**:87–90.

Cybulska, J., and Jeljaszewicz, J., 1966, Bacteriostatic activity of serum against staphylococci, *J. Bacteriol.* **91**:953–962.

Dack, G. M., 1956, The role of enterotoxin of *Micrococcus pyogenes* var. *aureus* in the etiology of pseudomembranous enterocolitis, *Am. J. Surg.* **92**:765–769.

Davison, A. L., and Baddiley, J., 1963, The distribution of teichoic acids in staphylococci, *J. Gen. Microbiol.* **32**:271–276.

Dobrin, R. S., Day, N. K., Quie, P. G., Moore, H. L., Vernier, R. L., Michael, A. F., and Fish, A. J., 1975, The role of complement, immunoglobulin and bacterial antigen in coagulase negative staphylococcal shunt nephritis, *Am. J. Med.* **59**:660–673.

Dorval, G., Welsh, K. I., and Wigzell, H., 1974, Labeled staphylococcal protein A as an immunological probe in the analysis of cell surface markers. *Scand. I. Immunol.* **3**:405–411.

Dossett, J. H., Kronvall, G., Williams, R. C., Jr., and Quie, P. G., 1969, Antiphagocytic effects of staphylococcal protein A, *J. Immunol.* **103**:1405–1410.

Downey, J. R., and Kejima, M., 1967, Influence of serum on intracellular digestion of *Staphylococcus aureus* by polymorphonuclear neutrophils from the guinea pig, *J. Reticuloendothel. Soc.* **4**:168–176.

Easmon, C. S. F., and Glynn, A. A., 1975, Complement and staphylococcal skin infection in mice, *J. Med. Microbiol.* **8**:Piii.

Easmon, C. S. F., and Glynn, A. A., 1976, Comparison of subcutaneous and intraperitoneal staphylococcal infections in normal and complement deficient mice, *Infect, Immun.* **13**:399–406.

Editorial, Levamisole, 1975, *Lancet* **1**:151–152.

Eistenstein, T. K., Winston, S. H., and Berry, L. J., 1968, Ribosomal extracts as protective antigens against *Salmonella typhimurium* and *Staphylococcus aureus* infections, *Bacteriol. Proc.* **87**:87.

Ekstedt, R. D., 1963a, Studies on immunity to staphylococcal infection in mice. I. Effect of dosage, viability, and interval between immunization and challenge on resistance to infection following injection of whole cell vaccines, *J. Infect. Dis.* **112**:143–151.

Ekstedt, R. D., 1963b, Studies on immunity to staphylococcal infection in mice. II. Effect of immunization with fractions of *Staphylococcus aureus* prepared by physical and chemical methods, *J. Infect. Dis.* **112**:152–157.

Ekstedt, R. D., 1972, Immunity to the staphylococci, in: *The Staphylococci* (J. Cohen, ed.), pp. 385–418, Wiley-Interscience, New York.

Ekstedt, R. D., 1974, Immune response to surface antigens of *Staphylococcus aureus* and their role in resistance to staphylococcal disease, *Ann. N.Y. Acad. Sci.* **236**:203–219.

Finland, M., 1972, Changing patterns of susceptibility of common bacterial pathogens to antimicrobial agents, *Ann. Intern. Med.* **76**:1009–1036.

Fischer, G. W., Podgore, J. K., and Bass, J. W., 1975, Immunopotentiation by Levamisole, *Lancet* **1**:1137.

Fisher, S., 1960, A heat-stable protective staphylococcal antigen, *Aust. J. Exp. Biol. Med. Sci.* **38**:479–485.

Forsgren, A., 1969, Protein A from *Staphylococcus aureus*. VIII. Production of protein A by bacterial and L-forms of *Staphylococcus aureus*, *Acta Pathol. Microbiol. Scand.* **75**:481–490.

Forsgren, A., 1970, Significance of protein A production by staphylococci, *Infect. Immun.* **2**:672–673.

Forsgren, A., 1973, Pathogenicity of protein A mutants of *Staphylococcus aureus*, *Contrib. Microbiol. Immunol.* **1**:102–108.

Forsgren, A., and Nordstrom, K., 1974, Protein A from *Staphylococcus aureus*: The biological significance of its reaction with IgG, *Ann. N.Y. Acad. Sci.* **236**:252–256.

Forsgren, A., and Quie, P. G., 1974a, Effects of staphylococcal protein A on heat labile opsonins, *J. Immunol.* **112**:1177–1180.

Forsgren, A., and Quie, P. G., 1974b, Influence of the alternate complement pathway on opsonization of several bacterial aspects, *Infect. Immun.* **10**:402–404.

Forsgren, A., and Sjöquist, J., 1966, "Protein A" from *S. aureus*. I. Pseudoimmune reaction with human γ-globulin, *J. Immunol.* **97**:822–827.

Forsgren, A., Schmeling, D., and Quie, P. G., 1974, Effect of tetracycline on the phagocytic function of human leukocytes, *J. Infect. Dis.* **130**:412–415.

Forsgren, A., Svedjelund, A., and Wigzell, H., 1976, Lymphocyte stimulation by protein A of *Staphylococcus aureus*, *Eur. J. Immunol.* **6**:207–213.

Firedman, H., and Warrren, G. H., 1974, Enhanced susceptibility of penicillin-resistant staphylococci to phagocytosis after *in vitro* incubation with low doses of nafcillin (38177), *Proc. Soc. Exp. Biol. Med.* **146**:707–711.

Friend, P., Repine, J. E., Kim, Y., Clawson, C. C., and Michael, A. F., 1975, Deficiency of the second component of complement (C2) with chronic vasculitis, *Ann. Intern. Med.* **83**:813–816.

Ghetie, V., Fabricius, H. A., Nilsson, K., and Sjöquist, J., 1974, Movement of IgG receptors on the lymphocyte surface induced by protein A of *Staphylococcus aureus*, *Immunology* **26**:1081–1091.

Gilbert, I., 1931, Dissociation in an encapsulated staphylococcus, *J. Bacteriol.* **21**:157–160.

Gillespie, W. A., Pope, R. C., and Simpson, K., 1957, Pemphigus neonatorum caused by *Staphylococcus aureus* type 71, *Br. Med. J.* **1**:1044–1046.

Gladstone, G. P., Walton, E., and Kay, U., 1974, The effect of cultural conditions on the susceptibility of staphylococci to killing by cationic proteins from rabbit polymorphonuclear leukocytes, *Br. J. Exp. Pathol.* **55**:427–447.

Goldman, J. M., and Th'ng, K., 1973, Phagocytic function of leucocytes from patients with acute myeloid and chronic granulocytic leukaemia. *Br. J. Haematol.* **25**:299–308.

Greenberg, L., and Cooper, M. Y., 1960, Polyvalent somatic antigen for the prevention of staphylococcal infection, *Can. Med. Assoc. J.* **83**:143–157.

Greenberg, L., Cooper, M. Y., and Healy, G. M., 1961, Staphylococcus polyvalent somatic antigen vaccine. II. An improved method of preparation, *Can. Med. Assoc. J.* **84**:945–947.

Grov, A., 1975, Human IgM interacting with staphylococcal protein A, *Acta Pathol. Microbiol. Scand.* **83B**:173–176.

Grov, A., and Rude, S., 1967, Immunochemical characterization of *Staphylococcus aureus* cell walls, *Acta Path. Microbiol. Scand.* **71**:409–416.

Gustafson, G. T., Ståalenheim, G., Forsgren, A., and Sjöquist, J., 1968, "Protein A" from *Staphyloccus aureus*. IV. Production of anaphylaxis-like cutaneous and systemic reactions in nonimmunized guinea pigs, *J. Hematol.* **100**:530–534.

Hale, J. H., and Smith, W., 1945, The influence of coagulase on the phagocytosis of staphylococci, *Br. J. Exp. Pathol.* **26**:209–217.

Hanessian, S., and Haskell, T. H., 1964, Structural studies on staphylococcal polysaccharide antigen, *J. Biol. Chem.* **239**:2758–2764.

Harvey, R. L., Kronvall, G., Troup, G. M., Anderson, R. E., and Williams, R. C., Jr., 1970, Chemotaxis of polymorphonuclear leukocytes by protein A of the *Staphylococcus*, *Soc. Exp. Biol. Med.* **135**:453–456.

Haukenes, G., 1967, Serological typing of *Staphylococcus aureus*, *Acta Pathol. Microbiol. Scand.* **70**:590–600.

Hawiger, J., Horn, R. G., Koenig, M. G., and Collins, R. D., 1969, Activation and release of lysosomal enzymes from isolated leukocytic granules by liposomes: A proposed model for degranulation in polymorphonuclear leukocytes, *Yale J. Biol. Med.* **42**:57–70.

Hayes, W., 1968, *The Genetics of Bacteria and Their Viruses*, Wiley, New York.

Hill, H. R., and Quie, P. G., 1974, Raised serum-IgE levels and defective neutrophil chemotaxis in three children with eczema and recurrent bacterial infections, *Lancet* **1**:183–187.

Hill, H. R., Quie, P. G., Pabst, H. F., Ochs, H. D., Clark, R. A. Klebanoff, S. J., and Wedgwood, R. J., 1974, Defect in neutrophil granulocyte chemotaxis in Job's syndrome of recurrent "cold" staphylococcal abscesses, *Lancet* **2:**617–619.

Hill, M. J., 1968, A staphylococcal agressin, *J. Med. Microbiol.* **1:**33–43.

Hirsch, J. G., 1964, Demonstration by fluorescence microscopy of adsorption onto bacteria of a heat-labile factor from guinea pig serum, *J. Immunol.* **92:**155–158.

Humphreys, D. W., Wheat, L. J., and White, A., 1974, Staphylococcal heat-stable opsonins, *J. Lab. Clin. Med.* **84:**122–128.

Jagicza, A., 1973, Immunochemical investigation of the antigens of drug-resistant staphylococcal strains, *Contrib. Microbiol. Immunol.* **1:**180–182.

Jasin, H. E., 1972, Human heat-labile opsonins: Evidence for their mediation via the alternate pathway of complement activation, *J. Immunol.* **109:**26–31.

Jeljaszewicz, J., 1972, Toxins (hemolysin), in: *The Staphylococci* (J. Cohen, ed.), pp. 249–280, Wiley-Interscience, New York.

Jeljaszewicz, J., Smigielski, S., and Grojec, P., 1976, Staphylococcal leukocidin: Stimulatory effect on granulopoiesis by cytostatic agent and review of the literature, in: *Staphylococci and Staphylococcal Diseases* (J. Jeljaszewicz, ed.), pp. 639–656, Fischer-Verlag, New York.

Jensen, K., 1958, A normally occurring staphylococcus antibody in human serum, *Acta Pathol. Microbiol. Scand.* **44:**421–428.

Johnsen, G. S., Grov, A., and Oeding, P., 1975, Studies on polysaccharide C of *Staphylococcus epidermidis, Acta Pathol. Microbiol. Scand.* **83:**235–239.

Johnson, F. R., Agnello, V., and Williams, R. C., Jr., 1972, Opsonic activity in human serum deficient in C2, *J. Immunol.* **109:**141–145.

Johnston, R. B., Wilfert, C. M., Buckley, R. H., Webb, L. S., DeChatelet, L. R., and McCall, C. E., 1975, Enhanced bactericidal activity of phagocytes from patients with chronic granulomatous disease in the presence of sulphisoxasole. *Lancet* **1:**824–827.

Jozefczyk, Z., 1974, Specific human antibodies to enterotoxins A, B, and C1 of staphylococcus: Their increased synthesis in staphylococcal infection, *J. Infect. Dis.* **130:**1–7.

Kagan, B. M., 1972, L-forms, in: *The Staphylococci* (J. Cohen, ed.), pp. 65–74, Wiley-Interscience, New York.

Kapral, F. A., and Miller, M. M., 1971, Product of *Staphylococcus aureus* responsible for the scalded-skin syndrome, *Infect. Immun.* **4:**541–545.

Kapral, F. A., and Shayegani, M. C., 1959, Intracellular survival of staphylococci, *J. Exp. Med.* **110:**123–128.

Karakawa, W. W., and Kane, J. A., 1975, Immunochemical analysis of a Smith-like antigen isolated from two human strains of *Staphylococcus aureus, J. Immunol.* **115:**565–568.

Keys, T. F., and Hewitt, W. L., 1973, Endocarditis due to micrococci and *Staphylococcus epidermidis, Arch. Intern. Med.* **182:**215–220.

Koch, C., 1975, Heterogeneity of phagocytic malfunction in myeloid leukaemia, *Acta Pathol. Microbiol. Scand.* **83**(c):383–389.

Koenig, M. G., 1962, Factors relating to the virulence of staphylococci. I. Comparative studies on two colonial variants, *Yale J. Biol. Med.* **34:**537–558.

Koenig, M. G., Melly, M. A., and Rogers, D. A., 1962, Factors relating to the virulence of staphylococci. II. Observations on four mouse-pathogenic strains, *J. Exp. Med.* **116:**589–599.

Kowalski, J. J., and Berman, D. T., 1971, Immunobiological activity of cell wall antigens of *Staphylococcus aureus, Infect. Immun.* **4:**205–211.

Kronvall, G., and Williams, R. C., Jr., 1969, Differences in anti-protein A activity among IgG subgroups, *J. Immunol.* **103:**828–833.

Kronvall, G., and Williams, R. C., Jr., 1971, The star phenomenon, a three component immunoprecipitation involving protein A, *Immunochemistry* **8:**577–584.

Kronvall, G., Quie, P. G., and Williams, R. C., Jr., 1970, Quantitation of staphylococcal protein A: Determination of equilibrium constant and number of protein A residues on bacteria, *J. Immunol.* **104:**273–278.

Kronvall, G., Dossett, J. H., Quie, P. G., and Williams, R. C., Jr., 1971, Occurrence of protein A in staphylococcal strains: Quantitative aspects and correlation to antigenic and bacteriophage types, *Infect. Immun.* **3:**10–15.

Lacey, R. W., and Chopra, I., 1975, Effect of plasmid carriage on the virulence of *Staphylococcus aureus, J. Med. Microbiol.* **8:**137–147.

Lacey, R. W., and Richmond, M. H., 1974, The genetic basis of antibiotic resistance in *S. aureus:* The importance of gene transfer in the evolution of this organism in the hospital environment. *Ann. N.Y. Acad. Sci.* **236:**395–412.

Lack, C. H., and Towers, A. G., 1962, Serological tests for staphylococcal infection, *Br. Med. J.* **2:**1227–1231.

Larson, H. E., and Blades, R., 1976, Impairment of human polymorphonuclear leukocyte function by influenza virus, *Lancet* **2:**283.

Laxdal, T., Messner, R. P., Williams, R. C., Jr., and Quie, P. G., 1968, Opsonic, agglutinating and complement-fixing antibodies in patients with subacute bacterial endocarditis, *J. Lab. Clin. Med.* **71:**638–653.

Lay, W. H., and Nussenzweig, V., 1968, Receptors for complement on leukocytes, *J. Exp. Med.* **128:**991–1009.

Lazarus, G. M., and Neu, H. C., 1975, Agents responsible for infection in chronic granulomatous disease of childhood, *J. Pediatr.* **86:**415–417.

Li, I. W., and Mudd, S., 1965, The heat-labile serum factor associated with intracellular killing of *Staphylococcus aureus, J. Immunol.* **94:**852–857.

Li, I. W., Mudd, S., and Kapral, F. A., 1963, Dissociation

of phagocytosis and intracellular killing of *Staphylococcus aureus* by human blood leukocytes, *J. Immunol.* **90**:804–809.

Lidwell, O. M., Towers, A. G., Ballard, J., and Gladstone, B., 1974, Transfer of microorganisms between nurses and patients in a clean air environment, *J. Appl. Bacteriol.* **37**:649–656.

Lind, I., 1972, Correlation between the occurrence of protein A and some other properties in *Staphylococcus aureus*, *Acta Path. Microbiol. Scand.* **80**(c):702–708.

Lind, I., 1973, Occurrence of protein A in strains of *Staphylococcus aureus* demonstrated by means of labeled globulins, *Contrib. Microbiol. Immunol.* **1**:93–97.

Lind, I., and Mansa, B., 1974, Immunochemical study of the interaction between staphylococcal protein A, rabbit antistaphylococcal sera, and selected sera from nonimmunized animals, *Scand. J. Immunol.* **3**:147–156.

Lind, I., Live, I., and Mansa, B., 1970, Variation in staphylococcal protein A reactivity with G-globulins of different species, *Acta Pathol. Microbiol. Scand.* **78B**:673–682.

Linnemann, C. C., Jr., Watanakunakorn, C., and Bakie, C., 1973, Pathogenicity of stable L-phase variants of *Staphylococcus aureus:* Failure to colonize experimental endocarditis in rabbits, *Infect. Immun.* **7**:715–730.

Liu, T. Y., and Gotschlich, E. C., 1967, Muramic acid phosphate as a component of the mucopeptide of grampositive bacteria, *J. Biol. Chem.* **242**:471–476.

Löfkvist, T., and Sjöquist, J., 1962, Chemical and serological analysis of antigen preparations from *Staphylococcus aureus*, *Acta Pathol. Microbiol. Scand.* **56**:295–304.

Lyell, A., 1967, A review of toxic epidermal necrolysis in Britain, *Br. J. Dermatol.* **79**:662–667.

McCabe, W. R., 1968, Role of the reticuloendothelial system in bacterial interference in embryonated eggs, *J. Lab. Clin. Med.* **72**:318–328.

McDermott, W., 1969, Microbial persistence, *Harvey Lect. Ser.* **63**:1–31.

Mandell, G. L., 1975, Catlase, superoxide dismutase, and virulence of *Staphylococcus aureus*, *J. Clin. Invest.* **55**:561–566.

Martin, R. R., Daugharty, H., and White, A., 1966, Staphylococcal antibodies and hypersensitivity to teichoic acids in man, *Antimicrob. Agents Chemother.* **965**:91–96.

Melish, M. E., Glasgow, L. A., Turner, M. D., and Lillibridge, C. B., 1974, The staphylococcal epidermolytic toxin: Its isolation, characterization, and site of action, *Ann. N.Y. Acad. Sci.* **236**:317–342.

Melly, M. A., Thomison, J. B., and Rogers, D. B., 1960, Fate of staphylococci within human leukocytes, *J. Exp. Med.* **112**:1121–1129.

Melly, M. A., Duke, L. J., Liau, D.-F., and Hash, J. H., 1974, Biological properties of the encapsulated *Staphylococcus aureus* M, *Infect. Immun.* **10**:389–397.

Messner, R. P., Laxdal, T., Quie, P. G., and Williams, R. C., Jr., 1968, Serum opsonin, bacteria and poly-

morphonuclear leukocyte interactions in subacute bacterial endocarditis, *J. Clin. Invest.* **47**:1109–1120.

Miller, D., and Beck, S., 1975, Polymorphonuclear leukocyte phagocytosis: Quantitation by a rapid radioactive method, *J. Lab. Clin. Med.* **86**:344–348.

Miller, M. E., Seals, J., Kaye, R., and Levitsky, L. C., 1969, A familial plasma associated defect of phagocytosis, *Lancet* **2**:60–61.

Morrice, J. J., and Young, D. G., 1974, Bacterial colonization of Holter valves: A ten-year survey, *Developmental Med. Child. Neurol.* **16**(32):85–90.

Morse, S. I., 1960, Isolation of a phagocytosis-inhibiting substance from culture filtrates of an encapsulated *Staphylococcus aureus*, *Nature (London)* **186**:102–103.

Morse, S. I., 1962, Isolation and properties of a surface antigen of *Staphylococcus aureus*, *J. Exp. Med.* **115**:295–311.

Morse, S. I., 1963, Isolation and properties of a group antigen of *Staphylococcus albus*, *J. Exp. Med.* **117**:19–26.

Morse, S. I., 1965, Biological attributes of staphylococcal cell walls, *Ann. N.Y. Acad. Sci.* **128**:191–213.

Movitz, J., 1974, A study on the biosynthesis of protein A in *Staphylococcus aureus*, *Eur. J. Biochem.* **48**:131–136.

Mudd, S., 1970, A successful parasite: Infection by *Staphylococcus aureus*, in: *Infectious Agents and Host Reactions* (S. Mudd, ed.), pp. 197–227, Saunders, Philadelphia.

Mudd, S., 1971, Resistance against *Staphylococcus aureus*, *J. Am. Med. Assoc.* **218**:1671–1673.

Mudd, S., Yoshida, K., Li, I. W., and Lenhart, N. A., 1963, Identification of a somatic antigen of *Staphylococcus aureus* critical for phagocytosis by human blood leukocytes, *Nature (London)* **199**:1200–1201.

Mudd, S., Taubler, J. H., and Baker, A. G., 1970, Delayed-type hypersensitivity to *Staphylococcus aureus* in human subjects, *J. Reticuloendothel. Soc.* **8**:493–498.

Nagel, J. G., Tuazon, C. U., Cardella, T. A., and Sheagren, J. N., 1975, Teichoic acid serologic diagnosis of staphylococcal endocarditis, *Ann. Intern. Med.* **82**:13–17.

Novick, R. P., 1969, Extra chromosomal inheritance in bacteria, *Bacteriol. Rev.* **33**:210–263.

Oeding, P., 1967, Antigenic studies on micrococcus strains, *Acta Pathol. Microbiol. Scand.* **70**:120–128.

Oeding, P., 1974, Cellular antigens of staphylococci, *Ann. N.Y. Acad. Sci.* **236**:15–21.

Oeding, P., and Grov, A., 1972, Cellular antigens, in: *The Staphylococci* (J. Cohen, ed.), pp. 333–356, Wiley-Interscience, New York.

Olcen, P., Danielsson, D., and Kjellsander, J., 1975, The use of protein A-containing staphylococci sensitized with anti-meningococcal antibodies for grouping *Neisseria meningitidis* and demonstration of meningococcal antigen in cerebrospinal fluid, *Acta Pathol. Microbiol. Scand* **83**(B):387–396.

Paevy, D. L., Adler, W. H., and Smith, R. T., 1970, The mitogenic effects of endotoxin and staphylococcal enterotoxin B on mouse spleen cells and human peripheral lymphocytes, *J. Immunol.* **105**:1453–1458.

Peterson, P. K., Verhoef, J., Sabath, L. D., and Quie, P. G., 1977a, Effect of protein A on staphylococcal opsonization, *Infect. Immun.* **15**:760–764.

Peterson, P. K., Laverdiere, M., Quie, P. G., and Sabath, L. D., 1977b, Abnormal neutrophil chemotaxis and T-lymphocyte function in staphylococcal scalded skin syndrome in an adult patient, *Infection* **5**:128–131.

Pryjma, J., Pryjma, K., Grov, A., and Heczko, P. B., 1976, Immunological activity of staphylococcal cell wall antigens, in: *Staphylococi and Staphylococcal Diseases* (J. Jeljaszewicz, ed.), pp. 873–881, Fischer-Verlag, New York.

Pulverer, G., and Jeljaszewicz, J., 1976, Staphylococcal micrococcins, in: *Staphylococi and Staphylococcal Diseases* (J. Jeljaszewicz, ed.), pp. 599–621, Fischer-Verlag, New York.

Queneau, P., Lejeune, E., Bertoye, A., Bouview, M., Bertrand, J., and Perrier, J., 1972, Interet du dosage des antistaphylolysines en pathologie osteoarticulaire, *Lyon Med.* **228**:345–350.

Quie, P. G., 1969, Microcolonies (G-variants) of *Staphylococcus aureus, Yale J. Biol. Med.* **41**:394–403.

Quie, P. G., and Wannamaker, L. W., 1962, Demonstration of an inhibitor of the Müller phenomenon in human sera, its identification as antistaphylokinase, *J. Clin. Invest.* **41**:92–100.

Quie, P. G., White, J. G., Holmes, B., and Good, R. A., 1967, *In vitro* bactericidal capacity of human polymorphonuclear leukocytes; diminished activity in chronic granulomatous disease of childhood, *J. Clin. Invest.* **46**:668–679.

Quie, P. G., Messner, R. P., and Williams, R. C. Jr., 1968, Phagocytosis in subacute bacterial endocarditis: Localization of the primary opsonic site to Fc fragment, *J. Exp. Med.* **128**:553–570.

Quie, P. G., Hill, H. R., and Davis, A. T., 1974, Defective phagocytosis of staphylococci, *Ann. N.Y. Acad. Sci.* **236**:233–243.

Reid, L. H., Weston, W. L., and Humbert, J. R., 1974, Staphylococcal scalded skin syndrome, *Arch. Dermatol.* **109**:239–241.

Ribble, J. C., and Shinefield, H. R., 1967, Bacterial interference in chick embryos, *J. Clin. Invest.* **46**:446–452.

Rogers, D. E., and Melly, M. A., 1960, Further observations on the behavior of staphylococci within human leukocytes, *J. Exp. Med.* **111**:533–558.

Rotta, J., 1975, Endotoxin-like properties of the peptidoglycan, *Z. Immun.-Forsch. Bd.* **149s**:230–244.

Rudin, L., Sjostrom, J.-E., Lindberg, M., and Philipson, L., 1974, Factors affecting competence for transformation in *Staphylococcus aureus, J. Bacteriol.* **118**:155–164.

Sall, T., Mudd, S., and Taubler, J., 1960, Concerning the surfaces of cells of *Staphylococcus pyogenes, J. Exp. Med.* **113**:693–700.

Salton, M. R. J., 1964, *The Bacterial Cell Wall*, Elsevier, Amsterdam.

Schleifer, K. H., 1973, Chemical composition of staphylococcal cell walls, *Contrib. Microbiol. Immunol.* **1**:13–23.

Schmidt, J., 1966, Untersuchungen über Staphylokokken-Hyaluronidase. VII. Chemisch definierte Hemmstoffe und spezifische inhibitoren, *Zentralbkt. Bakteriol. (Orig. B)* **199**:483–490.

Schoenbaum, S. C., Gardner, P., and Shittlito, J., 1975, Infections of cerebrospinal fluid shunts: Epidemiology, clinical manifestations, and therapy, *J. Infect. Dis.* **131**:543–552.

Scribner, D. J., and Fahrney, D., 1976, Neutrophil receptors for IgG and complement: Their role in the attachment and ingestion phases of phagocytosis, *J. Immunol.* **116**:892.

Sevag, M. G., 1964, Prevention of the emergence of antibiotic-resistant strains of bacteria by atabrine, *Arch. Biochem. Biophys.* **108**:85–88.

Shayegani, M., Hitsatsune, K., and Mudd, S., 1970, Cell wall component which affects the ability of serum to promote phagocytosis and killing of *Staphylococcus aureus, Infect. Immun.* **2**:750–756.

Shayegani, M., DeCourcy, S. J., and Mudd, S., 1973, Cell-mediated immunity in mice infected with *S. aureus* and elicited with specific bacterial antigens, *J. Reticuloendothel. Soc.* **14**:44–51.

Shinefield, H. R., Ribble, J. C., Boris, M., and Eichenwald, H. F., 1972, Bacterial interference, in: *The Staphylococci* (J. Cohen, ed.), pp. 503–515, Wiley-Interscience, New York.

Shinefield, H. R., Ribble, C., Boris, M. J., Eichenwald, H. F., Aly, R., and Maibach, H., 1974, Bacterial interference between strains of *S. aureus, Ann. N.Y. Acad. Sci.* **236**:444–455.

Shurtleff, D. B., Foltz, E. L., Weeks, R. D., and Loeser, J., 1974, Therapy of *Staphylococcus epidermidis:* Infections associated with cerebrospinal fluid shunts, *Pediatrics* **53**:55–62.

Sjöquist, J., 1973, Structure and immunology of protein A, *Contrib. Microbiol. Immunol.* **1**:83–92.

Sjöquist, J., and Stålenheim, G., 1969, Protein A from *Staphylococcus aureus.* IX. Complement-fixing activity of protein A–IgG complexes, *J. Immunol.* **103**:467–473.

Sjöquist, J., Melour, B., and Hjelur, H., 1972, Protein A isolated from *Staphylococcus aureus* after digestion with lysostaphin, *Eur. J. Biochem.* **29**:572–578.

Stålenheim, G., Gotze, O, Cooper, N. R., Sjöquist, J., and Muller-Eberhard, H. J., 1973, Consumption of human complement components by complexes of IgG with protein of *Staphylococcus aureus, Immunochemistry* **10**:501–507.

Targowski, S. P., and Berman, D. T., 1975, Cell-mediated immune reactions *in vitro* to cell walls and peptidoglycan from *Staphylococcus aureus, Z. Immun.-Forsch. Bd.* **149s**:295–301.

Taylor, A. G., and Plommet, M., 1973, Anti-gamma haemolysin as a diagnostic test in staphylococcal osteomyelitis, *J. Clin. Pathol.* **26:**409–412.

Thompson, E. N., and Williams, R., 1974, Bactericidal capacity of peripheral blood leukocytes in relation to bacterial infections in acute lymphoblastic leukaemia in childhood, *J. Clin. Pathol.* **27:**906–910.

Towers, A. G., and Gladstone, G. P., 1958, Two serological tests for staphylococcal infection, *Lancet* **2:**1192–1195.

van der Vijver, J. C. M., Van Es-Boon, M. M., and Michel, M. F., 1975, A study of virulence factors with induced mutants of *Staphylococcus aureus, J. Med. Microbiol.* **8:**279–287.

Verhoef, J., van Boven, C. P. A., and Holtriger, B., 1972, Host-controlled modification and restriction of phages in coagulase-negative staphylococci, *J. Gen. Microbiol.* **71:**231–239.

Verhoef, J., Peterson, P. K., Kim, Y., Sabath, L. D., and Quie, P. G., 1977a, Opsonic requirements for staphyloccoal phagocytosis: Heterogeneity among strains, *Immunology* **33:**191–198.

Verhoef, J., Peterson, P. K., and Quie, P. G., 1977b, Human polymorphonuclear leukocyte receptors for staphylococcal opsonins, *Immunology* **33:**231–240.

Wadstrom, T., Thelestam, M., and Mollby, R., 1974, Biological properties of extracellular proteins from staphylococci, *Ann. N.Y. Acad. Sci.* **236:**343–361.

Warren, R., Rogolsky, M., Wiley, B. B., and Glasgow, L. A., 1975, Isolation of extrachromosomal deoxyribonucleic acid for exfoliative toxin production from phage group II *Staphylococcus aureus, J. Bacteriol.* **122:**99–105.

Watanakunakorn, C., and Bakie, C., 1974, Pathogenicity of stable L-phase variants of *Staphylococcus aureus:* Failure to colonize normal and oxamide-induced hydronephrotic renal medulla of rats, *Infect. Immun.* **9:**766–768.

Wiley, B. B., 1963, The incidence of encapsulated staphylococci and anticapsular antibodies in normal humans, *Can. J. Microbiol.* **9:**27–33.

Wiley, B. B., 1972, Capsules and pseudocapsules of *Staphylococcus aureus,* in: *The Staphylococci* (J. Cohen, ed.), pp. 41–64, Wiley-Interscience, New York.

Wiley, B. B., and Maverakis, N. H., 1968, Virulent and avirulent encapsulated variants of Staphylococcus aureus, *J. Bacteriol.* **95:**998–1003.

Wiley, B. B., and Maverakis, N. H., 1974, Capsule production and virulence among strains of *Staphylococcus aureus, Ann. N.Y. Acad. Sci.* **236:**221–232.

Wiley, B. B., Allman, S., Rogolsky, M., Norden, C. W., and Glasgow, L. A., 1974, Staphylococcal scalded skin syndrome: Potentiation by immunosuppression in mice: Toxin-mediated exfoliation in a healthy adult, *Infect. Immun.* **9:**636–640.

Williams, R. C., Jr., and Quie, P. G., 1971, Opsonic activity of agammaglobulinemic human sera, *J. Immunol.* **106:**51–55.

Williams, R. E. O, Blowers, R., Garrod, L. P., and Shooter, R. A., 1966, *Hospital Infections,* Lloyd-Luke Ltd., London.

Winblad, S., and Ericson, C., 1973, Sensitized sheep red cells as a reactant for *Staphylococcus aureus* protein A, *Acta Pathol. Microbiol. Scand* **81(B):**150–156.

Winkler, K. C., DeWaart, J., and Grootsen, C. (with collaboration of Zegers, J. M., Tellier, N. F., and Vertregt, C. D.), 1964, Lysogenic conversion of staphylococci to loss of beta-toxin, *J. Gen. Microbiol.* **39:**321–333.

Woodin, A. M., 1972, Staphylococcal leucocidin, in: *The Staphylococci* (J. Cohen, ed.), pp. 281–300, Wiley-Interscience, New York.

Wright, A. E., and Douglas, S. R., 1904, An experimental investigation of the role of the blood fluids in connection with phagocytosis. *Proc. R. Soc. London* **72:**357–370.

Wysokinska, T., 1973, The immunologic value of some staphylococcal antigens, *Contrib. Microbiol. Immunol.* **1:**281–282.

Yoshida, K., 1971, Demonstration of serologically different capsular types among strains of *Staphylococcus aureus* by the serum-soft agar technique, *Infect. Immun.* **3:**535–539.

Yoshida, K., and Takeuchi, Y., 1970, Comparison of compact and diffuse variants of strains of *Staphylococcus aureus, Infect. Immun.* **9:**523–527.

Yoshida, K., Nakamura, A., Toshichika, O., and Iwani, S., 1974, Detection of capsular antigen production in unencapsulated strains of *Staphylococcus aureus, Infect. Immun.* **9:**620–623.

Yotis, W. W., and Fitzgerald, T., 1974, Hormonally induced alterations in *S. aureus, Ann. N.Y. Acad. Sci.* **236:**187–202.

Zen-Yoji, H., Terayama, T., Benoki, M., and Kuwahara, S., 1961, Studies on staphylococcal coagulase. I. Antigenic difference of coagulase and distribution of the anticoagulase in human sera, *Jpn. J. Microbiol.* **5:**237–247.

5

Immunology of *Haemophilus influenzae* Infections

E. RICHARD MOXON

1. Introduction

Haemophilus influenzae is a leading cause of acute bacterial infections in infancy and childhood and an important agent of chronic pulmonary infections in children and adults. The bacillus was so named because it was observed in the purulent sputum of individuals stricken with influenzal infection in the European outbreak of 1889–1892 (Pfeiffer, 1892). The erroneous conclusion that this bacterium was the cause of influenza prevailed until the studies of Smith *et al.* (1933) established beyond doubt that influenza is caused by viruses. By that time, however, its nomenclature had been firmly established.

The significance of *H. influenzae* as a cause of life-threatening or fatal disseminated sepsis in childhood was first comprehensively documented in a report by Ritchie (1910), who described three cases of meningitis and reviewed 17 examples of disseminated sepsis reported in the literature.

The mortality rate of untreated *H. influenzae* infections with meningeal involvement is 92% (Rivers, 1922). Antimicrobial therapy reduced mortality dramatically, but deaths from meningitis still represent a significant problem in the United States and elsewhere (Table 1). Also of great concern, disabling and appar-

ently permanent CNS residua occur with high frequency among individuals who survive meningitis, despite the appropriate use of antibiotics (Table 2). In the last decade recognition of continuing mortality and morbidity has spurred an explosion of interest in the immunobiology and pathogenesis of *H. influenzae* infections. In addition to meningitis, *H. influenzae* causes serious, occasionally fatal infections such as pneumonitis, epiglottitis, septic arthritis, and pericarditis; it is a leading cause of otitis media in children and is associated with exacerbations of bronchitis in individuals with chronic lung disease. Thus the goal of preventing *H. influenzae* infections is a high priority of biomedical research.

2. Microbiology

2.1. Biosynthesis

Bacteria of the genus *Haemophilus*, species *influenzae*, are pleomorphic gram-negative coccobacilli. They are indigenous to the upper respiratory tract of man, who is the only host in which the organisms are known to be naturally prevalent. *H. influenzae* is unable to synthesize some essential metabolites, including tetrapyrrole, which must be supplied in the form of protoporphyrin (factor X) and diphosphopyridine nucleotide (factor V) (Davis, 1921). Factor X is apparently required for formation of the cytochromes, peroxidases, and catalases essential to aerobic respiration (Lwolff

E. RICHARD MOXON • Eudowood Division of Infectious Diseases, Department of Pediatrics, The Johns Hopkins University School of Medicine, Baltimore, Maryland 21205.

TABLE 1. Crude Mortality Rates
per Year among 100,000 Persons
in the United States[a]

Pertussis	(1932–1936)	3.92
Tetanus	(1939–1941)	0.45
Poliomyelitis	(1950–1954)	1.21
Measles	(1950–1954)	0.24
H. influenzae meningitis	(1966–1976)	0.40

[a] After Mortimer (1973).

and Lwolff 1937; Granick and Gilder, 1946). Under anaerobic conditions the majority of strains do not require factor X, but factor V is essential. The minimum concentrations of hemin and nicotinamide adenine dinucleotide necessary for growth of *H. influenzae* were found to be 2–10 µg/ml and 0.2–1.0 µg/ml (Evans *et al.*, 1974).

2.2. Immunochemistry

Many strains are mucoid and display a characteristic irridescence owing to elaboration of an extracellular slime layer consisting of acidic, negatively charged polysaccharide polymers (Pittman, 1931), while other strains form non-irridescent colonies (Fig. 1) which lack a detectable capsule and possess surface colonial characteristics varying from finely granular to deeply serrated. The latter variants are readily produced in the laboratory when mucoid strains are repeatedly subcultured. Following nomenclature in use at the time for *S. pneumoniae*, Pittman designated the smooth (encapsulated) and rough (unencapsulated) *H. influenzae* as S and R forms, respectively.

Six chemically distinct encapsulated variants exist, designated types a, b, c, d, e, and f (Pittman, 1931). Some confusion regarding

TABLE 2. Long-Term Neurological
Residua from *H. influenzae* Meningitis

	Sell (n = 86)	Feigin (n = 50)
Significant residua[a]	30.2%	8.0%
Possible residua[b]	14.0%	28.0%
None detected	43.0%	64.0%

[a] IQ <70, seizures, hearing loss (severe), motor deficits, or partial blindness.
[b] IQ 70–90, hearing loss (mild), speech problems, or behavior problems.

subdivision of type e was clarified by Williamson and Zinneman (1951), who found that most type e strains had two capsular antigenic components, e_1 and e_2, while some had only the e_2 component. Strains having composite capsules containing two polysaccharide antigens (e.g., ab, ad) do not occur naturally but can be induced in the laboratory by the process of transformation—the transfer of heritable traits by exposure of one cell to the DNA obtained from another bacterial cell of the same species (Alexander and Leidy, 1951). When type b organisms were exposed to the DNA of type a organisms, bacteria having both type a and type b antigens resulted. These variants were capable of introducing the "ab" trait into an unencapsulated type-d-derived strain. Transformation is a useful laboratory tool since the facility with which a strain is transformed indicates how close its serotype is to that of the transforming cell. This approach has been used to support the concept that many unencapsulated strains of *H. influenzae* are variants of encapsulated strains (Ravin, 1961).

Some strains lack detectable capsule but elaborate polysaccharide antigen (MacPherson, 1948; May, 1965). Recently, ultrastructural studies were performed on a mucoid, encapsulated type b strain and two of its mutants which lacked demonstrable capsules (Doern and Buckmire, 1976). The cells were exposed to type-specific antiserum and deposited on grids by suspension overlay. Electron microscopy identified the capsule around the mucoid strain as a broad electron-dense zone approximately 200 nm in width. Studies of the mutants showed that these variants lacked capsule, although the cells elaborated detectable type-specific polysaccharide which was thought to be located within the bacterial cell. These observations are consistent with the idea that many strains of *H. influenzae* lose the power to form capsules, but continue to elaborate type-specific polysaccharide.

Extraction and purification of the type-specific capsular polysaccharides have permitted definition of their chemical composition. Types a, b, c, and f are sugar phosphates (Zamenhof and Leidy, 1954; Rosenberg *et al.*, 1961) whereas types d and e do not contain phosphate (Rosenberg *et al.*, 1961; Egan and Tsui, 1979). The structure of the type b polysaccharide was shown by chemical and spectro-

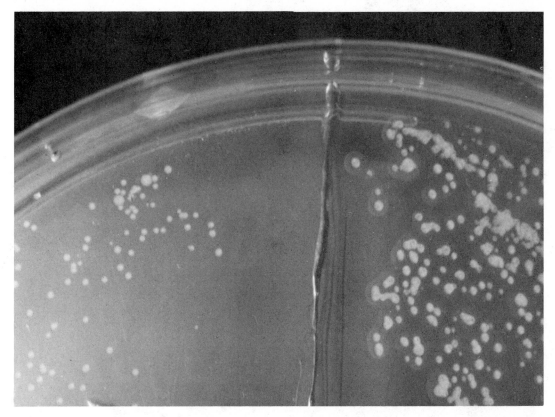

Figure 1. An unencapsulated (left) and an encapsulated, type b (right) strain of *H. influenzae*. The bacteria were streaked onto growth medium containing anti-type b, hyperimmune serum (gift from J. B. Robbins, M.D.). Note halos around encapsulated, type b colonies and absence of these halos around the unencapsulated organisms. Photograph by S. Buescher, M.D.

scopic analyses to be a phosphodiester-linked ribose–ribitol copolymer (Crisel *et al.*, 1975) (Fig. 2); this structure has been subsequently confirmed by Branefors-Helander *et al.* (1976). The structure of the type a polysaccharide has been elucidated by Branefors-Helander *et al.* (1976) and has the structure shown. The type c polysaccharide is an *O*-acetylated copolymer of *N*-acetylglucosamine and galactose containing phosphodiester linkages (Egan *et al.*, 1979). The structure of the type f polysaccharide has recently been elucidated by Egan *et al.* (1979); it is a phosphodiester-linked *N*-acetylgalactosamine polymer whose structure is given in Fig. 2. The structures of the d and e polysaccharides have not yet been elucidated. Both the type d and e polysaccharides contain *N*-acetylglucosamine (Rosenberg *et al.*, 1961; Egan *et al.*, 1979); the second sugar component (both d and e are based on disac-

charide repeating units) is still unidentified. It is perhaps interesting to note that the type d polysaccharide is neutral while the type e is acidic (Egan *et al.*, 1979).

Since strains elaborating the type b polysaccharide cause the majority of invasive *H. influenzae* infections in humans, its isolation and purification have been studied in detail. The production of immunologically active preparations of type b antigen (PRP*) has proved of value in the study of host responses to, and immunization against, *H. influenzae*. Early methodology used fractional precipitation of liquid culture filtrates with organic solvents, following which the antigen was precipitated out or separated by electrophoresis (Dingle and Fothergill, 1939; Zamenhof *et al.*,

*Polyribophosphate. The type b capsular polysaccharide is a polymer consisting of equimolecular portions of ribose, ribitol, and phosphate.

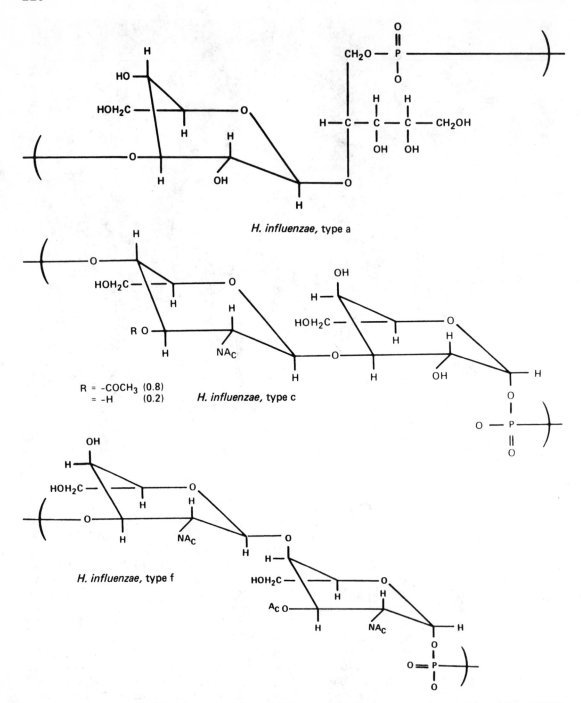

Figure 2. Chemical composition of capsular polysaccharide from *H. influenzae* type a, b, c, and f, and *E. coli* K100.

1953). Zamenhof and Leidy (1954) extracted the antigen from cells suspended in solid phase, thus eliminating contamination by the growth media. Rodriguez *et al.* (1972) isolated antigen by ion exchange and chloroform extraction. Improved methodology—resulting in optimal yields of immunologically active material largely free of endotoxin and other con-

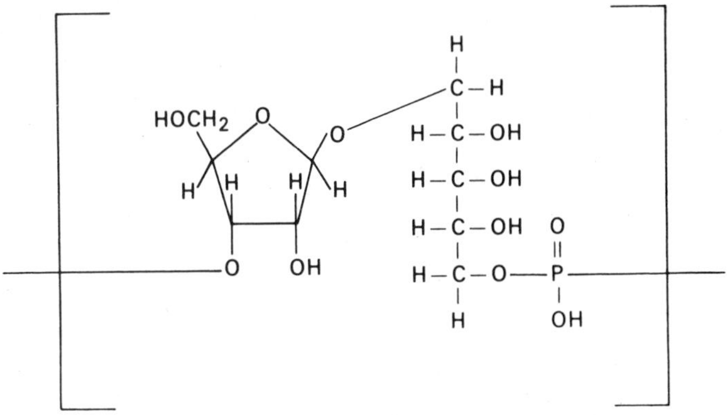

H. influenzae, type b

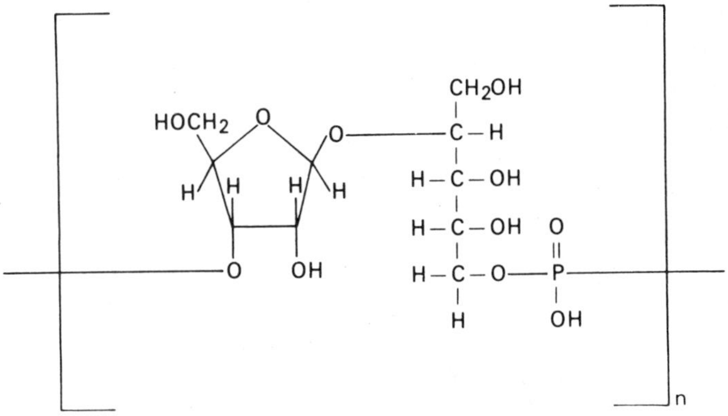

E. coli, K100

Figure 2. (*Continued*)

taminating nucleic acids, protein, and polysaccharides—became possible when it was recognized that PRP is synthesized throughout growth and in early stationary phase (Anderson *et al.*, 1976). Furthermore, the majority of the polysaccharide is released from the cell in 6–8 hr. The use of quaternary nitrogen detergents for isolation of anionic polysaccharides (Jacques *et al.*, 1949; Scott, 1960; Gotschlich *et al.*, 1969) permitted the isolation of relatively pure capsular polysaccharide. Such preparations were free of the numerous contaminating products of bacterial metabolism as well as the components of the complex media required for growth of *H. influenzae*.

The cell envelope of *H. influenzae* appears to be similar to that of other gram-negative bacteria. Recently, *H. influenzae* lipopolysaccharide has been purified; its composition and biological properties are similar to the lipopolysaccharide of enteric bacilli (Flescher and Insel, 1978).

Cell wall (somatic) antigens of *H. influenzae* have not been chemically characterized. Early investigations, using agglutination reactions, suggested an enormous diversity of antigenic determinants (Park *et al.*, 1918; Rivers and Kohn, 1921). Platt (1939) reported that saline extracts of nine randomly selected *H. influenzae* strains (which included encapsulated and unencapsulated strains) possessed a common antigen demonstrable by precipitin reaction with crude antisera. The component (called M substance) was unstable if heated to 55°C, cooled to 0°C, or subjected to a pH greater than 7.2 or less than 6.4. It was very toxic to mice, resulting in severe congestion and petechiae of the lungs and pleura. Tunevall (1953) was unable to confirm these observations; however, using gel precipitation techniques, he demonstrated species-specific antigens which were present in sodium carbonate extracts of two "rough" and two encapsulated *H. influenzae* strains. In contrast, a more comprehensive study of 52 typable and 21 untypable strains was performed by Omland (1964), who disrupted the bacterial cells by sonication. The antigenic extracts thus obtained were examined by electrophoresis and, with very few exceptions, exhibited marked heterogeneity.

3. Host–Microbe Interactions

3.1. Surface and Invasive Infections

H. influenzae bacilli commonly colonize the upper respiratory tract of man and are also well-documented occupants of the conjunctival and vaginal mucosae. At these sites, infection may be initiated with the potential to cause a spectrum of pathological conditions. A catalogue of these differing entities invites an obvious distinction between infections in which *H. influenzae* remains confined to the surface of epithelial tissues and those where there is invasion of subepithelial tissues. In the latter instance dissemination may occur by contiguous, lymphatic, or hematogenous spread (Table 3). Encapsulated *H. influenzae* cause either variety of infection and are notorious, particularly in the case of type b strains, for their potential to cause invasive disease. Some workers have questioned the primary pathogenic role of unencapsulated *H. influenzae,* suggesting that isolates obtained from infected respiratory tract sites (sinus, middle ear, lung) might represent dissociated forms of encapsulated *H. influenzae* (MacPherson, 1948; May, 1965). However, in a study of 300 middle ear isolates (Harding *et al.,* 1973), 83% were untypable by slide agglutination; when further examined using the more sensitive indirect fluorescent antibody (IFA) and hemagglutination-inhibition techniques, The percentage of untypable strains was 77%. These workers had previously demonstrated that their techniques would identify dissociated forms of encapsulated *H. influenzae*. Thus it was concluded that unencapsulated *H. influenzae* is often the

TABLE 3. Infections Caused by *H. influenzae*

Surface
Otitis media
Paranasal sinusitis
Conjunctivitis
Nasopharyngitis
Deep tissue
Cellulitis (orbital, facial)
Epiglottitis
Glossitis
Pneumonitis
Metastatic
Meningitis
Arthritis
Osteomyelitis
Subcutaneous abscess
Pericarditis
Epididymitis
Peritonitis

primary pathogen in acute otitis media of children.

3.2. Epithelial Attachment

In order to initiate infection, *H. influenzae* must colonize or invade mucosal tissue and replicate despite competition by indigenous microorganisms and clearance or killing of bacteria by mucus trapping, ciliary activity, and phagocytosis. These considerations suggest that infection by *H. influenzae* would be unlikely unless the bacterium has some device for attaching firmly to respiratory epithelial cells or that host defenses, such as mucociliary clearance, are defective. The selective adherence of *H. influenzae* to human respiratory epithelial cells has not been directly studied. Recent investigation of the attachment by *Neisseria meningitidis* to human buccal epithelial cells indicates that encapsulated strains adhere less well than strains lacking capsule (Craven and Frasch, 1978). Since capsule production is thought to be a virulence factor, these observations are provocative and suggest that similar studies of *H. influenzae* should prove valuable in defining the relationship of adherence to invasive disease. In suckling rats the observations that (1) a very small inoculum of type b *H. influenzae* (less than five bacteria) may initiate colonization (Moxon and Murphy, 1978) and (2) type b organisms more readily cause invasive infection via the respiratory as opposed to gastrointestinal mucosa (Glode *et al.*, 1977) suggest preferential attachment of *H. influenzae* to respiratory epithelial cells.

3.3. Ciliostasis

A proposed mechanism facilitating respiratory tract colonization by *H. influenzae* is production of ciliostatic factor (Denny, 1974). When cell-free supernatants from cultures of various strains of encapsulated and unencapsulated *H. influenzae* were incubated with isolated tracheal rings, ciliostasis was observed. The ciliostatic substance was produced early in the growth cycle of *H. influenzae*, although significant ciliostasis was not observed earlier than 3 days after exposure of the ciliated epithelium. The ciliostatic factor was not fully characterized, but its properties were consistent with an endotoxin. Although these observations merit further study, other bacterial species were not studied, and it is therefore not clear whether the effect was unique to *H. influenzae*.

3.4. Viral–Bacterial Synergism

Potentiation of *H. influenzae* infection by concomitant viral infection has been the subject of a number of clinical and experimental studies. The association of fatal respiratory tract infections was observed during the influenza outbreaks of 1889–1892 and 1918–1919. Later studies indicated that a serious pneumonitis of pigs required simultaneous infection by influenza virus and a bacterial species closely related to *H. influenzae*, *H. suis* (Shope, 1931). Further observations concerned two outbreaks of a "common cold" syndrome which occurred in a colony of chimpanzees (Dochez *et al.*, 1932). On each occasion, more than 50% of the stricken animals were found to harbor large numbers of *H. influenzae* in the nasopharynx, although these bacteria were virtually never observed in the absence of viral infection. Indeed, during covalescence and between outbreaks, *H. influenzae* was not detected. Importantly, *H. influenzae* isolates at the peak of viral illness were encapsulated strains, identified as types a and b. As the chimpanzees convalesced, the bacteria dis-

sociated to unencapsulated forms. This suggestion that concurrent viral infections increased host susceptibility to infection with *H. influenzae* and facilitated capsule production was further investigated by Buddingh (1963). Influenza C and *H. influenzae* b were inoculated into the allantoic sac of chick embryos. A significantly higher incidence and severity of *H. influenzae* sepsis were observed among embryos inoculated with virus and *H. influenzae*, as compared to bacteria alone. Bacterial growth was more rapid and associated with greater quantities of capsular polysaccharide. *In vivo* synergism between influenza virus and *H. influenzae* b has also been observed experimentally in suckling rats (Michaels *et al.*, 1977) in which prior infection with influenza virus resulted in a significantly increased incidence of bacteremia and meningitis. A plausible explanation for the altered susceptibility observed following influenza infection might include interference with bacterial clearance, since the virus attaches to respiratory epithelial cells and impairs mucociliary clearance of bacteria. However, the observations of Dochez and Buddingh also suggested that influenza infection may provide an environment favorable to replication and capsule production. Additional effects of the influenza virus might include infection of lymphocytes, thus blunting the immune response, or alterations in the chemotactic and metabolic functions of phagocytes, thus diminishing bacterial clearance.

3.5. Local Antibody

A direct correlation between the concentration of locally produced IgA antibody and decreased isolation of *H. influenzae* has been noted (Sloyer *et al.*, 1975). These studies employed an indirect fluorescent technique which detected IgA antibody to unspecified determinants of encapsulated *H. influenzae*. Culture-proven episodes of acute otitis media apparently resulted in synthesis of IgA antibody by cells of the middle ear mucosa, since local IgA levels were higher than those in serum. (Secretory piece was also demonstrated in middle ear exudates.) However, the presence of secretory IgA, which may have been short lived, did not protect against subsequent episodes of otitis media, although clearing of exudate was hastened. In fact, these authors suggested that a decreased incidence of recurrent episodes of *H. influenzae* otitis media correlated best with the presence of serum IgM antibody.

3.6. Serum Antibody to Capsular Antigen

For many years studies of serological response to *H. influenzae,* although numerous, proved difficult to interpret owing to the wide variety of techniques employed and the antigenic heterogeneity of the different strains studied. However, following the recognition that some strains were encapsulated and that type b strains were responsible for virtually all life-threatening infections, it was shown that blood from children aged 3 months to 3 years lacked bactericidal activity against a type b strain (Fothergill and Wright, 1933). In contrast, the blood of most neonates, older children, and adults was bactericidal (Fig. 3A). Parallel studies also showed that blood from individuals of all ages possessed bactericidal activity to an unencapsulated strain. The bactericidal activity of fresh blood *in vitro* was due mainly to antibody and complement, with only modest activity attributable to antibody-dependent phagocytosis (Ward and Wright, 1932). However, Alexander *et al.* (1944) observed that when type-specific antiserum was administered during the treatment of *H. influenzae* b meningitis, phagocytosis of organisms in CSF increased dramatically. She suggested that the capsule of *H. influenzae,* like that of *Streptococcus pneumoniae,* was antiphagocytic, and that enhancement of phagocytosis (opsonization) by type-specific antibody played a major role in immunity. During the last decade this hypothesized role for anti-PRP antibody has been critically reinvestigated, and its role in immunity has been firmly established.

Using hemagglutination and radioimmune assays, serum anti-PRP antibody concentrations in humans of different ages have been shown to conform rather closely to age-related distribution of serum bactericidal activity noted by Fothergill and Wright (Anderson *et al.,* 1972, 1977; Schneerson *et al.,* 1971; Peltola *et al.,* 1977). Inspection of recent data (Fig. 3B) indicates the striking inverse relationship of serum anti-PRP antibody to the incidence of invasive *H. influenzae* b infection (meningitis) at different ages. In fact, the "mirror image"

fit is even more striking than the original data that led Wright and Fothergill to postulate the existence of serum antibody to *H. influenzae* b. Using a spectrophotometric assay, it was demonstrated that anti-PRP antibody effectively promoted phagocytosos of *H. influenzae* b (Johnston *et al.,* 1973). Following immunization of adult humans with purified PRP, a prompt and sustained rise in bactericidal and opsonizing activity was elicited.

Further circumstantial evidence consistent with a protective role for anti-PRP antibodies in humans includes (1) the inverse relationship between the (age-related) incidence of systemic *H. influenzae* b infections, other than meningitis, and the serum concentrations of anti-PRP antibody (Schneerson *et al.,* 1971) and (2) low or undetectable levels of serum anti-PRP antibodies in serum samples from individuals in the acute phase of type b but increased serum concentrations in convalescence (O'Reilly *et al.,* 1975). To these observations can be added more evidence obtained from animal experiments. Type-specific hyperimmune serum protected rabbits against invasive infection; this effect was abolished by adsorption of the antiserum with purified capsular antigen (Alexander *et al.,* 1944). In rats protection against a lethal dose of *H. influenzae* was consistently associated with anti-PRP antibody levels of ≥ 40 ng/ml (Smith *et al.,* 1973).

An important question concerns the source of antigenic stimulation for the production of anti-PRP antibodies. Surveys of the prevalence of *H. influenzae* b carriage among infants and children suggest that exposure to this bacterium alone is insufficient to explain the acquisition of serum anti-PRP antibody among the majority of individuals aged more than 3–4 years (Sell *et al.,* 1973). A similar age-related development of anti-PRP antibodies was observed in laboratory rabbits and primates from which *H. influenzae* could not be cultured (Schneerson and Robbins, 1971). However, cultures of the respiratory and gastrointestinal tracts revealed several species of commensal bacteria with capsules cross-reactive with *H. influenzae* b (Bradshaw *et al.,* 1971) (Table 4). In subsequent studies one such cross-reactive bacterium, *Escherichia coli* 075.K.100 H5 (Fig. 2), was fed to humans (Schneerson and Robbins, 1975) and animals (Handzel *et al.,*

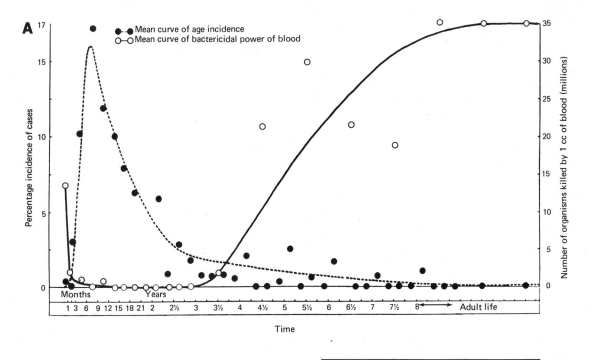

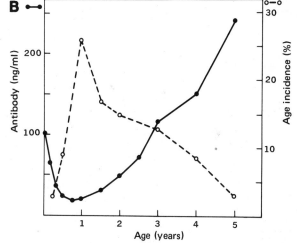

Figure 3.(A) Relation of the age incidence of *H. influenzae* meningitis to bactericidal antibody titers in the blood. From Fothergill and Wright (1933). (B) Age distribution of naturally acquired antibody to *H. influenzae* type b in healthy children and of meningitis due to *H. influenzae* type b. The antibody data are the geometric mean titers, and the incidence data are the percentages of 397 patients admitted to the Children's Hospital Medical Center (Boston) during 1961–1973.

1975) and resulted in induction of bactericidal and opsonizing anti-PRP antibodies. Observations such as these not only are important in understanding the mechanisms by which natural immunity may be acquired but also have implications with regard to immunization against invasive *H. influenzae* b infections (see Section 4).

Asymptomatic colonization of individuals with any of the six serotypes of *H. influenzae* results in production of the homologous type-

specific serum antibodies (Sell and Shapiro, 1960; Turk and Green, 1964). Because of the significantly higher prevalence of infections caused by type b strains, the immune response to colonization or acute infection with this serotype has been intensively studied, particularly among individuals aged 3 months to 3 years who are most susceptible to these systemic infections. In one study, among 35 individuals with documented systemic *H. influenzae* b infections, all seroconverted as

TABLE 4.   Survey of Bacteria Cross-Reactive with the
Capsular Polysaccharide of *Haemophilus influenzae* Type B[a]

Source[b]	Number[b]	Number and species with cross-reacting antigen (CRA)
Children	70	14 *Staphylococcus aureus*
		8 *Staphylococcus epidermidis*
		1 β-hemolytic *Streptococcus* (group A)
		1 *Escherichia coli*
Adult rabbits	60	7 *Staphylococcus epidermidis*
Young adults	17	9 *Staphylococcus epidermidis*
		8 *Streptococcus viridans*
		3 *Bacillus* species
		1 diphtheroid
		1 *Pseudomonas*
Total		
Cultures	294	
Isolates with CRA		53 (18%)

[a] After Bradshaw *et al.* (1971).
[b] Throat and stool cultures.

evidenced by formation of anti-PRP antibodies (Schneerson *et al.*, 1971). The study population included 11 children aged less than 12 months and five children aged 12–24 months. Subsequent reports failed to detect measurable anti-PRP antibody in the majority of children aged less than 2 years who had contracted invasive *H. influenzae* b meningitis and epiglottitis (Norden *et al.*, 1972; Feigin *et al.*, 1976). These questions raised the important issues of whether these children were immunologically unresponsive to PRP and, if so, on what basis. Subsequent studies indicated that the majority of individuals did synthesize at least some antibody in response to natural infection. The intensity of the response, however, required consideration of several variables. These included the age of the patient, the timing of the serum sample in relation to the acute infection, the rate of clearance of free antigen (PRP), and the method of antibody assay. Thus O'Reilly *et al.* (1975) measured the concentrations of PRP in serial serum samples obtained from 45 children with *H. influenzae* b meningitis. Free antigen was generally detected for periods ranging from 1 to 30 days after initiation of effective therapy (Fig. 4). Complexes of PRP, dissociable by acid and pepsin, were detected in serum samples of 17 patients; one individual demonstrated the PRP complex for 5 months following the onset of the acute infection. Anti-PRP antibody, measured by RIA, was detected in 79% of individuals during the first 100 days of convalescence. Sixty percent of these children were aged 1 year or less. The intensity of the anti-PRP antibody response was related both to age and to efficiency of antigen clearance. Thus antibody levels were invariably low when antigenemia was prolonged, irrespective of age. Those who failed to develop anti-PRP antibodies also showed impaired antigen clearance.

In summary, the majority of individuals contracting systemic *H. influenzae* b infections possess low or undetectable levels of anti-PRP antibody. Following infection, most individuals produce anti-PRP antibodies, although the amount of free antibody is dependent on such factors as age and the rate of antigen clearance. A rare individual, usually aged less than 2 years, may contract two or more episodes of systemic *H. influenzae* b sepsis. Apparently, invasive infection with *H. influenzae* b is not always a sufficient stimulus to induce protective amounts of antibody. There have been attempts to estimate the minimum serum concentration of anti-PRP antibody associated with protection against *H. influenzae* b sepsis (Robbins *et al.*, 1973). However, such an estimate must take into account the functionally different protective properties of the various classes and subclasses of immunoglobulins, as well as the undetermined contribution of other serum components, including antibodies to noncapsular (somatic) antigens.

3.7. Serum Antibody to Somatic Antigen

Otitis media, paranasal sinusitis, and pneumonitis are frequently caused by unencapsulated or non-type b *H. influenzae*. Tunevall (1953) looked for complement-fixing serum antibodies to a sodium carbonate extract of unencapsulated *H. influenzae*. These studies were prompted by earlier findings which suggested the existence of an antigen common to all strains, whether encapsulated or not (Platt, 1939). Complement-fixing antibodies were found in most newborns and individuals older than 4 years; the titers in young children were substantially lower. Thus Tunevall concluded that an age-related distribution of antibodies to somatic antigen existed which was similar to that of antibodies to type b capsular antigen. In a later study (Anderson *et al.*, 1972) it was clearly shown that adult sera often contained substantial bactericidal and opsonizing activity that could not be adsorbed out with purified PRP. It was concluded that antibodies to unspecified somatic antigen (or antigens) often occurred in human sera in the presence or absence of anti-PRP antibodies. Whereas much evidence suggests that the latter is important in protection against *H. influenzae* b sepsis, the significance of antibodies to somatic antigens is poorly understood. Studies performed on individuals with chronic bronchitis have shown that antibodies to somatic antigens are higher among patients with purulent sputum than among those without bacterial invasion of their bronchial tissues (May, 1952). These findings seem to discourage the conclusion that such antibodies are protective (Turk and May, 1967). It is also noteworthy that acute sera from individuals with suppurative *H. influenzae* infections frequently demonstrate bactericidal activity that is not abolished by adsorption with purified capsular antigen; indeed, bacteremia apparently persists in the

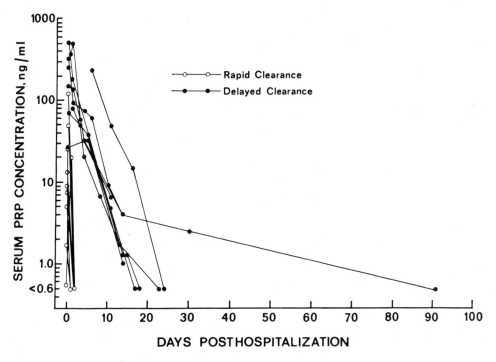

Figure 4. Kinetics of clearance of PRP from serum. The data represent the results of assays for PRP in sequential serum specimens from 33 patients sampled with sufficient frequency to allow examination of clearance patterns and rates.

presence of these antibodies (Table 5). How-ever, assays for bactericidal activity must be interpreted with caution since there are phen-otypic differences between "broth grown" and "*in vivo* grown" *H. influenzae* (Shaw *et al.*, 1976). Some evidence suggesting a pro-tective role for antibodies to somatic antigen has been demonstrated in rats experimentally infected with *H. influenzae* b (Granoff and Rockwell, 1978). Following bacterial chal-lenge, one-third of the rats did not respond with detectable levels of anti-PRP antibody. However, their sera did contain opsonizing and bactericidal activity which protected against rechallenge with the homologous *H. influen-zae* strains.

3.8. Complement Components

A role for complement components in host defense against *H. influenzae* infections was intimated by the studies of Fothergill and Wright (1933), who found that the bactericidal activity of human serum for *H. influenzae* b was decreased by heating to 56°C. Further evidence of the biological relevance of acti-vation of terminal complement components is suggested by the increased susceptibility to pyogenic infections of patients with congenital deficiencies of complement function (see later). More recently, the role of complement com-ponents was investigated in the suckling rat model (Crosson *et al.*, 1976). After intranasal challenge with *H. influenzae* b, rats depleted of C3 and C5 by cobra venom factor demon-strated a greater incidence of bacteremia and a higher mortality rate (Fig. 5). In contrast to the effects on bacteremia, complement deple-tion did not apparently directly influence the occurrence of meningitis or the rate of bac-terial multiplication within the cerebrospinal fluid.

The interaction of complement, antibody, and phagocytic cells has been studied *in vitro*

TABLE 5.　Antibody Activity and Bacteremia in Children with *H. influenzae* Meningitis[a]

| | Preadmission | | Data on admission blood sample | | | Convalescent bactericidal titer[c] |
| | | | Bactericidal titer[c] (ng/ml) | Anti-PRP titer (ng/ml) | *H. influenzae* b cultured | |
Case	Days ill	Antibiotics[b]				
1	4	—	8	ND[d]	+	64
2	1	—	2	ND	+	2
3	7	Am, Cf	1.2	<7.0	+	ND
4	2	—	1.2	ND	+	ND
5	7	—	1.2	<7.0	+	4
6	2	—	1.2	60	+	2
7	3	P	1.2	ND	+	1.2
8	14	Am	1.2	34	—	2
9	3	—	1.2	59	—	64
10	4	Am, P	1.2	<7.0	—	2
11	1	—	1.2	34	—	8
12	3	Am	1.2	ND	—	1.2
13	1	—	1.2	<7.0	—	4
14	1	—	<1.2	<7.0	+	2
15	1	—	<1.2	<7.0	+	1.2
16	7	—	<1.2	<7.0	+	2
17	7	Am, P	<1.2	<7.0	+	<1.2
18	3	—	<1.2	ND	+	<1.2
19	3	Am	<1.2	18	—	8
20	1	Am	<1.2	<7.0	—	1.2
21	1	—	<1.2	12	—	>64
22	1	—	<1.2	<7.0	—	ND

[a] After Shaw *et al.* (1976).
[b] Am, Ampicillin; Cf, cephalothin; P, penicillin.
[c] Against patient's CSF isolate.
[d] ND, Not determined.

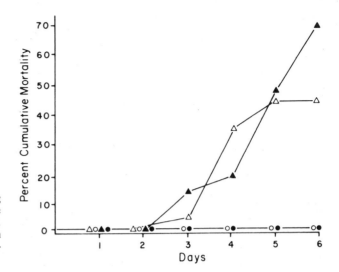

Figure 5. Percent cumulative mortality among infant rats treated with CoVF (△) or saline (○) and inoculated intranasally with 4×10^6 *H. influenzae* b, and among infant rats treated with CoVF (▲) or saline (●) and inoculated intranasally with 2×10^7 *H. influenzae* b.

(Johnston *et al.*, 1973). In the presence of high concentrations of anti-PRP antibody, phagocytosis of *H. influenzae* b occurred in the absence of complement components. However, optimal opsonization by serum apparently requires fixation of C3 to bacteria. Fixation may occur through the activity of specific antibody and complement or through the alternative pathway of complement activation which bypasses C1, 4, 2; the relative contribution of each of these pathways, *in vivo*, has not been elucidated. However, normal phagocytosis of *H. influenzae* occurred in the presence of C2-deficient serum, suggesting that opsonization does proceed by activation of C3 through the alternative pathway; this observation was further supported by the demonstration that *in vitro* unencapsulated and encapsulated (type b) *H. influenzae* activated C3 through both the alternative and classical pathways (Quinn *et al.*, 1977).

3.9. Phagocytosis

In the above discussion of serum antibody and complement, there is an assumption that clearance or killing of *H. influenzae* involves the cooperation of serum components and phagocytes. However, in experiments to date, the effect of serum and phagocytes, acting together, has not been differentiated from the bactericidal effect of serum alone. Although Fothergill *et al.* (1937) found prolonged survival of type b *H. influenzae* in CSF leuko-

cytes, Johnston *et al.* (1973) found that peripheral leukocytes killed *H. influenzae* within minutes when the bacteria were incubated in the presence of serum containing type-specific antibody. Current concepts concerning host defense against extracellular bacteria endorse a critical role for phagocytic clearance. In the case of encapsulated bacteria, studies performed on *Streptococcus pneumoniae* (Wood, 1960) and *Escherichia coli* (Howard and Glynn, 1971) have indicated that the bacterial capsule enhances the resistance of these organisms to phagocytic ingestion. *In vitro* studies of the phagocytosis of *H. influenzae* (discussed above) used polymorphonuclear leukocytes obtained from peripheral blood—a convenient and practical source of human phagocytes. However, removal of *H. influenzae* from the bloodstream is predominantly effected through the fixed phagocytes of the reticuloendothelial system (Weller *et al.*, 1978). Interestingly, in contrast to the pattern observed with *S. pneumoniae* (Schulkind *et al.*, 1967), splenic clearance of *H. influenzae* (on a weight basis) was equal to the hepatic uptake in the nonimmune animal and exceeded hepatic clearance in the presence of type-specific antibody. The importance of the spleen in defense against *H. influenzae* b was further emphasized by the demonstration that splenectomy increases the frequency of meningitis and fatal sepsis (Moxon *et al.*, 1980; Weller *et al.*, 1977). The type b capsule was evidently a key factor in retarding intravascular clearance. Following (intravenous) inoculation of an encapsulated type b strain, rats lacking anti-PRP antibodies cleared bacteria at an exponential rate for 10 min; thereafter, the bacteremia plateaued and persisted for several days. In contrast, unencapsulated *H. influenzae* was completely removed in 30 min. A mutant strain, containing 0.1% as much capsular polysaccharide as its fully encapsulated "parent," was also rapidly cleared. Addition of a solution of PRP to an inoculum of the capsule-deficient mutant did not alter its rate of clearance; apparently, the capsule and the bacteria must be integrated in order to resist clearance. However, the virtual monopoly exercised by type b strains in causing systemic *H. influenzae* infections in humans remains poorly understood. Of interest, Leidy *et al.* (1963) found that a type d strain was more virulent for mice than a type b strain. The type d strain gave rise to noncapsulated variants that were also more virulent than the type b strain. When this noncapsulated type-d-derived strain was exposed to type b DNA, the transformed organism was more virulent than the strain produced by exposing the unencapsulated type b variant to the identical DNA. These observations suggest that virulence may not be solely dictated by the type specificity of the capsule. Recently, the relative virulence of encapsulated strains (types a–f) has been investigated in infant rats. Most encapsulated strains, irrespective of type, resulted in bacteremia and meningitis when inoculated intraperitoneally in large numbers. However, type b strains were substantially more virulent than all of the others. Following intranasal inoculation, only type b strains consistently resulted in bacteremia and meningitis (Moxon, 1979).

4. Pathogenesis

Spread of *H. influenzae* from one individual to another occurs by airborne droplets or by way of inanimate objects contaminated by respiratory secretions of individuals who carry the organism. Nasopharyngeal carriage is very common. The upper respiratory tract of 60–80% of persons harbor *H. influenzae* (mostly unencapsulated strains), and associated infection is rare. However, unencapsulated strains may cause otitis media, paranasal sinusitis, and

exacerbations of lung infections in individuals with chronic lung disease. In children less than 5 years, approximately 25% of strains removed from the upper respiratory tract have capsules. At any one time, only about 3% of such children are colonized with type b strains, but these are the individuals most likely to manifest evidence of systemic infections. In older children and adults, less than 1% harbor type b organisms. The relative frequency with which non-type b encapsulated strains cause locally or systemically invasive infection is not known. Holdaway and Turk (1967) found that type e strains were commonly isolated from purulent sputum and that type a strains were particularly common in patients with acute paranasal sinusitis. However, more than 95% of encapsulated strains isolated from normally sterile body fluids (e.g., blood, CSF) are type b. Type b strains may invade any region of the upper or lower respiratory tract (e.g., otitis media, epiglottitis, acute pneumonitis, and empyema). Cellulitis of the face or orbit may occur secondary to lymphatic spread from an upper respiratory focus, or by autoinoculation of the skin or mucosa with infected respiratory tract secretions (Nelson and Ginsburg, 1976; Granoff, 1977). In the above infections secondary bloodstream invasion is very common, but bacteremia may also occur in the absence of such obvious primary foci of infections (Marshall, 1979). In either circumstance, hematogenous spread may result in metastatic infection, typically meningitis or septic arthritis.

This synoptic view of *H. influenzae* infections owes much to the observations of Alexander (1953), details of which were never published; subsequent reports have merely substantiated and extended her descriptions. Nonetheless, many features remain poorly understood. The pathogenesis of epiglottitis offers a good example of the limitations of existing knowledge. Epiglottitis differs from meningitis in a number of clinical and epidemiological features, the most obvious of which is the significantly higher mean age of affected individuals. Comparison of serum anti-PRP antibody levels also reveals a significantly higher concentration among epiglottitis patients when compared to unaffected persons or individuals with meningitis (Robbins *et al.*, 1973). It has been suggested that these differences in susceptibility can be related to genetic factors, since individuals contracting epiglottitis showed a different distribution of erythrocyte phenotypes and frequencies of HLA antigens compared to meningitis patients (Whisnant *et al.*, 1973).

Experimental infection of laboratory animals has contributed usefully to knowledge of the pathogenesis of *H. influenzae* infections. Despite the lack of susceptibility of many species of laboratory animal, successful investigations have been conducted using monkeys (Scheifle *et al.*, 1980), chimpanzees (Dochez *et al.*, 1932), rabbits (Schneerson *et al.*, 1971), rats (Smith *et al.*, 1973; Moxon *et al.*, 1974), and chick embryos (Gallovan, 1937; Buddingh, 1963). In general, adult animals have proved unsatisfactory since most species of mammals seem to develop substantial immunity as they mature.

Experimental infection of 12- to 14-day-old embryonated chicken eggs has indicated the pathogenic sequence occurring during infection of the chorioallantoic membrane (Buddingh *et al.*, 1956). During the first 6–12 hr following inoculation, unencapsulated *H. influenzae* proliferated rapidly, following which lesions similar to those seen in human infection were demonstrated. Surface infection of the membrane was characterized by accumulation of phagocytes, macrophages, mononuclear cells, red cells, and thrombocytes. Bacteria tended to segregate to the outer edges of the layer of surface exudate. This exudate limited the spread of bacteria into the underlying membranal tissue space and circulation. On histological examination, sinusitis, pneumonitis, and purulent tracheobronchitis occurred in 50% of embryos inoculated with unencapsulated *H. influenzae*, but disseminated infection (e.g., meningitis) did not occur, and few embryos died. Degeneration of the inflammatory cells rapidly ensued, with coagulation, a shift to acid pH, and hyalinization. Following inoculation of encapsulated type b *H. influenzae*, considerable phagocytosis occurred, but many bacteria remained extracellular. In some embryos—depending on inoculum size, capsule formation, and rate of bacterial growth in allantoic fluid—ulceration of the membrane occurred, with bacterial invasion of the bloodstream, metastatic infec-

tion, and death of the embryo. The occurrence of disseminated sepsis in the chick embryo was greatly facilitated by prior inoculation of influenza C virus.

The induction of bacteremia and meningitis in suckling rats has also proved a valuable experimental model of invasive *H. influenzae* infection (Smith *et al.*, 1973; Moxon *et al.*, 1974). Meningitis ranks as the most serious complication of systemic *H. influenzae* disease in humans and has been the major stimulus for investigating the basis of protective immunity to this organism. The induction of meningitis by intranasal inoculation of *H. influenzae* b has permitted sequential studies of the pathogenesis of meningitis from nasopharyngeal colonization to invasion and inflammation of the meninges (Fig. 6).

Inoculation of as few as ten *H. influenzae* b organisms may be sufficient to result in sustained nasopharyngeal colonization with large numbers of encapsulated *H. influenzae*. Despite this fact, bloodstream invasion rarely occurs following intranasal challenge with less than 10^3 organisms. Several hours are necessary for the small inoculum to proliferate, during which time polymorphonuclear leukocytes congregate in the mucosa. Thus, when challenged with relatively few bacteria, the defenses of the nasopharynx are equal to the task, and only nasopharyngitis results.

Following larger challenge doses (10^7) of *H. influenzae* b, bacteria may be detected in the blood within minutes. Many extracellular bacteria are found in the lumen of the nasopharynx and on the surfaces of oral and nasopharyngeal mucosa. Some bacteria penetrate deep into the submucosa of the nasopharynx and can be visualized in the perineural spaces of olfactory neurons beneath the cribriform plate. However, *H. influenzae* b does not invade the leptomeninges by this direct route (Ostrow *et al.*, 1979). Bacteria apparently penetrate into the subepithelial nasopharyngeal tissues. In many rats the RES removes these bacteria and the infection is rapidly terminated. However, in a proportion of rats—depending on the age of the animal and the size of the inoculum— a second phase of bacteremia occurs which is intense ($>10^3$ organism/ml) and sustained. Several features of this "late" bacteremia are remarkable. First, the thousands of bacteria

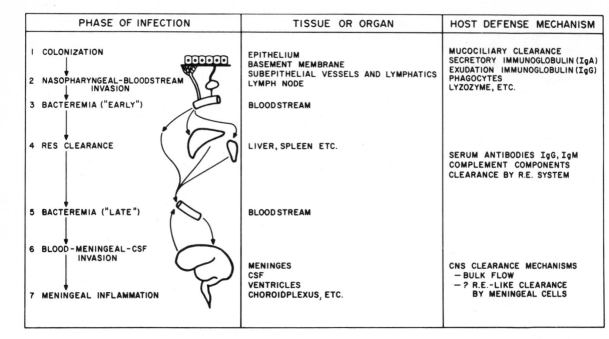

PHASE OF INFECTION	TISSUE OR ORGAN	HOST DEFENSE MECHANISM
1 COLONIZATION	EPITHELIUM BASEMENT MEMBRANE SUBEPITHELIAL VESSELS AND LYMPHATICS LYMPH NODE	MUCOCILIARY CLEARANCE SECRETORY IMMUNOGLOBULIN (IgA) EXUDATION IMMUNOGLOBULIN (IgG) PHAGOCYTES LYZOZYME, ETC.
2 NASOPHARYNGEAL-BLOODSTREAM INVASION		
3 BACTEREMIA ("EARLY")	BLOODSTREAM	
4 RES CLEARANCE	LIVER, SPLEEN ETC.	SERUM ANTIBODIES IgG, IgM COMPLEMENT COMPONENTS CLEARANCE BY R.E. SYSTEM
5 BACTEREMIA ("LATE")	BLOODSTREAM	

6 BLOOD-MENINGEAL-CSF
    INVASION
	MENINGES
	CSF
	VENTRICLES
	CHOROIDPLEXUS, ETC.
		CNS CLEARANCE MECHANISMS
		—BULK FLOW
		—? R.E.-LIKE CLEARANCE
		    BY MENINGEAL CELLS

7 MENINGEAL INFLAMMATION		

Figure 6. Pathogenesis of experimental *H. influenzae* meningitis.

in the blood are the progeny of a very few organisms—perhaps a single bacterium (Moxon and Murphy, 1978). Second, bacteremia is associated with invasion of the meninges, an event related to the magnitude of bacteremia. Third, bacteremia is totally prevented by small quantities of anti-PRP antibodies (Moxon *et al.*, 1977). Finally, RES clearance of bacteria remains extremely efficient, so that persistence of bacteremia is dependent on continuous seeding of the bloodstream from extravascular foci (Shaw *et al.*, 1976). Once invasion of the meninges has occurred, the repository of bacteria in the CNS may also seed the bloodstream, but the primary focus or foci responsible for initial bloodstream dissemination of bacteria to the meninges is not known.

Little is known of how or where *H. influenzae* invades the meninges. In one study an early histopathological feature was margination of bacteria on the vascular endothelium of the superior sagittal sinus (Moxon *et al.*, 1974). Additional observations in monkeys have indicated that bacteria may actually enter via the choroid plexus (Daum *et al.*, 1978).

Experimental models have thus provided valuable insight into the pathogenesis of invasive *H. influenzae* infections. However, the extraordinary proclivity of this bacterium for tissues such as the meninges remains very much a mystery.

If the experimental findings in rats relating the magnitude of bacteremia to occurrence of meningitis pertain in humans, invasive sepsis (e.g., meningitis) should occur more frequently among individuals in whom clearance of intravascular bacteria is defective. In fact, a number of congenital and/or acquired diseases which increase the susceptibility of humans to infections have provided valuable insights into the relative importance of humoral and cellular defenses against *H. influenzae*. Thus individuals with congenital asplenia demonstrate increased susceptibility to *H. influenzae* sepsis and meningitis (Waldman *et al.*, 1977), as do persons who have been splenectomized (Eraklis *et al.*, 1967) or who have functional hyposplenia due to sickle cell disease (Barrett-Connor, 1971; Ward and Smith, 1976). In contrast, isolated neutropenia has not been clearly associated with increased susceptibility to *H. influenzae* infections (Howard *et al.*, 1977; Chilcote *et al.*, 1976).

The central importance of antibody and

complement in facilitating phagocytic ingestion of encapsulated *H. influenzae* is supported by the natural history of persons with congenital deficiencies of these proteins. Thus males with X-linked agammaglobulinemia well illustrate the importance of serum antibody. Such individuals are usually infection free during the first 6–9 months of life, owing to passive protection by maternal γ-globulin. Subsequently, undue susceptibility to infection with pyogenic organisms, including *H. influenzae,* becomes evident, usually during the second year of life. By this time, their sera contains >100 mg/100 ml, and serum IgA and IgM concentrations are less than 1% of adult values (Janeway and Gitlin, 1957). Therapy with injections of γ-globulins effectively counters the increased susceptibility to bacterial infection (see later). Schur *et al.* (1970) have described two individuals with deficiency of immunoglobulin subclasses who were subject to repeated pulmonary infections with *H. influenzae.* The subclasses implicated were those important to fixation of complement (IgG1) and opsonization of polysaccharide antigens (IgG2). Inborn areas of metabolism resulting in deficiency of complement components C3 and C6 have also been associated with increased susceptibility (Alper *et al.,* 1969; Leddy *et al.,* 1974).

In the treatment of individuals with Hodgkin's lymphoma, aggressive chemotherapy, combined with radiotherapy, impaired humoral defenses against systemic *H. influenzae* infections and increased the risk of fatal septicemia, particularly when splenectomy was also performed (Weitzman *et al.,* 1977). Prior to treatment many of these patients suffering from Hodgkin's lymphoma contracted infections typical of the host deficient in cell-mediated immune functions, and *H. influenzae* sepsis did not occur.

Taken together, these observations are in accord with the notion that the pathogenicity of *H. influenzae* in both normal and immunodeficient patients is that typical of an extracellular pathogen. The bacteria are rapidly killed once phagocytosed, but are not ingested efficiently if antibody, C3, or reticuloendothelial phagocytes are deficient. It would appear that cell-mediated immunity does not play an essential role in defense against systemic *H.* *influenzae* infections, but direct evidence bearing on this matter is lacking.

5. Immunodiagnosis

During the last decade a number of methods have been modified or devised for detecting *H. influenzae* type-specific antigen and antibody. Precipitin and Quellung reactions for detecting capsular antigen have given way to more sensitive techniques, such as counter-immunoelectrophoresis (CIE). Similarly, bactericidal and passive hemagglutination assays for antibody have been superseded by highly specific and sensitive radioimmune assays.

5.1. Detection of Antigen

5.1.1. CIE

Several studies have documented the usefulness of CIE for routine microbiological procedures such as serotyping (Myhre, 1974) and in establishing the clinical diagnosis, course, and prognosis in individuals with meningitis (Ingram *et al.,* 1972; Coonrod and Rytel, 1972), epiglottitis (Smith and Ingram, 1975), and other systemic *H. influenzae* b infections (Ward *et al.,* 1978). False-positive results occur infrequently, although theoretically these would be expected in samples containing cross-reacting antigens (e.g., *Escherichia coli* K.100, *S. pneumoniae,* type 6). Predictably, the sensitivity of the test can be enhanced using techniques which increase the concentration of antigen in the sample (e.g., polysaccharide gels, negative pressure dialysis, ultrafiltration).

5.1.2. Latex Particle Agglutination (LPA)

In the LPA assay commercially prepared latex particles (0.8 μm diameter) are coated with antibody. The suspension can be stored at 4°C (not frozen) for as long as it remains uncontaminated. Samples thought to contain antigen are mixed with the suspension of antibody-coated latex spheres and observed for agglutination. The procedure is rapid, is simpler than CIE, and has been successfully used to identify individuals with systemic *H. influenzae* b infections (Ward *et al.,* 1978).

5.1.3. Enzyme-Linked Immunoadsorbent Assay (ELISA)

In the ELISA test the wells in polyvinyl plates are coated with antibody, following which test solutions thought to contain antigen are incubated in the sensitized wells. After washing, an enzyme-linked antibody conjugate is added and reacts with any antigen already captured by antibody on the well surface. Finally, enzyme substrate is added; its rate of degradation is proportional to the enzyme-labeled antibody present, which in turn depends on the amount of antigen in the test sample. Crosson *et al.* (1978) found that this technique was as sensitive as CIE and had the additional advantages of yielding an exact end point and providing immediate quantitation of antigen concentration.

Recently, an indirect method, using two unlabeled antibodies and an enzyme-labeled antiglobulin, has provided a more sensitive assay than previously described ELISA systems (Yolken *et al.*, 1977). Utilizing this approach, Pepple *et al.* (1980) developed an indirect ELISA system capable of detecting 0.1 ng/ml PRP. Data indicating the sensitivity and specificity of this assay as compared to LPA and CIE are shown in Table 8. While all three methods were highly specific, the ELISA system has proved more sensitive.

5.2. Detection of Antibody

5.2.1. Passive Hemagglutination

In the passive hemagglutination assay erythrocytes are coated with antigen and incubated with the sample thought to contain antibody; the latter causes agglutination of the erythrocytes. At 37°C, purified IgM fractions from human sera are roughly a hundredfold more active than IgG. Thus this assay is not suitable for measurements of, for example, placentally transmitted antibodies. It has proved useful in evaluating antibody responses to PRP in adults but is insufficiently sensitive for use in young children. The test must be used with careful attention to the possibility of nonspecific agglutination, non-PRP-sensitized cell control tests should be run with every serum sample.

5.2.2. Radioimmune Assay

The radioimmune assay measures binding of radiolabeled antigen to precipitated globulins. Antigen is either externally labeled with ^{125}I or internally labeled with tritium. The extent of binding is determined using the double label technique of Gotschlich (1971). The assay is subject to less nonspecific interference than passive hemagglutination and is approximately a hundredfold more sensitive when antigen of high specific activity is used.

6. Immunization

6.1. Passive

Prior to specific therapy, 92% of individuals contracting *H. influenzae* meningitis died. The first attempts at specific therapy used intrathecal administration of equine hyperimmune serum. The results were not favorable; indeed, toxic reactions were often severe. Intrathecal or intravenous injections of hyperimmune rabbit serum (Alexander *et al.*, 1944) were well tolerated and reduced mortality to about 70% (Alexander, 1953). However, the availability of antibiotics rendered this serum therapy obsolete in the late 1940s.

Passive immunization of individuals with congenital deficiencies of γ-globulin remains one of the mainstays of their management. An effective prophylactic dose of γ-globulin was found empirically to be that which raised the serum value by 200 mg/100 ml (Janeway and Rosen, 1966). To maintain this level, monthly injections of 300 mg of γ-globulin per kilogram of body weight must be given. Smaller doses are ineffective (Medical Research Council Working Party, 1969). The average level of anti-PRP antibodies in commercially available immunoglobulin preparations is approximately 40 μg/ml (range 20–73 μg/ml) (Robbins *et al.*, 1973). On this basis, it has been calculated that the minimal protective level of anti-PRP antibodies in these patients is 0.06–0.1 μg/ml. However, it should be emphasized that the protective efficacy of passively administered γ-globulin may include the influence of serum components other than type-specific antibody; if so, this estimate may be invalid.

6.2. Active

The dramatic impact of antibiotics on mortality temporarily quenched interest in the immunobiology of *H. influenzae* infections. However, in the last decade several concerns have prompted consideration of active immunization against type b infections. In addition to a persisting mortality (~5%) from meningitis, survivors are frequently afflicted with serious and apparently permanent CNS dysfunction (Table 2) these sequelae occur in spite of appropriate management, including optimal administration of antibiotics (Sproles *et al.*, 1969; Sell *et al.*, 1973; Feigin *et al.*, 1976). The population at risk involves primarily infants and young children. Forty percent are younger than 12 months and 32% are aged 12–23 months. Thus an effective immunization program must induce immunity in infants.

Because of the evidence indicating the protective capacity of anti-PRP antibodies and also the successful results obtained by immunizing susceptible individuals with purified capsular antigens of *Streptococcus pneumoniae* (MacLeod *et al.*, 1945), PRP was a logical choice for active immunization. The candidate immunogen promised to be virtually free of toxicity. A predictable problem with this approach was the poor immunogenicity characteristic of some polysaccharide antigens, together with the need to induce an antibody response in very young children. Purified preparations of PRP were injected into adults and children in a number of trials (Schneerson *et al.*, 1971; Anderson *et al.*, 1972; Smith *et al.*, 1973). The vaccine proved to be very well tolerated. Local erythema and tenderness were common, but not severe; general reactions were limited to some irritability and temperature rise not exceeding 38.5°C. Adults generally demonstrated a substantial rise in titer, maximum levels occurring within 3 weeks. These levels persisted for years (Schneerson

et al., 1971). Infants and children were immunized according to various schedules. The most frequent observation in infants immunized before 6 months of age was a decline in titer of antibody, presumably representing natural decay of maternal acquired antibody and absence of response to PRP. Through 18 months of age, antibody levels were not different from those of unvaccinated children (Table 6) (Anderson *et al.*, 1977; Peltola *et al.*, 1977). After 2 years of age, the incidence of positive responses was ≥80% (Smith *et al.*, 1973; Anderson *et al.*, 1977; Peltola *et al.*, 1977). No change in these results was apparent when either the dose of PRP was varied or booster doses were given. These results suggested that purified PRP was unlikely to be an effective immunogen in infants—the population at highest risk of *H. influenzae* b infections. This prediction was confirmed in a superbly executed trial in Finland which showed conclusively that a single subcutaneously administered dose of purified PRP did not protect children aged less than 17 months against systemic *H. influenzae* b disease (Mäkelä *et al.*, 1977) (Table 7). However, vaccination did induce significant protection among children aged greater than 17 months.

These results mandate the consideration of alternative methods of immunization, although it is still conceivable that modifications in methods of preparing purified PRP, such as those affecting molecular size, could enhance its immunogenicity. Since the antigens of *Bordetella pertussis* often affect the antibody response to other antigens, studies were performed to determine the occurrence of favorable (or unfavorable) interactions when DPT vaccine and PRP were simultaneously administered. It was concluded that DPT produced no

TABLE 6. Anti-PRP Antibody Status of Children 1–5 Years after Vaccination[a]

Age (mo) at Vaccination	Number of children		Mean antibody level (γg/ml)		Children with <0.15 μg/ml (%)	
	Vaccine	Control	Vaccine	Control	Vaccine	Control
3–17[b]	30	175	0.36	0.34	50	37
18–23	10	121	0.72	0.40	10	31
24–71	125	338	2.51[c]	0.51	2[c]	21

[a] After Peltola *et al.* (1977).
[b] This age group received two doses of *H. influenzae* type b vaccine.
[c] Significant difference (*p* < 0.001) between vaccine and control groups.

TABLE 7. Cases of Bacteremic Disease Caused by *H. influenzae* B[a] among 130,178 Children[b]

	H. influenzae type b vaccine	Group A meningococcal vaccine	Not vaccinated
Children vaccinated at age 3–17 mo			
Number	11,584	10,864	approx. 6000
H. influenzae type b cases (number)			
1st yr	7	1	2
2nd yr	1	3	2
Children vaccinated at age 18–71 mo			
Number	37,393	38,431	approx. 26,000
H. influenzae type b cases (number)			
1st yr	0	11	5
2nd yr	2	5	1

[a] Typed as b in 38 cases, while in two the strain was lost before typing and only assumed to be type b.
[b] After Peltola *et al.* (1977).

increment in the immune response to PRP (Anderson *et al.*, 1977; Moxon *et al.*, 1975).

Since evidence from animals has indicated that purified polysaccharides are T-cell-independent antigens, a logical approach to enhancing the immunogenicity of PRP is to make it T-cell dependent. To this end, Anderson and Smith (1977) isolated a polysaccharide–protein complex from culture supernatants of *H. influenzae* b. This immunogen appears to consist of PRP combined with protein (about 7%). In weanling rabbits, which do not respond to PRP, the complex induced high titers of anti-PRP antibody. Another approach, suggested by Gotschlich (1977), proposes the use of electrostatic complexing agents to form a pro-

tein–polysaccharide complex bound by noncovalent bonds. Injection of such complexes into mice induced high levels of serum antibodies. Priming of the animal with the carrier protein elicited a booster response to subsequent injection of the complexes, evidence that the polysaccharide–protein complex was acting as a thymus-dependent T-cell immunogen. The application of this approach has not been investigated in humans.

It has been proposed by Robbins *et al.* (1973) that anti-PRP antibodies could be induced by colonization with genetically unrelated but immunologically cross-reactive bacteria, such as *Escherichia coli* (serotype K100). Strains of *E. coli* K100 colonize the gastroin-

TABLE 8. Comparison of Rapid Diagnostic Techniques in the Detection of *Haemophilus influenzae* b Antigen (PRP)[a]

	Source	Number of specimens	Culture ⊕	LPA	CIE	ELISA
H. influenzae b meningitis	CSF	Initial 6	6/6	4/6	4/6	5/6,
		Subsequent 15	0/15	4/15	3/15	11/15
	Urine[b]	44	NC[c]	23/44	31/44	44/44
Other[d]	CSF	34	0/34	0/34	0/34	0/34
	Urine	21	NC	1/21	2/21	0/21

[a] J. M. Pepple *et al.*, 1980.
[b] Urine data include 44 specimens from eight patients with positive CSF cultures for *H. influenzae* b.
[c] Not cultured.
[d] All patients were culture negative for *H. influenzae* b. CSF data includes 34 specimens from 34 patients, nine with positive cultures (*H. influenzae* a, one; *N. meningitidis* b, two; *S. pneumoniae*, three; enterovirus, one; herpes hominis, one; Epstein–Barr virus, one). Urine data include 21 specimens from 21 patients without *H. influenzae* b infection.

testinal tract of 1% of humans from early infancy onward. When adult humans or several species of laboratory animals are fed large numbers of these *E. coli,* no untoward effects have been noted, and the gastrointestinal tract becomes colonized for several weeks (Handzel *et al.,* 1975; Schneerson and Robbins, 1975). Following colonization, antibodies (bactericidal and opsonizing) to *H. influenzae* b were induced. The protective efficacy of this approach has been investigated in suckling rats, which lack anti-PRP antibodies and are highly susceptible to experimental infection with *H. influenzae* b. After colonization of neonatal rats with *E. coli* K100, significant protection against bacteremia (Myerowitz and Norden, 1977) and meningitis (Moxon and Anderson, 1979) was demonstrated. Protection was associated with priming of serum anti-PRP antibodies. The protective activity of these sera could be removed by adsorption with PRP. Despite these promising preliminary observations, objections to this approach to immunization have been put forward. There are obvious concerns about the safety of feeding live bacteria to healthy young children, particularly since strains of *E. coli* K100 have been known to cause urinary tract infections. Further anxieties were engendered by a report that children with systemic *H. influenzae* b infection were significantly more frequently intestinal carriers of the cross-reacting *E. coli* K100 than an appropriately matched control group (Ginsberg *et al.,* 1976). The explanation for this latter observation is not known; it has been suggested that prior colonization with the cross-reactive bacteria might increase, rather than decrease, the susceptibility of humans to invasive *H. influenzae* b infections (Griffiss and Bertram, 1977).

A number of other alternative approaches to prevention of *H. influenzae* b infection of childhood are being investigated in animal studies. These include (1) use of a ribosomal vaccine (Lynn *et al.,* 1977), (2) protection induced by immunization with "core antigen" (endotoxin) using the J-5 *E. coli* mutant (Marks *et al.,* 1978), and (3) protection induced through antibodies to somatic antigen (Granoff and Rockwell, 1978).

In summary, initial optimism that a successful vaccine for systemic *H. influenzae* b infection would be achieved during the present decade has been dampened. Nonimmune infants produce inadequate quantities of protective antibody in response to immunization with PRP. However, PRP seems to act as a good secondary stimulus of memory cells already primed by exposure to natural immunogens.

7. Conclusion

H. influenzae is an important cause of infections in humans. Encapsulated, type b strains are a leading cause of bacterial meningitis, arthritis, pneumonitis, and other septicemic infections of childhood. Unencapsulated *H. influenzae* commonly causes otitis media in children and is also implicated frequently in chronic infections of the paranasal sinuses and exacerbations of pneumonitis among children and adults.

Clinical and experimental experience indicates that reticuloendothelial phagocytes and humoral immunity are the pivotal elements of host defense. Thus the pathogenic characteristics of *H. influenzae* are those typical of an extracellular pathogen. *H. influenzae* is rapidly killed once phagocytosed; however, in the absence of complement and antibody, serious localized and generalized infections occur. Antibiotic therapy substantially reduces morbidity and mortality compared to untreated infections, but deaths or serious disabilities continue to occur with unacceptable frequency. Thus the prevention of *H. influenzae* infections remains a challenging and high-priority goal of biomedical research.

ACKNOWLEDGMENTS

Research reported herein was supported in part by Grant NS-12554 from the National Institutes of Health and in part by the Hospital for Consumptives of Maryland (Eudowood), Baltimore, Maryland

References

Alexander, H. E., 1953, in: *Holt's Pediatrics* (L. E. Holt and R. McIntosh, eds.), p. 1200, Appleton-Century-Crofts, New York.

Alexander, H. E., and Leidy, G., 1951, Induction of heritable new type in type-specific strains of *H. influenzae*, *Proc. Soc. Exp. Biol. Med.* **78**:626–626.

Alexander, H. E., Heidelberger, M., and Leidy, G., 1944, The protective or curative element in type b *H. influenzae* rabbit serum, *Yale J. Biol. Med.* **16**:425–430.

Alper, C. A., Propp, R. P., Klemperer, M. R., and Rosen, F. S., 1969, Inherited deficiency of the third component of human complement, *J. Clin. Invest.* **48**:553–557.

Anderson, P., and Smith, D. H., 1977, Immunogenicity in weanling rabbits of a polyribophosphate complex from *Haemophilus influenzae* type b, *J. Infect. Dis.* **136**:S63–70.

Anderson, P., Johnston, R. B., and Smith, D. H., 1972, Human serum activities against *Haemophilus influenzae* type b, *J. Clin. Invest.* **51**:31–38.

Anderson, P., Pitt, J., and Smith, D. H., 1976, The synthesis and release of polyribophosphage by *Haemophilus influenzae* type b *in vitro*, *Infect. Immun.* **13**:581–589.

Anderson, P., Smith, D. H., Ingram, D. L., Wilkins, J., Wehrle, P. F., and Howie, V. M., 1977, Antibody to polyribophosphate of *Haemophilus influenzae* type b in infants and children: Effect of immunization with polyribophosphate, *J. Infect. Dis.* **136**:S57–62.

Barrett-Connor, E., 1971, Bacterial infections and sickle cell anemia: An analysis of 250 infections in 166 patients and a review of the literature, *Medicine* **50**:97–112.

Bradshaw, M. W., Schneerson, R., Parke, J. C., and Robbins, J. B., 1971, Bacterial antigens cross-reactive with the capsular polysaccharide of *Haemophilus influenzae* type b, *Lancet* **1**:1095–1096.

Branefors-Helander, P., Erbing, C., Kenne, L., and Lindberg, B., 1976, Structural studies of the capsular antigen from *Haemophilus influenzae* type b, *Acta Chem. Scand.* **30**:276–277.

Buddingh, G. J., 1963, Bacterial dynamics in combined infection; a study of population dynamics of strains of *Haemophilus influenzae* type b in combined infection with influenza C virus in embryonated eggs, *Am. J. Pathol.* **43**:407–418.

Chilcote, R. R., Baehner, R. L., Hammond, D., and the Investigation and Special Studies Committee of the Children's Cancer Study Group, 1976, Septicemia and meningitis in children splenectomized for Hodgkin's disease, *N. Engl. J. Med.* **295**:798–800.

Coonrod, J. D., and Rytel, M. W., 1972, Determination of etiology of bacterial meningitis by counterimmunoelectrophoresis, *Lancet* **1**:1154–1157.

Craven, D. E., and Frasch, C. E., 1978, Pili-mediated and nonmediated adherence of *Neisseria* meningitidis and its relationship to invasive disease, in: *Immunobiology of Neisseria gonorrhoeae: Proceedings of a Conference held in San Francisco, Ca.* (G. F. Brooks, E. C. Gotschlich, K. K. Holmes, W. D. Sawyer, and F. E. Young, eds.), pp. 250–252, American Society for Microbiology, Washington, D.C.

Crisel, R. M., Baker, R. S., and Dorman, D. E., 1975, Capsular polymer of *Haemophilus influenzae* type b.

I. Structural characterization of the capsular polymer of strain Eagan, *J. Biol. Chem.* **250**:4926–4930.

Crosson, F. J., Winkelstein, J. A., and Moxon, E. R., 1976, Participation of complement in the non-immune host defense against experimental *Haemophilus influenzae* type b septicemia and meningitis, *Infect. Immun.* **14**:882–887.

Crosson, F. J., Winkelstein, J. A., and Moxon, E. R., 1978, Enzyme-linked immunosorbent assay for detection and quantitation of capsular antigen of *Haemophilus influenzae* type b, *Infect. Immun.* **22**:617–619.

Daum, R. S., Schiefele, D. W., Syriopoulou, V., Averill, D., and Smith, A. L., 1978, Ventricular involvement in experimental *Haemophilus influenzae* meningitis, *J. Pediatr.* **93**:927–930.

Davis, D. J., 1921, Food accessory factors in bacterial growth. III. Further observation on the growth of Pfeiffer's bacillus, *J. Infect. Dis.* **29**:171–189.

Denny, F. W., 1974, Effect of a toxin produced by *Haemophilus influenzae* on ciliated respiratory epithelium, *J. Infect. Dis.* **129**:93–100.

Dingle, J. H., and Fothergill, L. D., 1939, Purification of the type specific polysaccharide from *Haemophilus influenzae* type b, *J. Immunol.* **37**:53–68.

Dochez, A. R., Mills, K. C., and Kneeland, Y., Jr., 1932, Variation of *H. influenzae* during acute respiratory infection in the chimpanzee, *Proc. Soc. Exp. Biol. Med.* **30**:314–316.

Doern, G. V., and Buckmire, F. L., 1976, Ultrastructural characterization of capsulated *Haemophilus influenzae* type b and two spontaneous non-typable mutants, *Infect. Immun.* **127**:523–535.

Egan, W., 1978, personal communication.

Egan, W., and Tsui, F. P., 1979, unpublished.

Egan, W., Tsui, P. A., Climensen, P. A., and Schneerson, R., 1979, unpublished.

Eraklis, A. J., Kevy, S. V., Diamond, L. K., and Cross, R., 1967, Hazard of overwhelming infection after splenectomy in childhood, *N. Engl. J. Med.* **276**:1225–1229.

Evans, M. N., Smith, D. D., and Wicken, A. J., 1974, Haemin and nicotinamide adenine dinucleotide requirements of *Haemophilus influenzae* and *Haemophilus parainfluenzae*, *J. Med. Microbiol.* **7**:359–365.

Feigin, R. D., Stechenberg, B. W., Chang, M. J., Dunkle, L. M., Wang, M. L., Palkes, H., Dodge, P. R., and Davis, H., 1976, Prospective evaluation of treatment of *Haemophilus influenzae* meningitis, *J. Pediatr.* **88**:542–548.

Fildes, P., 1921, The nature of the effect of blood-pigment upon the growth of *B. influenzae*, *Br. J. Exp. Pathol.* **2**:16–25.

Flesher, A. R., and Insel, R. A., 1978, Characterization of lipopolysaccharide of *Haemophilus influenzae*, *J. Infect. Dis.* **138**:719–729.

Fothergill, L. D., and Wright, J., 1933, Influenzal meningitis: The relation of age incidence to the bactericidal power of blood against causal organism, *J. Immunol.* **24:**273–284.

Fothergill, L. D., Chandler, C. A., and Dingle, J. H., 1937, The survival of virulent *H. influenzae* in phagocytes, *J. Immunol.* **32:**335–339.

Gallovan, M., 1937, Encephalitis and meningitis in the chick embryo following inoculation of the chorio-allantoic membrane with *Haemophilus influenzae, Am. J. Pathol.* **13:**911–926.

Ginsberg, C. M., Schneerson, R., McCracken, G. H., and Robbins, J. B., 1976, Prog. Abstr. Intersci. Conf. Antimicrob. Agent Chemother. 16th, Chicago, Abstr. No. 148.

Glode, M. P., Sutton, A., Moxon, E. R., and Robbins, J. B., 1977, Pathogenesis of neonatal *Escherichia coli* meningitis: Induction of bacteremia and meningitis in infant rats fed *E. coli* K.1, *Infect. Immun.* **16:**75–80.

Gotschlich, E. C., 1971, A simplification of the radioactive antigen binding test by a double label technique, *J. Immunol.* **107:**910–911.

Gotschlich, E. C., 1977, cited in: Current status and prospects for improved and new bacterial vaccines, *J. Infect. Dis.* **136:**S92.

Gotschlich, E. C., Liu, T. Y., and Artenstein, M. S., 1969, Preparation and immunochemical properties of the group A, group B and group C meningococcal polysaccharides, *J. Exp. Med.* **129:**1349–1365.

Granick, S., and Gilder, H., 1946, The porphyrin requirements of *Haemophilus influenzae* and some functions of the vinyl propionic acid side chains of heme, *J. Gen. Physiol.* **30:**1–13.

Granoff, D., 1977, *Haemophilus influenzae* cellulitis following soft tissue injury, *J. Pediatr.* **91:**679–680.

Granoff, D. M., and Rockwell, R., 1978, Experimental *Haemophilus influenzae* type b meningitis: Immunological investigation of the infant rat model, *Infect. Immun.* **20:**705–713.

Griffiss, J. M., and Bertram, M. A., 1977, Immunoepidemiology of meningococcal disease in military recruits. II. Blocking of serum bactericidal activity by circulating IgA early in the course of invasive disease, *J. Infect. Dis.* **136:**733–739.

Handzel, Z. T., Argaman, M., Parke, J. C., Schneerson, R., and Robbins, J. B., 1975, Heteroimmunization to the capsular polysaccharide of *Haemophilus influenzae* type b induced by enteric cross-reacting bacteria, *Infect. Immun.* **11:**1045–1051.

Harding, A. L., Anderson, P., Howie, V. M., Ploussard, J. H., and Smith, D. H., 1973, *Haemophilus influenzae* isolated from children with otitis media, in: *Haemophilus influenzae* (S. H. Sell and D. T. Karzon, eds.), pp. 21–28, Vanderbilt University Press, Nashville, Tenn.

Holdaway, M. D., and Turk, D. C., 1967, in: *Haemophilus influenzae: Its Clinical Importance* (D. C. Turk and J. R. May, eds.), p. 69, English University Press, London.

Howard, C. J., and Glynn, A. A., 1971, Some physical properties of K antigens of *Escherichia coli* related to their biological activity, *Infect. Immun.* **4:**6–11.

Howard, M. W., Strauss, R. G., and Johnston, R. B., 1977, Infections in patients with neutropenia, *Am. J. Dis. Child.* **131:**788–790.

Ingram, D. L., Anderson, P., and Smith, D. H., 1972, Countercurrent immunoelectrophoresis in the diagnosis of systemic diseases caused by *Haemophilus influenzae* type b, *J. Pediatr.* **81:**1156–1159.

Janeway, C. A., and Gitlin, D., 1957, Gamma globulins, *Adv. Pediatr.* **9:**65–136.

Janeway, C. A., and Rosen, F. S., 1966, The gamma globulins. IV. Therapeutic uses of gamma globulins, *N. Engl. J. Med.* **275:**826–831.

Jaques, L. B., Monkhouse, F. C., and Stewart, M., 1949, A method for the determination of heparin in blood, *J. Physiol.* **109:**41–43.

Johnston, R. B., Anderson, P., and Newman, S., 1973, Opsonization and phagocytosis of *Haemophilus influenzae* type b, in: *Haemophilus influenzae* (S. H. Sell and D. T. Karzon, eds.), pp. 99–112, Vanderbilt University Press, Nashville, Tenn.

Leddy, J. P., Frank, M. M., Gaither, T., Baum, J., and Klemperer, M. R., 1974, Hereditary deficiency of the sixth component of complement in man, *J. Clin. Invest.* **53:**544–553.

Leidy, G., Hahn, E., Zamenhof, S., and Alexander, H. E., 1963, Biochemical aspects of virulence of *Haemophilus influenzae, Ann. N.Y. Acad. Sci.* **88:**1195–1202.

Lindberg, B., 1978, unpublished studies.

Lwolff, A., and Lwolff, M., 1937, Role physiologique de l'hémine pour *Haemophilus influenzae* Pfeiffer, *Ann. Inst. Pasteur* **59:**129–136.

Lynn, M., Tewari, R. P., and Solotorovsky, M., 1977, Immunoprotective activity of ribosomes from *Haemophilus influenzae, Infect. Immun.* **15:**453–460.

MacLeod, C. M., Hodges, R. G., Heidelberger, M., and Bernhard, W. G., 1945, Prevention of pneumococcal pneumonia by immunization with specific capsular polysaccharides, *J. Exp. Med.* **82:**445–465.

MacPherson, C. F. C., 1948, A method of typing *Haemophilus influenzae* by the precipitin reaction, *Can. J. Res.* **26:**197–199.

Mäkelä, H., Peltola, H., Käyhty, H., Jousimies, H., Pettay, O., Ruoslahti, E., Sivonen, A., and Renkonen, O. V., 1977, Polysaccharide vaccines of Group A *Neisseria meningitidis* and *Haemophilus influenzae* type b: A field trial in Finland, *J. Infect. Dis.* **136:**S43–50.

Marks, M. I., Ziegler, E. J., Douglas, H., and Braude, A. I., 1978, Prog. Abstr. Intersci. Conf. Antimicrob. Agent Chemother. 18th, Atlanta, Ga., Abstr. No. 503.

Marshall, R. E., Teele, D. W., and Klein, J. O., 1979, Unsuspecting bacteremia due to Haemophilus influenzae; outcome in children not initially admitted to hospital (abstr. 833), *Pediatr. Res.* **13:**464.

May, J. R., 1952, The bacteriology of chronic bronchitis, *Lancet* **2:**1206–1207.

May, J. R., 1965, The bacteriology and chemotherapy of chronic bronchitis, *Br. J. Dis. Chest* **59**:57–65.

Medical Research Council Working Party, 1969, Hypogammaglobulinemia in the United Kingdom, *Lancet* **1**:163–168.

Michaels, R. H., Myerowitz, R. L., and Klaw, R., 1977, Potentiation of experimental meningitis due to *Haemophilus influenzae* by Influenza A virus, *J. Infect. Dis.* **135**:641–645.

Mortimer, E. A., 1973, Immunization against *Haemophilus influenzae, Pediatrics* **52**:633.

Moxon, E. R., 1979, unpublished studies.

Moxon, E. R., and Anderson, P., 1979, Meningitis caused by *Haemophilus influenzae* in infant rats; protective immunity and antibody priming by gastrointestinal colonization with *Escherichia coli, J. Infect. Dis.* **140**:471–478.

Moxon, E. R., and Murphy, P. A., 1978, *Haemophilus influenzae* bacteremia and meningitis resulting from survival of a single organism, *Proc. Natl. Acad. Sci. USA* **75**:1534–1536.

Moxon, E. R., Smith, A. L., Averill, D. R., and Smith, D. H., 1974, *Haemophilus influenzae* meningitis in infant rats after intranasal inoculation, *J. Infect. Dis.* **129**:154–162.

Moxon, E. R., Anderson, P., Smith, D. H., Adrienzen, B., Graham, G. G., and Baker, R. S., 1975, Antibody responses to a combination vaccine against *Haemophilus influenzae* type b, diphtheria, pertussis and tetanus, *Bull. WHO* **52**:87–90.

Moxon, E. R., Glode, M. P., Sutton, A., and Robbins, J. B., 1977, The infant rat as a model of bacterial meningitis, *J. Infect. Dis.* **136**:S186–190.

Moxon, E. R., Goldthorn, J., and Schwartz, A. D., 1980, The effect of splenectomy on intravenous and intranasal challenge with *Haemophilus influenzae* type b, *Infect. Immun.* (in press).

Myerowitz, R. L., and Norden, C. W., 1977, Effect of neonatal gastrointestinal colonization with cross-reacting *Escherichia coli* on anticapsular antibody production and bacteremia in experimental *Haemophilus influenzae* type b disease of rats, *Infect. Immun.* **17**:83–90.

Myhre, E. B., 1974, Typing of *Haemophilus influenzae* by counterimmunoelectrophoresis, *Acta Pathol. Microbiol. Scand.* **82**:164–166.

Nelson, J. C., and Ginsburg, C. M., 1976, An hypothesis on the pathogenesis of *Haemophilus influenzae* buccal cellulitis, *J. Pediatr.* **88**:709.

Norden, C. W., Melish, M., Overall, J. C., and Baum, J., 1972, Immunologic responses to *Haemophilus influenzae* meningitis, *J. Pediatr.* **80**:209–214.

Omland, T., 1964, Serological studies on *Haemophilus influenzae* and related species. 8. Examination of ultrasonically prepared *Haemophilus* antigens by means of immuno-electrophoresis, *Acta Pathol. Microbiol. Scand.* **62**:89–106.

O'Reilly, R. J., Anderson, P., Ingram, D. L., Peter, G.,

and Smith, D. H., 1975, Circulating polyribophosphate in *Haemophilus influenzae* type b meningitis, *J. Clin. Invest.* **56**:1012–1022.

Ostrow, P. T., Moxon, E. R., Vernon, N., and Kapko, R. J., 1979, Pathogenesis of bacterial meningitis; studies on the route of meningeal invasion following *Haemophilus influenzae* inoculation of infant rats, *Lab. Invest.* **40**:678–685.

Park, W. H., Williams, A. W., and Cooper, G., 1918, The results of the use of agglutinin in the identification of strains of influenzae bacilli, *Proc. Soc. Exp. Biol. Med.* **16**:120.

Peltola, H., Kähty, H., Sivonen, A., and Makälä, P. H., 1977, *Haemophilus influenzae* type b capsular polysaccharide vaccine in children: A double-blind field study of 100,000 vaccines 3 months to 5 years of age in Finland, *Pediatrics* **60**:730–737.

Pepple, J., Moxon, E. R., and Yolken, R. H., 1980, Indirect enzyme-linked immunosorbent assay for the quantitation of the type-specific antigen of *Haemophilus influenzae* b: A preliminary report, *J. Pediatr.* **97**:233–237.

Pfeiffer, R., 1892, Vorlaufige mittheilungen uber die erreger der influenzae, *Dtsch. Med. Wochenschr.* **18**:284.

Pittman, M., 1931, Variation and type specificity in the bacterial species *Haemophilus influenzae, J. Exp. Med.* **53**:471–492.

Platt, A. E., 1939, A serological study of *Haemophilus influenzae*. 2. Two serologically active protein fractions isolated from Pfeiffer's bacillus, *Aust. J. Exp. Biol. Med. Sci.* **17**:19–24.

Quinn, P. H., Crosson, F. J., Winkelstein, J. A., and Moxon, E. R., 1977, Activation of the alternative complement pathway by *Haemophilus influenzae* type b, *Infect. Immun.* **16**:400–402.

Ravin, A. W., 1961, The genetics of transformation, *Adv. Genet.* **10**:61–163.

Ritchie, J., 1910, On meningitis associated with an influenza-like bacillus, *J. Pathol. Bacteriol.* **14**:615–627.

Rivers, T. M., 1922, Influenzal meningitis, *Am. J. Dis. Child.* **24**:102–124.

Rivers, T. M., and Kohn, L. A., 1921, The biological and the serological reactions of influenza bacilli producing meningitis, *J. Exp. Med.* **34**:477–493.

Robbins, J. B., Schneerson, R., Argaman, M., and Handzel, Z. T., 1973, *Haemophilus influenzae* type b: Disease and immunity in humans, *Ann. Intern. Med.* **78**:259–269.

Rodriguez, L. P., Schneerson, R., and Robbins, J. B., 1972, The isolation and some physicochemical, serologic, and biologic properties of the capsular polysaccharide of *Haemophilus influenzae* type b, *J. Immunol.* **107**:1071–1079.

Rosenberg, E., Leidy, G., Jaffee, I., and Zamenhof, S., 1961, Studies on type-specific substances of *Haemophilus influenzae*, types e and f, *J. Biol. Chem.* **236**:2841–2849.

Scheifle, D. W., Daum, R. S., Syriopoulou, V. P., Averill,

D. R., and Smith, A. L., 1980, A primate model of *Haemophilus influenzae* meningitis, *J. Lab. Clin. Invest.* (in press).

Schneerson, R., and Robbins, J. B., 1971, Age-related susceptibility to *Haemophilus influenzae* type b disease in rabbits, *Infect. Immun.* **4**:397–401.

Schneerson, R., and Robbins, J. B., 1975, Induction of serum *Haemophilus influenzae* type b capsular antibodies in adult volunteers fed cross-reacting *Escherichia coli* 075.K.100.H5, *N. Engl. J. Med.* **292**:1093–1096.

Schneerson, R., Rodriguez, L. P., Parke, J. C., and Robbins, J. B., 1971, Immunity to disease caused by *Haemophilus influenzae* type b. II. Specificity and some biologic characteristics of "natural" infection acquired and immunization induced antibodies to the capsular polysaccharide of *Haemophilus influenzae* type b, *J. Immunol.* **107**:1081–1089.

Schulkind, M. L., Ellis, E. F., and Smith, R. T., 1967, Effect of antibody upon clearance of I^{125} labeled pneumococci by the spleen and liver, *Pediatr. Res.* **1**:178–184.

Schur, P. H., Borel, H., Gelfand, E. W., Alpert, C. A., and Rosen, F. S., 1970, Gamma-C globulin deficiencies in patients with recurrent pyogenic infections, *N. Engl. J. Med.* **283**:631–634.

Scott, J. E., 1960, Aliphatic ammonium salts in the assay of acidic polysaccharides from tissues, *Methods Biochem. Anal.* **8**:145–197.

Sell, S. H., and Shapiro, J. L., 1960, Interstitial pneumonitis induced by experimental infection with *Hemophilus influenzae*, *Am. J. Dis. Child.* **100**:16–22.

Sell, S. H., Merrill, R. E., Doyne, E. O., and Zimshy, E. P., 1972, Long-term sequelae of *Haemophilus influenzae* meningitis, *Pediatrics.* **49**:206–211.

Sell, S. H., Turner, D. J., and Federspick, C. F., 1973, Natural infections with *Haemophilus influenzae* in children. I. Types identified, in: *Haemophilus influenzae* (S. H. Sell and D. T. Karzon, eds.), pp. 3–11, Vanderbilt University Press, Nashville, Tenn.

Shaw, S., Smith, A. L., Anderson, P., and Smith, D. H., 1976, The paradox of *Haemophilus influenzae* type b bacteremia in the presence of serum bactericidal activity, *J. Clin. Invest.* **58**:1019–1029.

Shope, R. E., 1931, Swine Influenza. I. Experimental transmission and pathology, *J. Exp. Med.* **54**:349–359.

Sloyer, J. L., Cate, C. C., Howie, V. M., Ploussard, J. H., and Johnston, R. B., 1975, The immune response to acute otitis media in children. II. Serum and middle ear fluid antibody in otitis media due to *Haemophilus influenzae*, *J. Infect. Dis.* **132**:685–688.

Smith, A. L., Smith, D. H., Averill, D. R., Marino, J., and Moxon, E. R., 1973, Production of *Haemophilus influenzae* b meningitis in infant rats by intraperitoneal inoculation, *Infect. Immun.* **8**:278–290, 1973.

Smith, D. H., Peter, G., Ingram, D. L., Harding, A. L., and Anderson, P., 1973, Response of children immu-

nized with capsular polysaccharide of *Haemophilus influenzae* type b, *Pediatrics* **52**:637–644.

Smith, E. W. P., and Ingram, D. L., 1975, Counterimmunoelectrophoresis in *Haemophilus influenzae* type b epiglottitis and pericarditis, *J. Pediatr.* **86**:571–573.

Smith, W., Andrewes, C. H., and Laidlaw, P. P., 1933, A virus obtained from influenza patients, *Lancet* **2**:66–68.

Sproles, E. T., Azerrad, J., Williamson, C., and Merrill, R. E., 1969, Meningitis due to *Haemophilus influenzae*; long-term sequelae, *J. Pediatr.* **75**:752–788.

Tunevall, G., 1953, Studies on *Haemophilus influenzae*: *Haemophilus influenzae* antigens studied by the gel precipitation method, *Acta Pathol. Microbiol. Scand.* **32**:193–197.

Turk, D. C., and Green, C. A., 1964, Measurement of antibodies reacting with capsular antigens of *Haemophilus influenzae*, *J. Clin. Pathol.* **17**:294–296.

Turk, D. C., and May, J. R., 1967, *Haemophilus influenzae: Its Clinical Importance*, p. 104, English University Press, London.

Waldman, J. D., Rosenthal, A., Smith, A. L., Shurin, S., and Nadas, A. S., 1977, Sepsis and congenital asplenia, *J. Pediatr.* **90**:555–559.

Ward, H. K., and Wright, J., 1932, Studies on influenzal meningitis. I. The problem of specific therapy, *J. Exp. Med.* **55**:223–234.

Ward, J., and Smith, A. L., 1976, *Haemophilus influenzae* bacteremia in children with sickle cell disease, *J. Pediatr.* **88**:261–263.

Ward, J. L., Siber, G. R., Scheifle, D. W., and Smith, D. H., 1978, Rapid diagnosis of *Haemophilus influenzae* type b infections by latex particle agglutination and counterimmunoelectrophoresis, *J. Pediatr.* **93**:37–42.

Weitzman, S. A., Aisenberg, A. C., Siber, G. R., and Smith, D. H., 1977, Impaired humoral immunity in treated Hodgkin's disease, *N. Engl. J. Med.* **297**:245–248.

Weller, P. F., Smith, A. L., Anderson, P., and Smith, D. H., 1977, The role of encapsulation and host age in the clearance of *Haemophilus influenzae* bacteremia, *J. Infect. Dis.* **135**:34–41.

Weller, P. F., Smith, A. L., Smith, D. H., and Anderson, P., 1978, Role of immunity in the clearance of bacteremia due to *Haemophilus influenzae*, *J. Infect. Dis.* **138**:427–436.

Whisnant, J. K., Rogentine, G. N., and Robbins, J. B., 1973, Studies on mechanism of susceptibility to *Haemophilus influenzae* type b disease; Relationship of erythrocytes and histocompatibility antigens with *Haemophilus influenzae* type b meningitis and epiglottitis, in: *Haemophilus influenzae* (S. H. Sell and D. T. Karzon, eds.), pp. 197–202, Vanderbilt University Press, Nashville, Tenn.

Williamson, G. M., and Zinneman, K., 1951, The occurrence of two distinct capsular antigens in *H. influenzae* type e strains, *J. Pathol. Bacteriol.* **63**:695–698.

Wood, W. B., Jr., 1960, Phagocytosis with particular reference to encapsulated bacteria, *Bacteriol. Rev.* **24:**41–49.

Yolken, R. H., Greenberg, H. B., and Merson, M., 1977, Enzyme-linked immunosorbent assay for detection of *E. coli* heat labile enterotoxin, *J. Clin. Microbiol.* **6:**439–443.

Zamenhof, S., and Leidy, G., 1954, Further studies on poly-ribophosphate and other poly-sugarphosphates, *Fed. Proc.* **13:**327.

Zamenhof, S. G., Leidy, P. L., Fitzgerald, P. L., Alexander, H. E., and Chargaff, E., 1953, Polyribophosphate, the type specific substance of *Haemophilus influenzae,* type b, *J. Biol. Chem.* **203:**695–704.

6

Immunology of *Neisseria meningitidis*

MARTHA L. LEPOW and RONALD GOLD

1. Introduction

Meningococcal disease has been a worldwide problem for many centuries. The meningococcus, *Neisseria meningitidis,* first described by Weichselbaum in 1887, is a gram-negative, kidney-bean-shaped organism found both intra- and extracellularly.

The portal of entry is usually respiratory, through the nasopharynx, but nothing is known of mechanism of attachment of the organism. For reasons to be elaborated on in subsequent sections, it is likely that the majority of natural immunizing infections are subclinical.

1.1. Spectrum of Infection

Several clinical types of systemic infections are recognized. The septicemic form is characterized by a fulminant course, with severe purpura, intravascular coagulopathy, shock, and very high fatality rate. More commonly the bacteremia leads to meningitis without shock or other features of the fulminating disease. A purpuric rash is present in about 60% of cases of meningitis, presumably the result of the predilection of the meningococcal exotoxin for cutaneous blood vessels (Davis and Arnold, 1974) leading to the development of local Shwartzman-type reactions.

MARTHA L. LEPOW ● Department of Pediatrics, Albany Medical College, Albany, New York 12208. RONALD GOLD ● Hospital for Sick Children, Toronto, Canada.

Other forms of meningococcal disease have been reported, including pneumonia, conjunctivitis, otitis media, cellulitis, arthritis, and pericarditis. In addition, chronic meningococcemia has been described in which fever with or without rash, joint manifestations, or meningitis can recur at different times. There is no information on HLA typing related to clinical disease manifestations.

In the preantibiotic era the case fatality rate of systemic meningococcal disease was over 80%. With the discovery of sulfonamides and penicillin for treatment, the overall mortality rate was lowered to 10% or less. Central nervous system sequelae are uncommon when treatment is initiated early. Because of the widespread prevalence of sulfonamide-resistant strains, penicillin is the drug of choice for treatment of the disease. Unfortunately, penicillin will not affect the carrier state and cannot be used to control transmission.

1.2. Epidemiology

Meningococcal disease is endemic throughout the world and periodically becomes epidemic. In the United States, epidemics had occurred at 7–10 year intervals until the mid-1940s (Branham, 1956). Since then there has not been a major outbreak despite the occurrence of epidemics in many other parts of the world (Pfair, 1958; McCormick *et al.,* 1974). During the period 1962–1968, the incidence of meningococcal disease per year was approximately 6000 (Feldman *et al.,* 1976). However, the annual number of reported cases fell to less than 2000 between 1971 and 1975, the lowest incidence since reporting began in 1920 (Morbidity and Mortality Weekly Report, 1976).

Meningococcal meningitis and meningoccemia are diseases primarily of early childhood. Over half of all cases occur in children less than 5 years of age, with the peak incidence at 6–8 months of life (Fraser *et al.*, 1973). During epidemics there is a tendency for increased frequency of disease among older children and teenagers. Morbidity and mortality rates are higher in males than females; they are also greater in blacks and American Indians than in whites, perhaps because the disease is more common among the poor (Feldman *et al.*, 1976).

Prior to 1960 most epidemics were associated with group A meningococci (Branham, 1956). Since then the epidemic potential of group B and group C strains has been recognized. Outbreaks of group B disease have occurred among U.S. military recruits (Artenstein *et al.*, 1971a), in Belgium (Weekly Epidemiological Record, 1976), in Norway (Peltola, 1977), and in the Sudan (Erwa *et al.*, 1971). Group C epidemics have occurred among U.S. military recruits (Artenstein *et al.*, 1971a), in Brazil (de Morais *et al.*, 1974), in Argentina (Weekly Epidemiological Record, 1975), and in Nigeria (Whittle and Greenwood, 1976).

At the present time, group B and C strains cause 80–90% of meningococcal disease in the United States. However, disease caused by group Y meningococci has been increasing in frequency (Meningococcal Surveillance Group, 1976). Group A strains have rarely been isolated in the United States in the past 20 years, except during very localized outbreaks in Oregon, Washington, and Alaska (Morbidity and Mortality Weekly Report, 1977).

2. Serological Classification

Meningococci can be classified serologically by means of agglutination reactions into at least nine groups: A, B, C, D, X, Y, Z, 29E, and W135. Group specificities are determined by the capsular polysaccharides, the chemical compositions of which are indicated in Table 1. Group C meningococci have also been subdivided on the basis of differences in the structure of the capsular polysaccharide (Apicella, 1974). The neuraminic acid polymer of most group C strains has both *N*- and *O*-acetyl groups and is resistant to enzymatic degradation by neuraminidase. The variant C polysaccharide lacks *O*-acetyl groups and is neuraminidase sensitive (Gotschlich, 1975).

Meningococci can also be divided into serotypes on the basis of antigenic differences detected originally by bactericidal reactions (Gold and Wyle, 1970; Frasch and Chapman, 1972a). Subsequently, a variety of methods have been developed to identify serotypes, including precipitin techniques (Frasch and Chapman, 1972b), bactericidal inhibition (Frasch and Chapman, 1973), and polyacrylamide gel electrophoresis (Frasch and Gotschlich, 1974). Serotype specificity is de-

TABLE 1. Chemical Structure of Capsular Polysaccharides of *Neisseria meningitidis*

Serotype	Chemistry of repeating unit	Linkage	Location of *O*-acetyl groups	References
A	*N*-Acetyl, *O*-acetyl mannosamine-6-phosphate	α-1,6	C3	Liu *et al.* (1971a), Bundle *et al.* (1974)
B	*N*-Acetyl neuraminic acid	α-2,8	None	Liu *et al.* (1971b), Bhattacharjee *et al.* (1975)
C	*N*-Acetyl, *O*-acetyl neuraminic acid	α-2,9	C7 and C8	Liu *et al.* (1971b), Bhattacharjee *et al.* (1975)
X	*N*-Acetyl glucosamine-4-phosphate	α-1,4	None	Bundle *et al.* (1974)
Y	*N*-Acetyl, *O*-acetyl neuraminic acid: glucose	α-2,6	Unknown	Bhattacharjee *et al.* (1976)
W135	*N*-Acetyl neuraminic acid: galactose	α-2,6	None	Bhattacharjee *et al.* (1976)
29E	3-Deoxyoctulosonic acid (KDO): 2-deoxygalactosamine	Unknown	Unknown	Bhattacharjee *et al.* (1974)

termined by the major proteins in the outer cell membrane of the bacteria (Frasch and Gotschlich, 1974). Serotype-specific proteins are common to groups B, C, and Y meningococci (Kasper *et al.,* 1973; Frasch, 1977), but group A strains have a unique serotype protein different from those of the other serotypes. Twelve serotype proteins have been identified and more are under investigation (Frasch, 1977).

During epidemics of group C disease in the U.S. Army (Gold *et al.,* 1971) and Brazil (Munford *et al.,* 1975), over 80% of strains isolated from cases were found to be serotype 2. Serotype 2 also accounts for most cases of group B disease and is also commonly found in many group Y and W135 cases (Frasch, 1977). The outer membrane proteins of serotype 2 groups B and C meningococci are chemically and serologically identical (Frasch and Gotschlich, 1974; Munford *et al.,* 1975). Griffiss *et al.* (1977) found that strains of groups B, C, and Y isolated from concurrent cases of meningococcal disease in U.S. Army recruits were predominantly serotype 2.

Differences in the antigenic determinants of the lipopolysaccharide (LPS) in the outer cell membrane also contribute to the antigenic diversity of meningococci (Zollinger *et al.,* 1974; Frasch *et al.,* 1976; Bertram *et al.,* 1976). The LPS antigens have not yet been investigated systematically as a means of classifying strains of meningococci.

3. Factors Contributing to Pathogenicity

Group C meningococcal disease has been shown to have a significantly higher case fatality rate than group A disease because of the higher frequency of fulminant meningococcemia in the former (Evans-Jones *et al.,* 1977). Group B disease appears to share with group C the propensity to produce more severe disease (Peltola, 1977). The factors responsible for the more frequent occurrence of fulminant disease with group C strains, especially in infants and young children, are not known. There does not appear to be a difference in endotoxin content among the three types. It is not known whether factors other than endotoxin contribute to the coagulopathy. Antige-

nemia is more common with group C than with group A disease (Evans-Jones *et al.,* 1977). Moreover, anti-A polysaccharide antibody concentrations are higher in infants and young children than anti-C levels (Gold and Lepow, 1976). As will be described subsequently, some organisms in the pharynx or intestine of infants contain antigens that cross-react with group A which contribute significantly to anti-A antibodies during early life. The lack of naturally acquired anti-C antibody may contribute to the frequency of fulminant disease by allowing more rapid growth of group C strains, while the higher, but not protective, levels of anti-A antibody may impede growth of group A meningococci sufficiently to prevent fulminant meningococcemia. Whether differences in the virulence of strains of meningococci play a role in the severity of human disease is not known.

Allergic reactions, consisting of allergic vasculitis and arthritis, are also more common after group C than group A disease (Evans-Jones *et al.,* 1977). The frequency of allergic complications correlates with the frequency of antigenemia at the time of admission to hospital (Whittle *et al.,* 1973). Moreover, there is a fall in the concentration of $C'3$ coincident with the onset of the rash and/or arthritis (Greenwood *et al.,* 1973). Examination of skin and synovial membrane biopsies reveals deposition of immune complexes containing the capsular polysaccharide, immunoglobulin, and complement.

The mechanisms accounting for endemic and epidemic spread of meningococci in either closed or open populations are not understood. Some outbreaks have been temporally related to influenza A infections (Eickhoff, 1971; Young *et al.,* 1972), but no association between meningococcal acquisitions or disease and other viral respiratory infections has been found (Artenstein *et al.,* 1967).

4. The Immune Response in Man

4.1. Antibody Assays

Antibodies induced in humans as the result of the carrier state, disease, or immunization can be detected by a variety of serological methods (Artenstein *et al.,* 1971c).

4.1.1. Bactericidal Assay

The bactericidal assay measures complement-mediated lysis of viable organisms by whole serum. Bactericidal activity is mediated predominantly by IgG (Gotschlich et al., 1969b). Standardization of the assay is difficult because of the variability of the human or animal sera used as complement sources.

4.1.2. Indirect Hemagglutination Assay

The indirect hemagglutination assay (IHA) has been much easier to standardize than the bactericidal assay. Erythrocytes can be sensitized with the purified polysaccharides (Gotschlich et al., 1969b). Most of the hemagglutinating activity resides in the IgM fraction of antibody (Gotschlich et al., 1969b).

4.1.3. Indirect Immunofluorescence

Indirect immunofluorescence, utilizing whole organisms as the antigen, has been used to measure antibodies present in the three major immunoglobulin classes, IgG, IgM, and IgA (Goldschneider et al., 1969a).

The IHA assay, because of its simplicity, has proven to be extremely useful in studies of group-specific serological responses of adults to disease and immunization (Artenstein et al., 1971b). The IFA and bactericidal assays, while considerably more tedious and difficult to standardize, have been invaluable in analyzing the cross-reactive antibodies stimulated by carrier infections with meningococci and N. lactamica (Goldschneider et al., 1969b; Gold et al., 1978a), as will be discussed in detail in a subsequent section.

4.1.4. Radioimmunoassay

The most sensitive method of detecting antibody to the meningococcal polysaccharides is the radioactive antigen-binding assay (Gotschlich et al., 1972). The lower limits of detectability of anti-A and anti-C with this assay have been approximately 0.1–0.2 μg/ml (Gold et al., 1976). Results of the radioactive binding assay can be expressed in terms either of percentage of antigen bound (Brandt et al., 1972) or of micrograms of antibody protein per milliliter of serum. The former values are measured directly by the assay; the latter are extrapolated from standard curves relating percentage of antigen bound to the antibody concentration in standard sera as determined by quantitative precipitation. In the range of 10–90% antigen binding, there is a linear relationship between percentage of antigen bound and logarithm of the antibody concentration (Gotschlich et al., 1972). This assay has been used extensively in studies of the antibody responses of infants to immunization with the groups A and C polysaccharide vaccines because of the low antibody concentration found in infants.

4.1.5. Human Antibody Response to Infection

The antibody response of adults and children over 2 years of age to systemic meningococcal disease is very rapid and very intense. Antibody can be detected by the 4th to 7th day after onset of disease by means of bactericidal, hemagglutinating, immunofluorescent, and radioactive antigen-binding assays (Goldschneider et al., 1969b; Artenstein et al., 1971b; Wyle et al., 1972). The antigens inducing the antibody following disease include the cell membrane protein and lipopolysaccharide as well as the group-specific capsular polysaccharide. Zollinger et al. (1974) demonstrated that although the titers of hemagglutinating antibody to the protein and lipopolysaccharide antigens are equivalent after groups B and C disease, very little antibody is induced by the B polysaccharide in comparison to the C polysaccharide.

Asymptomatic carriage of groups B, C, or Y meningococci by army recruits has also been shown to be immunogenic (Goldschneider et al., 1969b). Bactericidal titers increase as do fluorescent antibody titers with IgG, IgA, and IgM against the homogeneous strain. Zollinger et al. (1974) found that most of the antibody resulting from carriage of group B meningococci was directed against the cell membrane protein, with little antibody found against either the lipopolysaccharide or capsular polysaccharide.

Infants under 1 year of age may not respond to systemic disease in the same way as adults. Baltimore and Hammerschlag (1977) studied three infants with meningococcal bacteremia, none of whom developed demonstrable bactericidal antibody against the infecting strain. However, Gold et al. (1978a) found that infants did develop cross-reacting bactericidal antibody against groups B and C meningococci following carriage of *N. lactamica* (see Section 4.2). The difference in responsiveness of infants to disease may parallel the age-dependent response to purified polysaccharide vaccines. It is not known whether the differences observed are due to differences in clearance of antigen.

4.2. Development of Natural Immunity

4.2.1. Role of Virulent Organisms

In closed population groups, such as military recruit camps, outbreaks of meningococcal disease are associated with high rates of acquisition of the virulent strain (Gotschlich *et al.,* 1969c; Artenstein *et al.,* 1970b). However, during civilian epidemics the carrier rate of the epidemic strain is often very low in the general population, although carriage is common among household contacts of cases (Munford *et al.,* 1974; Peltola, 1977). As a result of extensive experience with surveillance of meningococcal carriage in U. S. Army recruits, Artenstein *et al.* (1974) concluded that "for practical purposes, *routine* carrier surveys have not provided any predictive information concerning incidence of disease and, therefore, have been deleted from control programs in the U. S. Army."

Longitudinal studies of acquisition of meningococci by infants and 6- to 8-year-old school children under endemic disease conditions indicate that such acquisition is very infrequent. The annual acquisition rate was found to be 2.5% in infants and 3.9% in older children (Gold *et al.,* 1978a).

The age-related development of natural immunity, as defined by the presence of bactericidal antibody, appears to be the result of exposure to a variety of antigens. Immunity in the newborn infant depends on transplacental passage of antimeningococcal IgG from the mother to fetus (Goldschneider *et al.,* 1969a). These passively acquired antibodies are lost during the first few months of life, resulting in marked susceptibility of young infants to disease.

4.2.2. Role of *Neisseria lactamica*

Carriage of *Neisseria lactamica,* a bacterium closely related to the meningococcus, results in the development of cross-reacting bactericidal antibody to groups A, B, and C meningococci in infants and children (Goldschneider, 1969b; Gold *et al.,* 1978a). Since most infants acquire *N. lactamica* during the first 2 years of life (Gold *et al.,* 1978a), these organisms may be a major source of natural immunization. In adults carriage of both groupable (encapsulated) and nongroupable (unencapsulated) meningococci results in the development of cross-reactive bactericidal antibody to groups A, B, and C (Goldschneider *et al.,* 1969b; Reller *et al.,* 1973). Other neisserial strains have not been studied for cross-reacting antibodies.

The antigens responsible for the cross-reacting antibodies induced by the carriage of *N. lactamica* and *N. meningitidis* in infants, children, and adults have not been identified. The serotype-specific proteins present in the outer cell membrane are the most likely candidate antigens. Frasch (1977) has shown that children under 2 years of age make antibody to serotype 2 after recovery from group B or group C sterotype 2 disease. Moreover, adult levels of antibody to serotype 2 are reached by age 10. In addition, guinea pigs develop specific immunity to serotype 2 infection after the development of antibody to serotype 2.

4.2.3. Role of Normal Bacterial Flora

Antibodies against the capsular polysaccharides of groups A and C meningococci are also acquired in early childhood, although at markedly different rates. Most infants have detectable anti-A antibody by 1 year of age but do not have detectable anti-C antibody until 2–3 years of age (Gold *et al.,* 1976; Gold and Lepow, 1976). These antipolysaccharide antibodies are acquired in the absence of detectable carriage of groups A or C meningococci (Gold *et al.,* 1978c). Possible sources of the antigens responsible for the anti-A and anti-C antibodies are members of the normal throat and fecal bacterial flora with capsular polysaccharides similar or identical to the meningococci. A variety of such bacteria have been identified (Table 2), but which ones are responsible for natural immunization remains to be determined. The use of *N. lactamica* or other normal flora as immunogens will not be prudent until their degree of pathogenicity is defined.

TABLE 2. Bacteria with Antigens Cross-Reactive with Groups A, B, and C Meningococci

Antigen cross-reactive against serogroup	Organism	References
A	*Bacillus pumilis*	Robbins *et al.* (1975)
	Staphylococcus aureus	Gold *et al.* (1978c)
	Staphylococcus epidermidis	Gold *et al.* (1978c)
B	*Escherichia coli* K1	Robbins *et al.* (1975)
	Streptococcus viridans	Gold *et al.* (1978c)
C	*Escherichia coli* K92	Robbins *et al.* (1975)
	Streptococcus viridans	Gold *et al.* (1978c)

4.3. Evidence That Immunity Is Antibody Mediated

Goldschneider *et al.* (1969a) have summarized the evidence that immunity to invasive meningococcal disease depends on specific antibody:

1. The age-specific incidence of meningococcal disease is inversely related to the age-specific prevalence of bactericidal antibody. The peak incidence of disease occurs at 6–12 months of age and 50% of cases occur in infants under 2 years of age, at a time when the proportion of infants with detectable bactericidal antibody is at a minimum.
2. Only 5.6% of Army recruits who developed group C disease had detectable bactericidal antibody at the time of arrival at recruit training camp compared to 82% of controls without disease.
3. Thirty-eight percent of recruits who acquired a group C strain, against which they lacked bactericidal antibody, developed meningococcal disease compared to lack of disease in recruits with prior antibody.
4. Group-specific horse antiserum administered intrathecally reduced the case fa-

tality rate of meningococcal disease (Flexner, 1913).
5. It was shown by Goldschneider *et al.* (1969b) that antipolysaccharide antibody composes the major component of the bactericidal response to the group C meningococcus. The other contributing antigens to the bactericidal response have not been completely identified.

Subsequent experience with the groups A and C meningococcal polysaccharide vaccines confirmed the importance of antibody directed against specific polysaccharides in preventing meningococcal disease.

The minimum concentration of antipolysaccharide antibody to be associated with protection has not been determined directly. Peltola *et al.* (1977) have estimated that 2 μg/ml of anti-A antibody is required for protection, based on the observations that 60% of adults had ≥2 μg/ml and 60% of adults also had protective levels of bactericidal antibody. In addition, acute phase sera of patients with group A meningococcal disease had anti-A concentrations of less than 2 μg/ml (Makala *et al.*, 1977). Furthermore, protection was seen in immunized infants in whom vaccine induced geometric mean anti-A or anti-C concentrations of approximately 2 μg/ml (Peltola *et al.*, 1977; Amato Neto *et al.*, 1974). Data are not available for minimal protective levels in agammaglobulinemic children treated with γ-globulin because of the low incidence of meningococcal disease.

4.4. Mechanisms of Killing Meningococci *in Vivo*

Bactericidal antibodies present in human sera are directed against a variety of antigens, including the capsular polysaccharide, the serotype-specific protein, and, perhaps, the lipopolysaccharide. Group-specific opsonic antibodies have also been demonstrated in human sera (Roberts, 1970). Although antibodies to the capsular polysaccharide have been shown to be protective against groups A and C meningococci, the group B polysaccharide is poorly immunogenic in man (Wyle *et al.*, 1972), suggesting that antibody to the serotype proteins or other antigens in the outer cell membrane is also involved in protection. The occurrence of recurrent meningococcal meningitis or chronic meningococcemia (Lim *et al.*, 1976) and gonococcemia (Petersen *et al.*, 1976) in patients with specific deficiencies in terminal components of complement (C6–C9) necessary for cell lysis suggests that bactericidal reactions may be important *in vivo* in defense against invasive meningococcal disease. Deficiency in terminal complement components does not affect phagocytosis or intracellular killing of meningococci by human leukocytes (Nicholson and Lepow, 1978). Disease develops in such patients despite the presence of circulating bactericidal antibody to the invading meningococcus. The defective bactericidal activity can be restored by the addition of exogenous complement or the purified missing complement component to the patient's sera.

4.5. Infection in Special Hosts

4.5.1. Splenectomy

Splenectomized persons are at special risk of overwhelming infections with encapsulated organisms including pneumococci, meningococci, and *Hemophilus influenzae* b. Eraklis and Filler (1972) reviewed 1413 patients who had had splenectomy. The patients at highest risk for serious infection were those whose splenectomy was secondary to underlying hematological disease. Dickerman (1976) established that the risk of infection in persons with splenectomy due to trauma was greater than in the general population. Patients with Hodgkin's disease who have splenectomy as part of a staging laparotomy and who receive radiation and chemotherapy have a greater risk of severe infection (Chilcote *et al.*, 1976).

Patients with sickle cell disease undergo autosplenectomy during the first years of life (Seeler *et al.*, 1972) and may have defects in opsonization (Winklestein and Drachman, 1968). Low IgM levels (Gavrilis *et al.*, 1974) and a defect in the alternative pathway of the complement system (Johnston *et al.*, 1973) have been suggested as contributing factors in the increased risk of overwhelming sepsis in children with sickle cell disease, especially with pneumococcal disease. Again, because of low incidence of meningococcal disease, similar data have not been forthcoming.

Studies of Ammann *et al.* (1977) indicate that splenectomized patients (exclusive of those with Hodgkin's disease) who are over 2 years of age are capable of responding to pneumococcal polysaccharide vaccines with high titers of circulating antibodies. Protection with the polyvalent vaccine has been demonstrated in patients with sickle cell disease, and the implication is that similar results could be expected with meningococcal A and C vaccines.

The association of chronic meningococcemia with IgM deficiency has been suggested by reports of Hobbs *et al.* (1967) and Fass and Saslaw (1972). In the Hobbs report, there was a family constellation. None of these patients was studied for complement deficiencies.

4.5.2. Agammaglobulinemia

Agammaglobulinemic children have increased susceptibility to invasion with encapsulated organisms (Rosen and Janeway, 1966). The low incidence of meningococcal disease, including fulminating disease, probably accounts for the lack of reports of an increased risk of such children to the meningococcus. In addition, passively administered IgG may be therapeutic.

No data are available on response of the neutropenic host—largely because of rarity of neutropenia and meningococcal disease.

5. Immunoprevention

5.1. Development of Groups A and C Meningococcal Polysaccharide Vaccines

The impetus for renewed interest in vaccines to prevent meningococcal disease was the emergence of widespread resistance to sulfonamides among groups B and C (Artenstein *et al.*, 1971a; Millar *et al.*, 1963) and later group A meningococci (Vassiliades *et al.*, 1969). Sulfonamides had been the major tool for control of meningococcal outbreaks in military camps and other closed population groups. The lack at that time of any equally effective chemotherapeutic agent to control the carrier state and thereby interrupt transmission spurred the development of vaccines. Once it had been demonstrated that immunity to meningococcal disease was associated with the presence of circulating antibody and that antibody to the capsular polysaccharide was a major component of the bactericidal activity of serum for groups A and C, the next step was to prepare vaccines from the capsular polysaccharides. Gotschlich *et al.* (1969a) developed a relatively simple procedure permitting extraction and purification of the groups A and C meningococcal polysaccharides in high molecular weight form. The molecular size of the polysaccharides has proven to be a major determinant of immunogenicity, as was expected from the work of Kabat and Bezer (1958) on the immunogenicity of dextran in man.

The currently used manufacturing processes for the groups A and C polysaccharide vaccines involve purification by cold phenol or chloroform–ethanol, respectively (Wong *et al.*, 1977). Standardization of these vaccines is unique, since there is no known animal model which can be used to assess clinical potency. A variety of physicochemical, serological, and biological assays have been developed as indicators of immunogenicity in man in order to avoid having to test each vaccine lot in human volunteers. The chemical, physical, serological, and biological specifications of clinically acceptable vaccines are summarized in Table 3.

The immunogenicity of purified capsular polysaccharide of group A meningococci had been first studied by Kabat *et al.* (1944). The vaccine proved to be nonimmunogenic in man, probably because the method of preparation resulted in material with molecular weight less than 50,000 (Liu *et al.*, 1971a).

5.1.1. Immunogenicity and Efficacy in Adults

A series of field trials conducted by Artenstein and coworkers of the Walter Reed Army Institute of Research in U.S. Army recruit volunteers established the safety and immunogenicity of the groups A and C polysaccharide vaccines in adults (Gotschlich *et al.*, 1969b; Artenstein *et al.*, 1970a; Gold and Artenstein, 1971). When administered intracutaneously, most recipients developed local reactions consisting of erythema and rarely swelling and tenderness. The size of the local erythema was dose related. Following subcutaneous administration with needle and sy-

TABLE 3. Specifications for Groups A and C Meningococcal Polysaccharide Vaccines[a]

Chemical analysis (dry weight)	A: Mannosamine phosphate minimum 60% or inorganic phosphorus minimum 7.5% C: Sialic acid minimum 80% O-Acetyl content minimum 2 μmol/mg Residual protein: maximum 1% Residual nucleic acids: maximum 1%
Physical analysis	Molecular size: Minimum of 50% of the antigen recovered from Sepharose 4B column with a K_d of 0.5 or smaller Residual moisture in final container: maximum 1%
Serological analysis	Purity: No inhibition of hemagglutination by the vaccine at a minimum final concentration of 100 μg (dry weight)/ml in the presence of heterologous antibody and erythrocytes sensitized with heterologous antigen Specificity: Inhibits hemagglutination of erythrocytes sensitized with homologous antigen in the presence of homologous antibody
Biological analysis	Clinical potency: Injection of 50 μg induces a fourfold or greater rise in bactericidal antibody titer in at least 80% of adult human volunteers Pyrogenicity: Vaccine in a test dose of 2.5–0.25 μg/ml per kg body weight of the rabbit meets the pyrogenicity standard of Section 610.13 of the U.S. Food and Drug Regulations (1974)

[a] From Wong *et al.* (1977).

ringe or jet-injector, local reactions were significantly less frequent than after intracutaneous injection. No significant systemic reactions were observed (Artenstein *et al.*, 1970a).

Antibody was detectable as early as 6 days after immunization and peaked in 10–14 days. Following a 50-μg dose, fourfold or greater increases in bactericidal titer were observed in over 90% of recipients. Significant antibody rises could also be detected by hemagglutination and immunofluorescence. Increases in IgG, IgA, and IgM were detectable by the latter assay, all in large quantities. The antibody response to the group C polysaccharide was dose related: although no difference was observed between doses of 50 and 100 μg, both of these doses induced greater titers than 10 μg. Subsequent studies have shown that 50 μg of A or C vaccine results in peak antibody concentrations of 20–40 µg/ml of specific antipolysaccharide antibody in adults.

Studies of the group C vaccine in military recruit populations during epidemics of group C disease showed that significant local immunity was induced in the nasopharynx as a result of immunization. The acquisition rate of the group C carrier state during the 8 weeks for basic training was reduced by 50% or more (Gotschlich *et al.*, 1969c; Artenstein *et al.*, 1970b; Devine *et al.*, 1970). Two large-scale field trials in the U.S. Army were undertaken in 1968–1970 involving 28,390 recruits (Gold and Artenstein, 1971). The incidence of group C meningococcal disease was significantly reduced, consistent with a protective efficacy of almost 90%. The protection was group specific in that the incidence of group B disease was the same in the vaccine and control groups. Since October 1971 all U.S. Army recruits entering basic training have received the group C vaccine, and group C disease has disappeared from the recruit training centers (Artenstein *et al.*, 1974).

The group A vaccine was also tested for safety and efficacy in U.S. Army recruits in small-scale trials (Gotschlich *et al.*, 1969c; Artenstein *et al.*, 1971b). During an epidemic of group A disease in Finland, the group A vaccine was evaluated in the Finnish Army and found to be 90% effective in preventing disease (Makela *et al.*, 1975).

The persistence of the antibody response in adults has been examined in only a few individuals. Antibody titers persist with little significant change over 14–18 months (Artenstein, 1971; Brandt and Artenstein, 1975). Persistence of antibody amongst various immunoglobulin classes is not known.

5.1.2. Immunogenicity in Children over 2 Years

Since responses of older children as well as infants to the group A and group C vaccines are different, results are summarized in Table 4 as well as explained in the text. Initial studies of the groups A and C polysaccharide vaccines in small groups of children 2–10 years of age clearly indicated that the vaccines were safe and immunogenic (Goldschneider *et al.*, 1972; Monto *et al.*, 1973). However, the geometric mean antibody concentrations measured by the radioactive antigen-binding assay after im-

TABLE 4. Antibody Responses of Infants and Children to Primary and Booster Immunizations with Group A and C Meningococcal Polysaccharide Vaccines

| Age | Dose[b] | Geometric mean antibody concentration (µg/ml)[a] | | | |
| | | Anti-A | | Anti-C | |
		Pre[c]	Post[d]	Pre[c]	Post[d]
3 mo	1°	0.34	0.32	0.11	0.29
7 mo	1°	0.17	0.34	0.09	0.80
	2°	0.22	2.09	0.14	0.23
12 mo	1°	0.17	0.93	0.12	1.69
	2°	0.28	4.00	0.12	0.94
18 mo	1°	0.56	3.04	0.20	2.98
2–6 yr	1°	4.28	13.23	0.36	10.13
	2°	2.73	14.16	0.35	9.98
6–8 yr	1°	1.68	9.35	0.33	9.12

[a] Each age group consisted of ≥25 subjects.
[b] Dose: 25 µg of A or C polysaccharide at 3, 7, and 12 months of age, 50 µg at 18 months and 2–6 and 6–8 years of age. 1°, Primary immunization; 2°, booster immunization with 3–4 months between 1° and 2° doses of vaccine except at 12 months of age, when 1° was given 9 months previously.
[c] Pre, preimmunization sera.
[d] Post, 1-month-postimmunization sera.

munization with 25–50 µg of A or C vaccine were only 50% of the levels seen in adults. Persistence of anti-A and anti-C in these children also differed from the pattern in adults. The rate of decline was linear, although more rapid for anti-C than for anti-A, and reached baseline levels in 3–4 years (Goldschneider *et al.*, 1972). A second dose of A vaccine administered 3 years after the primary immunization resulted in anti-A levels comparable to those following the primary inoculation, but the antibody concentration showed no significant decline during the 3 years of observation after the booster (Lepow *et al.*, 1977). The booster response among the three immunoglobulin classes has not been determined. All of the children had anti-A concentration ≥2.0 µg/ml at 3 years after booster compared to 25% of unimmunized children of the same age.

Antibody responses were followed over a 4-year period in a larger group of 6- to 8-year-old school children immunized successfully with a jet injector (Lepow *et al.*, 1977). The preimmunization concentrations of anti-A and anti-C antibody were 1.68 and 0.33 µg/ml, respectively. One month after administration of 50 µg of either A or C vaccine, the mean anti-

A and anti-C concentrations were both approximately 9 μg/ml, and 95% of children had ≥2.0 μg/ml of anti-A or anti-C antibody. The rate of decline of anti-C was significantly greater than anti-A during the first year after immunization, but between 1 and 4 years the antibody concentrations declined at the same rate. Thus anti-A concentrations declined 32% to 5.5 μg/ml while anti-C fell 68% of 3.6 μg at 1 year. At 4 years the anti-A and anti-C concentrations were 3.6 and 1.5, respectively, while the proportions of children with >2.0 μg of anti-A and anti-C were 80% and 40%, respectively. By contrast, unimmunized children of the same age as the study children 4 years after immunization had anti-A and anti-C concentrations of 1.17 and 0.45 μg/ml, respectively.

5.1.3. Immunogenicity in Infants

Since the peak age incidence of meningococcal disease occurs in the first year of life, detailed investigations of the safety and immunogenicity of the vaccines in infants have been necessary in order to define the optimal dose and schedule of immunizations. Both the A and C vaccines have been well tolerated by infants as young as 2–3 months of age. Transient local erythema at the injection site and increased irritability have been observed in 8–10% of infants (Goldschneider *et al.*, 1973; Gold *et al.*, 1976). During the field trial of the A vaccine in Finland, reaction rates were significantly higher including fever >38.5°C in 3.8% of infants (Peltola *et al.*, 1977). Analyses of the lots of A vaccine used in the Finnish trials showed significant correlation between endotoxin contamination and reaction rates (Kuronen *et al.*, 1977), indicating the importance of strict quality control in vaccine production.

The responses of infants to the A and C vaccines are significantly different and are also summarized in Table 4. The factors determining the immunogenicity of the vaccines in infants include age of infant, amount of vaccine, molecular size of polysaccharide in the vaccine, number of doses of vaccine, and prior experience with meningococcal or cross-reacting polysaccharides.

At 2–3 months of age almost all infants have less than 0.08 μg/ml of anti-C polysaccharide antibody, and approximately 90% will respond

to primary immunization at 3 months of age with significant rises in anti-C (Gold *et al.*, 1976). In contrast, most infants have detectable anti-A antibody at 3 months of age, but less than 5% have any rise in anti-A concentration after primary immunization. With increasing age there is an almost linear increase in the immunogenicity of both the A and C vaccines. Indeed, if age and peak antibody concentration are plotted on a log-log scale, the relationship between age and anti-A and anti-C concentration is linear between 6 months and 20 years of age (Gotschlich *et al.*, 1976).

The response of infants is also dose dependent. At 3, 7, and 12 months of age, there are significant differences in the responses to 10, 25, or 100 μg/ml of C vaccine. However, 200 μg is no more effective than lower doses at 3 months of age (Gold *et al.*, 1976). Similar findings are obtained after primary immunization with the A vaccine at 3, 7, and 12 months of age, although the differences are not statistically significant.

The availability of lots of group A vaccine which differ in molecular weight has permitted elucidation of the relationship between molecular size and immunogenicity. Gotschlich *et al.* (1972) showed that a vaccine with molecular weights of less than 50,000 induced significantly less anti-A antibody than lots of vaccine greater than 84,000 molecular weight. The dependence of the immunogenicity on molecular size of the A vaccine has been confirmed by Gold *et al.* (1976) in infants. More recently, studies of a group C vaccine having molecular weight greater than 1 million indicate that this very large vaccine is significantly more immunogenic than the standard vaccine in children 2–10 years of age (Gold *et al.*, 1977a) and in infants (Gold, unpublished results).

The most striking difference in the response of infants to the A and C vaccines was the presence of anamnestic responses to booster doses of A vaccine and their absence with the C vaccine (Gold *et al.*, 1976). When infants who had received primary immunization with A vaccine at 3 months of age were given booster doses at 7 or at 12 months of age, geometric mean anti-A concentrations of approximately 2 and 4 μg/ml were achieved. Primary immunization at 7 and 12 months of age resulted in significantly lower anti-A concentrations—approximately 0.4 and 1.0 μg/ml, respectively. In contrast, booster injections of 25 or 100 μg of C vaccine at 7 or 12 months of age resulted in decreased anti-C concentrations compared to the effect of primary immunization at these ages. Such suppression of the anti-C responses was not observed when the primary dose of C vaccine was 10 μg. Moreover, when the primary was given at 7 months of age followed by a booster at 12 months of age, no suppression occurred. Similar hyporesponsiveness to repeated doses of C vaccine was noted in adults by Artenstein and Brandt (1975). Army recruits who were immunized with a lot of A vaccine containing trace amounts of C polysaccharide (approximately 0.03 μg per 50 μg dose of A vaccine) showed lower anti-C responses to the C vaccine administered 2 weeks later than recruits who received only the C vaccine. This same lot of A vaccine (lot A7) did not induce any depression of responsiveness to C vaccine in infants when it was administered at least 4 months before the C vaccine (Gold *et al.,* 1976). Although the mechanism of the decreased responsiveness to C vaccine is not understood, there is no evidence that a single dose of C vaccine increases the susceptibility of infants to group C disease (Taunay *et al.,* 1974). When children 2–10 years of age were given two doses of C vaccine at an interval of 2–3 months, neither enhancement or suppression of the antibody response was observed (Gold *et al.,* 1977a). Moreover, infants who had received two doses of C vaccine at 3 and at 7 or 12 months of age and who had displayed hyporesponsiveness to the second dose, had normal responses to a third dose of C vaccine administered at 2 years of age (Gold *et al.,* 1977a). Lack of an animal model makes studies of T-cell responses difficult to undertake with meningococcal polysaccharides, although work is in progress with other polysaccharide antigens.

In an attempt to enhance the anti-A concentrations achieved by immunization of infants, Gold *et al.* (1978b) immunized infants with three doses of A vaccine at 2, 4, and 6 months of age. The geometric mean anti-A concentrations achieved 1 month after the third dose of vaccine were significantly lower than those observed in infants immunized with two doses of vaccine at 3 and 7 months of age. Whether the reduced response was the result of the shorter interval between doses or the greater total quantity of polysaccharide administered is unknown. The optimal schedule of immunization of infants with the A vaccine, in terms of antigen dose, interval between doses, the molecular size of vaccine, remains to be determined.

No cross-reactions between the A and C vaccines have been observed at any age, except in A vaccines contaminated with trace amounts of C vaccine (Artenstein and Brandt, 1975; Gold *et al.,* 1976). The vaccines can be administered as a combined bivalent preparation without any interference in the antibody responses to either polysaccharide (Gold *et al.,* 1977a). Administration of DPT vaccine at the same time as the bivalent A/C meningococcal vaccine had no effect on the response of 18-month-old children to the latter (Gold and Lepow, 1976).

Persistence of antibody following immunization of infants with A or C vaccine is relatively short. The rate of decline of anti-C antibody is more rapid than anti-A, but both anti-A and anti-C concentration reach baseline values by 24 months of age following immunization at 12 months or earlier (Gold *et al.,* 1977a). Thus booster immunization at 18–24 months of age will probably be necessary in order to maintain protective antibody levels. Persistence of antibody after a booster immunization at 2 years of age is currently under study in order to determine the need for additional boosters.

5.1.4. Efficacy in Preventing Disease in Infants and Children

The group A vaccine has been shown to be 100% effective in preventing group A disease in Egyptian school children 6–15 years of age for at least 2 years (Wahden *et al.,* 1973). Another field trial in the Sudan, involving primarily school children, also demonstrated protection against disease (Erwa *et al.,* 1973). Efficacy in Finnish infants and children 3 months to 5 years of age has been reported by Peltola *et al.* (1977). Infants 3–18 months to 5 years received a single immunization. In a double-blind field trial, no cases of group A disease occurred among the vaccines during the 1-year follow-up period, compared to six cases in 40,000 control children who received *Hemophilus influenzae* type b vaccine and 13 cases in 30,000 children who received no vaccine. Vaccine studies were carried out in other areas of Finland, in which 80% of children under 5 years of age were immunized, also showed complete protection against the group A meningococcal strains causing disease concurrently in unimmunized older children and adults. Antibody responses of the Finnish infants were similar to those observed in American infants.

The situation with the group C vaccine in infants differs significantly from the efficacy demonstrated with the A vaccine. During the group C meningococcal epidemic in Sao Paolo Brazil in 1971, 67,000 children 6–35 months of age received 50 µg of the group C vaccine and an equal number received DPT (Taunay *et al.*, 1974). Although the vaccine was 75% effective in preventing disease in children 24–35 months old, no protection was observed in infants 6–24 months of age. The geometric mean antibody response in the older group of children was 2.0 µg/ml (Amato Neto *et al.*, 1974). The antibody responses of the Brazilian children were significantly lower than those in American children of the same age. Whether the lower response in Brazilian children resulted from host factors (e.g., malnutrition) or vaccine factors (smaller molecular weight) has not been determined.

5.2. Current Recommendations for Uses of Meningococcal A and C Vaccines

The Advisory Committee on Immunization Practices of the U.S. Public Health Service has published recommendations on the uses of groups A and C meningococcal vaccines which have been licensed by the Food and Drug Administration (Morbidity and Mortality Weekly Report 1975). The results of vaccine field trials with the group A vaccine suggest that control of epidemic group A disease is feasible. Although the current official recommendations restrict the use of the vaccines to children over 6 years of age, the results of the Finnish and Brazilian field trials indicate that significant protection can be expected against group A disease at all ages and against group C disease in children over 2 years of age. Children under 2 years should receive two doses of 50 µg of A vaccine at an interval of 3 months, while older children and adults should

receive a single dose of A vaccine. A single dose of C vaccine is recommended for children over 2 and adults in the event of epidemic group C disease.

Routine immunization of children cannot yet be recommended with either the group A or the group C vaccine until studies of antibody persistence are completed. Such data are necessary in order to determine the immunization schedule needed to maintain protective antibody levels during childhood.

In addition to use in epidemic control, the bivalent A/C meningococcal vaccine should be considered for all travelers going to areas of the world where epidemic meningococcal disease is occurring, especially the meningitis belt in Africa (Whittle and Greenwood, 1976).

The A/C vaccine should also be considered for household contacts in cases of A or C disease, since 20–30% of secondary cases occur more than 1 week after the index case. Prompt use of the vaccine might provide protection against the risk of late secondary disease. Although there are insufficient data on susceptibility of children with sickle cell disease to fulminating meningococcal disease, the increased susceptibility to pneumococcal disease suggests that these vaccines would be useful should epidemic meningococcal disease occur.

5.3. Future Goals of Immunoprophylaxis of Meningococcal Disease

Control of meningococcal disease will not be attained by immunoprophylaxis until several major problems are solved. The immunogenicity of the group C vaccine in infancy must be improved, in terms both of peak anti-C concentrations induced and of persistence of anti-C antibodies. Studies of the very large molecular weight C polysaccharide currently in progress are very promising. The variant C polysaccharide also must be evaluated to determine whether it is a better immunogen.

Another possibility of enhancing immunogenicity might be to complex the purified polysaccharide to a carrier protein. Such complexes have been shown to be significantly more immunogenic than purified polysaccharides with *H. influenzae* type b in animal models (Anderson and Smith, 1977).

The lack of any vaccine for group B meningococcal disease must be remedied, especially in light of the recently described epidemics of group B disease. The group B capsular polysaccharide does not appear to be immunogenic in man, either after natural exposure resulting from group B disease (Zollinger *et al.*, 1974) or after immunization with the purified polysaccharide (Wyle *et al.*, 1972). Attempts are under way to prepare the serotype 2 protein as a vaccine. Much more work on the epidemiology of the serotypes of group B disease is needed in order to provide the knowledge needed to use serotype-specific vaccines. For example, serotype 9 strains have been associated with group B disease in England as well as serotype 2 (Munford and Gorman, 1974).

The increasing incidence of group Y meningococcal disease has stimulated development of a group Y polysaccharide vaccine (Farquhar *et al.*, 1977). A study of the Y vaccine in a small number of adults found it to be safe and immunogenic. Field trials to demonstrate the protective efficacy of the Y vaccine will be very difficult if not impossible to carry out, since the incidence of Y disease is too low, even in military recruit camps. If studies of the safety, immunogenicity, and antibody persistence of the Y vaccine in infants, children, and adults indicate that anti-Y concentrations similar to those found to be protective against group A and C disease (i.e., approximately 2 µg/ml) can be induced by the vaccine, then the Y vaccine may be recommended for use in the absence of direct field trials demonstrating protection.

The need for vaccines against the other groups of meningococci (X, Z, 29E, W135) remains unknown.

Studies are under way to determine optimal dosage schedules for children less than 5 years of age for A and C vaccines in order to make mass immunization practical.

6. Immunotherapy

Intrathecal horse serum containing antimeningococcal antibody was used to treat meningococcal disease for nearly 25 years following the demonstration of its efficacy by Flexner (1913). With the development of sulfonamides and antibiotics, such treatment was no longer continued.

Passive antibody transmitted from mother to fetus is protective in the infants for the early months. Immunization of pregnant women has been considered to boost their antibody titers and thus increase period of passive protection of young infants. A recent study from Brazil suggested that passage of maternal antibody to the fetus after immunization of pregnant women with C vaccine was irregular and that the titers in the infant were frequently lower than those of the mother (Carvalho *et al.*, 1977). However, since antibody levels were determined by hemagglutination, which measures primarily IgM, the results of this study are difficult to evaluate. Because of the transient partial tolerance induced by the C vaccine when administered at 3 months of age, further studies of immunization of pregnant women should be approached with caution until it can be shown that polysaccharides do not pass from mother to fetus.

7. Summary and Prospects

Meningococcal disease remains one of the major epidemic infectious diseases of man. Although sulfonamides allowed for containment of epidemic disease for 25 years, emergence of resistant strains in the mid-1960s made another approach mandatory.

Vaccine development followed the demonstration that antibody to the capsular polysaccharides formed the major portion of the bactericidal antibody associated with naturally acquired immunity to disease. The group A vaccine has been successful in epidemic disease control in all age groups, while the group C vaccine has been effective in persons over 2 years of age. The lack of an effective group B vaccine is a major problem in the control of meningococcal disease. The use of outer membrane proteins associated with serotype specificity is under investigation. Polysaccharide vaccines against group Y meningococci have been developed, but the need for this and vaccines against other serogroups remains to be determined.

Although control of epidemic groups A and C meningococcal disease is now feasible, routine immunization will depend on the development of immunization schedules which provide protective antibody levels throughout childhood.

Even with available immunizing agents, further understanding of the mechanism of disease production, genetic factors which may affect host response, and the role of T cells in host response to disease as well as vaccine will contribute to ultimate disease control.

References

Amato Neto, V., Finger, H., Gotschlich, E. C., Feldman, R. A., Avila, C. A. de, Konicki, S. R., and Laus, W. C., 1974, Serologic response to serogroup C meningococcal vaccine in Brazilian preschool children, *Rev. Inst. Med. Trop. Sao Paulo* **16**:149–153.

Ammann, A. J., Addiego, J., Wara, D. W., Lubin, B., Smith, W. B., and Mentzer, W. C., 1977, Polyvalent pneumococcal-polysaccharide immunization of patients with sickle-cell anemia and patients with splenectomy, *N. Engl. J. Med.* **297**:897–900.

Anderson, P., and Smith, D. H., 1977, Immunogenicity in weanling rabbits of a polyribophosphate complex from *Haemophilus influenzae* Type b, *J. Infect. Dis.* **136**:S63–S70.

Apicella, M. A., 1974, Identification of a subgroup antigen on the *Neisseria meningitidis* group C capsular polysaccharide, *J. Infect. Dis.* **129**:147–153.

Artenstein, M. S., 1971, Meningococcal infections. 5. Duration of polysaccharide-vaccine-induced antibody. *Bull. WHO* **45**:291–293.

Artenstein, M. S., and Brandt, B. L., 1975, Immunologic hyporesponsiveness in man to group C meningococcal polysaccharide, *J. Immunol.* **115**:5–7.

Artenstein, M. S., Rust, J. H., Hunter, D. H., Lamson, T. H., and Buescher, E. L., 1967, Acute respiratory disease and meningococcal infection in Army recruits, *JAMA* **201**:1004–1008.

Artenstein, M. S., Gold, R., Zimmerly, J. G., Wyle, F. A., Branche, W. C., Jr., and Harkins, C., 1970a, Cutaneous reactions and antibody responses to meningococcal group C vaccines in man, *J. Infect. Dis.* **121**:372–377.

Artenstein, M. S., Gold, R., Zimmerly, J. G., Wyle, F., Schneider, H., and Harkin, C., 1970b, Prevention of meningococcal disease by group C polysaccharide vaccine, *N. Engl. J. Med.* **282**:417–420.

Artenstein, M. S., Schneider, H., and Tingley, M. D., 1971a, Meningococcal infections. 1. Prevalence of serogroups causing disease in U.S. Army personnel in 1964–1970, *Bull. WHO* **45**:275–278.

Artenstein, M. S., Branche, W. C., Jr., Zimmerly, J. G., Cohen, R. L., Tramont, E. C., Kasper, D. L., and Harkins, C., 1971b, Meningococcal infections. 3. Studies of the group A polysaccharide vaccines, *Bull. WHO* **45**:283–286.

Artenstein, M. S., Brandt, B. L., Tramont, E. C., Branche, W. C., Jr., Fleet, H. D., and Cohen, R. L., 1971c, Serologic studies of meningococcal infection and polysaccharide vaccination, *J. Infect. Dis.* **124**:277–288.

Artenstein, M. S., Winter, P. E., Gold, R., and Smith, C. D., 1974, Immunoprophylaxis of meningococcal infection, *Milit. Med.* **139**:91–95.

Baltimore, R. S., and Hammerschlag, M., 1977, Meningococcal bacteremia—Clinical and serologic studies of infants with mild illness, *Am. J. Dis. Child.* **131**:1001–1004.

Bertram, M. A., Griffiss, J. M., and Brand, D. D., 1976, Response to antigenic determinants on *Neisseria meningitidis* lipopolysaccharide investigated with a new radioactive antigen-binding assay, *J. Immunol.* **116**:842–846.

Bhattacharjee, A. K., Jennings, H. J., and Kenny, C. P., 1974, Characterization of 3-deoxy-D-manno octulosonic acid as a component of the capsular polysaccharide antigen from *Neisseria meningitidis* serogroup 29E, *Biochem. Biophys. Res. Commun.* **61**:489–493.

Bhattacharjee, A. K., Jennings, H. J., Kenny, C. P., Martin, A., and Smith, I. C. P., 1975, Structural determinations of the sialic acid polysaccharide antigens of *Neisseria meningitidis* serogroups B and C with carbon 13 nuclear magnetic resonance, *J. Biol. Chem.* **250**:1926–1932.

Bhattacharjee, A. K., Jennings, H. J., Kenny, C. P., Martin, A., and Smith. I. C. P., 1976, Structural determination of the polysaccharide antigens of *Neisseria meningitidis* serogroups Y, W-135, and BO, *Can. J. Biochem.* **54**:1–8.

Brandt, B. L., and Artenstein, M. S., 1975, Duration of antibody responses after immunization with Group C *Neisseria meningitidis* polysaccharide, *J. Infect. Dis.* **131**:S69–S75.

Brandt, B. L., Wyle, F. A., and Artenstein, M. S., 1972, A radioactive antigen-binding assay for *Neisseria meningitidis* polysaccharide antibody, *J. Immunol.* **108**:913–920.

Branham, S. E., 1956, Milestones in the history of the meningococcus, *Can. J. Microsec.* **2**:175–188.

Bundle, D. R., Smith, I. C. P., and Jennings, H. J., 1974, Determination of the structure and conformation of bacterial polysaccharides by C13 nuclear magnetic resonance: Studies on the group-specific antigens of *Neisseria meningitis* serogroups A and X, *J. Biol. Chem.* **249**:2275–2281.

Carvalho, A., Giampaglia, C., Kimura, H., Pereira, O., Farhat, C., Neves, J., Prandini, R., Carvalho, E., and Zarvos, A. M., 1977, Maternal and infant antibody response to meningococcal vaccination in pregnancy, *Lancet* **2**:809–811.

Chilcote, R. R., Baehner, R. L., and Hammond, D., 1976, Septicemia and meningitis in children splenectomized for Hodgkin's disease, *N. Engl. J. Med.* **295**:798–800.

Davis, C. E., and Arnold, K., 1974, Role of meningococcal endotoxin in meningococcal purpura, *J. Exp. Med.* **140:**159–171.

DeMorais, J. S., Munford, R. S., Risi, J. B., Antezana, E., and Feldman, R. A., 1974, Epidemic disease due to serogroup C *Neisseria meningitidis* in Sao Paolo, Brazil, *J. Infect. Dis.* **129:**568–571.

Devine, L. F., Pierce, W. E., Floyd, T. M., Rhode, S. L., Edwards, E. A., Siess, E. E., and Peckingpaugh, R. O., 1970, Evaluation of group C meningococcal polysaccharide vaccine in marine recruits, San Diego, California, *Am. J. Epidemiol.* **92:**25–32.

Dickerman, J. D., 1976, Bacterial infection and the asplenic host: A review, *J. Trauma* **16:**662–668.

Eickhoff, T. C., 1971, Sero-epidemiologic studies of meningococcal infections with the indirect hemagglutination test, *J. Infect. Dis.* **123:**519–526.

Eraklis, A. J., and Filler, R. M., 1972, Splenectomy in childhood: A review of 1413 cases, *J. Pediatr. Surg.* **7:**382–388.

Erwa, H. H., Satti, M. H., and Abbas, A. M., 1971, Cerebrospinal meningitis in the Sudan, *Sudan Notes Rec.* **52:**101–109.

Erwa, H. H., Haseeb, M. A., Idris, A. A., Lapeyssonie, L., Sanborn, W. R., and Sippel, J. E., 1973, A serogroup A meningococcal polysaccharide vaccine, *Bull. WHO* **49:**301–305.

Evans-Jones, L. G., Whittle, H. C., Onyewotu, I. I., Egler, L. J., and Greenwood, B. M., 1977, Comparative study of group A and group C meningococcal infection, *Arch. Dis. Child.* **52:**320–323.

Farquhar, J. D., Hankens, W. A., DeSanctis, A. N., DeMeio, J. L., and Metzgar, D. P., 1977, Clinical and serological evaluation of purified polysaccharide vaccines prepared from *Neisseria meningitidis* group Y (39828), *Proc. Soc. Exp. Biol. Med.* **155:**453–455.

Fass, R. J., and Saslaw, S., 1972, Chronic meningococcemia: Possible pathogenic role of IgM deficiency, *Arch. Intern. Med.* **130:**943–946.

Feldman, R. A., Koehler, R. E., and Fraser, D. W., 1976, Race-specific differences in bacterial meningitis death rates in the United States 1962–1968, *Am. J. Publ. Health* **66:**392–396.

Flexner, S., 1913, The results of the serum treatment in 1300 cases of epidemic meningitis, *J. Exp. Med.* **17:**553–576.

Frasch, C. E., 1977, Role of protein serotype antigens in protection against disease due to *Neisseria meningitidis*, *J. Infect. Dis.* **136:**S84–S90.

Frasch, C. E., and Chapman, S. S., 1972a, Classification of *Neisseria meningitidis* group B into distinct serotypes. I. Serological typing by a microbacterial method, *Infect. Immun.* **5:**98–102.

Frasch, C. E., and Chapman, S. S., 1972b, Classification of *Neisseria* group B into distinct serotypes. II. Extraction of type-specific antigens for serotyping by precipitin techniques, *Infect. Immunol.* **6:**127–133.

Frasch, C. E., and Chapman, S. S., 1973, Classification of *Neisseria meningitidis* group B into distinct serotypes. III. Application of a new bactericidal inhibition technique to distribution of serotypes among cases and carriers, *J. Infect. Dis.* **127:**149–154.

Frasch, C. E., and Gotschlich, E. C., 1974, An outer membrane protein of *Neisseria meningitidis* group B responsible for serotype specificity, *J. Exp. Med.* **140:**87–104.

Frasch, C. E., McNelis, R. M., and Gotschlich, E. C., 1976, Strain specific variation in the protein and lipopolysaccharide composition of the group B meningococcal outer membrane, *J. Bacteriol.* **127:**973–981.

Fraser, D. W., Darby, C. P., Koehler, R. E., Jacobs, C. F., and Feldman, R. A., 1973, Risk factors in bacterial meningitis: Charleston County, South Carolina, *J. Infect. Dis.* **127:**271–277.

Gavrilis, P., Rothenberg, S. P., and Guy, R., 1974, Correlation of low serum IgM levels with absence of functional splenic tissue in sickle cell disease syndromes, *Am. J. Med.* **57:**542–545.

Gold, R., and Artenstein, M. S., 1971, Meningococcal infections. 2. Field trial of group C meningoccocal polysaccharide vaccine in 1969–70, *Bull WHO* **45:**279–282.

Gold, R., and Lepow, M. L., 1976, Present status of polysaccharide vaccines in the prevention of meningococcal disease, *Adv. Pediatr.* **23:**71–93.

Gold, R., and McLean, R. H., 1978, Absence of the sixth component of complement in a child with chronic meningococcemia, *Pediatr. Res.* **12:**480 (abstr.).

Gold, R., and Wyle, F. A., 1970, New classification of *N. meningiditis* by means of bactericidal reactions, *Infect. Immun.* **1:**479–484.

Gold, R., Winklehake, J. L., Mars, R. S., and Artenstein, M. S., 1971, Identification of an epidemic strain of group C *Neisseria meningitidis* by bactericidal serotyping, *J. Infect. Dis.* **124:**593–597.

Gold, R., Lepow, M. L., Goldschneider, I., Draper, T. L., and Gotschlich, E. C., 1976, Clinical evaluation of group A and group C meningococcal polysaccharide vaccines in infants, *J. Clin. Invest.* **56:**1536–1547.

Gold, R., Lepow, M. L., Goldschneider, I., Gotschlich, E. C., DeSanctis, A. N., and Metzgar, D. P., 1977a, Immunogenicity of groups A and C meningococcal polysaccharides of differing molecular weights, *Pediatr. Res.* **11:**500.

Gold, R., Lepow, M. L., Goldschneider, I., and Gotschlich, E. C., 1977b, Immune response of human infants to polysaccharide vaccines of groups A and C *Neisseria meningitidis*, *J. Infect. Dis.* **136:**S31–S35.

Gold, R., Goldschneider, I., Lepow, M. L., Draper, T. F., and Randolph, M., 1978a, Carriage of *Neisseria meningitidis* and *Neisseria lactamica* in infants and children, *J. Infect. Dis.* **137:**112–121.

Gold, R., Lepow, M. L., Goldschneider, I., and Gotschlich, E. C., 1978b, Antibody responses of human infants to 3 doses of group A meningococcal polysaccharide vaccine administered at 3, 4 and 6 months of age, *J. Infect. Dis.* **138:**731–735.

Gold, R., Lepow, M. L., and Randolph, M., 1978c, Natural immunity to pyogenic bacteria, *Pediatr. Res.* **12**:492 (abstr.).

Goldschneider, I., Gotschlich, E. C., and Artenstein, M. S., 1969a, Human immunity to the meningococcus. I. Role of humoral antibodies, *J. Exp. Med.* **129**:1307–1326.

Goldschneider, I., Gotschlich, E. C., and Artenstein, M. S., 1969b, Human immunity to the meningococcus. II. Development of natural immunity, *J. Exp. Med* **129**:1327–1348.

Goldschneider, I., Lepow, M. L., and Gotschlich, E. C., 1972, Immunogenicity of the group A and group C meningococcal polysaccharides in children, *J. Infect. Dis.* **125**:509–519.

Goldschneider, I., Lepow, M. L., Gotschlich, C., Mauck, F. T., Bachl, F., and Randolph, M., 1973, Immunogenicity of group A and group C meningococcal polysaccharides in human infants, *J. Infect. Dis.* **128**:769–776.

Gotschlich, E. C., 1975, Development of polysaccharide vaccines for the prevention of meningococcal diseases, *Monogr. Allergy* **9**:245–248.

Gotschlich, E. C., Liu, T. Y., and Artenstein, M. S., 1969a, Human immunity to the meningococcus. III. Preparation and immunochemical properties of the group A, group B and group C meningococcal polysaccharides, *J. Exp. Med.* **129**:1349–1365.

Gotschlich, E. C., Goldschneider, I., and Artenstein, M. S., 1969b, Human immunity to the meningococcus. IV. Immunogenicity of group A and group C meningococcal polysaccharides in human volunteers, *J. Exp. Med.* **129**:1367–1384.

Gotschlich, E. C., Goldschneider, I., and Artenstein, M. S., 1969c, Human immunity to the meningococcus. V. The effect of immunization with meningococcal group C polysaccharide on the carrier state, *J. Exp. Med.* **129**:1385–1395.

Gotschlich, E. C., Rey, M., Triau, R., and Sparks, K. J., 1972, Quantitative determination of the human immune response to immunization with meningococcal vaccines, *J. Clin. Invest* **51**:89–96.

Gotschlich, E. C., Goldschneider, I., Lepow, M. L., and Gold, R., 1976, Immune response to bacterial polysaccharides in man, in: *Antibodies in Human Diagnosis and Therapy* (E. Habar and R. M. Krause, ed.), pp. 391–403, Raven Press, New York.

Greenwood, B. M., Whittle, H. C., and Bryceson, A. D. M., 1973, Allergic complications of meningococcal disease. II. Immunological investigations, *Br. Med. J.* **2**:737–740.

Griffiss, J. M., Broud, D. M., Silver, C. A., and Artenstein, M. S., 1977, Immunoepidemiology of meningococcal disease in military recruits. I. A model for serogroup independency of epidemic potential as determined by serotyping, *J. Infect. Dis.* **136**:176–186.

Hobbs, J. R., Milner, R. D. G., and Watt, P. J., 1967, Gamma-M deficiency predisposing to meningococcal septicaemia, *Br. Med. J.* **4**:583–586.

Johnston, R. B., Jr., Newman, S. L., and Struth, A. G., 1973, An abnormality of the alternative pathway of complement activation in sickle cell disease, *N. Engl. J. Med.* **288**:803–808.

Kabat, E. A., and Bezer, A. E., 1958, The effect of variation in molecular weight in the antigenicity of dextran in man, *Arch. Biochem. Biophys.* **78**:306–318.

Kabat, E. A., Kaiser, H., and Sikorski, H., 1944, Preparation of type-specific polysaccharide of the type 1 meningococcus and a study of its effectiveness as an antigen in human beings, *J. Exp. Med.* **80**:299–307.

Kasper, D. L., Winkelhake, J. L., Brandt, B. L., and Artenstein, M. S., 1973, Antigenic specificity of bactericidal antibodies in antisera to *Neisseria meningitidis*, *J. Infect. Dis.* **127**:378–387.

Kuronen, T., Peltola, H., Nors, T., Haque, H., and Makela, P. H., 1977, Adverse reactions and endotoxin content of polysaccharide vaccines, *Dev. Biol. Stand.* **34**:117–125.

Lepow, M. L., Goldschneider, I., Gold, R., Randolph, M., and Gotschlich, E. C., 1977, Persistence of antibody following immunization of children with groups A and C meningococcal polysaccharide vaccines, *Pediatrics* **60**:673–680.

Lim, D., Gewurz, A., Lint, T. F., Ghaze, M., Sepheri, B., and Gewurz, H., 1976, Absence of the sixth component of complement in a patient with repeated episodes of meningococcal meningitis, *J. Pediatr.* **89**:42–47.

Liu, T. Y., Gotschlich, E. C., Jonssen, E. K., and Wysocki, J. R., 1971a, Studies on the meningococcal polysaccharides. I. Composition and chemical properties of the group A polysaccharide, *J. Biol. Chem.* **246**:2849–2858.

Liu, T. Y., Gotschlich, E. C., Dunne, F. T., and Jonssen, E. K., 1971b, Studies on the meningococcal polysaccharides. II. Composition and chemical properties of the group B and C polysaccharides, *J. Biol. Chem.* **246**:4703–4712.

Makela, P. H., Kayhty, H., Weckstrom, P., Sivonen, A., and Renkonen, O.-V., 1975, Effect of group A meningococcal vaccine in Army recruits in Finland, *Lancet* **2**:883–886.

Makela, P. H., Peltola, H., Kayhty, H., Jousimies, H., Pettay, O., Ruoslahti, E., Sivonen, A., and Renkonen, O.-V., 1977, Polysaccharide vaccines of group A *Neisseria meningitidis* and *Haemophilus influenzae* type b: A field trial in Finland, *J. Infect. Dis.* **136**:S43–S50.

McCormick, J. B., Weaver, R. E., Thornsberry, C., and Feldman, R. A., 1974, Trends in disease caused by *Neisseria meningitidis:* 1972 and 1973, *J. Infect. Dis.* **130**:212–214.

Meningococcal Surveillance Group, 1976, Analysis of endemic meningococcal disease by serogroup and evaluation of chemoprophylaxis, *J. Infect. Dis.* **134**:201.

Millar, J. W., Siess, E. E., and Feldman, H. A., Silberman, C., and Frank, P., 1963, *In vivo* and *in vitro* resistance to sulfadiazine in strains of *Neisseria meningitidis, JAMA* **186**:139–141.

Monto, A. S., Brandt, B. L., and Artenstein, M. S., 1973,

Response of children to *Neisseria meningitidis* polysaccharide vaccines, *J. Infect. Dis.* **127**:394–400.

Morbidity Mortality Weekly Report, 1975, Meningococcal polysaccharide vaccines, *Morbid. Mortal. Wkly. Rep.* **25**:381–382.

Morbidity Mortality Weekly Report, 1976, Reported morbidity and mortality in the United States, *Morbid. Mortal. Wkly. Rep.* **25**(53):50.

Morbidity Mortality Weekly Report, 1977, Follow-up on meningococcal disease—Alaska, Oregon, Washington, *Morbid. Mortal. Wkly. Rep.* **26**:101–102.

Munford, R. S., and Gorman, G. W., 1974, Serotyping *Neisseria meningitidis, Lancet* **2**:177.

Munford, R. S., Taunay, A. deE., deMorais, J. S., Fraser, D. W., and Feldman, R. A., 1974, Spread of meningococcal infection within households, *Lancet* **1**:1275–1278.

Munford, R. S., Patton, C. M., and Gorman, G. W., 1975, Epidemiological studies of antigens common to groups B and C *Neisseria meningitidis, J. Infect. Dis.* **131**:286–290.

Nicholson, A., and Lepow, J. H., 1978, Role of complement in defense against *N. meningiditis, Clin. Res.* **26**:525A.

Peltola, H., 1977, Group A meningococcal and *Haemophilus influenzae* type b capsular polysaccharide vaccines in infants and children under school age, Ph.D. thesis, 72 pp., Helsinki, Finland.

Peltola, H., Makela, P. H., Kayhty, H., Jousimies, H., Herva, E., Hallstrom, H., Sivonen, A., Renkonen, O.-V., Pettay, O., Karanko, V., Ahvonen, P., and Sarna, S., 1977, Clinical efficacy of meningococcus group A capsular polysaccharide vaccine in children 3 months to 5 years of age, *N. Engl. J. Med.* **297**:686–691.

Petersen, B. H., Graham, J. A., and Brooks, G. E., 1976, Human deficiency of the eighth component of complement: The requirement for C8 for serum Neisseria gonorrhoeae bactericidal activity, *J. Clin. Invest.* **57**:283–290.

Pfair, J. J., 1958, Meningococcal meningitis, in: *Preventive Medicine in World War II*, Vol. IV: *Communicable Diseases Transmitted Chiefly through Respiratory and Alimentary Tracts* (J. B. Coates, Jr., ed.), pp. 191–209, Office of the Surgeon General Department of the Army, Washington, D.C.

Reller, L. B., MacGregor, R. R., and Beaty, H. N., 1973, Bactericidal antibody after colonization with *Neisseria meningitidis, J. Infect. Dis.* **127**:56–62.

Robbins, J. B., Schneerson, R., Glode, M. P., Vann, W., Schiffer, M. S., Liu, T. Y., Parke, J. C., and Huntley, C., 1975, Cross-reactive antigens and immunity to diseases caused by encapsulated bacteria, *J. Allergy Clin. Immunol.* **56**:141–151.

Roberts, R. B., 1970, The relationship between group A and C meningococcal polysaccharides and serum opsonins in man, *J. Exp. Med.* **131**:499–513.

Rosen, F. S., and Janeway, C. A., 1966, The gammaglobulins. III. The antibody deficiency syndromes, *N. Engl. J. Med.* **275**:709–715, 769–775.

Seeler, R. A., Metzger, W., and Mufson, M. A., 1972, *Diplococcus pneumoniae* infections in children with sickle cell anemia, *Am. J. Dis. Child.* **123**:8–10.

Taunay, A. de E., Galvao, P. A., deMorais, J. A., Gotschlich, E. C., and Feldman, R. A., 1974, Disease prevention by meningococcal serogroup C polysaccharide vaccine in preschool children, *Pediatr. Res.* **8**:429.

Vassiliades, P., Kanellakis, A., and Papadakis, J., 1969, Sulfadiazine-resistant group A meningococci isolated during the 1968 meningitis epidemic in Greece, *J. Hyg.* **67**:279–288.

Wahdan, M. H., Rizk, F., El-Akkad, A. M., El Ghoroury, A. A., Hablas, R., Girgis, N. I., Amer, A., Boctar, W., Sippel, J. E., Gotschlich, E. C., Triau, R., Sanborn, W. R., and Cvjetanovic, B., 1973, A controlled field trial of a serogroup A meningococcal polysaccharide vaccine, *Bull. WHO* **48**:667–673.

Weekly Epidemiological Record, 1975, Meningitis, Argentina, *Wkly. Epidemiol. Rec.* **50**:161.

Weekly Epidemiological Record, 1976, Meningococcal meningitis, *Wkly. Epidemiol. Rec.* **51**:333–334.

Whittle, H. C., and Greenwood, B. M., 1976, Meningococcal meningitis in the norther savannah of Africa, *Trop. Doc.* **6**:99–104.

Whittle, H. C., Abdullahi, M. T., Fakunle, F. A., Greenwood, B. M., Bryceson, A. D. M., Parry, E. H. O., and Turk, J. L., 1973, Allergic complications of meningococcal disease. I. Clinical aspects, *Br. Med. J.* **2**:733–737.

Winkestein, J. A., and Drachman, R. H., 1968, Deficiency of pneumococcal serum opsonizing activity in sickle-cell disease. *N. Engl. J. Med.* **279**:459–466.

Wong, H. H., Barrera, O., Sutton, A., May, J., Hochstein, D. H., Robbins, J. D., Robbins, J. B., Parkman, P. D., and Seligman, E. B., Jr., 1977, Standardization and control of meningococcal vaccines, group A and group C polysaccharides, *J. Biol. Stand.* **5**:197–215.

Wyle, F. A., Artenstein, M. S., Brandt, B. L., Tramont, E. C., Kasper, D. L., Altieri, P. L., Berman, S. L., and Lowenthal, L. P., 1972, Immunologic response of man to group B meningococcal polysaccharide vaccines, *J. Infect. Dis.* **126**:514–522.

Young, L. S., LaForce, F. M., Head, J. J., Feely, J. C., and Bennett, J. V., 1972, A simultaneous outbreak of meningococcal and influenzae infections, *N. Engl. J. Med.* **287**:5–9.

Zollinger, W. D., Pennington, C. L., and Artenstein, M. S., 1974, Human antibody response to three meningococcal outer membrane antigens: Comparison by specific hemagglutination assays, *Infect. Immun.* **10**:975–984.

7

Immunology of *Bordetella pertussis*

STEPHEN I. MORSE

1. Introduction

The importance of whooping cough as a cause of childhood morbidity and mortality has markedly decreased since the beginning of this century as the result of improved supportive care, introduction of antimicrobials, and effective immunization. The advances in therapy and prevention have been achieved without concomitant knowledge of many of the determinants of the host–parasite interaction. For example, unlike with most specific acute childhood infections, the newborn is highly susceptible, even if the mother has either been immunized or contracted natural disease in childhood. In susceptible populations an attack rate startlingly high for a bacterial disease may occur, yet the first events of pathogenesis are uncertain. It is known that the disease is not invasive and that the localization of the organisms in the respiratory tract is on the ciliated epithelim, but only now is information being uncovered which may reveal the precise nature of the receptor–bacterial complex responsible for this striking tropism. A curious phenomenon in whooping cough is the occurrence of the most severe symptoms at a time when it is difficult to recover viable organisms. The causative agent, *Bordetella pertussis*, produces a wide array of effects in experimental animals. But in most cases the responsible

bacterial substances have not been isolated, nor is it known whether they play a primary or secondary role in human disease. Whether the mechanisms of elimination of viable organisms and clinical recovery involve phagocytic cells, opsonic antibody, bactericidal antibody, antitoxic antibody, or a process involving neither conventional cellular nor humoral defenses is a question that still receives only speculative and unproven responses. At the same time, we maintain our ignorance of the protective antigen contained in pertusses vaccine as well as of the immunological response which confers specific resistance in artificially or naturally immunized individuals. There are even those, particularly in the United Kingdom, who believe that pertussis vaccine has too little protective effect, compared to the incidence of adverse reactions, to warrant its use. Consequently, vaccine acceptance has fallen markedly in the British Isles and there has been an associated rise in the incidence of whooping cough.

1.1. Clinical Picture of Whooping Cough

The incubation period of whooping cough (pertussis) is usually between 7 and 14 days. A prodromal catarrhal phase then develops which takes the form of an undifferentiated, nonspecific upper respiratory disease. After 1–2 weeks the paroxysmal stage begins and the clinical diagnosis is usually obvious. The patient develops episodes of severe paroxysmal coughing terminated by a crowing inspiratory

STEPHEN I. MORSE • State University of New York, Downstate Medical Center, Brooklyn, New York 11203.

"whoop" from which the picturesque and accurate name of the disease derives. Up to 20 paroxysms a day may occur, and during the paroxysms cyanosis and evidence of increased intravascular pressure, e.g., epistaxis and conjunctival hemorrhage, may appear. The paroxysmal stage lasts 2–4 weeks and convalescence is gradual (Lapin, 1943).

Patients with uncomplicated pertussis are afebrile, and the only striking laboratory abnormality is leukocytosis, or occasionally hyperleukocytosis, which occurs in approximately 70% of patients and parallels in degree the clinical course, i.e., it is maximal during the paroxysmal state (Thelander et al., 1933; Lagergren, 1963). The differential leukocyte count is striking in that the majority of cells are mature-appearing small lymphocytes. Although polymorphonuclear leukocytosis may also occur, a predominance of these cells, as well as fever, suggests a secondary bacterial complication.

It must be remembered that very young infants, older children, and adults (irrespective of prior clinical disease or immunization) often do not exhibit the typical clinical picture of whooping cough.

In susceptible closed populations there is extensive spread of pertussis, and the attack rate may be 90%, exceeding that of other bacterial illnesses and approaching the communicability of measles and varicella. Spread is by direct droplet transmission via the respiratory tract. Given the distinct clinical manifestations of whooping cough and the tendency for local epidemics, pertussis should be relatively easy to identify in records from the past. Yet the earliest written description of pertussis appears to be that of de Baillou (Major, 1939), who wrote of an epidemic in Paris in 1578. Thus as Olson (1975) has pointed out, "it might well be that Parisians of the mid-sixteenth century witnessed the birth of a disease previously unknown to man."

1.2. Etiology

Although minute coccobacillary organisms had often been seen in stained preparations of sputum from patients with whooping cough, *B. pertussis* was not isolated until 1906, when Bordet and Gengou succeeded in culturing the agent from Bordet's son, who had clinical whooping cough (Olson, 1975). The complex

Bordet–Gengou solid medium contains blood, glycerine, and potato extract and still enjoys popularity as the medium of choice for primary isolation of *B. pertussis*. Fulfilling Koch's postulates proved difficult because analogous experimental disease is difficult to induce in common laboratory animals. However, convincing evidence that *B. pertussis* causes whooping cough was obtained by the Macdonalds (Macdonald and Macdonald, 1933), who deliberately infected their four children with *B. pertussis*; two of the children developed clinical whooping cough and *B. pertussis* was isolated from each. The other two children, who had been previously injected with killed organisms, did not develop the disease. In addition, Shibley and Hoelscher (1934) induced a disease in chimpanzees with *B. pertussis* in which the findings closely resembled those of human pertussis.

Bordetella parapertussis was isolated in the late 1930s from patients with whooping cough, and, although isolated less frequently than *B. pertussis*, it is a significant etiological agent in some regions of the world, including Denmark, Czechoslovakia, and the Soviet Union. *Bordetella bronchiseptica*, unlike the other two species, which have been found only in man, is an enzootic pathogen for some animals and is rarely responsible for clinical whooping cough.

The possibility of a viral etiology of whooping cough had long been suggested, and in recent years there have been a number of reports suggesting that certain viruses, particularly adenoviruses, may cause the pertussis syndrome (Connor, 1970; Pereira and Candeias, 1971; Nelson et al., 1975). These viruses have been isolated from some patients with the clinical picture of whooping cough, including lymphocytosis, in which there was no bacteriological or serological evidence of *B. pertussis* infection. The evidence remains clear, however, that in most instance the causative agent of the whooping cough syndrome is *B. pertussis*.

1.3. Characteristics of *B. pertussis*

The three species in the genus *Bordetella* were formerly classified as species of *Hemophilus* because of similarities in microscopic morphology and a requirement for medium containing blood for the primary isolation of *B. pertussis*. Reclassification of the organisms into the genus *Bordetella* is justified because they are antigenically unrelated to *Hemophilus* and because the requirement for blood for growth of *B. pertussis* is not for nutritional purposes but rather to neutralize unknown toxic materials, perhaps fatty acids, produced during growth. Liquid and solid growth media containing charcoal, albumin, starch, or anion exchange resins instead of blood are quite satisfactory.

In fresh isolates *B. pertussis* is a minute (0.5-μm diameter) gram-negative coccobacillus that is nonmotile and does not form spores. It has little fermentative capacity for sugars, nor does it possess urease or reduce nitrates. When the organisms are subcultured on artificial media, a number of changes occur in their physiological and biological attributes. Leslie and Gardner (1931) denoted these changes as transitions from phase I to phase IV, although the intermediate phases II and III are difficult to define. In many respects this transition is analogous to the smooth-to-rough (S → R) variation seen in many gram-negative organisms, but virtually nothing is known of the genetics and biochemical mechanisms involved in the phase changes of *B. pertussis*.

Phase I organisms will not grow in simple media; blood or other substances which neutralize compounds inimical to the survival of the organism are required. In microscopic appearance phase I organisms are uniform and the shiny "bisected pearl" colonies develop slowly. In contrast, phase IV organisms grow well in conventional media and there is marked pleomorphism.

Of greatest significance in the differential properties of phase I and phase IV strains are the contrasts in virulence, antigenic structure, and biological effects. Phase I cells are virulent, whereas phase IV organisms are not, and, most importantly, effective vaccines can be made only from phase I strains. A variety of biological effects are caused by the injection of phase I *B. pertussis* cells or products into experimental animals (see below) but not by phase IV organisms.

Phase I *B. pertussis* cells are hemagglutinating and possess 2.0–2.5 nm × 60–100 nm pili (Morse and Morse, 1970), which are believed to be the hemagglutinating component (Sato *et al.*, 1974; Morse and Morse, 1976). Although the other species of *Bordetella*, *B. par-*

apertussis and *B. bronchiseptica*, possess pili, phase IV *B. pertussis* strains do not (Morse and Morse, 1970). Phase I cells also possess a poorly defined capsule which is less prominent in phase IV strains (Lawson, 1940).

2. Biological Effects of *B. pertussis* and Its Products

2.1. *In Vivo* Effects

2.1.1. Adjuvanticity

B. pertussis cells or cell products produce a variety of effects in experimental animals (Table 1) (reviewed in Morse, 1976), and a number of these influence the immune response. *B. pertussis* is a potent adjuvant for many immune responses to heterologous antigens. When T-cell-dependent antigens such as sheep erythrocytes are used as immunogens, both IgG and IgM antibody production may be increased, and, depending on the dose, *B. pertussis* may act directly on T cells or directly on B cells (Dresser, 1972). *B. pertussis* cells also potentiate *in vitro* antibody responses (Maillard and Bloom, 1972; Murgo and Athanassiades, 1975).

When T-independent antigens such as type 3 pneumococcal polysaccharide are injected into mice, *B. pertussis* causes a qualitative shift in antibody formation (Kong and Morse, 1976). Instead of the usual IgM response, IgG antibody is also present. Quantitative changes depend on the dose of the polysaccharide.

Cell-mediated immunity is enhanced by injection of killed *B. pertussis* cells, as in the

TABLE 1. **Biological Effects of *B. pertussis***

In vivo
1. Adjuvanticity
   a. IgG and IgM antibody
   b. Cell-mediated immunity
   c. Reaginic antibody
2. Endotoxic reactions
3. Lethality and dermal necrosis
4. Leukocytosis with predominating lymphocytosis[a]
5. Histamine sensitization[a]
6. Inhibition of epinephrine-induced hyperglycemia[a]

In vitro
1. Adjuvant activity
2. Mitogenicity for mouse T cells and human peripheral blood lymphocytes (? T cells)[a]
3. Decreased cyclic AMP response

[a] Produced by purified lymphocytosis-promoting factor.

production of experimental allergic encephalomyelitis (Levine *et al.*, 1966).

B. pertussis also causes increased production of reaginic antibody (Mota, 1958, 1964). Whereas the adjuvant activity of *B. pertussis* for IgG and IgM production and for cell-mediated immunity is independent of, and indeed may be suppressed by, pertussis-induced lymphocytosis, the enhanced production of reaginic antibody may be directly related to lymphocytosis (Tada *et al.*, 1971, 1972; Okumura and Tada, 1971). It is postulated by Tada and co-workers that suppressor T cells which regulate the reaginic antibody response are in the blood during the lymphocytosis and no longer exert control of IgE antibody production in lymphoid tissues. However, direct experimental proof that isolated, purified lymphocytosis-promoting factor can induce enhanced reaginic antibody formation has yet to be obtained. The ability of *B. pertussis* to cause heightened sensitivity to both active and passive anaphylaxis may also be related to increased levels of reaginic antibody.

Demonstration of reaginic antibody in the pertussis system has been performed only with PCA reactions, and levels of IgE antibody, or its equivalent, have not been directly measured. Thus it is possible that enhanced effector mechanisms may play a role in enhanced reactivity.

2.1.2. Endotoxin

Like other gram-negative bacteria, *B. pertussis* contains heat-stable lipopolysaccharide endotoxin (LPS), which is a structural component of the cell wall. *B. pertussis* endotoxin has the same general biological properties as other endotoxins. It is probable that the adjuvant effects of whole organisms are caused by the LPS since, as with endotoxins from other organisms, *B. pertussis* LPS is itself an adjuvant (Nakase *et al.*, 1970). However, a heat-labile component has also been implicated (Levine *et al.*, 1966). Other endotoxic effects include pyrogenicity in animals; leukopenia followed by polymorphonuclear leukocytosis; preparation and elicitation of the Shwartzman reaction; and, in appropriate doses, lethality for certain experimental animals. Although the immunochemical aspects of the lipopolysaccharide have not been completely elucidated, it seems to be a complex antigen (Aprile and Wardlaw, 1973).

2.1.3. Heat-Labile Toxin(s)

B. pertussis also produces a lethal heat-labile toxin that may be identical to the material which causes dermal necrosis. This toxin has been neither isolated nor characterized, although it is most likely a protein (Munoz, 1971). It is not a true exotoxin as are tetanus and diphtheria toxins, since it is not freely liberated into the extracellular growth medium. Instead, the bulk of the activity resides within the cells and is released when the cells lyse.

2.1.4. Induction of Lymphocytosis

The striking phenomenon of lymphocytosis in clinical whooping cough is mimicked in animals by the injection of killed *B. pertussis* cells or culture supernatants as well as in experimental disease. Purified lymphocytosis-promoting factor (LPF) has been isolated from culture supernatants. It is a protein, free of lipid and carbohydrate, which has a molecular weight of approximately 74,000 and consists of four subunits detected by polyacrylamide electrophoresis using SDS and 2-mercaptoethanol (Morse and Morse, 1976). Isolated LPF is immunogenic, and specific antiserum has been prepared. When 0.5 μg of LPF is injected intravenously into mice, lymphocyte counts averaging 120,000 lymphocytes per 10^{-3} ml are reached 3–5 days later. As in the case of clinical whooping cough, the cells are mature. The reaction is not due to increased lymphocyte proliferation; rather, the extraordinary increase in circulating lymphocytes is caused by an aberration of the normal pattern of lymphocyte recirculation (Morse and Riester, 1967). It is not entirely clear whether lymphocytes from the lymphoid organs, other than the spleen, enter the blood at a faster rate, but they are not able to leave the blood and enter into the traffic areas of lymph nodes at a normal rate (Taub *et al.*, 1972). The number of circulating B lymphocytes as well as T lymphocytes (Morse and Morse, 1976) is increased, and there is a reciprocal decrease of these cells in the spleen.

The mechanism of lymphocytosis in clinical pertussis is likely to be the same as in experimental animals, although this has not been proven. In human disease there is also an increase in both circulating T and B cells (Bernales *et al.*, 1976).

It is not surprising that during the time of peak lymphocytosis there is a decrease in the ability of animals to respond to many antigens, because the lymphoid organs are depleted of lymphocytes. It is unlikely that impairment in function, as opposed to abnormal compartmentalization, is responsible for the lack of immunolgical responsiveness, since, by a number of criteria, the isolated blood lymphocytes can function normally (Phanuphak *et al.*, 1972).

Polymorphoculcear leukocytosis is also induced by purified LPF, and the time course of the response parallels that for lymphocytosis. It is, however, of far less magnitude.

LPF is responsible for two other effects of *B. pertussis* in experimental animals: (1) histamine sensitization and (2) insensitivity to the hyperglycemic effect of epinephrine (Morse and Morse, 1976).

a. Histamine Sensitization. The ability of phase I *B. pertussis* cells and supernatant fluids to sensitize experimental animals to the lethal effects of histamine has been ascribed to histamine-sensitizing factor or HSF (reviewed by Munoz, 1971). It is now clear that LPF and HSF are identical. It is also probable that LPF sensitizes mice to the lethal effects of serotonin and to such nonspecific factors as stress and cold which develop concomitantly with histamine sensitization. The mechanism responsible for histamine sensitization has not been clarified, although it probably bears a relationship to the β-adrenergic nervous system. For example, β-adrenergic blocking agents such as propranolol also induce histamine sensitization and, conversely, exogenous epinephrine inhibits the lethal response to histamine of pertussis-sensitized mice. The effects of β-adrenergic agents also indicate a role for cyclic nucleotides in the reaction. There is no evidence that decreased catabolism of histamine occurs.

b. Unresponsiveness to Epinephrine-Induced Hyperglycemia. Mice injected with *B. pertussis* do not undergo the expected hyperglycemia when epinephrine, histamine, or serotonin is administered (Szentivanyi *et al.*, 1963). Inoculation of purified LPF into mice also results in inhibition of epinephrine-induced hyperglycemia, and, in addition, fasting blood glucose levels are often reduced (Morse and Morse, 1976). The causation of these effects is most likely complex and may involve both decreased muscle glycogenolysis and increased levels of biologically active insulin (Gulbenkian *et al.*, 1968; Katada and Ui, 1977).

2.2. *In Vitro* Effects

2.2.1. Depression of Induced Cellular Cyclic AMP

In human lymphocytes LPF prevents the accumulation of intracellular cyclic AMP, which normally occurs in response to β-adrenergic agents such as isoproterenol (Parker and Morse, 1973). This *in vitro* finding is mirrored by the apparent decrease in levels of cyclic AMP in various tissues after the injection of *B. pertussis* cells (Ortez *et al.*, 1975). The reason for cyclic AMP unresponsiveness has not been delineated. It is unlikely that specific receptors are blocked, since the *in vitro* inhibition affects both isoproterenol and prostaglandin E_1, which have different receptors. It is more likely that the effect is on the adenylate cyclase system or on the activity of cyclic nucleotide phosphodiesterases which destroy cyclic AMP.

2.2.2. Mitogenic Effect of LPF on Lymphocytes

LPF is a potent mitogen for murine lymphocytes *in vitro* (Kong and Morse, 1977a,b). Lymph node and spleen lymphocytes are fully reactive, whereas bone marrow cells or spleen cells from congenitally athymic mice lacking mature T cells do not respond. Further proof that LPF specifically activates T cells was shown by the inhibition of thymidine uptake by Thy-1 (anti-Θ) antiserum. Moreover, the electron microscopic appearance of the blast cells was that of T-cell-derived blasts rather than antibody-secreting cells generated from B lymphocytes. Lymphocytes from germ-free animals also responded to LPF, suggesting that proliferation was not dependent on prior T-cell sensitization. The responsiveness of lymphocytes from germ-free mice and the similarity of the proliferative reaction of cells from mice of a wide range of inbred strains and sources, the lack of antibody reacting with

LPF in normal mice, and the peak time of thymidine incorporation at 3 days all suggest that LPF is a nonspecific T-cell mitogen and is not inducing antigen-specific stimulation of presensitized cells.

The mechanism of stimulation is uncertain but conceivably could be related to the effects of LPF on cyclic nucleotide metabolism. The fact that LPF binds to B lymphocytes without inducing proliferation suggests, however, that activation is more complex.

In contrast to the activity of the mitogen Con A, normal mouse thymocytes do not proliferate in response to LPF. The same is true for the mitogen PHA, although both PHA and LPF stimulate cortisone-resistant thymocytes. There is, however, considerable evidence that LPF does not affect the same population of T cells as does PHA.

Although it is the T cell which responds to LPF, an accessory cell is required. The accessory cell adheres to nylon wool columns but is not a mononuclear phagocyte. It does possess surface Ig and appears to be a B cell (Ho *et al.*, 1977; M. K. Ho, unpublished data).

As noted previously, the lymphocytosis evoked by LPF *in vivo* is not the result of lymphocyte proliferation. The apparent discrepancy between the *in vivo* and *in vitro* findings is readily explained by the doses required. *In vitro* mitogenesis requires relatively more LPF than the dose needed for optimal lymphocytosis. Furthermore, the mitogenic response occurs only within narrow confines of LPF concentration which would be difficult to achieve predictably in animals.

Human peripheral blood lymphocytes (PBL) also are markedly stimulated by LPF (Morse *et al.*, 1975, 1977; Andersen *et al.*, 1977). The responsiveness bears no relationship to prior exposure either to clinical whooping cough or to immunization against the disease, and PLBs from all normal subjects tested respond, whether the test is carried out in AB serum or in fetal calf serum. When homologous serum is employed, the PBLs from occasional individuals do not respond, because of circulating anti-LPF antibody. In addition to the uniformity of response, the finding that cord blood lymphocytes are stimulated is evidence that the proliferation is not due to the effect of LPF as an antigen on presensitized cells. PBLs from

patients with chronic lymphocytic leukemia, a B-cell malignancy, does not respond to LPF.

Although the weight of evidence indicates, but does not prove, that LPF is a mitogen for human T cells, the interaction of more than one cell type is necessary for the mitogenic effect, as it is in the murine system.

3. Pathogenesis of Whooping Cough

Whooping cough is a noninvasive surface disease. The organisms are specifically localized to the ciliated epithelial cells of the tracheobronchial tree, where they proliferate to high numbers and cause desquamation of these cells. A tenacious mucous exudate is usually found. Peribronchial and peribronchiolar infiltration with lymphocytes is common. Although interstitial pneumonitis and bronchopneumonia have been described, extensive involvement makes it likely that secondary bacterial or viral infection has occurred.

3.1. Establishment of the Infection

The mechanism of the pathogenesis of pertussis is unknown, but it is worthwhile to consider questions that may be framed in the light of what is known about the disease and about the organism. The primary question is the reason for the strict cellular tropism. The organisms are found only in relation to ciliated epithelium; adjacent cells are uninfected (Collier *et al.*, 1977; Muse *et al.*, 1977). It is controversial whether the attachment is to the cilia *per se* or to the microvilli between them (Hopewell *et al.*, 1972). (One of the curiosities in this field is the ability to produce fatal disease in mice by the intracerebral injection of small numbers of phase I *B. pertussis*. Indeed, protection against this type of infection is used to assay the efficacy of vaccines. Although it appears that the principles of strict tropism and lack of invasiveness are violated, it turns out that the organisms are localized to the ciliated ependymal cells lining the ventricles.)

The recognition sites on the bacterium and host cell have not been delineated. Far more detailed structural analysis of infected ciliated cells is required, and experiments with chick embryo tracheas and hamster tracheal rings may be particularly informative.

It is known that *B. pertussis* cells will attach to a variety of tissue culture cells and to erythrocytes (Holt, 1972). Thus, although *B. pertussis* may attach to nonciliated cells, there may be far more specificity for ciliated epithelium and tighter binding to receptors on these cells.

In recent years there has been great interest in the mechanism by which bacteria selectively adhere to surfaces. The possible role of pili in mucosal adherence of *N. gonorrheae* and certain streptococci, for example, has evoked a number of studies. The pili of *B. pertussis* have yet to be purified, but although they attach to erythrocytes of a number of species their ability to attach to other host cells has not been established. Nor is it known whether the pili of phase I *B. pertussis* bear an antigenic or a chemical relationship to the pili of *B. parapertussis* or *B. bronchiseptica*, an important point because there is no cross-protection between the species.

3.2. Induction of the Disease

Following an incubation period of 7–14 days, upper respiratory symptoms appear that are indistinguishable from those of an undifferentiated viral infection. It is during this catarrhal stage, which usually lasts 1–2 weeks, that the disease is most contagious and organisms are most readily isolated. However, because of the nonspecific nature of the clinical picture the diagnosis of whooping cough is not entertained, unless an epidemic is in progress, until the paroxysmal stage.

The paroxysmal stage is characterized by episodes of paroxysmal coughing, which consist of a long series of repetitive, severe coughs terminating in a profound inspiratory effort and a crowing "whoop". More than 20 paroxysms a day may occur, and the episodes are often followed by vomiting, making alimentation difficult. Increased venous pressure may result in epistaxis or conjunctival hemorrhages. Encephalopathy occurring during whooping cough is the result of anoxia or hemorrhages of the brain rather than a primary effect of the organism or its products. Unlike most other bacterial diseases, uncomplicated whooping cough is unaccompanied by fever; the presence of fever signifies a secondary infection.

The primary causation of the changes in the respiratory tract and the characteristic clinical picture is not fully known. Experimental work using cultured hamster tracheal rings has shown that *B. pertussis* not only specifically attaches to ciliated cells but also causes their death without affecting neighboring, nonciliated cells (Collier *et al.*, 1977; Muse *et al.*, 1977). Presumably the organism produces a toxin which kills the cells, as in the case of *H. influenzae* (Denny, 1974), but formal proof is lacking.

Viable organisms are either absent or present only in low numbers during the paroxysmal stage of pertussis, and it is therefore possible that some of the clinical findings are due to sensitization, particularly since *B. pertussis* is known to sensitize some species of experimental animals to histamine, serotonin, and a variety of nonspecific stresses. *B. pertussis* also causes a heightened homocytotropic antibody response to heterologous antigens, and such responses might result in pulmonary symptoms if the appropriate antigen interacted with mast cells coated with the corresponding IgE. None of these possibilities has been proved or disproved in respect to the clinical findings in whooping cough.

Lymphocytosis is a prominent feature of clinical pertussis, but there is little evidence that this phenomenon plays a role in pathogenesis. Pertussis-induced lymphocytosis in experimental animals results in suppression of cell-mediated immunity, and it has been reported that patients with whooping cough have depressed tuberculin reactions (Pieroni *et al.*, 1972). Although hypoglycemia is found in patients with pertussis, this may be a manifestation of reduced caloric intake rather than an abnormality of the β-adrenergic system or increased insulin secretion.

Nevertheless, since the responsible bacterial product, LPF, does produce overt manifestations, the possibility exists of histamine sensitization, β-adrenergic blockade, enhanced IgE formation, and alterations of cyclic AMP metabolism occurring in patients with whooping cough. In contrast, there is no febrile response in pertussis, and therefore little evidence for endotoxemia.

3.3. Pathology and Immunology of Infection Resolution

The paroxysmal stage gradually subsides over a period of 2–4 weeks and a convalescent phase lasting a few weeks then occurs. The pathological changes that occur during resolution are poorly understood, for a number of reasons. In patients, the usual cause of death is secondary infection, which makes it difficult to assign specific pathology to *B. pertussis*. In addition, too few detailed pathological studies in primates have been performed, and studies on the pathology in mice following intranasal infection are not entirely germane to human disease since pneumonia is frequent. Nevertheless, it is likely that some of the findings in mice may be extrapolated to human disease.

Initially, the organisms are found free in the increased bronchiolar mucus. Then polymorphonuclear leukocytes are present in high numbers, free bacteria become rare, and the viable count of *B. pertussis* decreases rapidly. In mice viable organisms may persist in low numbers within lung macrophages, the complaisant phase (Cheers and Gray, 1969), and then also disappear concomitant with the appearance of protective humoral antibodies (Gray and Cheers, 1969). Resolution of the lesions then occurs.

Antibodies to *B. pertussis* can be found in the sera of patients convalescent from whooping cough. These are measured by complement fixation, agglutination, precipitation, hemagglutination inhibition, complement-dependent bactericidal capacity, opsonic activity, and passive protection against lethal intranasal or intracerebral infection of the mouse. Winter (1953) found that all of 20 convalescent patients tested produced mouse-protective antibody, whereas antibacterial agglutinins appeared in 62% and antihemagglutinins in only 12%. The mouse protection antibody did not rise until 4 weeks after the onset of the whoop and declined sharply within a few months; demonstrable titers persisted for a few years.

Aftandelians and Connor (1973a) studied the development of complement-dependent bactericidal antibodies in patients with whooping cough. In approximately half a demonstrable increase in titer occurred, and the rise was more prominent in those who gave no prior history of pertussis immunization. The bacteriocidins attained high titer in some patients in the paroxysmal stage and in others during the convalescent phase. Bactericidal antibody persisted for at least 10 months after the illness. IgG was found to have bactericidal antibody whereas IgM did not. This is in accord with the finding by Dolby and Dolby (1969) that the bactericidal activity of rabbit anti-*B. pertussis* IgG was more potent.

Aftandelians and Connor (1973b) also studied the appearance of precipitins in patients with whooping cough using a crude unstandardized sonic extract of *B. pertussis* as antigen. Seroconversion occurred in 86% of patients whereas only 42% developed agglutinins.

4. Bacteriological and Serological Diagnosis

Bordetella pertussis can be isolated most frequently during the catarrhal and early paroxysmal stages of the disease and only infrequently thereafter. The sample for culture is best obtained by the pernasal swab technique. A sterile swab is mounted on a thin flexible copper wire which is passed over the floor of the nares and into the pharynx and is then plated on Bordet–Gengou or other suitable medium. Penicillin is usually incorporated into the medium to prevent overgrowth of other organisms before the slow-growing *B. pertussis* colonies appear, usually after 48–72 hr. Problems in bacteriological diagnosis arise because during the catarrhal stage when cultures are more likely to be positive the physician often does not suspect whooping cough and cultures are simply not taken. In addition, the medium used for culture may not be suitable and the laboratory personnel inexperienced.

To overcome disadvantages inherent in the isolation and recognition of *B. pertussis* and to provide more rapid diagnosis, a fluorescent antibody test (FAT) (Whitaker *et al.*, 1960) has been introduced in which fluorescein-tagged *B. pertussis* antiserum is overlaid on a slide on which the sample has been streaked and suitably fixed. There are some false positives, perhaps as many as 10%, as well as false negatives. In general, however, the FAT is satisfactory, although it is not much more sensitive than culture techniques (Linnemann *et al.*, 1968). The FAT is also useful in identifying colonies suspected of being *B. pertussis*. The *B. pertussis* antisera currently employed will not recognize *B. parapertussis*.

Serological tests are not useful for the primary diagnosis of whooping cough in the acute phase because, as previously noted, they are not positive until late in the disease. They can be important, however, in the retrospective diagnosis, as well as in epidemiological and surveillance studies. Tests for the presence of agglutinins are most often employed. The organisms to be used as antigen should be "from a young, actively growing phase I culture of representative and/or broad antigenic coverage" (Manclark, 1976). The surface of *B. pertussis* is a mosaic of at least seven heat-labile antigens (factors, serotype antigens, agglutinogens), none of which has been isolated or characterized. Thus, if one is examining the agglutinin response to a particular pertussis vaccine, the test organism should be either the vaccine strain or a strain in which antigens of the vaccine strain are represented. If one is evaluating whether natural infection of immunization with an unknown strain has occurred, broad antigen coverage is required and often mixtures of strains are used (Manclark, 1976).

Similarly, the agglutination test with appropriately adsorbed antisera can be employed to identify strains for epidemiological purposes or to ensure that a particular strain is antigenically stable. With respect to unknown strains, they may vary greatly in agglutinin adsorption, and evaluation of their ability to evoke specific agglutinins should also be carried out.

The antigen used for complement-fixation tests is crude material prepared by treating organisms with NaOH and heat. Using both agglutination and complement-fixation tests, the Combined Scottish Study (1970) found that in children under 6 months of age with whooping cough, positive serological tests occurred in 19%, whereas cultures were positive in 42%. In older children it appeared that the converse was true.

5. Immunization against Pertussis

It is difficult at this time for many to appreciate the dramatic decrease in both the morbidity and mortality from whooping cough that has occurred in the United States during the past few decades. In 1930 there were 166,914 cases and 5707 deaths reported; in 1975 there were 1738 cases and 14 deaths reported. As shown in Fig. 1, the mortality from whooping cough began to decline before the introduction of active immunization. It is reasonable to assume that this decline was related to improved measures of supportive care, including fluid and electrolyte therapy, respiratory assistance, and alimentation. In contrast to the finding with respect to mortality, the decline in incidence of pertussis in the United States clearly

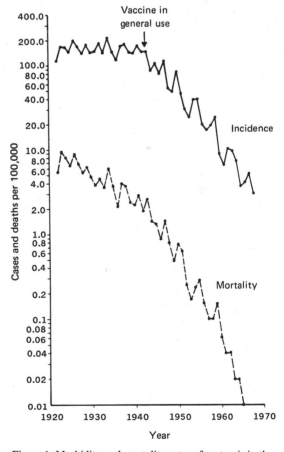

Figure 1. Morbidity and mortality rates of pertussis in the United States, 1922–1968.

coincided with the mass introduction of *B. pertussis* vaccine (Fig. 1).

5.1. Efficacy of Pertussis Vaccine

Although the marked decrease in the incidence of whooping cough in the United States, as shown in Fig. 1, was related to the introduction of petussis vaccine, there are some workers in the United Kingdom who suggest that the reduction in incidence of whooping cough was a natural occurrence independent of vaccine and that immunization against whooping cough is unnecessary and ineffective. These conclusions are at variance with the results and interpretations of a study by a committee in the United Kingdom formed to examine this question (Joint Committee on Vaccination and Immunization, 1975) and the findings that appropriately prepared vaccines can afford approximately 90% protection of exposed, susceptible children (reviewed in Pittman, 1970).

There is abundant evidence that immunization does not engender lifelong protection (Lambert, 1965; Morse, 1968; Kurt *et al.*, 1972; Linnemann *et al.*, 1975), and the same is probably true for clinical disease. The true incidence of whooping cough in later life is difficult to ascertain because the disease tends to be milder and is often difficult to recognize. It would be important to determine accurately by serological and/or bacteriological methods the exact incidence of pertussis in a large adult population in which a history of prior immunization or disease can be obtained. An ancillary question is whether there is a reservoir of *B. pertussis*. Healthy carriers have not been uncovered (Linnemann *et al.*, 1968), nor has an animal reservoir been found; certainly this fragile organism does not sustain itself as an environmental contaminant. It is unlikely that a reservoir does not exist; perhaps the organism is carried in a nonculturable form or in the rough phase and therefore is not recognizable as *B. pertussis*.

The impermanence of immunity against whooping cough probably accounts for the susceptibility of newborns, rather than inability of protective antibody to cross the placenta or cell-mediated immunity as a major factor. This situation is in marked contrast to that of *H. influenzae*, where maternal antibody protects the newborn. Greater than 70% of deaths associated with whooping cough occur in infants under 1 year of age, with the majority in infants less than 6 months. For this reason the current recommendation is that immunization begin at 2–3 months or even 6 weeks, and two more doses be given at 4–6 week intervals. The pertussis vaccine consists of killed phase I cells or crude extracts and is usually combined with alum-precipitated diphtheria and tetanus toxoids (DPT). The *B. pertussis* component has an adjuvant effect enhancing the response to these toxoids. A reinforcing dose of DPT is administered approximately 1 year after the third injection, and a "booster" is given at the time of entry into school. As discussed below, pertussis vaccine is generally not recommended for older individuals.

Administration of human hyperimmune γ globulin has little or no demonstrable effect as either a prophylactic or a therapeutic measure.

5.2. Toxicity of Pertussis Vaccine

In addition to the question of efficacy, proponents of the discontinuation of pertussis vaccine claim that the vaccine's side effects are unacceptable. Pain at the site, fever, and irritability are the more common side effects seen. Convulsions and even a fatal encephalopathy have been reported (Kulenkampff *et al.*, 1974). The true incidence of serious neurological complications *directly* related to pertussis vaccination is uncertain, but it is reasonable to defer immunization of an infant with a previous history of convulsion and perhaps also where there is a family history.

Whooping cough in adults may occur in localized epidemics in hospitals, and two recent episodes in pediatric staff members have been described fully (Kurt *et al.*, 1972; Linnemann *et al.*, 1975). In these outbreaks the problem of protecting adults at risk must be addressed because, although the disease is often mild in older individuals, it can be incapacitating. It has been generally accepted, without definitive data, that pertussis immunization in adults presents more risks of serious side effects, although both Volk *et al.* (1964) and Kendrick *et al.* (1969) found only local reactions without serious complications. In their studies Linnemann *et al.* (1975) injected over 800 adults with 0.2 ml of pertussis vaccine. A rise in agglutinin titers occurred in 77% of 286 whose sera were tested. Local reactions, e.g., erythema, swelling, and pain, were frequent. Short-term fever occurred in approximately 10%. Two of the vaccinees had a generalized rash, and one required steroid therapy. Another vaccinee with a history of a childhood febrile convulsion had a transient episode of memory impairment. Their conclusion was that "pertussis vaccine given parenterally in reduced dosage will induce an antibody response in most adults, but local reactions and occasional systemic reactions are a problem." Chemoprophylaxis with erythromycin or the development of less toxic vaccines may prove more satisfactory in these situations.

5.3. Protective Component of Pertussis Vaccine

With due apologies to Baroness D'Orczy, there is a quality to the search for the specific protective component of pertussis vaccine reminiscent of the search for the elusive Scarlet Pimpernel. A number of antigens or ill-defined clusters of antigens have been reported as "the protective antigen," including agglutinogens, HSF, the substrate for bactericidal antibody, capsule, hemagglutinin, and lethal toxin (Pittman, 1970). It is not surprising that the protective antigen has not been identified, since the mechanism of pathogenicity has not been established and few of the antigens have been isolated, characterized, and used as purified immunogens.

Although the protective antigen is not identified, the efficacy of a given lot of vaccine in man is well correlated with the degree of protection produced against intracerebral challenge in mice. In the United States, no less than 4 and no more than 12 mouse-protective units must be in a single human dose which contains no more than 16–20×10^9 organisms. Toxicity is determined by injecting mice with one-half of a human dose. With a nontoxic vaccine, following an initial weight loss the mice must regain their starting weight by 72 hr after injection and then gain a further 3 g by 7 days. Testing for efficacy and toxicity is a cumbersome time- and animal-consuming procedure.

The "magic" that makes a vaccine effective and nontoxic has not been revealed. Vaccine failures in the past have generally been attributed to inappropriate organisms which lack potency in the mouse protection test. The variations may be related to the heterogeneity of morphology and serotype of any *B. pertussis* strain (Cameron, 1976), so that a clone not containing protective antigen may become the predominating organism. Preston and co-workers (Preston, 1963; Preston and Stanbridge, 1972) also attributed what they viewed as vaccine failure to the appearance in the population of disease-producing organisms which contained an agglutinogen (factor 3) not represented in the vaccine. When organisms possessing factor 3 were incorporated into the vaccine, protection appeared to increase. However, there is considerable dispute regarding the cause-and-effect relationship of these findings (Eldering *et al.*, 1966, 1967).

The presence in serum of agglutinins, precipitins, complement-fixing antibodies, or bacteriocidins directed against *B. pertussis* does not necessarily correlate with protection (e.g., see Olson, 1975), although all may appear after immunization as well as infection. However, these tests are useful for epidemiological studies. For example, they can indicate whether populations have been exposed to pertussis, and it is of interest that the prevalence of antibodies to pertussis, whether induced by natural disease or immunization, is only 25–35% after childhood. The relatively low prevalence of *B. pertussis* antibodies in later life undoubtedly accounts for the occurrence of pertussis in adults (Linnemann and Nasenbeny, 1977), which often goes unrecognized, and the susceptibility of newborns. The presence in sera of antibodies which can passively protect mice is taken as *prima facie* evidence of immunity, but here too there is controversy (Dolby and Stephens, 1973). A skin test has also been used to distinguish between susceptible and immune subjects, but general experience holds it to be unsatisfactory.

In sum, the protective antigen remains to be identified and isolated, and the mode of pathogenicity of whooping cough must be clearly understood if pertussis immunization is to be put on a rational basis. Correlative studies on the nature of humoral protection and the possible role of cell-mediated immunity are also needed. In this regard, the hypothesized attachment of *B. petussis* to cilia has generated great interest (Geller and Pittman, 1973) in determining whether secretory IgA antibodies, perhaps directed against the pili, are protective.

References

Aftandelians, R., and Connor, J. D., 1973a, Bactericidal antibody in serum during infection with *Bordetella pertussis*, *J. Infect. Dis.* **128:**555–558.

Aftandelians, R., and Connor, J. D., 1973b, Immunologic studies of pertussis: Development of precipitins, *J. Pediatr.* **83:**206–214.

Andersen, V., Hertz, J. B., Sørensen, S. F., Baekgaard, P., Christensen, P. E., Ramhoj, W., Hansen, G. A., Wardlaw, A. C., and Sato, Y., 1977, In vitro stimulation of human lymphocytes by *Bordetella pertussis, Acta Pathol. Microbiol. Scand. Sect. C* **85:**65–72.

Aprile, M. A., and Wardlaw, A. C., 1973, Immunochemical studies on the lipopolysaccharides of *Bordetella pertussis, Can. J. Microbiol.* **19:**231–239.

Bernales, R., Eastman, J., and Kaplan, J., 1976, Quantitation of circulating T and B lymphocytes in children with whooping cough, *Pediatr. Res.* **10:**965–967.

Cameron, J., 1976, Problems associated with the control testing of pertussis vaccine, *Applied Microbiol.* **20:**9–26.

Cheers, C., and Gray, D. F., 1969, Macrophage behaviour during the complaisant phase of murine pertussis, *Immunology* **17:**875–887.

Collier, A. M., Peterson, L. P., and Baseman, J. B., 1977, Pathogenesis of *Bordetella pertussis* infection in hamster tracheal organ culture, *J. Infect. Dis.* **136:**S196–S203.

Combined Scottish Study, 1970, Diagnosis of whooping cough: Comparison of serological tests with isolation of *Bordetella pertussis, Br. Med. J.* **4:**637–659.

Connor, J. D., 1970, Evidence for an etiologic role of adenoviral infection in pertussis syndrome, *N. Engl. J. Med.* **283:**390–394.

Denny, F. W., 1974, Effect of a toxin produced by *Haemophilus influenzae* on ciliated respiratory epithelium, *J. Infect. Dis.* **129:**93–100.

Dolby, J. M., and Dolby, D. E., 1969, The antibody activities of 19 S and 7 S fractions from rabbit antisera to *Bordetella pertussis, Immunology* **16:**737–747.

Dolby, J. M., and Stephens, S., 1973, Pertussis antibodies in the sera of children exposed to *Bordetella pertussis* by vaccination or infection, *J. Hyg.* **71:**193–207.

Dresser, D. W., 1972, The role of T cells and adjuvant in the immune response of mice to foreign erythrocytes, *Eur. J. Immunol.* **2:**50–57.

Eldering, G., Holwerda, J., and Baker, J., 1966, *Bordetella pertussis* culture having only species factor 1, *J. Bacteriol.* **91:**1759–1762.

Eldering, G., Holwerda, J., and Baker, J., 1967, Mouse-protective properties of *Bordetella pertussis* serotypes in passive tests, *J. Bacteriol.* **93:**1758–1761.

Geller, B. D., and Pittman, M., 1973, Immunoglobulin and histamine-sensitivity response of mice to live *Bordetella pertussis, Infect. Immun.* **8:**83–90.

Gray, D. F., and Cheers, C., 1969, The sequence of enhanced cellular activity and protective humoral factors in murine pertussis immunity, *Immunology* **17:**889–896.

Gulbenkian, L. S., Schobert, L., Nixon, C., and Tabachnick, I. I. A., 1968, Metabolic effects of pertussis sensitization in mice and rats, *Endocrinology* **83:**885–892.

Ho, M.-K., Kong, A. S., and Morse, S. I., 1977, Influence of non-responding cells on the mitogenic response of murine T cells to the lymphocytosis-promoting factor of *Bordetella pertussis, Fed. Proc.* **36:**1323.

Holt, L. B., 1972, The pathology and Immunology of *Bordetella pertussis* infection, *J. Med. Microbiol.* **5:**407–424.

Hopewell, J. W., Holt, L. B., and Desombre, T. R., 1972, An electron microscope study of intracerebral infection of mice with low-virulence *Bordetella pertussis, J. Med. Microbiol.* **5:**154–157.

Joint Committee on Vaccination and Immunization of the Central Health Services Council and the Scottish Health Service Planning Council, 1975, *Br. Med. J.* **3:**687–688.

Katada, T., and Ui, M., 1977, Spontaneous recovery from streptozotocin-induced diabetes in rats pretreated with pertussis vaccine or hydrocortisone, *Diabetologia* **13:**521–525.

Kendrick, P. L., Gottshall, R. Y., Anderson, H. D., Volk, V. K., Bunney, W. E., and Top, F. H., 1969, Pertussis agglutinins in adults, *Public Health Rep.* **84:**9–15.

Kong, A. S., and Morse, S. I., 1976, The effect of *Bordetella pertussis* on the antibody response in mice to type III pneumococcal polysaccharide, *J. Immunol.* **116:**989–993.

Kong, A. S., and Morse, S. I., 1977a, The *in vitro* effects of *Bordetella pertussis* lymphocytosis-promoting factor on murine lymphocytes. I. Proliferative response, *J. Exp. Med.* **145:**151–162.

Kong, A. S., and Morse, S. I., 1977b, The *in vitro* effects of *Bordetella* pertussis lymphocytosis-promoting factor on murine lymphocytes. II. Nature of the responding cells, *J. Exp. Med.* **145:**163–172.

Kulenkampff, M., Schwartzman, J. S., and Wilson, J., 1974, Neurological complications of pertussis inoculation, *Arch. Dis. Child.* **49:**46–49.

Kurt, T. L., Yeager, A. S., Guenette, S., and Dunlop, S., 1972, Spread of pertussis by hospital staff, *JAMA* **221:**264–267.

Laergren, J., 1963, The white blood cell count and the erythrocyte sedimentation rate in pertussis, *Acta Paediatr.* **52:**405–409.

Lambert, H. J., 1965, Epidemiology of a small pertussis outbreak in Kent County, Mich., *Public Health Rep.* **80:**365–369.

Lapin, J. H., 1943, *Whooping Cough*, Thomas, Springfield, Ill.

Lawson, G. M., 1940, Modified technique for staining capsules of *Haemophilus pertussis, J. Lab. Clin. Med.* **25:**435–438.

Leslie, P. H., and Gardner, A. D., 1931, The phases of *Haemophilus pertussis, J. Hyg.* **31:**423–434.

Levine, S., Wenk, E. J., Devlin, H. B., Pieroni, R. E.,

and Levine, L., 1966, Hyperacute allergic encephalomyelitis: Adjuvant effect of pertussis vaccines and extracts, *J. Immunol.* **97:**363–368.

Linnemann, C. C., Jr., and Nasenbery, J., 1977, Pertussis in the adult, *Annu. Rev. Med.* **28:**179–185.

Linnemann, C. C., Jr., Bass, J. A., and Smith, M. H., 1968, The carrier state in pertussis, *Am. J. Epidemiol.* **88:**422–427.

Linnemann, C. C., Jr., Perlstein, P. H., Ramundo, N., Minton, S. D., Englender, G. S., McCormick, J. B., and Hayes, P. S., 1975, Use of pertussis vaccine in an epidemic involving hospital staff, *Lancet* **2:**540–543.

Macdonald, H., and Macdonald, E. J., 1933, Experimental pertussis, *J. Infect. Dis.* **53:**328–330.

Maillard, J., and Bloom, B. R., 1972, Immunological adjuvants and the mechanism of cell cooperation, *J. Exp. Med.* **136:**185–190.

Major, R. H., 1939, *Classic Descriptions of Disease,* 2nd ed., Thomas, Springfield, Ill.

Manclark, C. R., 1976, Serological response to *Bordetella pertussis,* in: *Manual of Clinical Immunology* (N. R. Rose and H. Friedman, eds.), pp. 312–314, American Society for Microbiology, Washington, D.C.

Morse, J. H., and Morse, S. I., 1970, Studies on the ultrastructure of *Bordetella pertussis.* I. Morphology, origin, and biological activity of structures present in the extracellular fluid of liquid cultures of *Bordetella pertussis, J. Exp. Med.* **131:**1342–1357.

Morse, J. H., Kong, A. S., Arden, J., and Morse, S. I., 1975, The mitogenic response of human lymphocytes to the lymphocytosis-promoting factor (LPF) of *Bordetella pertussis, Proc. 18th Meet. Am. Soc. Hematol.,* p. 187.

Morse, J. H., Kong, A. S., Lindenbaum, J., and Morse, S. I., 1977, The mitogenic effect of the lymphocytosis promoting factor from *Bordetella pertussis* on human lymphocytes, *J. Clin. Invest.* **60:**683–692.

Morse, S. I., 1968, Pertussis in adults, *Ann. Intern. Med.* **68:**953–954.

Morse, S. I., 1976, Biologically active components and properties of *Bordetella pertussis, Adv. Appl. Microbiol.* **20:**9–26.

Morse, S. I., and Morse, J. H., 1976, Isolation and properties of the leukocytosis- and lymphocytosis-promoting factor of *Bordetella pertussis, J. Exp. Med.* **143:**1483–1502.

Morse, S. I., and Riester, S. K., 1967, Studies on the leukocytosis and lymphocytosis induced by *Bordetella pertussis.* I. Radioautographic analysis of the circulating cells in mice undergoing pertussis-induced hyperleukocytosis, *J. Exp. Med.* **125:**401–408.

Mota, I., 1958, Mast cell and histamine in rat anaphylaxis: The effect of *Haemophilus pertussis, Nature (London)* **182:**1021–1022.

Mota, I., 1964, The mechanism of anaphylaxis. I. Production and biological properties of mast cell sensitizing antibody, *Immunology* **7:**681–699.

Munoz, J., 1971, Protein toxins from *Bordetella pertussis,* in: *Bacterial Toxins,* Vol. IIA (S. Kadis, T. C. Montie,

and S. J. Ajl, eds.), pp. 271–300, Academic Press, New York.

Murgo, A. J., and Athanassiades, T. J., 1975, Studies on the adjuvant effect of *Bordetella pertussis* vaccine to sheep erythrocytes in the mouse. I. *In vitro* enhancement of antibody formation with normal spleen cells, *J. Immunol.* **115:**928–931.

Muse, K. E., Collier, A. M., and Baseman, J. B., 1977, Scanning electron microscopic study of hamster tracheal organ cultures infected with *Bordetella pertussis, J. Infect. Dis.* **136:**768–777.

Nakase, Y., Tateisi, M., Sekiya, K., and Kasuga, T., 1970, Chemical and biological properties of the purified O antigen of *Bordetella pertussis, Jpn. J. Microbiol.* **14:**1–8.

Nelson, K. E., Gavitt, F., Batt, M. D., Kallick, C. A., Reddi, K. T., and Levin, S., 1975, The role of adenoviruses in the pertussis syndrome, *J. Pediatr.* **86:**335–341.

Okumura, K., and Tada, T. 1971, Regulation of homocytotropic antibody formation in the rat. III. Effect of thymectomy and splenectomy, *J. Immunol.* **106:**1019–1025.

Olson, L. C., 1975, Pertussis, *Medicine* **54:**427–469.

Ortez, R. A., Seshachalam, D., and Szentivanyi, A., 1975, Alterations in adenyl cyclase activity and glucose utilization of *Bordetella pertussis*-sensitized mouse spleen, *Biochem. Pharmacol.* **24:**1297–1302.

Parker, C. W., and Morse, S. I., 1973, The effect of *Bordetella pertussis* on lymphocyte cyclic AMP metabolism, *J. Exp. Med.* **137:**1078–1090.

Pereira, M. S., and Candeias, J. A. N., 1971, The association of viruses with clinical pertussis, *J. Hyg.* **69:**399–403.

Phanuphak, P., Moorhead, J. W., and Claman, H. N., 1972, Immunologic activities of pertussis treated lymphocytes, *Int. Arch. Allergy* **43:**305–316.

Pieroni, R. E., Stevens, D. L., Stojanović, A., and Levine, L., 1972, Investigation of the responsiveness of BCG vaccinated children with whooping cough to tuberculin, *Int. Arch. Allergy* **42:**583–589.

Pittman, M., 1970, *Bordetella pertussis*—bacterial and host factors in the pathogenesis and prevention of whooping cough, in: *Infectious Agents and Host Reactions* (S. Mudd, ed.), pp. 239–270, Saunders, Philadelphia.

Preston, N. W., 1963, Type-specific immunity against whooping cough, *Br. Med. J.* **2:**724–726.

Preston, N. W., and Stanbridge, T. N., 1972, Efficacy of pertussis vaccines: A brighter horizon, *Br. Med. J.* **3:**448–451.

Sato, Y., Arai, H., and Suzuki, K., 1974, Leukocytosis-promoting factor of *Bordetella pertussis.* III. Its identity with protective antigen, *Infect. Immun.* **9:**801–810.

Shibley, G. S., and Hoelscher, H., 1934, Studies on whooping cough. I. Type-specific (S) and dissociation (R) forms of *Hemophilus pertussis, J. Exp. Med.* **60:**403–418.

Szentivanyi, A., Fishel, C. W., and Talmage, D. W., 1963, Adrenalin mediation of histamine and serotonin hyperglycemia in normal mice and the absence of adrenal in-induced hyperglycemia in pertussis-sensitized mice, *J. Infect. Dis.* **113:**86–98.

Tada, T., Taniguchi, M., and Okumura, K., 1971, Regulation of homocytotropic antibody formation in the rat. II. Effect of x-irradiation, *J. Immunol.* **106:**1012–1018.

Tada, T., Okumura, K., Ochiai, T., and Iwasa, S., 1972, Effect of lymphocytosis-promoting factor of *Bordetella pertussis* on the immune response. II. Adjuvant effect for the production of reaginic antibody in the rat, *Int. Arch. Allergy* **43:**207–216.

Taub, R. N., Rosett, W., Adler, A., and Morse, S. I., 1972, Distribution of labelled lymph node cells in mice during the lymphocytosis induced by *Bordetella pertussis*, *J. Exp. Med.* **136:**1581–1593.

Thelander, H. E., Henderson, H. G., and Kilgariff, K., 1933, The blood picture in pertussis: A graphic study, *J. Pediatr.* **2:**288–298.

Volk, V. K., Gottshall, R. Y., Anderson, H. D., Top, F. H., Bunney, W. E., and Serfling, R. E., 1964, Antibody response to booster dose of diphtheria and tetanus toxoids and pertussis vaccine, *Public Health Rep.* **79:**424–434.

Whitaker, J. A., Donaldson, P., and Nelson, J. D., 1960, Diagnosis of pertussis by fluorescent antibody method, *N. Engl. J. Med.* **263:**850–851.

Winter, J. L., 1953, Development of antibodies in children convalescent from whooping cough, *Proc. Soc. Exp. Biol. Med.* **83:**866–870.

8

Immunobiology of Diphtheria

LANE BARKSDALE

1. Introduction

Between 1821 and 1826 Pierre Fidèle Breton-neau (1826) established the clinical entity diphtheria. Its hallmark was the pseudomembrane or diphtheritic membrane. By 1869 Trendelenberg had shown that pseudomembranes could be produced in rabbits and in pigeons following the injection of pseudomembranous material from human cases of diphtheria. Bretonneau conceived of diphtheria as a disease of singular etiology comparable in its uniqueness to the causes of measles and of variola. This unitarian view was soon lost to some students of the disease. In methylene-blue-stained smears of material taken from pseudomembranes, more than one shape of bacterium could be observed. In fact, Klebs (1875) found diphtheria from one locality to be caused by a fungus, *Microsporon diphtheri-cum,* and later he described a bacillary type of diphtheria from another locality (Klebs, 1883). When Friedrich Loeffler tackled the problem of the etiology of diphtheria, he accepted the concept of a single etiology as promulgated by Bretonneau. Working in Koch's laboratory, he designed a program for direct microscopic examination of methylene-blue-stained material from pseudomembranes, cultivation of such materials on solid media, and inoculation of animals with bacterial cultures (Loeffler, 1884). This remarkable investigator was the first to distinguish the probable role

of streptococci in diphtheria associated with scarlatinal infections from that of occasional chains of streptococci (normal flora) found associated with frank cases of diphtheria.[*] He was able to demonstrate diphtheria bacilli in smears of only 13 out of 22 cases of clinical diphtheria. From six of these he isolated *Corynebacterium diphtheriae.* He isolated diphtheria bacilli from one normal child. Because of the lack of a one-to-one correlation in these findings, he was not adamant in claiming to have established the etiology of the disease. But he had in fact clearly established its etiology. From the time of Loeffler, it has been evident that harboring diphtheria bacilli is not synonymous with diphtheria and that Koch's postulates cannot be fulfilled in every case of

[*] Some 30 years ago the writer and his co-workers became concerned with certain unorthodox manifestations of diphtheria. This led to a study of equally unorthodox diphtheria bacilli. In the early part of that period there were several thousand cases of diphtheria available to us. We made it a practice that we, ourselves, examined and took culture material from each pseudomembrane of cases with which we were concerned. To our surprise, typical membranes often yielded no *C. diphtheriae* and very atypical membranes sometimes yielded almost pure cultures of diphtheria bacilli. An early conflict between our findings and clinical impressions involved a young soldier from whom we had isolated *C. diphtheriae* but whose outpatient status remained "streptococcal pharyngitis." He died days later while waiting on sick call. Like many patients with diphtheria, he did not look so ill but felt miserable. Of course, he had both a streptococcal pharyngitis and diphtheria. Histopathological findings in sections from his heart confirmed the latter. Now, 30 years later, we realize that, with a few exceptions, none of the manifestations of diphtheria seen by us was any different from what Friedrich Loeffler carefully described in 1884.

LANE BARKSDALE • Department of Microbiology, New York University School of Medicine and Medical Center, New York, New York 10016.

diphtheria. Loeffler's experimental infections in animals led to the discovery that diphtheria bacilli tended to remain at the site of injection, although autopsy revealed damage to organs far from that site. Roux and Yersin (1888) demonstrated that the connection between diphtheria bacilli at one site and damage to distant internal organs was a soluble poison, diphtherial toxin. These observations have given rise to the concept that diphtheria bacilli *always* remain at the superficial site of colonization, the pseudomembrane or the cutaneous lesion.* Further, since Roux and Yersin pointed out that toxin itself could be responsible for many of the signs of the disease, in the legend of diphtheria there has been a tendency to confuse intoxication with infection. The discovery of antibodies capable of neutralizing the toxicity of diphtherial toxin (Behring and Kitasato, 1890) and their apparent effects in reducing case fatality rates in epidemics of diphtheria obscured for many the need for investigating antibacterial immunity toward *C. diphtheriae.* As a result, textbook presentations of the immunology of diphtheria are often confused. In fact, it has been implied that immunization with toxoid has got rid of diphtheria bacilli in some societies. Bonventre (1975) has called this sort of assertion a manifestation of arrogance and has suggested that there are still many questions about diphtheria which remain unanswered. The discussion of the immunology of diphtheria that follows indicates a number of aspects of the interaction of diphtheria bacilli and human beings which merit further study.

2. Diphtheria and Diphtheria Bacilli

Diphtheria, a communicable disease of man caused by the growth of any one of a number of types of *C. diphtheriae* on the mucous membranes or, less commonly, in cutaneous tissues, occurs sporadically throughout the world. Although it is often held that diphtheria has

disappeared from civilized countries (Pappenheimer and Gill, 1973), contemporary public health reports are not in accord with this view. Every year, in populations living under crowded and other conditions indicative of relative poverty and/or poor hygiene, there occur outbreaks of diphtheria: e.g., Miami, 1969 (Hennekens and Saslaw, 1976), San Antonio, 1970 (Marcuse and Grand, 1973; McCloskey *et al.,* 1971), Manchester, 1971 (Butterworth *et al.,* 1974), Wurzburg, 1975 (Ströder, 1976), Seattle, 1972–1975 (Pedersen *et al.,* 1977), Montreal, 1974 (Gauvreau *et al.,* 1977). The data in Table 1 indicate that prior to immunization there was a decline in deaths due to diphtheria. In the San Antonio outbreak the case fatality rate was 1%.

Most of the information found in textbooks regarding immunity to diphtheria was gathered prior to 1951 and deals primarily with immun-

Table 1. Diphtheria Death Returns, Metropolitan Asylums Boards[a]

Year	Case mortality (%)	Year	Case mortality (%)
1889	40.7	1909	9.4
1890	33.5	1910	7.8
1891	30.6	1911	8.4
1892	29.3	1912	6.2
1893	30.4	1913	6.2
1894	29.3	1914	7.9
1895	22.8	1915	8.4
1896	21.2	1916	6.8
1897	17.7	1917	6.7
1898	15.4	1918	7.7
1899	13.9	1919	9.3
1900	12.3	1920	8.6
1901	11.1	1921	8.8
1902	11.0	1922	8.7
1903	9.7	1923	6.8
1904	10.0	1924	7.0
1905	8.3	1925	5.0
1906	8.8	1926	4.9
1907	9.6	1927	4.0
1908	9.7		

[a] These data, adapted from Wilson and Miles (1955), indicate a general decline in case fatality rates for diphtheria in England. The use of antitoxin was routine after about 1895. Mass immunization with diphtherial toxoid did not take place in England until 1941. In the following decade deaths per million from diphtheria dropped from 60 to 0.7. In the United States the attack rate per hundred thousand in 1920 was 151, and in 1958 was 0.5. A limited study (1969–1970) of diphtheria among the immunized (three or more injections of toxoid) revealed 1.5% deaths in 203 cases and 12.8% deaths in 1300 nonimmunized cases (Brooks *et al.,* 1974).

---

* In nature there seems to be very little that is invariant. Thus, in early studies of diphtheria in which tracheotomies were performed, there was evidence for invasion of the deeper tissues by diphtheria bacilli (Andrewes *et al.,* 1923). In addition, certain strains, when inoculated intracutaneously or subcutaneously into guinea pigs, could be isolated from the heart blood of six of 14 animals (Coleman, 1949; Maitland *et al.,* 1952).

ity to diphtherial toxin. While diphtherial toxin causes toxemia that may lead to death, it does not (see Table 2), as is sometimes implied (Davis *et al.*, 1973), cause diphtheria. Diphtheritic infections involve a wide variety of strains of *C. diphtheriae,* much as streptococcal infections may be caused by any of several types of *Streptococcus pyogenes.* Before the 1950s the orthodox view* held that diphtheria bacilli which made toxin were true diphtheria bacilli and those which did not were "diphtheroids," along with other species as *C. pseudodiphtheriticum* and *C. xeroxis.* Freeman (1951) discovered that nontoxinogenic *C. diphtheriae* in the process of being lysed by a temperate phage B produced diphtherial toxin. The production of toxin was subsequently shown to be under the control of a phage gene(s) called *tox.* It is now known that the gene *tox* is present in the genomes of a number of, but by no means all, corynebacteriophages and that it can gain expression in any strain of *C. diphtheriae* which can be lysed or lysogenized by such a phage. Figure 1 makes it clear that both toxinogenic and nontoxinogenic diphtheria bacilli are infectious. That toxin itself is not essential to infectivity has long been a matter of record, because of the existence of toxin-producing strains which are incapable of multiplying in animal tissues. While the two strains shown in Fig. 1 are equally invasive, only C7(ϕ), carrying *tox*, can cause toxemic diphtheria. The infection caused by the nontoxinogenic strain is of consequence mainly in infants, where overgrowth of the trachea by a pseudomembrane can lead to obstruction of breathing and to death (Edward and Allison, 1951; Barksdale *et al.*, 1960). The capacity to colonize mucous membranes (invasiveness)† exhibited by the pair of toxino-

Table 2. Effect of Early Administration of Antitoxin on Case Fatality Rate[a]

Day[b] of disease antitoxin administered	Number of cases treated	Case fatality rate (%)
1	225	0
2	1441	4.2
3	1600	11.1
4	1276	17.3
5 or >5	1645	18.7

[a] From Russell (1943). There appears to be a saturation point at 4 days, beyond which fatality remains constant and the fatality of the disease is unaffected by antitoxin. During the first days of the disease the amount of toxin produced will be related rather directly to the increase in numbers of diphtheria bacilli. Toxin must penetrate cells of the patient in order to exert its lethal effect. Antitoxin can prevent penetration but is without effect on toxin that has reached an intracellular location. While antibiotic therapy is without effect on toxin action, if offered soon enough it can, by killing diphtheria bacilli, markedly limit the final amounts of toxin produced. In the San Antonio outbreak (McCloskey *et al.*, 1971) penicillin or erythromycin was used as a part of the treatment of patients with diphtheria and of carriers. In a recently reported 598 cases of diphtheria in Delhi (Dutta *et al.*, 1976) the case fatality rate was 17%. About 16% of strains of *C. diphtheriae* from 223 bacteriologically positive cases were resistant to penicillin; fewer to ampicillin. The only antibiotic to which all strains (337 strains accumulated from 1972–1975) were sensitive was gentamycin.
[b] Determining the exact day of disease is difficult.

genic and nontoxinogenic strains shown in Fig. 1 may be related to the production of corynebacterial cord factor (an α,α'-trehalose dimycolate), a neuraminidase (capable of cleaving *N*-acetylneuraminic acid (NAN) residues from mucins and from cell surfaces), NAN lyase (capable of splitting *N*-acetyl neuraminic acid into *N*-acetyl mannosamine and pyruvate), and diphthin (a putative protease which hydrolyzes certain immunoglobulins).

Diphtheria bacilli may be divided into three major groups‡ on the basis of the shapes and sizes assumed by their colonies on certain solid media (Fig. 2). Those forming medium-sized smooth colonies are termed *mitis.*

---

* "Diphtheroid" was from the start a bad term: (1) Etymologically it means "like diphtheria." Of course, a bacterium cannot be like a disease. (2) The creation of the term was a way of begging the question of what is *C. diphtheriae.* The writer once traveled a long, long distance to discuss nontoxinogenic diphtheria bacilli with an eminent authority whose considered opinion was that "organisms which fail to make diphtheria toxin cannot be called *C. diphtheriae.*"
† As employed here "invasiveness" is equivalent to "virulence." Specifically with regard to *C. diphtheriae,* the term "virulence" was early perverted to mean toxinogenicity as in the name of the intradermal test for detecting toxin, the intradermal "virulence test."

‡ While McLeod and his co-workers referred to these three groups as "types" and others have referred to them as "biotypes" (Marcuse and Grand, 1973), they mainly represent groupings according to shape of colony. Such variation in colonial properties is manifested by many bacteria (e.g.. *Streptococcus pneumoniae, Salmonella typhimurium, Shigella sonnei*). The manner in which bacteria pile up to form a colony is dependent on the properties of their surfaces, the chemical bases for which are peculiar to each taxon. Actual typing of *Corynebacterium diphtheriae* is based on serological identification of surface antigens (serological typing) and sensitivity to corynebacteriophages (phage typing).

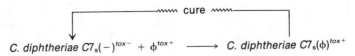

$$C.\ diphtheriae\ C7_s(-)^{tox-} + \phi^{tox+} \longrightarrow C.\ diphtheriae\ C7_s(\phi)^{tox+}$$

Invasive
Nontoxinogenic
Sensitive to phage φ

May cause nontoxemic diphtheria

Invasive
Toxinogenic
Immune to phage φ
Lysogenic for phage φ
May cause toxemic diphtheria

Figure 1. Changes brought to *Corynebacterium diphtheriae*, strain $C7_s(-)^{tox-}$, after lysogenization by a bacteriophage carrying the *tox* gene. Presumably the indicator strain $C7_s$ is nonlysogenic, hence the designation $(-)$, and is nontoxinogenic, *tox⁻*. When nontoxinogenic, nonlysogenic $C7_s$ is lysed by a phage carrying the *tox⁺* marker, such as ϕ^{tox+}, toxin is produced during the course of phage multiplication and lysis of the cell. When lysogenized by ϕ^{tox+}, the genome of $C7_s(\phi)^{tox+}$ includes phage genes which endow it with immunity to homologous phage (lysogenic immunity = synthesis of specific repressor) and the ability to synthesize diphtherial toxin. The subscript s refers to the smooth (surface) antigen of the strain. Once the K antigens of Lautrop (see text) are systematized, s would be replaced with a more specific designation, e.g., $C7_{K15}(-)^{tox-}$. See also Fig. 5, where K antigens are shown as "surface protein." From Barksdale (1970). Reproduced with permission of the publisher. For additional data concerning lysogeny and genetic changes in bacteria, see Barksdale and Arden (1974). Furthermore, the closely related "species" of *Corynebacterium*, *C. pseudotuberculosis (ovis)* and *C. ulcerans,* when lysed or lysogenized by *tox*-carrying bacteriophages, produce diphtherial toxin.

$C7_s(-)^{tox-}$ and $C7_s(\phi)^{tox+}$ are typical *mitis* strains. Another group of diphtheria bacilli forms dwarf-smooth colonies, and still another forms medium-sized rough colonies. McLeod, working only with toxinogenic strains, established a correlation between the clinical severity of toxemic diphtheria and the colonial morphology assumed by the causal toxinogenic diphtheria bacilli. The more severe infections (grave = *gravis*) were caused by diphtheria bacilli that grew as rough colonies and to some extent by those that grew as dwarf-smooth colonies (intermediate = *intermedius*). The milder infections (*mitis*) were associated with smooth strains. Soon after the discovery of an association between clinical severity of diphtheria and the colonial type of *C. diphtheriae* isolated from the cases, the terms *gravis, mitis,* and *intermedius* came to be regarded literally. However, as more and more data were gathered, it became evident that infections attributed to *intermedius* strains were sometimes milder than infections associated with *mitis* strains. Figure 2 presents the correlations found between clinical severity and colony-form group of causal bacilli among 25,000 cases of diphtheria examined by J. W. McLeod and his associates (McLeod, 1943;

see also Wilson and Miles, 1955). These groups of corynebacteria and their nontoxinogenic homologues can more specifically be identified by serological typing and phage typing. Thus any consideration of the immunology of diphtheria must encompass antibacterial as well as antitoxic immunity.

Immunofluorescence and Problems in the Laboratory Diagnosis of Diphtheria. There are more than 20 phage types of *C. diphtheriae,* a number of serological types, and the colonial types mentioned in Fig. 2. These various types are primarily of epidemiological significance, and, for obvious reasons, their delineation cannot be considered here. Any laboratory dealing with cultures from cases of diphtheria, however, will be dealing with one or more of these types of *C. diphtheriae.* Efforts have been made to find a means for rapidly identifying *C. diphtheriae* in exudates from patients. Those diphtheria bacilli which are toxinogenic all synthesize a biologically and immunologically identical toxin. Thus there is available an antigen which specifically identifies toxinogenic *C. diphtheriae* (for the exception(s), see caption of Fig. 1). Elsewhere in this chapter the problem of freeing toxin of other antigens is discussed, and it is made clear that antitoxin which lacks antibacterial antibodies is very rare. Despite the longstanding problem of the specificities of antibodies in antitoxin, there were reports some years ago suggesting that fluorescing antitoxic sera could be employed for specifically singling out cells of toxinogenic *C. diphtheriae* with the aid of a fluorescence microscope (Whitaker *et al.*, 1961). Unfortunately, adequate controls were not employed in those studies. Had they been, it would have become apparent to the authors that commercial fluorescing antitoxic sera also react with nontoxinogenic *C. diphtheriae* (Allen

and Cluff, 1961; Moody and Jones, 1963). From Fig. 1 it is clear that toxinogenic and nontoxinogenic strains of *C. diphtheriae* may be very closely related. Most, if not all, commercially available fluorescing antitoxic antibody binds to toxinogenic and nontoxinogenic strains as well. In a recent study of 310 patients, 77 of whom were diagnosed clinically as having diphtheria, commercially available fluorescent antiserum (prepared against somatic antigens of *C. diphtheriae*) was used (McCracken and Mauney, 1971). Two findings of these writers are worthy of note: (1) Slides

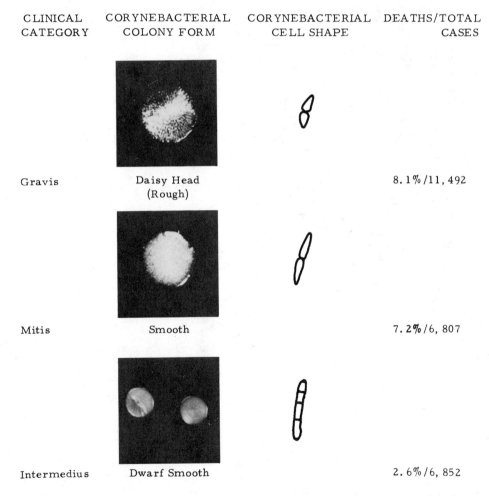

CLINICAL CATEGORY	CORYNEBACTERIAL COLONY FORM	CORYNEBACTERIAL CELL SHAPE	DEATHS/TOTAL CASES
Gravis	Daisy Head (Rough)		8. 1%/11, 492
Mitis	Smooth		7. 2%/6, 807
Intermedius	Dwarf Smooth		2. 6%/6, 852

Figure 2. Separation of toxinogenic strains of *Corynebacterium diphtheriae* on the basis of the forms assumed by their colonies, which in turn are related to the shapes and surface properties of individual corynebacterial cells. In a series of 25,000 cases of diphtheria, McLeod (1943) and co-workers found a rough correlation between colony form and clinical severity of the disease.

prepared directly from throat swabs proved unsatisfactory for examination, whereas slides prepared from swabs which had incubated in a growth medium for 3–4 hr yielded positive fluorescence and gave a 95% agreement with definitive bacteriological identification. (2) There was no relationship between the degree of fluorescence and the particular strain coated with fluorescent antibody. The strains of *C. diphtheriae* examined included nontoxinogenic and toxinogenic strains. The authors noted that "examples of *gravis, intermedius* and *mitis* strains were included in the bacterial isolates obtained throughout the epidemic."

The laboratory identification of *C. diphtheriae* may be considerably facilitated by the use of Tinsdale's tellurite agar on which the cystine desulfhydrase activity of the species can be detected as brown halos around the colonies. It has recently been suggested that the species complex, *C. diphtheriae*, actually includes the varieties *gravis, intermedius, mitis,* and *ulcerans* and probably should include *C. pseudotuberculosis* (*C. ovis*) as well. This cluster of organisms shares a number of properties not found in other members of the genus *Corynebacterium*. They are singular in that they cannot deamidate pyrazinamide (Sulea *et al.,* 1980). Furthermore, they share with all members of the genus the incapacity to ferment either lactose or xylose. Like all corynebacteria, they produce a catalase. All five varieties are capable of bringing about the hydrolysis of Tween 60 (polyoxyethylene sorbitan monopalmitate), which attests to their general lipolytic capacities. They all ferment glucose, mannose, and maltose. Singular properties by which each may be distinguished are as follows:

1. *Gravis* strains produce rough ("daisy head") colonies on tellurite agar and, in addition to the fermentation of the above three carbohydrates, ferment starch. They fail to hydrolyze gelatin or casein. They are urease negative. Their cells do not appear to contain multiple compartments when viewed under the light microscope.
2. *Intermedius* strains produce dwarf, smooth colonies on tellurite agar. They do not ferment starch nor do they hydrolyze either gelatin, urea, or casein. The individual cells appear under the light

microscope to contain multiple compartments. This property is very striking when the cells are viewed in the presence of dilute methylene blue by phase contrast microscopy.

3. *Mitis* strains form raised, smooth, glistening colonies on tellurite agar. They fail to ferment starch and show no proteolytic action on gelatin or casein. (Sucrose-fermenting stains have been reported.) They do not hydrolyze urea. Their cells (stained) do not exhibit multiple compartments when viewed with the light microscope.
4. *Ulcerans* strains form smooth, glistening colonies on tellurite agar. They are biochemically the most active members of the species. Most of them ferment starch and trehalose; they hydrolyze gelatin, urea, and sphingomyelin. They produce no caseinase. Their stained cells do not appear to contain multiple compartments when viewed under the light microscope. Cells in old cultures are small and ovoid to coccal in shape.
5. *Pseudotuberculosis* (*C. ovis*) strains form medium-sized (larger than *intermedius* and smaller than *mitis* colonies) on tellurite agar. Their fermentation and proteolytic pattern is similar to that of *mitis* strains except for the hydrolysis of urea and sphingomyelin. Sphingomyelinase (phospholipase D) activity was first reported for a few strains of *C. pseudotuberculosis* by Soucek *et al.* (1967) and of *C. ulcerans* by Souckova and Soucek (1972). These phospholipases D have been extensively studied by Linder and Bernheimer (1978), who with the author have demonstrated their presence in a large number of certified strains of *C. ulcerans* and *C. pseudotuberculosis.*

Any of the above five entities may, when carrying a *tox*$^+$ prophage (see Fig. 1), produce diphtherial toxin. Furthermore, properties such as colonial morphology may vary. For example, colonies of rough strains of *mitis* may be indistinguishable from *gravis* strains. Another commonly variable property is the capacity to ferment galactose.

Among each of the five varieties of *C. diphtheriae* are serologically distinct races and sublines showing characteristic sensitivities to batteries of corynebacteriophages, the phage types. Such subdivisions according to serological type or phage type are of considerable value for epidemiology. They are the only means we have for identifying specific lines of *C. diphtheriae* (McCloskey *et al.*, 1972). At present only phage typing is practiced and that only in Romania (Saragea and Maximescu, 1966) and to a lesser degree in Alberta, Canada (Toshach *et al.*, 1977). When epidemiologists use "biotype" unsupplemented with phage typing, they are simply naming a variety of *C. diphtheriae*, e.g., "biotype *gravis*," and that indicates very little (Marcuse and Grand, 1973; Brooks *et al.*, 1974).

3. Diphtherial Toxin

Diphtherial toxin is a protein of molecular weight around 62,000 (Kato *et al.*, 1960; Raynaud *et al.*, 1965), lethal for man (see Table 2) in amounts of about 130 ng/kg body weight (Barksdale *et al.*, 1960; Wilson, 1967). The control of sensitivity to toxin appears to be located in the long arm of human chromosome V (Creagan *et al.*, 1975; Lalley *et al.*, 1976; George and Francke, 1977). Since toxin is an antigen with a specific biological activity, the capacity to kill cells, and since antitoxin neutralizes that activity, it has long been possible to study toxin–antitoxin reactions without confusion from the other antigens and antibodies which were present (as discussed in the preceding section). This is especially true of titrations of either toxin or antitoxin in the skins of sensitive animals. For example, crystalline toxin, when assayed in the rabbit, contains about 5×10^4 minimum reactive doses (MRD) per μg of toxin protein. The neutralization of this toxicity by antitoxin provides a very sensitive method for assessing low levels of antitoxin.

3.1 Toxin, a Corynebacterial Adenosine Diphosphoribosyl Transferase

Diphtherial toxin consists of a single polypeptide chain containing two disulfide bridges. Following mild treatment with trypsin and exposure to dithiothreitol, it can be separated into two fragments, an N-terminal fragment A

(molecular weight 24,000) and a C-terminal fragment B (molecular weight 39,000) (see Fig. 3). While toxin itself exhibits no biological ac-

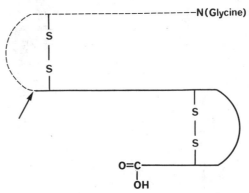

Figure 3. Diagrammatic representation of diphtherial toxin, a single polypeptide chain, molecular weight 62,000, cross-bonded by two disulfide bridges. At the bend, indicated by the arrow, is a trypsin-sensitive region containing three arginines. While the amino-terminal amino acid is known to be glycine, the carboxyl-terminal amino acid has not been determined. Nicking the peptide chain by trypsin action at the arrow point, followed by reduction of the disulfide bonds in the presence of dithiothreitol, liberates the dotted portion of the molecule, the A fragment. The solid line represents the B fragment. Fragment A is capable of removing the adenosine diphosphoribosyl moiety from nicotinamide adenine dinucleotide and covalently linking it to an acceptor molecule. It consists of 193 amino acids, position 1 being occupied by glycine and position 193 by an arginine (DeLange *et al.*, 1976). Its active site involves a tryptophan residue at position 153 (Michel and Dirkx, 1977). It is responsible for the following group transfer reactions: (1) $NAD^+ + EF-2 \rightleftharpoons ADP$-ribosyl $EF-2$ + nicotinamide + H^+, (2) $NAD^+ + HOH \rightleftharpoons ADP$-ribose + nicotinamide + H^+, and (3) NAD^+ + toxin $\rightleftharpoons ADP$-ribosyl-toxin + nicotinamide + H^+; EF-2 = elongation factor 2 (see text). Fragment B carries the specificity required for attaching the toxin molecule to sensitive mammalian cells (Pappenheimer and Gill, 1973; Collier, 1975; DeLange *et al.*, 1976). Burgoyne *et al.* (1976) have reported the successful isolation of the notoriously hydrophobic B fragment, the coupling of it to a vaccinia-virus-related protein, and the uptake by HeLa cells of the B-coupled vaccinia protein. Pietrowski and Stephen (1978) have succeeded in bringing about the sulfonation of fragment B (BSSO₃); the sulfonated fragment showed a capacity to bind to HeLa cells. Employing reduced fragment A (ASH) they were able—by mixing ASH with BSSO₃ (in 0.4 Tris-HCl, pH 6.5, containing 0.5 M SrCl₂ as a sulfite trap), deaerating and purging with oxygen-free nitrogen gas, incubating in the cold (4°C), and purifying on Sephadex in two stages—to reconstitute whole toxin from the fragments. Zanen *et al.* (1976) have reported the production of a nitrated toxin molecule following treatment of toxin with tetranitromethane. The nitrated toxin was of insignificant toxicity but retained its capacity to bind to cell receptors.

tivity other than its capacity to attach to and kill cells, fragment A behaves as a diphospho-pyridine nucleotidase (NADase) and an adenosine diphosphoribosyl transferase. Through the latter function, fragment A is capable of blocking protein synthesis *in vitro* by covalently linking the adenosine diphosphoribose moiety of nicotinamide adenine dinucleotide to eukaryotic elongation factor 2 (EF2). Because of the enzymatic activity of fragment A, toxin has been called a proenzyme. Fragment A has been said to be nontoxic for animal cells. Whether or not the secondary effects of the ADP-ribosylation of EF2 can account for all of the pathology that precedes diphtherial death in intoxicated guinea pigs has been questioned by Bonventre (1975).

3.2. Fixation of Toxin to Animal Cells

Since almost everything that is interesting about diphtherial toxin and the genes that code for its synthesis seems an accident of nature, one would expect that the means by which toxin enters cells would be fortuitous. Whatever the receptors for toxin on animal cells, their presence is undoubtedly for some purpose other than the binding of diphtherial toxin. The idea that some cells had receptors for toxin and others did not was early bolstered by the fact that rats and mice (and their cells in culture) are relatively resistant to toxin, whereas rabbits, guinea pigs, and humans and their cells in culture are 10,000 times as sensitive (see Collier, 1975; Pappenheimer, 1977). (For a consideration of resistant cell lines derived from sensitive ones, see Moehring and Moehring, 1976.)

Kim and Groman (1965) demonstrated that ammonium salts as well as glutamine and prolamine inhibited the toxicity of diphtherial toxin (DT-in) for HeLa cells. Subsequently, it was found that multivalent cations were required for binding of toxin (Duncan and Groman, 1969). In the case of the interaction of toxin with Vero cells such binding could be blocked by nucleotides, the triphosphates of which were more powerful in blocking than monophosphates (Middlebrook *et al.*, 1978). In binding studies employing [135]I-labeled DT-in and membrane-enriched fractions from rat,

rabbit, or guinea pig cells, Chang and Neville (1978) have shown that the binding of DT-in by each of the three membrane-enriched cell fractions is similar. Similar cofactors were required for binding to each, and similar nucleotides competitively inhibited that binding of DT-in. These authors have concluded that both rats and mice have binding sites for diphtherial toxin but that the lack of a transporting mechanism is responsible for their relative insensitivity to toxin. They have suggested, therefore, that sensitive cells such as those of man genetically would be *binding* + and *transport* + for diphtherial toxin, whereas rats would be *binding* + and *transport* − . They point out that, whereas Creagan *et al.* (1975) have suggested that human chromosome V might code for the toxin receptor (= sensitivity to toxin), in fact the information missing from the toxin-resistant mouse–human hybrid with a mouse chromosome V is the information expressed as the capacity to transport toxin.

Despite the fact that lack of receptors may not be the basis for the relative resistance of rat and mouse cells to DT-in, characterization of the receptor to which toxin fixes remains a worthwhile goal. Draper *et al.* (1978) have looked at DT-in as a lectin. They have found that the lectins, concanavalin A (Con A), wheat germ agglutinin (WGA), and succinyl Con A (Suc Con A), were potent in blocking the inhibition of protein synthesis in Chinese hamster V79 cells by DT-in. Con A and WGA appeared to compete for the site on the V79 cells to which toxin fixes. These investigators have interpreted this as a competition resulting from binding of Con A, for example, to carbohydrate terminals on cell surfaces to which DT-in also binds. In agreement with this line of reasoning, they found that the cell wall polysaccharide of *Salmonella cholera suis* and glycopeptide from ovalbumin were also effective inhibitors of DT-in. Their tentative conclusion was that the lectin-binding properties of DT-in might involve a specificity for *N*-acetylglucosamine and mannose. Subsequent information (Proia *et al.*, 1979) indicates that the toxin-sensitive hamster cell appears to carry a few toxin-binding glycoproteins (0.1 to 0.2%) among its surface glycoproteins (receptors?) of molecular weight ± 150,000.

3.3. Antigenic Structure of Toxin

Fragments A and B are immunologically distinct. Antisera prepared against fragment A are incapable of neutralizing the toxicity of diphtherial toxin. All evidence suggests that the effectiveness of toxin-neutralizing antibodies can be attributed to their capacity to combine with the carboxyl end (B portion) of diphtherial toxin (see Fig. 3). High-avidity antitoxin apparently contains antibody directed principally against the B portion. Most crude toxin preparations contain some A fragments. In fact, it was through the ADP-ribosylating and NADase activities of so-called purified preparations of toxin that the A fragment was originally discovered. Thus preparations of antitoxin and even immune human sera contain some antibody directed against A fragments (Ittelson and Gill, 1973; Pappenheimer *et al.,* 1972; Uchida *et al.,* 1972, 1973a,b).

Diphtherial toxin is an excellent protein antigen having, besides antigenicity, an additional biological activity, the killing of mammalian cells. The latter is easily assessed in the skins of animals and in cell cultures. In the early years of the development of a means of immunizing against diphtherial toxin, two kinds of immunogens were used: (1) small repeated doses of toxin and (2) toxin–antitoxin mixtures devoid of detectable free toxin (i.e., uncombined with antitoxin). Each of these methods involved problems not inherent in the use of toxoid. Following a suggestion made by Glenny and Hopkins (1923), Ramon (1923, 1928) tried the capacity of formaldehyde to render toxin into immunogenic, nontoxic toxoid. The result was the discovery of a means of preparing an antigen which offered satisfactory protection against diphtheritic intoxication.

3.4. Toxoid as Formalinized Toxin

Toxin treated with formalin under slightly alkaline conditions becomes innocuous toxoid. If the neutralizing effect of antitoxin synthesized in response to toxoid stems from its capacity to combine with the B portion of diphtherial toxin, the effectively immunogenic toxoid must contain the required antigenic configuration at its B end. Yet toxoid lacks the capacity to fix to the receptors on animal cells or to compete with toxin in such fixation. Most probably, the formalinization of toxin, through the tying up of the ϵ-amino groups of lysine and the methylene bridging of lysines to tyrosines or histidines, renders the toxin molecule insusceptible to the processes which normally convert it into separate fragments. The structure of this formalinized molecule not only precludes "proenzyme-to-enzyme conversion" but also destroys the fitness to bind to the mammalian cell. Yet antibody synthesized in response to toxoid satisfactorily neutralizes toxicity (Pappenheimer and Gill, 1973; Collier, 1975).

A necessary adjunct for the successful implementation of a toxoid production program was a strain of *C. diphtheriae* which produced large amounts of toxin. Most strains of diphtheria bacilli produce only small amounts of this protein. The problem this fact posed for immunization programs was solved by William Hallock Park, a clinician and microbiologist. He was directly responsible for the development of the first program of immunization against diphtheria in the United States. In 1896 he and Williams had isolated a peculiar diphtheria bacillus, the Park-Williams No. 8 strain, which was a hyperproducer of diphtherial toxin (>300 μg/ml/10^9 bacilli = 10,000 molecules/cell) and was relatively noninvasive. This came to be the strain of *C. diphtheriae* used for the production of diphtherial toxin in those parts of the world where immunization with toxoid was practiced.

Once a method of producing large batches of toxin and toxoid became available, attention was turned to the matter of standardizing toxin and antitoxin. Since toxin is a soluble antigen, toxin and antitoxin interaction could be examined over a wide range of concentrations. These precipitin reactions were termed "flocculation reactions"; 1 flocculating unit of toxin was and is that amount of toxin which combines with one unit of antitoxin. That amount is the Lf unit (flocculating unit) of toxin $\approx$ ± 55 guinea pig MLDs $\approx$ ± 1.55 μg toxin protein nitrogen.

3.5. Toxoid, a Complex of Antigens

Diphtherial toxoid is often regarded as a highly specific antigen, and there is a tendency to interpret a positive response to skin testing with toxoid as directly related to previously injected toxoid (e.g., see Franz *et al.*, 1976). The fact that toxoid is a complex of antigens was established about 20 years ago. It had been known for over half a century that when patients were immunized with diphtherial toxoid (see Section 3.6) some of them responded by developing a variety of antibodies (humoral immunity) and some of them, in addition, developed delayed hypersensitivity (cell-mediated immunity, CMI) (Andrewes *et al.*, 1923; Neill and Fleming, 1929). This happened even when "purified" toxoid was employed as an immunizing agent (Lawrence and Pappenheimer, 1948; Pappenheimer and Lawrence, 1948a,b). The range of skin test reactions elicited by purified toxoid is diagrammed in Fig. 4. Finger and Kabat (1958) and Kuhns and Dukstein (1957) have shown that such purified toxoid contains other corynebacterial antigens, and Arden (1970) has shown that some of these unidentified antigens occur in both nontoxinogenic and toxinogenic *C. diphtheriae, C. pseudotuberculosis ovis, C. diphtheriae* variety *ulcerans, C. diphtheriae gravis, C. diphtheriae intermedius,* and to a lesser degree *C. xerosis.* It was Pope who first showed that crystalline toxin was a mixture of antigens (Pope and Stevens, 1958; Pope *et al.*, 1966), and Raynaud (1965) confirmed this by demonstrating the heterogeneity of antibodies formed in response to purified diphtherial toxoid.

From the foregoing it should be clear that a positive skin test response to diphtherial toxoid may involve the elicitation of cells and/or antibodies previously primed either by toxoid or by agents which share antigens with toxoid (and which have previously had a priming relationship with the subject whose skin is being tested with toxoid). See also Section 3.6.

3.6. The Schick Test

The intracutaneous test introduced by Bela Schick in 1913 for the detection of circulating antitoxin, now known as the Schick test, has been of immeasurable value in detecting individuals with circulating antibody against diphtherial toxin. It is one of the few skin tests which detects, on the one hand, the actual biological activity of an antigen—the capacity to kill cells of the skin (the Schick-positive state)—and, on the other, the capacity of circulating antibody to neutralize that activity (the Schick-negative state). Furthermore, it discriminates between those individuals whose antitoxic antibody includes high levels of IgE from those in whom the neutralization of antitoxin involves principally IgG and other isotypes. In addition, the Schick test can reveal the existence of states of delayed hypersensitivity to a number of corynebacterial products. For over 30 years at New York University School of Medicine, Dr. Sherwood Lawrence has been administering the Schick test to medical students at the time they are concerned in the microbiology laboratory with diphtheria and diphtheria bacilli. In any class of 40 students the various reactions to the Schick test which are diagrammed in Fig. 4 develop. Thus in each class there is available for discussion the immunological basis for those reactions which are "cell mediated" and those which involve principally antigen–antibody reactions, including the very circumscribed anaphylactic reactions which develop in the skins of atopic individuals. The understanding the student derives from this exercise equips him to comprehend the differences and similarities between the Schick test and the tuberculin test.

In a number of states, materials for the Schick test are not available. Massachusetts is one of those states which does make available to its physicians the required materials. In most countries in which diphtheria occurs, Schick tests are carried out when needed (Häuser, 1972; Marcuse and Grand, 1973). Aside from the practical application of the test, an understanding of it is germaine to the most elementary grasping of the immunobiology of diphtheria.

3.7. The (Immunologic) Nonresponder to Diphtherial Toxin

In a survey of immune responses to diphtherial toxoid by young adults, Edsall in 1954 found that about 2% failed to develop circulating antitoxin (Edsall *et al.*, 1954). Bazaral and co-workers confirmed this finding (Bazaral *et al.*, 1973). In their study, approximately 2%

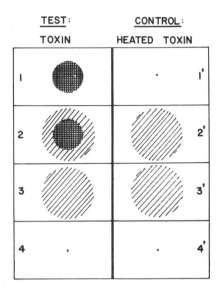

TEST: CONTROL:

TOXIN   HEATED TOXIN

Figure 4. Diagrammatic representation of four reactions to the Schick test. Approximately 0.0006 μg of toxin protein N (one-fiftieth the minimal amount, MLD, required to kill a guinea pig weighing 250 g) is injected into the forearm, the test site; 0.0124 μg formalinized toxoid is injected at a control site. Readings are made at 48 and at 96 hr. Necrosis at the test site, shown as a cross-hatched circle in box 1, indicates insufficient circulating antitoxin to neutralize the test dose of toxin. The dot at site 1′ represents the scar from the initial injection needle. This reaction (site 1 and 1′) is referred to as a Schick-positive reaction. The reactions shown at sites 4 and 4′ indicate that there is enough circulating antitoxin to neutralize the injected toxin. These define the Schick-negative state. The parallel lines shown in sites 3 and 3′ indicate a delayed hypersensitive reaction accompanying a Schick-negative response; i.e., there is enough circulating antitoxin to neutralize the test dose of toxin but there is delayed allergy to some corynebacterial products. This has been called "the pseudoreaction." At sites 2 and 2′ there is necrosis due to the injected toxin accompanied by delayed allergy: a "combined reaction" indicating a state of delayed hypersensitivity to corynebacterial products unaccompanied by circulating antitoxin sufficient to neutralize the killing action of diphtherial toxin. About 2–5% of immunized populations give an immediate hypersensitivity reaction at both sites from 20 to 45 min after receiving the injections. This reaction, induced by circulating IgE specific for the injected material, is almost always followed at 48–96 hr by the reaction shown at 4 and 4′ but sometimes the immunity is accompanied by delayed hypersensitivity reactions as shown at sites 3 and 3′. For information on antigens other than toxin in purified preparations of toxin, see text. For a discussion of this modified Schick test, see Pappenheimer (1958) and Brochure 3–5, The Commonwealth of Massachusetts, Department of Public Health, Massachusetts Public Health Biologic Laboratories, Boston, Massachusetts 02130. For information concerning the United States Standard Reagents for the Schick test, see Barile *et al.* (1971).

of adult males failed to make an antidiphtherial toxin response following two booster doses of 1.5 Lf (approximately 4.5 μg protein nitrogen) of adsorbed diphtheria tetanus toxoid, although these nonresponders made precipitating antibody to tetanus toxoid and had normal levels of immunoglobulins. Recently evidence has been obtained that suggests that the immune response to diphtherial toxin in humans is partially controlled by a dominant gene that is not closely linked to HLA (major histocompatibility antigens) (McMichael *et al.*, 1977). It should be noted here that low responders to tetanus toxoid have been shown to have a significant association with the locus coding for HLA-B5 in man (Sasazuki *et al.*, 1978). These are two of a growing number of reports in the literature of failure in immunological responsiveness that apparently involves "single" antigens (Vaz *et al.*, 1970; Convit *et al.*, 1972; DeVries *et al.*, 1976). The hypertoxic case of diphtheria (the bullneck syndrome) may turn out to be the reaction of the nonresponder to infection with toxinogenic *gravis* and *intermedius,* or even *mitis,* types of diphtheria bacilli.

4. Colonization by *C. diphtheriae*

4.1. Colonization in the Presence of Circulating "Antitoxin"

Those healthy individuals whose throat flora include one or more strains of *C. diphtheriae* are termed "carriers." In the San Antonio outbreak the carrier rate of 16.6% for the fully immunized (with diphtherial toxoid) was not significantly different from that of 10.5% for the nonimmunized (Marcuse and Grand, 1973). It is well established that average antitoxin levels among carriers and among noncarriers from immunized (with toxoid) populations are the same (Kostyukovskaya, 1966). Thus, levels of circulating antitoxin seem to have no bearing on the establishment of the carrier state or, in other words, on the colonization or failure of colonization of the throat by *C. diphtheriae.* In fact, carriage of toxinogenic or nontoxinogenic *C. diphtheriae* may occur in the presence of high levels of circulating antitoxin. While the work of Huang (1942a) does suggest the specific antibacterial immunity can negatively influence the growth of diphtheritic membranes, there is no evidence that carriers lack antibacterial immunity.

4.2. Colonization in the Presence of Nasopharyngeal Pathology

Kostyukovskaya (1966) studied the capacity of leukocytes from normal (immunized with toxoid) and carrier (immunized with toxoid) persons to interact with *C. diphtheriae*. The phagocytic indexes of adult carriers and adult normals were essentially equal. For children (2–12 years), the phagocytic index was 0.79 for carriers (145 individuals) and 0.42 for normals (55 individuals). Among 108 children subdivided into those exhibiting acute disturbance in the nasopharynx (33), those showing chronic nasopharyngeal pathology (62), and those showing no disturbance in the nasopharynx (13), the respective phagocytic indexes were 1.3, 0.57, and 0.44. It is clear that the degree of phagocytic activity found correlated with acute aggravation in the nasopharynx. When quantitative measurements were made of circulating antitoxin in carriers, the highest number of children with circulating levels above 0.03 antitoxin unit (au)/ml were among those showing nasopharyngeal pathology. When the antitoxin levels in 60 of these were checked at zero observation time and at 3–6 months, increases in levels of circulating antitoxin were found. Thus, at zero time, 21 had less than 0.05 au/ml, 5 had 0.05–0.1 au/ml, 16 had 0.1–0.4 au/ml, and 18 had 0.4–0.8 au/ml, whereas at 3–6 months 2 had 0.05–0.1 au/ml, 15 had 0.1–0.4 au/ml, and 43 had 0.4–0.8 au/ml. It is clear, then, that among children carriers (1) there are appreciable numbers of persons prone to nasopharyngeal pathology and (2) in such individuals manifesting such pathology there is an enhanced immune response as evidenced by (a) elevated phagocytosis of *C. diphtheriae* and (b) increasing levels of circulating antitoxin.

It is common practice to render carriers "free" of corynebacteria by giving them a course of antibiotics. However, when these individuals are subjected to serious bacteriological examination over a protracted period of time, a number of them are found to be no longer free of their corynebacteria (Barksdale

et al., 1960; Gray and James, 1973). Much remains to be learned about the factors involved in the carriage of *C. diphtheriae.* Elsewhere herein, mention is made of the suitability of tonsillar crypts to colonization by diphtheria bacilli. Platts-Mills and Ishizaka (1975), employing a lymphocyte culture system derived from tonsils of immunized individuals, have shown that synthesis of IgG, IgA, and sometimes IgM is stimulated in some of the lymphocyte cultures following the addition of toxoid. The amounts of antibody made were impressive. The IgA lacked a secretory piece but was heavier than 7 S, suggesting that a number of dimers were formed. Diphtheria bacilli growing in crypts would be expected to release stimulating antigens continually, thus providing a continuous local antibody response. This release should facilitate local phagocytosis as well as provide local antitoxin when toxinogenic strains are present.

4.3. Colonization in the Presence of Streptococci, Staphylococci, and Other Organisms

In the throats and/or skin lesions in which diphtheria develops may be found impressive numbers of Group A hemolytic streptococci (*Streptococcus pyogenes*) (Loeffler, 1884), Group B streptococci, *Staphylococcus aureus* (Cockcroft *et al.,* 1973), or the misnamed streptococcus, *C. pyogenes* (Liebow *et al.,* 1946; Barksdale *et al.,* 1957). Further, diphtheria bacilli may be found in lesions that develop following insect bites (Liebow *et al.,* 1946) and in a number of skin conditions seen in clinics of dermatology (Thaung *et al.,* 1978). In these situations, the clinical decision as to whether the *C. diphtheriae* present is or is not associated with diphtheritic pathology is sometimes difficult to make.

In large outbreaks of diphtheria, so-called hypertoxic cases are often seen. In such cases, following a swelling in and tenderness of the cervical glands there develops a massive edema of the tissues of the neck ("bullneck") and chest. It had occurred to Updyke and Frobisher (1947) that some additional factor might be operating in infections which led to such hypertoxemia. Updyke and Frobisher investigated in experimental animals the possibility that hypertoxic diphtheria (malignant diphtheria) might result from the synergistic action between *C. diphtheriae* and *Streptococcus pyogenes*. Their findings were negative. As stated in the preceeding section, perhaps the basis for diphtherial hypertoxemia is to be found in a genetic peculiarity of the patient.

5. Antibacterial Immunity in Diphtheria

In this section the antibacterial immune response in diphtheria will be considered to be those immune reactions of the host to corynebacterial products other than diphtherial toxin. Complement-dependent opsonins were early demonstrated in certain antitoxic sera from human subjects, and their titers were found to be independent of those of antitoxin (Andrewes *et al.*, 1923, pp. 168–169). Filosofova has recently shown that in experimental infections with *C. diphtheriae* the level of leukocytosis was related to the duration of the infectious process. The highest levels were attained in animals infected with nontoxinogenic strains (see Fig. 1). The phagocytic capacity was also most highly developed in animals infected with nontoxinogenic strains and was more or less directly related to the size of the infecting dose (Filosofova *et al.*, 1977).

Corynebacterial cells are characterized by superficial, heat-labile, type-specific protein antigens, the K antigens (Huang, 1942a; Cummins, 1954; Lautrop, 1950), by a number of common antigens, including rabinogalactanmycolate and muramyl peptides (the O antigens of Lautrop, 1950), and by such enzymes as nitrate-reductase, glucan-phosphorylase, and neuraminidase (Arden and Barksdale, 1974, 1976; Arden *et al.*, 1972). Except for the type-specific protein antigens which make possible the serotyping of corynebacteria, immune responses to selected corynebacterial antigens other than toxin and toxoid have not been investigated. However, a role of antibacterial immunity in recovery from diphtherial infections has been adduced from immunizations employing toxoids prepared from different types of *C. diphtheriae*, as discussed below.

5.1. Serotypes and Infection with *C. diphtheriae*

Agglutinins for *C. diphtheriae* have been on record since 1896 (Andrewes *et al.*, 1923), and Durand and Guérin (1921) were among the first to demonstrate the value of serological typing in the epidemiology of diphtheria. Serological typing of corynebacteria* has never been practiced to an extent comparable to the typing of *Streptococcus pneumoniae*, *Streptococcus pyogenes*, or the salmonellae and shigellae. Nor have the antigenic determinants responsible for serological specificities of corynebacteria been chemically defined. Whereas, for example, in the case of *Salmonella typhimurium* (and numerous other salmonellae), specific sugars (dideoxyhexoses) which determine O-antigen serotypes are known, and their contributions to the virulence of particular salmonellae have been well documented (Mäkelä, *et al.*, 1973), no such level of sophistication has been attained in the analysis of corynebacterial antigens. Nevertheless, the epidemiological significance of corynebacterial serotypes has been well established. While a number of the surface K antigens of corynebacteria are distinct, there are cross-reactions between others. The PW8 strain (Park and Williams, 1896; Lampidis and Barksdale, 1971), now universally used for the production of diphtherial toxoid, belongs to serotype K(D5). Huang (1942b) found that patients infected with organisms belonging to type K(D5) and treated with antitoxin derived from animals immunized with toxoid synthesized (as toxin) by the PW8 strain [also of serotype K(D5)] showed a more rapid clearance of K(D5) organisms from the throat than did patients infected with heterologous strains.

This beneficial effect of antibacterial im-

---

* Although working systems for serological typing of *C. diphtheriae* have been described by several investigators (e.g., Ewing, 1933, described five serotypes of 106 starch-fermenting isolates of *C. diphtheriae gravis* from different localities), no system for international use has yet been established. Instead, phage typing has seemed the more economical means for sorting *C. diphtheriae*, and Saragea and Maximescu (1964) have assembled a group of 24 corynebacteriophages with which they have been able to distinguish 19 phage types of *C. diphtheriae*. They have found it possible to type 75% of 12,000 strains of *C. diphtheriae* from various parts of the world (Saragea and Maximescu, 1966).

munity on the course of diphtherial infections was examined experimentally and clinically by Maitland *et al.* (1952) in diphtheria of the *gravis* category. These investigators observed that, in 40% of guinea pigs inoculated subcutaneously with a specific strain of *C. diphtheriae gravis,* the inoculated bacillus could be isolated from the heart blood of the infected animals. There were no positive blood cultures from animals receiving homologous anti-*gravis* serum along with the injections. These and other animal experiments led to trials of a particular anti-*gravis* serum as an adjunct to antitoxin treatment in severe cases of diphtheria. The effect of such antiserum was to upgrade the clinical course of the disease. In other words, those patients receiving antiserum "did much better" than those receiving antitoxin alone.

5.2. Humoral and Delayed Hypersensitivity Responses to Corynebacterial Products Injected into the Guinea Pig

The employment of diphtherial toxoid (DT) for basic studies in immunology using the guinea pig and rabbit has a long history. Newer information stems from the work of Uhr *et al.* (1957), Uhr and Baumann (1961a,b), and, more recently, Kostiala and Kosunen (1972a,b). Most of these studies have employed DT or DT-antitoxin precipitates, each in complete Freund's adjuvant (CFA). The antibody response has been measured as (1) skin test read at 4 hr (Arthus reaction), (2) passive hemagglutination of erythrocytes coated with antigen, (3) hemolytic antibody (hemolysins), and (4) cytophilic antibody. Mercaptoethanol treatment has been employed to qualitatively distinguish a predominantly IgM response from a predominantly IgG response. The cell-mediated response (CMI) has been measured as (1) a 24-hr delayed hypersensitivity reaction in the skin and (2) the inhibition of the migration of macrophages. In earlier experiments (Uhr and Baumann, 1961a,b) antibody was measured by its capacity to neutralize diphtherial toxin in the skin of rabbits or guinea pigs.

Following the injection of 1–2 μg DT-antitoxin mixtures into guinea pigs, delayed hypersensitivity to DT develops 2–3 weeks before there is a measurable antibody response. While CFA enhances such a response, it is,

of course, not required for the development of specific DH (Uhr *et al.,* 1957). DH in response to DT or DT-antitoxin correlates directly with inhibition of migration of macrophages by DT in immunized animals and does not correlate with the development of anti-DT passive hemagglutinins, hemolysins, or cytophilic antibody on peritoneal exudate cells (PE). DT-antitoxin precipitates have been employed not only for priming for DH but also for its elicitation.

Antibodies developing 3 weeks after the administration of DT have been mostly sensitive to mercaptoethanol (and therefore are, presumably, IgM) but antibodies developing later were shown to be resistant (and therefore, presumably, mostly IgG) (Kostiala and Kosunen, 1972a,b). The value of minute amounts of DT-antitoxin precipitates in priming for an IgG response was demonstrated by Uhr and Baumann (1961b). Kostiala and Kosunen (1972b) administered to guinea pigs, already immunized with DT in CFA, three separate boosting doses of DT in saline. It was apparent that boosting increased anti-DT passive hemagglutinins, hemolysins, and cytophilic antibody on the surface of peritoneal exudate cells (PE), but skin reactions to DT became negative and migration of PE was no longer inhibited by DT. The animals employed for boosting showed DH to PPD and to DT prior to the start of the experiment. Those animals which lost their DH to DT retained their DH to PPD. When normal peritoneal macrophages were incubated in the sera of boosted DT-negative animals, their migration was not inhibited by antigen, although they had (cytophilic) antibody on their surfaces as indicated by rosette formation. When sera from the boosted animals were used as final media in chambers where PE cells of actively immunized guinea pigs were migrating, antigen inhibited those PE cells. This seemed to the authors to rule out the presence of a blocking factor in the sera of the boosted animals. Rather, the findings seemed to indicate that, in suppressed delayed hypersensitivity, mediator cells either do not react with antigen or were not present in peritoneal exudate. Whether suppressor T cells (e.g., see Asherson and Zembala, 1975) or suppressor adherent cells (macrophages? see Klimpel and Henney, 1978) are responsible for this particular suppression remains to be seen.

It is clear from the experiments discussed above, from the experiments of Platts-Mills and Ishizaka (1975) employing plasma cells from tonsillar tissue (see later), from the caption of Fig. 4, and from the discussions of antibacterial immunity and of diphtherial carriers that the immune response to corynebacterial infections includes the production of at least the immunoglobulin isotypes IgA, IgM, IgG, and IgE, migration inhibition factor, and its corollary, delayed hypersensitivity. In cellular terms, this translates as involving the triad of the immune response: B cells from the plasma cell arm of the immune system, T cells, and macrophages. The suppression of DH in those guinea pigs immunized with DT in CFA and boosted with DT in saline probably involved a subset of T cells or macrophages. These responses, together with the various immunopathologies mentioned in the section on active immunization, indicate the usefulness of corynebacterial antigens for studies in immunobiology.

5.3. Adjuvant Action of *C. diphtheriae*

A number of bacterial cells and/or their products stimulate mammalian immune systems to increased responses, either to an increased yield of antibody and/or to an earlier and more intense delayed hypersensitivity reaction. Bacteria and other agents so affecting cells of the immune system have been termed "adjuvants." Mycobacterial cells contained in water-in-oil emulsions (mannide monooleate, 1.5 parts; paraffin oil, 8.5 parts), known as complete Freund's adjuvant (CFA), have been classed as primarily T-cell-oriented adjuvants, whereas *Propionibacterium parvum**

---

* The organisms called *Corynebacterium parvum*, widely used for stimulating the reticuloendothelial systems of experimental animals, are, for the most part, *Propionibacterium acnes*, type I. Interest in *P. acnes* has been widespread, following the discovery that intraperitoneal and intravenous administration of it (as vaccines in experimental animals) has led to such effects as increased clearance of foreign material (e.g., carbon particles) from the circulation, increased resistance to various protozoan and microbial infections *in vivo*, enhanced antibody production, increased sensitivity to endotoxin and histamine, and protection against graft vs. host diseases (Wolstenholme and Knight, 1973). Further, a number of reports concerning the antitumor activity of vaccines of *P. acnes* suggest that in those vaccines lies a potential for anticancer therapy (Woodruff and Boak,

has been classed as a B-cell adjuvant and the lipopolysaccharide of *Escherichia coli* has been reported to stimulate both B- and T-cell activity (Allison, 1973).

Diphtheria bacilli belong to the CMN (*Corynebacterium, Mycobacterium,* and *Nocardia*; Barksdale, 1970) group, and it is characteristic of those mycolic-acid-containing microbes that they can effect an adjuvant action on the immune response of animals infected with or given injections of them. Members of the CMN group share a common rigid muramyl layer of the cell wall and the lipopolysaccharide, arabinogalactan mycolate, but differ as to the means by which this and mannose-containing polysaccharides are conjugated to the muramyl peptides, the types of mycolic acids present, etc. (see Fig. 5). Only recently have the dimycolates of trehalose (cord factor = α,α'-trehalose dimycolate) produced by *C. diphtheriae* received the investigative attention shown the dimycolates of *Mycobacterium tuberculosis* (Bloch, 1950; Noll *et al.*, 1956; Goren, 1972; Barksdale and Kim, 1977). They were known by their structure and certain of their activities (Kato, 1970) to be very similar to mycobacterial cord factor (Yarkoni *et al.*, 1973). When mycobacterial cord factors are conjugated with such carriers as serum albumin, they serve as a hapten, and antibody capable of neutralizing their toxicity can be formed toward them (Kato, 1972).

1966; Israeli and Halpern, 1972; Milas and Mujagic, 1972; Baum and Breese, 1976; McBride *et al.*, 1976). Cummins and Linn (1977) have systematically investigated the reticulostimulating ability of vaccines (prepared from 155 strains of *P. acnes*, types I and II, *P. avidum*, types I and II, *P. granulosum*, and other related and unrelated bacteria) as judged by the degree of spleen hypertrophy which followed their intraperitoneal injection into mice. Vaccines from most of the strains tested caused a statistically significant increase in spleen weight, but the ability to produce spleen ratios (test mean weight/control mean weight) of 4 or more was confined to *P. acnes* and *P. avidum* strains. *P. acnes,* type II, gave high spleen ratios more frequently than strains of any other type. Recently, Ferguson and Cummins (1978) determined the nutritional requirements of several of these propionibacteria, thus making it possible to grow the organisms in media free of complex substances. These studies by Cummins and associates (1) provide technical data essential to immunologists working with *P. acnes* and (2) open the way for the isolation and purification of those molecular species responsible for the capacity of propionibacteria to stimulate the reticuloendothelial system.

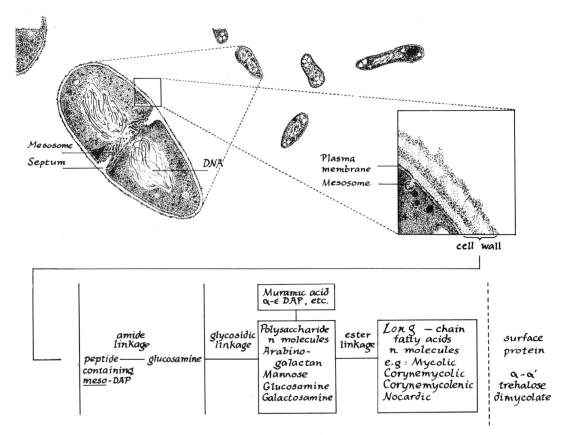

Figure 5. Diagram of a bacterial cell from the *Corynebacterium–Mycobacterium–Nocardia* (CMN) group. Specific antigen(s) distinctive for different serotypes is indicated as surface protein(s). Common antigens within the CMN group, capable of giving a rise to serological cross-reactions, include arabinogalactans and arabinomannans. The adjuvant action exhibited by CMN organisms can be accounted for by the fatty acids covalently bound to various macromolecules of the cell wall. From Barksdale (1970). Reprinted with permission of the publishers.

Whereas the mycobacterial dimycolates contain mycolic acids of chain lengths ranging from C_{80} to C_{90}, those of *Corynebacterium* range from C_{28} to C_{36}. Parant *et al.* (1978) have found that either natural or synthetic trehalose dicorynomycolates were as effective in protecting mice against infection with either *Klebsiella pneumoniae* or *Listeria monocytogenes* as were the longer-chain mycobacterial dimycolates. Since *C. diphtheriae* produces the "ultimate mycobacterial adjuvant" (Barksdale and Kim, 1977), *N*-acetylmuramyl-L-alanyl-D-isoglutamine (Audibert *et al.*, 1976; Kotani *et al.*, 1975), and since the adjuvanticity of its cord factors is equivalent to those of *M. tuberculosis* and other mycobacteria, it, like other members of the CMN group, has the capacity to enhance the antibody response and the delayed hypersensitivity response to any antigen X with which it is combined in an immunization procedure.

6. Infection in Experimental Animals as Related to Infection in Man

6.1. Experimental Infections of Guinea Pigs and Rabbits

In 1959 Murata, Hirose, and associates, on the assumption that the use of syringes and needles for experimentally infecting animals is most unnatural, decided to study diphtheritic infections of the guinea pig by inoculating onto the conjuctiva (Murata *et al.*, 1959; see also Bormann and Scheurer, 1933, and Kaga

1951). They reviewed and confirmed the finding of Kaga (1951) that diphtheria bacilli placed on healthy conjuctiva failed to cause disease; and injured conjuctiva was a prerequisite for the development of a diphtheritic lesion. Injury was produced with a hot bacteriological loop. Care was taken not to injure the cornea. Severity of infection varied with the strain used and was not related to the amounts of toxin each strain produced *in vitro*. Thus the PW8 strain, which yields highest levels of toxin *in vitro*, caused a very mild infection. Once the experimental lesion cleared up, *C. diphtheriae* could still be recovered from the area of the conjuctiva. Hirose, Murata, and others (Hirose *et al.*, 1962) extended these experiments in an effort to assess the role in the prevention of conjuctival diphtheria of (1) passively administered antitoxic antibodies, (2) passively administered antibacterial antibodies, (3) vaccination with toxoid, and (4) vaccination with formalinized bacteria. Their experiments clearly showed that animals receiving intraperitoneal injections of antibacterial serum (rabbit) and challenged 24 hr later with doses of *C. diphtheriae* in the injured (seared) conjuctiva failed to resist diphtheritic infection. On the other hand, animals actively immunized with formalin-killed *C. diphtheriae* (6 weekly injections totaling 180 mg) were well protected against conjunctival infection (while two injections totaling 200 mg were also satisfactory, one injection totaling 100 mg was not). Levels of antibacterial agglutinins found in the sera did not vary in relation to the protection found. Sera from the immunized animals were assayed for antitoxin and less than 0.001 unit was present per ml (the lower limit of detection). To further test the absence of circulating antitoxin, a group of guinea pigs was subjected to four weekly injections of formalin-killed bacteria (100 mg/injection). Schick testing of these animals and nonimmunized control guinea pigs failed to indicate the presence of circulating antitoxin. Thus, vaccines prepared from formalin-killed toxinogenic diphtheria bacilli protected guinea pigs against challenge with living *C. diphtheriae* administered to the seared conjuctiva. The protection does not involve circulating antitoxin, seems unrelated to levels of circulating antibacterial antibodies, and cannot be effected with passively administered antibacterial sera. Protec-

tion, then, appears to involve cell-mediated immunity (CMI). Some years earlier Frobisher (Frobisher and Updyke, 1947; Frobisher and Parsons, 1950) had demonstrated the protection of significant numbers of rabbits immunized with *nontoxinogenic C. diphtheriae* against challenge with toxinogenic strains. It now seems that Frobisher was correct in his speculation that this protection appeared to be like the "Koch phenomenon" (certainly the first-observed and probably the most well-known example of cell-mediated immunity). This reaction may be summarized as follows:

$$C.\ diphtheriae\ \xrightarrow{\text{CMI}}\ \begin{array}{l}\text{Protection concomitant}\\\text{with evolution}\\\text{of the carrier state}\end{array}$$

In this equation the role of antitoxin is infinitesimally small or nonexistent. In the preceding section we have spelled out at the molecular level the capacity of *C. diphtheriae* to induce "nonspecific antibacterial immunity" vs., e.g., *Klebsiella pneumoniae* or *Listeria monocytogenes*.

Before we relate these findings to certain unsolved problems concerning diphtheria in man, two other experiments of Hirose, Murata, and associates must be discussed. The first concerns toxoid. Guinea pigs were immunized with varying amounts of toxoid for four weeks, sample bleedings were taken for measurement of antitoxin, and the animals were challenged on the injured conjunctiva. Resistance in these animals appeared to be more or less directly related to the titer of circulating antitoxin. Groups of guinea pigs received varying amounts of intracardial doses of antitoxin "A" or antitoxin "B." Some were challenged with organisms used to produce the antitoxin ("A" or "B"), others with the heterologous organism. Those animals receiving more than 0.3 au/100 g body weight were fully protected. One tenth of that amount did not protect. It seemed in each case that homologous antitoxin was more effective than heterologous antitoxin. Ten days after injection, the eye secretions of the completely protected animals yielded viable *C. diphtheriae*. Ten days after the infection, then, symptomless animals carried *C. diphtheriae*. While the authors interpreted the results of the two types of experiments, immunization with toxoid and with passively administered antitoxin, to indicate that antitoxin protects against diphtheritic infection, other interpretations seem worthy of consideration. We have discussed at length the impurity of purified toxoid. Immunization with the toxoid leads to the production of primarily antitoxic antibodies but also some antibacterial antibodies, as well as to a degree of cell-mediated immunity (delayed hypersensitivity). Thus in the toxoid-immunized animal the challenging organism is confronted with antitoxin to neutralize any toxin it may have produced (thereby creating antigen–antibody complexes, themselves inducers of delayed hypersensitivity) as well as the other cell-mediated factors which serve to convert infection to carriage. In those challenged animals which were protected by passively administered antitoxin, the development of the carrier state may also have been augmented by toxin–antitoxin complexes.

6.2. Immunity to *C. diphtheriae*, Immunity to Diphtherial Toxin, and Carriage of *C. diphtheriae* in Humans

The results of the animal experiments of Murata, Hirose, and associates and those of Frobisher indicate that cell-mediated immunity is critical in the establishment of diphtherial immunity. Further, antitoxic immunity is of no more consequence in diphtherial immunity than is antiscarlatinal immunity in immunity to Group A streptococcal infections (despite the fact that antitoxin can protect one from death due to diphtherial toxin). The equating of immunity to toxin with immunity to diphtheria has generated confusion, and significant epidemiological findings have been overlooked. For example, Craig (1962), in a study of immunity (as determined by the Schick Test) in a Brooklyn community, found convincing, if circumstantial, evidence that infection with *C. diphtheriae* was endemic and that overt cases of disease were extremely rare. Further, since 20–25% of the children under 15 were Schick-positive (in half of whom tests for circulating antitoxin yielded negative results), the absence of detected disease could not be attributed to an absence of people susceptible to toxin. Although Craig's data led to the conclusion that there existed in the Brooklyn community a very high infection/case ratio, he had

no bacteriological data to support his conclusion. He postulated that the immunity he was seeing might be in some way related to the somatic antigens of *C. diphtheriae*. In order to examine this suggestion that there is more *C. diphtheriae* around than there appears to be, one needs an endemic area in which suitable bacteriology is practiced. For the past decade and half in the American Pacific Northwest there have been reports of groups of humans among whom *C. diphtheriae* is common. In certain communities in Alberta where a variety of phage types of *C. diphtheriae* had been isolated, the types remained fairly constant over the years 1968–1976. A total of 127 strains from residents of homes for the mentally retarded included two different phage types of *C. diphtheriae mitis* (nontoxinogenic), two phage types of *intermedius* (nontoxinogenic), and one phage type of *gravis* (toxinogenic). The diphtheria bacilli were isolated from swabs from throats, cutaneous lesions, and ears. No clinical cases of diphtheria were observed in this community for an 8-year period. In another community in which one phage type of *C. diphtheriae* (a nontoxinogenic *mitis* strain) prevailed for eight years with no clinical infections reported, there occurred in 1976 two mild cases involving a *gravis* strain, phage type 10, 11, 22. Subsequently, that strain became endemic in the community (Toshach *et al.*, 1977; see also Pedersen *et al.*, 1977). Toshach has compared 1871 strains of *C. diphtheriae* isolated from noses and throats and 1010 from cutaneous sites (50% from ears) and found no difference in phage type or biotype. Recently a search was made for *C. diphtheriae* in patients attending a venereal disease and dermatology clinic in Rangoon, Burma (Thaung *et al.*, 1978). Specimens were obtained from patients with dermatoses such as impetigo, pyoderma, ecthyma, and such skin lesions as scabies and eczema, etc. About 150 new patients a day attended the clinic. Ten cases (ages: infants to 19 years) were chosen each day. Of 493 patients, 64% had *C. diphtheriae* in their skin lesions. Of 108 strains tested, 18.5% were toxinogenic and most were var. *intermedius*. Cockcroft has pointed out that in cutaneous lesions harboring *C. diphtheriae* among a selected group of patients in the Vancouver area (Cockcroft *et al.*, 1973), Group A streptococci, Group B streptococci, and/or *Staphylococcus aureus* were commonly associated with the lesions. The above-mentioned findings in Rangoon extend the list of organisms and conditions which may provide diphtheria bacilli with a more nutritious environment and enhance their capacity to colonize man. More data are needed to provide us with a better understanding of the carriage of *C. diphtheriae*. As pointed out earlier, carefully followed cases among healthy medical personnel have demonstrated continuous carriage for at least 5 years (Barksdale *et al.*, 1960). In such cases *C. diphtheriae* would seem to be a bona fide part of the flora of the individual.

7. Diphtheria as a Medical Problem of Sporadic Occurrence

Contemporary reports of diphtheria in the United States and Canada and in Europe often stress the socioeconomic level of the persons associated with outbreaks of the disease. What seems crucial is the personal hygiene of the individuals concerned and whether or not they have retained their tonsils. *C. diphtheriae* is an efficient colonizer of tonsillar crypts, and it has long been known that carriers with tonsils harbor the bacilli longer than persons whose tonsils have been removed (Andrewes *et al.*, 1923). Despite all of the sophisticated information available concerning the immunology and bacteriology of diphtheria, it is appalling that, even today, the signal for the presence of diphtheria in a community is death of a victim of the disease. When one looks into how this happens in situations where the victims live in areas with available diagnostic bacteriology, it often turns out that the clinician and the laboratory were not looking for *C. diphtheriae*. In the 1971 outbreak in Manchester (Butterworth *et al.*, 1974) circumstances surrounding diphtherial death in a 9-year-old boy included delayed clinical and microbiological indentification.* McSwiggan and

* The difficulty in identification involved the laboratory personnel's belief that *C. diphtheriae* does not ferment sucrose. Sucrose fermentation has since 1900 been employed as a means of separating *C. diphtheriae* (supposedly sucrose negative) from *C. xerosis* (sucrose positive). In recent years sucrose-fermenting strains of *C. diphtheriae* have been involved in outbreaks of diphtheria in the United States and Europe (Barksdale, 1970).

Taylor (1975) have suggested that routine culture for *C. diphtheriae* in diagnostic laboratories is not advisable. They have advised that "the detection of diphtheria at an early stage will best be achieved by urging clinicians to voice their suspicions to the laboratory, and also to alert practitioners to the fact that not all laboratories *routinely* examine specimens for *C. diphtheriae*." Bezjak (1975), speaking from experience in Yugoslavia, has added the view that "in countries with a low diphtheria prevalence, there is no need for *routine* investigation for diphtheria bacilli in every patient with a sore throat." The view held by us is more in accord with that of other opinions provoked by the Manchester outbreak and expressed by E. J. Stokes (1975) writing from London:

Although the disease is rare, continued attempts to culture are, I think, necessary for several reasons.

The clinician tends to think of diphtheria when antibiotic treatment has failed. If he has had the forethought to submit a swab for culture before treatment, he will not unreasonably feel aggrieved if no opinion can be expressed by the laboratory, other than the absence of hemolytic streptococci. Cultures aimed at excluding this pathogen cannot be relied on to reveal diphtheria bacilli.

Unless selective medium for *Corynebacterium diphtheriae* is used routinely, it may not be available in good condition when urgently needed. Demands tend to be made late in the day, at weekends, and on Bank Holidays. Although a large number of negative cultures will be processed, the work is not excessive, expensive, or entirely without value. Staff learn to recognise common commensals on tellurite medium, which will help them to investigate cultures in clinically suspected cases.

We are at risk from people flown in from parts of the world where the disease is still common, and immunisation in this country against rare infections tends to be omitted. In this situation, alertness in the laboratory, and the ability to make a diagnosis, not only reliably but quickly, is, I think, essential.

Clinicians rarely encounter diphtheria, and their expertise in recognising it cannot now be relied on. We can keep our hand in by examining simulated specimens containing *C. diphtheriae* sent by the Quality-control Laboratory. I think it is for us to support the clinicians, not vice versa.

In accord with Stokes' expressed position, Hutchison and Geddes (1975) report a signal diphtheritic death of a child in Birmingham followed by the isolation of *C. diphtheriae* "from a routine throat-swab taken from a child admitted to one of the pediatric wards" of their hospital. They note that "In view of the significant number of children in England who are not immunised against diphtheria and the ready access to areas of the world where this infection is endemic, we cannot afford to be complacent."

The foregoing quotations from contemporary medical personnel make it clear that diphtheria is ever with us. A scan of current world medical literature indicates that in every society today there are segments in which diphtheria is endemic. An inspection of Table 1 offers a perspective on the disease which is worthy of comment. First, the case mortality (in England) shifted from 40% in 1889 down to 4.0% in 1927. Although antitoxin was available in England after 1890, no general program of prophylactic immunization was initiated until 1941. The decline in diphtheria must in part, then, be attributed to more accurate diagnosis, better sanitation, and improved standards of living. In the United States the most completely studied outbreak of diphtheria in recent years was that occurring in San Antonio (McCloskey *et al.,* 1971; Marcuse and Grand, 1973). For 25 years prior to the outbreak the median number of diphtheria cases reported per year from San Antonio was 14. In 1970, a total of 196 cases were reported. The disease occurred in persons having circulating antitoxin and in persons showing no immunity to toxin. Often the strain of *C. diphtheriae* associated with the epidemic was isolated in conjunction with what appeared to be resident endemic strain(s). Strains of *C. diphtheriae mitis,* both toxinogenic and nontoxinogenic, *C. diphtheriae gravis,* and *C. diphtheriae intermedius* were isolated. The case rate for the fully immunized was 6.6%, being significantly lower than that for those not having received toxoid, 14.4%. The efficacy of the toxoid immunization was calculated from the observed case rates for those with full immunization and those with none. Vaccine efficacy (%) = $U - I/U \times 100$, where U is attack rate in those with no immunization and I is attack rate in the fully immunized. In those households which could be followed, the efficacy of toxoid immunization was 54.2%.

Under ideal conditions, then, to limit outbreaks of diphtheria and to eliminate diphtheritic death, both antibacterial immunity and antitoxic immunity are required. To cope with outbreaks as they now occur, the minimum we can do would seem to be (1) to have mass immunization with toxoid and (2) to have guaranteed sources of antitoxin—human immune serum at best, equine antitoxin at least. (At present neither is manufactured in the United States.) It goes without saying that an awareness of the possible occurrence of diphtheria among us must be perpetuated and facilities for its diagnosis must be maintained.

8. Methods of Immunization Against Diphtheritic (Toxic) Death

8.1. Active Immunization with Diphtherial Toxoid

8.1.1. Immunization of Children

Children born of mothers who are naturally or artificially immune to diphtherial toxin have, at birth, circulating antitoxic IgG. For a while, in the early months, falling levels of this protective antibody can be replenished by breast feeding (see Fig. 6). Many pediatricians initiate diphtherial toxoid immunization (combined with tetanus toxoid and pertussis vaccine), as early as 2 months of age. In most states of the United States, children cannot enter public school unless they have completed such immunization. Despite the effectiveness of toxoid, many children in the developed countries, to say nothing of the developing countries, are susceptible to diphtheritic intoxication. There are two reasons for this: (1) failure to be adequately immunized and (2) inability to respond to toxoid by synthesizing neutralizing antibody. Individuals who specifically fail to respond to diphtherial toxin (producing less than 0.003 IU/ml), but who are capable of a normal response to tetanus toxoid, comprise about 2% of persons sampled in studies in the United States (see Section 3.7).

The triple antigen, generally referred to as DPT, is a combination of diphtherial toxoid, tetanus toxoid, and pertussis vaccine. The

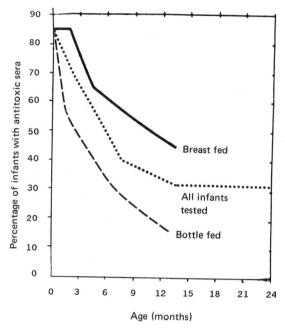

Figure 6. Influence of breast feeding on maintenance of circulating anticorynebacterial antibodies (measured as antitoxin) in the sera of infants. It is clear that antitoxin levels in breast-fed infants were augmented by antibodies from mother's milk. Adapted from von Gröer and Kassowitz (1919). Antitoxin levels in infants, soon after birth, are close to the antenatal titers found in the mothers and less than the levels found in cord blood. Antitoxin acquired from the mother has a half-life of about 4.5 weeks (Barr *et al.*, 1949). Above a certain critical level, IgG acquired from the mother may serve to suppress the primary response to diphtherial toxoid (discussed in Solomon, 1971). Data from a recently reported outbreak of diphtheria in Delhi (Dutta *et al.*, 1976) indicate the value these passively acquired antibodies may have for infants under 6 months of age. In the age group 6–11 months the fatalities were 31%. Clinical diphtheria was seen in only ten infants under 6 months (2.9% of 598 cases), all of whom survived.

diphtherial toxin is prepared from the culture fluid of a strain of *C. diphtheriae* grown on a modified casein hydrolysate medium (Mueller and Miller, 1941). The tetanus toxin is prepared from the culture fluid of a strain of *Clostridium tetani* grown in a semisynthetic medium (Latham *et al.*, 1962). Each toxin is rendered into toxoid by treatment with formaldehyde. Each contains, finally, no more than 0.02% free HCHO. The pertussis vaccine is prepared with cells of *Bordetella pertussis* grown on a casein hydrolysate medium supplemented with a dialysate of yeast extract (Cohen and Wheeler, 1946) and with 5% agar

and 4% charcoal (Wadsworth, 1947). The combined "triple antigen," adsorbed on aluminum phosphate, is preserved with 0.01% thimerosal (mercury derivative). The aluminum content of the final product does not exceed 0.85 mg/0.5-ml dose. The basic immunizing course for infants and children through 6 years of age consists of three (primary) doses of 0.5 ml each at 4- to 8-week intervals, followed by a fourth (reinforcing) dose, 0.5 ml, approximately 1 year after the third priming dose. The fourth (reinforcing) dose is an integral part of the immunization procedure. The plan of the immunization requires the fourth dose for completion of the basic immunization process. Doses are given intramuscularly (preferably the midlateral muscles of the thigh or deltoid). The same muscle site should not be injected more than once during the course of the immunization. It is recommended that immunization with DPT be initiated at 2 months of age (Public Health Service Advisory Committee on Immunization Practices, 1971; Steigman, 1977). Booster doses of tetanus and diphtherial toxoids for individuals over 6 years of age employ preparations of diphtherial toxoid and tetanus toxoid adsorbed on aluminum phosphate, labeled for adult use.

8.1.2. Immunization of Adults

When employing diphtherial toxoid (or tetanus toxoid) for the immunization of adults, it must be borne in mind that these are complex antigens which, in sufficient amounts, can give rise to illness when injected into immune individuals, either as priming injections or so-called booster injections. They can initiate local anaphylaxis in the atopic (allergic, asthmatic) individual whose levels of IgE specific for the injected antigen(s) are high. They have been known to provoke severe Arthus reactions in individuals having relatively high levels of circulating antibodies specific for components of the injected material [e.g., in a patient infected with $C7_s(-)^{tox^-}$ whose circulating antitoxin level was greater than 0.5 IU/ml, a severe Arthus reaction resulted from a booster dose of diphtherial toxoid (Barksdale *et al.*, 1960)]. In addition, many adults show intensive delayed hypersensitivity reactions to immunizing doses of diphtherial toxoid, reactions not often encountered in children. Edsall *et al.* (1954) has suggested that these reactions might be minimized in a population by either (1) immunizing only susceptibles as determined by the Schick testing, (2) using purified toxoid (see Section 3.5), or (3) reducing the dose of toxoid administered. He adds that the first method is tedious and time consuming and requires considerable organization and labor. Further, today, only an occasional public health laboratory has the necessary materials. The second method is of real value, but, as explained earlier (see Section 3.5), it will not eliminate all of the severe reactions. Edsall has shown that a small dose of 1 Lf (1.5–2.0 μg) can be used in immunization of young adult Americans without regard to Schick-positive status and with the occurrence of only a very occasional severe reaction.

8.2. Passive Immunization, Antitoxin Therapy

In reports on the San Antonio outbreak (McCloskey *et al.,* 1971; Marcuse and Grand, 1973) there was evidence of some difficulty in obtaining antitoxin for therapeutic use. [At this writing, no antitoxin is being manufactured by pharmaceutical companies in the United States. There is, however, a pool of previously manufactured antitoxin (horse) available from one drug company.] The physicians concerned with the San Antonio outbreak skin-tested their patients for sensitivity to antitoxin, subsequently putting those patients who needed such through a regimen of desensitization (see below). For treatment, large doses of antitoxin, 40,000–80,000 units, were used. The incidence of serum sickness was 8.6% for all patients treated and 20% among patients older than 15 years. This incidence of serum sickness is to be expected. The number of cases of anaphylactic shock encountered was not reported. These very real dangers of horse serum therapy are well known. For reasons which are obvious from the foregoing, Richard McCloskey (McCloskey and Smilack, 1972) has examined the possibility of having available in the United States human immune globulins carrying high levels of antidiphtherial toxin. Toward this end, he and Smilack obtained from commercial sources immune serum globulin, pertussis immune globulin, vaccinia immune globulin, and tetanus immune globulin. The level of diphtherial antitoxin in these preparations was on the order of 6 units (IU)/

ml compared with 2000 units (IU)/ml for commercially available antitoxin (horse). Thus none of the available human immunoglobulins contained diphtherial antitoxin in sufficient concentration to allow the use of human globulins for the antitoxic therapy of diphtheria. Since it is clear that diphtheria will continue to occur in the United States, there should be developed a specific human diphtherial immune serum globulin for intravenous use. As McCloskey has pointed out, this could afford antitoxic therapy without hypersensitivity reactions, an unavoidable risk with current equine diphtherial antitoxin.

The following guidelines for the administration of antitoxin (equine) in the therapy of diphtheritic infections are adapted from the 1977 and the 1964 reports of The American Academy of Pediatrics Committee on the Control of Infectious Diseases (Steigman, 1977) and the brochure accompanying Diphtherial Antitoxin (horse) Wyeth. Antitoxin should be administered on the basis of clinical diagnosis even before culture results are available. Site and size of membrane, degree of toxicity, and duration of illness are guides for estimating dose of antitoxin; the presence of soft, diffuse cervical lymphadenitis suggests moderate to severe toxin absorption. Dosage is purely empirical. Suggested ranges are listed in Table 3.

Larger doses are indicated if toxicity is marked or if the patient has been ill longer than 48 hr. Also, in such instances, intravenous administration is indicated.

8.2.1. Precautions

Before the administration of any product prepared from horse serum, appropriate measures must be taken to rule out the presence of dangerous sensitivity. Appropriate measures

Table 3. Dose Ranges of Diphtheria Antitoxin

Location of lesion	Dosage (units)	Route
Tonsils	20,000	Intramuscular
Anterior nose	10,000–20,000	Intramuscular
Pharynx or uvula	20,000–40,000	Intramuscular
Larynx	20,000–40,000	Intramuscular
Nasopharynx	40,000–75,000	Half intravenous, half intramuscular

include (1) a careful review of the patient's history and (2) a suitable test for detecting sensitivity to the product to be used. Important allergic historical information that demands utmost care with administration includes (1) a past history of asthma, hay fever, urticaria, or other allergic symptoms, (2) the occurrence of allergic symptoms on exposure to horses, and (3) prior injections of equine antiserum. Regardless of the clinical allergic history, a skin or conjuctival test should be performed in *every* patient prior to *each* administration of antiserum.

8.2.2.   Skin Test

The skin test consists of injecting intracutaneously enough to raise a small wheal (0.02 ml) of a 1 : 100 or 1 : 10 dilution (in Sodium Chloride Injection, U.S.P.) of Normal Horse Serum or the antiserum to be administered. A control test with Sodium Chloride Injection, U.S.P., facilitates interpretation of test results. The use of larger amounts for the skin test dose increases the likelihood of false-positive reactions and of systemic reaction in the hypersensitive patient. A 1 : 100 dilution should be used for preliminary skin testing if (1) sensitivity is suspected from the history or (2) therapeutic concentrations of antitoxin are indicated and the physician elects to use a dilution of the antitoxin to be administered for the skin test. An exquisitely hypersensitive individual may experience a severe and occasionally fatal reaction from the skin test dose alone. A positive reaction occurs within 5–30 min, and is manifested by a wheal, with or without pseudopodia and surrounding erythema. As a general rule, the shorter the interval between injection and the beginning of the skin reaction, the greater is the degree of sensitivity.

8.2.3.   Conjunctival Test

The conjuctival test consists of the instillation of one drop of diluted Normal Horse Serum or the antiserum to be given into the conjuctival sac. A drop of Sodium Chloride Injection, U.S.P., placed in the opposite conjuctival sac serves as a control. A positive reaction occurs within a few to 10 min. Mild positive reactions may be manifested by itching and slight dilation of the conjuctival vessels. More strongly positive reactions may include marked dilation of vessels, itching, and edema of the conjuctiva and eyelids. A 1 : 100 dilution should be used for preliminary testing if (1) sensitivity is suspected from the history or (2) therapeutic concentrations of antitoxin are indicated and the physician elects to use a dilution of the antitoxin to be administered for the conjuctival test. If a positive reaction occurs, it is advisable to instill a drop or two of epinephrine, 1 : 1000, into the affected eye.

8.2.4.   Interpretation of Sensitivity Tests and Administration of Antitoxin

If the clinical allergic history is negative and the result of a skin or conjuctival test is negative, it is very likely safe to proceed with administration of antiserum. If the allergic history is positive and either a skin or conjuctival test is strongly positive, administration may be extremely dangerous, especially if the positive sensitivity test is accompanied by systemic allergic manifestations. In such instances the risk of administering antiserum must be carefully weighed against the risk of withholding it. As a general rule, administration is contraindicated.

A negative allergic history and absence of reaction to a properly performed skin or conjunctival test do not rule out the possibility of occurrence of a severe immediate reaction on administration of the therapeutic or prophylactic dose. Also, a negative skin or conjunctival test has no bearing whatsoever on whether or not delayed serum reaction (serum sickness) will occur following administration of prophylactic or therapeutic doses.

In instances when the allergic history is negative and the result of a properly performed skin or conjunctival test is mildly or questionably positive, the following method of administration may be used to reduce the likelihood of occurrence of a severe immediate systemic reaction: (1) Prepare 1 : 100 and 1 : 10 dilutions (in Sodium Chloride Injection, U.S.P.) in separate sterile vials or syringes. (2) Allow at least 15 min, preferably 30, between injections, and proceed with the next dose only if no reaction follows the previous dose. (3) Inject subcutaneously, using a tuberculin-type syringe, 0.1, 0.2, and 0.5 ml of the 1 : 100 dilution at the aforementioned intervals, repeat with the 1 : 10 dilution and, finally, with undiluted antitoxin. (4) If a reaction occurs after any injection, place a tourniquet proximal to the site of injections and administer an appropriate dose of epinephrine, 1 : 1000, proximal to the tourniquet or into another extremity. Wait at least 30 min before giving another dose of antitoxin; the amount of the next dose shall be the same as the last one that failed to evoke a reaction. (5) If no reaction occurs after 0.5 ml of undiluted antiserum has been given, it is probably safe to continue doubling this dose at 15-min intervals until the entire predetermined prophylactic or therapeutic dose has been administered.

In those cases where intravenous administration is considered necessary or desirable, it is preferable to prepare a 1 : 10 dilution of antitoxin in Sodium Chloride Injection, U.S.P., or 5% Dextrose Injection, U.S.P. This should be run in slowly as an intravenous drip; administration of the first milliliter should take 2–3 min. Intravenous administration should not be started until the response to a test dose administered subcutaneously has been noted. Extreme care must be taken if intravenous administration is considered necessary in those individuals who have had to receive antiserum in gradually increasing doses because of a questionably positive or mildly positive sensitivity test response, as described in the previous paragraph.

References

Allen, J. C., and Cluff, L. E., 1961, Identification of toxinogenic *C. diphtheriae* with fluorescent antitoxin: Demonstration of nonspecificity, *Proc. Soc. Exp. Biol. (N.Y.)* 112:194–199.

Allison, A. C., 1973, Effects of adjuvants on different cell types and their interactions in immune responses, in: *Immunopotentiation* (G. E. W. Wolstenholme and J. Knight, eds.), pp. 73–94, Associated Scientific Publishers, Amsterdam.

Andrewes, F. W., Bulloch, W., Douglas, S. R., Dreyer, G., Gardner, A. D., Fildes, P., Ledingham, J. C. G., and Wolf, C. G. L., 1923, *Diphtheria: Its Bacteriology, Pathology and Immunology,* His Majesty's Stationery Office, London.

Arden, S. B., 1970, Comparative studies of *Corynebacterium diphtheriae, C. ovis, C. ulcerans* and related species, (New York University), University Microfilms, Ann Arbor, Mich., Order No. 71-15, 358.

Arden, S. B., and Barksdale, L., 1974, Glucose-1-phosphate-induced accumulation of intracellular starch: A

distinguishing feature of certain corynebacteria, *Int. J. Syst. Bacteriol.* 24:139–141.

Arden, S. B., and Barksdale, L., 1976, Nitrate reductase activities in lysogenic and nonlysogenic strains of *Corynebacterium diphtheriae* and related species, *Int. J. Syst. Bacteriol.* 26:66–73.

Arden, S. B., Chang, W.-H., and Barksdale, L., 1972, Distribution of neuraminidase and *N*-acetylneuraminate lyase activities among corynebacteria, mycobacteria, and nocardias, *J. Bacteriol.* 112:1206–1212.

Asherson, G. L., and Zembala, M., 1975, Inhibitory T cells, *Curr. Top. Microbiol. Immunol.* 72:55–100.

Audibert, F., Chédid, L., Lefrancier, P., and Choay, J., 1976, Distinctive adjuvanticity of synthetic analogs of mycobacterial water-soluble components, *Cell. Immunol.* 21:243–249.

Barile, M. F., Kolb, R. W., and Pittman, M., 1971, United States standard diphtheria toxin for the Schick test and the erythema potency assay for the Schick test dose, *Infect. Immun.* 4:295–306.

Barksdale, L., 1970, *Corynebacterium diphtheriae* and its relatives, *Bacteriol. Rev.* 34:378–422.

Barksdale, L., and Arden, S. B., 1974, Persisting bacteriophage infections, lysogeny, and phage conversions, *Annu. Rev. Microbiol.* 28:265–299.

Barksdale, L., and Kim, K.-S., 1977, *Mycobacterium, Bacteriol. Rev.* 41:217–372.

Barksdale, W. L., Li, K., Cummins, C. S., and Harris, H., 1957, The mutation of *Corynebacterium pyogenes* to *Corynebacterium haemolyticum, J. Gen. Microbiol.* 16:749–758.

Barksdale, L., Garmise, L., and Horibata, K., 1960, Virulence, toxinogeny, and lysogeny in *Corynebacterium diphtheriae, Ann. N.Y. Acad. Sci.* 88:1093–1108.

Barr, M., Glenny, A. T., and Randall, K. J., 1949, Concentration of diphtheria antitoxin in cord blood, *Lancet* 257(ii):324–326.

Baum, M., and Breese, M., 1976, Antitumor effect of *Corynebacterium parvum*: Possible mode of action, *Br. J. Cancer* 33:468–473.

Bazaral, M., Goscienski, P. J., and Hamburger, R. N., 1973, Characteristics of human antibody to diphtheria toxin, *Infect. Immun.* 7:130–136.

Behring and Kitasato, 1890, Ueber das Zustandekommen der Diphtherie-Immunität und der Tetanus-Immunität bei Thieren, *Dtsch. Med. Wochenschr.* 16:1113–1114.

Bezjak, V., 1975, Recognition of diphtheria, *Lancet* 1:924.

Bloch, H., 1950, Studies on the virulence of tubercle bacilli: Isolation and biological properties of a constituent of virulent organisms, *J. Exp. Med.* 91:197–218.

Bonventre, P. F., 1975, Diphtheria, in: *Microbiology— 1975* (D. Schlessinger, ed.), pp. 272–277, American Society for Microbiology, Washington, D.C.

Bormann, F., and Scheurer, O., 1933, Experimentelle Untersuchungen an der Schleimhautdiphtherie der Tiere. I. Die spezifische Wirksamkeit des Diphtherieserums bei bazillärer Tierinfektion, *Z. Kinderh.* 55:73–91.

Bretonneau, P., 1826, *Des Inflammations Spéciales du*

Tissu Muqueux et en Particulier de la Diphthérite (etc.), Prevot, Paris.

Brooks, G. F., Bennett, J. V., and Feldman, R. A., 1974, Diphtheria in the United States, 1959–1970, *J. Infect. Dis.* **129**:172–178.

Burgoyne, R. D., Wolstenholme, J., and Stephen, J., 1976, The preparation of stable, biologically active B fragment of diphtheria toxin, *Biochem. Biophys. Res. Commun.* **71**:920–925.

Butterworth, A., Abbott, J. D., Simmons, L. E., Ironside, A. G., Mandel, B. K., Williams, R. F., Brennand, J., Mann, N. M., and Simon, S., 1974, Diphtheria in the Manchester area, 1967–1971, *Lancet* **2**:1558–1561.

Chang, T.-M., and Neville, D. M., Jr., 1978, Demonstration of diphtheria toxin receptors on surface membranes from both toxin-sensitive and toxin-resistant species, *J. Biol. Chem.* **253**:6866–6871.

Cockcroft, W. H., Boyko, W. J., and Allen, D. E., 1973, Cutaneous infections due to *Corynebacterium diphtheriae, Can. Med. Assoc. J.* **108**:329–331.

Cohen, S. M., and Wheeler, M. W., 1946, Pertussis vaccine prepared with phase-I cultures grown in fluid medium, *Am. J. Public Health* **36**:371–376.

Coleman, M. B., 1949, Unusual strains of diphtheria bacilli from throat cultures, *J. Bacteriol.* **58**:712–713.

Collier, R. J., 1975, Diphtheria toxin: Mode of action and structure, *Bacteriol. Rev.* **39**:54–85.

Convit, J., Avila, J. L., Goihman, M., and Pinardi, M. E., 1972, A test for the determination of competency in clearing bacilli in leprosy patients, *Bull. WHO* **46**:821–826.

Craig, J. P., 1962, Diphtheria: Prevalence of inapparent infection in a nonepidemic period, *Am. J. Publ. Health* **52**:1444–1452.

Creagan, R. P., Chen, S., and Ruddle, F. H., 1975, Chromosome assignments of genes in man using mouse-human somatic cell hybrids: Association of diphtheria toxin sensitivity with chromosome 5, *Cytogenet. Cell Genet.* **14**:279–281.

Cummins, C. S., 1954, Some observations on the nature of the antigens in the cell wall of *Corynebacterium diphtheriae, Br. J. Exp. Pathol.* **35**:166–180.

Cummins, C. S., and Linn, D. M., 1977, Reticulostimulating properties of killed vaccines of anaerobic coryneforms and other organisms, *J. Natl. Cancer Inst.* **59**:1697–1708.

Davis, B. D., Dulbecco, R., Eisen, H. N., Ginsberg, H. S., Wood, W. B., Jr., and McCarty M. (eds.), 1973, *Microbiology including Immunology and Molecular Genetics*, 2nd ed., Harper and Row, New York.

Delange, R. J., Drazin, R. E., and Collier, R. J., 1976, Amino-acid sequence of Fragment A, an enzymically active fragment from diphtheria toxin, *Proc. Natl. Acad. Sci. USA* **73**:69–72.

DeVries, R. R. P., Lai, R. F. M., Fat, A., Nijenhuis, L. E., and van Rood, J. J., 1976, HLA-linked genetic control of host response to *Mycobacterium leprae, Lancet* **2**:1328–1330.

Draper, R. K., Chin, D., and Simon, M. I., 1978, Diph-

theria toxin has the properties of a lectin, *Proc. Natl. Acad. Sci. USA* **75**:261–265.

Duncan, J. L., and Groman, N. B., 1969, Activity of diphtheria toxin. II. Early events in the intoxication of HeLa cells, *J. Bacteriol.* **98**:963–969.

Durand, P., and Guérin, J., 1921, Types de Bacilles diphtériques et épidémiologie, *C. R. Soc. Biol.* **84**:980–981.

Dutta, J. K., Ayyagari, A., Guatum, A. P., Chadha, S. K., and Ray, S. N., 1976, A comparative study of bacteriologically proved and clinically diagnosed (culture negative) cases of diphtheria, *J. Indian Med. Assoc.* **67**:241–245.

Edsall, G., Altman, J. S., and Gaspar, A. J., 1954, Combined tetanus-diphtheria immunization of adults: Use of small doses of diphtheria toxid, *Am. J. Public Health* **44**:1537–1545.

Edward, D. G., and Allison, V. D., 1951, Diphtheria in immunized persons with observations on a diphtheria-like disease associated with non-toxigenic *C. diphtheriae, J. Hyg.* **49**:205–219.

Ewing, J. O., 1933, The serological grouping of the starch fermenting strains of *C. diphtheriae, J. Pathol. Bacteriol.* **37**:345–351.

Ferguson, D. A., and Cummins, C. S., 1978, Nutritional requirements of anaerobic coryneforms, *J. Bacteriol.* **135**:858–867.

Filosofova, T. G., Kolisnichenko, N. I., and Bliznjuk, G. I., 1977, Cellular immunity with "healthy diphtheritic" carriage (in Ukranian), *Mikrobiol. Zh. (Kiev)* **39**:637–640.

Finger, I., and Kabat, E. A., 1958, A comparison of human antisera to purified diphtheria toxoid with antisera to other purified antigens by quantitative precipitin and gel diffusion techniques, *J. Exp. Med.* **108**:453–474.

Franz, M. L., Carella, J. A., and Galant, S. P., 1976, Cutaneous delayed hypersensitivity in a healthy pediatric population: Diagnostic value of diphtheria-tetanus toxoids, *J. Pediatr.* **88**:975–977.

Freeman, V. J., 1951, Studies on the virulence of bacteriophage-infected strains of *Corynebacterium diphtheriae, J. Bacteriol.* **61**:675–688.

Frobisher, M., Jr., and Parsons, E. I., 1950, Studies on type-specific protection with somatic antigens of *C. diphtheriae, Am. J. Hyg.* **52**:239–246.

Frobisher, M., Jr., and Updyke, E. L., 1947, Further studies on the immunization of rabbits to toxigenic *Corynebacterium diphtheriae* by injection of non-toxigenic diphtheria bacilli, *J. Bacteriol.* **54**:609–617.

Gauvreau, L., Breton, J. P., Bergeron, M. G., Dorval, J., Martineau, G., and Frenette, G., 1977, Epidemie de diphterie survenue sur la Cote Nord du St-Laurent a l'automne de 1974, *Can. Med. Assoc. J.* **116**:1279–1283.

George, D. L., and Francke, U., 1977, Regional mapping of human genes for hexosaminidase B and diphtheria toxin sensitivity on chromosome 5 using mouse x human hybrid cells, *Somat. Cell Genet.* **3**:629–638.

Glenny, A. T., and Hopkins, B. E., 1923, Diphtheria toxoid as an immunising agent, *Br. J. Exp. Pathol.* **4**:283–288.

Goren, M. B., 1972, Mycobacterial lipids: Selected topics, *Bacteriol. Rev.* **36**:33–64.

Gray, R. D., and James, S. M., 1973, Occult diphtheria infection in a hospital for the mentally subnormal, *Lancet* **1**:1105–1106.

Häuser, H. F., 1972, Zur Immunitätslage der Diphtheriae. I. Untersuchung bei 613 Rekruten der Jahrgänge 1946–1951, *Z. Immunitaetsforsch.* **143**:271–279.

Hennekens, C. H., and Saslaw, M. S., 1976, A diphtheria outbreak in Dade County, Florida, *South. Med. J.* **69**:759–761.

Hirose, S.-I., Akama, K., Kameyama, S., and Murata, R., 1962, Virulence and immunity of *Corynebacterium diphtheriae*. II. Evidence of the different mechanisms in the protection of the conjunctival diphtheria, *Jpn. J. Med. Sci. Biol.* **15**:9–17.

Huang, C. H., 1942a, Studies on the antibacterial property in diphtheria, *Am. J. Hyg.* **35**:317–324.

Huang, C. H., 1942b, Further studies on the serological classification of *C. diphtheriae, Am. J. Hyg.* **35**:325–336.

Hutchison, J. G. P., and Geddes, A. M., 1975, Recognition of diphtheria, *Lancet* **1**:1377.

Israeli, L., and Halpern, B., 1972, *Corynbacterium parvum* in advanced cancers: First evaluation of therapeutic activity of this immunostimulin, *Nouv. Presse Med.* **1**:19–23.

Ittelson, T. R., and Gill, D. M., 1973, Diphtheria toxin. Specific competition for cell receptors, *Nature (London)* **242**:330–332.

Kaga, N., 1951, Studies on experimental diphtheria, especially concerning the production of diphtheria toxin [in Japanese], *Keio-Igaku* **28**:111–122.

Kato, M., 1970, Action of a toxic glycolipid of *Corynebacterium diphtheriae* on mitochondrial structure and function, *J. Bacteriol.* **101**:709–716.

Kato, M., 1972, Antibody formation to trehalose-6,6′-dimycolate (cord factor) of *Mycobacterium tuberculosis, Infect. Immun.* **5**:203–212.

Kato, I., Nakamura, H., Uchida, T., Koyama, J., and Katsura, T., 1960, Purification of diphtheria toxin. II. The isolation of crystalline toxin-protein and some of its properties, *Jpn. J. Exp. Med.* **30**:129–145.

Kim, K., and Groman, N. B., 1965, *In vitro* inhibition of diphtheria toxin action by ammonium salts and amines, *J. Bacteriol.* **90**:1552–1556.

Klebs, E., 1875, Beiträge zur Kenntniss der pathogen Schistomyceten, *Arch. Exp. Pathol. Pharmakol.* **4**:207–247.

Klebs, E., 1883, Ueber Diphtherie, *Verh. Congr. Inn. Med. Wiesb.* **2**:139–154.

Klimpel, G. R., and Henney, C. S., 1978, BCG-induced suppressor cells. I. Demonstration of a macrophage-like suppressor cell that inhibits cytotoxic T cell generation *in vitro, J. Immunol.* **120**:563–569.

Kostiala, A. A. I., and Kosunen, T. U., 1972a, Delayed hypersensitivity, macrophage migration, and antibodies in guinea-pigs immunized with diphtheria toxoid. I. Immunization with antigen–antibody precipitates. *Scand. J. Immunol.* **1**:143–151.

Kostiala, A. A. I., and Kosunen, T. U., 1972b, Delayed hypersensitivity, macrophage migration, and antibodies in guinea-pigs immunized with diphtheria toxoid. II. Macrophage cytophilic antibody to diphtheria toxoid, in desensitized animals, *Scand. J. Immunol.* **1**:153–159.

Kostyukovskaya, O. N., 1966, Characteristics of the immunity of diphtheria bacilli carriers (in Russian), *Vopr. Immunol.* **2**:99–104.

Kotani, S., Watanabe, Y., Kinoshita, F., Shimono, T., Morisaki, I., Shiba, T., Kusumoto, S., Tarumi, Y., and Ikenaka, K., 1975, Immunoadjuvant activities of synthetic *N*-acetylmuramyl-peptides or -amino acids, *Biken J.* **18**:105–111.

Kuhns, W. J., and Dukstein, W., 1957, Multiple antibody responses following immunization of human subjects with diphtheria toxoid, *J. Immunol.* **79**:154–161.

Lalley, P. A., Brown, J. A., and Shows, T. B., 1976, Assignment of hexosaminidase-B to chromosome 5, its segregation after diphtheria toxin selection and the linkage of hexosamidase-A, mannose phosphate isomerase, and pyruvate kinase (M2), *Cytogenet. Cell Genet.* **16**:188–191.

Lampidis, T., and Barksdale, L., 1971, Park–Williams number 8 strain of *Corynebacterium diphtheriae, J. Bacteriol.* **105**:77–85.

Latham, W. C., Bent, D. F., and Levine, L., 1962, Tetanus toxin production in the absence of protein, *Appl. Microbiol.* **10**:146–152.

Lautrop, H., 1950, Studies on antigenic structure of *Corynebacterium diphtheriae, Acta Pathol. Microbiol. Scand.* **27**:443–447.

Lawrence, H. S., and Pappenheimer, A. M., Jr., 1948, Immunization of adults with diphtheria toxoid. I. Immunological properties of formalinized diphtherial protein fractions from culture filtrates, *Am. J. Hyg.* **47**:226–232.

Liebow, A. A., MacLean, P. D., Bumstead, J. H., and Welt, L. G., 1946, Tropical ulcers and cutaneous diphtheria, *Arch. Intern. Med.* **78**:255–295.

Linder, R., and Bernheimer, A. W., 1978, Effect on sphingomyelin-containing liposomes of phospholipase D from *Corynebacterium ovis* and the cytolysin from *Stoichactis helianthus, Biochim. Biophys. Acta* **530**:236–246.

Loeffler, F., 1884, Untersuchungen über die Bedeutung der Mikroorganismen für die Entstehung der Diphtherie beim Menschen, bei der Taube und beim Kalbe, *Mitt. Klin. Gesundh. Berlin* **2**:421–499.

McBride, W. H., Dawes, J., and Tuach, S., 1976, Antitumor activity of *Corynebacterium parvum* extracts, *J. Natl. Cancer Inst.* **56**:437–439.

McCloskey, R. V., and Smilack, J., 1972, Diphtheria antitoxin content of human immune serum globulins, *Ann. Intern. Med.* **77**:757–758.

McCloskey, R. V., Eller, J. J., Green, M., Mauney, C. U., and Richards, S. E. M., 1971, The 1970 epidemic of diphtheria in San Antonio, *Ann. Intern. Med.* **75:**495–503.

McCloskey, R. V., Saragea, A., and Maximescu, P., 1972, Phage typing in diphtheria outbreaks in the Southwestern United States, 1968–1971, *J. Infect. Dis.* **126:**196–199.

McCracken, A. W., and Mauney, C. U., 1971, Identification of *Corynebacterium diphtheriae* by immunofluorescence during a diphtheria epidemic, *J. Clin. Pathol.* **24:**641–644.

McLeod, J. W., 1943, The types mitis, intermedius and gravis of *Corynebacterium diphtheriae*, a review of observations during the past ten years, *Bacteriol. Rev.* **7:**1–41.

McMichael, A. J., Sasazuki, T., and McDevitt, H. D., 1977, The immune response to diphtheria toxoid in humans, *Transplant. Proc.* **9:**191–194 (Suppl. 1).

McSwiggan, D. A., and Taylor, C. E. D., 1975, Recognition of diphtheria, *Lancet* **1:**515.

Maitland, H. B., Marshall, F. N., Petrie, G. F., and Robinson, D. T., 1952, Diphtheria anti-*gravis* serum: Its action on experimental infection and in the treatment of patients, *J. Hyg.* **50:**97–106.

Mäkelä, P. H., Valtonen, V. V., and Valtonen, G., 1973, Role of O-antigen (lipopolysaccharide) factors in the virulence of *Salmonella*, in: *Bacterial Lipopolysaccharides* (E. H. Kass and S. M. Wolff, eds.), pp. 73–77, University of Chicago Press, Chicago.

Marcuse, E. K., and Grand, M. G., 1973, Epidemiology of diphtheria in San Antonio, Tex., 1970, *J. Am. Med. Assoc.* **224:**305–310.

Michel, A., and Dirkx, J., 1977, Occurrence of tryptophan in the enzymically active site of diphtheria toxin fragment A, *Biochim. Biophys. Acta* **491:**286–295.

Middlebrook, J. L., Dorland, R. B., and Leppla, S. H., 1978, Association of diphtheria toxin with Vero cells: Demonstration of a receptor, *J. Biol. Chem.* **253:**7325–7330.

Milas, L., and Mujagic, H., 1972, Protection by *Corynebacterium parvum* against tumour cells injected intravenously, *Rev. Eur. Etud. Clin. Biol.* **17:**498–500.

Moehring, T. J., and Moehring, J. M., 1976, Interaction of diphtheria toxin and its active subunit, fragment A, with toxin-sensitive and toxin-resistant cells, *Infect. Immun.* **13:**1426–1432.

Moody, M. D., and Jones, W. L., 1963, Identification of *Corynebacterium diphtheriae* with fluorescent antibacterial reagents, *J. Bacteriol.* **86:**285–293.

Mueller, J. H., and Miller, P. A., 1941, Production of diphtheria toxin of high potency (100 Lf) on a reproducible medium, *J. Immunol.* **40:**21–32.

Müller, H. E., 1972, Der immunelektrophoretische Nachweis von Neuraminidase und Diphthin bei der Diagnose von *Corynebacterium diphtheriae*, *Zbl. Bakt. Hyg. I. Abt. Orig.* **A221:**550–554.

Murata, R., Akama, K., Hirose, S.-I., Kameyama, S., Nakano, T., and Yamamoto, A., 1959, Virulence and immunity of *Corynebacterium diphtheriae*. I. General

pictures of infection and immunity in the conjunctival diphtheria, *Jpn. J. Med. Sci. Biol.* **12:**319–330.

Neill, J. M., and Fleming, W. L., 1929, Hypersensitiveness to diphtheria bacilli. A hypersensitive reaction associated with toxin content of test material, *J. Immunol.* **17:**419–440.

Noll, H., Bloch, H., Asselineau, J., and Lederer, E., 1956, The chemical structure of the cord factor of *Mycobacterium tuberculosis*, *Biochim. Biophys. Acta* **20:**299–309.

Pappenheimer, A. M., Jr., 1958, The Schick test, 1913–1958, *Int. Arch. Allergy Appl. Immunol.* **12:**35–41.

Pappenheimer, A. M., Jr., 1977, Diphtheria toxin, *Annu. Rev. Biochem.* **46:**69–94.

Pappenheimer, A. M., Jr., and Gill, D. M., 1973, Diphtheria: Recent studies have clarified the molecular mechanisms involved in its pathogenesis, *Science* **182:**353–358.

Pappenheimer, A. M., Jr., and Lawrence, H. S., 1948a, Immunization of adults with diphtheria toxoid. II. An analysis of the pseudoreactions to the Schick test, *Am. J. Hyg.* **47:**233–240.

Pappenheimer, A. M., Jr., and Lawrence, H. S., 1948b, Immunization of adults with diphtheria toxoid. III. Highly purified toxoid as an immunizing agent, *Am. J. Hyg.* **47:**241–246.

Pappenheimer, A. M., Jr., Uchida, T., and Harper, A. A., 1972, An immunological study of the diphtheria toxin molecule, *Immunochemistry* **9:**891–906.

Parant, M., Audibert, F., Parant, F., Chedid, L., Soler, E., Polonsky, J., and Lederer, E., 1978, Nonspecific immunostimulant activities of synthetic trehalose-6,6'-diesters (lower homologs of cord factor), *Infect. Immun.* **20:**12–19.

Park, W. H., and Schroder, M. C., 1932, Diphtheria toxin–antitoxin and toxoid: A comparison, *Am. J. Public Health* **22:**7–16.

Park, W. H., and Williams, A. W., 1896, The production of diphtheria toxin, *J. Exp. Med.* **1:**164–185.

Pedersen, A. H. B., Spearman, J., Tronca, E., Bader, M., and Harnisch, J., 1977, Diphtheria on skid road, Seattle, Wash., 1972–75, *Public Health Rep.* **92:**336–342.

Pietrowski, R. A., and Stephen, J., 1978, Reconstitution of fully active diphtheria toxin from purified fragments A and B, *FEBS Lett.* **87:**311–314.

Platts-Mills, T. A. E., and Ishizaka, K., 1975, IgG and IgA diphtheria antitoxin responses from human tonsil lymphocytes, *J. Immunol.* **114:**1058–1064.

Pope, C. G., and Stevens, M. F., 1958, The purification of diphtheria toxin and the isolation of crystalline toxin-protein, *Br. J. Exp. Pathol.* **39:**139–149.

Pope, C. G., Stevens, M. F., and Thomas, D., 1966, Observations on crystalline diphtheria toxin: The optical density per Lf unit at 276 mμ, *Br. J. Exp. Pathol.* **47:**45–51.

Proia, R. L., Eidels, L., and Hart, D. A., 1979, Diphtheria-binding glycoproteins on hamster cells: Candidates for diphtheria toxin receptors, *Infect. Immun.* **25:**786–791.

Public Health Service Advisory Committee on Immunization Practices, 1971, Diphtheria and tetanus toxoids and pertussis vaccine, *Morbidity and Mortality Week. Rep. (U.S.)* **20:**396–397.

Ramon, G., 1923, Pouvoir floculant et pouvoir toxique de la toxine diphtérique, *C. R. Soc. Biol. Paris* **89:**2–4.

Ramon, G., 1928, L'anatoxine diphtérique: Ses propriétés—Ses applications, *Ann. Inst. Pasteur (Paris)* **42:**959–1009.

Raynaud, M., 1965, Heterogeneity of diphtheria antibodies, *Proc. 2nd Meet. Fed. Eur. Biochem. Soc.* **1:**197–251.

Raynaud, M., Bizzini, B., and Relyveld, E., 1965, Composition en amino-acides de la toxine diphtérique purifiée, *Bull. Soc. Chim. Biol.* **47:**261–266.

Roux, E., and Yersin, A., 1888, Contribution a l'étude de la diphtérie, *Ann. Inst. Pasteur (Paris)* **2:**629–661.

Russell, W. T., 1943, The epidemiology of diphtheria during the last forty years, *Med. Res. Coun. Spec. Rep.Ser.* **247:**6–52.

Saragea, A., and Maximesco, P., 1964, Schéma provisoire de lysotypie pour *Corynebacterium diphtheriae, Arch. Roum. Pathol. Exp. Microbiol.* **23:**817–838.

Saragea, A., and Maximescu, P., 1966, Phage typing of *Corynebacterium diphtheriae*: Incidence of *C. diphtheriae* phage types in different countries, *Bull. WHO* **35:**681–689.

Sasazuki, T., Kohno, Y., Iwamoto, I., Tanimura, M., and Naito, S., 1978, Association between an HLA haplotype and low responsiveness to tetanus toxin, *Nature (London)* **272:**359–361.

Schick, B., 1913, Die Diphtherietoxin-Hautreaktion des Menschen als Vorprobe der prophylaktischen Diphtherieheilseruminjektion, *Muench. Med. Wochenschr.* **60:**2608–2610.

Solomon, J. B., 1971, *Foetal and Neonatal Immunology*, North-Holland, Amsterdam.

Soucek, A., Michalec, C., and Souckova, A., 1967, Enzymic hydrolysis of sphingomyelins by a toxin of *Corynebacterium ovis, Biochim. Biophys. Acta* **144:**180–182.

Souckova, A., and Soucek, A., 1972, Inhibition of the hemolytic action of alpha and beta lysins of *Staphylococcus pyogenes* by toxigenic strains of *Corynebacterium haemolyticum, Corynebacterium ovis* and *Corynebacterium ulcerans, Toxicon* **10:**501–509.

Steigman, A. J. (ed.), 1977, *Report of the Committee on Infectious Diseases*, 18th ed., American Academy of Pediatrics, Evanston, Ill.

Stokes, E. J., 1975, Recognition of diphtheria, *Lancet* **1:**1235–1236.

Ströder, J., 1976, Diphtherie im Verzug—Alarm für alle Ärzte! *Muench. Med. Wochenschr.* **118**(31):[7]–[8].

Sulea, I. T., Pollice, M. C., and Barksdale, L., 1980, Pyrazine carboxylamidase activity in the genus *Corynebacterium, Int. J. Syst. Bacteriol.* **30** (in press).

Thaung, U., Naung, T., Khine, K. S., and Ming, C. K., 1978, Epidemiological features of skin diphtheria infection in Rangoon, Burma, *S. E. Asian J. Trop. Med. Publ. Health* **9:**4–10.

Toshach, S., Valentine, A., and Sigurdson, S., 1977, Bacteriophage typing of *Corynebacterium diphtheriae, J. Infect. Dis.* **136:**655–660.

Trendelenburg, 1869, Ueber die Contagiosität und local Natur der Diphtheritis, *Arch. Klin. Chir.* **10:**720–742.

Uchida, T., Pappenheimer, A. M., Jr., and Harper, A. A., 1972, Reconstitution of diphtheria toxin from two nontoxic cross-reacting mutant proteins, *Science* **175:**901–903.

Uchida, T., Pappenheimer, A. M., Jr., and Harper, A. A., 1973a, Diphtheria toxin and related proteins. II. Kinetic studies on intoxication of HeLa cells by diphtheria toxin and related proteins, *J. Biol. Chem.* **248:**3845–3850.

Uchida, T., Pappenheimer, A. M., Jr., and Harper, A. A., 1973b, Diphtheria toxin and related proteins. III. Reconstitution of hybrid "diphtheria toxin" from nontoxic mutant proteins, *J. Biol. Chem.* **248:**3851–3854.

Uhr, J. W., and Baumann, J. B., 1961a, Antibody formation. I. The suppression of antibody formation by passively administered antibody, *J. Exp. Med.* **113:**935–957.

Uhr, J. W., and Baumann, J. B., 1961b, Antibody formation. II. The specific anamnestic antibody response, *J. Exp. Med.* **113:**959–970.

Uhr, J. W., Salvin, S. B., and Pappenheimer, A. M., Jr., 1957, Delayed hypersensitivity. II. Induction of hypersensitivity in guinea pigs by means of antigen-antibody complexes, *J. Exp. Med.* **105:**11–24.

Updyke, E. L., and Frobisher, M., Jr., 1947, A study of bacterial synergism with reference to the etiology of malignant diphtheria, *J. Bacteriol.* **54:**619–632.

Vaz, N. M., Vaz, E. M., and Levine, B. B., 1970, Relationship between histocompatibility (H-2) genotype and immune responsiveness to low doses of ovalbumin in the mouse, *J. Immunol.* **104:**1572–1574.

von Gröer, F., and Kassowitz, K., 1919, Studien über die normale Diphtherieimmunität des Menschen. IV. Die normale Diphtherieimmunität im Kindesalter. *Z. Immunitaetsforsch. Exp. Ther. 1. Orig.* **28:**327–367.

Wadsworth, A. B., 1947, *Standard Methods of the Division of Laboratories and Research of the New York State Department of Health*, 3rd ed., p. 200, Williams and Wilkins, Baltimore.

Whitaker, J. A., Nelson, J. D., and Fink, C. W., 1961, The fluorescent antitoxin for the immediate diagnosis of diphtheria, *Pediatrics* **27:**214–218.

Wilson, G. S., 1967, *The Hazards of Immunization*, pp. 39–42, Athlone Press, University of London.

Wilson, G. S., and Miles, A. A. (eds.), 1955, *Topley and Wilson's Principles of Bacteriology and Immunity*, Vol. II, 4th ed., p. 1565, Williams and Wilkins, Baltimore.

Wolstenholme, G. E. W., and Knight J. (eds.), 1973, *Immunopotentiation*, Associated Scientific Publishers, Amsterdam.

Woodruff, M. F., and Boak, J. L., 1966, Inhibitory effect

of *Corynebacterium parvum* on growth of tumour transplants in isogenic hosts, *Br. J. Cancer* **20:**345–355.

Yarkoni, E., Bekierkunst, A., Asselineau, J., Toubiana, R., Toubiana, M. J., and Lederer, E., 1973, Suppression of growth of Ehrlich ascites tumor cells in mice pretreated with synthetic analogs of trehalose-6, 6-dimycolate (cord factor), *J. Natl. Cancer Inst.* **51:**717–720.

Zanen, J., Muyldermans, G., and Beugnier, N., 1976, Competitive antagonists of the action of diphtheria toxin in HeLa cells, *FEBS Lett.* **66:**261–263.

9

Immunity of
Listeria monocytogenes

ROBERT J. NORTH

1. *Listeria* and Listeriosis

The bacterium *Listeria monocytogenes* was originally isolated as the disease-causing agent from the livers, spleens, and myocardia of clinically ill rabbits and guinea pigs by Murray *et al.* (1926). The finding that it causes a very pronounced monocytosis when inoculated into rabbits is responsible for its specific name. It has been known for many years that *Listeria* is responsible for economically important outbreaks of disease in sheep flocks and cattle herds. Indeed, there is little doubt that the veterinary profession is more familiar with the organism than the medical profession is, in spite of the steadily increasing number of reported cases of listeriosis in humans.

In this chapter current information about the immunopathology of listeriosis will be presented. However, in view of the large amount of information gained about cell-mediated immunity in general from study of listeriosis in rodents, emphasis will be given to mechanisms of immunity in rodents. There is every reason for believing that the same mechanisms of immunity operate in humans.

1.1. *Listeria*

Listeria monocytogenes is a small, nonspore-forming, flagellated, gram-positive bacterium which, when examined in smears, may

display a typical diphtheroid morphology. It is classified in Bergey as a genus of uncertain affilation, and there is probably only one species.

Gray and Killinger (1966) list 11 serotypes of *Listeria monocytogenes* which are distinguished on the basis of different somatic (O) and flagellar (H) antigens. Most isolates from recent cases of human listeriosis in the United States are of serotype 4b, with 1b being the next most common. All serotypes, however, are potentially pathogenic in man and animal (Seeliger, 1957), and the relative frequency with which they are isolated may vary from year to year.

The presence of one of the O antigens causes antisera to *Listeria* to cross-react with a range of common bacteria. Neter *et al.* (1960) showed, in addition, that *Listeria* possesses the Rantz antigen, which is shared with other gram-positive bacteria. More recent evidence (Pease *et al.*, 1972) suggests, however, that a different antigen may be responsible.

As with other infectious agents, the pathogenicity of *Listeria* depends on its capacity to avoid destruction by the host's first line of cellular defenses. Its short generation time gives it the potential, furthermore, to overwhelm a developing mechanism of acquired immunity if it initially gains entry to the tissues in large enough numbers. There is convincing evidence to show (Mackaness, 1962; Fauve *et al.*, 1966; Ratzan *et al.*, 1972) that *Listeria* is a facultative intracellular parasite and that it can survive and multiply in mammalian mac-

ROBERT J. NORTH • Trudeau Institute, Inc., Saranac Lake, New York 12983.

rophages, destroying these cells in a relatively short time.

Most strains produce a hemolysin (Harvey and Faber, 1941), and culture filtrates of the organism were shown by Liu and Bates (1961) to be highly toxic for rabbits and mice. Njoko-Obi and Osebold (1962) suggested that the toxin is responsible for the destruction of macrophages: a suggestion supported by the demonstration (Kingdon and Sword, 1970a) that a purified preparation of the hemolysin is toxic for macrophages *in vitro* and can lyse isolated lysosomes. The toxicity of the hemolysin for macrophages was later confirmed by Watson and Lavizzo (1973), who showed, in addition, that *Listeria* also produces a lipolysin that is toxic for macrophages. The hemolysin appears to be responsible for the *in vivo* toxocity of the organism (Kingdon and Sword, 1970b) and causes death, at least partly as a result of its toxicity for cardiac muscle. Mice infected with the organism also show a generalized imbalance of energy metabolism (McCullum and Sword, 1972). It is highly likely that the hemolysin and lipolysin are responsible for the local tissue necrosis that surrounds foci of infection.

1.2. Epidemiology

Listeria has a worldwide distribution and is ubiquitous in nature. It has been isolated from at least 35 species of wild mammals and 17 species of birds, as well as from domestic, zoo, and laboratory animals and house pets (Gray, 1963). In addition, it is commonly found as a saprophyte in feces, silage, and vegetable matter (Weis and Seeliger, 1975).

Unfortunately, little is known about the epidemiology and epizoology of the disease. Outbreaks of listeriosis have been reported in groups of children in hospital wards (Line and Cherry, 1952; Levy and Nassau, 1960), and Seeliger (1957) has discussed the epidemiological significance of a large outbreak that occurred in a nursing school in East Germany. There are also documented examples of direct transfer of the disease from infected animals to man (Seeliger, 1957). Bojsen-Móller (1972) has drawn on the literature, as well as on his own extensive studies in Denmark, to show that a surprisingly high percentage of humans carry *L. monocytogenes* in their urogenital

tract and intestine, and excrete the organism in their feces. Indeed, the relatively low incidence of listeriosis in spite of the ubiquitous presence of *Listeria* in nature, and its presence in symptom-free animals and humans, is indicative of an opportunistic infection. The possibility should be kept in mind, furthermore, that the puzzling outbreaks of listeriosis in groups of apparently healthy individuals may be a consequence of "contagious immunosuppression." There is ample evidence to show (Woodruff and Woodruff, 1975) that subclinical infection with relatively benign viruses can cause severe suppression of the immune response. In fact, recent unpublished experiments by McGregor and collaborators in this Institute have shown that subclinical infection with Newcastle disease virus can cause a greatly increased susceptibility to *Listeria* infection in the rat, a species that is normally highly resistant to *Listeria* (Gray and Killinger, 1966).

1.3. Listeriosis in Animals

That listeriosis is responsible for commercial losses of livestock has been known for many years and is well documented by Jones and Woodbine (1961). The disease in ruminants causes encephalitis and abortion.

Listeria encephalitis in sheep was first reported by Gill in New Zealand in 1931, and by Jones and Little in cattle in New Jersey in 1934. Outbreaks have since been reported with great frequency from all parts of the world. The disease causes destruction of the meninges and the brain and is characterized by localized sites of infection and necrosis in both sites. Perivascular cuffing of small blood vessels by mononuclear cells is common. More extensive zones of necrosis develop as the disease progresses, and at this stage the pathogen can generally be isolated from the liver and other organs. Except for intracranial inoculation, most experimental attempts to produce encephalitis in laboratory animals have been unrewarding (Gray and Killinger, 1966).

Abortion commonly occurs late in gestation in sheep and during midterm in cattle. The aborted fetuses invariably are heavily infected. Liveborn young generally die of septicemia and of heavily infected internal organs. The mother, however, may show no apparent signs of illness, although the organism can be found in her reproductive tract. It has proved relatively easy to produce experimental abortion with *Listeria* in farm and laboratory animals. In appraising the published results obtained with cattle, sheep, goats, rabbits, rats, and guinea pigs, Gray and Killinger state (1966) that "regardless of animal species, stage of gestation, type of placenta, or route of exposure, the uterine contents quickly became infected." Their description (1966) of the results obtained with pregnant rabbits inoculated conjuctivally reveals that the doe may show no signs of symptoms except for a vaginal discharge that occurs after 2–4 days, depending on the stage of gestation. This is rapidly followed by either abortion or birth of heavily infected young. The finding that abortion may sometimes occur within 24 hr of conjunctival inoculation indicates that *Listeria* is well equipped to cross the placenta.

1.4. Human Listeriosis

It is generally agreed by those who have devoted years of work to the subject that human listeriosis is a greatly underrated disease. Gray and Killinger (1966) suggest that the apparent incidence of the disease is in direct proportion to the level of familiarity with the causative agent. Polk (1970) has pointed out that even though reporting listeriosis is not mandatory, the 125 cases of human listeriosis reported to the Center for Disease Control in 1969 outnumbered the number of cases of anthrax, botulism, leptospirosis, poliomyelitis, murine typhus, or trichinosis. It is significant that 20–30% of the cases reported in the United States involve infants in the first 4 weeks of life with most other cases occurring in people over 40 years. Busch (1971) quotes figures to show that the overall mortality rate between 1967 and 1969 was at least 18%, which means that listeriosis causes more deaths than many notifiable diseases. Similar statistics have been obtained in Great Britain, where 72 cases were reported between 1967 and 1969, of which 50% were in children less than 12 months of age. The mortality rate was 23%.

Busch (1971) lists the most common clinical manifestations of the disease in the United States as meningoencephalitis, abortion, conjunctivitis, endocarditis, pneumonitis, pyo-

derma, septicemia, and urethritis. Of the 104 clinical descriptions reported in 1971 in the United States, 75% dealt with cases of meningitis (Moore and Zehmer, 1973).

The pathology of listeriosis in humans is similar to that seen in animals and is adequately described by Seeliger (1957), Gray and Killinger (1966), and by Bojsen-Móller (1972) in particular. Listeriosis of the central nervous system can be meningitic, or encephalitic and myelitic. According to Gray and Killinger (1966) encephalitis is an extension of primary infection of the meninges. As in animals, the pathology is characterized by numerous foci of infection with surrounding zones of necrosis. Necrosis becomes more extensive as the disease progresses.

Listeria-induced abortion can occur in symptom-free women either early or late in gestation, but most commonly after the 4th month when the placenta is formed. The aborted fetuses display miliary listeriosis with extensive numbers of granulomas and areas of necrosis in internal organs, particularly in the liver. Liveborn infants may already show signs of the disease, including disseminated papules on the skin. Septicemia and involvement of the central nervous system are common. There seems general agreement that this form of the disease is contracted *in utero,* and in many cases the mothers of aborted fetuses show the presence of the organism in their cervix and vagina. It is interesting in this regard that Saxbe (1972) both on the basis of the evidence which shows that *Listeria* can be a cause of habitual abortion and from detailed readings of historical accounts has speculated that the failure of Queen Anne to produce a Protestant heir to the throne of England, in spite of 17 pregnancies, was the result of the persistent presence of *Listeria* in her reproductive tract.

Meningitis is the most common form of the disease during the first weeks of life. A recent paper by Visintine *et al.* (1977) describing a series of 22 cases of neonatal *Listeria* meningitis over a 14-year period lists fever, irritability, and anorexia as the most common symptoms. In almost all cases *Listeria* was cultured from the CSF. These workers emphasize the finding that the disease was associated, in most cases, with a pronounced increase in the number of monocytes circulating in blood, a symptom that was said to characterize the disease when it was first described in rabbits by Murray *et al.* in 1926. Unlike gram-negative bacterial meningitis of neonates, *Listeria* meningitis occurs predominantly after the 1st week of life, and sometimes as late as the 2nd month. This brings up the question of the mode of transmission from mother to offspring, and the possibility that the disease is contracted after birth.

Many investigators contend that listeriosis is an opportunistic infection, in that it mostly occurs in the very young, the aged, and patients with an underlying primary disease. Listeriosis has been reported as a complication in patients with Hodgkin's disease, malignant histiocytoma, lymphosarcoma, carcinoma of the breast and colon, acute and chronic leukemias, multiple myeloma, lupus erythematosus, cirrhosis, myocardial disease, and diabetes mellitus, and in patients given organ transplants (Buchner and Schneierson, 1968; Busch, 1971). Corticosteroid therapy also lowers resistance to *Listeria* infection (Johnson and Colley, 1969). However, Medoff *et al.* (1971) have questioned the opportunistic nature of liste- riosis on the basis of their experience with 11 patients, six of whom showed no signs of an underlying primary disease. Reports from the U.S. Disease Control Center also show that a large percentage of cases involved apparently healthy individuals.

1.5. Diagnosis

It is generally agreed that there is no satisfactory immunodiagnostic test for listeriosis. Distrust in serological tests is based on the numerous reports of false positives caused by antigens that are shared with a spectrum of other bacteria and also on numerous reports of high antibody titers in humans who have had no history of listeriosis.

Isolation and bacteriological identification are the only safe diagnostic procedures. The bacteriological procedures for identifying *Listeria* are set out in detail by Gray and Killinger (1966), Buchner and Schneierson (1968), and Bojsen-Moller (1972). Lack of familiarity with the bacteriological characteristics of the organism is blamed for underestimates of the frequency of the disease. This was well illustrated by Croft (1962), who sent cultures of *Listeria* as unknowns to 46 diagnostic laboratories with the result that 26 of them confused *Listeria* with other bacteria.

1.6. Immunity and Vaccination

Little is known about immunity to listeriosis in humans. Uncertainty about the meaning of a positive agglutination test makes it impossible to speculate about the possible importance of antibodies. Vaccines composed of killed bacteria have not been used in humans. If they had, it is highly likely that they would not have afforded any protection. A review of the veterinary literature led Jones and Woodbine (1961) to conclude that all attempts to protect animals with either "killed vaccines" or "immune serum" have been unsuccessful. The reasons for the ineffectiveness of vaccines now seems clear from the results of detailed studies of anti-*Listeria* immunity in rodents: studies that were performed with the primary aim of understanding the basic mechanisms of cell-mediated immunity to infection in general, with the goal of finding knowledge applicable to the disease in humans.

2. Rodent Listeriosis as a Model of Cell-Mediated Immunity to Infection

2.1. Immunity in Response to Infection

A review of the literature shows that all attempts to protect animals against *Listeria* infection with "killed" vaccines have failed. In contrast, laboratory animals that survive a living infection acquire a powerful mechanism of immunity that can protect against challenge with many lethal doses of the parasite (Osebold and Sawyer, 1957; Mackaness, 1962; Coppel and Youmans, 1969; North, 1975). An important property of this acquired immunity in the mouse, moreover, is that it is of relatively long duration. It was shown by Mackaness (1962), for instance, that mice which survive an immunizing infection remain immune to lethal challenge infection for about 3 months or more, although the immunity progressively wanes with time. These results were confirmed by North (1975), who showed, in addition, that the long-lived immunity is specific for the homologous organism. It is important to realize, furthermore, the anti-*Lis-*

teria immunity in the mouse lasts for a long time after the immunizing organism is completely eliminated from the tissues. Rodent listeriosis is an acute infection which does not result in a "carrier state" as does infection with certain other facultative, intracellular, bacterial parasites. Immunity persists, therefore, in the apparent absence of continuous antigenic stimulation.

Immunity that results from active infection is not mediated by humoral antibody. It has been shown convincingly that infusions of serum from immune mice have no effect on the capacity of normal recipients to modify the growth of a *Listeria* challenge infection (Osebold and Sawyer, 1957; Mackaness, 1962; Miki and Mackaness, 1964; Mackaness, 1969). Perhaps this is not surprising in view of the knowledge (Mackaness, 1962; North, 1975) that primary immunizing infection does not result in the generation of antibodies that can be detected by either direct agglutination or passive hemagglutination. Secondary infection, on the other hand, can result in the production of antibody (Mackaness, 1962; North, 1975), but of relatively low titer. In the case of the mouse, furthermore, it is apparent that all of the antibody produced in response to secondary infection is mercaptoethanol sensitive (North, 1975), thus indicating that it is all 19 S globulin. Failure to demonstrate a significant level of antibody production in response to primary infection has also been reported by those who have employed guinea pigs to study immunity to listeriosis (Fulton *et al.*, 1975). Nevertheless, primary infection in both species does result in the generation of an acquired, long-lasting state of specific immunological reactivity to the parasite, as evidenced by the development of a state of delayed-type hypersensitivity to its antigens. The significance of this functional indicator of cell-mediated immunity will be dealt with at a later stage of the discussion.

2.2. Macrophages as the Expressors of Immunity

Failure to demonstrate a role for humoral antibodies in anti-*Listeria* immunity prompted Mackaness (1962) to propose that the immunity is cellular in nature. This proposal was made against a background of evidence which favored the view that immunity to tuberculosis also is not mediated by humoral antibodies but is dependent instead on the acquisition of macrophages with greatly enhanced antibacterial resistance. Indeed, it was logical to hypothesize that the most likely way for a host to overcome infection with those bacteria that parasitize its phagocytic cells would be for it to acquire phagocytes with an intracellular environment that is hostile to the growth of these parasites. The evidence that such macrophages were acquired during *Mycobacteria* infection was supplied by Lurie (1942), Suter (1953), and Berthrong and Hamilton (1959), who showed that macrophages harvested from BCG-vaccinated animals could inhibit the growth of tubercle bacilli ingested *in vitro*.

The role of the macrophage in immunity to listeriosis in the mouse was revealed by an *in vitro* plaquing technique (Mackaness, 1962) which involved a comparison between listericidal activity of monolayers of peritoneal macrophages from immune and normal mice. The technique involved the preparation of pure macrophage monolayers and the complete removal of extracellular bacteria from the cultures after phagocytosis. The appearance in stationary 24-hr cultures of normal macrophages of large numbers of discrete plaques representing foci of infected cells showed that *Listeria* could survive in macrophages, multiply intracellularly, and infect neighboring cells. In contrast, very few plaques were seen to develop in immune macrophages. This evidence, together with the knowledge that both types of cells initially ingested the same number of bacteria, allowed the conclusion that the macrophages from immune animals had acquired potent intrinsic listericidal activity. It was also shown that the addition of "immune" serum to the cultures made no difference to bacterial inactivation (Mackaness, 1962; Ratzan *et al.*, 1972). These findings were essentially confirmed later in the guinea pig by Armstrong and Sword (1964) and in the mouse by Fauve *et al.* (1966), who followed the fate of *Listeria* by direct bacterial enumeration. The findings of Armstrong and Sword, however, revealed an additional important characteristic of the enhanced antibacterial mechanism of "immune" macrophages: that these cells had also acquired the capacity to destroy *Salmonella typhosa*. This led them to suggest that the immunity generated in response to *Listeria* infection is nonspecific and that the term "cellular resistance" rather than "cellular immunity" be used to describe it. The nonspecificity of the enhanced antibacterial activity of macrophages was later confirmed *in vitro* by others (Blanden, 1968).

In vivo experiments have also demonstrated that *Listeria*-immune mice display increased nonspecific resistance to heterologous bacteria. It was shown by North (1975) and North and Deissler (1975), for instance, that the acquisition by mice of the capacity to eliminate *Listeria* from their tissues is associated with a greatly enhanced capacity to inactivate intravenously injected *Salmonella enteritidis* and *Yersinia enterocolitica*. The nonspecific nature of anti-*Listeria* resistance, therefore, likens it to the nonspecific resistance generated in response to infection with *Mycobacteria, Brucella, Salmonella,* and other intracellular bacteria (see North, 1974b). The fact that mice infected with these organisms show a greatly increased resistance to *Listeria* infection represents additional evidence that macrophages play the key role in the expression of anti-*Listeria* immunity itself, since macrophages are the only cells known to be capable of expressing this type of enhanced nonspecific bactericidal activity.

It is noteworthy, however, that the increased bactericidal activity of macrophages acquired during *Listeria* infection is short-lived in relation to the length of time that the host remains immune to secondary infection. It was shown by North and Deissler (1975) that although very high levels of macrophage-expressed nonspecific resistance to heterologous bacteria are acquired during immunizing *Listeria* infection, this nonspecific resistance is lost soon after the immunizing infection is terminated. The timing of the decay of *in vivo* nonspecific resistance, furthermore, is concordant with the disappearance from the host of macrophages that can destroy *Listeria in vitro* (Mackaness, 1962). The significance of the short-lived nature of macrophage activation in terms of the overall response to infection will be discussed later.

It is also important to realize that increased bactericidal activity is not the only adaptive change that occurs in macrophages during *Listeria* infection. As might be expected, an increased capacity to destroy *Listeria* intracellularly is associated with a greatly enhanced capacity for phagocytosis. It was shown (North, 1969a) that peritoneal macrophages harvested from *Listeria*-infected mice display a greatly increased *in vitro* capacity for ingesting polystyrene latex particles. That this increased ingestive capacity was demonstrable with inert particles in the presence of heterologous serum shows that it is not dependent on serum opsonins but is dependent instead on an intrinsic physiological change in the cells. Again, the greatly increased phagocytic capacity of macrophages from *Listeria*-infected mice is at least partly related to their greatly increased capacity for spreading on either a glass or a plastic surface (North, 1969a, 1970a). Indeed, the striking speed at which *Listeria*-resistant macrophages spread on a substratum *in vitro* is one of their most notable characteristics. The fact that increased capacities for inactivating bacteria, phagocytosis, and spreading are acquired coincidentally (North, 1969a; Ratzan *et al.* 1972) has led to the choice of the general term "macrophage activation" to describe the adaptive modulatory changes that occur in these cells during infection. Needless to say, macrophage activation occurs in response to infection with a range of intracellular parasites (Ruskin *et al.,* 1969; North, 1974b). The fact that this equips the host to resist infection nonspecifically with a range of unrelated parasites is of obvious survival value.

2.3. Mobilization of Macrophages

While increased bactericidal activity of macrophages is ultimately responsible for the elimination of *Listeria* from the host, this end is greatly aided by augmentation of macrophage numbers in infected tissues. It is well to realize, moreover, that in order for immunity to be expressed it is necessary that macrophages be focused in adequate numbers at sites of bacterial implantation. The evidence suggests that the host increases the number of macrophages in infected tissues in two ways: (1) by increasing the rate of replication of those macrophages already resident in its tissues and (2) by directing the entry into the tissues of its pool of mobile macrophages from blood. These two events have been studied in the liver; the organ which becomes most heavily infected.

That macrophages of the liver (Kuppfer cells) possess a large potential for division was clearly shown by Kelly *et al.* (1962), who employed tritiated thymidine ([^{3}H]-TdR) to radiolabel specifically macrophages synthesizing DNA *in situ* in response to injections of endotoxin and other agents. That this potential for replication is expressed vigorously during the course of *Listeria* infection was revealed by North (1969b), who followed changes in the level of [^{3}H]-TdR incorporated into liver DNA at progressive times of infection. It was found that a large increase in [^{3}H]-TdR incorporation occurred in the liver between 24 and 48 hr of infection and that the amount of radiolabel incorporated from a single pulse of the compound slowly decayed thereafter. Autoradiographs of sections of the same livers revealed that increased [^{3}H]-TdR incorporation was associated with a striking increase in the number of labeled cells in sinusoids. The labeled cells, moreover, were relatively large and closely opposed to the walls of sinusoids, thus indicating that they were Kuppfer cells. Their identity as Kuppfer cells was further evidenced by the demonstration that they were phagocytic and were resident in the liver long before infection was initiated. It was shown, for instance, that most of the cells dividing on the 2nd day of infection could be physiologically marked 2 weeks before infection by an intravenous injection of colloidal carbon. Electron microscopy of autoradiographs (North, 1974b) of liver sections furnished additional evidence that the dividing cells were resident macrophages in that they all possessed a mature cytoplasm with phagosomes containing large quantities of colloidal carbon. It was clear that the labeled cells were structurally different from the poorly phagocytic, fenestrated, endothelial cells which line the walls of sinusoids.

Macrophages in the peritoneal cavity also demonstrate a burst of mitotic activity during *Listeria* infection. Pulse labeling with [^{3}H]-TdR (North, 1969a) revealed that macrophages in the peritoneal cavity showed a large increase in division between 24 and 48 hr of infection, i.e., at the same time as macrophages in the liver. It was possible to conclude, furthermore, that the replicating peritoneal cells were resident macrophages by showing that they could be physiologically marked by an intraperitoneal injection of polystyrene latex particles given 2 weeks before infection.

It is clear, then, that the response to listeriosis in the mouse includes a striking augmentation in the number of macrophages in infected tissues as a result of division by tissue macrophages. The possible importance of this source of new macrophages to the expression of acquired resistance is indicated by the knowledge (North, 1969a) that increased macrophage division precedes immediately the onset of elimination of *Listeria* from the tissue and is associated with the acquisition of nonspecific resistance to other infectious agents. It occurs, moreover, at a time when the host is first capable of expressing delayed-type hypersensitivity to the antigens of the parasite.

It is doubtful, nevertheless, whether the expansion of the liver macrophage population by local division is essential for the elimination of a low-level immunizing infection from this organ. This is indicated by the additional finding (North, 1970b) that suppression of macrophage replication by local X irradiation of the liver did not result in a slower rate of bacterial elimination from this organ. The expansion of the resident macrophage population undoubtedly represents an adaptive change that serves to guard against the threat of bacteremia and concurrent infections with other bacteria. Macrophage division can be considered an additional parameter of macrophage activation.

Even so, an increase in the number of tissue macrophages is not in itself enough to eliminate *Listeria* from the tissues. In order for the host to achieve this end it is essential that it focus its macrophages at sites of bacterial implantation and multiplication. Rodent listeriosis, like the disease in humans, is characterized by the development of large numbers of infective foci in internal organs. Presumably, these discrete but expanding areas of infection represent the sites of initial bacterial implantation in susceptible fixed macrophages. In the liver, the most heavily infected organ, it is apparent that the parasite escapes from susceptible fixed phagocytes and rapidly crosses the sinusoid wall to infect neighboring parenchymal cells in which it multiplies extensively (North, 1970b). By 24 hr, infective foci are characterized by areas of heavily infected and disintegrating parenchymal cells infiltrated with polymorphonuclear leukocytes. However, these latter cells, in spite of their large numbers, appear to serve little purpose in restricting bacterial growth. This is evidenced by the findings that they also become replete with bacteria and are present during the time when the bacterial load in the liver is increasing rapidly. It is not until about 48 hr of infection that the host shows signs of controlling bacterial growth, an event associated with a progressive accumulation in infective foci of mononuclear phagocytes. A knowledge of the properties of these particular macrophages, therefore, is important for an understanding of the expression of resistance to *Listeria*.

It is known from pulse-labeling studies with [³H]-TdR (Volkman and Gowans, 1965) that blood monocytes are the progeny of a rapidly dividing population of precursor cells in bone marrow. They are constantly released into blood, where they circulate with a half-life of 22 hr in the mouse (van Furth and Cohn, 1968) and 72 hr in the rat (Volkman, 1966), before being lost randomly by mechanisms that remain unknown. A single pulse of [³H]-TdR given to mice (van Furth and Cohn, 1968) results in a rapid and progressive release of radiolabeled monocytes into the blood, in that by 48 hr as many as 60% of the total circulating monocytes are labeled. By timing correctly the injection of a pulse of [³H]-TdR with the induction of an inflammatory response, it can be shown that blood monocytes are the major source of macrophages that populate sites of inflammation (Volkman and Gowans, 1965; Spector and Coote, 1965; van Furth and Cohn, 1968). On the basis of this information, it was predicted that blood monocytes would be found to be the source of macrophages that populate sites of *Listeria* infection in the liver.

North (1970b) showed that an intravenous pulse of [³H]-TdR given several hours before intravenous infection with *Listeria* resulted 48 hr later in a progressive accumulation of radiolabeled DNA in the infected liver. It was obvious from the design of the experiment that this DNA came from an extrahepatic source. Autoradiographs of sections of the same livers revealed that most of the label was associated with large numbers of typical macrophages in infective foci, although some labeled cells were also present in the sinusoids at large. The

progessive accumulation of labeled macrophages at infective sites, moreover, was associated with the onset of progressive elimination of bacteria from the liver. Thus it was concluded that blood monocytes are the antecedents of the majority of macrophages which express anti-*Listeria* immunity at infective foci.

It should be realized, in this connection, that all of the published *in vitro* studies which show that anti-*Listeria* immunity is expressed by macrophages were performed with tissue macrophages that, under normal circumstances, may never be given the opportunity to express immunity *in vivo*. In all cases the macrophages were harvested from the unstimulated peritoneal cavity, a compartment in the mouse that rarely contains bacteria during sublethal intravenous infection. In view of the knowledge that the mediation of macrophage activation is likely to be a local rather than a systemic event (see later), it is probable that the most highly activated macrophages exist in infective foci.

In summary, then, the expression of resistance to experimental infection with *Listeria monocytogenes* relies on the generation of adaptive changes in macrophages. These changes include the acquisition of enhanced antibacterial mechanisms by individual macrophages which enable these cells to ingest bacteria at a faster rate and to destroy them rapidly after they are interiorized. The acquisition of these antibacterial properties is associated, furthermore, with a striking augmentation in the number of macrophages in infected tissues. This is achieved both by vigorous division of resident macrophages in the tissues and by the emigration and accumulation of monocytes from blood. Because of their superior numbers in infective foci, it is almost certain that monocyte-derived macrophages are the actual effectors of immunity. On the other hand, the large buildup of macrophages in the tissues at large represents almost surely a reserve mechanism that serves to protect against possible increases in bacterial numbers. Nevertheless, without a continuous mobile source of blood monocytes, the host is unable to express resistance, in spite of the presence of increased numbers of activated macrophages in its reticuloendothelial system. Recent unpublished observations in this laboratory provide evidence which shows that interruption of blood monocyte production as a result of sublethal γ-irradiation results in an immediate resumption of bacterial growth in the liver. This occurs, even though the enhanced antibacterial activity of fixed macrophages, as measured by the initial kill of an intravenous *Listeria* challenge, remains essentially intact.

2.4. Immunological Basis of Acquired Immunity

The nonspecific resistance to heterologous bacteria that is associated with the acquisition of anti-*Listeria* resistance has led some investigators to suggest that anti-*Listeria* resistance is acquired nonimmunologically. Of course, if this suggestion is correct, then it would also apply to the resistance generated against other intracellular parasites including *M. tuberculosis*. Until fairly recently, moreover, the only evidence for hypothesizing that cellular immunity to infection is based on an underlying immune response was that its generation is invariably associated with the development of a state of delayed-type hypersensitivity to antigens of the infecting organisms. The functional role of delayed sensitivity, however, still remains obscure, in spite of the current favored practice of equating it with cellular immunity.

It was not until Mackaness (1964) examined the question of specificity that the immunological basis of anti-*Listeria* immunity was revealed. This worker showed that although the acquisition of immunity in mice is accompanied by the development of an enhanced capacity to resist infection with heterologous bacteria nonspecificially, this nonspecific resistance decays rapidly and can be regenerated only in an accelerated fashion by reinfecting the host with the homologous organism. This was interpreted to mean that nonspecific resistance, as expressed by macrophages, is a by-product of an underlying specific immune response that can be regenerated anamnestically only by reexposure to specific bacterial antigens. A similar conclusion was reached later by Coppel and Youmans (1969), who showed that although immunizing infection with *Listeria* resulted in an increased nonspecific resistance to heterologous bacteria, it was only resistance to the homologous organism which was long-lived. The meaning of these results in terms of immunological memory will be discussed later.

2.5. Thymus-Derived Lymphocytes as the Mediators of Immunity

The direct demonstration that anti-*Listeria* immunity is cell mediated was accomplished by Mackaness (1969), who showed that a high level of anti-*Listeria* immunity could be passively transferred to normal recipient mice with spleen cells, but not with serum, from convalescing donors. It was found, in addition, that the spleen cells needed to be viable and that they were no longer protective after incubation with heterologous antilymphocyte serum and complement (Mackaness and Hill, 1969). This demonstration led to the conclusion that although anti-*Listeria* immunity is expressed by activated macrophages, the activation of these effector cells is mediated by a population of specifically sensitized lymphocytes. The expression of adoptive immunity within 24 hr of cell transfer indicated, furthermore, that the mediation of macrophage activation by sensitized lymphocytes is a rapid process. This evidence for the cell-mediated nature of anti-*Listeria* immunity was strongly supported by the subsequent demonstration (McGregor *et al.*, 1971) of its passive transfer with thoracic duct lymphocytes in the rat.

That sensitized, thymus-derived lymphocytes (T cells) are the mediators of anti-*Listeria* immunity has been demonstrated in three separate laboratories with the use of AKR anti-C3Hθ serum, which, in the presence of complement, specifically lyses the T cells of most strains of mice. It was shown (Lane and Unanue, 1972; Blanden and Langman, 1972; North, 1973a) that the capacity of immune spleen cells from *Listeria*-immune mice to immunize normal recipients adoptively was completely ablated by incubating the spleen cells with anti-θ serum and complement. Thus, in keeping with the present-day accepted definition, anti-*Listeria* immunity is T cell-mediated.

In view of this information, it was surprising to find that adult mice (North, 1973a) and rats (McGregor *et al.*, 1973) which had been made substantially T cell-deficient as a result of thymectomy and lethal ionizing radiation, and protected with bone marrow cells, could handle a sublethal *Listeria* infection as efficiently as normal mice. A partial explanation for this apparent contradiction is represented by the additional finding that these same animals contained a residual T-cell population, in that a relatively low level of adoptive immunity to normal recipients could still be transferred passively with cells. Indeed, it has been reported (Cheers and Waller, 1975) that T-cell-deficient mice can display a compensatory "nonspecific" activation of their macrophage systems that gives them an even greater than normal capacity for inactivating *Listeria*. It should be noted, however, that those workers (Emmerling *et al.*, 1975) who had the foresight to carry experimentation over an adequate period of time have shown that although T-cell-deficient mice display normal or above normal anti-*Listeria* activity during the early period of infection, they are unable to completely eliminate *Listeria* from their tissues. This results in an otherwise acute infection developing into a chronic infection. It should be pointed out, in addition, that the increased anti-*Listeria* activity possessed by T-cell-deficient mice, as well as by lethally irradiated, bone-marrow-restored mice (Campbell *et al.*, 1974; Cheers and Waller, 1975), is nonspecific. For this reason its presence is no more surprising than the increased anti-*Listeria* activity that exists in mice infected with *M. tuberculosis* or other microorganisms. Any procedure that results in macrophage activation also results in nonspecific resistance to *Listeria* as well as other bacteria. It is known, furthermore, that this nonspecific component of resistance cannot be passively transferred with lymphocytes. Because *Listeria* is exquisitely sensitive to inactivation by macrophages, T-cell-deficient mice with compensatory macrophage activation may not be suitable tools for analyzing anti-*Listeria* immunity or immunity to other parasites that are easily destroyed by macrophages.

2.6. Kinetics of Production of Mediator T Cells

An analytical investigation of the fundamental nature of the mechanisms of cellular immunity must be based on a knowledge of the rate of its generation and decay. In the absence of such points of reference there is no way of determining the stage of the immune response that is being analyzed. The time course of production of the cells that mediate active immunity to an immunizing *Listeria* infection was followed by North (1973b). Based on the knowledge that the level of adoptive immunity expressed by recipient mice is directly proportional to the number of mediator cells infused (North and Spitalny, 1974), North showed that cells capable of adoptively immunizing normal recipients against lethal challenge appeared in the spleen as early as day 2 of infection, rapidly increased in number to peak on day 6, and then progressively declined in number over the following 2 weeks. A small number of protective cells persisted in the spleen after this time. It was further shown (North, 1973b) that the phase of progressive production of protective lymphocytes over the first 6 days was associated with corresponding progressive increases in the cellularity of the spleen, the number of θ-positive T cells, and the number of T cells engaged in DNA synthesis. The subsequent progressive decay of production of protective T cells, on the other hand, was associated with a concordant decay of all of these parameters. It was logical to propose, therefore, that the production of protective T cells is based on vigorous cell division and that these cells are not sustained in adequate numbers in the absence of cell division.

2.7. Properties and Functions of Mediator T Cells

The characteristics of the T cells that mediate anti-*Listeria* immunity have been studied in both the mouse and the rat. Because of the relative ease of cannulating the thoracic duct of the rat, it is in this species that the recirculating properties of mediator cells have been studied. It was revealed by McGregor *et al.* (1971), for instance, that cells capable of immunizing normal recipients adoptively appear in the thoracic duct lymph by the 7th day of subcutaneous immunizing infection. It was further shown that the entry of these cells into central lymph is associated with the simultaneous entry of large lymphoid blast cells. Again, by employing intermediate recipient rats, it was possible to demonstrate that intravenously infused mediator cells do not return from blood back to central lymph. These cells appear to differ, therefore, from the majority of small lymphocytes which are known to constantly circulate between these two fluid compartments.

Another property of the mediator cells is their sensitivity to corticosteroids. North (1972) demonstrated that an injection of cortisone acetate at the time of peak production of these cells in the spleen results in a rapid, striking loss from this organ of cells capable of immunizing normal recipients adoptively. The loss of protective cells was associated, moreover, with an equally striking reduction in the total cellularity of the spleen. It is highly likely, therefore, that the increased susceptibility of corticosteroid-treated mice to *Listeria* infection (Miller and Heberg, 1965; North, 1971), as well as to infection with other intracellular parasites, is the result of destruction of the T cells that mediate immunity. The recent claim by Zinkernagel and Doherty (1975) that mediator T cells in the spleen are resistant to corticosteroids must be considered with the realization that their assay system was not based on a comparison between the immunity transferred with the total number of mediator cells in the spleens of control and cortisone-treated animals but rather on immunity transferred per given number of cells. Consequently, a huge loss of cortisone-sensitive T cells could have gone undetected.

A further characteristic of the cellular mediators of immunity is that most of them are actively dividing. Direct evidence that the mediator cells belong to a replicating population was obtained by employing the antimitotic drug vinblastine, which is known to ablate resistance to *Listeria* infection in mice (North, 1970c) and to destroy selectively cells dividing *in vivo*. It was shown in the rat (McGregor and Logie, 1973) that an *in vivo* pulse of vinblastine resulted in a rapid depletion of protective lymphocytes from thoracic duct lymph of 5-day-infected donors. Likewise, a 15-hr pulse of vinblastine was found to eliminate almost completely protective T cells from the spleens of infected mice at peak response (North, 1973b).

This rapidly dividing population of protective T cells also has a short functional life span.

Such a short life span is suggested by the observation that their number in the spleen (North, 1973b) and elsewhere (North and Spitalny, 1974) declines rapidly and progressively after they reach peak production, when *Listeria* is being eliminated efficiently from the tissues. Their short life span is best evidenced, however, by the short-lived nature of adoptive anti-*Listeria* immunity. North (1974a) showed that while an intravenous infusion of mediator T cells results in the adoptive transfer to normal recipients of high levels of immunity to a *Listeria* challenge, this immunity decays rapidly over a 48-hr period and all but disappears by 96 hr. Although the fate of passively transferred protective T cells is not known, it seems reasonable to conclude that, as far as host immunity is concerned, most of these cells become functionally inert within 4 days. A similar conclusion has been reached about the mediators of antiallograft immunity (Sprent, 1976).

A remaining functional characteristic of mediator T cells that needs to be discussed is their propensity for entering sites of inflammation. Indeed, it is becoming increasingly evident (Asherson and Allwood, 1972) that the T cells that mediate all examples of cellular immunity possess the capacity to detect and enter those sites of tissue injury which contain the target antigens to which the T cells have been sensitized. In the case of listeriosis it is generally believed that sensitized T cells must enter foci of infection in order to mediate the local activation of the monocyte-derived macrophages that express immunity.

The propensity of the T-cell mediators of anti-*Listeria* immunity for entering sites of inflammation was studied by Koster *et al.* (1971), who showed that there was an enrichment of protective cells in sterile peritoneal exudates of infected rats. They also showed that the entry of these cells was nonspecific. Some of the factors that govern the emigration of mediator T cells into peritoneal inflammation were revealed in the mouse by North and Spitalny (1974), who showed that their entry into exudates was proportional to the prevailing level of their production in the spleen, with the largest number of cells accumulating in exudates induced at the time of peak production on day 6 of infection. It was also found that an intraperitoneal injection of casein at any stage of infection resulted in the continuous accumulation of protective T cells for a 3-day period, after which their number in the peritoneal cavity declined progressively. The 3-day period of accumulation, however, was shown not to be the result of continuous entry of protective T cells for the whole of this period. It was caused, instead, by the division of a small number of dividing cells that entered only during the first 24 hr. Presumably, then, these cells cross the endothelium of small blood vessels only during the acute phase of the inflammatory response.

That inflammation acts to attract and concentrate protective T cells is also well illustrated by the finding (North and Spitalny, 1974) that, at any given time after infection, the total number of protective T cells present in a 48-hr inflammatory exudate is capable of transferring passively the samel level of adoptive immunity as the total number of protective T cells in the spleen. On a cell-for-cell basis, moreover, peritoneal exudate cells were shown to be at least 6 times more efficient than spleen cells. It should be pointed out, however, that the peritoneal cavities of infected mice receive a small number of protective T cells in the apparent absence of either inflammation or local infection. The cells are present in numbers that are proportional to the prevailing level of their production in the spleen. It is possible, therefore, that these cells are physiologically adapted to pervade constantly all tissues in small numbers in the absence of inflammation.

2.8. T-Cell Mediation of Macrophage Activation

The most important function of *Listeria*-sensitized T cells is to mediate the mobilization and activation of macrophages. There is no evidence to show that sensitized T cells by themselves possess the capacity to inactivate *Listeria*. Indeed, the many unpublished attempts in this laboratory to demonstrate such a capacity *in vitro* have been completely unsuccessful. On the other hand, there is convincing *in vitro* evidence that macrophages from *Listeria*-immune animals possess potent listericidal activity. The need for macrophages in the expression of immunity is also indicated by experiments with adoptive immunization

which have shown that adoptive immunity cannot be expressed in recipients that have been treated with agents known to suppress the recipients' production of mobile macrophages (Tripathy and Mackaness, 1969; McGregor and Koster, 1971; North and Mackaness, 1973).

Direct evidence for the lymphocyte mediation of macrophage activation *in vivo* comes from experiments (North and Mackaness, 1973) demonstrating that infusion of *Listeria*-sensitized T cells into *Listeria*-challenged recipients results in a strikingly accelerated increase in the onset of macrophage division in the recipient's livers. This type of increased macrophage division *in vivo* was examined later by Izumi *et al.* (1975) in mice with delayed hypersensitivity to soluble protein antigens. These workers showed that increased macrophage division could be achieved by infusing normal mice with the by-products (lymphokines) of an *in vitro* reaction between sensitized lymphocytes and specific antigen. More recently, Hadden *et al.* (1975) have demonstrated that lymphokines produced in a similar way can trigger macrophages to divide *in vitro*.

In fact, there is now ample *in vitro* evidence to support the hypothesis that the activation of macrophages by specifically sensitized lymphocytes is achieved by way of the action of soluble mediators. It is perhaps unfortunate for the sake of this discussion, however, that although *Listeria* has been used as a tool for detecting macrophage activation *in vitro*, none of the experiments was designed with the primary aim of analyzing anti-*Listeria* immunity *per se*. The basic finding of Simon and Sheagren (1972) that lymphocytes from animals with delayed sensitivity, when incubated with specific antigen *in vitro*, secrete soluble factors that trigger the acquisition of enhanced listericidal activity by macrophages *in vitro* has been confirmed on many occasions (Krahenbuhl *et al.*, 1973; Middlebrook *et al.*, 1974; Jones and Youmans, 1974, Bast *et al.*, 1974; Cole, 1975). This type of experimentation has also been used to show (Nathan *et al.*, 1973) that the *in vitro* activation of macrophages is associated with an increase in their metabolic activity. It was found in all of the cases, moreover, that the production and secretion of soluble mediators do not take place in the absence of specific antigen. It seems reasonable to propose, therefore, that the greatest concentrations of lymphokines in the *Listeria*-infected host are present within foci of infection, since it is only at these sites that replicating antigen, lymphocytes, and macrophages exist in close proximity.

2.9. Immunological Memory

A major adaptive function of the primary response to a pathogenic microorganism is to equip the host for a protracted period of time with a heightened immunological potential for responding more vigorously to a second encounter with the same or antigenically related microorganisms. The characteristics of this state of immunological memory have been fairly well characterized for humoral immunity, where it is known that immunological memory can be carried by both T cells and B cells and that memory cells are functionally distinct from antibody-forming cells. The adaptive significance of antibody memory is well illustrated by the proven efficacy of many antiviral vaccines.

The nature of memory in cell-mediated immunity, however, is not so well defined. The demonstration that a memory system is generated during the primary immune response to allografts has required the use of *in vitro* models. It was shown by Cerottini *et al.* (1974), for instance, that the generation of cytotoxic effector T lymphocytes that results from a mixed lymphocyte reaction *in vitro* occurs earlier, and reaches higher levels sooner, when the responding lymphocytes are obtained from the spleens of mice that have been specifically immunized to alloantigens 2–4 months previously. These workers showed, in addition, that memory cells are produced as a result of *in vitro* exposure of lymphocytes to alloantigens. In this cell-mediated system, then, immunological memory can be defined as the acquired capacity to respond to a second encounter with antigen by a more rapid and vigorous production of sensitized, cytotoxic, effector T cells. It is analogous, therefore, to antibody memory, which is expressed as an accelerated production of antibody-forming (effector) B cells.

The expression of memory in cell-mediated anti-*Listeria* immunity appears to be similar to the expression of memory in cell-mediated antiallograft immunity. It was shown convincingly, by the technique of adoptive immunization (North, 1975), that the protracted period of specific immunity to lethal secondary infection displayed by mice surviving a primary immunizing infection is based on an acquired capacity to generate protective mediator T cells faster, and, if need be, in much larger numbers than normal mice do. The mediator cells generated in response to secondary infection were shown to possess the same characteristics as those produced in response to primary infection. In both cases they were replicating θ-positive T cells. An important finding (North, 1975) was that the magnitude of expression of memory depends on the size of the secondary challenge infection, and hence on the level of secondary antigenic stimulation. Indeed, it was found that although immunized mice challenged with a sublethal immunizing infection showed an accelerated production of protective T cells, they actually produced fewer of these cells in the long run than did nonimmunized mice. An examination of the growth curves of the challenge organism in these two groups of mice revealed, however, that while it grew appreciably for 48 hr in normal mice to supply adequate antigenic stimulation before being progressively eliminated, it did not grow at all in immunized mice. This can be interpreted to mean that the generation of mediator T cells is driven by specific antigen and that the generation of these cells ceases when the level of antigenic stimulation falls below a threshold level.

2.10. Active Immunity and Immunological Memory

It was shown by North and Deissler (1975) that primary immunizing infection with *L. monocytogenes* results in the sequential generation of two distinct states of immunological reactivity (Fig. 1). There are generated (1) a short-lived state of active immunity that functions to eliminate urgently the infecting organism from the tissues and (2) a long-lived state of heightened immunological potential (memory) which enables the host to generate a more vigorous and protective state of active immunity in response to secondary infection. It is the state of primary active immunity to infection which has involved most of the

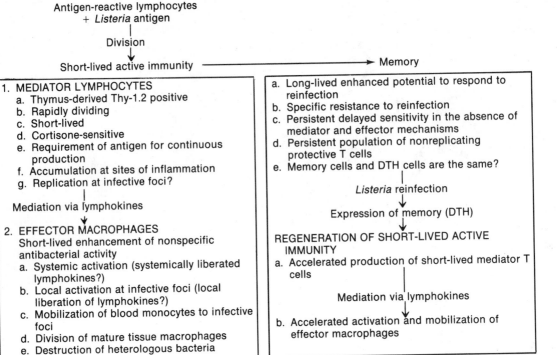

Figure 1. Cell-mediated anti-*Listeria* immunity.

preceding pages of this chapter. This state is characterized by the production of adequate numbers of mediator T cells and effector macrophages which function to eliminate *Listeria* from the tissues completely in about 10 days or more. Active immunity ends, then, when it is no longer needed, and its termination is characterized by the loss of those cells which mediate and express it. Indeed, the short functional life span of mediator T cells would ensure their rapid disappearance soon after the antigen that stimulates their production is destroyed. Moreover, in the absence of mediator T cells there is no mechanism to sustain macrophage activation, which rapidly decays in turn to normal levels (North and Deissler, 1975).

The generation of a secondary state of active immunity involves the production of the same types of cells, except that peak production is reached 2 days earlier and the infecting organism is consequently eliminated much sooner. Because the host already possesses large numbers of mediator and effector cells, it ob-

viously possesses the greatest capacity to resist a secondary infection during the state of active immunity. In fact, a *Listeria* challenge inoculum given during active immunity is immediately eliminated without having a chance to multiply, in contrast to the same challenge inoculum given during the state of memory when a brief period of growth occurs before a secondary state of active immunity is generated to sterilize the tissues. It is only during the state of active immunity that the host displays resistance to infection with heterologous bacteria.

The state of memory is not associated with the presence of a population of replicating mediator T cells or an activated macrophage system. It is associated, instead, with the presence of a small and persistent population of nonreplicating protective T cells that can transfer passively the capacity to respond anamnestically to normal recipients (North and Deissler, 1975). It is also associated with a persistent state of delayed cutaneous sensitivity to *Listeria* antigens.

2.11. Delayed-Type Hypersensitivity

The close association between immunity to certain disease-forming microorganisms and a state of specific delayed sensitivity to antigens of these organisms has been known for many years. That a delayed-sensitivity reaction is characterized by a mononuclear cell infiltration dependent on the generation of an inflammatory response qualitatively distinct from that which results in acute sensitivity reactions has also been appreciated for a long time (Bloom and Chase, 1967). Indeed, the demonstration in 1942 by Landsteiner and Chase that delayed sensitivity, unlike immediate sensitivity, can be passively transferred with living lymphoid cells, but not with serum, represented the first evidence for the existence of a mechanism of cell-mediated immunity as distinct from humoral immunity. However, in spite of the very large number of publications on the subject since that time, the functional significance of delayed sensitivity remains obscure, in spite of the favored practice of employing the term as a synonym for cell-mediated immunity. Indeed, the earlier claim by Rich (1941) that delayed sensitivity to the tubercle bacillus aids the disease process rather than host immunity has not been disproved, despite claims to the contrary. In the same vein, the flood of publications which claim that *in vitro* correlates of delayed sensitivity represent evidence for the possession of a state of cellular immunity are devoid of functional explanation.

As is the case with immunity to most intracellular bacterial parasites, the generation of anti-*Listeria* immunity is associated with the concordant generation of a state of delayed sensitivity. This capacity to express delayed reactions to cutaneous injections of soluble *Listeria* antigens occurs, moreover, in the apparent absence of circulating antibodies (Mackaness, 1962; North and Deissler, 1975) and can be transferred passively from immunized mice to normal recipients with θ-positive T cells (Youdim *et al.,* 1973), but not with serum. It has been shown in addition (North, 1973b) that the generation of delayed sensitivity parallels exactly the generation of the T cells that can transfer passively anti-*Listeria* immunity to normal recipients. Thus it peaks at the time of peak active immunity. Unlike active immunity, however, the state of delayed sensitivity is relatively long-lived both in the mouse (North and Deissler, 1975) and in the guinea pig (Fulton *et al.,* 1975). Indeed, it persists for the duration of immunological memory, and it can be transferred passively (North, unpublished) with nonreplicating T cells, as has been shown with other models of delayed sensitivity (Lagrange and Mackaness, 1975; Bloom *et al.,* 1964). This is not to say, however, that it cannot be transferred with the replicating T cells that are present during the state of active immunity. Instead, it appears that unlike active immunity, which can be transferred only with dividing, short-lived T cells, delayed sensitivity can also be transferred with both types of T cells. It seems reasonable to propose, therefore, that the cells which carry immunological memory are the same cells that are responsible for delayed sensitivity and that a delayed-sensitivity reaction is a local manifestation of immunological memory of the T-cell-mediated type. This seems to be the only adaptive function that this protracted state of sensitivity would have evolved to serve.

3. Summary and Conclusions

Evidence has been presented to show that active immunity in rodents to infection with the facultative intracellular parasite *Listeria monocytogenes,* although expressed by activated macrophages, is mediated by a population of short-lived, replicating, thymus-derived lymphocytes (T cells). The evidence is consistent with the hypothesis that the adaptive modulatory changes that result in the enhanced listericidal activity of macrophages are mediated by sensitized T cells by way of soluble mediators. Moreover, the macrophage component of the response not only involves the acquisition of enhanced antibacterial mechanisms by individual macrophages but also involves a striking augmentation in the number of these cells in infected tissues. This is achieved by an increase in the rate of replication of resident tissue macrophages and by an influx of monocytes from blood. It is the mobile monocyte-derived macrophages, however, which are mainly responsible for the expression of immunity at infective foci.

The complete elimination of *Listeria* from the tissues by activated macrophages within 2 weeks is followed by a protracted state of heightened resistance to reinfection which lasts for at least 3 months. It was shown that this state of long-lived immunity does not depend on the persistence of activated macrophages but depends instead on an acquired capacity of the host to reactivate its macrophage system immunologically in an accelerated fashion. It was suggested that the anti-*Listeria* response can be interpreted as resulting in two distinct states of immunological reactivity: (1) a short-lived state of active immunity that is mediated by short-lived T cells and expressed by activated macrophages and that functions to eliminate rapidly the infecting organism from the tissues and (2) a long-lived state of immunological memory that is carried by nonreplicating, long-lived T cells and that enables the host to regenerate a state of active immunity more vigorously and at a faster tempo. Since activated macrophages are present only during active immunity, it is only during this short-lived state that the host displays nonspecific resistance to infection with heterologous bacteria—hence the futility of using macrophage-mediated, nonspecific antibacterial resistance alone as a measure of specific cell-mediated immunity (Schell *et al.*, 1974). It is suggested that failure to appreciate the existence of a state of immunological memory as distinct from active immunity, when designing *in vivo* and *in vitro* experiments to analyze cell-mediated immunity, can result in the publication of conflicting results from different laboratories. The existence of these two immune states should also be taken into account when designing procedures for testing the efficacy of antibacterial vaccines. Again, it seems highly likely that some of the confusion about the functional significance of delayed-type hypersensitivity (Lefford, 1975) is the result of a failure to realize that, like immunological memory, the state of delayed sensitivity persists long after the cells that mediate and effect active immunity have disappeared. Indeed, it is suggested on this basis that the capacity to express cutaneous delayed sensitivity is an indicator of the possession of immunological memory of the T-cell-mediated type.

While a relatively large amount is known about immunity to listeriosis in rodents, practically nothing is known about immunity to the disease in humans. In the light of the increasing pragmatic nature of basic research, therefore, it may well be asked whether knowledge about rodent listeriosis is applicable to man. Obviously, those who would pose this question would also be questioning most of the basic knowledge about immunology, since it has been mainly obtained from experiments in rodents. It could be suggested on the basis of the evidence which points to listeriosis as being an opportunistic infection, however, that most humans are innately resistant to the organism. But so are laboratory animals. Even mice, in which most experiments have been performed, show no outward clinical signs of the disease during infection, even during the time when *Listeria* is multiplying rapidly in their tissues. In fact, normal mice possess enough innately resistant macrophages to inactivate 50–60% of an intravenous *Listeria* inoculum in less than 12 hr (North *et al.*, 1976). Rats are even more resistant (Gray and Killinger, 1966) and can be killed only by inoculating them with a ridiculously large number of bacteria (North, unpublished). Yet both species eliminate *Listeria* by generating sensitized T cells and activated macrophages. It seems reasonable to propose, therefore, that most humans who contract listeriosis overcome the disease by generating T-cell-mediated immunity before clinical signs become manifest and that it is only in those individuals who are unable to generate this type of immunity that the disease takes on a progressive course.

References

Armstrong, A. S., and Sword, C. P., 1964, Cellular resistance in listeriosis, *J Infect. Dis.* **114:**258–264.

Asherson, G. L., and Allwood, G. G., 1972, Inflammatory lymphoid cells in immunized lymph nodes that move to sites of inflammation, *Immunology* **22:**493–502.

Bast, R. C., Cleveland, R. P., Littman, B. H., Zbar, B., and Rapp, H. J., 1974, Acquired cellular immunity: Extracellular killing of *Listeria monocytogenes* by a product of immunologically activated macrophages, *Cell. Immunol.* **10**:248–259.

Berthrong, M., and Hamilton, M. A., 1959,Tissue culture studies on resistance in tuberculosis. II. Monocytes from normal and immunized guinea pigs infected with virulent human tubercle bacilli, *Am. Rev. Tuberc.* **79**:221–230.

Blanden, R. V., 1968, Modification of macrophage function, *J. Reticuloendothel. Soc.* **5**:179–202.

Blanden, R. V., and Langman, R. E., 1972,Cell-mediated immunity to bacterial infection in the mouse: Thymus-derived cells as effectors of acquired resistance to *Listeria monocytogenes, Scand. J. Immunol.* **1**:379–391.

Bloom, B. R., and Chase, M. W., 1967, Transfer of delayed-type-hypersensitivity: A critical review, *Progr. Allergy* **10**:151–255.

Bloom, B. R., Hamilton, L. D., and Chase, M. W., 1964, Effects of mitomycin C on the cellular transfer of delayed-type-hypersensitivity in the guinea pig, *Nature (London)* **201**:689–691.

Bojsen-Móller, J., 1972, Human listeriosis: Diagnstic epidemiological and clinical studies, *Acta Pathol. Microbiol. Scand. Sect. B,* Suppl. No. 229, pp. 12–157.

Buchner, L. H., and Schneierson, S. S., 1968, Clinical and laboratory aspects of *Listeria monocytogenes* infections, *Am. J. Med.* **45**:904–921.

Busch, L. A., 1971, Human listeriosis in the United States, 1967–1969, *J. Infect. Dis.* **123**:328–331.

Campbell, P. A., Martens, B. L., Cooper, H., and McClatchy, J. K., 1974, Requirement for bone marrow-derived cells in resistance to *Listeria, J. Imunnol.* **112**:1407–1414.

Cerottini, J.-C., Enger, H. D., MacDonald, H. R., and Brunner, K. T., 1974, Generation of cytotoxic T lymphocytes *in vitro.* I. Response of normal and immune mouse spleen cells in mixed leukocyte culture, *J. Exp. Med.* **140**:703–717.

Cheers, C., and Waller, R., 1975, Activated macrophages in cogenitally athymic nude mice and lethally-irradiated mice, *J. Immunol.* **115**:844–847.

Cole, P., 1975, Activation of mouse peritoneal macrophages to kill *listeria monocytogenes* by T-lymphocyte products, *Infect. Immun.* **12**:36–41.

Coppel, S., and Youmans, G. P., 1969, Specificity of acquired resistance produced with *Listeria monocytogenes* and *Listeria* fractions, *J. Bacteriol.* **97**:121–126.

Croft, C. C., 1962, Listeric infections in Ohio, in: *Second Symposium on Listeric Infection* (M. L. Gray, ed.), p. 284, Montana State College, Boseman, Mont.

Emmerling, P., Finger, H., and Bockemühl, J., 1975, *Listeria monocytogenes* infection in nude mice, *Infect. Immun.* **12**:437–439.

Fauve, R. M., Bouanchaud, D., and Delaunay, A., 1966, Resistance cellulaire a l'infection bacterienne. IV. Immunization active et résistance des macrophages de souris N. C. S. a la multiplication intracellulaire de *Listeria monocytogenes, Corynebacterium kutscheri,* et

Brucella melitensis, Ann. Inst. Pasteur **110**:106–117 (Suppl. 3).

Fulton, A. M., Dustoor, M. M., Kansinski, J. E., and Blazkovec, A. A., 1975, Blastogenesis as an *in vitro* correlate of delayed hypersensitivity in guinea pigs infected with *Listeria monocytogenes, Infect. Immun.* **12**:647–665.

Gill, D. A., 1931, Bovine bacterial encephalitis (circling disease) and the bacterial genus *Listerella, Aust. Vet. J.* **13**:46–56.

Gray, M. L., 1963, Epidemiological aspects of listeriosis, *Am. J. Public Health* **55**:554–569.

Gray, M. L., and Killinger, A. H., 1966, *Listeria monocytogenes* and listeric infections, *Bacteriol. Rev.* **30**:309–382.

Gray, M. L., Stafseth, H. J., and Thorp, F., 1951, A four year study of listeriosis in Michigan, *J. Am. Vet. Med. Assoc.* **188**:242–252.

Hadden, J. W., Sadilk, J. R., and Hadden, E. M., 1975, Macrophage proliferation induced *in vitro* by a lymphocyte factor, *Nature (London)* **257**:483–485.

Harvey, P. C., and Faber, J. E., 1941, Some biochemical reactions of the *listerella* groups, *J. Bacteriol.* **1**:45–46.

Izumi, S., Penrose, J. M., More, D. G., and Nelson, D. S., 1975 further observations on the immunological induction of DNA synthesis in mouse peritoneal macrophages: Role of products of activated lymphocytes, *Int. Arch. Allergy App. Immunol.* **49**:573–584.

Johnson, M. L., and Colley, E. W., 1969, *Listeria monocytogenes* encephalitis associated with cortocosteroid therapy, *J. Clin. Pathol.* **22**:465–469.

Jones, F. S., and Little, R. B., 1934, Sporadic encephalitis in cows, *Arch. Pathol.* **18**:580.

Jones, S. M., and Woodbine, M., 1961, Microbiological aspects of *Listeria monocytogenes* with special reference to listeriosis in animals, *Vet. Rev. Annot. U.K. Common. Bur. Anim. Health* **7**:39–68.

Jones, T., and Youmans, G. P., 1974 Nonspecific inhibition of growth of intracellular *Listeria monocytogenes* by lymphocyte culture products, *Infect. Immun.* **9**:472–474.

Kelly, L. S., Brown, B. A., and Dobson E. L., 1962, Cell division and phagocytic activity in liver reticuloendothelial cells, *Proc. Soc. Exp. Biol. Med.* **110**:555–562.

Kingdon, G. C., and Sword, C. P., 1970a, Effects of *Listeria monocytogenes* hemolysin on phagocytic cells and lysosomes, *Infect. Immun.* **1**:356–362.

Kingdon, G. C., and Sword, C. P., 1970b, Cardiotoxic and lethal effects of *Listeria monocytogenes* hemolysin, *Infect. Immun.* **1**:373–379.

Koster, F. T., McGregor, D. D., and Mackaness, G. B., 1971, The mediator of cellular immunity. II. Migration of immunologically committed lymphocytes into inflammatory exudates, *J. Exp. Med.* **133**:400–409.

Krahenbuhl, J. L., Rosenberg, L. T., and Remington, J. S., 1973, The role of thymus-derived lymphocytes in the *in vitro* activation of macrophages to kill *Listeria monocytogenes, J. Immunol.* **111**:992–995.

Lagrange, P. H., and Mackaness, G. B., 1975, A stable form of delayed type hypersensitivity, *J. Exp. Med.* **141**:82–96.

Landsteiner, K., and Chase, M. W., 1942, Experiments on transfer of cutaneous sensitivity to simple chemical compounds, *Proc. Soc. Exp. Biol. Med.* **49**:688–690.

Lane, F. C., and Unanue, E. R., 1972, Requirement of thymus (T) lymphocytes for resistance to listeriosis, *J. Exp. Med.* **135**:1104–1112.

Lefford, M. J., 1975, Delayed sensitivity and immunity to tuberculosis, *Am. Rev. Resp. Dis.* **111**:243–246.

Levy, E., and Nassau, E., 1960, Experience with listeriosis in the newborn: An account of a small epidemic in a nursery ward, *Ann. Pediat.* **194**:321–326

Line, F. G., and Cherry, W. B., 1952, Meningitis due to *Listeria Monocytoenes, JAMA* **148**:366–369.

Liu, P. V., and Bates, J. L, 1961, An extracellular haemorrhagic toxin produced by *Listeria monocytogenes, Can. J. Microbiol.* **7**:107–108.

Lurie, M. B., 1942, Studies on the mechanisims of immunity in tuberculosis: The fate of tubercle bacilli ingested by mononuclear phagocytes derived from normal and immunized animals, *J. Exp. Med.* **75**:247–267.

McCullum, R. E., and Sword, C. P., 1972, Mechanisms of pathogenesis in *Listeria monocytogenes* infection. V. Early imbalance in host energy metabolism during experimental listeriosis, *Infect. Immun.* **5**:863–871.

McGregor, D. D., and Koster, F. T., 1971, The mediator of cellular immunity. IV. Cooperation between lymphocytes and mononuclear phagocytes, *Cell. Immunol.* **2**:317–325.

McGregor, D. D., and Logie, P. S., 1973, The mediator of cellular immunity. VI. Effect of antimitotic drug vinblastine on the mediator of cellular resistance to infection, *J. Exp. Med.* **137**:660–674.

McGregor, D. D., Koster, F. T., and Mackaness, G. B., 1971, The mediator of cellular immunity. I. The lifespan and circulation dynamics of the immunologically committed lymphocyte, *J. Exp. Med.* **133**:389–399.

McGregor, D. D., Hahn, H. H., and Mackaness, G. B., 1973, The mediator of cellular immunity. V. Development of cellular resistance to infection in thymectomized irradiated rats, *Cell. Immunol.* **6**:186–199.

Mackaness, G. B., 1962, Cellular resistance to infection, *J. Exp. Med.* **116**:381–406

Mackaness, G. B., 1964, The immunological basis of acquired cellular resistance, *J. Exp. Med.* **120**:105–120.

Mackaness, G. B., 1969, The influence of immunologically committed lymphoid cells on macrophage activity *in vivo, J. Exp. Med.* **129**:973–992.

Mackaness, G. B., and Hill, W. C., 1969, The effect of anti-lymphocyte globulin on cell-mediated resistance to infection, *J. Exp. Med.* **129**:993–1012.

Medoff, G., Kunz, L. J., and Weinberg, A. N., 1971, Listeriosis in humans: An evaluation, *J. Infect. Dis.* **123**:247–250.

Middlebrook, G., Salmon, B. J., and Kreisberg, J. I., 1974, Sterilization of *Listeria monocytogenes* by guinea pig peritoneal exudate cell cultures, *Cell. Immunol.* **14**: 270–283.

Miki, K., and Mackaness, G. B., 1964, The passive transfer of acquired resistance to *Listeria monocytogenes, J. Exp. Med.* **120**:93–103.

Miller, J. F. A. P., and Osoba, D., 1967, Current concepts of the immunological functions of the thymus, *Physiol. Rev.* **47**:437–450.

Miller, J. K., and Heberg, M., 1965, Effects of cortisone on susceptibility of mice to *Listeria monocytogenes, Am. J. Clin. Pathol.* **43**:248–253.

Moore, R. M., and Zehmer, R. B., 1973, Listeriosis in the United States—1971, *J. Infect. Dis.* **127**:610–611.

Murray, E. G. D., Webb, A., and Swann, M. B. R., 1926, A disease of rabbits characterized by large mononuclear leukocytosis, caused by a hitherto undescribed bacillus, *Bacterium monocytogenes, J. Pathol. Bacteriol.* **29**: 407–439.

Nathan, C. F., Remold, H. G., and David, J. R., 1973, Characterization of a lymphocyte factor which alters macrophage function, *J. Exp. Med.* **137**:275–290.

Neter, E., Anzai, H., and Gorzyniski, E. A., 1960, Identification of an antigen common to *Listeria monocytogenes* and other bacteria, *Proc. Soc. Exp. Biol. Med.* **105**:131–134.

Njoko-Obi, A. M., and Osebold, J. W., 1962, Studies on mechanisms of immunity of listeriosis. I. Interaction of peritoneal exudate cells from sheep with *Listeria monocytogenes, J. Immunol.* **89**:187–194.

North, R. J., 1969a, Cellular kinetics associated with the development of acquired cellular resistance, *J. Exp. Med.* **130**:299–314.

North, R. J., 1969b, Mitotic potential of fixed phagocytes in the liver during the development of cellular immunity, *J. Exp. Med.* **130**:315–326.

North, R. J., 1970a, Endocytosis, *Sem. Hematol.* **7**:161–171.

North, R. J., 1970b, The relative importance of blood monocytes and fixed macrophages to the expression of cell-mediated immunity to infection, *J. Exp. Med.* **132**:521–534.

North, R. J., 1970c, Suppression of cell-mediated immunity to infection by an antimitotic drug: Evidence that migrant macrophages express immunity, *J. Exp. Med.* **132**:535–545.

North, R. J., 1971, The action of cortisone acetate on cell-mediated immunity to infection. Suppression of host cell proliferation and alteration of cellular composition of infective foci, *J. Exp. Med.* **134**:1485–1500.

North, R. J., 1972, The action of cortisone acetate on cell-mediated immunity to infection: Histogenesis of the lymphoid cell response and selective elimination of committed lymphocytes, *Cell. Immunol.* **3**:501–515.

North, R. J., 1973a, Importance of thymus-derived lymphocytes in cell-mediated immunity to infection, *Cell. Immunol.* **7**:166–176.

North, R. J., 1973b, The mediators of anti-*Listeria* immunity as an enlarged population of short-lived, replicating T cells: Kinetics of their production, *J. Exp. Med.* **138**:342–355.

North, R. J., 1974a, T cell-dependent macrophage activation in cell-mediated anti-*Listeria* immunity, in: *Activation of Macrophages* (W.-H. Wagner and H. Hahn, eds.), pp. 210–220, Excerpta Medica Amsterdam, American Elsevier, New York.

North, R. J., 1974b, Cell mediated immunity and the response to infection, in: *Mechanisms of Cell-Mediated Immunity* (R. T. McClusky and S. Cohen, eds.), pp. 185–219, Wiley, New York.

North, R. J., 1975, Nature of memory in T cell-mediated antibacterial immunity: Anamnestic production of mediator T cells, *Infect. Immun.* **12**:754–760.

North, R. J., and Deissler, J. F., 1975, Nature of memory in T cell-mediated immunity: Cellular parameters that distinguish between the active immune response and a state of memory, *Infect. Immun.* **12**:761–767.

North, R. J., and Mackaness, G. B., 1973, Immunological control of macrophage proliferation *in vivo, Infect. Immun.* **8**:68–73.

North, R. J., and Spitalny, G., 1974, The inflammatory lymphocyte in cell-mediated antibacterial immunity: Factors governing the accumulation of mediator T cells in peritoneal exudates, *Infect. Immun.* **10**:489–498.

North, R. J., Kirstein, D. P., and Tuttle, R. L., 1976, Subversion of host defense mechanisms by murine tumors. I. A circulating factor that suppresses macrophage-mediated resistance to infection, *J. Exp. Med.* **143**:559–573.

Osebold, J. W., and Sawyer, M. T., 1957, Immunization studies on listeriosis in mice, *J. Immunol.* **78**:262–268.

Pease, P. E., Nicholls, L., and Stuart, M. R., 1972, Evidence that precipitin cross-reactions between *Listeria, Erysipelothrix,* and *Bacillus licheniformis* are not due to the Rantz antigen, *J. Gen. Microbiol.* **73**:567–569.

Polk, L. D., 1970, Listeriosis—Rare or rarely recognized, *Clin. Pediatr.* **9**:635.

Ratzan, K. R., Musher, D. M., Keusch, G. T., and Weinstein, L., 1972, Correlation of increased metabolic activity, resistance to infection, enhanced phagocytosis, and inhibition of bacterial growth by macrophages from *Listeria*- and BCG-infected mice, *Infect. Immun.* **5**:499–504.

Rich, A. R., 1941, The significance of hypersensitivity to infection, *Physiol. Rev.* **21**:70–111.

Ruskin, J., McIntosh, J., and Remington, J. S., 1969, Studies on the mechanisms of resistance to phylogenetically diverse intracellular organisms, *J. Immunol.* **103**:252–259.

Saxbe, W. B., 1972, *Listeria monocytogenes* and Queen Anne, *Pediatrics* **49**:97–101.

Schell, R. F., Ealey, W. F., Harding, G. E., and Smith, D. W., 1974, The relationship between listericidal and mycobacteriostatic activity of BCG-vaccinated mice, *J. Reticuloendothel. Soc.* **16**:139–149.

Seeliger, H. P. R., 1957, *Some New Aspects of Human Listeriosis,* pp. 1–29, Publication of the U.S. Communicable Disease Center, Atlanta, Ga.

Simon, H. B., and Sheagren, J. N., 1972, Enhancement of macrophage bactericidal capacity by antigenically stimulated immune lymphocytes, *Cell. Immunol.* **4**:163–174.

Spector, W. G., and Coote, E., 1965, Differentially labelled blood cells in the reaction to paraffin oil, *J. Pathol. Bacteriol.* **90**:589–598.

Sprent, J., 1976, Fate of *H2*-activated T lymphocytes in syngeneic hosts. I. Fate in lymphoid tissues and intestines traced with ^{3}H-thymidine, ^{125}I-deoxyuridine and ^{51}chromium, *Cell. Immunol.* **21**:278–302.

Suter, E., 1953, Multiplication of tubercle bacilli within mononuclear phagocytes in tissue cultures derived from normal animals and animals vaccinated with BCG, *J. Exp. Med.* **97**:235–245.

Sword, C. P., and Wilder, M. S., 1967, Plasma enzyme changes in Listeria monocytogenes infected mice, *J. Infect. Dis.* **117**:387–392.

Tripathy, S. P., and Mackaness, G. B., 1969, The effect of cytotoxic agents on the passive transfer of cell-mediated immunity, *J. Exp. Med.* **130**:17–25.

van Furth, R., and Cohn, Z. A., 1968, The origin and kinetics of mononuclear phagocytes, *J. Exp. Med.* **128**:415–433.

Visintine, A. M., Oleske, J. M., and Nahmias, A. J., 1977, *Listeria monocytogenes* infection in infants and children, *Am. J. Dis. Child.* **131**:393–397.

Volkman, A., 1966, The origin and turnover of mononuclear cells in peritoneal exudates in the rat, *J. Exp. Med.* **124**:2411–2419.

Volkman, A., and Gowans, J. L., 1965, The origin of macrophages from bone marrow in the rat, *Br. J. Exp. Pathol.* **46**:62–70.

Watson, B. B., and Lavizzo, J. C., 1973, Extracellular antigens from *Listeria monocytogenes.* II. Cytotoxicity of hemolytic and lipolytic antigens for cultured mouse macrophages, *Infect. Immun.* **7**:753–758.

Weis, J., and Seeliger, H. P. R., 1975, Incidence of *Listeria monocytogenes* in nature, *Appl. Microbiol.* **30**:29–32.

Woodruff, J. F., and Woodruff, J. J., 1975, T lymphocyte interaction with viruses and virus-infected tissues, *Progr. Med. Virol.* **9**:120–160.

Youdim, S., Stutman, O., and Good, R. A., 1973, Thymus dependence of cells involved in transfer of delayed hypersensitivity to *Listeria monocytogenes* in mice, *Cell. Immunol.* **8**:395–402.

Zinkernagel, R. M., and Doherty, P. C., 1975, Coritsone-resistant effector T cells in acute lymphocytic choriomeningitis and *Listeria monocytogenes* infection in mice, *Aust. J. Exp. Biol. Med.* **53**:297–304.

10

Immunology of Enterobacterial Infections

W. LEE HAND and JAMES W. SMITH

1. Introduction

This chapter will be devoted to a discussion of immunological mechanisms relevant to infection caused by the Enterobacteriaceae. There is considerable debate concerning the proper categorization of these enterobacteria.* However, the usual clinical microbiological classification indicates that the family Enterobacteriaceae is composed of aerobic (facultative anaerobic) gram-negative rods which can be placed in the following divisions or tribes (and genera): Escherichieae (*Escherichia, Shigella*), Edwardsielleae (*Edwardsiella*), Salmonellae (*Salmonella, Arizona, Citrobacter*), Klebsiellae (*Klebsiella, Enterobacteria, Serratia*), Proteeae (*Proteus, Providencia*), and Erwineae (*Erwinia, Pectobacterium*) (Ewing and Martin, 1974). The immune responses related to systemic (disseminated) and local (urinary tract and respiratory tract) extraintestinal infections due to Enterobacteriaceae will be discussed here. Enteric disease caused by certain pathogenic enterobacteria (such as *Salmonella, Shigella*, and *Escherichia coli*) will be covered in Chapter 11.

Enterobacteria have long been recognized as a major cause of certain extraintestinal infections, such as urinary tract infections. However, in the past 20–30 years a striking increase in the frequency of serious infections caused by aerobic gram-negative bacilli, especially Enterobacteriaceae and *Pseudomonas*, has occurred. The opportunistic aerobic gram-negative bacilli are the leading cause of nosocomial (hospital-acquired) infections, which are associated with substantial morbidity, mortality, and excess financial cost in hospitalized patients (Stamm *et al.*, 1977; Sanford, 1975; Feingold, 1970; Rogers, 1959). As we shall see, an understanding of the immunology of these organisms is crucial to efforts at controlling such infections.

2. Microbial Characteristics

Many of the Enterobacteriaceae are normal inhabitants of the human intestinal tract (Donaldson, 1964). *Escherichia coli* is the predominant aerobic organism in the large intestine and feces. Some members of this family are pathogenic for animals or plants while other strains are free-living saprophytes.

---

* For the purposes of this chapter, the words "enterobacteria" and "enterobacterial" will refer to the Enterobacteriaceae.

W. LEE HAND • V.A. Medical Center (Atlanta), Decatur, Georgia 30033, and Department of Medicine, Emory University School of Medicine, Atlanta, Georgia 30303. JAMES W. SMITH • V.A. Medical Center and Department of Medicine, University of Texas (Southwestern) Medical School at Dallas, Dallas, Texas 75216.

2.1. Normal Flora Interactions

2.1.1. GI Tract

Interactions of the Enterobacteriaceae with other intestinal organisms are discussed in Chapter 11.

2.1.2. Respiratory Tract

Small numbers of Enterobacteriaceae are occasionally recovered from the normal upper respiratory tract (Rosenthal and Tager, 1975; Johanson *et al.*, 1969; Julianelle and Siegel, 1945). However, in one study 35% of moderately ill and 73% of critically ill hospitalized patients had aerobic gram-negative bacilli (mostly Enterobacteriaceae) in their oropharynx (Johanson *et al.*, 1969). Changes in pharyngeal flora were apparently independent of antibiotic usage. This appearance of gram-negative bacilli in the upper respiratory tract precedes the development of hospital-associated pneumonia with these same organisms (Johanson *et al.*, 1972). The recent observation that gram-negative bacilli (especially *Klebsiella–Enterobacter*) are present in the oropharynx of many nonhospitalized chronic alcoholic subjects may relate to the apparent increase in gram-negative rod pneumonias seen in these individuals (Mackowiak *et al.*, 1978). The mechanisms responsible for increased carriage of aerobic gram-negative bacilli in the upper respiratory tract remain speculative. Normal oropharyngeal defenses against Enterobacteriaceae appear to be very efficient and may include both physical clearance and bactericidal mechanisms (LaForce *et al.*, 1976). Salivary glycoproteins and specific immunoglobulins can prevent colonization of the upper respiratory tract by certain gram-positive organisms, presumably by inhibiting attachment of the bacteria to mucosal cells (Gibbons, 1975; Gibbons and van Houte, 1975; Williams and Gibbons, 1975, 1972). Whether alterations in these or other local factors lead to oropharyngeal colonization with enterobacteria and similar organisms is currently unknown.

Colonization of the respiratory tract with aerobic gram-negative bacilli is sometimes a consequence of treatment with antibiotics which eradicate the organisms normally found in the upper respiratory tract (e.g., treatment of pneumonia with penicillin). In this instance simple colonization with no evidence of disease is usually the only consequence. However, this antibiotic-induced alteration in flora may be one factor which predisposes to gram-negative rod pneumonia in compromised patients (Tillotson and Finland, 1969).

2.2. Antigenic Composition of Enterobacteriaceae

Several enterobacterial antigens have been studied for evidence of activity in determination of microbial pathogenicity or in stimulation of the host immune response. Three enterobacterial surface antigenic components, termed H, O, and K, have been rather well defined. The H antigen is a heat-labile protein component of flagella. The K (or capsular) antigen is usually polysaccharide in nature, and is an outer layer, which may or may not form a distinct capsule. O (or somatic) antigen is a heat-stable lipopolysaccharide component of the bacterial cell wall. The O antigen has been studied extensively because of its immunological importance and because the molecule possesses the endotoxin activity. The lipopolysaccharide (LPS) has three components: O-specific polysaccharide side chain of repeating units (oligosaccharide), core polysaccharide, and lipid A (Westphal, 1975; Luderitz, *et al.*, 1966a,b). The polysaccharide side chain accounts for the antigenic specificity of the strain, whereas lipid A is responsible for the endotoxin activity of this molecule (Rietschel *et al.*, 1975; Luderitz *et al.*, 1973; Galanos *et al.*, 1972). Several hundred different O polysaccharides have been identified in the family Enterobacteriaceae. At least 164 O groups are described for *E. coli* alone (Ørskov *et al.*, 1977). In contrast, only five different core polysaccharides (one in *Salmonella* and four in *E. coli*) have been identified (Ørskov *et al.*, 1977). Lipid A preparations from various enterobacteria are similar (Rietschel *et al.*, 1975). The lipid A–core polysaccharide complex has been referred to as "core glycolipid" or "LPS core antigen."

The so-called enterobacterial common antigen (or common antigen of Enterobacteriaceae), as the name implies, is shared by the Enterobacteriaceae (Kunin, 1963; Kunin *et al.*, 1962). The precise composition and cellular location of enterobacterial common antigen (ECA) remain unknown. ECA apparently exists in two forms. In most organisms the antigen is in a free form, not tightly linked to other cellular components, and located on the cell surface. In some bacteria [rough (R) mutants, lacking the O polysaccharide], ECA is bound to LPS core polysaccharide (Makela and Mayer, 1976). Recent evidence suggests that ECA is at least in part an amino sugar heteropolymer of *N*-acetyl-D-glucosamine and *N*-acetyl-D-mannosaminuronic acid units, which are partly esterified by palmetic acid (Mannel and Mayer, 1978).

Other enterobacterial antigens have been described, but their role in the pathogenesis or immunology of infection is poorly defined. These antigens include cell wall protein closely associated with LPS (Ahlstedt and Holmgren, 1975; Wober and Alaupovic, 1971a,b), lipoprotein of the outer membrane (Melchers *et al.*, 1975), and ribosomes, including RNA and protein constituents (Eisenstein, 1975; Berry *et al.*, 1975; Johnson, 1973; Smith and Bigley, 1972a,b; Venneman, 1972; Venneman and Berry, 1971; Venneman *et al.*, 1970; Venneman and Bigley, 1969).

2.3. Factors Contributing to Invasiveness and Pathogenesis of Disease

2.3.1. Bacterial Antigens

As we have already indicated, enterobacterial infections are often opportunistic in nature. Those factors promoting invasiveness of the Enterobacteriaceae are poorly defined. Recent studies indicate that K antigen may be an important virulence factor in certain extraintestinal infections (Ørskov, 1978; Cheasty *et al.*, 1977; Kaijser *et al.*, 1977; Ørskov *et al.*, 1963, 1971, 1977; Glynn and Howard, 1970, 1971; Sjostedt, 1946; Vahlne, 1945). K1 antigen, which is very similar to or identical with meningococcal group B capsular polysaccharide (Kasper *et al.*, 1973; Grados and Ewing, 1970), is found in 80% of *E. coli* strains causing neonatal meningitis (Glode *et al.*, 1977a, Schiffer *et al.*, 1976; Sarff *et al.*, 1975; McCracken *et al.*, 1974; Robbins *et al.*, 1974). The severity of disease is greater in those meningeal infections caused by organisms with K1 antigen than in meningitis due to other *E. coli*. Furthermore, strains of *E. coli* bearing K antigen are more commonly isolated from patients with upper urinary tract infection than from

the stool of the same individuals or from urine of patients with infection limited to the lower urinary tract (Kaijser *et al.*, 1977; McCabe *et al.*, 1975; Kaijser, 1973; Glynn *et al.*, 1971). The apparent ability of K1 antigen to confer the property of invasiveness to *E. coli* (in newborns) and to group B meningococci may, in part, be related to the poor immunogenicity of the cross-reacting polysaccharide (*N*-acetyl neuraminic acid). In addition, *E. coli* with K antigen is more resistant to phagocytosis and to complement-mediated killing than are organisms lacking K antigen (Bortoussi *et al.*, 1978; Weinstein *et al.*, 1978; Glynn and Howard, 1971; Glynn and Howard, 1970).

The O antigen also plays a role in virulence, Rough (R) strains of Enterobacteriaceae (e.g., *Salmonella*) lacking the O-specific polysaccharide side chain have little or no capacity to cause disease. Semirough forms, in which the length of the polysaccharide side chains is shortened, also have reduced virulence (Valtonen, 1969; Nakano and Saito, 1969; Medearis *et al.*, 1968). In addition, it has been shown that small changes in the O antigen (lipopolysaccharide) of *S. typhimurium* will significantly alter virulence for animals (Makela *et al.*, 1973). Certain O antigenic groups of *E. coli* (1, 2, 4, 6, 7, 11, 18, 39, and 75) are more commonly associated with urinary tract infections than other serogroups. These common O serogroups also predominate in stool isolates from the same individuals (Holmgren and Smith, 1975), but the percentages of recovery from the feces are lower (Hanson *et al.*, 1977; Ørskov *et al.*, 1977).

The possibility that ECA serves as a virulence factor has been considered. Valtonen *et al.* (1976) found that certain *E. coli* and *S. typhimurium* strains which contained ECA were more virulent for mice than the comparable organisms without ECA.

Vosti (1969) evaluated a number of characteristics of *E. coli* isolated from infected urinary tracts and from other sources. There were no differences in motility, utilization of carbohydrates, antibiotic sensitivities, or production of colicins between O serogroups commonly causing urinary tract infection and strains of other serogroups. However, strains frequently recovered from the urinary tract were likely to produce hemolysis and to resist the action of colicins. Minshew *et al.* (1978)

reported that *E. coli* recovered from extraintestinal sites of human infection was more likely than fecal isolates to (1) cause hemolysis (hemolysin production), (2) produce colicin V, (3) agglutinate human erythrocytes in the presence of D-mannose, and (4) kill 13-day-old chick embryos. It was suggested that the hemolysin is a cytotoxic factor, that colicin V protects against defense mechanisms of the host, and that the hemagglutinin plays a role in specific tissue adherence.

2.3.2. Endotoxin Activity

The literature concerning the effects of endotoxin on the host is vast and can be only briefly summarized here. It has been assumed that the biological activity of LPS (endotoxin) plays a role in the pathogenesis, if not the initiation, of enterobacterial infections (e.g., Berry, 1975; Braude *et al.,* 1973; Nowotny, 1969). In experimental animals the effects of the intact lipopolysaccharide or of solubilized lipid A include fever, hypotension, leukopenia followed by leukocytosis, disseminated intravascular coagulation, complement activation, and a number of metabolic alterations (Elin and Wolff, 1976; Westphal, 1975; Rietschel *et al.,* 1975; Nowotny, 1969). Some of these endotoxin effects have been documented in humans (Wolff, 1973). Similar findings may be observed in human gram-negative rod septicemia. However, there is no conclusive evidence that these manifestations of human enterobacterial infection are primarily due to endotoxin (Shands, 1975; Kass *et al.,* 1973).

In addition to these "toxic" effects, LPS also has a number of effects on host immune responses and defense mechanisms. Endotoxin may suppress the *in vivo* immune response (antibody formation) if given at an appropriate time prior to antigen administration (Schwab, 1975; Franzl and McMaster, 1968). However, cell wall components (? LPS–protein complex) of enterobacteria enhance the production of O-specific IgG antibody (while suppressing IgM antibody production) in animals when the organisms are administered prior to challenge with *E. coli* of an unrelated O serotype (Ahlstedt and Lindholm, 1977; Ahlstedt and Holmgren, 1975; Holmgren and Ahlstedt, 1974). Furthermore, endotoxin serves as an adjuvant (enhanced antibody response) when administered at the same time as or following

antigen presentation (Chedid and Audibert, 1977; Johnson, 1975; Neter, 1969; Franzl and McMaster, 1968). It is believed that these manifestations of endotoxin activity are due to a direct effect of LPS on lymphocytes and macrophages (Rosenstreich *et al.,* 1977; Rosenstreich and Mergenhagen, 1975; Johnson, 1975; Allison *et al.,* 1973). The most striking of these cellular effects is the ability of LPS to act as a mitogen and polyclonal antibody stimulator for B lymphocytes (Peavy *et al.,* 1974; Moller *et al.,* 1973; Andersson *et al.,* 1973; Andersson *et al.,* 1972; Peavy *et al.,* 1970). Mitogenic activity is separable from LPS antigenic properties (Poe and Michael, 1976; Johnson, 1975; Coutinho and Moller, 1973; Peavy *et al.,* 1973; Moller *et al.,* 1973). This direct stimulation of B-lymphocyte proliferation is independent of T-cell function and may be one means by which LPS serves as an adjuvant (Skidmore *et al.,* 1976; Johnson, 1975). However, reported studies disagree on whether or not LPS is mitogenic for human B lymphocytes (Rickles *et al.,* 1977; Gale *et al.,* 1977; Hsu, 1975; Chess *et al.,* 1974). There is some evidence that endotoxin has a direct action on T as well as B lymphocytes. For example, LPS may act synergistically with phytohemagglutinin to activate T cells (Rosenstreich and Mergenhagen, 1975). Furthermore, LPS may substitute for or augment helper T-cell activity (Armerding and Katz, 1974; Watson *et al.,* 1973) Endotoxin also has an effect on macrophages (Weinberg *et al.,* 1978; Rosenstreich *et al.,* 1978; Rosenstreich and Mergenhagen, 1975; Johnson, 1975; Wahl *et al.,* 1974; Allison *et al.,* 1973). LPS can interact directly with macrophages to produce at least some characteristics of macrophage activation. In addition, LPS may indirectly induce macrophage activation by stimulation of lymphokine release from lymphocytes. To complete the cycle of lymphocyte–macrophage interactions, LPS-exposed macrophages produce factors with profound effects on lymphocytes and other cells (reviewed by Hoffman *et al.,* 1978; Unanue, 1976; see also Wood and Cameron, 1978; Hoffman *et al.,* 1976, 1977).

In addition to these effects on cells involved in the immune response, endotoxin influences other host defense mechanisms. Activation by endotoxin or by gram-negative bacilli of the complement system in normal serum is in part accomplished through the alternative pathway of complement activation (Morrison and Kline, 1977; Fine, 1974; Reed and Albright, 1974; Mergenhagen *et al.*, 1973; Kane *et al.*, 1973; Root *et al.*, 1972; Phillips *et al.*, 1972; Gotze and Muller-Eberhard, 1971; Gewurz *et al.*, 1968). This mechanism for complement activation may be an important "normal" host defense mechanism, mediating serum bactericidal or opsonizing activity, in the absence of specific antibacterial antibody. However, it has also been suggested that LPS-mediated complement activation may be an initating factor in certain "toxic" effects (e.g., disseminated intravascular coagulation) of endotoxin (reviewed by Brown, 1974). Other recent studies indicate that endotoxin-mediated complement activation, intravascular coagulation, and hypotension may not be so closely interrelated (Ulevitch *et al.*, 1975, 1978; Ulevitch and Cochrane, 1978; Muller-Berghaus and Lohmann, 1974).

Endotoxin has both direct and indirect effects on migration of phagocytes. *In vitro* and *in vivo* exposure of granulocytes to LPS inhibits chemotaxis (Issekutz and Biggar, 1977; Territo and Golde, 1976) and increases adherence (MacGregor, 1977). Similarly, LPS inhibits macrophage migration (Heilman and Bast, 1967). However, LPS interacts with serum to yield C5a, a cleavage product of C5 with chemotactic activity for granulocytic and mononuclear phagocytes (Snyderman *et al.*, 1968, 1975).

In animal models the administration of endotoxin leads to a short-lived increase in nonspecific resistance to infection (Cluff, 1970). This phenomenon is probably due to changes in reticuloendothelial macrophage function ("activation") and to increased serum antibacterial activity (Kochan and Berendt, 1974; Elin and Wolff, 1974; Allison *et al.*, 1973). LPS-unresponsive animals (C3H/HeJ mice) have a defect in the macrophage activation process and fail to exhibit an increase in nonspecific resistance to infection after exposure to endotoxin (Chedid *et al.*, 1976). One mechanism for the enhanced serum antibacterial effect is an endotoxin-induced fall in serum iron level (with a corresponding decrease in percent saturation of serum iron binding capacity) (Elin and Wolff, 1974). Since iron is required for bacterial metabolism, this de-

creased saturation of iron binding capacity (with decreased availability of iron to bacteria) will increase the ability of serum factors to inhibit or kill organisms. LPS also causes an increase in serum bactericidal activity as a result of elevated serum fatty acid levels (Kochan and Berendt, 1974). It is believed that these fatty acids are released by macrophages in response to endotoxin stimulation (or an active infectious process).

In summary, it is apparent that endotoxin has many points of interaction with host defense mechanisms and immunological responses. From the standpoint of the host, this interaction may be either beneficial or detrimental, depending on the dosage and timing of exposure to endotoxin.

2.3.3. Other Factors Which Influence Host Defenses

Components of the enterobacterial cell other than LPS are B-cell mitogens and polyclonal activators. A cell wall protein that is usually complexed to LPS is a potent stimulator of murine B cells, including those of LPS-unresponsive C3H/HeJ mice (Goodman *et al.*, 1978; Staber *et al.*, 1978; Betz and Morrison, 1977; Sultzer and Goodman, 1976). The lipoprotein of the outer membrane of *E. coli* was recently shown to be a mitogen for mouse B lymphocytes (Melchers *et al.*, 1975). The biological significance of these activities is unknown.

Enterobacteriaceae (*E. coli*) produce both low- and high-molecular-weight substances which are chemotactically active for neutrophils and mononuclear leukocytes, including alveolar macrophages (Tainer *et al.*, 1975; Yoshida *et al.*, 1975; Lynn *et al.*, 1975; Schiffman *et al.*, 1975; Ward *et al.*, 1968). In addition, some enterobacteria produce proteases which release leukotactic fragments from C3 and C5 (Ward *et al.*, 1973). Furthermore, synthesis and release by *E. coli* of substances with macrophage migration inhibitory activity, blastogenic activity for lymphocytes, and cytotoxicity for fibroblasts have been described (Yoshida *et al.*, 1975). The relationship of these substances to the endotoxin molecule requires clarification. The similarity of these biologically active factors, or cytokines, to the lymphokines produced by stimulated lymphocytes is obvious. The possible role of enterobacterial cytokines in stimulation of host defense mechanisms is of interest and deserves further study.

3. Host Characteristics

As already noted, Enterobacteriaceae in the host are usually restricted to the lumen of the GI tract. Enterobacterial infections in the "normal" host are limited to certain definite categories. Specifically, urinary tract infections (due usually to *E. coli*) are frequent in females throughout life but are uncommon in males without anatomical abnormalities of the urinary tract until prostatism, surgery, and other urinary tract instrumentation intervene in older males (for recent review, see Kunin, 1974). Enteric infections caused by those Enterobacteriaceae (*Salmonella, Shigella,* and *E. coli*) which are pathogenic for the normal host are covered in Chapter 11.

It is especially in the compromised host that enterobacterial infections have become such an important problem. Enterobacteriaceae and other aerobic gram-negative bacilli are now the principal causes of hospital-acquired infections (Stamm *et al.*, 1977; Sanford, 1975; Bennett *et al.*, 1971; Feingold, 1970). Major types of hospital-associated infections due to these organisms include urinary tract infections, wound infections, respiratory tract infections, phlebitis due to indwelling intravenous catheters, and bacteremia secondary to one of these other infections. Recent estimates of the incidence of gram-negative rod bacteremia range from 71,000 to 300,000 cases per year in the United States (Wolff and Bennett, 1974; McCabe *et al.*, 1972).

In general, certain aspects of the hospital environment, including antibiotic usage (Finland, 1970; Tillotson and Finland, 1969) and defects in host defense mechanisms, predispose to these infections (Sanford, 1975; Feingold, 1970; Klainer and Beisel, 1969). Examples of defects in host defenses which may lead to infection include

1. Impaired skin and mucous membrane barriers—tracheostomy and endotracheal intubation, bladder catheterization, indwelling intravenous catheters, inhalation of infected aerosols from contaminated inhalation therapy equipment,

surgical procedures, burns, and alterations of indigenous microbial flora by antibiotics.
2. Deficient phagocytic cells—leukopenia and/or altered phagocyte function as a result of neoplasia and cytotoxic or immunosuppressive drug therapy; primary leukocyte defects.
3. Abnormal humoral factors
   a. Immunoglobulin (antibody)—hypogammaglobulinemia secondary to underlying disease and immunosuppressive therapy.
   b. Complement—alterations of complement activity due to decreased synthesis or increased utilization of complement components in cirrhosis, sickle cell disease, etc. (Hand and King, 1978, 1977; Johnston *et al.*, 1973; Ruddy *et al.*, 1972).
4. Defective cell-mediated immunity—abnormalities predisposing to systemic salmonellosis in animals (Mackaness and Blanden, 1967).

Not only the predisposition to infection but also the outcome of serious gram-negative bacillus infection (bacteremia) is related to the gravity of underlying disease in the host (McCabe and Jackson, 1962). That is, the mortality rate rises with increasing severity and deteriorating prognosis of the underlying disease.

4. Microbe–Host Interactions

4.1. Colonization vs. Disease

Under ordinary circumstances the enterobacterial inhabitants of the intestinal tract are confined to the lumen of the bowel and cause no disease. With the exception of illness due to enterotoxigenic *E. coli,* it is only when normal host defenses fail that these enterobacterial organisms become invasive and produce overt disease. In females, colonization of the perineum with Enterobacteriaceae is thought to precede actual infection of the urinary tract (Stamey *et al.*, 1971). However, even spread of these organisms to urethra and bladder may not lead to overt clinical disease ("asymptomatic bacteriuria") (reviewed by Kunin, 1974).

Similarly, there are usually no Enterobacteriaceae in the normal upper respiratory tract (Mackowiak *et al.*, 1978; Johanson *et al.*, 1969; Julianelle and Siegel, 1945). Under special conditions, such as alcoholism or hospitalization for serious disease, the upper respiratory tract may harbor significant numbers of gram-negative bacilli (Mackowiak *et al.*, 1978; Johanson *et al.*, 1969, 1972). Likewise, colonization of the respiratory tract with gram-negative bacilli follows treatment with antibiotics which eradicate the normal upper respiratory flora (Tillotson and Finland, 1969). In any of these circumstances, respiratory tract colonization with no evidence of disease is the usual outcome, but serious gram-negative rod pneumonia may occur (Johanson *et al.*, 1972; Tillotson and Finland, 1969).

4.2. "Normal" Host Defense Mechanisms

It is discouraging to note that we still know little about the relative importance of various normal host defenses in protection against enterobacterial infection. It is true, of course, that various mucous membrane defense mechanisms (physical barriers, enzymes, gastric acid, antibody, microbial antagonism, etc.) limit the Enterobacteriaceae to their location in the lumen of the intestinal tract (Cohn, 1973).

In the absence of specific acquired immunity, it is probable that protection against systemic enterobacterial infection is dependent on the presence of certain serum factors and phagocytes acting in concert. Heat-stable factors (antibody) and heat-labile factors (complement) are involved in both the direct bactericidal activity and phagocytosis-promoting function of normal serum (Winkelstein, 1973; Quie, 1972; Austen and Cohn, 1963; Mackie and Finkelstein, 1932). "Natural" antibodies, especially of IgM class, against Enterobacteriaceae are found in sera of most individuals (Michael, 1969; Michael and Rosen, 1963; Michael *et al.*, 1962; Lovell, 1934). These antibodies, which can be directed against any of several bacterial antigens, are apparently the result of exposure to certain widely shared (similar or identical) bacterial antigens. The bactericidal activity of normal serum can be mediated by this "natural" antibody via classical pathway activation of the complement

system. Many gram-negative bacilli and endotoxin preparations are able to activate the complement system by means of the alternative complement pathway (Morrison and Kline, 1977; Fine, 1974; Reed and Albright, 1974; Mergenhagen *et al.*, 1973; Kane *et al.*, 1973; Root *et al.*, 1972; Phillips *et al.*, 1972; Gotze and Muller-Eberhard, 1971), but there is considerable variation in this capability. The activation of alternative pathway, and probably classical pathway, function may take place in the absence of specific antibody. At least part of the capacity of normal serum to kill enterobacteria is mediated by the alternative pathway mechanism (Hand and King, 1977; Reed and Albright, 1974; Root *et al.*, 1972; Gotze and Muller-Eberhard, 1971). However, it should be noted that the majority of gram-negative bacilli isolated from the blood of patients with bacteremia are resistant to the bactericidal effect of serum (Simberkoff *et al.*, 1976; Vosti and Randall, 1970; Roantree and Rantz, 1960). It has been suggested that the major function of serum bactericidal activity is to prevent bloodstream invasion by susceptible organisms.

The ability of normal serum to promote ingestion of Enterobacteriaceae by phagocytes is also mediated by "natural" antibody and complement activity. Opsonization of gram-negative bacilli by normal serum often utilizes both the classical and alternative pathways of complement activation (Hand and King, 1978; Reed, 1975; Forsgren and Quie, 1974a,b; Bjornson and Michael, 1973; Root *et al.*, 1972; Johnson *et al.*, 1972; Jasin, 1972). Alternative complement pathway function may be especially important as a normal host defense mechanism since opsonization due to activation of this system does not require the presence of antibody.

There is substantial recent evidence that the complement system is activated during human gram-negative rod bacteremia (Palestine and Klemperer, 1976; Füst *et al.*, 1976; Fearon *et al.*, 1975). This complement system activation appears to be mediated largely via the alternative pathway. The most impressive findings occur in patients with bacteremic shock, in whom levels of certain alternative pathway factors, C3, and terminal complement components (C5, C6, and C9) were lower than in bacteremic patients without shock and/or normal controls (Fearon *et al.*, 1975; McCabe, 1973).

On the basis of indirect evidence, it appears that both polymorphonuclear neutrophils (PMNs) and mononuclear phagocytes are important in protection against enterobacterial infection. With the possible exception of certain *Salmonella* strains, Enterobacteriaceae are extracellular organisms and are rapidly inactivated following phagocytosis. Impaired function of the reticuloendothelial system (macrophages of liver and spleen) in animal models (Kaye and Hook, 1963), and probably in humans (Pearson *et al.*, 1969, 1970), predisposes to infection with various organisms, including some Enterobacteriaceae. PMNs are crucial for normal resistance to these organisms. Drug-induced neutropenia in experimental animals leads to bloodstream invasion by organisms colonizing the intestinal tract (Ziegler *et al.*, 1973; Braude *et al.*, 1969). Similarly, neutropenia induced by cytoxic agents in treatment of human malignancy predisposes to gram-negative rod bacteremia (Quie, 1975). Abnormal PMN function also predisposes to bacterial infections, including those caused by Enterobacteriaceae (Quie, 1975; Lazarus and Neu, 1975; Quie, 1973). However, no defect in intrinsic neutrophil bactericidal activity was found in nonleukopenic, bacteremic patients without preexisting granulocyte abnormalities or treatment with cytotoxic drugs (Weinstein and Young, 1976).

4.3. Immune Response

4.3.1. Urinary Tract

Studies of the immune response in urinary tract infections have usually concentrated on production of antibody to the specific O antigen (lipopolysaccharide) of the infecting organism (Holmgren and Smith, 1975). Traditionally, studies of antibody in serum and other body fluids utilized direct agglutination tests with heat-killed organisms, which contain the heat-stable lipopolysaccharide as the antigen. The indirect hemagglutination test, which uses purified lipopolysaccharide as antigen, has largely replaced the direct agglutination method. In comparison with the direct agglutination procedure, the indirect hemagglutination test is more sensitive for detection of IgM antibody but less satisfactory for eval-

uation of IgG antibody. Recent development of primary binding methods, such as the enzyme-linked immunosorbent assay, permits the highly sensitive analysis of antibody in all immunoglobulin classes (Smith *et al.*, 1974; Engvall and Perlmann, 1972).

In experimental infection the serum immune response to the lipopolysaccharide or O antigen resembles the response to other antigens. The immunoglobulin class sequence of antibody is IgM initially, followed by IgG antibody. An increase in antibody avidity occurs with time after infection, and the immunoglobulin class expression of the antibody response relates to the quantity of antigen injected (Holmgren and Smith, 1975). During the primary immune response IgM is the major antibody against the O antigen of *E. coli*, whereas increasing quantities of IgG antibody follow repeated immunization. Memory appears to exist for both IgM and IgG antibody after repeated injections of organisms in experimental animals.

K antigen also is immunogenic in experimental animals. The antibody response is predominantly of IgM class, although small quantities of IgG antibody are detected in serum in a small number of animals (Smith and Kaijser, 1976a; Kaijser *et al.*, 1973). Exposure to purified K antigen prior to infection with a K-containing enterobacterial strain may prevent the development of antibody to K antigen. In contrast, antibody response to the O antigen is enhanced by prior administration of O antigen (Kaijser *et al.*, 1973). It has been postulated that tolerance to the polysaccharide may play a role in suppression of the antibody response to K antigen.

Studies of the human serum immune response to urinary tract infection have been reviewed by Holmgren and Smith (1975), Hanson (1973), Cobbs (1972), and Sanford (1968). When infection is limited to the bladder, no antibody or only an IgM antibody response to the O antigen of the infecting organism is detected in serum. On the other hand, an IgG antibody response occurs after infection of the upper urinary tract. If sequential studies are performed following upper tract infection, a rise in antibody titers may be detected (Jodal *et al.*, 1975). It has been suggested that the IgG antibody response in humans is related to the tissue invasion which accompanies kidney infection, whereas little tissue invasion or inflammatory reaction occurs with uncomplicated bladder infection in humans. Significant determinants of the antibody response include clinical activity of the disease, age, type of organism, and number of previous infections.

Individuals with active clinical disease have an elevated serum antibody response more frequently than those with asymptomatic bacteriuria of the upper urinary tract (Holmgren and Smith, 1975; Lindberg *et al.*, 1975). The serum antibody response appears to be an especially useful manifestation of renal involvement in infected children, except in infants less than 2 months of age, who mount little antibody response. Urinary tract isolates of *E. coli* rich in K antigen were found to induce a higher serum antibody response to the O antigen of the infecting organism than did those organisms with less or no K antigen (Glynn *et al.*, 1971). This observation is related to the finding that K-containing *E. coli* are more likely to involve the upper urinary tract than are organisms without K antigen.

In vitro tests have been employed to evaluate the local immune response in experimental animals (Holmgren and Smith, 1975). When pyelonephritic rabbit kidneys were studied for antibody production by means of the hemolytic plaque technique, only IgM production was detected (Miller and North, 1973). However, studies utilizing the incorporation of radiolabeled amino acids into protein and immunoglobulin have shown synthesis of IgG, IgM, and IgA in the infected rabbit kidney (Lehmann *et al.*, 1968). The local synthesis of specific IgG antibody against O antigen occurred by day 9 of infection, whereas IgM antibody was not detected until day 20 (Smith *et al.*, 1974). Local production of IgA antibody against the infecting organism was variably noted 14–24 days after infection.

Little local response to the K antigen was detected after infection with an *E. coli* containing K antigen, in contrast to the significant antibody response to O antigen (Smith and Kaijser, 1976a). Local antibody (IgG and IgM) against the murein-lipoprotein of the outer membrane has also been detected (J. W. Smith, 1977). Studies of a few surgically removed human pyelonephritic kidneys have shown significant synthesis of IgG, including antibody to the LPS of the infecting organism

(Holmgren and Smith, 1975). The detection of antibody which coats bacteria in urine appears to be an indirect test for locally produced antibody (Thomas *et al.*, 1974; Jones *et al.*, 1974). Experimental studies indicate that antibody coating bacteria is present at the initiation of local antibody synthesis 9–11 days after onset of infection (Smith *et al.*, 1977). These IgG and IgM antibodies are directed against the O antigen and the murein-lipoprotein of outer membrane and are detectable earlier than free urinary antibody.

Free antibody to LPS has been demonstrated in urine from both humans and experimental animals with urinary tract infection (Holmgren and Smith, 1975; Vosti and Remington, 1968). This free urinary antibody activity has been detected in IgA, IgG, and IgM classes of immunoglobulin. Experimental studies indicate that the appearance of antibody in urine follows shortly after the onset of local antibody synthesis but is not detectable in animals with high-titer serum antibody in the absence of local antibody production (Smith and Hand, 1972). These studies support the contention that antibody in urine represents local antibody.

Little information is available concerning the cell-mediated immune response in human urinary tract infection. Circulating lymphocytes from rabbits with urinary tract infection are stimulated by the LPS (O antigen) of the infecting *E. coli*, but little response has been detected to the K antigen of this organism (Smith, 1975; Smith and Kaijser, 1976b). At the local site of infection (kidney), lymphocytes exhibit a blastogenic response to LPS of the infecting organism at approximately 3 weeks after infection but lose this response by 5 weeks after infection. Local (kidney) lymphocytes fail to respond to PHA or to elaborate mediators of cellular immunity, although the presence of uropod-bearing lymphocytes indicates that T cells are present at the infected site (Smith *et al.*, 1975). Recent studies also suggest that kidney cells inhibit the responsiveness of lymphocytes to phytohemagglutinin (Miller *et al*, 1976). Thus it is possible that T lymphocytes found in the kidney soon after the onset of infection play a role in modulating the antibody response, rather than in producing mediators of cellular immunity (Smith *et al.*, 1975). However, the course of experimental pyelonephritis is not appreciably altered if animals are depleted of T lymphocytes prior to induction of infection (Miller *et al.*, 1975).

Experimental pyelonephritis induces a suppressor cell population within the spleen from 2 hr through 3 days of infection. The suppressor cell appears to be a macrophage which suppresses T-lymphocyte response to concanavalin A and results in a reduced host-vs.-graft response (Miller *et al.*, 1978). The suppressor effects can be reversed by indomethacin (J. W. Smith, unpublished).

The role of specific immunity in protection against enterobacterial urinary tract infection has been studied in experimental animal models. Immunization of animals with either heat-killed organisms, LPS (O antigen), or polysaccharide (K antigen) will protect against hematogenous induction of urinary tract infection (Kaijser and Olling, 1973; Sanford *et al.*, 1962). However, antibody to the H antigen does not provide protection in experimental studies (Kaijser and Olling, 1973). There exists little evidence that induction of serum antibody by immunization with heat-killed organisms or by passive administration of immune serum will protect against retrograde infection. In this regard it is of interest that hypogammaglobulinemic or T-cell-deficient patients have no more frequent or severe urinary tract infections than normal individuals. The only proven protection against retrograde urinary infection is observed after prior infection with the homologous organism (Holmgren and Smith, 1975; Montgomerie *et al.*, 1972). Thus the available studies would indicate that circulating antibody will protect against hematogenous urinary tract infection but is of minor importance in protection against retrograde infection. In contrast, local protection against retrograde urinary tract infection does occur following previous homologous infection, suggesting that local immunity may play a role in prevention of infection. There is no definitive information to establish whether antibody to the enterobacterial common antigen or LPS core antigen will protect against retrograde urinary tract infection.

4.3.2. Respiratory Tract

The normal "clearance" of bacteria from the lower respiratory tract (LRT) depends on mucociliary and alveolar macrophage function (Green, 1968; Green and Kass, 1964a). The actual killing of organisms which arrive in pulmonary alveoli is accomplished by alveolar macrophages. This antibacterial capacity is adversely affected by a number of factors, such as hypoxia and hyperoxia, ethanol, alveolar fluid, acute starvation, acidosis, renal failure, noxious gases, corticosteroids, and immunosuppressive agents (Harris *et al.*, 1977; Green, 1970; Huber *et al.*, 1970a,b; Goldstein *et al.*, 1969; Green 1968; Goldstein and Green, 1966, 1967; Green and Goldstein, 1966; Green and Kass, 1964a,b). Certain experimentally induced viral respiratory tract infections or chronic pulmonary diseases in animals are associated with impairment of pulmonary bactericidal activity against a variety of bacteria (Jakab and Dick, 1973; Goldstein *et al.*, 1969, 1973; Jakab and Green, 1972; Green and Goldstein, 1966; Green, 1968). The clinical implications of these findings are obvious. Morphological evidence of ciliary epithelial and other respiratory tract damage occurs in human and experimental viral infection (Jakab and Green, 1972; Hers, 1966), but physical transport of bacteria from the lung may be normal even though phagocyte antibacterial function is depressed (Jakab and Green, 1972). Hospitalized patients with severe underlying disease often have respiratory tract colonization with aerobic gram-negative bacilli (Johanson *et al.*, 1969, 1972). These patients are predisposed to development of gram-negative rod pneumonia, especially in the presence of the above predisposing factors or compromised mucociliary function (endotracheal intubation or tracheostomy) (Sanford, 1975; Pierce and Sanford, 1974; Tillotson and Finland, 1969).

Older studies demonstrated that local resistance to infection develops in the respiratory tract after a variety of bacterial infections or appropriate immunization (Gotschlich *et al.*, 1969; Goldschneider *et al.*, 1969; Hornich and Eigelsbach, 1966; Middlebrook, 1961; MacLeod *et al.*, 1945; Cannon and Walsh, 1937; Walsh and Cannon, 1936; Bull and McKee, 1928, 1929). However, none of these studies established a relationship between local immunity (resistance to infection) and any particular defense mechanism. Obviously, one means by which the specific immune response (antibody and cell-mediated immunity) might increase LRT antibacterial activity is through an effect on alveolar macrophage function.

IgG and secretory IgA are normally present in human tracheobronchial secretions and sputum (Waldman *et al.*, 1973; Masson *et al.*, 1965; Keimowitz, 1964). Antibody of both IgA and IgG classes has been reported after stimulation of the LRT with various antigens, including bacterial antigens (Reynolds and Thompson, 1973a; Kaltreider *et al.*, 1974; Waldman and Henney, 1971). There is no available information concerning LRT production of antibody against Enterobacteriaceae. However, LRT synthesis and secretion of antibody after induction of local infection with other bacteria have been studied in rabbits (Hand and Cantey, 1974). Secretions from infected animals contained IgG and/or IgA antibody against the infecting organism. Furthermore, in these same animals there was a marked increase in local synthesis of immunoglobulin (especially IgG) and production of specific antibody against the infecting organism. The data suggested that locally synthesized immunoglobulin was secreted into the LRT lumen. The biological activity of LRT antibody has not been completely studied, but IgG, and to a lesser extent secretory IgA, antibody against *Pseudomonas aeruginosa* will promote phagocytosis by rabbit and human alveolar macrophages (Reynolds *et al.*, 1975; Reynolds and Thompson, 1973b).

Local cell-mediated immunity (CMI) has been documented after LRT stimulation with various antigens (including bacterial antigen) and after LRT bacterial infection (Cantey and Hand, 1974; Reynolds *et al.*, 1974; Spencer *et al.*, 1974; Jurgensen *et al.*, 1973; Nash and Holle, 1973; Waldman and Henney, 1971; Galindo and Myrvik, 1970; Yamamoto *et al.*, 1970; Yamamoto and Anacker, 1970; Henney and Waldman, 1970). The cell-mediated immune response is known to produce marked changes (activation) in systemic macrophages (e.g., Mackaness, 1970). Although acquired immunity to systemic infections with many intracellular organisms depends on the activation of systemic mononuclear phagocytes, it had been suggested that alveolar macrophages are incapable of undergoing activation (Mackaness, 1974). However, it was recently documented that *in vitro* activation of normal al-

veolar macrophages can be induced by products of sensitized antigen-stimulated lymphocytes from animals with bacterial LRT infection (Johnson *et al.*, 1975). Macrophages obtained from the LRT of these same infected animals also were activated (*in vivo* activation). Both the *in vivo* and *in vitro* activated macrophages manifested an increased bactericidal activity against a variety of bacteria, including one of the Enterobacteriaceae (*S. typhimurium*). Whether enterobacterial LRT infection will also induce a local cell-mediated immune response remains to be evaluated.

It should be noted that certain gram-negative bacilli (e.g., *P. mirabilis, K. pneumoniae,* and *E. coli*) are inactivated at a slow rate by normal pulmonary antibacterial mechanisms in some experimental animals (Jay *et al.*, 1976; Jakab and Green, 1975; Kass *et al.*, 1966). Thus development of a specific immune response in the LRT may be especially crucial in protection against or recovery from infections with these organisms (Jakab and Green, 1973). Aerosol immunization of mice with a rough strain of *S. minnesota,* whose cell wall contains core glycolipid but no O polysaccharide, enhanced pulmonary bactericidal activity against other enterobacteria. Lung washings from immunized animals contained opsonizing activity for the challenge organism (*Serratia marcescens*) (LaForce, 1977).

4.3.3. Systemic Immune Response

Both strain-specific and cross-reactive antigens of Enterobacteriaceae provoke an immune response on the part of the host. Type-specific antibodies against O, H, and K antigens after challenge are well documented, and their protective value has been examined. In recent years there has been a great deal of interest in the immune response to various cross-reactive antigens of Enterobacteriaceae. Some of these antigens are cross-reactive within the family Enterobacteriaceae (enterobacterial common antigen, core glycolipid, and lipid A) (Domingue and Johnson, 1975; Westphal, 1975), whereas other antigens cross-react with nonenterobacterial organisms or host tissues (Lyampert and Danilova, 1975). Furthermore, some enterobacterial K antigens have a marked similarity to or identify with polysaccharide antigens of unrelated organisms (Robbins *et al.*, 1975a).

Production of type-specific antibody to superficial antigens of the Enterobacteriaceae occurs after systemic exposure to intact organisms (or purified antigen). Antibody to specific O antigens of enterobacterial organisms provides strain-specific protection against systemic infections, including hematogenous pyelonephritis, in animal models (Kaijser and Ahlstedt, 1977; Hanson et al., 1977; Kaijser and Olling, 1973; Kaijser et al., 1972; Kyriakos and Ikari, 1969; Sanford et al., 1962). IgG antibody to O antigen of P. mirabilis was shown to have greater opsonizing activity than IgM antibody against this organism in the absence of complement function (Smith et al., 1967). This finding is probably related to the observation that phagocytic cells have specific surface receptors for IgG but not IgM (Stossel, 1974; Quie, 1972; Huber and Fudenberg, 1968).

Recent studies indicate that antibody to capsular (K) antigen is also protective against infectious challenge in experimental animals (Hanson et al., 1977; Kaijser and Ahlstedt, 1977; Kaijser and Olling, 1973; Kaijser et al., 1972; Wolberg and Dewitt, 1969). Unfortunately, many K antigens (acidic polysaccharides) are poor immunogens, a fact which may be related to their role as virulence factors. There is little evidence to suggest a role for anti-H antibody in protection against enterobacterial infection. In fact, a recent study showed that antibody to H antigen provides no protection in a rabbit model of hematogenous pyelonephritis (Kaijser and Olling, 1973). Relatively little is known of the role which antibody to these specific antigens plays in protection of humans against enterobacterial infections. However, it is of interest that in gram-negative rod bacteremia patients with high titers of IgG antibody against specific O antigen or antibody to core glycolipid had a greater survival than individuals with low levels of these antibodies (Zinner and McCabe, 1976; McCabe et al., 1972).

Two antigens shared by most Enterobacteriaceae have been described. The so-called common antigen of Enterobacteriaceae (ECA) was described by Kunin (1963; Kunin et al., 1962). The biological significance of antibody to this enterobacterial cell wall antigen is still not clear. Some studies with antibody to ECA have demonstrated in vitro opsonizing activity (Domingue and Neter, 1966) and slight in vivo

protection against systemic enterobacterial infection (Domingue and Johnson, 1975; Frentz and Domingue, 1973; Gorzynski et al., 1971). In contrast, other studies found no in vitro biological activity for antibody to ECA (Kunin and Beard, 1963) and no protection against intravenous challenge with E. coli or K. pneumoniae after immunization with ECA (McCabe and Greely, 1973). Furthermore, McCabe and co-workers reported that levels of anti-ECA antibody were similar in control subjects and in patients with gram-negative rod bacteremia. Correlation of antibody titers with frequency of shock and death in patients with gram-negative rod bacteremia showed no obvious protective effect due to anti-ECA antibody (McCabe et al., 1972, 1973).

Evaluation of rough enterobacterial organisms has indicated that the core portion of cell wall LPS is common to most Enterobacteriaceae (Westphal, 1975; Luderitz et al., 1966a,b). This core glycolipid consists of 2-keto-3-deoxyoctonate (KDO) linked to lipid A. The LPS core, or even lipid A, appears to retain the biological activity of the intact endotoxin (LPS) complex (Rietschel et al., 1975; Luderitz et al., 1973; Galanos et al., 1972). Thus the possibility that antibody against this core glycolipid might provide broad protection against enterobacterial infection has been considered. In some animal studies antibody to the core antigen was found to provide protection against both the effects of endotoxin (Greisman et al., 1973; Greisman and Hornick, 1973; Braude et al., 1973; Braude and Douglas, 1972) and enterobacterial infection (Bruins et al., 1977; Ziegler et al., 1973; McCabe, 1972; Chedid et al., 1968). In contrast, Greisman et al. (1978) reported that sera from rabbits immunized with rough Enterobacteriaceae, and containing high titers of antibody against core LPS, afforded no more protection than the corresponding preimmune sera to mice challenged with other enterobacterial organisms. Similarly, antibody to lipid A was reported to protect against the effects of endotoxin (Rietschel and Galanos, 1977; Rietschel et al., 1975), but in at least two studies such antibody failed to offer any protection against enterobacterial challenge in animals (Bruins et al., 1977; Mullan et al., 1974). Young et al. (1975) found that in dogs antibody against LPS core antigen provided protection against the hemodynamic sequellae of bacteremia but did not enhance clearance of serum-resistant organisms from blood. Survival was increased in animals immunized with core antigen, as compared to controls, but was less than in animals immunized with specific bacterial vaccines (O antigen preparation). On the basis of these findings, and the observations that opsonizing and bactericidal activity of antibody against the core antigen was much less than that of type-specific antibody, it was suggested that antibody against core antigen might function primarily as an antitoxin (against endotoxin). As already noted, high titers of antibody against core antigen were associated with decreased frequency of shock and death in one group of patients with gram-negative rod bacteremia (McCabe *et al.*, 1972).

An interesting immunological phenomenon involving cross-reactivity between certain enterobacterial antigens and capsular antigens of pyogenic organisms (meningococci, pneumococci, and *Hemophilus influenzae*) has been defined (reviewed by Robbins *et al.*, 1975a,b) (Table 1). It is likely that protective antibody against these encapsulated pathogens is not always related to clinical infection or colonization with specific organism. Rather, it appears that at least some of this antibody is the result of exposure to cross-reacting antigens of other organisms, expecially Enterobacteriaceae. For instance, an *E. coli* capsular polysaccharide antigen (K100), which is similar to *H. influenzae* type b capsular polysaccharide (Schneerson *et al.*, 1972), elicits production of antibody protective against type b *H. influenzae* when animals are given cross-reacting *E. coli* by intravenous or oral administration (Handzel *et al.*, 1975; Robbins *et al.*, 1973). Similar results were observed in human volunteers who were fed *E. coli* with K100 antigen (Schneerson and Robbins, 1975). Other cross-reacting antigen combinations include pneumococcus type III polysaccharide and *E. coli* K7 (acidic capsular polysaccharide) (Robbins *et al.*, 1975a,b; Robbins *et al.*, 1972); other *E. coli* antigens and pneumococcal capsular polysaccharides (Heidelberger *et al.*, 1968); various *Streptococcus pneumoniae* and *Klebsiella pneumoniae* capsular polysaccharides (Heidelberger and Dutton, 1973; Heidelberger and Nimmich, 1972); meningococcus group A capsular polysaccharide and *N*-acetyl monosamine phosphate antigen of *Bacillus pumilus* (an enteric organism) (Robbins *et al*, 1975a,b; Myerowitz *et al.*, 1973; Robbins *et al.*, 1972); meningococcus group C capsular polysaccharide and a newly described *E. coli* capsular polysaccharide (K92) consisting of polyneuraminic acid (Glode *et al.*, 1977b; Liu *et al.*, 1977; Robbins *et al.*, 1972, 1975a,b; Myerowitz *et al.*, 1972). Indirect evidence suggesting that protective antibody against encapsulated pyogenic organisms is often stimulated by exposure to cross-reacting antigens includes infrequent colonization or disease due to the pathogenic organism and frequent carriage of the "nonpathogenic" cross-react-

TABLE 1. Cross-Reactions of Enterobacterial Antigens with Other Bacterial Antigens

Enterobacterial antigen	Cross-reacting antigen	Cross-reactive factor
Common antigen (ECA)	ECA of other Enterobacteriaceae	?
LPS core antigen	Core antigen of other Enterobacteriaceae	Lipid-A-core polysaccharide
E. coli K1	*N. meningitidis* group B capsular polysaccharide	*N*-Acetyl neuraminic acid
E. coli K92	*N. meningitidis* group C capsular polysaccharide	Polyneuraminic acid
E. coli K7	*S. pneumoniae* III capsular polysaccharide	? Uronic acid
E. coli K antigens (multiple)	*S. pneumoniae* capsular polysaccharides (multiple)	Various
E. coli K100	*H. influenzae* type b capsular polysaccharide	?
K. pneumoniae K polysaccharides (multiple)	*S. pneumoniae* capsular polysaccharides (multiple)	Various

ing organism, and elicitation of protective antibody against the pathogen in animals and humans by exposure to the cross-reacting organism or antigen (Robbins *et al.*, 1975a,b; Schneerson and Robbins, 1975).

E. coli K1 antigen is quite similar or identical to meningococcus group B capsular polysaccharide (Kaijser *et al.*, 1973; Grados and Ewing, 1970). Antibody to group B polysaccharide is protective against *E. coli* K1 infection in laboratory animals (Robbins *et al.*, 1974, 1975a,b). Unfortunately, neither of these antigens reliably induces antibody production in humans (Robbins *et al.*, 1975a,b; Kasper *et al.*, 1973).

The role of cell-mediated immunity as a systemic response to enterobacterial infection is poorly characterized. Intradermal inoculation of endotoxin in healthy adult volunteers elicited a delayed hypersensitivity reaction, suggesting previous development of CMI to this antigen (Greisman and Hornick, 1972). On the other hand, endotoxin has been reported to inhibit the cell-mediated immune response to other antigens (reviewed by Schwab, 1975).

It has been suggested that systemic CMI is important in protection against some of the enterobacteria. In animal models resistance to infection with *Salmonella,* a facultative intracellular organism, is at least in part mediated by CMI (Collins, 1974; Mackaness and Blanden, 1967). Crude ribosomes, as well as RNA and protein containing extracts of ribosomes, from *S. typhimurium* will provide protection against this organism (Angerman and Eisenstein, 1978; Hoops *et al.*, 1976; Eisenstein, 1975; Berry *et al.*, 1975; Johnson, 1973; Smith and Bigley, 1972a,b; Venneman, 1972; Venneman and Berry, 1971; Venneman *et al.*, 1970; Venneman and Bigley, 1969). Immunogenic ribosomal RNA preparations may contain specific *Salmonella* O antigen (endotoxin) components (Lin and Berry, 1978; Hoops *et al.*, 1976; Eisenstein, 1975; Berry *et al.*, 1975). Thus some of these RNA preparations may represent a "super antigen," with the RNA serving an adjuvant function. However, there are conflicting reports on the role of the O antigen in the protective effect elicited by ribosomal vaccines (Lin and Berry, 1978; Misfeldt and Johnson, 1977). Other ribosomal preparations appear to elicit cross-protection among *Salmonella* strains by means of a shared immunogen (? protein, ? core LPS) (Eisenstein, 1975). With the present state of knowledge it is impossible to be certain of the means by which *Salmonella* ribosomal preparations induce protection. There is evidence to suggest that both CMI (Berry *et al.*, 1975; Venneman and Berry, 1971) and antibody (? cytophilic) (Margolis and Bigley, 1972) may play a role in protection.

Enterobacterial antigens which are similar to, and elicit cross-reacting antibody to, mammalian tissue antigens have been described. Perhaps the best known of these interactions is that between human blood group ABO substances (glycoproteins) and enterobacterial O antigen oligosaccharides (Springer, 1975; Springer *et al.*, 1961). Human kidney antigens are known to cross-react with at least three enterobacterial antigens: *E. coli* O2 antigen, an unrelated *E. coli* component, and the common antigen of Enterobacteriaceae (Holmgren *et al.*, 1975). Furthermore, enterobacterial CA cross-reacts with colon antigens of humans and germ-free rats (Lagercrantz *et al.*, 1968; Perlmann *et al.*, 1967) and with human liver, muscle, and heart tissues (Morgenstern and Gorzynski, 1977). The role of antibody elicited by these bacterial antigens in the pathogenesis of any human renal, intestinal, or other disease process is speculative at the moment.

Persistence of enterobacterial antigen(s) in the kidneys after resolution of the actual infectious process has been suggested as a potential basis for immunologically mediated renal disease. Provocation of an injurious immune response by this retained antigen has been postulated as a cause of culture-negative "chronic pyelonephritis." Studies designed to determine the presence of enterobacterial antigen in such kidneys have yielded conflicting and inconclusive results (Schwartz and Cotran, 1973; Aoki *et al.*, 1969). At present the role of enterobacteria-induced immunopathology in the pathogenesis of chronic renal disease can only be described as uncertain.

5. Immunodiagnosis

5.1. Serum Antibody

Detection of serum antibody against the infecting organism (particularly antibody to the

O antigen) represents an indirect test for localization of urinary tract infection in humans (Hanson *et al.,* 1977, Holmgren and Smith, 1975; Cobbs, 1972; Reeves and Brumfitt, 1968). The presence of serum antibody correlates with infection involving the upper urinary tract or kidney. Up to 90% of children with clinical evidence of active upper urinary tract infection developed O antibody, which was principally IgG in nature, whereas only 5% of patients with cystitis developed such antibody (Jodal *et al.,* 1975). Studies using direct tests (such as ureteral catheterization and bladder washout procedure) for localization of infection have detected antibody more frequently in individuals with upper tract infection (Hewstone and Whitaker, 1969; Bremner *et al.,* 1969; Reeves and Brumfitt, 1968). Variables which influence the frequency of antibody in individuals with upper tract infection include clinical activity at time of study, age of patient, pregnancy, and the species and serotype of the organism (Holmgren and Smith, 1975). Asymptomatic individuals have serum antibody less often than symptomatic cases. Hanson has suggested that persons with asymptomatic bacteriuria have organisms which contain less O antigen and induce less inflammatory reaction than organisms in individuals with clinically active infection (Hanson, 1973, 1976). In summary, the serum antibody test is not so definitive as direct localization tests and remains primarily a research tool for correlating multiple factors in human infection.

5.2. Urinary Antibody

A more definitive test for localization of infection in the urinary tract is the test for antibody-coated bacteria (ACB) in urine sediment (Thomas *et al.,* 1974; Jones *et al.,* 1974). This test, which is more sensitive than determination of serum antibody (Jones *et al.,* 1974), correlates with infection of the upper urinary tract or of the kidney. An occasional patient with prostatitis alone also will be ACB positive (Jones, 1974). The test has excellent external validity, since multiple observers agreed on first reading of 88% of specimens (Schaberg *et al.,* 1977). A review of all studies in adults concerning internal validity indicated that the sensitivity of the test has been 91% and that the specificity and predictive value

were 100% (Jones, 1978). Hence the test appears to be an adequate, reproducibly accurate diagnostic serological determination. A positive ACB test also was a predictor of patients with a high probability of failing a standard course of therapy for urinary tract infection (Fang *et al.,* 1978). Thus this procedure is an indirect, noninvasive, and rapid test that has validity for localization of urinary tract infection.

6. Immunoprevention

Attempts at specific immunization against enteric pathogens are covered elsewhere (Chapter 11). In recent years an increasing interest in active immunization against the Enterobacteriaceae has developed. Obviously, this interest is a consequence of the frequency with which serious gram-negative rod infections (especially bacteremia) occur in hospitalized patients with compromised host defenses. One possible means of decreasing the number and/or consequences of such infections would be through appropriate immunization procedures. As we have discussed, antibody to certain enterobacterial antigens will protect animals against subsequent challenge. Antibody against O antigen determinants usually offers good protection against the specific organism (Kaijser and Ahlstedt, 1977; Kaijser and Olling, 1973; Kaijser *et al.,* 1972; Kyriakos and Ikari, 1969; Sanford *et al.,* 1962). However, the large number of O antigens found among Enterobacteriaceae causing human infection indicates that type-specific immunization would be a virtually impossible task.

Of greater current interest is the possibility that LPS core antigen, or possibly solubilized lipid A, could be used as an immunogen in compromised patients at risk for enterobacterial infections (Braude *et al.,* 1977; McCabe *et al.,* 1977; Young and Stevens, 1977; McCabe, 1976; Sanford, 1972). We have already observed that various core antigen preparations will stimulate production of protective antibody in experimental animals (Young *et al.,* 1975; Ziegler *et al.,* 1973; McCabe, 1972; Chedid *et al.,* 1968). Such antibody appears to be cross-protective against infection with many if not all Enterobacteriaceae. There is some clinical evidence that this antibody protects against shock and death in human gram-negative rod bacteremia (Zinner and McCabe, 1976; McCabe *et al.*, 1972). This "antiendotoxin" antibody probably offers less protection against intravenous challenge with enterobacterial organisms than does O specific antibody (Young *et al.*, 1975, 1977; McCabe, 1972). However, the possibility that some protection against gram-negative rod bacteremia (or at least the postulated endotoxin-mediated component) might be obtained by immunization of high-risk patients is an attractive concept. Obviously, additional toxicity and efficacy studies with various core antigen preparations in animals are needed before human studies are contemplated.

As we noted earlier, exposure of animals to enterobacterial organisms, or antigens which are cross-reactive with encapsulated pyogenic organisms (pneumococcus, meningococcus, *Hemophilus*) will often result in formation of protective antibody against the latter (Robbins *et al.*, 1975a,b). Furthermore, serum antibody to *H. influenzae* type b capsular polysaccharide was elicited in adult human volunteers after feeding of cross-reactive *E. coli* with K100 antigen (Schneerson and Robbins, 1975). Transient (3–8 weeks) intestinal colonization with this *E. coli* occurred in all volunteers and was without adverse effects. Whether such exposure to cross-reacting "nonpathogenic" enterobacteria will prove to be relevant, safe, and effective for human immunization against *H. influenzae* and other encapsulated pathogens remains to be determined.

The reverse aspects of this cross-protective phenomenon are also of potential importance. Many pneumococcal capsular polysaccharides are known to cross-react with *E. coli* or *K. pneumoniae* K antigens (Robbins *et al.*, 1975a; Heidelberger and Dutton, 1973; Heidelberger and Nimmich, 1972; Heidelberger *et al.*, 1968). The possibility that immunization with pneumococcal antigens might protect against enterobacterial infections has been investigated in an experimental animal model (Young and Stevens, 1977; Young *et al.*, 1977). Prior immunization with type III pneumococcus protected leukopenic rabbits against bacteremia with certain *Klebsiella* and *E. coli* strains. It is conceivable that use of the current pneumococcal vaccine will provide some protection against infection with cross-reacting Enterobacteriaceae (*E. coli* and *Klebsiella*).

7. Immunotherapy

There is no currently available immunotherapy for enterobacterial infections. Passive immunity to enterobacterial challenge can be transferred to animals by means of antiserum to LPS core antigen (Ziegler *et al.*, 1973; McCabe, 1972; Chedid *et al.*, 1968). Whether such antiserum would have protective value when administered after the onset of overt clinical septicemia and shock is unknown. The possibility that specific human immune globulin, when added to other therapeutic measures, might improve survival in gram-negative rod bacteremia deserves study.

References

Ahlstedt, S., and Holmgren, J., 1975, Alteration of the antibody response to *Escherichia coli* O antigen in mice by prior exposure to various somatic antigens, *Immunology* 29:487–496.

Ahlstedt, S., and Lindholm, L., 1977, Antibody response to *Escherichia coli* O antigens and influence of the protein moiety of the endotoxin, *Immunology* 33:629–633.

Allison, A. C., Davies, P., and Page, R. C., 1973, Effects of entodoxin on macrophages and other lymphoreticular cells, *J. Infect. Dis.* 128:S212–S219.

Andersson, J., Sjoberg, O., and Moller, G., 1972, Induction of immunoglobulin and antibody synthesis *in vitro* by lipopolysaccharides, *Eur. J. Immunol.* 2:349–353.

Andersson, J., Melchers, F., Galanos, C., and Luderitz, O., 1973, The mitogenic effect of lipopolysaccharide on bone marrow-derived mouse lymphocytes: Lipid A as the mitogenic part of the molecule, *J. Exp. Med.* 137:943–953.

Angerman, C. R., and Eisenstein, T. K., 1978, Comparative efficacy and toxicity of a ribosomal vaccine, acetone-killed cells, lipopolysaccharide, and a live cell vaccine prepared from *Salmonella typhimurium*, *Infect. Immun.* 19:575–582.

Aoki, S., Imamura, S., Aoki, M., and McCabe, W. R., 1969, "Abacterial" and bacterial pyelonephritis: Immunofluorescent localization of bacterial antigen, *N. Engl. J. Med.* 281:1375–1382.

Armerding, D., and Katz, D. H., 1974, Activation of T and B lymphocytes *in vitro*. I. Regulatory influence of bacterial lipopolysaccharide (LPS) on specific T-cell helper function, *J. Exp. Med.* 139:24–43.

Austen, K. F., and Cohn, Z. A., 1963, Contribution of serum and cellular factors in host defense reactions, *N. Engl. J. Med.* **268**:933–938, 994–1000, 1056–1064.

Bennett, J. V., Scheckler, W. E., Maki, D. G., and Brachman, P. S., 1971, Current national patterns—United States, in: *Proceedings of the International Conference on Nosocomial Infections* (P. S. Brachman and T. C. Eickhoff, eds.), pp. 42–49, Waverly Press, Baltimore.

Berry, L. J., 1975, Metabolic effects of endotoxin, in: *Microbiology—1975* (D. Schlessinger, ed.), pp. 315–319, American Society for Microbiology, Washington, D.C.

Berry, L. J., Douglas, G. N., Hoops, P., and Prather, N. E., 1975, Immunization against salmonellosis, in: *The Immune System and Infectious Diseases* (E. Neter and F. Milgrom, eds.), pp. 388–398, Karger, Basel.

Betz, S. J., and Morrison, D. C., 1977, Chemical and biologic properties of a protein-rich fraction of bacterial lipopolysaccharides. I. The *in vitro* murine lymphocyte response, *J. Immunol.* **119**:1475–1481.

Bjornson, A. B., and Michael, J. G., 1973, Factors in normal human serum that promote bacterial phagocytosis, *J. Infect. Dis.* **128**:S182–S186.

Bortolussi, R., Low, R., Ferrieri, P., and Quie, P. G., 1978, K1 capsular antigen production in *Escherichia coli* and relationship to opsonization, *Abstr. 18th Intersci. Conf. Antimicrob. Agents Chemother.*, Abstr. No. 505.

Braude, A. I., and Douglas, H., 1972, Passive immunization against the local Schwartzman reaction, *J. Immunol.* **108**:505–512.

Braude, A. I., Douglas, H., and Jones, J., 1969, Experimental production of lethal *Escherichia coli* bacteremia of pelvic origin, *J. Bacteriol.* **98**:979–991.

Braude, A. I., Douglas, H., and Davis, C. E., 1973, Treatment and prevention of intravascular coagulation with antiserum to endotoxin, *J. Infect. Dis.* **128**:S157–S164.

Braude, A. I., Ziegler, E. J., Douglas, H., and McCutchan, J. A., 1977, Antibody to cell wall glycolipid of gram-negative bacteria: Induction of immunity to bacteremia and endotoxemia, *J. Infect. Dis.* **136**:S167–S173.

Bremner, D. A., Fairley, K. F., and Kincaid-Smith, P., 1969, The serum antibody response in renal and bladder infections, *Med. J. Aust.* **1**:1069–1071.

Brown, D. L., 1974, Complement and coagulation, in *Progress in Immunology II*, Vol. 1 (L. Brent and J. Holborow, eds.), pp. 191–200, North-Holland, Amsterdam.

Bruins, S. C., Stumacher, R., Johns, M. A., and McCabe, W. R., 1977, Immunization with R mutants of *Salmonella minnesota*. III. Comparison of the protective effect of immunization with lipid A and the Re mutant, *Infect. Immun.* **17**:16–20.

Bull, C. G., and McKee, C. M., 1928, Respiratory immunity in rabbits. VI. The effects of immunity on the carrier state of the pneumococcus and *Bacillus bronchisepticus*, *Am. J. Hyg.* **8**:723–729.

Bull, C. G., and McKee, C. M., 1929, Respiratory immunity in rabbits. VII. Resistance to intranasal infection in the absence of demonstrable antibodies, *Am. J. Hyg.* **9**:490–499.

Cannon, P. R., and Walsh, T. E., 1937, Studies on the fate of living bacteria introduced into the upper respiratory tract of normal and intranasally vaccinated rabbits, *J. Immunol.* **32**:49–62.

Cantey, J. R., and Hand, W. L., 1974, Cell-mediated immunity after bacterial infection of the lower respiratory tract, *J. Clin. Invest.* **54**:1125–1134.

Cheasty, T., Gross, R. J., and Rowe, B., 1977, Incidence of K1 antigen in *Escherichia coli* isolated from blood and cerebrospinal fluid of patients in the United Kingdom, *J. Clin. Pathol.* **30**:945–947.

Chedid, L., and Audibert, F., 1977, Chemically defined bacterial products with immunopotentiating activity, *J. Infect. Dis.* **136**:S246–S251.

Chedid, L., Parant, M., Parant, F., and Boyer, F., 1968, A proposed mechanism for natural immunity to enterobacterial pathogens, *J. Immunol.* **100**:292–301.

Chedid, L., Parant, M., Damais, C., Parant, F., Juy, D., and Galelli, A., 1975, Failure of endotoxin to increase nonspecific resistance to infection of lipopolysaccharide low-responder mice, *Infect. Immun.* **13**:722–727.

Chess, L., MacDermott, R. P., and Schlossman, S. F., 1974, Immunologic functions of isolated human lymphocyte subpopulations. I. Quantitative isolation of human T and B cells and response to mitogens, *J. Immunol.* **113**:1113–1121.

Cluff, L. E., 1970, Effects of endotoxins on susceptibility to infections, *J. Infect. Dis.* **122**:205–212.

Cobbs, G. B., 1972, Localization of urinary tract infection, in: *Urinary Tract Infection and Its Management* (D. Kaye, ed.), pp. 52–64, Mosby, St. Louis.

Cohn, Z. A., 1973, Host–parasite relations in bacterial diseases, in: *Microbiology* (B. D. Davis, R. Dulbecco, H. N. Eisen, H. S. Ginsberg, W. B. Wood, and M. McCarty, eds.), pp. 627–665, Harper and Row, Hagerstown, Md.

Collins, F. M., 1974, Vaccines and cell-mediated immunity, *Bacteriol. Rev.* **38**:371–402.

Coutinho, A., and Moller, G., 1973, B cell mitogenic properties of thymus-independent antigens, *Nature (London), New Biol.* **245**:12–14.

Domingue, G., and Johnson, E., 1975, The common antigen of *Enterobacteriaceae* and its biological significance, in: *The Immune System and Infectious Diseases* (E. Neter and F. Milgrom, eds.), pp. 242–262, Karger, Basel.

Domingue, G. J., and Neter, E., 1966, Opsonizing and bactericidal activity of antibodies against common antigen of *Enterobacteriaceae*, *J. Bacteriol.* **91**:129–133.

Donaldson, R. M., Jr., 1964, Normal bacterial populations of the intestine and their relation to intestinal function, *N. Engl. J. Med.* **270**:938–945, 994–1001, 1050–1056.

Eisenstein, T. K., 1975, Evidence for O antigens as the

antigenic determinants in "ribosomal" vaccines prepared from *Salmonella, Infect. Immun.* **12**:364–377.

Elin, R. J., and Wolff, S. M., 1974, The role of iron in nonspecific resistance to infection induced by endotoxin, *J. Immunol.* **112**:737–745.

Elin, R. J., and Wolff, S. M., 1976, Biology of endotoxin, *Annu. Rev. Med.* **27**:127–141.

Engvall, E., and Perlmann, P., 1972, Enzyme-linked immunosorbent assay, ELISA. III. Quantitation of specific antibodies by enzyme-labeled anti-immunoglobulin in antigen-coated tubes, *J. Immunol.* **109**:129–135.

Ewing, W. H., and Martin, W. J., 1974, *Enterobacteriaceae*, in: *Manual of Clinical Microbiology, 2nd ed.* (E. H. Lennette, E. H. Spaulding, and J. P. Truant, eds.), pp. 189–221, American Society for Microbiology, Washington, D.C.

Fang, L. S. T., Tolkoff-Rubin, N. E., and Rubin, R. H., 1978, Efficacy of single-dose and conventional amoxicillin therapy in urinary-tract infection localized by the antibody-coated bacteria technic, *N. Engl. J. Med.* **298**:413–416.

Fearon, D. T., Ruddy, S., Schur, P. H., and McCabe, W. R., 1975, Activation of the properdin pathway of complement in patients with gram-negative bacteremia, *N. Engl. J. Med.* **292**:937–940.

Feingold, D. S., 1970, Hospital-acquired infections, *N. Engl. J. Med.* **283**:1384–1391.

Fine, D. P., 1974, Activation of the classic and alternate complement pathways by endotoxin, *J. Immunol.* **112**:763–769.

Finland, M., 1970, Changing ecology of bacterial infections as related to antibacterial therapy, *J. Infect. Dis.* **122**:419–431.

Forsgren, A., and Quie, P. G., 1974a, Influence of the alternate complement pathway on opsonization of several bacterial species, *Infect. Immunol.* **10**:402–404.

Forsgren, A., and Quie, P. G., 1974b, Opsonic activity in human serum chelated with ethylene glycoltetra-acetic acid, *Immunology* **26**:1251–1256.

Franzl, R. E., and McMaster, P. D., 1968, The primary immune response in mice. I. The enhancement and suppression of hemolysin production by a bacterial endotoxin, *J. Exp. Med.* **127**:1087–1107.

Frentz, G., and Domingue, G., 1973, Effects of immunization with ethanol-soluble enterobacterial common antigen on *in vivo* bacterial clearance and hematogenous pyelonephritis, *Proc. Soc. Exp. Biol. Med.* **142**:246–252.

Füst, G., Petras, G., and Ujhelyi, E., 1976, Activation of the complement system during infections due to gram-negative bacteria, *Clin. Immunol. Immunopathol.* **5**:293–302.

Galanos, C., Rietschel, E. T., Luderitz, O., Westphal, O., Kim, Y. B., and Watson, D. W., 1972, Biological activities of lipid A complexed with bovine serum albumin, *Eur. J. Biochem.* **32**:230–233.

Gale, R. P., Opelz, G., and Golde, D. W., 1977, The effect of endotoxin on circulating lymphocytes in normal man, *Br. J. Haematol.* **36**:49–58.

Galindo, B., and Myrvik, Q. N., 1970, Migratory response of granulomatous alveolar cells from BCG-sensitized rabbits, *J. Immunol.* **105**:227–237.

Gewurz, H., Shin, H. S., and Mergenhagen, S. E., 1968, Interactions of the complement system with endotoxic lipopolysaccharide: Consumption of each of the six terminal complement components, *J. Exp. Med.* **128**:1049–1057.

Gibbons, R. J., 1975, Attachment of oral streptococci to mucosal surfaces, in: *Microbiology—1975* (D. Schlessinger, ed.), pp. 127–131, American Society for Microbiology, Washington, D.C.

Gibbons, R. J., and van Houte, J., 1975, Bacterial influence in oral microbial ecology, *Annu. Rev. Microbiol.* **29**:19–44.

Glode, M. P., Sutton, A., Robbins, J. B., McCracken, G. H., Gotschlich, E. C., Kaijser, B., and Hanson, L. A., 1977a, Neonatal meningitis due to *Escherichia coli* K1, *J. Infect. Dis.* **136**:S93–S97.

Glode, M. P., Robbins, J. B., Liu, T.-Y., Gotschlich, E. C., Ørskov, I., and Ørshov, F., 1977b, Cross-antigenicity and immunogenicity between capsular polysaccharides of group C *Neisseria meningitidis* and of *Escherichia coli* K92, *J. Infect. Dis.* **135**:94–102.

Glynn, A. A., and Howard, C. J., 1970, The sensitivity to complement of strains of *Escherichia coli* related to their K antigens, *Immunology* **18**:331–346.

Glynn, A. A., and Howard, C. J., 1971, The virulence for mice of strains of *Escherichia coli* related to the effects of K antigens on their resistance to phagocytosis and killing by complement, *Immunology* **20**:767–777.

Glynn, A. A., Brumfitt, W., and Howard, C. J., 1971, K antigens of *Escherichia coli* and renal involvement in urinary-tract infections, *Lancet* **1**:514–516.

Goldschneider, I., Gotschlich, E. C., and Artenstein, M. S., 1969, Human immunity to the meningococcus. II. Development of natural immunity, *J. Exp. Med.* **129**:1327–1348.

Goldstein, E., and Green, G. M., 1966, The effect of acute renal failure on the bacterial clearance mechanisms of the lung, *J. Lab. Clin. Med.* **68**:531–542.

Goldstein, E., and Green, G. M., 1967, Alteration of the pathogenicity of *Pasteurella pneumotropica* for the murine lung caused by changes in pulmonary antibacterial activity, *J. Bacteriol.* **93**:1651–1656.

Goldstein, E., Green, G. M., and Seamans, C., 1969, The effect of silicosis on the antibacterial defense mechanisms of the murine lung, *J. Infect. Dis.* **120**:210–216.

Goldstein, E., Akers, T., and Prato, C., 1973, Role of immunity in viral-induced bacterial superinfections of the lung, *Infect. Immun.* **8**:757–761.

Goodman, M. G., Parks, D. E., and Weigle, W. O., 1978, Immunologic responsiveness of the C3H/HeJ mouse: Differential ability of butanol-extracted lipopolysaccharide (LPS) to evoke LPS-mediated effects, *J. Exp. Med.* **148**:800–813.

Gorzynski, E. A., Ambrus, J. L., and Neter, E., 1971, Effect of common enterobacterial antiserum on experimental *Salmonella typhimurium* infection of mice, *Proc. Soc. Exp. Biol. Med.* **137**:1209–1212.

Gotschlich, E. C., Goldschneider, I., and Artenstein, M. S., 1969, Human immunity to the meningococcus. V. The effect of immunization with meingococcal group C polysaccharide on the carrier state, *J. Exp. Med.* **129**:1385–1395.

Gotze, O., and Muller-Eberhard, H. J., 1971, The C3-activator system: An alternate pathway of complement activation, *J. Exp. Med.* **134**:905–1085.

Grados, O., and Ewing, W. H., 1970, Antigenic relationship between *Escherichia coli* and *Neisseria meningitidis*, *J. Infect. Dis.* **122**:100–103.

Green, G. M., 1968, Pulmonary clearance of infectious agents, *Annu. Rev. Med.* **19**:315–336.

Green, G. M., 1970, The J. Burns Amberson lecture—In defense of the lung, *Am. Rev. Resp. Dis.* **102**:691–703.

Green, G. M., and Goldstein, E., 1966, Nonspecific resistance to bacterial infection in laboratory models of chronic pulmonary disease, *Am. Rev. Resp. Dis.* **94**:491–492 (Abstr).

Green, G. M., and Kass, E. H., 1964a, The role of the alveolar macrophage in the clearance of bacteria from the lung, *J. Exp. Med.* **119**:167–176.

Green, G. M., and Kass, E. H., 1964b, Factors influencing the clearance of bacteria by the lung, *J. Clin. Invest.* **43**:769–776.

Greisman, S. E., and Hornick, R. B., 1972, Cellular inflammatory responses of man to bacterial endotoxin: A comparison with PPD and other bacterial antigens, *J. Immunol.* **109**:1210–1222.

Greisman, S. E., and Hornick, R. B., 1973, Mechanisms of endotoxin tolerance with special reference to man, *J. Infect. Dis.* **128**:S265–S276.

Greisman, S. E., Young, E. J., and DuBuy, B., 1973, Mechanisms of endotoxin tolerance. VIII. Specificity of serum transfer, *J. Immunol.* **111**:1349–1360.

Greisman, S. E., DuBuy, J. B., and Woodward, C. L., 1978, Experimental gram-negative bacterial sepsis: Reevaluation of the ability of rough mutant antisera to protect mice, *Proc. Soc. Exp. Biol. Med.* **158**:482–490.

Hand, W. L., and Cantey, J. R., 1974, Antibacterial mechanisms of the lower respiratory tract. I. Immunoglobulin synthesis and secretion, *J. Clin. Invest.* **53**:354–362.

Hand, W. L., and King, N. L., 1977, Deficiency of serum bactericidal activity against *Salmonella typhimurium* in sickle cell anemia, *Clin. Exp. Immunol.* **30**:262–270.

Hand, W. L., and King, N. L., 1978, Serum opsonization of Salmonella in sickle cell anemia, *Am. J. Med.* **64**:388–395.

Handzel, Z. T., Argaman, M., Parke, J. C., Jr., Schneerson, R., and Robbins, J. B., 1975, Heteroimmunization to the capsular polysaccharide of *Haemophilus influenzae* type B induced by enteric cross-reacting bacteria, *Infect. Immun.* **11**:1045–1052.

Hanson, L. A., 1973, Host-parasite relationships in urinary tract infections (Editorial), *J. Infect. Dis.* **127**:726–730.

Hanson, L. A., 1976, *Escherichia coli* infections in childhood. Significance of bacterial virulence and immune defense, *Arch. Dis. Child.* **51**:737–742.

Hanson, L. A., Ahlstedt, S., Fasth, A., Jodal, U., Kaijser, B., Larsson, P., Lindberg, U., Olling, S., Sohl-Akerlund, A., and Svanborg-Eden, C., 1977, Antigens of *Escherichia coli*, human immune response, and the pathogenesis of urinary tract infections, *J. Infect. Dis.* **136**:S144–S149.

Harris, G. D., Johanson, W. G., Jr., and Pierce, A. K., 1977, Determinants of lung bacterial clearance in mice after acute hypoxia, *Am. Rev. Resp. Dis.* **116**:671–684.

Heidelberger, M., and Dutton, G. G. S., 1973, Cross-reactions of additional extracellular polysaccharides of *Klebsiella*, *J. Immunol.* **11**:857–859.

Heidelberger, M., and Nimmich, W., 1972, Additional immunochemical relationships of capsular polysaccharides of *Klebsiella* and pneumococci, *J. Immunol.* **109**:1337–1344.

Heidelberger, M., Jann, K., Jann, B., Ørskov, F., Ørskov, I., and Westphal, O., 1968, Relations between structures of three K polysaccharides of *Escherichia coli* and cross-reactivity in anti-pneumococcal sera, *J. Bacteriol.* **95**:2415–2417.

Heilman, D. H., and Bast, R. C., Jr., 1967, *In vitro* assay of endotoxin by the inhibition of macrophage migration, *J. Bacteriol.* **93**:15–20.

Henney, C. S., and Waldman, R. H., 1970, Cell-mediated immunity shown by lymphocytes from the respiratory tract, *Science* **169**:696–697.

Hers, J. F. Ph., 1966, Disturbances of the ciliated epithelium due to influenza virus, *Am. Rev. Resp. Dis.* **93**:162–171 (Suppl. 3).

Hewstone, A. S., and Whitaker, J., 1969, The correlation of ureteric urine bacteriology and homologous antibody titer in children with urinary infection, *J. Pediatr.* **74**:540–543.

Hoffman, M. K., Green, S., Old, L. J., and Oettgen, H. F., 1976, Serum containing endotoxin-induced tumor necrosis factor substitutes for helper T cells, *Nature (London)* **263**:416–417.

Hoffman, M. K., Galanos, C., Koenig, S., and Oettgen, H. F., 1977, B-cell activation by lipopolysaccharide: Distinct pathways for induction of mitosis and antibody production, *J. Exp. Med.* **146**:1640–1647.

Hoffman, M. K., Oettgen, H. F., Old, L. J., Mittler, R. S., and Hammerling, U., 1978, Induction and immunological properties of tumor necrosis factor, *J. Reticuloendothel. Soc.* **23**:307–319.

Holmgren, J., and Ahlstedt, S., 1974, Enhancement of the IgG antibody production to *Escherichia coli* O antigen by prior exposure to serologically different *E. coli* bacteria, *Immunology* **26**:67–76.

Holmgren, J., and Smith, J. W., 1975, Immunological aspects of urinary tract infections, *Progr. Allergy* **18**:289–352.

Holmgren, J., Goldblum, R. M., Blomberg, J., Hanson, L. A., Hermodsson, S., Holm, S., and Kaijser, B., 1975,

Antigenic relationships between kidney and enteric bacteria, in: *The Immune System and Infectious Diseases* (E. Neter and F. Milgrom, eds.), pp. 263–271, Karger, Basel.

Hoops, P., Prather, N. E., Berry, L. J., and Ravel, J. M., 1976, Evidence for an extrinsic immunogen in effective ribosomal vaccines from *Salmonella typhimurium*, *Infect. Immun.* **13**:1184–1192.

Hornich, R. B., and Eigelsbach, H. T., 1966, Aerogenic immunization of man with live tularemia vaccine, *Bacteriol. Rev.* **30**:532–538.

Hsu, S. H., 1975, Blastogenesis of human lymphocytes by endotoxin, *Immunol. Commun.* **4**:407–417.

Huber, G., LaForce, M., and Mason, R., 1970a, Impairment and recovery of pulmonary antibacterial defense mechanisms after oxygen administration, *J. Clin. Invest.* **49**:47a (Abstr.).

Huber, G. L., LaForce, F. M., Mason, R. J., and Monaco, A. P., 1970b, Impairment of pulmonary bacterial defense mechanisms by immuno-suppressive agents, *Surg. Forum* **21**:285–286.

Huber, H., and Fudenberg, H. H., 1968, Receptor sites of human monocytes for IgG, *Int. Arch. Allergy Appl. Immunol.* **34**:18–31.

Issekutz, A. C., and Biggar, W. D., 1977, Influence of serum-derived chemotactic factors and bacterial products on human neutrophil chemotaxis, *Infect. Immun.* **15**:212–220.

Jakab, G. J., and Dick, E. C., 1973, Synergistic effect in viral–bacterial infection: Combined infection of the murine respiratory tract with Sendai virus and *Pasturella pneumotropica*, *Infect. Immun.* **8**:762–768.

Jakab, G. J., and Green, G. M., 1972, The effect of Sendai virus on bactericidal and transport mechanisms of the murine lung, *J. Clin. Invest.* **51**:1989–1998.

Jakab, G. J., and Green, G. M., 1973, Immune enhancement of pulmonary bactericidal activity in murine virus pneumonia, *J. Clin. Invest.* **52**:2878–2884.

Jakab, G. J., and Green, G. M., 1975, Variations in pulmonary antibacterial defenses among experimental animals, *Infect. Immun.* **11**:601–602.

Jasin, H. E., 1972, Human heat labile opsonins: Evidence for their mediation through the alternate pathway of complement activation, *J. Immunol.* **109**:26–31.

Jay, S. J., Johanson, W. G., Jr., Pierce, A. K., and Reisch, J. S., 1976, Determinants of lung bacterial clearance in normal mice, *J. Clin. Invest.* **57**:811–817.

Jodal, U., Lindberg, U., and Lincoln, K., 1975, Level diagnosis of symptomatic urinary tract infections in childhood, *Acta Paediatr. Scand.* **64**:201–208.

Johanson, W. G., Pierce, A. K., and Sanford, J. P., 1969, Changing pharyngeal bacterial flora of hospitalized patients, *N. Engl. J. Med.* **281**:1137–1140.

Johanson, W. G., Jr., Pierce, A. K., Sanford, J. P., and Thomas, G. D., 1972, Nosocomial respiratory infections with gram-negative bacilli, *Ann. Intern. Med.* **77**:701–706.

Johnson, A. G., 1975, Endotoxins as adjuvants, in: *The Immune System and Infectious Diseases* (E. Neter and F. Milgrom, eds.), pp. 183–190, Karger, Basel.

Johnson, F. R., Agnello, V., and Williams, R. C., Jr., 1972, Opsonic activity in human serum deficient in C2, *J. Immunol.* **109**:141–145.

Johnson, J. D., Hand, W. L., King, N. L., and Hughes, C. G., 1975, Activation of alveolar macrophages after lower respiratory tract infection, *J. Immunol.* **115**:80–84.

Johnson, W., 1973, Ribosomal vaccines. II. Specificity of the immune response to ribosomal ribonucleic acid and protein isolated from *Salmonella typhimurium*, *Infect. Immun.* **8**:395–400.

Johnston, R. B., Jr., Newman, S. L., and Struth, A. G., 1973, An abnormality of the alternate pathway of complement activation in sickle-cell disease, *N. Engl. J. Med.* **288**:803–808.

Jones, S. R., 1974, Bacterial prostatitis and antibody-coated bacteria in the urine sediment, *N. Engl. J. Med.* **291**:365.

Jones, S. R., 1978, The current status of urinary tract infection localization by the detection of antibody-coated bacteria in the urine sediment. in: *Infectious Diseases: Current Topics* (D. Gilbert and J. P. Sanford, eds.), Vol. 1, pp. 97–106, Grune and Stratton, Inc., New York.

Jones, S. R., Smith, J. W., and Sanford, J. P., 1974, Localization of urinary-tract infections by detection of antibody-coated bacteria in urine sediment, *N. Engl. J. Med.* **290**:591–593.

Julianelle, L. A., and Siegel, M., 1945, The epidemiology of acute respiratory infections conditioned by sulfonamides. II. Gross alterations in the nasopharyngeal flora associated with treatment, *Ann. Intern. Med.* **22**:10–20.

Jurgensen, P. F., Olsen, G. N., Johnson, J. E., III, Swenson, E. W., Ayoub, E. M., Henney, C. S., and Waldman, R. H., 1973, Immune response of the human respiratory tract. II. Cell-mediated immunity in the lower respiratory tract to tuberculin and mumps and influenza viruses, *J. Infect. Dis.* **128**:730–735.

Kaijser, B., 1973, Immunology of *Escherichia coli*: K antigen and its relation to urinary-tract infection, *J. Infect. Dis.* **127**:670–677.

Kaijser, B., and Ahlstedt, S., 1977, Protective capacity of antibodies against *Escherichia coli* O and K antigens, *Infect. Immun.* **17**:286–289.

Kaijser, B., and Olling, S., 1973, Experimental hematogenous pyelonephritis due to *Escherichia coli* in rabbits: The antibody response and its protective capacity, *J. Infect. Dis.* **128**:41–49.

Kaijser, B., Holmgren, J., and Hanson, L. A., 1972, The protective effect against *E. coli* of O and K antibodies of different immunoglobulin classes, *Scand. J. Immunol.* **1**:27–32.

Kaijser, B., Jodal, U., and Hanson, L. A., 1973, Studies on antibody response and tolerance to *E. coli* K antigens in immunized rabbits and in children with urinary tract infections, *Int. Arch. Allergy Appl. Immunol.* **44**:260–273.

Kaijser, B., Hanson, L. A., Jodal, U., Lidin-Janson, G., and Robbins, J. B., 1977, Frequency of *E. coli* K antigens in urinary-tract infections in children, *Lancet* 1:663–664.

Kaltreider, H. B., Kyselka, L., and Salmon, S. E., 1974, Immunology of the lower respiratory tract. II. The plaque-forming response of canine lymphoid tissues to sheep erythrocytes after intrapulmonary or intravenous immunization, *J. Clin. Invest.* 54:263–270.

Kane, M. A., May, J. E., and Frank, M. M., 1973, Interactions of the classical and alternate complement pathway with endotoxin lipopolysaccharide, *J. Clin. Invest.* 52:370–376.

Kasper, D. L., Winkelhake, J. L., Zollinger, W. D., Brandt, B. L., and Artenstein, M. S., 1973, Immunological similarity between polysaccharide antigens of *Escherichia coli* 07:K1 (L): NM and Group B *Neisseria meningitidis*, *J. Immunol.* 110:262–268.

Kass, E. H., Green, G. M., and Goldstein, E., 1966, Mechanisms of antibacterial action in the respiratory tract, *Bacteriol. Rev.* 30:488–496.

Kass, E. H., Porter, P. J., McGill, M. W., and Vivaldi, E., 1973, Clinical and experimental observations on the significance of endotoxemia, *J. Infect. Dis.* 128:S299–S302.

Kaye, D., and Hook, E. W., 1963, The influence of hemolysis or blood loss on susceptibility to infection, *J. Immunol.* 91:65–75.

Keimowitz, R. I., 1964, Immunoglobulins in normal human tracheobronchial washings: A qualitative and quantitative study, *J. Lab. Clin. Med.* 63:54–59.

Klainer, A. S., and Beisel, W. R., 1969, Opportunistic infection: A review, *Am. J. Med. Sci.* 258:431–456.

Kochan, I., and Berendt, M., 1974, Fatty acid-induced tuberculoidal activity in sera of guinea pigs treated with bacillus Calmette-Guerin and lipopolysaccharide, *J. Infect. Dis.* 129:696–704.

Kunin, C. M., 1963, Separation, characterization, and biological significance of a common antigen in Enterobacteriaceae, *J. Exp. Med.* 118:565–586.

Kunin, C. M., 1974, *Detection, Prevention and Management of Urinary Tract Infections*, 2nd ed., Lea and Febiger, Philadelphia.

Kunin, C. M., and Beard, M. V., 1963, Serological studies of O antigens of *Escherichia coli* by means of the hemagglutination test, *J. Bacteriol.* 85:541–548.

Kunin, C. M., Beard, M. V., and Halmagyi, N. E., 1962, Evidence for a common hapten associated with endotoxin fractions of *E. coli* and other *Enterobacteriaceae*, *Proc. Soc. Exp. Biol. Med.* 111:160–166.

Kyriakos, M., and Ikari, N. S., 1969, The role of antibody in experimental pyelonephritis, *J. Pathol.* 97:513–525.

LaForce, F. M., 1977, Effect of aerosol immunization with RE595 *Salmonella minnesota* on lung bactericidal activity against *Serratia marcescens*, *Enterobacter cloacae*, and *Pseudomonas aeruginosa*, *Am. Rev. Resp. Dis.* 116:241–249.

LaForce, F. M., Hopkins, J., Trow, R., and Wang, W. L. L., 1976, Human oral defenses against gram-negative rods, *Am. Rev. Resp. Dis.* 114:929–935.

Lagercrantz, R., Hammarstrom, S., Perlmann, P., and Gustafsson, B. E., 1968, Immunological studies in ulcerative colitis. IV. Origin of autoantibodies, *J. Exp. Med.* 128:1339–1352.

Lazarus, G. M., and Neu, H. C., 1975, Agents responsible for infection in chronic granulomatous disease of childhood, *J. Pediatr.* 86:415–417.

Lehmann, J. D., Smith, J. W., Miller, T. E., Barnett, J. A., and Sanford, J. P., 1968, Local immune response in experimental pyelonephritis, *J. Clin. Invest.* 47:2541–2550.

Lin, J.-H., and Berry, L. J., 1978, The use of strain LT2-M1 in identifying the protective antigens in a *Salmonella typhimurium*-derived ribosomal vaccine, *J. Reticuloendothel. Soc.* 23:135–143.

Lindberg, U., Jodal, U., Hanson, L. A., and Kaijser, B., 1975, Asymptomatic bacteriuria in school girls. IV. Difficulties of level diagnosis and the possible relation to the character of infecting bacteria, *Acta Paediatr. Scand.* 64:574–580.

Liu, T.-Y., Gotschlich, E. C., Egan, W., and Robbins, J. B., 1977, Sialic acid-containing polysaccharides of *Neisseria meningitidis* and *Escherichia coli* strain Bos-12: Structure and immunology, *J. Infect. Dis.* 136:S71–S77.

Lovell, R., 1934, The presence and significance of agglutinins for some members of the *Salmonella* group occurring in the sera of normal animals, *J. Comp. Pathol. Ther.* 47:107–124.

Luderitz, O., Galanos, C., Risse, H. J., Ruschmann, E., Schlecht, S., Schmidt, G., Schulte-Holthausen, H., Wheat, R., Westphal, O., and Schlosshardt, J., 1966a, Structural relationships of *Salmonella* O and R antigens, *Ann. N.Y. Acad. Sci.* 133:349–374.

Luderitz, O., Staub, A. M., and Westphal, O., 1966b, Immunochemistry of O and R antigens of *Salmonella* and related *Enterobacteriaceae*, *Bacteriol. Rev.* 30:192–255.

Luderitz, O., Galanos, C., Lehmann, V., Nurminen, M., Rietschel, E. T., Rosenfelder, G., Simon, M., and Westphal, O., 1973, Lipid A: Chemical structure and biological activity, *J. Infect. Dis.* 128:S17–S29.

Lyampert, I. M., and Danilova, T. A., 1975, Immunological phenomena associated with cross-reactive antigens of micro-organisms and mammalian tissues, *Progr. Allergy* 18:423–477.

Lynn, W. S., Turner, S. R., and Tainer, J. A., 1975, Nonpeptide chemotaxins isolated from bacterial growth media, in: *Microbiology—1975* (D. Schlessinger, ed.), pp. 202–205, American Society for Microbiology, Washington, D.C.

McCabe, W. R., 1972, Immunization with R mutants of *S. minnesota*. I. Protection against challenge with heterologous gram-negative bacilli, *J. Immunol.* 108:601–610.

McCabe, W. R., 1973, Serum complement levels in bacteremia due to gram-negative organisms, *N. Engl. J. Med.* **288**:21–23.

McCabe, W. R., 1976, Immunoprophylaxis of gram-negative bacillary infections, *Annu. Rev. Med.* **27**:335–341.

McCabe, W. R., and Greely, A., 1973, Common enterobacterial antigen. II. Effect of immunization on challenge with heterologous bacilli, *Infect. Immun.* **7**:386–392.

McCabe, W. R., and Jackson, G. G., 1962, Gram-negative bacteremia I. Etiology and ecology, *Arch. Intern. Med.* **110**:847–855.

McCabe, W. R., Kreger, B. E., and Johns, M., 1972, Type-specific and cross-reactive antibodies in gram-negative bacteremia, *N. Engl. J. Med.* **287**:261–267.

McCabe, W. R., Greely, A., DiGenio, T., and Johns, M. A., 1973, Humoral immunity to type-specific and cross-reactive antigens of gram-negative bacilli, *J. Infect. Dis.* **128**:S284–S289.

McCabe, W. R., Carling, P. C., Bruins, S., and Greely, A., 1975, The relation of K-antigen to virulence of *Escherichia coli*, *J. Infect. Dis.* **131**:6–10.

McCabe, W. R., Bruins, S. C., Craven, D. E., and Johns, M., 1977, Cross-reactive antigens: Their potential for immunization-induced immunity to gram-negative bacteria, *J. Infect. Dis.* **136**:S161–S166.

McCracken, G. H. Jr., Sarff, L. D., Glode, M. P., Mize, S. G., Schiffer, M. S., Robbins, J. B., Gotschlich, E. C., Ørskov, I., Ørskov, F., and the Cooperative Neonatal Meningitis Study Group, 1974, Relation between *Escherichia coli* K1 capsular polysaccharide antigen and clinical outcome in neonatal meningitis, *Lancet* **2**:246–250.

MacGregor, R. R., 1977, Granulocyte adherence changes induced by hemodialysis, endotoxin, epinephrine, and glucocorticoids, *Ann. Intern. Med.* **86**:35–39.

Mackaness, G. B., 1970, The monocyte in cellular immunity, *Semin. Haematol.* **7**:172–184.

Mackaness, G. B., 1974, Delayed hypersensitivity in lung disease, *Ann. N.Y. Acad. Sci.* **221**:312–316.

Mackaness, G. B., and Blanden, R. V., 1967, Cellular immunity, *Progr. Allergy* **11**:89–140.

Mackie, T. J., and Finkelstein, M. H., 1932, The bactericidins of normal serum: Their characters, occurrence in various animals and the susceptibility of different bacteria to their action, *J. Hyg.* **32**:1–24.

Mackowiak, P. A., Martin, R. M., Jones, S. R., and Smith, J. W., 1978, Pharyngeal colonization by gram-negative bacilli in aspiration-prone persons, *Arch. Intern. Med.* **138**:1224–1227.

MacLeod, C. M., Hodges, R. G., Heidelberger, M., and Bernhard, W. G., 1945, Prevention of pneumococcal pneumonia by immunization with specific capsular polysaccharides, *J. Exp. Med.* **82**:445–465.

Makela, P. H., and Mayer, H., 1976, Enterobacterial common antigen, *Bacteriol. Rev.* **40**:591–632.

Makela, P. H., Valtonen, V. V., and Valtonen, M., 1973, Role of O-antigen (lipopolysaccharide) factors in the virulence of *Salmonella*, *J. Infect. Dis.* **128**:S81–S85.

Mannel, D., and Mayer, H., 1978, Isolation and chemical characterization of the enterobacterial common antigen, *Eur. J. Biochem.* **86**:361–370.

Margolis, J. M., and Bigley, N. J., 1972, Cytophilic macroglobulin reactive with bacterial protein in mice immunized with ribonucleic acid-protein fractions of virulent *Salmonella typhimurium*, *Infect. Immun.* **6**:390–397.

Masson, P. L., Heremans, J. F., and Prignot, J., 1965, Studies on the proteins of human bronchial secretions, *Biochim. Biophys. Acta* **111**:466–478.

Medearis, D. N., Jr., Camitta, B. M., and Heath, E. C., 1968, Cell wall composition and virulence in *Escherichia coli*, *J. Exp. Med.* **128**:399–414.

Melchers, F., Braun, V., and Galanos, C., 1975, The lipoprotein of the outer membrane of *Escherichia coli*: A B-lymphocyte mitogen, *J. Exp. Med.* **142**:473–482.

Mergenhagen, S. E., Synderman, R., and Phillips, J. K., 1973, Activation of complement by endotoxin, *J. Infect. Dis.* **128**:S86–S90.

Michael, J. G., 1969, Natural antibodies, *Curr. Top. Microbiol. Immunol.* **48**:43–62.

Michael, J. G., and Rosen, F. S., 1963, Association of "natural" antibodies to gram-negative bacteria with the γ1-macroglobulins, *J. Exp. Med.* **118**:619–626.

Michael, J. G., Whitby, J. L., and Landy, M., 1962, Studies on natural antibodies to gram-negative bacteria, *J. Exp. Med.* **115**:131–146.

Middlebrook, G., 1961, Immunological aspects of airborne infection: Reactions to inhaled antigens, *Bacteriol. Rev.* **25**:331–346.

Miller, T., and North, D., 1973, Studies of the local immune response to pyelonephritis in the rabbit, *J. Infect. Dis.* **128**:195–201.

Miller, T., Burnham, S., and Simpson, G., 1975, Selective deficiency of thymus-derived lymphocytes in experimental pyelonephritis, *Kid. Int.* **8**:88–97.

Miller, T. E., Scott, L., Simpson, G., and Ormrod, D. J., 1976, Depression of the T lymphocyte response to phytohaemagglutinin by renal cells, *Clin. Exp. Immunol.* **24**:442–500.

Miller, T., Scott, L., Stewart, E., and North, D., 1978, Modification by suppressor cells and serum factors of the cell-mediated immune response in experimental pyelonephritis, *J. Clin. Invest.* **61**:964–972.

Minshew, B. H., Jorgensen, J., Swanstrum, M., Grootes-Reuvecamp, G. A., and Falkow, S., 1978, Some characteristics of *Escherichia coli* strains involved from extraintestinal infections of humans, *J. Infect. Dis.* **137**:648–654.

Misfeldt, M. L., and Johnson, W., 1977, Role of endotoxin contamination in ribosomal vaccines from *Salmonella typhimurium*, *Infect. Immun.* **17**:98–104.

Moller, G., Sjoberg, O., and Andersson, J., 1973, immunogenicity, tolerogenicity, and mitogenicity of lipopolysaccharides, *J. Infect. Dis.* **128**:S52–S56.

Montgomerie, J. Z., Kalmanson, G. M., Hubert, E. G., and Guze, L. B., 1972, Pyelonephritis. XIV. Effect of immunization on experimental *Escherichia coli* pyelonephritis, *Infect. Immun.* **6**:330–354.

Morgenstern, M. A., and Gorzynski, E. A., 1977, Immunogenic cross-reactivity between human tissues and the enterobacterial common antigen, *Infect. Immun.* **17**:36–42.

Morrison, D. C., and Kline, L. F., 1977, Activation of the classical and properdin pathways of complement by bacterial lipopolysaccharides (LPS), *J. Immunol.* **118**:362–368.

Mullan, N. A., Newsome, P. M., Cunnington, P. G., Palmer, G. H., and Wilson, M. E., 1974, Protection against gram-negative infections with antiserum to lipid A from *Salmonella minnesota* R595, *Infect. Immun.* **10**:1195–1201.

Muller-Berghaus, G., and Lohmann, E., 1974, The role of complement in endotoxin-induced disseminated intravascular coagulation: Studies in congenitally C_6-deficient rabbits, *Br. J. Haematol.* **28**:403–418.

Myerowitz, R. L., Schneerson, R., Robbins, J. B., and Turck, M., 1972, Urinary tract *Escherichia coli* with cross-reactive antigens to encapsulated pyogenic bacteria, *Lancet* **2**:250–253.

Myerowitz, R. L., Gordon, R. E., and Robbins, J. B., 1973, Polysaccharides of the genus *Bacillus* cross-reactive with the capsular polysaccharides of *Diplococcus pneumoniae* type III, *Haemophilus influenzae* type b, and *Nisseria meningitidis* group A, *Infect. Immun.* **8**:896–900.

Nakano, M., and Saito, K., 1969, Chemical components in the cell wall of *Salmonella typhimurium* affecting its virulence and immunogenicity in mice, *Nature (London)* **222**:1085–1086.

Nash, D. R., and Holle, B., 1973, Local and systemic cellular immune responses in guinea-pigs given antigen parenterally or directly into the lower respiratory tract, *Clin. Exp. Immunol.* **13**:573–583.

Neter, E., 1969, Endotoxins and the immune response, *Curr. Top. Microbiol. Immunol.* **47**:82–124.

Nowotny, A., 1969, Molecular aspects of endotoxic reactions, *Bacteriol. Rev.* **33**:72–98.

Ørskov, F., 1978, Virulence factors of the bacterial cell surface, *J. Infect. Dis.* **137**:630–633.

Ørskov, F., Ørskov, I., Jann, B., and Jann, K., 1971, Immunoelectrophoretic patterns of extracts from all *Escherichia coli* O and K antigen test strains: Correlation with pathogenicity, *Acta Pathol. Microbiol. Scand. Ser. B* **79**:142–152.

Ørskov, I., Ørskov, F., Jann, B., and Jann, K., 1963, Acidic polysaccharide antigens of a new type from *E. coli* capsules, *Nature (London)* **200**:144–146.

Ørskov, I., Ørskov, F., Jann, B., and Jann, K., 1977, Serology, chemistry, and genetics of O and K Antigens of *Escherichia coli, Bacteriol. Rev.* **41**:667–710.

Palestine, A. G., and Klemperer, M. R., 1976, In vivo activation of properdin factor B in normotensive bacteremic individuals, *J. Immunol.* **117**:703–705.

Pearson, H. A., Spencer, R. P., and Cornelius, E. A., 1969, Functional asplenia in sickle-cell anemia, *N. Engl. J. Med.* **281**:923–926.

Pearson, H. A., Cornelius, E. A., Schwartz, A. D., Zelson, J. H., Wolfson, S. L., and Spencer, R. P., 1970, Transfusion-reversible functional asplenia in young children with sickle-cell anemia, *N. Engl. J. Med.* **283**:334–337.

Peavy, D. L., Adler, W. H., and Smith, R. T., 1970, The mitogenic effects of endotoxin and staphylococcal enterotoxin B on mouse spleen cells and human peripheral lymphocytes, *J. Immunol.* **105**:1453–1458.

Peavy, D. L., Shands, J. W., Adler, W. H., and Smith, R. T., 1973, Selective effects of bacterial endotoxins on various subpopulations of lymphoreticular cells, *J. Infect. Dis.* **128**:S91–S99.

Peavy, D. L., Adler, W. H., Shands, J. W., and Smith, R. T., 1974, Selective effects of mitogens on subpopulations of mouse lymphoid cells, *Cell. Immunol.* **11**:86–98.

Perlmann, P., Hammarstrom, S., Lagercrantz, R., and Campbell, D., 1967, Antibodies to colon in rats and human ulcerative colitis: Cross-reactivity with *Escherichia coli* O:14 antigen, *Proc. Soc. Exp. Biol. Med.* **125**:975–980.

Phillips, J. K., Snyderman, R., and Mergenhagen, S. E., 1972, Activation of complement by endotoxin: A role for γ_2 globulin, C1, C4 and C2 in the consumption of terminal complement components by endotoxin-coated erythrocytes, *J. Immunol.* **109**:334–341.

Pierce, A. K., and Sanford, J. P., 1974, Aerobic gram-negative bacillary pneumonias, *Am. Rev. Resp. Dis.* **110**:647–658.

Poe, W. J., and Michael, J. G., 1976, Separation of the mitogenic and antigenic responses to bacterial lipopolysaccharide, *Immunology* **30**:241–248.

Quie, P. G., 1972, Bactericidal function of human polymorphonuclear leukocytes, *Pediatrics* **50**:264–270.

Quie, P. G., 1973, Infections due to neutrophil malfunction, *Medicine* **52**:411–417.

Quie, P. G., 1975, Pathology of bactericidal power of neutrophils, *Semin. Hematol.* **12**:143–160.

Reed, W. P., 1975, Serum factors capable of opsonizing *Shigella* for phagocytosis by polymorphonuclear neutrophils, *Immunology* **28**:1051–1059.

Reed, W. P., and Albright, E. L., 1974, Serum factors responsible for killing of *Shigella, Immunology* **26**:205–215.

Reeves, D. S., and Brumfitt, T. W., 1968, Localization of urinary tract infection: A comparative study of methods, in: *Urinary Tract Infection* (F. O'Grady and W. Brumfitt, eds.), pp. 53–67, Oxford University Press, London.

Reynolds, H. Y., and Thompson, R. E., 1973a, Pulmonary host defenses. I. Analysis of protein and lipids in bronchial secretions and antibody responses after vaccination with *Pseudomonas aeruginosa, J. Immunol.* **111**:358–368.

Reynolds, H. Y., and Thompson, R. E., 1973b, Pulmonary host defenses. II. Interaction of respiratory antibodies with *Pseudomonas aeruginosa* and alveolar macrophages, *J. Immunol.* **111**:369–380.

Reynolds, H. Y., Thompson, R. E., and Devlin, H. B., 1974, Development of cellular and humoral immunity in the respiratory tract of rabbits to *Pseudomonas* lipopolysaccharide, *J. Clin. Invest.* **53**:1351–1358.

Reynolds, H. Y., Kazmierowski, J. A., and Newball, H. H., 1975, Specificity of opsonic antibodies to enhance phagocytosis of *Pseudomonas aeruginosa* by human alveolar macrophages, *J. Clin. Invest.* **56**:376–385.

Rickles, F. R., Levin, J., Hardin, J. A., Barr, C. F., and Conrad, M. E., 1977, Tissue factor generation by human mononuclear cells: Effects of endotoxin and dissociation of tissue factor generation from mitogenic response, *J. Lab. Clin. Med.* **89**:792–803.

Rietschel, E. T., and Galanos, C., 1977, Lipid A antiserum-mediated protection against lipopolysaccharide- and lipid A-induced fever and skin necrosis, *Infect. Immun.* **15**:34–49.

Rietschel, E. T., Galanos, C., and Luderitz, O., 1975, Structure, endotoxicity, and immunogenicity of the lipid A component of bacterial lipopolysaccharides, in: *Microbiology—1975* (D. Schlessinger, ed.), pp. 307–314, American Society for Microbiology, Washington, D.C.

Roantree, R. J., and Rantz, L. A., 1960, A study of the relationship of the normal bactericidal activity of human serum to bacterial infection, *J. Clin. Invest.* **39**:72–81.

Robbins, J. B., Myerowitz, R. L., Whisnant, J. K., Argaman, M., Schneerson, R., Handzel, Z. T., and Gotschlich, E. C., 1972, Enteric bacteria cross-reactive with *Neisseria meningitidis* groups A and C and *Diplococcus pneumoniae* types I and III, *Infect. Immun.* **6**:651–656.

Robbins, J. B., Schneerson, R., Argaman, M., and Handzel, Z. T., 1973, *Haemophilus influenzae* type b: Disease and immunity in humans, *Ann. Intern. Med.* **78**:259–269.

Robbins, J. B., McCracken, G. H., Jr., Gotschlich, E. C., Ørskov, F., Ørskov, I., and Hanson, L. A., 1974, *Escherichia coli* K1 capsular polysaccharide associated with neonatal meningitis, *N. Engl. J. Med.* **290**:1216–1220.

Robbins, J. B., Schneerson, R., Liu, T. Y., Schiffer, M. S., Schiffman, G., Myerowitz, R. L., McCracken, G. H., Jr., Ørskov, I., and Ørskov, F., 1975a, Cross-reacting bacterial antigens and immunity to disease caused by encapsulated bacteria, in: *The Immune System and Infectious Diseases* (E. Neter and F. Milgrom, eds.), pp. 218–241, Karger, Basel.

Robbins, J. B., Schneerson, R., Glode, M. P., Vann, W., Schiffer, M. S., Liu, T. Y., Parke, J. C., Jr., and Huntley, C., 1975b, Cross-reactive antigens and immunity to diseases caused by encapsulated bacteria, *J. Allergy Clin. Immunol.* **56**:141–151.

Rogers, D. E., 1959, The changing pattern of life-threatening microbial disease, *N. Engl. J. Med.* **261**:677–683.

Root, R. K., Ellman, L., and Frank, M. M., 1972, Bactericidal and opsonic properties of C4-deficient guinea pig serum, *J. Immunol.* **109**:477–486.

Rosenstreich, D. L., and Mergenhagen, S. E., 1975, Interaction of endotoxin with cells of the lymphoreticular system: Cellular basis of adjuvanticity, in: *Microbiology—1975* (D. Schlessinger, ed.), pp. 320–326, American Society for Microbiology, Washington, D.C.

Rosenstreich, D. L., Glode, L. M., and Mergenhagen, S. E., 1977, Action of endotoxin on lymphoid cells, *J. Infect. Dis.* **136**:S239–S245.

Rosenstreich, D. L., Vogel, S. N., Jacques, A., Wahl, L. M., Scher, I., and Mergenhagen, S. E., 1978, Differential endotoxin sensitivity of lymphocytes and macrophages from mice with an X-linked defect in B cell maturation, *J. Immunol.* **121**:685–690.

Rosenthal, S., and Tager, I. B., 1975, Prevalence of gram-negative rods in the normal pharyngeal flora, *Ann. Intern. Med.* **83**:355–357.

Ruddy, S., Gigli, I., and Austen, K. F., 1972, The complement system of man, *N. Engl. J. Med.* **287**:489–495, 545–549, 592–596, 642–646.

Sanford, J. P., 1968, Management of urinary tract infections, *Med. Times* **96**:715–730.

Sanford, J. P., 1972, The Jennerian approach to gram-negative bacillary bacteremia? (Editorial), *N. Engl. J. Med.* **287**:304–305.

Sanford, J. P., 1975, Pathogenetic mechanisms in opportunistic gram-negative bacillary infections: Epidemiological and host factors, in: *Microbiology—1975* (D. Schlessinger, ed.), pp. 302–306, American Society for Microbiology, Washington, D.C.

Sanford, J. P., Hunter, B. W., and Souda, L. L., 1962, The role of immunity in the pathogenesis of experimental hematogenous pyelonephritis, *J. Exp. Med.* **115**:383–410.

Sarff, L. D., McCracken, G. H., Jr., Schiffer, M. S., Glode, M. P., Robbins, J. B., Ørskov, I., and Ørskov, F., 1975, Epidemiology of *Escherichia coli* K1 in healthy and diseased newborns, *Lancet* **2**:1099–1104.

Schaberg, D. R., Haley, R. W., Terry, P. M., and McGowan, J. E., 1977, Reproducibility of interpretation of the test for antibody-coated bacteria in urinary sediment, *J. Clin. Microbiol.* **6**:359–361.

Schiffer, M. S., Oliveira, E., Glode, M. P., McCracken, G. H., Jr., Sarff, L. M., and Robbins, J. B., 1976, A review: Relation between invasiveness and the K1 capsular polysaccharide of *Escherichia coli*, *Pediatr. Res.* **10**:82–87.

Schiffman, E., Showell, H. V., Corcoran, B. A., Ward, P. A., Smith, E., and Becker, E. L., 1975, The isolation and partial characterization of neutrophil chemotactic factors from *Escherichia coli*, *J. Immunol.* **114**:1831–1837.

Schneerson, R., and Robbins, J. B., 1975, Induction of serum *Haemophilus influenzae* type b capsular antibodies in adult volunteers fed cross-reacting *Escherichia coli* 075:K100:H5, *N. Engl. J. Med.* **292**:1093–1096.

Schneerson, R., Bradshaw, M., Whisnant, J. K., Myerowitz, R. L., Parke, J. C., Jr., and Robbins, J. B., 1972, An *Escherichia coli* antigen cross-reactive with the capsular polysaccharide of *Haemophilus influenzae* type B: Occurrence among known serotypes, and immunochemical and biologic properties of *E. coli* antisera toward *H. influenzae* type b, *J. Immunol.* **108**:1551–1562.

Schwab, J. H., 1975, Suppression of the immune response by micro-organisms, *Bacteriol. Rev.* **39**:121–143.

Schwartz, M. M., and Cotran, R. S., 1973, Common enterobacterial antigen in human chronic pyelonephritis and interstitial nephritis, *N. Engl. J. Med.* **289**:830–835.

Shands, J. W., Jr., 1975, Endotoxin as pathogenetic mediator of gram-negative infection, in: *Microbiology—1975* (D. Schlessinger, ed.), pp. 302–306, American Society for Microbiology, Washington, D.C.

Simberkoff, M. S., Ricupero, I., and Rahal, J. J., Jr., 1976, Host resistance to *Serratia marcescens* infection: Serum bactericidal activity and phagocytosis by normal blood leukocytes, *J. Lab. Clin. Med.* **87**:206–217.

Sjostedt, S., 1946, Pathogenicity of certain serological types of B. coli, *Acta Pathol. Microbiol. Scand. Suppl.* **63**:1–148.

Skidmore, B. J., Chiller, J. M., Weigle, W. O., Riblet, R., and Watson, J., 1976, Immunologic properties of bacterial lipopolysaccharide (LPS). III. Genetic linkage between the in vitro mitogenic and in vivo adjuvant properties of LPS, *J. Exp. Med.* **143**:143–150.

Smith, J. W., 1975, Local immune response in experimental pyelonephritis in the rabbit. II. Lymphocyte stimulation by lipopolysaccharide of infecting organism, *Immunology* **29**:1077–1085.

Smith, J. W., 1977, Local immune response to lipoprotein of the outer membrane of *Escherichia coli* in experimental pyelonephritis, *Infect. Immun.* **17**:366–370.

Smith, J. W., and Hand, W. L., 1972, Immunoglobulin content and antibody activity in urine in experimental urinary tract infection, *J. Immunol.* **108**:861–866.

Smith, J. W., and Kaijser, B., 1976a, The local immune response to *Escherichia coli* O and K antigen in experimental pyelonephritis, *J. Clin. Invest.* **58**:276–281.

Smith, J. W., and Kaijser, B., 1976b, Local immune response in experimental pyelonephritis in the rabbit. III. Lymphocyte responsiveness to O and K antigens of *Escherichia coli*, *Immunology* **31**:233–237.

Smith, J. W., Barnett, J. A., May, R. P., and Sanford, J. P., 1967, Comparison of the opsonic activity of γ-G- and γ-M-anti-*Proteus* globulins, *J. Immunol.* **98**:336–343.

Smith, J., Holmgren, J., Ahlstedt, S., and Hanson, L. A., 1974, Local antibody production in experimental pyelonephritis: Amount, avidity and immunoglobulin class, *Infect. Immun.* **10**:411–415.

Smith, J. W., Adkins, M. J., and McCreary, D., 1975, Local immune response in experimental pyelonephritis in the rabbit. I. Morphological and functional features of the lymphocytic infiltrate, *Immunology* **29**:1067–1076.

Smith, J. W., Jones, S. R., and Kaijser, B., 1977, Significance of antibody-coated bacteria in urinary sediment in experimental pyenonephritis, *J. Infect. Dis.* **135**:577–581.

Smith, R. A., and Bigley, N. J., 1972a, Detection of delayed hypersensitivity in mice injected with ribonucleic acid–protein fractions of *Salmonella typhimurium*, *Infect. Immun.* **6**:384–389.

Smith, R. A., and Bigley, N. J., 1972b, Ribonucleic acid–protein fractions of virulent *Salmonella typhimurium* as protective immunogens, *Infect. Immun.* **6**:377–383.

Snyderman, R., Gewurz, H., and Mergenhagen, S. E., 1968, Interaction of the complement system with endotoxic lipopolysaccharide: Generation of a chemotactic factor for polymorphonuclear leukocytes, *J. Exp. Med.* **128**:259–275.

Snyderman, R., Pike, M. C., McCarley, D., and Lang, L., 1975, Quantification of mouse macrophage chemotaxis *in vitro*: Role of C5 for the production of chemotactic activity, *Infect. Immun.* **11**:488–492.

Spencer, J. C., Waldman, R. H., and Johnson, J. E., III, 1974, Local and systemic cell-mediated immunity after immunization of guinea pigs with live or killed *M. tuberculosis* by various routes, *J. Immunol.* **112**:1322–1328.

Springer, G. F., 1975, The role of blood group-active substances, in: *The Immune System and Infectious Diseases* (E. Neter and F. Milgrom, eds.), pp. 202–217, Karger, Basel.

Springer, G. F., Williamson, P., and Brandes, W. C., 1961, Blood group activity of gram-negative bacteria, *J. Exp. Med.* **113**:1077–1093.

Staber, F. G., Gisler, R. H., Schumann, G., Tarcsay, L., Schlafli, E., and Dukor, P., 1978, Modulation of myelopoiesis by different bacterial cell-wall components: Induction of colony-stimulating activity (by pure preparations, low-molecular-weight degradation products, and a synthetic low-molecular analog of bacterial cell-wall components) *in vitro*, *Cell. Immunol.* **37**:174–187.

Stamey, T. A., Timothy, M., Millar, M., and Mihara, G., 1971, Recurrent urinary infections in adult women: The role of introital enterobacteria, *Calif. Med.* **115**:1–19.

Stamm, W. E., Martin, S. M., and Bennett, J. V., 1977, Epidemiology of nosocomial infections due to gram-negative bacilli: Aspects relevant to development and use of vaccines, *J. Infect. Dis.* **136**:S151–S160.

Stossel, T. P., 1974, Phagocytosis, *N. Engl. J. Med.* **290**:717–723, 774–780, 833–839.

Sultzer, B. M., and Goodman, G. W., 1976, Endotoxin protein: A B-cell mitogen and polyclonal activator of C3H/HeJ lymphocytes, *J. Exp. Med.* **144**:821–827.

Tainer, J. A., Turner, S. R., and Lynn, W. S., 1975, New aspects of chemotaxis: Specific target-cell attraction by lipid and lipoprotein fractions of *Escherichia coli* chemotactic factor, *Am. J. Pathol.* **81**:401–410.

Territo, M. C., and Golde, D. W., 1976, Granulocyte function in experimental human endotoxemia, *Blood* **47**:539–544.

Thomas, V., Shelokov, A., and Forland, M., 1974, Antibody-coated bacteria in the urine and the site of urinary-tract infection, *N. Engl. J. Med.* **290**:588–590.

Tillotson, J. R., and Finland, M., 1969, Bacterial colonization and clinical superinfection of the respiratory tract complicating antibiotic treatment of pneumonia, *J. Infect. Dis.* **119**:597–624.

Ulevitch, R. J., and Cochrane, C. G., 1978, Role of complement in lethal bacterial lipopolysaccharide-induced hypotensive and coagulative changes, *Infect. Immun.* **19**:204–211.

Ulevitch, R. J., Cochrane, C. G., Henson, P. M., Morrison, D. C., and Doe, W. F., 1975, Mediation systems in bacterial lipopolysaccharide-induced hypotension and disseminated intravascular coagulation, *J. Exp. Med.* **142**:1570–1590.

Ulevitch, R. J., Cochrane, C. G., Bangs, K., Herman, C. M., Fletcher, J. R., and Rice, C. L., 1978, The effect of complement depletion on bacterial lipopolysaccharide (LPS)-induced hemodynamic and hematologic changes in the rhesus monkey, *Am. J. Pathol.* **92**:227–240.

Unanue, E. R., 1976, Secretory function of mononuclear phagocytes, *Am. J. Pathol.* **83**:396–417.

Vahlne, G., 1945, Serological typing of the colon bacillus, with special reference to the occurrence of *B. coli* in man under normal and pathological conditions, particularly in appendicitis, *Acta Pathol. Microbiol. Scand. Suppl.* **62**:1–127.

Valtonen, V., 1969, Virulence of salmonella strains with a reduced amount of O-antigen, *J. Gen. Microbiol.* **57**:28–29.

Valtonen, M. V., Larinkari, U. M., Plosila, M., Valtonen, V. V., and Makela, P. H., 1976, Effect of enterobacterial common antigen on mouse virulence of *Salmonella typhimurium, Infect. Immun.* **13**:1601–1605.

Venneman, M. R., 1972, Purification of immunogenically active ribonucleic acid preparations of *Salmonella typhimurium:* Molecular-sieve and anion-exchange chromatography, *Infect. Immun.* **5**:269–282.

Venneman, M. R., and Berry, L. J., 1971, Cell-mediated resistance induced with immunogenic preparations of *Salmonella typhimurium, Infect. Immun.* **4**:381–387.

Venneman, M. R., and Bigley, N. J., 1969, Isolation and partial characterization of an immunogenic moiety obtained from *Salmonella typhimurium, J. Bacteriol.* **100**:140–148.

Venneman, M. R., Bigley, N. J., and Berry, L. J., 1970, Immunogenicity of ribonucleic acid preparations obtained from *Salmonella typhimurium, Infect. Immun.* **1**:574–582.

Vosti, K. L., 1969, Biological characterization of *Escherichia coli.* Common vs. uncommon serotypes, in: *Urinary Infections in the Male,* Proceedings for Workshop, pp. 101–116, National Research Council, Washington, D.C.

Vosti, K. L., and Randall, E., 1970, Sensitivity of serologically classified strains of *Escherichia coli* of human origin to the serum bactericidal system, *Am. J. Med. Sci.* **259**:114–119.

Vosti, K. L., and Remington, J. S., 1968, Host–parasite interaction in patients with infections due to *Escherichia coli.* III. Physicochemical characterization of O-specific

antibodies in serum and urine, *J. Lab. Clin. Med.* **72**:71–84.

Wahl, L. M., Wahl, S. M., Mergenhagen, S. E., and Martin, G. R., 1974, Collagenase production by endotoxin-mediated macrophages, *Proc. Natl. Acad. Sci. USA* **71**:3598–3601.

Waldman, R. H., and Henney, C. S., 1971, Cell-mediated immunity and antibody responses in the respiratory tract after local and systemic immunization, *J. Exp. Med.* **134**:482–494.

Waldman, R. H., Jurgensen, P. F., Olsen, G. N., Ganguly, R., and Johnson, J. E., III, 1973, Immune response of the human respiratory tract. I. Immunoglobulin levels and influenza virus vaccine antibody response, *J. Immunol.* **111**:38–41.

Walsh, T. E., and Cannon, P. R., 1936, Studies on acquired immunity in rabbits to intranasal infection with type I pneumococcus, *J. Immunol.* **31**:331–346.

Ward, P. A., Lepow, I. H., and Newman, L. J., 1968, Bacterial factors chemotactic for polymorphonuclear leukocytes, *Am. J. Pathol.* **52**:725–736.

Ward, P. A., Chapitis, J., Conroy, M. C., and Lepow, I. H., 1973, Generation by bacterial proteinases of leukotactic factors from human serum, and human C3 and C5, *J. Immunol.* **110**:1003–1009.

Watson, J., Trenkner, E., and Cohn, M., 1973, The use of bacterial lipopolysaccharide to show that two signals are required for the induction of antibody synthesis, *J. Exp. Med.* **138**:699–714.

Weinberg, J. B., Chapman, H. A., Jr., and Hibbs, J. B., Jr., 1978, Characterization of the effects of endotoxin on macrophage tumor cell killing, *J. Immunol.* **121**:72–80.

Weinstein, R. J., and Young, L. S., 1976, Neutrophil function in gram-negative rod bacteremia: The interaction between phagocytic cells, infecting organisms, and humoral factors, *J. Clin. Invest.* **58**:190–199.

Weinstein, R., Stevens, P., and Chu, C., 1978, Relationship between resistance to phagocytosis and content of *E. coli* K-1 capsular antigen, *Abstr. 18th Intersci. Conf. Antimicrob. Agents Chemother.,* Abstr. No. 506.

Westphal, O., 1975, Bacterial endotoxins, *Int. Arch. Allergy Appl. Immunol.* **49**:1–43.

Williams, R. C., and Gibbons, R. J., 1972, Inhibition of bacterial adherence by secretory immunoglobulin A: A mechanism of antigen disposal, *Science* **177**:697–699.

Williams, R. C., and Gibbons, R. J., 1975, Inhibition of streptococcal attachment to receptors on human buccal epithelial cells by antigenically similar salivary glycoproteins, *Infect. Immun.* **11**:711–718.

Winkelstein, J. A., 1973, Opsonins: Their function, identity, and clinical significance, *J. Pediatr.* **82**:747–753.

Wober, W., and Alaupovic, P., 1971a, Studies on the protein moiety of endotoxin from gram-negative bacteria: Characterization of the protein moiety isolated by phenol treatment of endotoxin from *Serratia marcescens* 08 and *Escherichia coli* 0141:K85 (B), *Eur. J. Biochem.* **19**:340–356.

Wober, W., and Alaupovic, P., 1971b, Studies on the protein moiety of endotoxin from gram-negative bacteria: Characterization of the protein moiety isolated by acetic acid hydrolysis of endotoxin from *Serratia marcescens* 08, *Eur. J. Biochem.* **19:**357–367.

Wolberg, G., and DeWitt, C. W., 1969, Mouse virulence of K (L) antigen-containing strains of *Escherichia coli, J. Bacteriol.* **100:**730–737.

Wolff, S. M., 1973, Biological effects of bacterial endotoxins in man, *J. Infect. Dis.* **128:**S259–S264.

Wolff, S. M., and Bennett, J. V., 1974, Gram-negative-rod bacteremia (Editorial), *N. Engl. J. Med.* **291:**733–734.

Wood, D. D., and Cameron, P. M., 1978, The relationship between bacterial endotoxin and human B-cell-activating factor, *J. Immunol.* **121:**53–60.

Yamamoto, K., and Anacker, R. L., 1970, Macrophage migration inhibition studies with cells from mice vaccinated with cell walls of *Mycobacterium* bovis BCG: Characterization of experimental system, *Infect. Immun.* **1:**587–594.

Yamamoto, K., Anacker, R. L., and Ribi, E., 1970, Macrophage migration inhibition studies with cells from mice vaccinated with cell walls of *Mycobacterium bovis* BCG: Relationship between inhibitory activity of lung cells and resistance to airborne challenge with *Myco-bacterium tuberculosis* H37RV, *Infect. Immun.* **1:**595–599.

Yoshida, T., Cohen, S., Bigazzi, P. E., Kurasuji, T., and Amsden, A., 1975, Inflammatory mediators in culture filtrates of *Escherichia coli, Am. J. Pathol.* **81:**389–400.

Young, L. S., and Stevens, P., 1977, Cross-protective immunity to gram-negative bacilli: Studies with core glycolipid of *Salmonella* minnesota and antigens of *Streptococcus pneumoniae, J. Infect. Dis.* **136:**S174–S180.

Young, L. S., Stevens, P., and Ingram, J., 1975, Functional role of antibody against "core" glycolipid of *Enterobacteriaceae, J. Clin. Invest.* **56:**850–861.

Young, L. S., Martin, W. J., Meyer, R. D., Weinstein, R. J., and Anderson, E. T., 1977, Gram-negative rod bacteremia: Microbiologic, immunologic, and therapeutic considerations, *Ann. Intern. Med.* **86:**456–471.

Ziegler, E. J., Douglas, H., Sherman, J. E., Davis, C. E., and Braude, A. I., 1973, Treatment of *E. coli* and *Klebsiella* bacteremia in agranulocytotic animals with antiserum to a UDP-Gal epimerase-deficient mutant, *J. Immunol.* **111:**433–438.

Zinner, S. H., and McCabe, W. R., 1976, Effects of IgM and IgG antibody in patients with bacteremia due to gram-negative bacilli, *J. Infect. Dis.* **133:**37–45.

11

Immunology of Enteric Pathogens
Salmonella, Shigella, and Escherichia coli

MYRON M. LEVINE and RICHARD B. HORNICK

1. Introduction

1.1. General

From the moment of birth the human gastrointestinal tract is assaulted daily with bacterial organisms; the lower ileum and colon are permanently and heavily colonized with bacterial flora. Certain bacteria when ingested have the ability to cause enteric disease; these include *Shigella, Salmonella,* and certain *Escherichia coli*. In this chapter the virulence properties and pathogenetic mechanisms of these agents will be discussed as well as their interaction with the host and the host's defenses.

1.2. Known Pathogenic Mechanisms of Bacterial Enteric Pathogens

Bacterial enteric pathogens may be loosely categorized into two groups according to the pathogenic mechanism by which they cause disease. One group, typified by *Vibrio cholerae* and certain strains of *Escherichia coli,* produces enterotoxins (Finkelstein and Lo-Spalluto, 1969; Smith and Halls, 1967; Sack

et al., 1971). These organisms colonize the upper small bowel of a susceptible host (Gorbach *et al.,* 1971; DuPont *et al.,* 1971a), do not morphologically damage the intestinal mucosa (Gangarosa *et al.,* 1960), and cause disease by effects of absorbed enterotoxin on the adenylate cyclase–cyclic AMP system of intestinal epithelial cells (Chen *et al.,* 1971; Evans *et al.,* 1972; Kantor *et al.,* 1974a,b).

The second group of organisms causes disease by their capacity to invade intestinal epithelial cells (LaBrec *et al.,* 1964). Invasive organisms may be further subdivided into the more destructive invasive type, which includes shigellae (Takeuchi *et al.,* 1965, 1968; Takeuchi, 1971) and certain *E. coli* strains (DuPont *et al.,* 1971a; Ogawa *et al.,* 1968), and the less destructive samonella organisms (Takeuchi, 1971; Takeuchi and Sprinz, 1967).

As a prerequisite to disease causation, all of the above-mentioned bacteria must adsorb to intestinal mucosa, either to allow absorption of enterotoxin or as a preliminary step to subsequent overt invasion.

1.2.1. Description of Virulence Factors and Pathogenesis of Shigella Infections

The association between invasive capacity of shigella and virulence is indisputable (LaBrec *et al.,* 1964; Takeuchi *et al.,* 1965, 1968; Takeuchi, 1971; Formal *et al.,* 1965b; Levine *et*

MYRON M. LEVINE and RICHARD B. HORNICK ● Division of Infectious Diseases, University of Maryland School of Medicine, Baltimore, Maryland 21201.

al., 1973a). Three phenotypic virulence properties have been described which are prerequisites for complete virulence of shigellae: (1) the ability to survive gastric transit and proliferate in the intestinal lumen, (2) the capacity to invade intestinal epithelial cells (LaBrec *et al.*, 1964), and (3) the ability to proliferate within epithelial cells after invasion (Falkow *et al.*, 1963). Working in the guinea pig model with shigellae–*E. coli* hybirds obtained by conjugation, Formal *et al.* (1971a) have been able to identify the chromosomal loci associated with the last two mentioned virulence properties. When a hybrid is produced in which the purine E segment of the *E. coli* genome is incorporated into the virulent shigella chromosome, the resultant modified shigella strain loses its ability to invade epithelial cells (Formal *et al.*, 1971a). Similarly, incorporation of genome coding for the xylose–rhamnose portion of *E. coli* K12 into the chromosome of a virulent shigella modifies the shigella; the resultant hybrid retains the capacity to invade epithelial cells but loses the ability to multiply within the cells after invasion (Falkow *et al.*, 1963).

Invasive capacity of shigellae may be demonstrated in guinea pig (LaBrec *et al.*, 1964; Formal *et al.*, 1965b; LaBrec and Formal, 1961), monkey (Takeuchi *et al.*, 1968), and human intestine (Levine *et al.*, 1973a), rabbit ileal loop (Levine *et al.*, 1973a; Gemski *et al.*, 1972), HeLa cell culture (Levine *et al.*, 1973a; Gemski *et al.*, 1972), and guinea pig eye (Sereny, 1957). The ability of virulent shigellae to cause purulent keratoconjunctivitis in the guinea pig eye is a simple useful screening test for virulence of shigella strains (Sereny, 1957; Mackel *et al.*, 1961). After multiple passages in the laboratory, shigellae commonly lose their invasive potential (Mackel *et al.*, 1961), as do freshly isolated strains, if the inoculated cultures are more than 36 hr old (Cross and Nakamura, 1970).

Takeuchi *et al.* (1965, 1968) have used the electron microscope to document the pathological steps in invasion of guinea pig (Takeuchi *et al.*, 1965) and monkey (Takeuchi *et al.*, 1968; Takeuchi, 1971) intestine. Disease in monkeys closely resembles clinical disease in man; only man and higher apes are natural hosts. Shigellae in monkey, as in man, invade the terminal ileum (ileocecal valve) and the

length of the colon; fever, diarrhea, colitis, and dysentery (blood and mucus in stools) result. Considerable epithelial cell damage is obvious on both light and electron microscopic examination. The colitis is characterized by a gradient of inflammation, being most prominent at the luminal surface and diminishing toward the submucosa, which shows minimal reaction. Despite the striking colitis and formation of microulcers, bloodstream invasion with shigellae is a distinctly uncommon phenomenon (Barrett-Connor and Connor, 1970). A heavy polymorphonuclear leukocyte reaction is evoked, and leukocytes may be identified in the stool of patients with shigellae (Harris *et al.*, 1972).

The 39 shigella serotypes are divided into four groups: A (*S. dysenteriae*), B (*S. flexneri*), C (*S. boydii*), and D (*S. sonnei*). *S. sonnei* is the most common serotype isolated in the industrialized countries, while *S. flexneri* serotypes predominate in the less-developed world. There is a spectrum of clinical illness caused by the various serotypes; although any particular serotype can cause either mild diarrhea or fulminating dysentery, *S sonnei* tends to be associated with milder disease than *S. flexneri* serotypes. *Shigella dysenteriae* 1, Shiga's bacillus (Shiga, 1898), was the first serotype isolated and has always stood apart from other shigellae because of its clinical virulence (Levine *et al.*, 1973a; Block and Ferguson, 1940; Cahill *et al.*, 1966; Mujibur Rahaman *et al.*, 1975; Mata *et al.*, 1970), pandemic potential (Mata *et al.*, 1970; Shiga, 1906, 1936; Gangarosa *et al.*, 1970; Reller *et al.*, 1971; Mendizabal-Morris *et al.*, 1971), and elaboration of an exotoxin *in vitro* (Conradi, 1903; Olitsky and Kligler, 1920).

During the Central American Shiga dysentery pandemic of 1968–1970, it was shown that cell-free culture supernatants of the pandemic strain caused transudation of fluid in the isolated rabbit ileal loop (Keusch *et al.*, 1972a). Since the rabbit ileal loop model had been so instrumental in description of the enterotoxins of *V. cholerae* and *E. coli*, the term "enterotoxin" was suggested for the exotoxin of *S. dysenteriae* 1 (Keusch *et al.*, 1972a). The Shiga exotoxin had previously been referred to as "neurotoxin" because of its ability to cause limb paralysis following injection into rabbits (Conradi, 1903; Flexner and Sweet, 1906). It was also demonstrated that the Shiga exotoxin was cytotoxic for cells in tissue culture (Vicari *et al.*, 1960). Because of the toxin's ability to cause transudation of fluid in the rabbit ileal loop, as well as cause an inflammatory infiltration in mucosa of the jejunal loop (Keusch *et al.*, 1972b), Keusch (1973) suggested that *S. dysenteriae* 1 enterotoxin could wholly account for the pathophysiology and clinical disease resulting from shigella infection.

The role of the *S. dysenteriae* 1 enterotoxin/neurotoxin/cytotoxin in pathogenesis of human disease is still unclear. Other than in its ability to cause secretion in the isolated rabbit ileal loop, it does not resemble the well-characterized heat-labile toxins of *V. cholerae* and *E. coli* (Keusch and Donta, 1975). In contrast to these, Shiga toxin does not stimulate the adenylate cyclase system to cause increased production of cyclic AMP (Flores *et al.*, 1974). There is no immunological cross-reactivity of Shiga toxin with *E. coli* or cholera toxin (Flores *et al.*, 1974), while the last two are immunologically closely related (Smith and Sack, 1973; Gyles, 1974b; Nalin *et al.*, 1974a,b).

In studies designed to investigate the relative importance of enterotoxin v. invasive property in pathogenesis of *S. dysenteriae* 1 disease, adult volunteers were fed doses (10^6–10^{11}) of a proliferating noninvasive attenuated Shiga strain that retained its ability to produce enterotoxin (Levine *et al.*, 1973a). Eighty-five of eighty-six men tolerated this noninvasive enterotoxigenic strain without adverse reaction. In one man diarrhea and dysentery occurred; however, organisms recovered from this volunteer were clearly shown to be revertants that had regained the invasive capacity. Thus toxin production in the absence of invasive capacity is not associated with causation of disease in humans. It appears that shigellae must invade the intestinal mucosa before the shigella enterotoxin can initiate a pathophysiological response in the host.

Initially it was thought that the same protein was responsible for neurotoxicity, cytotoxicity, and enterotoxicity. Cytotoxicity (Keusch, 1973), the most quantifiable and readily demonstrable biological activity (Keusch *et al.*, 1972c), was used to assay for enterotoxicity by extrapolation. Keusch and Jacewicz (1973) observed that convalescent sera from individuals infected with other shigella serotypes exhibited neutralizing activity in the HeLa cell assay with *S. dysenteriae* 1 exotoxin; this observation prompted the suggestion that all shigella serotypes produce exotoxin *in vivo*, although until the work of O'Brien *et al.* (1977b), only *S. dysenteriae* 1 had been shown to produce toxin *in vitro*.

A semicontinuous fermenter system was adapted by McIver *et al.* (1975) in which broth culture filtrates of *S. dysenteriae* 1 gave relatively abundant yields of crude exotoxin which was active in test systems for enterotoxicity (rabbit ileal loop), neurotoxicity (parenteral inoculation of mice), and cytotoxicity (HeLa cell monolayers).

Polyacrylamide gel electrophoresis of the highly active crude toxin revealed that the exotoxin was a minor component in a mixture of proteins. This contrasts with gel electrophoresis of exotoxins of *V. cholerae*, *Corynebacterium diphtheriae*, and *Clostridium tetani*, where the toxins present prominent distinct bands (McIver *et al.*, 1975).

Chromatography of the crude exotoxin using Sephadex G-150 followed by G-100 gels revealed that there were two distinct peaks of HeLa cell cytoxicity activity; the lesser peak was associated with enterotoxicity and neurotoxicity in the rabbit ileal loop and mouse lethality assays, respectively (Keusch and Jacewicz, 1975). Crude and partially purified chromatographed exotoxins were further analyzed by polyacrylamide gel electrophoresis and isoelectric focusing (McIver *et al.*, 1975; Keusch and Jacewicz, 1975). Two regions with toxic activity were encountered. One region isoelectric at approximately pH 7.2–7.25 possessed neurotoxicity, enterotoxicity, and cytotoxicity. A second distinct region isoelectric at pH 6.0–6.1 exhibited much greater cytotoxicity in the HeLa cell assay but was virtually devoid of enterotoxic or neurotoxic activity. Thus it is apparent that at least two distinct exotoxins are produced by *S. dysenteriae* 1, one of which is purely a cytotoxin. The relationship, if any, between the two toxins is not yet known. The previously stated hypothesis that all shigellae produce enterotoxin (i.e., cytotoxin) *in vivo* (Keusch and Jacewicz, 1973), based on the observation that individuals infected with *S. sonnei* and *S. flexneri* developed serum neutralizing activity against Shiga HeLa cell cytotoxin, gained support from the report of O'Brien *et al.* (1977) that *S. flexneri* 2a elaborates a similar cytoxin. The identity of the cytotoxin moiety that stimulated this antibody response is unknown, but it may be a purely cytotoxic moiety devoid of enterotoxin activity similar to the *S dysenteriae* 1 toxin isoelectric at pH 6 or that described by Takeda *et al.* (1977).

Takeda *et al.* (1977) have described a cytotonic toxin produced by *S. dysenteriae* 1 that is distinct from the cytotoxin. This cytotonic toxin causes morphological changes in Chinese hamster ovary cells and exhibits vascular permeability factor activity in the rabbit skin test. In these properties it resembles cholera enterotoxin, *E coli* heat-labile enterotoxin, and the cytotonic toxin of *Salmonella typhimurium* described by Sandefur and Peterson (1976, 1977).

1.2.2. Description of Virulence Factors and Pathogenesis of Salmonella Infections

The genus *Salmonella* is exceedingly large, comprising approximately 1400 serotypes, most of which are widely distributed in nature as enterobacteria of animals. One particular serotype responsible for typhoid fever, *S. typhi*, is restricted to the human host reservoir.

Human disease caused by salmonellae may be divided into three clinical pathological classifications: (1) self-limited gastroenteritis, (2) enteric fever, and (3) septicemic and metastatic infections (Bornstein, 1943).

The serotypes responsible for enteric fever and septicemic/metastatic infections are rather limited. *S. typhi* and the paratyphoid bacilli A and B cause enteric fever, the first being responsible for more than 90% of all such infections. *S. chlolerasuis* (Rhame *et al.*, 1973) and *S. paratyphi* C are the serotypes classically identified with bacteremia followed by metastatic localized pyogenic infections. Many serotypes cause self-limited gastroenteritis. A number of serotypes usually associated with self-limited gastroenteritis in the adult, such as *S. typhimurium, S. heidelburg,* and *S. st. paul,* may cause bacteremic enteric fever in infants (Cherubin *et al.,* 1974).

The pathogenesis of salmonella infection has been well studied in lower animals (Takeuchi, 1967; Takeuchi and Sprinz, 1967; Powell *et al.,* 1971; Giannella *et al.,* 1973a) and primates (Kent *et al.,* 1966a; Rout *et al.,* 1974). Following ingestion and gastric transit, salmonellae invade the small intestine and colon. The bacteria first adsorb to the brush border of the cells and are then brought into the cell by a pinocytosislike mechanism, remaining in vacuoles. They migrate toward the lamina propria surface of the cell, where they are discharged. The mechanisms of extrusion into the lamina propria is not known. On arrival in the lamina propria the salmonella organisms incite a chemotactic response. Serotypes associated with self-limited gastroenteritis induce a polymorphonuclear response, while *S. typhi* is associated with a macrophage response. The former serotypes ordinarily remain confined to the intestinal wall. *S. typhi,* in contrast, is carried through the body by macrophages and seeds organs of the reticuloendothelial system.

In rats salmonellae produce an ileocecitis, while in primates striking diffuse colitis is seen in addition to ileitis. In monkeys with induced *S. typhimurium* diarrheal disease there were no morphological changes in jejunal mucosa while striking changes were noted in colonic and ileal mucosa. Monkeys with severe diarrhea exhibited fluid and electrolyte transport abnormalities in jejunum, ileum, and colon. Giannella *et al.* (1973a) studied eight *S. typhimurium* strains in the isolated rabbit ileal loop for their invasive properties and ability to invoke fluid secretion. Invasive and secretion-evoking properties were unrelated to the "virulence" of strains as determined by the mouse intraperitoneal inoculation assay (Jenkin and Rowley, 1963). Invasive property was a prerequisite for induction of fluid exsorption. However, not all invasive strains induced fluid secretion, and an invasive strain which elicited only minimal morphological mucosal changes evoked fluid exsorption comparable to exsorption evoked by invasive strains that induced considerable histopathological changes; furthermore, fluid secretion began before morphological changes could be identified. Giannella *et al.* were unable to demonstrate an enterotoxin, and the manner in which salmonellae evoked fluid exsorption after invasion was unclear. More recently an enterotoxin elaborated by *S. typhimurium* has been described that is related to cholera enterotoxin. This toxin resembles cholera and *E. coli* heat-labile enterotoxin in that it causes elongation of Chinese hamster ovary cells and exhibits permeability factor activity in rabbit skin. These effects are neutralized by cholera antitoxin (Sandefur and Peterson, 1977). Another report suggests that salmonellae may produce a heat-stable diarrheagenic enterotoxin (Koupal and Deibel, 1975).

The polysaccharide Vi antigen of *S. typhi* (*N*-acetyl aminohexuronic acid) (Clark *et al.*, 1958) was discovered by Felix (Felix and Pitt, 1934a,b) and shown to be associated with increased virulence of *S. typhi* in mice (Felix and Pitt, 1951). There are also epidemiological observations to support the concept that virulence of *S. typhi* strains for humans is correlated with content of Vi antigen (Felix and Anderson, 1951; Findlay, 1951). *S. typhi* strains from two outbreaks of typhoid fever were compared; one outbreak was characterized by mild illness, the other by clinically severe disease. The Vi content of the latter strain was richer in Vi. Perhaps the most direct evidence for the importance of Vi antigen was seen in challenge experiments in volunteers where attack rates for clinical typhoid fever were significantly higher following ingestion of 10^7 organisms of strains with Vi than without, 51% vs. 26% (Hornick *et al.*, 1970). Thus the Vi antigen does appear to be a significant virulence factor with respect to human disease.

It has been hypothesized that the Vi antigen protects the *S. typhi* cell wall lipopolysaccharide (O antigen) from lysis by serum bactericidal antibody (Felix and Bhatnagar, 1935; Felix and Pitt, 1951). Rough salmonella strains lacking O antigen (endotoxin) are avirulent in humans and most animal models.

1.2.3. Description of Virulence Properties and Pathogenesis of *Escherichia coli* Enteropathogens

In the 1940s and 1950s certain strains of *E. coli* were incriminated by epidemiological methods as important causes of infantile summer diarrhea and epidemic nursery diarrhea in Europe and North America (Bray, 1945; Giles and Sangster, 1948; Neter *et al.*, 1953; Neter, 1959; Taylor *et al.*, 1949). Particular *E. coli* serotypes could be cultured with high frequency from infants ill with diarrhea, while isolation from well control infants was uncommon. The most frequently incriminated serotypes came to be called "enteropathogenic *E.*

coli" or "EPEC." Volunteer studies carried out in the United Kingdom (Kirby *et al.*, 1950), the United States (Neter and Shumway, 1950; Ferguson and June, 1952; June *et al.*, 1953; Wentworth *et al.*, 1956), and Japan (Koya *et al.*, 1954) in the early 1950s clearly showed that EPEC strains from cases of infantile diarrhea could cause diarrhea when fed in high doses, while "normal flora" control strains did not. These early volunteer studies were carried out at a time when no laboratory tests existed to distinguish virulent from avirulent strains within a particular *E. coli* serotype.

In recent years it has become apparent that many other serotypes of *E. coli*, distinct from classic infant diarrhea "enteropathogenic" serotypes, are enteropathogens of adults and older children, as well as infants (De *et al.*, 1956; Sakazaki *et al.*, 1967; Ogawa *et al.*, 1968; Rowe *et al.*, 1970; DuPont *et al.*, 1971a; Gorbach and Khurana, 1972; Shore *et al.*, 1974; R. B. Sack *et al.*, 1975a; D. A. Sack *et al.*, 1975; Orskov *et al.*, 1976; Ryder *et al.*, 1976). These *E. coli* serotypes, many of which are of serotypes not previously associated with diarrheal disease, were shown to fall into two distinct categories on the basis of clinical and pathogenetic features (Sakazaki *et al.*, 1967; Ogawa *et al.*, 1968; DuPont *et al.*, 1971a). Members of the first group of *E. coli* are proximal small bowel pathogens that elaborate a choleralike enterotoxin and cause afebrile, watery diarrhea (DuPont *et al.*, 1971a; R. B. Sack *et al.*, 1971). Members of the second group are large bowel pathogens which produce febrile colitis and dysentery (bloody mucoid stools) and exhibit invasive properties resembling those of shigella (Sakazaki *et al.*, 1967; Ogawa *et al.*, 1968; Dupont *et al.*, 1971a; Guerrant *et al.*, 1975; Tullock *et al.*, 1973).

In the following paragraphs enterotoxigenic, invasive, and enteropathogenic *E. coli* associated with diarrheal disease will be discussed.

a. Enterotoxigenic *E. coli*. Enterotoxigenic *E. coli* is responsible for diarrheal disease among infants of many animal species as well as human infants, children, and adults (travelers' diarrhea). Two virulence properties appear to be prerequisites for disease causation by such bacteria under natural conditions: (1) ability of the strain to produce enterotoxin and (2) possession of colonization factors such as adhesion pili on the surface of the bacteria which enable them to attach to selected sites in the host's gastrointestinal tract (Bertschinger *et al.*, 1972; Smith and Linggood, 1971b, 1972; Jones and Rutter, 1972).

(1) Enterotoxin. E. *coli* can elaborate two types of enterotoxin, heat labile (LT) and heat stable (ST) (Gyles, 1971; Evans *et al.*, 1973; Nalin *et al.*, 1974b). LT has been more extensively studied and characterized. Genes for synthesis of LT are often found in transferable plasmids (Skerman *et al.*, 1972; Smith and Linggood, 1971a; Gyles *et al.*, 1974). LT resembles cholera toxin physiologically as well as immunologically. LT induces active ion-transported fluid secretion by stimulating the adenylate cyclase–cyclic AMP system of intestinal epithelial cells (Evans *et al.*, 1972; Kantor *et al.*, 1974). With low doses of LT there is a delayed onset of several hours before net accumulation of fluid is evident in isolated intestinal loops of dog or rabbit (Evans *et al.*, 1973; Nalin *et al.*, 1974b); in contrast, with higher doses of LT, onset of fluid accumulation is more rapid (Evans *et al.*, 1973). If LT is rinsed from the mucosal surface after 10 min contact time, fluid accumulation will nonetheless occur (Nalin *et al.*, 1974b). LT can be assayed in ligated intestinal loops of a number of animal species. Chinese hamster ovary (Guerrant *et al.*, 1974), Y1 adrenal (D. A. Sack and R. B. Sack, 1975), and Vero (Speirs *et al.*, 1977) cells in tissue culture have been found to undergo overt morphological alteration in the presence of LT, and these cell lines are utilized as sensitive assays for LT; ST does not alter these cells. LT is inactivated by boiling.

LT is of high molecular weight, with estimates ranging from 35,000 to 100,000 (Lariviere *et al.*, 1973; Evans *et al.*, 1974, Dorner, 1975; Finkelstein *et al.*, 1976), and is antigenic (R. B. Sack, 1973; Donta *et al.*, 1974; R. B. Sack *et al.*, 1974, 1975b); it is immunologically closely related to cholera toxin (Smith and Sack, 1973; Gyles, 1974a,b; Donta, 1974; Nalin *et al.*, 1974a) and its effects can be neutralized by cholera antitoxin (Guerrant *et al.*, 1974; Evans *et al.*, 1974; Smith and Sack, 1973; Gyles, 1974b) LTs of human and animal strains are closely related immunologically (Evans *et al.*, 1973; Gyles, 1974a,b). There is also striking similarity in the molecular weights, base ratios, and polynucleotide sequences of the plasmids responsible for LT production from diverse sources (Gyles *et al.*, 1974).

ST is a low molecular weight (4400–5100 D) (Alderete and Robinson, 1973; Mullan *et al.*, 1978) nonimmunogenic material that evokes fluid secretion immediately after exposure to intestinal mucosa (Evans *et al.*, 1973; Nalin *et al.*, 1974). Fluid accumulation is of lesser volume and duration than for LT (Evans *et al.*, 1973; Nalin *et al.*, 1974b). The fluid-evoking property of ST is diminished if mucosa is rinsed after 10 min contact time (Nalin *et al.*, 1974b). ST is resistant to boiling, induces secretion by activating guanylate cyclase, and is plasmid-mediated (Gyles, 1971; Skerman *et al.*, 1972; Hughes *et al.*, 1978, Field *et al.*, 1978).

E. *coli* strains may elaborate either ST or LT alone or both. Strains that produce LT, alone or with ST, have been shown to be enteropathogenic for man and animals. Recent evidence has also implicated ST-alone strains as pathogens for animals (Whipp *et al.*, 1975) and man (D. A. Sack *et al.*, 1975; Levine, *et al.*, 1977). E. *coli* strains that produce ST alone were isolated from five individuals with travelers' diarrhea in the course of a prospective study (D. A. Sack *et al.*, 1975). The ST-producing E. *coli* was not isolated before travel or in convalescence, and in three individuals no other pathogenic bacteria or protozoa were identified during the diarrheal episodes. One of these ST-alone strains induced typical travelers' diarrhea when fed to healthy adult volunteers (Levine *et al.*, 1977b). Stool culture isolates recovered from the volunteers elaborated only ST, and none of the volunteers had rises in LT antitoxin.

There has been considerable research to identify the tissue receptors to which LT attaches; this work was stimulated by the observation that certain gangliosides have the propensity to bind LT *in vitro*. It has been found that ganglioside G_{M1} can bind E. *Coli* LT (Holmgren, 1973; Pierce, 1973; Zenser and Metzger, 1974), although perhaps less avidly than cholera toxin (Holmgren, 1973), and can neutralize its secretion-promoting and enzyme-inducing activities (Holmgren, 1973; Pierce, 1973; Zenser and Metzger, 1974). Choleragenoid, the naturally occurring cholera toxoid, will saturate mucosal tissue receptors in an isolated rabbit intestinal loop and thus prevent fluid accumulation when cholera toxin is subsequently applied; prior treatment with choleragenoid will not inhibit fluid accumulation in a ligated intestinal loop when followed by application of *E. coli* LT (Holmgren, 1973; Pierce, 1973). These observations suggest that ganglioside G_{M1} possesses a receptor that is common for the active binding sites for both *E. coli* LT and cholera toxin but that the receptors on intestinal cells for the two toxins are quite distinct.

(2) Colonization Factors. Observations in man and animals have shown that possession of enterotoxin *per se* does not a priori render an *E. coli* strain virulent. The *E. coli* must also possess the ability to attach to mucosal cells of the upper small intestine (Bertschinger *et al.*, 1970). This active attachment enables the *E. coli* to overcome the effective defense mechanism of intestinal motility which would otherwise clear the *E. coli* from the upper small bowel. Attached to the intestinal mucosal cells, *E. coli* can release enterotoxin within proximity of the epithelial cell membrane.

Studies in animals have identified colonization factors in animal *E. coli* pathogens, of which the best characterized are adhesion pili. These are protein, hairlike organelles on the bacterial surface that enable *E. coli* to adhere to proximal small intestinal mucosal cells. Well-defined adhesion pili have been identified for enterotoxigenic porcine, lamb, and calf *E. coli*. These include K88 antigen (pig strains), K99 antigen (lamb, calf, and some pig strains), and 987-type pili (pig strains) (Orskov *et al.*, 1964, 1975; Orskov and Orskov, 1966; Stirm *et al.*, 1967a,b; Smith and Linggood, 1971b, 1972; Jones and Rutter, 1972; Hohmann and Wilson, 1975; Isaacson *et al.*, 1977; Moon *et al.*, 1977; Nagy *et al.*, 1977).

There are several different classes of adhesion pili associated with enterotoxigenic *E. coli* pathogens of animals. One class, typified by the K88 and K99 antigen pili, is associated with spontaneous hemagglutination of erythrocytes and intestinal cell attachment that is not inhibited by mannose (Stirm *et al.*, 1967; Jones and Rutter, 1974b; Nagy *et al.*, 1977); that is, the pili receptor on the cell is not mannose containing or mannoselike. Genes for production of K88 and K99 pili are coded in transferable plasmids (Orskov *et al.*, 1966,

1975; Smith and Linggood, 1971b, 1972; Jones and Rutter, 1972). Phenotypic expression of K88 and K99 genes is suppressed by growth at 18 C and is not suppressed by culture on solid medium.

Sellwood *et al.* (1975) and Rutter *et al.* (1975) found that K88-positive *E. coli* do not attach to intestinal tissue from all piglets. Rather, two distinct phenotypes exist, adhesive for K88 antigen (susceptible) and nonadhesive (nonsusceptible). The trait allowing adhesion of K88 pili appears to be transmitted along Mendelian lines as a chromosomal dominant gene (S).

Other animal *E. coli* strains are known to be virulent but lack K88 or K99 surface antigens. They possess different types of adhesion pili (Hohmann and Wilson, 1975; Isaacson *et al.*, 1977; Moon *et al.*, 1977; Nagy *et al.*, 1977), of which the best studied are *E. coli* 987 pili. These pili do not confer ability to hemagglutinate guinea pig erythrocytes (Nagy *et al.*, 1977). Mutants of *E. coli* 987 that lack pili are avirulent (Isaacson *et al.*, 1977). Nonpathogenic animal strains of *E. coli* examined by Isaacson *et al.* (1977) possessed type 1 somatic pili that caused mannose-sensitive hemagglutination. Although these pili structures were morphologically indistinguishable in electron photomicrographs from type 987 pili, they were immunologically distinct (Isaacson *et al.*, 1977).

Hohmann and Wilson (1975) have also found that K88-negative porcine *E. coli* strains virulent for piglets possess the ability to adhere to intestinal epithelial cells *in vivo*, particularly in the distal small intestine.

While a single or closely related heat-labile enterotoxin appears to be operative in *E. coli* strains pathogenic for human and various animal species, adhesion pili appear to be rather species specific. For example, K88 antigen allows *E. coli* to adhere to porcine intestinal cells but not to bovine cells (Wilson and Hohmann, 1974).

Colonization factors such as adhesion pili also appear to be necessary for enterotoxigenic *E. coli* to produce clinical illness in man. An enterotoxigenic *E. coli* strain, *E. coli* 263, that was highly virulent for piglets failed to induce diarrhea when fed to man (DuPont *et al.*, 1971a). The enterotoxin plasmid from porcine *E. coli* strain 263 was transferred to *E.*

coli HS, a normal human colonic flora strain. When large numbers (10^8–10^{10}) of the resultant enterotoxigenic HS strain were fed to adult volunteers, no disease occurred (DuPont and Hornick, unpublished data). This established that other virulence properties, in addition to enterotoxin production, are necessary for complete virulence of *E. coli* strains in humans.

E. coli strain H10407 is a known human enteropathogen strain that produces LT and ST (Evans *et al.*, 1975). Electron microscopic studies of this strain have revealed surface pili, some of which, presumably, are adhesion pili that enable the bacteria to adhere to human intestinal mucosa (Evans *et al.*, 1975, 1978a; Swaney *et al.*, 1977). Strain H10407P is a spontaneously derived mutant of H10407 that has lost the ability to cause fluid accumulation in the infant rabbit test (Evans *et al.*, 1975). *E. coli* H10407P did not cause diarrhea when fed to volunteers, in contrast to the parent strain H10407 (Evans *et al.*, 1978b).

Strain H10407 exhibits both mannose-resistant hemagglutination (MRHA) of human type A erythrocytes and mannose-sensitive hemagglutination (MSHA) of guinea pig erythrocytes, while H10407P shows only MSHA; H10407P also elaborates only LT. Evans *et al.* (1975, 1977, 1978a) and others (Orskov and Orskov, 1977) conclude that there exist two distinct types of pili on strain H10407, one associated with mannose-resistant and the other with mannose-sensitive hemagglutination. Evans *et al.* (1975, 1977, 1978a,b) propose that the mannose-resistant hemagglutinin represents a plasmid-mediated colonization factor for human enterotoxigenic *E. coli* strains (colonization factor antigen I, CFA/I) and that it is a piluslike structure analogous to the K88 and K99 adhesion pili of animal strains.

While mannose-resistant hemagglutination is commonly found in other *E. coli* strains of serogroup O78 (serogroup of H10407) isolated from individuals with diarrhea, it is rare in enterotoxigenic *E. coli* of many other serogroups (I. Orskov and F. Orskov, 1977; Gross *et al.*, 1978; Levine and Daya, 1978).

Evans *et al.* (1978c) identified a second piluslike structure, colonization factor antigen II, that causes MRHA of bovine but not human erythrocytes and is found in some enterotoxigenic *E. coli* of serogroups 06 and 08.

Type 1 somatic pili permit *E. coli* to adhere to epithelial cells; thus they may serve a role as colonization factors in some enterotoxigenic *E. coli* (Brinton, 1977; Salit and Gotschlich, 1977; Isaacson *et al.*, 1978). Type 1 somatic pili (associated with mannose-sensitive hemagglutination) antigenically similar to those of H10407, occur in approximately 35% of enterotoxigenic *E. coli* isolated from individuals with diarrhea, irrespective of O serogroup (C. C. Brinton, Jr., unpublished data). *E. coli* type 1 pili have also been implicated in pathogenesis of urinary tract infections wherein their attachment to human epithelial cells (which is inhibited by mannose) is deemed a critical step in initiation of infection (Fowler and Stamey, 1977; Ofek *et al.*, 1977). It is now known how many antigenic types of adhesion pili exist among human *E. coli* enteropathogens.

(3) O Antigen. In the early period following recognition of enterotoxigenic *E. coli* as a pathogen responsible for travelers' diarrhea and infantile diarrhea it was thought that there was no correlation between enterotoxigenicity and serotype. It was assumed that any *E. coli* serotype might become virulent if the organism received an enterotoxin plasmid by conjugation. It is now appreciated that there is a very intimate relationship among O serogroup, enterotoxigenicity, and diarrheagenic behavior of *E. coli* in humans (F. Orskov *et al.*, 1976; D. J. Evans *et al.*, 1977; Rowe *et al.*, 1977; D. Sack *et al.*, 1977).

Certain O serogroups have been identified with great frequency in far-flung parts of the world among enterotoxigenic *E. coli* serogroups associated with human diarrheal disease. These serogroups include O6, O8, O15, O20, O25, O78, O109, O115, O128, O148, and O159 (I. Orskov and F. Orskov, 1976; D. J. Evans *et al.*, 1977; Rowe *et al.*, 1977; D. A. Sack *et al.*, 1977). These serogroups are distinct from those referred to as "enteropathogenic" that were associated with infant diarrhea during the 1940s and 1950s.

The exact mechanism whereby the O lipopolysacchride serves as a virulence property is not known. Partial explanation resides in the relationship between certain O serogroups and stability of enterotoxin plasmids. Enterotoxin plasmids are exceedingly stable in *E. coli* strains of some of the abovementioned serogroups (D. J. Evans *et al.*, 1977).

b. Invasive *E. coli*. Another group of *E. coli* enteropathogens exists quite distinct from those that cause disease by dint of adsorption to proximal small bowel and enterotoxin effects. The second group comprises *E. coli* strains that possess an invasive potential mimicking that of shigellae (Sakazaki *et al.*, 1967; Ogawa *et al.*, 1968, DuPont *et al.*, 1971a; Guerrant *et al.*, 1975; Tulloch *et al.*, 1973). Indeed, these *E. coli* strains show some relation to shigellae in biochemical and immunological as well as biological patterns (Ogawa *et al.*, 1968; DuPont *et al.*, 1971a; Tulloch *et al.*, 1973). Invasive *E. coli* is a pathogen of the colon, like shigellae, where it invades mucosal cells and causes dysentery and colitis. In the guinea pig and rabbit ileal loop models, invasive *E. coli* causes destruction of mucosa and intense inflammatory reaction comparable to those seen with shigellae (Ogawa *et al.*, 1968; DuPont *et al.*, 1971a; Formal *et al.*, 1971b). Similarly it produces keratoconjunctivitis in the guinea pig eye model (Sakazaki *et al.*, 1967; Ogawa *et al.*, 1968; Formal *et al.*, 1974). Most invasive *E. coli* strains share somatic antigens with various shigella serotypes (DuPont *et al.*, 1971a; Tulloch *et al.*, 1973; Orskov *et al.*, 1971). The role, if any, of pili as a virulence factor in invasive *E. coli* infections is not known.

E. coli strains associated with bacteremia, meningitis, and other bacteremic diseases of man and animals have been associated with certain virulence characteristics such as K1 antigen (Robbins *et al.*, 1974), plasmid-controlled Vir$^+$ toxin (Smith, 1974), and lethality character (Smith, 1974), the last possibly identical with colicin V. None of these virulence traits has been shown to be associated with enterotoxigenic or other invasive-type *E. coli* intestinal pathogens.

Colicins are plasmid-mediated proteins elaborated by enterobacteria that have deleterious effects on competitive organisms. Colicins have not been shown to be virulence characteristics for *E. coli* enteropathogens.

c. Enteropathogenic *E. coli*. In the 1940s and 1950s certain strains of *E. coli* were incriminated by epidemiological methods as important causes of infantile summer diarrhea and epidemic nursery diarrhea (Bray, 1945; Giles and Sangster, 1948; Taylor *et al.*, 1949; Neter, 1959). Certain *E. coli* serotypes were cultured with high frequency from infants ill with diarrhea, while isolation from well control infants was uncommon (Bray, 1945; Giles and Sangster, 1948; Taylor *et al.*, 1949). The serotypes most frequently incriminated came to be called "enteropathogenic *E. coli*" or EPEC and included serotypes within serogroups O55, O86, O111, O127, O128, and O142 (Neter, 1959; F. Orskov, *et al.*, 1960; Ewing *et al.*, 1963; Olarte and Ramos-Alvarez, 1965; Hone *et al.*, 1973).

Volunteer studies carried out in the early 1950s established that EPEC strains were isolated virulent for man, but at the time of the studies there existed no laboratory tests to identify pathogenetic mechanisms or virulence properties.

The observation that *E. coli* strains that cause adult travelers' diarrhea usually produce LT or ST or are invasive (Dupont *et al.*, 1971a; Shore *et al.*, 1974; Gorbach *et al.*, 1975; Merson *et al.*, 1976) prompted an examination of EPEC strains for these virulence properties. With few exceptions, the classic EPEC serotypes isolated from sporadic infantile diarrhea or from nursery outbreaks of diarrhea failed to demonstrate invasiveness, LT, or ST by sensitive techniques (R. B. Sack *et al.*, 1975a,b; Echeverria *et al.*, 1976; Goldschmidt and DuPont, 1976; Gross *et al.*, 1976; R. B. Sack, 1976a,b; Gurwith *et al.*, 1977). The issue was further confused when it was seen that LT- and ST-producing *E. coli* from adults and children with diarrhea (F. Orskov *et al.*, 1976; Rowe *et al.*, 1977) and from some nursery outbreaks (Ryder *et al.*, 1976; Rowe *et al.*, 1977) rarely were of "classic" infant diarrhea EPEC serotypes. These observations stimulated an intensive scientific controversy. Some workers suggested that the classic EPEC serotypes were indeed pathogenic but only when they possessed enterotoxin plasmids, which were prone to be lost on storage, thus explaining the failure to find enterotoxin when sought (R. B. Sack, 1975, 1976a,b; French, 1976; Raska and Raskova, 1976). Other workers interpreted the failure to demonstrate enterotoxigenicity or invasiveness in classic EPEC strains to indicate that *E. coli* may possess additional pathogenic mechanisms, distinct from LT, ST, or invasiveness, that enable it to cause diarrhea (Gross *et al.*, 1976; Rowe *et al.*, 1977).

Recent volunteer studies resolved this controversy (Levine *et al.*, 1978a). Three EPEC strains (O127:K63:H6, O128:K67:H2, and

O142:K86:H6) isolated from outbreaks of infantile diarrhea and one "normal" colonic flora strain (*E. coli* HS) from a healthy adult were fed in doses of 10^6, 10^8, and 10^{10} organisms with NaHCO$_3$ to adult volunteers. The strains had been stored for 7–9 years and were negative in usual sensitive tests for enterotoxins and invasiveness. Two of the strains (O127 and O142) caused incontrovertible diarrheal illness in the healthy adults. The large inoculum (10^{10} organisms) required to induce a high attack rate, the short incubation, and the diarrheal syndrome encountered closely resembled those reported in volunteer studies employing EPEC strains (including O127:K63) carried out in the early 1950s (Kirby *et al.*, 1950; Ferguson and June, 1952; June *et al.*, 1953; Koya *et al.*, 1954; Wentworth *et al.*, 1956). Isolates recovered from volunteers ill with diarrhea failed to produce LT or ST, and no volunteers had rises in LT antitoxin.

Highly concentrated culture supernatants of the O142 and O127 challenge strains caused a significant decrease in absorption in acute canine and acute rat jejunal loops, demonstrating the presence of an uncharacterized enterotoxin (Levine *et al.*, 1978a). Concentrated supernatants of the strains that did not cause diarrhea in volunteers (O128 and HS) did not alter fluxes in this assay. Work is under way to determine if the uncharacterized EPEC enterotoxin is of the Shiga-like variety reported by O'Brien *et al.* (1977a).

2. Host Nonspecific Defense Mechanisms

2.1. Gastric Acidity

Normal acidic contents of the stomach form the initial and exceedingly important barrier to invasion by salmonellae, *V. cholerae*, and *E. coli* (Cash *et al.*, 1974; Giannella *et al.*, 1970, 1971a, 1973; Gray and Trueman, 1971; G. H. Sack *et al.*, 1972; Soni and Rajapaksa, 1973). These observations are most clear-cut with respect to cholera. Since the high number of infecting organisms required to cause clinical disease is similar for both *V. cholerae* and enterotoxigenic *E. coli*, one suspects that gastric acidity is an important barrier to infection with either. Indeed, volunteer studies have clearly demonstrated the enhancement of virulence of an inoculum of *V. cholerae* following neutralization of gastric contents with 2 g of sodium bicarbonate (Cash *et al.*, 1974).

Exceptionally severe clinical disease has been associated with salmonella infection in hypochlorhydric hosts (Gray and Trueman, 1971; Soni and Rajapaksa, 1973; Giannella *et al.*, 1971b; Axon and Poole, 1973).

The gastric contents defense mechanism does not appear to be so important with respect to shigellae since as few as ten organisms can cause disease (Levine *et al.*, 1973a) and 200 organisms of several serotypes have caused attack rates of 25–50% in healthy volunteers (Levine *et al.*, 1973a; DuPont *et al.*, 1972b).

2.2. Intestinal Motility

The normal peristaltic motion of the intestine is another remarkable nonspecific defense against salmonella, shigella, and *E. coli* enteropathogens. Healthy guinea pigs are normally quite resistant to infection with shigellae, apparently as a result of the rapid clearance by intestinal motility of organisms introduced into the intestine (Dixon, 1960; Formal *et al.*, 1963; Dixon and Paulley, 1963). However, if challenged guinea pigs are treated with an intraperitoneal injection of opium, which greatly impedes intestinal motility, severe and commonly fatal infection with salmonellae (Kent *et al.*, 1966a) and shigellae (Formal *et al.*, 1958, 1959) ensues.

There is evidence to corroborate the importance of intestinal motility as a clearing mechanism in humans; treatment of *Shigella flexneri* 2a dysentery with an antiperistaltic agent was associated with a prolonged febrile response in compared to the course of infection in control patients (DuPont and Hornick, 1973). Furthermore, it has been observed that systemic invasion can follow treatment of salmonella gastroenteritis with antiperistaltic agents (Sprinz, 1969). The common denominator in these instances is believed to be decrease in intestinal motility leading to proliferation of organisms and increased invasion.

Intestinal motility is also an important defense against disease due to enterotoxigenic *E. coli* in man and animals. The proximal small bowel in North Americans and Europeans is virtually devoid of enterobacteria in the normal state, despite the continual ingestion of *E.*

coli and other enterobacteria (Drasar and Hill, 1974). This is mainly a function of the intestinal motility clearing mechanism. As previously discussed, virulent enterotoxigenic *E. coli* usually is endowed with adhesion pili, or other colonization factors, which allow the organism to adsorb to the mucosa of the proximal small bowel and avoid clearance.

2.3. Normal Intestinal Flora

The normal gut flora are inhibitory for shigella and salmonella enteropathogens (Bohnhoff *et al.*, 1964b; Freter, 1956; Hentges, 1967a, 1969; Hentges and Freter, 1962; Hentges and Maier, 1970; Maier and Hentges, 1972; Maier *et al.*, 1972; Nakamura, 1972). Several investigators have demonstrated that the antagonism is mediated by volatile short-chain fatty acids, which are end products of metabolism of normal gut flora (Bohnhoff *et al.*, 1964a,b; Hentges, 1967a,b, 1969; Hentges and Maier, 1970; Maier and Hentges, 1972; Maier *et al.*, 1972; Baskett and Hentges, 1973). The fatty acids include acetic, butyric, and propionic among others. The inhibition is pH related (Bohnhoff *et al.*, 1964b; Hentges, 1967a,b; Hentges and Maier, 1970; Baskett and Hentges, 1973), increasing with lower pH, and apparently involves undissociated acid molecules (Hentges, 1967a,b; Hentges and Maier, 1970; Maier *et al.*, 1972). Undissociated fatty acids permeate the bacterial cell wall more readily, but once within the bacteria both ionized and associated acid molecules interfere with bacterial metabolism (Baskett and Hentges, 1973). Although the inhibition of salmonellae and shigellae by normal enteric flora has been studied most intensively *in vitro* or in animals, evidence of *in vivo* inhibition in humans exists. Lactulose, a nonabsorbable disaccharide, was used to decrease excretion of *S. sonnei* by a long-term chronic large bowel carrier (Levine and Hornick, 1975; Levine *et al.*, 1973b). This disaccharide is not hydrolyzed by human intestinal lactase but arrives in the large bowel intact, where it is metabolized by normal colonic flora (Dahlqvist and Gryboski, 1965; Avery *et al.*, 1972). The end products of metabolism of lactulose by colonic bacteria are increased amounts of short-chain fatty acids and a lowered pH (Avery *et al.*, 1972). Administration of this drug to the carrier was fol-

lowed by an obvious diminution of excretion of shigellae. Administration of certain antibiotics to man or experimental animals can upset intestinal flora balance and greatly increase susceptibility to infection and clinical disease due to salmonellae and shigellae (Hornick *et al.*, 1970; Bohnhoff *et al.*, 1964; Freter, 1956).

3. Microbe–Host Interactions

If shigella, salmonella, or *E. coli* enteropathogens successfully overcome the nonspecific defense mechanisms of the gastric barrier and inhibitory effects of normal intestinal flora, they may now interact with four other host defenses: (1) local mucosal antibody, (2) phagocytes, (3) circulating antibody, and (4) cell-mediated immune mechanisms.

3.1. Local Mucosal Antibody

In the absence of mucosal antibody bacterial pathogens may adsorb to intestinal mucosa as a preliminary step to elaboration of enterotoxin or invasion. It is believed that specific immunoglobulin locally produced in the intestine serves an important antibacterial function.

Specific intestinal antibody, mostly IgA but also IgG and IgM, has been identified against shigellae, salmonellae, *E. coli*, and *V. cholerae* in intestinal fluids, stools, extracts, breast milk, and mucosal scrapings in humans and experimental animals (Allardyce *et al.*, 1974; Eddie *et al.*, 1971; Fubara and Freter, 1972, 1973; Girard and de Kalbermatten, 1970; Goldblum *et al.*, 1975; Hill and Porter, 1974; McClelland *et al.*, 1972; Porter *et al.*, 1974; Reed and Cushing, 1975; Reed and Williams, 1971). Specific local antibody has been identified in humans following both infection with virulent organisms (Allardyce *et al.*, 1974; Reed and Williams, 1971; Davies, 1922; Harrison and Banvard, 1947) and administration of immunizing agents (Girard and de Kalbermatten, 1970; Goldblum *et al.*, 1975; Freter and Gangarosa, 1963; Mel *et al.*, 1965a).

Considerable convincing exists to support the contention that immunity to shigellae, salmonellae, and *E. coli* can exist at the mucosal level. Volunteer studies have demonstrated potent antibacterial immunity to shigellae

(DuPont *et al.,* 1972b) and *S. typhi* (DuPont *et al.,* 1970; Gilman *et al.,* 1976; Levine *et al.,* 1976a) following oral immunization with live attenuated vaccines; immunity could not be correlated with serum antibody (DuPont *et al.,* 1970, 1972b; Gilman *et al.,* 1976; Levine *et al.,* 1976a). Guinea pigs infected with shigellae in one eye develop resistance to homologous reinfection in the affected eye, while the contralateral eye remains susceptible to infection (Sereny, 1957; Cross and Nakamura, 1970). Piglets can be passively protected from enterotoxigenic *E. coli* disease with colostral antibody to the K88 antigen which prevents adsorption of K88 + *E. coli* to piglet intestinal mucosa (Rutter and Jones, 1973).

The identity of the immunoglobulin class in which protective antibody resides and the mechanisms of protection against bacterial enteropathogens are presently unclear. Since secretory IgA (SIgA) is the predominant immunoglobulin in intestinal and other surface fluids (Girard and de Kalbermatten, 1970; Tomasi and Zigelbaum, 1963; Plaut and Keonil, 1969; Tomasi, 1972) and is relatively resistant to proteolytic degradation (Brown *et al.,* 1970; Cederblad *et al.,* 1966), it has been suggested to be active in antibacterial immunity. This hypothesis was fostered by the proven biological protective capacity of SIgA against viruses (Ogra and Karzon, 1969; Ogra *et al.,* 1968; Akao *et al.,* 1971). SIgA does not fix complement by the classic pathway (Tomasi, 1972; Adinolfi *et al.,* 1966a; Ishizaka *et al.,* 1966; South *et al.,* 1966); however, three groups suggest that, in the presence of lysozyme and complement or a serum factor, SIgA can be bactericidal (Hill and Porter, 1974; Adinolfi *et al.,* 1966b; Burdon, 1973). Others have been unable to document this bactericidal action (Allardyce *et al.,* 1974; Eddie *et al.,* 1971), and complement is believed not to be present in intestinal fluids in a form or concentration to allow such bactericidal mechanisms to occur *in vivo* (South, 1971). It has been shown that aggregated IgA can activate complement by the alternate pathway (Tomasi, 1972; Gotze and Muller-Eberhard, 1971) and perhaps by the classic pathway (Iida *et al.,* 1976), and it has been hypothesized that this may have relevance with respect to SIgA in the gut (Hill and Porter, 1974). Secretory IgA has been observed to act as an opsonin (Girard and de

Kalbermatten, 1970; Wernet *et al.,* 1971; Kaplan *et al.,* 1972), and lysozyme and complement have been noted to increase the opsonic activity of intestinal IgA (Girard and de Kalbermatten, 1970). Other workers have found that SIgA does not demonstrate opsonic activity (Eddie *et al.,* 1971; Quie *et al.,* 1968). Nevertheless, recent work leads one to speculate that SIgA is indeed important in antibacterial immunity at the gut surface, at least, if not in the bowel lumen. Fubara and Freter (1972, 1973) demonstrated the capacity of SIgA to protect mice from infection with *V. cholerae;* the antibacterial effect occurred at the mucosal surface and caused a reduction in the vibrio population attached to the mucosa. Simple bacterial agglutination by SIgA has been repeatedly demonstrated (Allardyce *et al.,* 1974; Girard and de Kalbermatten, 1970; McClelland *et al.,* 1972). It may be that mere coating of bacterial enteropathogens by SIgA thereby preventing attachment to intestinal mucosa represents, in conjunction with other defense mechanisms such as peristalsis and normal enteric flora (Shedlofsky and Freter, 1974), a simple but important form of antibacterial immunity in the intestine.

3.2. Phagocytes

In the absence of a local immune barrier at the mucosal level, salmonellae, shigellae, and invasive *E. coli* can penetrate epithelial cells and proliferate in intestinal cells or the lamina propria. Shigella organisms induce a striking chemotactic response, resulting in heavy infiltration of the intestinal layers with polymorphonuclear neutrophilic leukocytes (PMNs) (Takeuchi *et al.,* 1965, 1968; Takeuchi, 1971). Salmonella serotypes that cause gastroenteritis also induce an influx of PMNs, but to a much lesser degree (Takeuchi, 1971; Ogawa *et al.,* 1968; Takeuchi and Sprinz, 1967). Shigellae and salmonellae are ingested by the PMNs. Low concentrations of purified endotoxin from *S. typhi, S. typhimurium,* and *E. coli* were found to elicit a mononuclear inflammatory response 3–6 hr after intradermal inoculation of volunteers (Greisman and Hornick, 1972). With increasing doses of endotoxin the relative importance of PMN leukocytes increased and at the highest doses PMNs predominated; at the periphery of the histopathological lesions mononuclear cells were common. Repetitive intradermal inoculation with low doses of *S. typhi* endotoxin resulted in a histopathological lesion indistinguishable from the rose spot of typhoid fever. It is the toxophore part of the endotoxin molecule that is responsible for the early mononuclear response to low doses of endotoxin, not the specific polysaccharide side chains, since endotoxin from rough mutants lacking side chains induced a comparable chemotactic response.

Virulent shigellae have more resistance to phagocytes and intracellular killing than do avirulent noninvasive shigellae (Yee and Buffenmyer, 1970). Similarly, normal guinea pig macrophages *in vitro* exhibit greater phagocytic capacity against avirulent *S. typhimurium* than against virulent strains (Wells and Hsu, 1970). Miller *et al.* (1972) demonstrated that human PMN leukocytes exhibit enhanced oxygen consumption during phagocytosis of *S. typhi* strains of low virulence; phagocytosis of virulent *S. typhi* organisms was not accompanied by augmented O_2 consumption. Furthermore, PMNs of patients with clinical typhoid fever, accompanied by bacteremia, do not manifest an increase in nitroblue tetrazolium dye reduction (Miller *et al.*, 1972).

Enterotoxigenic *E. coli* do not invade epithelial mucosa and do not elicit a PMN response, and interaction with phagocytes is not a recognizable phenomenon in this type of infection. Invasive *E. coli* elicits a PMN response comparable to shigella infection (Ogawa *et al.*, 1968; DuPont *et al.*, 1971a; Formal *et al.*, 1971b). The O antigens of invasive *E. coli* are negatively charged and may enhance their resistance to phagocytosis (Orskov *et al.*, 1971).

3.3. Circulating Antibody Response

Infection with shigellae results in appearance of circulating antibody to somatic antigens. The predominantly IgM antibodies (Cáceres and Mata, 1974) that appear are bactericidal and usually disappear within 1 year (Cáceres and Mata, 1974; Neter and Durphy, 1957). The frequency and height of circulating antibody response are proportional to the degree of clinical severity of the dysentery (DuPont *et al.*, 1969). There is no evidence that circulating antibodies are protective against shigella infection. The *in vivo* immunological response to *S. dysenteriae* 1 exotoxin has already been discussed.

Salmonellae also stimulate circulating antibody to their somatic, capsular, and flagellar antigens. That circulating antibody has some role in antibacterial immunity to salmonellae is borne out by the protective effect of some parenteral killed typhoid vaccines (Ashcroft *et al.*, 1964a, 1967; Yugoslav Typhoid Commission, 1964; Polish Typhoid Committee, 1965). It is not clear whether IgM antibody directed against somatic O antigen or IgG antibody against capsular Vi or flagellar H antigens is more important in antibacterial effect (Cvjetanovic and Uemura, 1965; Edsall *et al.*, 1959; Felix *et al.*, 1935; Felix and Olitzki, 1926; Felix and Pitt, 1934a,b; Standfast, 1960; Tully and Gaines, 1961; Tully *et al.*, 1963; Wong *et al.*, 1974a; Yugoslav Typhoid Commission, 1957).

In murine and guinea pig salmonellosis there is also great debate regarding the role of circulating antibody in protection (Jenkin *et al.*, 1964; Ornellas *et al.*, 1970; Herzberg *et al.*, 1972, MacKaness *et al.*, 1966; Blanden *et al.*, 1966; Collins *et al.*, 1966; Jenkin and Rowley, 1963). Some evidence suggests that circulating antibody is important and can be induced by killed parenteral vaccines (Jenkin *et al.*, 1964; Ornellas *et al.*, 1970; Herzberg *et al.*, 1972; Jenkin and Rowley, 1963). Others minimize the protective role of circulating antibody and killed parenteral vaccines in murine salmonellosis (Mackaness *et al.*, 1966; Blanden *et al.*, 1966; Collins *et al.*, 1966). The route of challenge may be crucial in this regard; oral or intragastric inoculation would appear to be more pertinent than the intraperitoneal route in challenge studies assessing protection (Blanden *et al.*, 1966; Collins, 1970; Collins and Carter, 1972).

Some studies in animals suggest that cytophilic macrophage-associated IgM antibody may be the mediator of immunity in salmonellosis (Rowley *et al.*, 1964; Hsu and Mayo, 1973).

Enterotoxigenic *E. coli* can induce an antitoxin response in infected adults with clinical and subclinical disease (Donta *et al.*, 1974; Sack *et al.*, 1974; Levine *et al.*, 1977; D. G. Evans *et al.*, 1978b). The role of the IgG antitoxin antibodies in protection against subsequent infections is not clear. Antisomatic antibody appears in response to enterotoxigenic or enteropathogenic *E. coli* infections (Levine *et al.*, 1957, 1978a, 1979). Evans *et al.* (1978b) have shown rises in antibody to colonization factor antigen I in volunteers infected with *E. coli* H10407.

3.4. Cell-Mediated Immunity

Little is known about cell-mediated immunity with respect to infections with *E. coli* enteropathogens or shigellae in man or animals.

Cell-mediated immunity forms the main basis of resistance in mouse typhoid (*Salmonella typhimurium*) infection (Mackaness *et al.*, 1966; Blanden *et al.*, 1966; Collins *et al.*, 1966). Shortly after infection of mice with small numbers of *S. typhimurium* intravenously, most of the organisms can be found in the liver and spleen. Although most of the inoculum is destroyed, some organisms survive and proliferate. Twenty-four hours after infection bacteremia is distinctly uncommon. However, 4–6 days later significant bacteremia appears, which continues for several days and is accompanied by peak bacterial counts in mouse spleen and liver. Beginning approximately 8 days after inoculation, bacteremia greatly diminishes and the number of salmonellae in liver and spleen progressively falls, although infection persists. Beyond day 14 of infection the mice develop the capability to completely eliminate organisms of rechallenge superinfection; this ability to prevent implantation of the superinfecting organisms occurs despite inability of the mouse host to eradicate persistent foci of the primary infection in liver and spleen (Mackaness *et al.*, 1966). Passive transfer to normal mice of immune serum from mice actively infected with *S. typhimirium* or immunized with heat-killed organisms results in increased ability of the recipient to clear organisms from the blood but inability to impede proliferation in the tissues.

The tissue immunity of infected mice, seen to develop beyond the 14th day, was found to be due to activated macrophages which develop enhanced microbiocidal properties (Blanden *et al.*, 1966). While it has been suggested that the increased microbiocidal activity of these macrophages is due to cell-bound antibody (Jenkin and Rowley, 1963; Rowley

et al., 1964; Hsu and Mayo, 1973), others have demonstrated that the macrophages are nonspecific in their increased antibacterial activity and will avidly destroy unrelated intracellular bacterial species (Blanden *et al.*, 1966). Lack of specificity argues against an antibody mechanism being responsible for enhanced macrophage activity. Macrophages from mice infected with *S. typhimurium* inactivated *Listeria monocytogenes*, and the mice were resistant to infection with the latter. Conversely, *listeria*-infected mice resisted *S. typhimurium* challenge. Cross-resistance between these bacteria was evident despite nonexistence of cross-reacting antibodies.

Activation of macrophages occurs under the influence of thymus-dependent (T) lymphocyte mediators (North, 1975; North and Deissler, 1975). Significant demonstrable active immunity, as measured by specific mediator T cells and activated macrophages, requires persistence of the living intracellular bacteria (Blanden *et al.*, 1966; Collins *et al.*, 1966; North and Deissler, 1975). In this regard salmonellae that are incapable of causing sustained intracellular infection appear incapable of eliciting cell-mediated immunity despite multiple inoculations (Collins *et al.*, 1966).

Mice that survive infection with an intracellular bacterial parasite retain protection against rechallenge with the organism for several months (North, 1975; North and Deissler, 1975). The long-lived immunity is not the result of persistent activated macrophages but is rather due to a long-lived capability of these mice to generate mediator T cells more rapidly and in greater quantity than normal mice (North, 1975; North and Deissler, 1975). While the short-lived active cell-mediated immunity seen in later stages of infection with intracellular bacteria is effected by activated macrophages and is directed by replicated short-lived T cells, the long-lived resistance that protects for several months against subsequent challenge infections exists despite the absence of replicating mediator T cells and activated macrophages (North, 1975; North and Deissler, 1975). In response to rechallenge many weeks after recovery from primary infection, mice were able to regenerate mediator T cells and activated macrophages in an accelerated manner, and effective antibacterial immunity was expressed in the short time required to limit and eliminate the rechallenge organisms. The long-lived state of increased resistance following initial infection was accompanied by a persistent level of delayed sensitivity to bacterial antigens and a small, stable population of nondividing protective T cells. Passive transfer of these nonreplicating T cells confers on normal mice resistance to lethal challenge infection (North and Deissler, 1975).

3.5. Host–Parasite Interaction in Typhoid Fever

Shigella, salmonella, and *E. coli* intestinal infections are all characterized by a spectrum of clinical illness ranging from asymptomatic infection to mild illness to fulminating disease. The host interactions involved in determining how the illness is expressed have been best observed in typhoid fever and will be discussed as a model.

Inocula containing about 10^5 virulent *S. typhi* are necessary to cause typhoid fever in 25–50% of healthy adult volunteers (Hornick *et al.*, 1970). Following ingestion, *S. typhi* organisms that survive gastric transit probably rapidly penetrate the intestinal mucosa. Excretion of *S. typhi* within 72 hr after ingestion of the organisms cannot be correlated with subsequent development of typhoid fever (Hornick *et al.*, 1970; Gilman *et al.*, 1976; Levine *et al.*, 1976a). Excretion at this time may represent intestinal transit of the organisms or intraluminal proliferation. Typically stool cultures become negative after excretion in the first 72 hr and often will not become positive again until clinical illness occurs. Some individuals can excrete *S. typhi* for several weeks without ever showing evidence of clinical illness.

S. typhi, after penetrating the intestinal mucosa, elicits a mononuclear response in the lamina propria. The bacilli are probably rapidly disseminated to the organs of the reticuloendothelial system. Onset of clinical disease begins after an incubation period of approximately 9 days and is manifested by fever, headache, and abdominal pain. Hornick *et al.* (1970) found the incubation period to vary inversely with size of inoculum ingested. Bacteremia was documented in some volunteers 1–2 days prior to onset of fever. The rapidity

with which *S. typhi* reaches its intracellular habitat in the reticuloendothelial system can be inferred by the observations that some volunteers who ingested an ID_{95} dose of organisms and who were given appropriate antibiotic therapy for 28 days beginning 24 hr after ingestion nevertheless developed bacteremia toward the end of the expected incubation period. Furthermore, one individual developed typhoid fever after a 7-day course of antibiotic therapy. Approximately 15–17 days after ingestion of an infective inoculum of *S. typhi*, serum O titers reach their peak.

After antibiotic therapy of acute typhoid fever, approximately 15–20% of individuals experience a relapse. Organisms can be cultured from bone marrow despite absence of bacteremia in patients with partially treated typhoid fever (Gilman *et al.*, 1975), which further attests to the presence of the bacilli within cells of the reticuloendothelial system. Relapse occurs at a time when circulating antibody is evident in high titer (Woodward *et al.*, 1954).

S. typhi has a predilection for infection of the gallbladder at the time of bacteremia. If cholecystitis or stones are present in the host, chronic biliary infection can occur.

Chronic biliary carriers of *S. typhi* represent a phenomenon in which host immune defenses are able to prevent development of typhoid fever, although the biliary infection cannot be eradicated. The intestinal tract of the carrier is bathed each day by billions of virulent *S. typhi*. Apparently mucosal antibody can prevent invasion by the bacilli and the shower of organisms serves to continuously booster the mucosal antibody. Furthermore, persistence of the *S. typhi* in the gallbladder may serve to ensure an activated state of cell-mediated immunity against the parasite.

4. Immunodiagnosis

4.1. Immunodiagnosis of Salmonellae

4.1.1. Immunodiagnosis of Enteric Fever

A definitive diagnosis of enteric fever requires isolation of *S. typhi* or *S. paratyphi* A or B from an appropriate culture site (Christie, 1974; Huckstep, 1962; Stuart and Krikorian, 1928; Wilson and Miles, 1964; Gilman *et al.*,

1975). However, in the absence of bacteriological facilities (a common situation in endemic areas of the Third World) or when a suspect patient has already received prior antibiotic therapy, serological tests for the diagnosis of typhoid or paratyphoid fever are helpful.

In 1896 Widal and Sicard and Grunbaum reported that serum of patients ill with clinical typhoid fever agglutinated the typhoid bacillus. Felix (1924, 1930) made a significant improvement in serological diagnosis by introducing the concept and techniques of qualitative receptor analysis. Felix stressed the distinction between O and H antibodies and demonstrated that both group (O) and specific (H) agglutinins of S. typhi could be measured by using as antigen a variant strain (O901) lacking H antigen (which agglutinates only O antibody) in addition to the parent strain (H901), which possesses both antigens. Strain O901 reacting with serum from a patient with typhoid fever results in fine granular flakes of agglutination; H901 gives a picture of coarse floccular agglutination, as a consequence of H antibody. Thus, by use of these two strains and observation of coarse and fine granular agglutination, Felix introduced differential measurement of somatic and flagellar antibody.

The next important advance in serodiagnosis was the discovery by Felix of the Vi antigen of S. typhi (Felix and Pitt, 1934a,b). As previously discussed, this antigen is a polysaccharide capsule that coats the somatic antigen of almost all virulent strains.

a. Clinical Uses of Serodiagnostic Tests for Typhoid Fever. Volunteer studies have shown that approximately 70% of individuals who develop typhoid fever will exhibit a fourfold or greater rise in antibody titer to O, H, or Vi antigen and that the rise is detectable by the 4th to 5th day after onset of clinical illness (Levine et al., 1978b). In natural disease most individuals also develop rises in antibody titer (Levine et al., 1978b), although early therapy with chloramphenicol may have a suppressive effect on antibody response (El-Rooby and Gohar, 1956; Watson, 1957; Colon et al., 1957; Levine et al., 1978b).

As originally conceived, serodiagnosis of enteric fever was proposed as a simple and rapid means of allowing the clinician to diagnose typhoid or paratyphoid fever when a patient presented with disease. In our experience the majority of individuals who present with acute typhoid fever already have elevated antibody titers (Levine et al., 1978b). However, the diagnostic significance of the titers varies greatly with the geographic origin, age, and immunization history of the patient.

In nonendemic areas significant titers of O, H, and Vi antibody are uncommon (Wilson and Miles, 1964; Levine et al., 1978b). Thus an acutely ill, febrile patient indigenous to the United States who has elevated O or H titer to S. typhi should be suspected of having enteric fever and appropriate cultures must be made, particularly a bone marrow culture if prior antibiotics have been administered (Gilman et al., 1975; Levine et al., 1978b).

In an endemic area a single Widal reaction in a febrile patient cannot be given any diagnostic significance (Wilson and Miles, 1964; Levine et al., 1978b; Alves, 1936a,b,c; Giglioli, 1933a; Levine, 1974). Antibodies to S. typhi can result from immunization (Christie, 1974; Huckstep, 1962; Stuart and Krikorian, 1928; Wilson and Miles, 1964; Ashcroft et al., 1964b; Beattie and Elliot, 1937; Giglioli, 1933b; Horgan, 1932; Olitzki, 1972) and from past infection (Giglioli, 1933a; Ashcroft, 1963) as well as recent infection. Similarly the antibodies may be the result of infection with other enteric organisms that share common antigens with S. typhi (Reynolds et al., 1970; Sansone and Saslaw, 1972). In areas of high endemicity repetitive antigenic stimulation by small inocula of S. typhi is believed to be common and to result in far more asymptomatic and mild cases than clinically obvious infections (Hornick et al., 1974; Alves, 1936a; Giglioli, 1933b; Peller, 1928; Ashcroft, 1964).

In order to determine the utility and reliability of a single Widal test as confirmatory evidence for typhoid fever in an endemic area, sera from four populations were compared (Levine, 1974; Levine et al., 1978b). These included (1) healthy individuals and surgical patients living in three areas of Peru where typhoid fever was endemic (2) individuals from an area where typhoid was nonendemic, Baltimore, Maryland, (3) Mexican patients with bacteriologically confirmed acute typhoid fever,

TABLE 1. *Salmonella typhi* O, H, and VI Antibodies in 42 Mexican Patients with Bacteriologically Confirmed Acute Typhoid Fever

Age group (yr)	Number examined	Mean duration of illness (days)	Percent of sera positive			
			O ≥40	H ≥40	H ≥80	VI ≥15
0–4	2	18	100	100	100	100
5–9	12	15	92	92	92	92
10–14	19	16	95	95	90	84
15–19	9	15	89	78	67	78

and (4) U.S. adult volunteers who developed typhoid fever in the course of vaccine efficacy studies.

The serological data of the Mexican patients with acute typhoid fever are seen in Table 1. More than 90% of children less than 14 years of age had reciprocal O titers of 40 or above and H titers of 80 or above. Among nine patients aged 15–19, only two-thirds had H titers of 80 or above. The prevalence of O titers (≥40) and H titers (≥40 and ≥80) on various days during clinical illness in 112 volunteers with induced typhoid fever is shown in Fig. 1. As early as days 4 and 5 of clinical typhoid fever, 70% of the men tested had O titers ≥40 and H titers ≥80. On days 12–13 of illness 80% of sera tested had O titers ≥40.

In contrast, few individuals from Baltimore, a nonendemic area, had antibodies to *S. typhi* (Table 2). The peak prevalence of O antibody at a titer of 40 or greater was 4% in the 10–19 age group. H antibody was most commonly seen in the 30 + age group, where 15% had titers of 40 or greater and 9% had titers of 80 or greater.

In Table 3 are summarized results with Peruvian sera. O antibody at low titer was common in all age groups. A rather distinctive pattern was seen with H antibody. The prevalence paralleled the pattern of age-specific incidence rates for typhoid fever. H antibody was rare in children less than 5 years old. Prevalence of H antibody increased with age through 19; 75% of 15- to 19-year-olds had H titer of 80 or greater. In one of the three areas (where typhoid vaccine is not used) 76% of the 15- to 19-year-olds had H titers of 160 or above, and titers of 640 and 1280 were common.

These data confirm that in endemic areas, where subclinical infection is widespread, a single Widal test cannot be used to confirm the diagnosis of enteric fever in persons over 10 years of age. However, the test is still quite useful in children less than 10 years old in endemic areas and in unvaccinated persons of any age from a nonendemic area (Levine *et al.*, 1978b).

b. **Serodiagnostic Tests for Chronic *S. typhi* Carriers.** Felix *et al.* (1935, 1938) first suggested that measurement of Vi antibodies might be used as a screening test for detection

TABLE 2. *Salmonella typhi* O, H, and VI Antibodies in 275 Residents of Baltimore with No History of Typhoid Fever

Age group (yr)	Number examined	Percent of sera positive			
		O ≥40	H ≥40	H ≥80	VI ≥15
0–9	101	1	0	0	0
10–19	23	4	4	4	13
20–29	58	0	10	0	5
30 +	93	0	15	9	0

TABLE 3. Prevalence of *Salmonella typhi* Antibody in Peruvian Sera by Age Group

Age group (yr)	Number tested	O titers, % positive		H titers, % positive		
		≥20	≥40	≥20	≥40	≥80
0–4	16	19	12	0	0	0
5–9	246	28	16	26	19	11
10–14	209	23	13	37	32	22
15–19	102	43	29	79	79	75
20–39	41	32	22	63	59	39

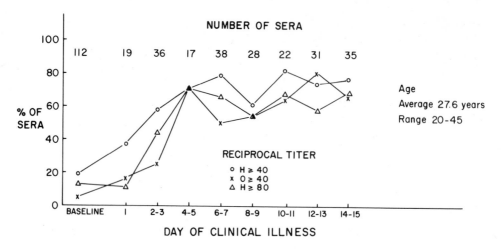

Figure 1. Immunology of enteric pathogens: *Salmonella, Shigella,* and *Escherichia coli.*

of chronic *S. typhi* carriers; the usefulness of this test is controversial and clarification is complicated by considerable disagreement in the literature with respect to methodology, as well as interpretation of results (Mackenzie and Windle Taylor, 1945; Landy and Lamb, 1953; Staack and Spaun, 1953; Schubert *et al.,* 1959; Anderson, 1960; Public Health Laboratory Service Working Pary, 1961; Bokkenheuser, 1964). Felix's (1938; Felix *et al.,* 1935) initial studies involved use of an *S. typhi* strain rich in Vi antigen; this strain, however, also contained O and H antigens, which interfered with the test. Use of an *S. typhi* strain, Vi I, possessing Vi but lacking O and H antigens, was an important breakthrough for bacterial agglutination tests (Bhatnager *et al.,* 1938). Somewhat later, several workers used crude (Staack and Spaun, 1953; Schubert *et al.,* 1959, Anderson, 1960) or purified (Landy and Lamb, 1953) Vi antigen extracted from *S. typhi, E. coli,* or citrobacter strains containing the Vi antigen, which was adsorbed to human (Landy and Lamb, 1953; Staack and Spaun, 1953; Anderson, 1960) or sheep (Schubert *et al.,* 1959; Anderson, 1960) red cells for hemagglutination (HA tests. Some workers continued to find success with bacterial agglutination (MacKenzie *et al.,* 1945; Public Health Laboratory Service Working Party, 1961) while others espoused the HA method (Schubert *et al.,* 1959), although the success of the later could not be repeated in all laboratories (Anderson, 1960).

Further disagreement exists on interpretation of results. While Felix and others felt that search for Vi antibodies was a helpful screening test, others disagreed (Bokkenheuser, 1964). It is obvious that methodology employed is crucial. In our own laboratory we do not find the HA test for Vi antibody useful in screening, since we find it positive in 5–13% of individuals aged 10–29 years, although it is rarely positive in young children or adults above age 30 (Levine, 1974). We use the HA microtiter method to screen for antibody, followed by the macrohemagglutination (tube) method. In our hands the microtiter assay appears to give considerable false-positive results. The disagreement on methodology and interpretation of results among some of the best enteric reference laboratories suggests that Vi antibody tests can probably not be relied on in most clinical laboratories and other methods should be used to search for chronic carriers.

c. Serodiagnosis of Paratyphoid Fever.
Measurement of antibodies to *S. paratyphi* A and B can be performed utilizing appropriate antigens. Paratyphoid A and B bacilli do not possess Vi antigen. Both paratyphoid A and B share common O antigens with *S. typhi,* while the flagellar H antigens of each serotype are distinct.

4.2. Immunodiagnosis of Shigellae

Kiyoshi Shiga (1898) first isolated dysentery bacilli by demonstrating that convalescent sera of a dysentery patient agglutinated organisms present in dysenteric fluxes of patients with acute disease. Bacteriological methods for detection of shigellae are so simple and widely available, even in the Third World, that serodiagnosis has all but disappeared as a clinical tool.

Hemagglutination tests for shigella antibody, utilizing passively adsorbed group or serotype-specific antigen (Neter and Walker, 1954; Young *et al.*, 1960; Lee *et al.*, 1966; Cáceres and Mata, 1970), have been employed with considerable success in epidemiological studies (Mata *et al.*, 1970; Gangarosa *et al.*, 1970; Neter, 1962; Gotoff *et al.*, 1963; Young *et al.*, 1967; Merson *et al.*, 1974), including investigation of outbreaks (Mata *et al.*, 1970; Gangarosa *et al.*, 1970; Gotoff *et al.*, 1963; Merson *et al.*, 1974). These tests have also been used to compare responses of various populations immunized with oral shigella vaccines (Mel *et al.*, 1965a; Levine *et al.*, 1972; DuPont *et al.*, 1972a; Levine *et al.*, 1974a); although the antibodies measured have no correlation with protection, they are useful in comparison of immune responses to vaccination among different groups (Levine *et al.*, 1972).

The propensity to develop circulating antibodies to shigella lipopolysaccharide has been found to correlate with the severity of clinical illness (DuPont *et al.*, 1969). Serological response of children immunized with oral attenuated shigella vaccines was noted to be related to the preimmunization titer (Levine *et al.*, 1972); children with significant preexistent titers did not develop fourfold rises in titer, in contrast to the increased frequency of seroconversion in children with minimal baseline titers.

Cáceres and Mata (1974) extracted an antigen of *S. dysenteriae* 1 which, in the passive HA test, gave high specificity and sensitivity for measurement of antibodies to Shiga's bacillus. Using this test in seroepidemiological studies, Mata *et al.* (1970) were able to demonstrate that the Shiga bacillus was endemic to Central America prior to the extensive

Shiga dysentery pandemic of 1968–1970, although it was an uncommon cause of dysentery in comparison with *S. flexneri* serotypes. They were also able to demonstrate evidence for widespread recent disease due to *S. dysenteriae* 1 in Guatemala by seroepidemiology.

4.2.1. Shigella Antitoxin Measurement

Discovery that the exotoxin elaborated by *S. dysenteriae* 1 induces transudation of fluid in the isolated rabbit ileal loop (Keusch *et al.*, 1972a) led to a resurgence of interest in measurement of toxin and antitoxin. Keusch *et al.* (1972c) developed a highly sensitive method for measuring minute quantities of neutralizing antibody based on the ability of the test sera to counteract the cytotoxic effect of Shiga toxin on HeLa cells. Some patients convalescent from *S. flexneri* and *S. sonnei* infections have also been found to possess this neutralizing antibody (Keusch and Jacewicz, 1973). The antibody is of the IgM class, is short lived, and is not followed by an IgG response, which makes it a unique immunological phenomenon as an antitoxin response to protein exotoxin (Keusch *et al.*, 1976). There is at present no clinical application for this assay.

4.3. Immunodiagnosis of *E. coli* Infections

4.3.1. Serodiagnosis

The HA technique utilizing antigen prepared from *E. coli* strains associated with epidemic outbreaks of diarrheal disease has been utilized for epidemiological purposes (Neter *et al.*, 1955). Presently measurement of antisomatic antibody to *E. coli* serotypes is rarely used.

Clinical infection with enterotoxigenic *E. coli* in adults is commonly followed by a fourfold or greater rise in antitoxin titer (Donta *et al.*, 1974; R. B. Sack *et al.*, 1974), although infected infants apparently develop rises less frequently (R. B. Sack *et al.*, 1975b). Antitoxin may be measured by the cumbersome rabbit ileal loop method (R. B. Sack *et al.*, 1974) or by titration using the adrenal cell assay (Donta *et al.*, 1974; D. A. Sack and R. B. Sack, 1975).

Small seroepidemiological studies of *E. coli* antitoxin comparing differing populations have been carried out (Donta *et al.*, 1974; Wallace and Donta, 1975; R. B. Sack *et al.*, 1975b). Prevalence of antitoxin was less in children and elderly adults (>50 years) than in adults aged 18–49 years. *E. coli* heat-stable enterotoxin appears to be nonimmunogenic in contrast to LT, and no serological tests exist for detection of ST.

4.3.2. Serotyping *E. coli* Isolates from Coproculture

In the years following recognition that certain strains of *E. coli* could be incriminated as agents responsible for epidemic infantile gastroenteritis and summer diarrhea, the only practical method available for diagnosis in the individual infant or for investigation of outbreaks was identification of the *E. coli* as an "enteropathogenic" serotype by agglutination with appropriate antisera. The "enteropathogenic" serotypes were biochemically identical to normal intestinal *E. coli* flora, and no practical laboratory test existed to distinguish pathogenic from nonpathogenic *E. coli* isolated from infants with diarrhea except serological methods. Ewing *et al.* (1963) determined the antigenic identity of 2279 *E. coli* isolates from cases of diarrhea within the United States and its territories which were received by the National Escherichia Center at the Center for Disease Control from 1950 to 1961. Of this number, 2019 isolates belonged to nine *E. coli* OB serogroups commonly associated with infantile diarrheal disease. Although 133 distinct serotypes were identified within these nine OB serogroups, 82% of the isolates fell within 20 serotypes and 13 of these 20 serotypes were associated with 75% of the cases of infantile diarrhea.

Serological screening of *E. coli* isolates from cases of sporadic as well as epidemic infantile diarrhea to determine if they fall within the serogroups associated with infantile diarrhea (Ewing *et al.*, 1963; Blair *et al.*, 1970) became routine in many hospital laboratories in the 1950s and 1960s, although the usefulness of such screening is under debate in the 1970s, with both detractors (Gangarosa and Merson, 1977; Goldschmidt and DuPont, 1976; R. B. Sack, 1976) and proponents (Rowe *et al.*, 1976, 1977; Gurwith *et al.*, 1977).

Kauffmann (1947) devised a scheme for classification of *E. coli* on the basis of O, H, and K antigens. Standard classification of *E. coli* is reviewed by Edwards and Ewing (1972). The term "K antigen" (K = Kapsel = capsule) refers collectively to surface envelope or capsular antigens found in *E. coli*, of which there are three types: L, A, and B. L antigens are envelope antigens, which are destroyed by heating to 100°C for 60 min. A antigens are capsular antigens whose agglutinability and antigenicity are destroyed by heating at 121°C for 120 min. B antigens have been described as envelope antigens whose antibody binding capacity is unaffected by heating at 121°C for 120 min.

In Kauffmann's original scheme *E. coli* organisms were divided into serogroups by O antigen. These were further subdivided by K and H antigens. Consecutive numbers were given to the O, K, and H antigens with the exception that B antigens were numbered separately from the other K antigens, e.g., O111:B4:H2. From 1956 (Kaufmann *et al.*, 1956) the B antigens have been given consecutive numbers as part of the K series and the type of K antigen is indicated in parentheses, e.g., O18:K75(B):H14. Where the number of the B antigen was changed in the modified system the old B number is included to avoid confusion, e.g., O111:K58(B4):H12.

The very existence of B antigens has been questioned for many years. Since the antigen binding capacity of B antigens in most instances cannot be inactivated, is has not been possible to prepare pure anti-B antisera by adsorption. Neither, generally, have strains been identified with the same O antigen but distinct B antigens (F. Orskov *et al.*, 1972). Thus the existence of B antigens has, with few exceptions, rested tenuously on a difference in titer of agglutination between heated and unheated suspensions of an *E. coli* strain tested with the same antiserum.

More recently, F. Orskov *et al.* (1971) presented evidence to suggest that neither the serotypes associated with infantile diarrhea nor those associated with dysenterylike disease possess thermostable K(B) antigens. Simple water extracts of *E. coli* O antigen (O1–O150) and K antigen (K1–K91) test strains were examined by immunoelectrophoresis with O and OK antisera. Serotypes associated with infantile diarrhea showed O antigen precipitation arcs that moved toward the cathode; K antigen lines were not seen. Serotypes associated with dysentery, in contrast, showed O antigen precipitation arcs on the anode aside; K antigens were not detected. F. Orskov *et al.* (1972) concluded that the B antigens previously thought to exist in many strains of *E. coli* are in fact part of the lipopolysaccharide O antigen.

5. Immunoprophylaxis

5.1. Vaccination against Typhoid and Paratyphoid Fever

5.1.1. Parenteral Killed Vaccine

Killed typhoid bacilli administered parenterally as immunizing agents have been available and used since the end of the nineteenth century, making typhoid vaccine one of the oldest of all vaccines. Parenteral typhoid vaccines were widely used in the armed forces of various countries since World War I. From these early mass applications certain impressions became evident: (1) the vaccine was highly reactogenic and (2) efficacy appeared to be quite variable. Despite the existence and use of parenteral killed typhoid vaccines over one-half century, it was not until the 1950s that careful well-controlled field trials were undertaken under auspices of the World Health Organization to evaluate efficacy of parenteral killed typhoid vaccines. Field trials were carried out in Yugoslavia (Yugoslav Typhoid Commission, 1964), Poland (Polish Typhoid Committee, 1965), Guyana (Ashcroft *et al.*, 1964a, 1967), and Tonga (Cvjetanovic, 1971). A summary of results of these field trials is contained in Table 4.

In summary, the acetone-killed vaccine was consistently shown to be superior to the heat-and-phenol-killed preparation, and both were more protective than the alcohol-killed vaccine. Alcohol-killed vaccine was advocated by Felix (1941a,b) because it contained better-preserved Vi antigen and induced a greater Vi antibody response than did heat-phenolized vaccines, a fact which Felix considered important; field trials contradicted this notion (Yugoslav Typhoid Commission, 1964; Ashcroft *et al.*, 1964a, 1967; Benenson, 1964). Wong *et al.* (1974b) showed that acetone was superior to heat–phenol treatment in preserving Vi antigen.

In the Guyana field trial, which involved school-aged children 5–15 years old, one dose

of typhoid vaccine was as protective as two doses and significant protection was documented for at least 7 years (Ashcroft *et al.*, 1964a, 1967), the period of observation. It has been suggested that in a hyperendemic area such as Guyana school-age children have already experienced multiple subclinical infections with *S. typhi* and the vaccine acts as a strong booster rather than as a primary immunogen (Ashcroft *et al.*, 1964a, 1967; Hornick *et al.*, 1970). In contrast, on the island of Tonga two doses of acetone-killed vaccine gave more protection than the single dose (Cvjetanovic, 1971). It has been suggested that in Tonga the numbers of virulent *S. typhi* ingested in the course of natural challenge in that environment are so high that they overcome the protective effect of a single dose of vaccine, and even with two doses protection is less than in other field trials.

Attempts have been made to correlate antigens, antibody, and protection with respect to parenteral vaccines. Such attempts have been largely frustrated. Edsall *et al.* (1959) and Standfast (1960) have shown that the ability to induce H antibody in rabbits was the only laboratory test to correlate with clinical protection in the Yugoslav field trials. Benenson (1964) found that recipients of acetone-inactivated vaccine in several World Health Organization field trials manifested significantly higher H antibody response than those who received heat-phenolized vaccine. However, clinical relapse in typhoid typically occurs when H antibody levels are quite high (Woodward *et al.*, 1954) and H antibody is not protective in the mouse or chimpanzee models (Tully and Gaines, 1961; Tully *et al.*, 1963). In contrast, unimmunized volunteers serving as controls in experimental challenge tests of typhoid vaccine who had preexistent "natural" H antibody at a titer of 20 or above had a significantly lower attack rate than control volunteers without H antibody (Gilman *et al.*, 1976; Levine *et al.*, 1976a). To further confuse the issue, this relationship between H antibody prior to challenge and protection did not exist for vaccinated volunteers. Neither O antibody or Vi antibody levels among vaccinees could be correlated with protection (Levine *et al.*, 1976a; DuPont *et al.*, 1970). Wong *et al.* (1974b) investigated the adhesion of Vi antigen to the bacterial cells in preparation of acetone

TABLE 4.   Results of WHO Field Trial with Parenteral Killed Typhoid Vaccines

Country	Period covered (yr)	Age range (yr)	Composition of group	Vaccine group[a]				Control		Efficacy[b]	
				K		L				K	L
				Cases of typhoid	Persons in trial	Cases of typhoid	Persons in trial	Cases of typhoid	Persons in trial		
Two doses of either vaccine K or L											
Yugoslavia	1960–1963	2–50	Mainly school children	16	5,028	37	5,068	75	5,039	79	51
Guyana	1960–1964	5–15	School children	6	24,046	26	23,431	99	24,241	94	73
Poland	1961–1964	5–14	School children	4	81,534	—	—	31	83,734	87	—
USSR	1962–1963	—	School children and young adults	—	—	13	36,112	50	36,999	—	73
One dose of either vaccine K or L											
Guyana	1960–1964	5–15	School children	0	3,319	3	3,371	14	3,515	100	78
Poland	1961–1964	5–14	School children	0	9,136	—	—	3	10,067	100	—
Two doses of either vaccine V or L				V		L				V	L
Yugoslavia	1954–1960	2–50	—	18	12,017	8	11,503	27	11,988	35	70
USSR	1962–1963	Most 7–16	School children	19	45,298	20	36,112	60	36,999	73	66

[a] Vaccines: K, acetone inactivated; L, heat and phenol inactivated; V, alcohol inactivated.

[b] Efficacy = $\dfrac{\text{Incidence in controls} - \text{incidence in vaccinees}}{\text{Incidence in controls}} \times 100$.

and heat-and-phenol-killed typhoid vaccines. It was found that acetone fixed Vi antigen to the bacteria, while heat-stable phenol preparation resulted in virtual complete loss of Vi antigen. Wong *et al.* (1974b) suggested that this discrepancy in Vi content between the two vaccines explained the difference in efficacy observed in field trials. However, the hypothesis is not borne out by serological studies of individuals vaccinated in these field trials; Vi antibody response was not superior in individuals who recieved acetone-inactivated vaccine than in those who received heat-and-phenol-killed vaccine (Benenson, 1964). While the mode by which parenteral killed vaccines protect is presumed to be circulating antibody, identity of the protective antibodies and antigens remains obscure (Benenson, 1964).

The protective effect of parenteral killed typhoid vaccines is closely correlated with challenge dose in the volunteer model (Hornick *et al.*, 1970). Against high inocula (10^7, 10^9) causing attack rates of 50–95% in unimmunized control volunteers, the vaccines conferred no protection. In contrast, against an ID_{25} of the challenge strain (10^5 organisms), 67% efficacy was measured. These studies clearly demonstrate that the protective capacity of vaccines is relative with respect to challenge dose.

Field trials to examine the efficacy of parenteral paratyphi A vaccines have been carried out (Joo, 1971). Some studies have suggested that paratyphoid B component of TAB (typhoid, paratyphi A and B) vaccine is not protective (Hejfec *et al.*, 1966). However, monovalent paratyphi B vaccines containing 5 times the amount of antigen of usual dosage regimens of TAB were found to offer protection (Hejfec *et al.*, 1968).

5.1.2. Cell-Free Extract Vaccines

An assortment of extract vaccines have been prepared from *S. typhi* (Joo, 1971). None is widely used as a practical immunizing agent.

Recently, the Vi antigen of *S. typhi* has been purified by Wong *et al.* (1974a) by modern methods for extraction of capsular polysaccharides and has undergone preliminary tests as a parenteral polysaccharide vaccine (Levin *et al.*, 1975). The Vi vaccine was administered to volunteers in doses of 25, 50, or 100 μgs; control volunteers received acetone-inactivated 6A vaccine. Both vaccines elicited

adverse reactions with comparable frequency, but the reactions were much milder with Vi vaccine. Vi antigen induced higher hemagglutinating antibody but lower bactericidal antibody responses than standard acetone-inactivated vaccine. Since clinical typhoid fever in man is a bacteremic disease and polysaccharide vaccines are notable for the long-lived antibody response that they elicit in adults, it is hoped that Vi vaccine will prove to be a successful immunizing agent of long duration. Field trials with this vaccine have not yet begun. Previously a less purified Vi antigen preparation (Webster *et al.*, 1952; Landy *et al.*, 1954, 1963) was employed as a parenteral vaccine in volunteers who were subsequently challenged with virulent organisms and the Vi vaccine gave only minimal protection (Hornick *et al.*, 1970).

5.1.3. Oral Killed Typhoid Vaccines

Much field experience has been gained with the use of killed typhoid bacilli administered as an oral vaccine in Eastern Europe (Mel *et al.*, 1974b; Joo, 1971), Chile (Borgoño *et al.*, 1972, 1976) and India (Chuttani *et al.*, 1971, 1972, 1973). These studies follow the original concept of Besredka (1919, 1927), who reported on vaccination against typhoid by the oral route and suggested that vaccine immunity should follow as closely as possible the pattern of natural infection-derived immunity. Although oral killed vaccine has been advocated by many workers, particularly those in Eastern Europe, controlled trials have not provided evidence to support efficacy. Two field trials undertaken in India (Chuttani *et al.*, 1971, 1972, 1973) failed to demonstrate protection from oral killed vaccine, even when administered in very high dosage. Studies undertaken in Chile have been equivocal. The preliminary study involved immunization of one endemic area with oral killed vaccine from the German Democratic Republic (Borgoño *et al.*, 1972). Another less endemic area was used as a control population. During this period of observation vaccine efficacy was 85% when incidence rates between the two groups were scrutinized. Since this field trial was not a randomized trial and risk of typhoid fever between vaccinated and control groups was not comparable, this study has been the object of criticism from an epidemiological design point of view. Borgoño et al. (1976) carried out two subsequent vaccine trials using oral killed vaccine from the German Democratic Republic in the first trial and vaccine from the German Federal Republic in the second trial. In the former trial the vaccine was protective (borderline statistical significance) with an efficacy of approximately 40%; in the second study vaccine was not protective.

In a carefully controlled challenge study involving volunteers, DuPont et al. (1971b) vaccinated men with oral killed typhoid vaccine (Taboral, Swiss Serum Vaccine Institutes). One group of men received six tablets (10^{11} S. typhi per tablet) and another group received 12 vaccine tablets. Vaccinees and comparable numbers of unimmunized control volunteers were challenged with 10^5 virulent Quailes strain S. typhi. Among the men who received six tablets, 40% developed typhoid fever vs. 43% of control volunteers, demonstrating no vaccine efficacy. The attack rate in men vaccinated with 12 tablets was 38%, in contrast to 54% in control volunteers; in this study the vaccine was 30% protective but the differences in attack rates were not statistically significant. In summary, controlled trials to date suggest that oral killed vaccine confers little or no clinical protection against typhoid fever in humans under either field or experimental conditions.

5.1.4. Oral Attenuated Typhoid Vaccines

Parenteral killed typhoid vaccines have proved to be protective for adults and older children living in endemic areas (Yugoslav Typhoid Commission, 1964; Ashcroft et al., 1964a, 1967; Polish Typhoid Committee, 1965; Hejfec et al., 1966). Nonetheless, these vaccines are unsatisfactory: (1) They frequently induce adverse reactions (fever, local inflammation) (Yugoslav Typhoid Commission, 1964; Ashcroft et al., 1964a; Polish Typhoid Committee, 1965). (2) Virgin (nonendemic) populations are less well protected (Hornick et al., 1970; Marmion et al., 1953; Edwards et al., 1962). (3) High infective inocula apparently overcome the protective effect, particularly in individuals from nonendemic areas (Hornick et al., 1970; Marmion et al., 1953; Edwards et al., 1962). (4) Local intestinal immunity is not stimulated.

A safe immunogenic oral typhoid vaccine could conceivably overcome many drawbacks of the parenteral killed vaccines. As already discussed, oral killed typhoid vaccines, although extremely well tolerated, have afforded minimal protection in well-designed volunteer and field trials. However, several live attenuated S. typhi strains have been investigated as possible oral immunizing agents with encouraging results.

Streptomycin-dependent (SmD) S. typhi strains have been developed by Cvjetanovic et al. (1970) and Reitman (1953, 1967). The former strain has been shown to be nonreactogenic, immunogenic, and protective in primates (Cvjetanovic et al., 1970). This strain has also been fed to several thousand Yugoslav adults and children without adverse effects (Mel et al., 1974b).

Reitman's SmD strain has been extensively examined for safety and efficacy in adult volunteers (DuPont et al., 1970; Levine et al., 1976a). This oral vaccine strain is noteworthy in its safety. Neither fever, vomiting, nor diarrhea was encountered following administration of multiple doses containing 30–100 billion organisms. SmD S. typhi is a noninvasive mutant incapable of proliferating in the absence of streptomycin or of penetrating intestinal epithelial cells. Even when fed concomitantly with streptomycin; which allows intraluminal proliferation of the organisms, the vaccine strain remains noninvasive.

Four studies were carried out to investigate the efficacy of SmD S. typhi as an oral attenuated vaccine (Levine et al., 1976a). Studies I and III employed freshly harvested vaccine while studies II and IV involved lyophilized vaccine. Five to eight doses (3×10^{10}–10^{11} organisms per dose) were given; oral streptomycin (1.0 g) was concomitantly administered in studies II and III, was administered with only two of the doses of vaccine in study I, and was not administered in study IV. In each of the four studies vaccinees and a comparable group of control volunteers were challenged with 10^5 virulent S. typhi organisms (Quailes strain). Freshly harvested vaccine was shown to be highly protective (66–78% efficacy) while lyophilized vaccine gave no clinical protection. Fresh vaccine also significantly interfered with intestinal proliferation of virulent *S. typhi*: only 17% of vaccinees excreted organisms vs. 75% of controls, signifying existence of local intestinal immunity.

Although freshly harvested SmD *S. typhi* vaccine was safe, was highly protective, and induced local immunity, to be realistically and economically employed in the field it would have to be available in lyophilized form and effective without streptomycin. The failure of the lyophilized preparation to confer clinical protection, even when fed with streptomycin, was disappointing, as well as enigmatic. Mouse protection studies showed no difference in immunogen content between the fresh and lyophilized vaccine. Field trials with this promising attenuated strain must await development of a lyophilized product that will retain the protective properties of the vaccine.

Another promising attenuated *S. typhi* strain is the gal E mutant, Ty 21a, isolated and characterized by Germanier and Furer (1975). This mutant has diminished or absent activity of several enzymes, particularly UDP-galactose-4-epimerase, responsible for incorporation of galactose into cell lipopolysaccharide.

In the absence of exogenous galactose the gal E. mutant is a rough strain. When the ambient environment contains galactose as a substrate, incomplete cell wall components are produced which are nonetheless immunogenic. As the intermediate products of galactose metabolism accumulate, such as galactose-1-phosphate and UDP-galactose, bacterial lysis occurs. Thus in animal and in *in vitro* studies addition of exogenous galactose to the gal E mutant results in formation of incomplete (but immunogenic and protective) cell wall antigens and bacteriolysis; the latter accounts for the *in vivo* avirulence of the strain.

The gal E. *S. typhi* attenuated mutant strain was tested for stability, safety, and efficacy as an oral vaccine in volunteers (Gilman *et al.,* 1977). One hundred and forty-four men received five to eight vaccine doses ($3–10 \times 10^{10}$ organisms per dose) in three trials; five vaccinees were given organisms grown in galactose-containing media. Significant adverse reactions were not seen. Vaccine organisms were recovered by stool culture from only half of vaccinees, usually just for 1 day. Fifty-five vaccinees and 64 control volunteers were challenged with 10^5 virulent *S. typhi* (Quailes

strain). Vaccinees who received vaccine grown in medium with exogenous galactose had significantly lower attack rates for typhoid fever than controls (2/28 vs. 23/43), demonstrating vaccine efficacy of 87%; these vaccinees excreted virulent *S. typhi* less frequently than controls (3/28 vs. 26/43), $p = 0.01$. Attack rates were not significantly different between men who received vaccine grown without galactose (5/27) and controls (8/21), $p = 0.24$. These results show that the epimeraseless gal E *S. typhi* mutant can synthesize protective cell wall lipopolysaccharide antigens in the presence of exogenous galactose. Instability and bacterial lysis, known to follow accumulation of galactose-metabolism intermediates *in vitro,* was reflected *in vivo* in avirulence and poor vaccine excretion.

Results obtained with SmD and gal E attenuated strains are very encouraging and suggest that a practical oral attenuated vaccine against typhoid fever may be available in the near future. Oral immunization may very well be the optimal form of immunoprophylaxis: (1) it most closely resembles natural infection, (2) oral attenuated strains are not associated with adverse reactions, (3) oral vaccines are highly protective even in the face of high inocula (ID_{50}), (4) oral attenuated vaccines induce local intestinal immunity. Furthermore, the immune intestinal barrier conferred on a vaccinated population in an endemic area would be expected to alter the ecology of *S. typhi* by interfering with transmission by asymptomatic excretors.

5.2. Shigella Vaccines

5.2.1. Parenteral Killed Vaccines

Circulating humoral antibodies are not the protective antibodies against shigella infection. Parenteral immunization with killed shigella organisms has failed to protect either man (Shaughnessy *et al.,* 1946; Hardy *et al.,* 1948; Higgins *et al.,* 1955) or monkey (Formal *et al.,* 1967) from natural or experimental infection despite induction of circulating antibody.

5.2.2. Shigella Toxoid

Shigella dysenteriae 1 exotoxin can be detoxified with formalin, ultraviolet light, and surface active agents (Engley, 1952). Shiga toxoid has not been utilized in man as an immunizing agent (Van Heynigan, 1971). Rhesus monkeys inoculated parenterally with two 125-μg doses of formalin-inactivated Shiga toxoid with aluminum hydroxide adjuvant developed extraordinarily high levels of circulating antitoxin but were as susceptible as control monkeys to development of shigellosis following experimental challenge (McIver et al., 1977).

5.2.3. Oral Attenuated Shigella Vaccines

The pioneer work of Formal et al. (1965b) established the virulence prerequisites common to all shigellae; as previously stated, these include (1) the ability to multiply in the intestinal lumen, (2) the capability to invade epithelial cells (LaBrec et al., 1964), and (3) the capability to proliferate within epithelial cells after invasion (Falkow et al., 1963). Elucidation of these virulence properties allowed the search for attenuated strains lacking one or more of these virulence attributes.

a. Mutant Attenuated Strains. Schneider and Formal (1963) described smooth colonial variants of a known virulent S. flexneri 2a strain which were readily identifiable by increased opacity (O) under oblique transmitted light in comparison with the smooth translucency (T) of the virulent parent strain. In contrast to the parent organism, the spontaneously derived mutant was nonpathogenic in the guinea pig model or guinea pig eye test (LaBrec et al., 1964; Formal et al., 1965b). The mutant was found to occur once in 10^4–10^5 cell divisions of the parent strain, bred true on subculture, and did not revert to the T form.

A spontaneously derived colonial mutant was found to be safe when fed to monkeys in high dosage (La Brec et al., 1964) and was proctective on subsequent experimental challenge (Formal et al., 1965c). When this strain was fed to adult volunteers (DuPont et al., 1972a), it was similarly well tolerated in doses of 10^8–10^9. When 10^{10} mutant organisms were fed to 47 volunteers, 45% developed diarrhea, 34% dysentery, and 32% fever. Revertant organisms which had regained the invasive capacity were abundant in stool cultures.

Istrati et al. (1961, 1964, 1967a) developed avirulent shigella mutants by serial passage on 2% nutrient agar slants. S. flexneri 2a mutant strain T_{32}, denoting 32 passages, has been shown to be noninvasive and negative in the

guinea pig eye test (Istrati et al., 1963; Istrati and Istrati, 1964). Multiple doses of this strain containing approximately 50 billion organisms have proved to be safe in adults and large numbers of children (Istrati et al., 1965, 1967a,b; Meitert et al., 1973). A controlled field trial of this vaccine in an institution with endemic dysentery demonstrated some evidence of efficacy (Meitert et al., 1973).

b. Streptomycin-Dependent Oral Shigella Vaccines. The attenuated shigella strains that have been most exhaustively studied are the streptomycin-dependent (SmD) strains of Mel et al. (1965a,b, 1968, 1971). SmD shigella vaccine organisms cannot proliferate in the absence of streptomycin; therefore, they are nonproliferating, as well as noninvasive. SmD vaccine strains have been prepared by Mel from several serotypes, including S. flexneri 1, 2a, 3, and 4 and S. sonnei. The safety of these strains has been demonstrated in healthy adults and children (Mel et al., 1965a,b, 1968, 1971, 1974a; Levine et al., 1972; DuPont et al., 1972) and debilitated institutionalized children (Levine et al., 1972, 1973c). Multiple doses of this nonproliferating strain, containing 20–50 billion organisms per dose, appear to be necessary for immunization (Mel et al., 1974a; DuPont et al., 1972b). Approximately 3–6% of vaccinees exhibit vomiting within hours of ingestion of vaccine (Mel et al., 1965a; Levine et al., 1972); this adverse effect is encountered almost exclusively following the first dose of vaccine and is uncommon thereafter.

As with all attenuated shigella and typhoid oral vaccines, vaccine organisms must be administered with some accompanying agent to enhance gastric transit and survival of vaccine organisms. Pretreatment with 2 g of $NaHCO_3$ in water was the standard method for enhancement of survival of vaccines during gastric transit in immunization of adults and some children (Mel et al., 1965, 1971; DuPont et al., 1972a). During pediatric studies in the United States, children refused to ingest the unpalatable $NaHCO_3$ solution (Levine et al., 1972). A vaccine "cocktail" was devised containing 4–8 oz of milk, a small but barely palatable amount of $NaHCO_3$ (0.8 g), and vaccine. This modification was shown to be as successful as the standard 2-g $NaHCO_3$ pretreatment in enhancement of survival of vaccine organisms (Levine et al., 1972), and all subsequent vaccine studies in the United States employed this method; Mel *et al.* (1974a) also adopted the "vaccine cocktail" for pediatric field trials in Yugoslavia.

In early field trials utilizing freshly harvested vaccine in adults, SmD vaccines were shown to be highly protective against natural challenge during one diarrheal season (Mel *et al.*, 1965b, 1968). In later studies involving children, lyophilized vaccine also showed protection but vaccine efficacy was less than in the earlier studies (Mel *et al.*, 1971, 1974a). Studies in children in Yugoslavia revealed that primary immunization conferred protection for more than 6 months but less than 12 months; yearly booster doses restimulated protective immunity to a degree comparable to that of primary vaccination (Mel *et al.*, 1974a).

Studies in the United States with Mel's SmD vaccines in adult volunteers (nonendemic area) revealed significant protective effects from vaccination in challenge studies, but vaccine efficacy was less than encountered among adults under conditions of natural challenge (DuPont *et al.*, 1972b). Immunized volunteers challenged with 180 shigella organisms exhibited vaccine efficacy of 60%, while among those challenged with 10^4 virulent organisms vaccine efficacy was 50%.

Shigellosis is endemic in many custodial institutions within the United States. Since neither antibiotics nor isolation techniques have been able to eradicate the infections, control by immunological means has been suggested employing oral attenuated shigella vaccines (Levine *et al.*, 1972, 1974a). Following preliminary studies demonstrating the safety of two types of attenuated shigella vaccine (Levine *et al.*, 1972), the SmD vaccines of Mel were selected for U.S. Public Health Service field trials because of the considerable experience with them (vaccination of more than 20,000 Yugoslav adults) and their proven efficacy.

In the United States more than two-thirds of institutional shigellosis is due to two serotypes, *S. flexneri* 2a and *S. sonnei*. Two institutions were selected for field trials, one with endemic *S. flexneri* 2a disease (Levine *et al.*, 1974a) and the other with *S. sonnei* infections (Levine *et al.*, 1975a, 1976b).

Vaccines were fed randomly to participants in the vaccine studies. Each vaccinated group was intended to serve as a control group for the other, since immunity to shigellae is serotype specific. In the institution with endemic *S. flexneri* 2a infections, attack rates were high and similar in both vaccinated groups, demonstrating no vaccine efficacy (Levine *et al.*, 1974a). All cases of symptomatic shigellosis occurred within 9 months of vaccination; despite clinical protection therafter, episodic asymptomatic excretion of shigellae was observed in one-third of the children. The level of immunity induced by SmD *S. flexneri* 2a oral vaccine was insufficient to prevent disease in this institutional environment; presumably this was due to the primitive level of hygiene existent in a coprophagic custodial population which resulted in ingestion of "unnaturally large" inocula capable of overcoming the local intestinal immunity induced by the vaccine.

In the *S. sonnei* endemic institution the controlled field trial design was complicated by some unexpected observations. Evidence of *in vivo* reversion of the *S. sonnei* vaccine to streptomycin-independent organisms was discovered (Levine *et al.*, 1975a). The revertants were associated with one of two distinct lots of lyophilized *S. sonnei* vaccine, were avirulent (noninvasive), and did not cause clinical adverse reactions. Furthermore, it was observed during vaccination in the course of this field trial that significant child-to-child transmission of vaccine strains was occurring (Levine *et al.*, 1975a). Following immunization in this institution, *S. sonnei* disease essentially disappeared despite the existence of several chronic asymptomatic carriers of virulent *S. sonnei* (Levine *et al.*, 1976b). Although it cannot be proven, it was hypothesized that because of child-to-child transmission of vaccine organisms, the controlled field trial more closely resembled a mass vaccination intervention trial; thus disappearance of *S. sonnei* disease from the institution could be attributed to the effect of the vaccine.

SmD shigella vaccines are safe and efficacious against low inocula encountered under many conditions of natural challenge. They require multiple doses for primary immunization, and booster doses must be given 6–12 months thereafter. In the face of extraordinarily high infective inocula, as encountered in some custodial populations, they are probably not effective. Immunity is serotype specific. Nonetheless, if most shigella morbidity can be shown to be due to just a few serotypes in a captive population (such as military units) exposed to low inocula, SmD shigella vaccines represent a practical control measure.

c. **Mutant–Hybrid Shigella Vaccines.** Another type of attenuated shigella organism that has been investigated as potential oral vaccine is the mutant–hybrid (MH) prototype developed by Formal *et al.* (1971c). Noninvasive shigella mutants are conjugated with *E. coli* K12 Hfr⁺ males. Shigella–*E. coli* hybrids are selected in which certain parts of the *E. coli* genome are incorporated into the shigella chromosome in stable form. The xylose–rhamnose (Falkow *et al.*, 1963; Formal *et al.*, 1965a) and purine E (Formal *et al.*, 1971a) portions of the *E. coli* genome are selected since they influence the phenotypic virulence of shigella after incorporation. The association is stable; approximately one in 10^9 hybrids spontaneously dissociates. Even if this should occur *in vivo*, the dissociated mutant is noninvasive and would have to reach high numbers to achieve the probability of reversion back to complete virulence. The theoretical impetus for development of MH strains was the development of a proliferating strain that would require only one of two doses for successful immunization, overcoming a major drawback of the SmD vaccines.

The MH *S. flexneri* 2a strain has the xylose–rhamnose segment of *E. coli* genome incorporated into an avirulent recipient shigella mutant. This vaccine strain has proven to be comparable in safety and efficacy to the SmD *S. flexneri* 2a vaccine when examined in volunteers (DuPont *et al.*, 1972a,b); it has also been shown to be as safe as SmD shigella vaccines when given to institutionalized children (Levine *et al.*, 1972). Bacteriological studies to investigate vaccine excretion showed that the *S. flexneri* 2a mutant–hybrid vaccine gave no evidence of being a proliferating strain; the percentage of vaccinees who excreted vaccine and duration of excretion were similar to those of individuals receiving nonproliferating SmD vaccines (DuPont *et al.*, 1972a; Levine *et al.*, 1972). For this reason field trials were not undertaken (Levine *et al.*, 1975).

Four mutant–hybrid strains of *S. dysenteriae* 1 were investigated in volunteers as pos-

sible oral vaccine candidates during the Central American Shiga dysentery pandemic (Levine *et al.*, 1974b). One strain was unsuitable because of genetic instability. Two other strains were genetically stable but reactogenic, causing diarrhea or fever; one of these strains was notable in that the shigella recipient had incorporated in its genome both the xylose–rhamnose and the purine E segments of *E. coli* chromosome but was nevertheless reactogenic. The remaining MH vaccine strain, 482-2E-1, was unique among all MH strains of shigella examined in that it was a proliferating strain. Following administration, most volunteer vaccinees excreted the strain for at least 7 days after a single oral dose of 10^8 or more organisms; several vaccinees shed the vaccine strain for more than 28 days after a single dose (Levine *et al.*, 1973a, 1974b). A total of 144 men were fed strain 482-2E-1; of these, 143 had no adverse reaction. In one volunteer given a 5×10^{10}-organism dose the MH strain completely reverted and the man developed Shiga dysentery (Levine *et al.*, 1973a). Organisms recovered from this individual could not ferment xylose or rhamnose and were invasive. Despite the genetic breakdown of the 482-2E-1 strain, it was an important landmark in oral shigella vaccine development because it demonstrated that a proliferating attenuated shigella strain could indeed be prepared.

d. *E. coli* **Bearing Shigella Surface Antigens.** Another generation of oral shigella vaccine candidates was prepared by genetic manipulation which had theoretical advantages over all previous oral shigella vaccines (Levine *et al.*, 1977a). In this instance shigellae and *E. coli* were conjugated; however, in constrast to the MH vaccines, the new strains utilized *E. coli* as the recipient (female) in conjugation experiments with an Hfr *S. flexneri* 2a (Formal *et al.*, 1970). It was found that loci for *S. flexneri* 2a group and type-specific surface antigens were associated with the *his*⁺ and *pro*⁺ loci, respectively. *E. coli* hybrids containing *his*⁺ and *pro*⁺ markers agglutinated in group- and type-specific antisera. These hybrids offered the theoretical advantages of complete safety, immunogenicity, and propensitv to proliferate.

E. coli hybrids bearing *S. flexneri* 2a surface antigens were fed to volunteers and found to be nonreactogenic; furthermore, evidence of proliferation was seen in excretion studies. Several groups of vaccinees and comparable numbers of control volunteers were involved in challenge studies with virulent *S. flexneri* 2a. The vaccine (multiple doses given in freshly harvested form) failed to protect against either high (10^4) or low (10^2) inocula of virulent organisms (Levine *et al.*, 1977a).

5.3. *E. coli* Vaccines

5.3.1. Vaccines against Enteropathogenic *E. coli* (EPEC)

Workers in Eastern Europe have developed formalinized corpuscular, sodium desoxycholate extract and Boivin extract vaccines from EPEC strains O111:K58, O55:K59, and O86: K61. These extract vaccines were administered orally in multiple doses to infants, following demonstration of their safety in adult volunteers. The extract vaccines were well tolerated by young infants, and circulating antibodies and coproantibodies were stimulated (Rauss *et al.*, 1972, 1974; Kubinyi *et al.*, 1972, 1974; Mochmann *et al.*, 1974). Nursery-acquired diarrheal infections due to EPEC continued as a problem in hospitals and infant nurseries in eastern Europe during the mid-1970s (Kubinyi *et al.*, 1972). Sporadic and epidemic infections were sufficiently common among infants immunized with vaccine or placebo to demonstrate vaccine efficacy of 30–65%, depending on age group (Rauss *et al.*, 1972, 1974; Kubinyi *et al.*, 1972, 1974).

5.3.2. Vaccines against Enterotoxigenic *E. coli*

Enterotoxigenic *E. coli* is the single most important etiological agent of travelers' diarrhea. Recent knowledge has generated optimism for the concept of immunological control of travelers' diarrhea due to enterotoxigenic *E. coli*. Epidemiological observations suggest that prior infections confer immunity (DuPont *et al.*, 1976). Travelers' diarrhea occured in 40% of newly arrived U.S. students in Mexico but in only 20% of long-term U.S. students and in only 11–14% of Venezuelan or Mexican students.

These findings were supported by volunteer studies. Volunteers challenged with an *E. coli* strain (O148:H28) that produces LT and ST were significantly protected against diarrhea

on subsequent rechallenge with the same strain, in comparison with control volunteers (Levine *et al.*, 1978). Clinical illness and immunological response to the O148:H28 strain did not, however, confer protection against challenge with a heterologous *E. coli* strain (O28:NM) that produces only LT.

Veterinary studies offer the most encouraging results to suggest that a vaccine to control enterotoxigenic *E. coli* infections in humans may not be far off. K88-, K99-, and 987-type pili have been purified from *E. coli* strains that cause *E. coli* diarrhea in piglets and have been used to parenterally immunize pregnant sows in the tests. Piglets suckled from immunized dams were significantly protected against diarrheal illness and death due to *E. coli* strains carrying the homologous pilus antigen (Rutter and Jones, 1973; Nagy *et al.*, 1978; Morgan *et al.*, 1978).

Studies examining the reactogenicity, immunogenicity, and efficacy in man of purified pili vaccines from human strains are currently underway (M. M. Levine and C. C. Brinton, Jr., unpublished data).

References

Adinolfi, M., Mollison, P. L., Polley, M. J., and Rose, J. M., 1966a, Gamma A-blood group antibodies, *J. Exp. Med.* **123:**951–967.

Adinolfi, M., Glynn, A. A., Lindsay, M., and Milne, C. M., 1966b, Serological properties of Gamma A antibodies to *Escherichia coli* present in human colostrum, *Immunology* **10:**517–526.

Akao, Y., Sasagawa, A., Shiga, S., and Kono, R., 1971, Comparative studies on the mode of neutralization reaction of poliovirus type 2 with serum IgG and secretory IgA from mother's milk and fecal extract, *Jpn. J. Med. Sci.* **24:**135–152.

Alderete, J. F., and Robertson, D. F., 1978, Purification and chemical characterization of the heat-stable enterotoxin produced by porcine strains of enterotoxigenic *Escherichia coli, Infect. Immun.* **19:**1021–1030.

Allardyce, A. R., Shearman, D. J. C., McClelland, D. B. L., Marwick, K., Simpson, A. J., and Laidlaw, R. B., 1974, Appearance of specific colostrum antibodies after infection with *Salmonella typhimurium, Br. Med. J.* **3:**307–309.

Alves, W. D., 1936a, "O" agglutinins for *B. typhosus* in an uninoculated native population, *S. Afr. Med. J.* **10:**6.

Alves, W. D., 1936b, T. A. B. and brucella agglutinins in an uninoculated native population, *S. Afr. Med. J.* **10:**7–8.

Alves, W. D., 1936c, "Normal" agglutinins and their bearing on the diagnosis of typhoid fever by agglutination tests, *S. Afr. Med. J.* **10**:9–10.

Anderson, E. S., 1960, Screening test for typhoid carriers, *Lancet* **1**:653.

Ashcroft, M. T., 1964, Typhoid and paratyphoid fever in the tropics. *J. Trop. Med. Hyg.* **67**:185–189.

Ashcroft, M. T., Nicholson, C. C., and Stuart, C. A., 1963, Typhoid antibodies in British Guiana school children, *W. Ind. Med. J.* **12**:247–252.

Ashcroft, M. T., Morrison-Ritchie, J., and Nicholson, C. C., 1964a, Controlled field trial in British Guiana school children of heat-killed phenolized and acetone-killed lyophilized typhoid vaccines, *Am. J. Hyg.* **79**:196–206.

Ashcroft, M. T., Morrison-Ritchie, J., and Nicholson, C. C., 1964b, Antibody responses to vaccination of British Guiana school children with heat-killed phenolized and acetone-killed lyophilized typhoid vaccines, *Am. J. Hyg.* **80**:221–228.

Ashcroft, M. T., Balwant, S., Nicholson, C. C., Ritchie, J. M., Sobryan, E., and Williams, F., 1967, A seven-year field trial of two typhoid vaccines in Guyana, *Lancet* **2**:1056–1059.

Avery, G. S., Davies, E. F., and Bragden, R. N., 1972, Lactulose: A review of its therapeutic and pharmacological properties with particular reference to human metabolism and its mode of action in portal systemic encepalopathy, *Drugs* **4**:7–48.

Axon, A. T., and Poole, D., 1973, Salmonellosis presenting with choleralike diarrhea, *Lancet* **1**:745–746.

Barrett-Connor, E., and Connor, J. D., 1970, Extraintestinal manifestations of shigellosis, *Am. J. Gastroenterol.* **53**:234–245.

Baskett, R. C., and Hentges, D. J., 1973, *Shigella flexneri* inhibition by acetic acid, *Infect. Immun.* **8**:91–97.

Beattie, C. P., and Elliot, J. S., 1937, Serologic diagnosis of enteric in the inoculated, *J. Hyg.* **37**:36–41.

Benenson, A. S., 1964, Serological responses of man to typhoid vaccines, *Bull. WHO* **30**:653–662.

Bertschinger, H. U., Moon, H. W., and Whipp, S. C., 1972, Association of *Escherichia coli* with the small intestinal Epithelium. I. Comparison of enteropathogenic and nonenteropathogenic porcine strains in pigs, *Infect. Immun.* **5**:595–605.

Besredka, A., 1919, De la vaccination contre les états typhoides par voie buccale, *Ann. Inst. Pasteur* **1919**:882–890.

Besredka, A., 1927, *Local Immunization,* Williams and Wilkins, Baltimore.

Bhatnagar, S. S., Speechly, C. C. G., and Singh, M., 1938, A Vi variant of *Salmonella typhi* and its application to the serology of typhoid fever, *J. Hyg.* **38**:663–672.

Blair, J. E., Lennette, E. H., and Truant, J. P., 1970, *Manual of Clinical Microbiology,* pp. 151–174, Williams and Wilkins, Baltimore.

Blanden, R. V., Mackaness, G. B., and Collins, F. M., 1966, Mechanisms of acquired resistance in mouse typhoid, *J. Exp. Med.* **124**:585–600.

Block, N. B., and Ferguson, W., 1940, An outbreak of Shiga dysentery in Michigan, 1938, *Am. J. Publ. Health* **30**:43–52.

Bohnhoff, M., Miller, C. P., and Martin, W. R., 1964a, Resistance of the mouse's intestinal tract to experimental salmonella infections. I. Factors which interfere with the initiation of infection by oral inoculation, *J. Exp. Med.* **120**:805–816.

Bohnhoff, M., Miller, C. P., and Martin, W. R., 1964b, Resistance of the mouse's intestinal tract to experimental salmonella infections. II. Factors responsible for its loss following streptomycin treatments, *J. Exp. Med.* **120**:817–828.

Bokkenheuser, V., 1964, Detection of typhoid carriers, *Am. J. Publ. Health* **54**:477–486.

Borgoño, J. M., Greiber, R., Baquedano, F., Carrillo, B., Concha, F., and Solari, G., 1972, Vacunación antitifica oral: Resultados preliminares, *Rev. Med. Chile* **100**:1129–1132.

Borgoño, J. M., Corey, O. G., and Engelhardt, H., 1976, Field trials with killed oral typhoid vaccines, *Dev. Biol. Stand.* **33**:80–84.

Bornstein, S., 1943, The state of the salmonella problem, *J. Immunol.* **46**:439–496.

Bray, J., 1945, Isolation of antigenically homogeneous strains of *Bact. coli* Neapolitanum from summer diarrhea of infants, *J. Pathol. Bacteriol.* **57**:239–247.

Brinton, C. C., Jr., 1977, The piliation phase syndrome and the uses of purified pili in disease control, in: *Proceedings of the XIIIth Joint U.S.–Japan Conference on Cholera,* Atlanta, Ga., September 1977, pp. 33–70, DHEW publication No. (NIH) 78–1590, NIH, Bethesda, Md.

Brown, W. R., Newcomb, R. W., and Ishizaka, K., 1970, Proteolytic degradation of exocrine and serum immunoglobulins, *J. Clin. Invest.* **49**:1374–1380.

Burdon, D. W., 1973, The bactericidal action of immunoglobulin A, *J. Med. Microbiol.* **6**:131–139.

Cáceres, A., and Mata, L. J., 1970, Hemaglutinación indirecta para la investigación de anticuerpos a enterobacteriaceaes, *Rev. Lat. Am. Microbiol. Parasitol.* **12**:137–144.

Cáceres, A., and Mata, L. J., 1974, Serologic response of patients with Shiga dysentery, *J. Infect. Dis.* **129**:439–443.

Cahill, K. M., Davis, J. A., and Johnson, R., 1966, Report on an epidemic due to *Shigella dysenteriae* type 1 in the Somali interior, *Am. J. Trop. Med. Hyg.* **15**:52–56.

Cash, R. A., Music, S. I., Libonati, J. P., Snyder, M. J., Wenzel, R. P., and Hornick, R. B., 1974, Response of man to infection with *Vibrio cholerae.* I. Clinical, serologic, and bacteriologic responses to a known inoculum, *J. Infect. Dis.* **129**:45–52.

Cederblad, G., Johansson, B. G., and Rymo, L., 1966, Reduction and proteolytic degradation of immunoglobulin A from human colostrum, *Acta. Chem. Scand.* **20**:2349–2357.

Chen, L. C., Rohde, J. E., and Sharp, G. W. G., 1971,

Intestinal adenyl-cyclase activity in human cholera, *Lancet* 1:939–941.

Cherubin, C. E., Neu, H. H., Imperato, P. J., Harvey, R. P., and Bellen, N., 1974, Septicemia with non-typhoid salmonella, *Medicine (Baltimore)* 53:365–376.

Christie, A. B., 1974, *Infectious Diseases: Epidemiology and Clinical Practice,* 2nd ed., E and S Livingstone, Ltd., Edinburgh.

Chuttani, C. S., Prakash, K., Vergese, A., Sharma, U., Singha, P., and Ghosh Ray, B., 1971, Effectiveness of oral killed typhoid vaccine, *Bull. WHO* 45:445–450.

Chuttani, C. S., Prakash, K., Vergese, A., Sharma, U., Singha, P., Ghosh Ray, R., and Agarwal, D. S., 1972, Controlled field trials of oral killed typhoid vaccines in India, *Int. J. Epidemiol.* 1:39–43.

Chuttani, C. S., Prakash, K., Vergese, A., Gupta, P., Chawla, R. K., Grover, V., and Agarwal, D. S., 1973, Ineffectiveness of an oral killed typhoid vaccine in a field trial, *Bull. WHO* 48:756–757.

Clark, W. R., McLaughlin, J., and Webster, M. E., 1958, An aminohexuronic acid as the principal hydrolytic component of the Vi antigen, *J. Biol. Chem.* 1958:81–89.

Collins, F. M., 1970, Immunity to enteric infection in mice, *Infect. Immun.* 1:243–250.

Collins, F. M., and Carter, P. B., 1972, Comparative immunogenicity of heat-killed and living oral salmonella vaccines, *Infect. Immun.* 6:451–458.

Collins, F. M., MacKaness, G. B., and Blanden, R. V., 1966, Infection-immunity in experimental salmonellosis, *J. Exp. Med.* 124:601–619.

Colon, A. R., Gross, D. R., and Tamer, M. A., 1975, Typhoid fever in children, *Pediatrics* 56:606–609.

Conradi, H., 1903, Ueber Iosliche, durch aseptische Autolyse erhaltene Gifstoffe von ruhr und typhus Bazillen, *Deutsch. Med. Wochenschr.* 29:26–28.

Cross, W. R., and Nakamura, M., 1970, Analysis of the virulence of *Shigella flexneri* by experimental infection of the rabbit eye, *J. Infect. Dis.* 122:394–400.

Cvjetanovic, B., 1971, Progress in the field study of acetone-dried vaccines against typhoid, in: *International Conference on the Application of Vaccines against Viral, Rickettsial and Bacterial Diseases of Man,* pp. 372–373, PAHO Sci. Publ. No. 226.

Cvjetanovic, B., and Uemura, K., 1965, The present status of field and laboratory studies of typhoid and paratyphoid vaccines, *Bull. WHO* 32:29–36.

Cvjetanovic, B., Mel, D. M., and Felsenfeld, O., 1970, Study of live typhoid vaccine in chimpanzees, *Bull. WHO* 42:499–507.

Dahlqvist, A., and Gryboski, J. D., 1965, Inability of the human small intestinal lactase to hydrolyze lactulose, *Biochim. Biophys. Acta* 110:635–636.

Davies, A., 1922, An investigation into the serological properties of dysentery stools, *Lancet* 2:1009–1010.

De, S. N., Bhattacharya, K., and Sarkar, J. K., 1956, A study of the pathogenicity of strains of Bacterium coli from acute and chronic enteritis, *J. Pathol. Bacteriol.* 71:201–209.

DeLorenzo, F., Soscia, M., Manzillo, G., and Balestrieri, G. G., 1974, Epidemic of cholera El Tor in Naples, 1973, *Lancet* 1:669.

Dixon, J. M. S., 1960, The fate of bacteria in the small intestine, *J. Pathol. Bacteriol.* 79:131–140.

Dixon, J. M. S., and Paulley, J. W., 1963, Bacteriological and histological studies of the small intestine of rats treated with mecamylamine, *Gut* 4:169–173.

Donta, S. T., 1974, Neutralization of cholera enterotoxin-induced steroidogenesis by specific antibody, *J. Infect. Dis.* 129:284–288.

Donta, S. T., Sack, D. A., Wallace, R. B., DuPont, H. L., and Sack, R. B., 1974, Tissue-culture assay of antibodies to heat-labile *Escherichia coli* enterotoxins, *N. Engl. J. Med.* 291:117–121.

Dorner, F., 1975, *Escherichia coli* enterotoxin purification and partial characterization, *J. Biol. Chem.* 250:8712–8719.

Drasar, B. S., and Hill, M. J., 1974, *Human Intestinal Flora,* Academic Press, London.

DuPont, H. L., and Hornick, R. B., 1973, Adverse effect of lomotil therapy in shigellosis, *JAMA* 226:1525–1528.

DuPont, H. L., Hornick, R. B., Dawkins, A. T., Snyder, M. J., and Formal, S. B., 1969, The response of man to virulent *Shigella flexneri* 2a, *J. Infect. Dis.* 119:296–299.

DuPont, H. L., Hornick, R. B., Snyder, M. J., Libonati, J. P., and Woodward, T. E., 1970, Immunity in typhoid fever: Evaluation of live streptomycin-dependent vaccine, *Antimicrob. Agents Chemother.,* pp. 236–239.

DuPont, H. L., Formal, S. B., Hornick, R. B., Snyder, M. J., Libonati, J. P., Sheehan, D. G., LaBrec, E. H., and Kalas, J. P., 1971a, Pathogenesis of *Escherichia coli* diarrhea, *N. Engl. J. Med.* 285:1–9.

DuPont, H. L., Hornick, R. B., Snyder, M. J., Dawkins, A. T., Heiner, G. G., and Woodward, T. E., 1971b, Studies of immunity in typhoid fever: Protection induced by killed oral antigens or by primary infection, *Bull. WHO* 44:667–672.

DuPont, H. L., Hornick, R. B., Snyder, M. J., Libonati, J. P., Formal, S. B., and Gangarosa, E. J., 1972a, Immunity in shigellosis. I. Response of man to attenuated strains of *Shigella, J. Infect. Dis.* 125:5–11.

DuPont, H. L., Hornick, R. B., Snyder, M. J., Libonati, J. P., Formal, S. B., and Gangarosa, E. J., 1972b, Immunity in shigellosis. II. Protection induced by oral live vaccine or primary infection, *J. Infect. Dis.* 125:12–16.

DuPont, H. L., Olarte, J., Evans, D. G., Pickering, L. K., Galindo, E., and Evans, D. J., 1976, Comparative susceptibility of Latin American and United States students to enteric pathogens, *N. Engl. J. Med.* 295:1520–1521.

Echeverria, P. D., Chang, C. P., Smith, D., and Anderson, G. L., 1976, Enterotoxigenicity and invasive capacity of "enteropathogenic" serotypes of *Escherichia coli, J. Pediatr.* 89:8–10.

Eddie, D. S., Schulkind, M. L., and Robbins, J. B., 1971, The isolation and biologic activities of purified secretory IgA and IgG anti-*Salmonella typhimurium* "O" antibodies from rabbit intestinal fluid and colostrum, *J. Immunol.* **106**:181–190.

Edsall, G., Carlson, C., Formal, S. B., and Benenson, A. S., 1959, Laboratory tests of typhoid vaccines used in a controlled field study, *Bull WHO* **20**:1017–1032.

Edwards, P. R., and Ewing, W. H., 1972, *Identification of Enterobacteriaceae*, 3rd ed., Burgess, Minneapolis.

Edwards, W. M., Crone, R. I., and Harris, J. F., 1962, Outbreak of typhoid fever in previously immunized persons traced to a common carrier, *N. Engl. J. Med.* **267**:742–751.

El-Rooby, A., and Gohar, M. A., 1956, Effect of chloramphenicol on agglutinin titre in enteric fevers, *J. Trop. Med. Hyg.* **59**:47–51.

Engley, F. B., Jr., 1952, The neurotoxin of Shigella dysenteriae (Shiga), *Bacteriol. Rev.* **16**:153–178.

Evans, D. G., and Evans, D. J., Jr., 1978, New surface-associated heat-labile colonization factor antigen (CFA/II) produced by enterotoxigenic *Escherichia coli* of serogroups O6 and O8, *Infect. Immun.* **21**:638–647.

Evans, D. G., Evans, D. J., Jr., and Pierce, N. F., 1973, Differences in the response of rabbit small intestine to heat-labile and heat-stable enterotoxins of *Escherichia coli, Infect. Immun.* **7**:873–880.

Evans, D. G., Silver, R. P., Evans, D. J., Jr., Chase, D. G., and Gorbach, S. L., 1975, Plasmid-controlled colonization factor associates with virulence in *Escherichia coli* enterotoxigenic for humans, *Infect. Immun.* **12**:656–667.

Evans, D. G., Evans, D. J., Jr., and Tjoa, W., 1977, Hemagglutination of human group A erythrocytes by enterotoxigenic *Escherichia coli* isolated from adults with diarrhea: Correlation with colonization factor, *Infect. Immun.* **18**:330–337.

Evans, D. G., Evans, D. J., Jr., Tjoa, W. S., and DuPont, H. L., 1978a, Detection and characterization of colonization factor of enterotoxigenic *Escherichia coli* isolated from adults with diarrhea, *Infect. Immun.* **19**:727–736a.

Evans, D. G., Satterwhite, T. K., Evans, D. J., Jr., and DuPont, H. L., 1978b, Differences in serological responses and excretion patterns of volunteers challenged with enterotoxigenic *Escherichia coli* with and without the colonization factor antigen, *Infect Immun.* **19**:883–888.

Evans, D. J., Jr., Chen, L. C., Curlin, G. T., and Evans, D. G., 1972, Stimulation of adenyl cyclase by *Escherichia coli* enterotoxin, *Nature (London), New Biol.* **236**:137–138.

Evans, D. J., Jr., Evans, D. G., and Gorbach, S. L., 1974, Polymixin B-induced release of low-molecular weight heat-labile enterotoxin from *Escherichia coli, Infect. Immun.* **10**:1010–1017.

Evans, D. J., Jr., Evans, D. G., DuPont, H. L., Orskov, F., and Orskov, I., 1977, Patterns of loss of enterotoxigenicity by *Escherichia coli* isolated from adults with diarrhea: Suggestive evidence for an interrelationship with serotype, *Infect. Immun.* **17**:105–111.

Ewing, W. H., Tatum, H. W., and Davis, B. R., 1957, The occurrence of *Escherichia coli* serotypes associated with diarrheal diseases in the United States, *Publ. Health Lab.* **15**:118–138.

Ewing, W. H., Davis, B. R., and Montague, T. S., 1963, Studies on the occurrence of *Escherichia coli* serotypes associated with diarrheal disease, in: *Center for Disease Control, U.S. Department of Health, Education, and Welfare Report*.

Falkow, S., Schneider, H., Baron, L. S., and Formal, S. B., 1963, Virulence of Escherichia–Shigella genetic hybrids for the guinea pig, *J. Bacteriol.* **86**:1251–1258.

Felix, A., 1924, The qualitative receptor analysis in its application to typhoid fever, *J. Immunol.* **9**:115–192.

Felix, A., 1930, The qualitative serum diagnosis of enteric fevers: Directions for its performance, *Lancet* **1**:505–507.

Felix, A., 1938, The detection of chronic typhoid carriers by agglutination tests, *Lancet* **2**:738–741.

Felix, A., 1941, New type of typhoid and paratyphoid vaccine, *Br. Med. J.* **1**:391–395.

Felix, A., and Anderson, E. S., 1951, Bacteriophage, virulence and agglutination tests with a strain of *Salmonella typhi* of low virulence, *J. Hyg.* **49**:349–364.

Felix, A., and Bhatnagar, S. S., 1935, Further observations on the properties of the Vi antigen of *B. typhosus* and its corresponding antibody, *Br. J. Exp. Pathol.* **16**:422–434.

Felix, A., and Olitzki, L., 1928, The use of preserved bacterial suspensions for the agglutination test: With especial reference to the enteric fevers and typhus fevers, *J. Hyg.* **28**:55–66.

Felix, A., and Pitt, R. M., 1934a, A new antigen of *B. typhosus:* Its relation to virulence and to active and passive immunisation, *Lancet* **2**:186–191.

Felix, A., and Pitt, M., 1934b, Virulence of *B. typhosus* and resistance to O antibody, *J. Pathol. Bacteriol.* **38**:409–420.

Felix, A., and Pitt, R. M., 1951, The pathogenic and immunogenic activities of *Salmonella typhi* in relation to its antigenic constituents, *J. Hyg.* **49**:92–110.

Felix, A., Krikorian, K. S., and Rietter, R., 1935, The occurrence of typhoid bacilli containing Vi antigen in cases of typhoid fever and of Vi antibody in their sera, *J. Hyg.* **35**:421–427.

Felix, A., Rainsford, S. G., and Stokes, E. J., 1941, Antibody response and systemic reactions after inoculation of a new type T.A.B.C. vaccine, *Br. Med. J.* **1**:435–440.

Ferguson, W. W., and June, R. C., 1952, Experiments on feeding adult volunteers with *Escherichia coli* III, B4, a coliform organism associated with infant diarrhea, *Am. J. Hyg.* **55**:155–169.

Field, M., Graf, L. H., Jr., Laird, W. J., and Smith, P. L., 1978, Heat-stable enterotoxin of *Escherichia coli: In vitro* effects on guanylate cyclase activity, cyclic GMP concentration and ion transport in small intestine, *Proc. Natl. Acad. Sci. USA* **75**:2800–2804.

Findlay, T. H., 1951, Mouse virulence of strains of *Sal-*

monella typhi from a mild and a severe outbreak of typhoid fever, *J. Hyg.* **49**:111–113.

Finkelstein, R. A., and LoSpalluto, J. J., 1969, Pathogenesis of experimental cholera: Preparation and isolation of choleragen and choleragenoid, *J. Exp. Med.* **130**:185–202.

Finkelstein, R. A., LaRue, M. K., Johnston, D. W., Vasil, M. L., Cho, G. J., and Jones, J. R., 1976, *J. Infect. Dis. Suppl.* **133**:S120–137.

Flexner, S., and Sweet, J. E., 1906, The pathogenesis of experimental colitis and the relation of colitis in animals and man, *J. Exp. Med.* **8**:514–535.

Flores, J., Grady, G. F., McIver, J., Witkum, P., Beckman, B., and Sharp, G. W. G., 1974, Comparison of the effects of enterotoxins of *Shigella dysenteriae* and *Vibrio cholerae* on the adenylate cyclase system, *J. Infect. Dis.* **130**:374–379.

Formal, S. B., Dammin, G. J., LaBrec, E. H., and Schneider, E. H., 1958, Experimental shigella infections: Characteristics of a fatal infection produced in guinea pigs, *J. Bacteriol.* **75**:604–610.

Formal, S. B., Dimmin, G. J., Schneider, H., and LaBrec, E. H., 1959, Experimental shigella infections. II. Characteristics of a fatal enteric infection in guinea pigs following the subcutaneous inoculation of carbon tetrachloride, *J. Bacteriol.* **78**:800–804.

Formal, S. B., Abrams, G. D., Schneider, H., and Sprinz, H., 1963, Experimental shigella infections. VI. Role of the small intestine in an experimental infection in guinea pigs, *J. Bacteriol.* **85**:119–125.

Formal, S. B., LaBrec, E. H., Kent, T. H., and Falkow, S., 1965a, Abortive intestinal infection with an *Escherichia coli–Shigella flexneri* hybrid strain, *J. Bacteriol.* **89**:1374–1382.

Formal, S. B., LaBrec, E. H., and Schneider, H., 1965b, Pathogenesis of bacillary dysentery in laboratory animals, *Fed. Proc.* **24**:29–34.

Formal, S. B., LaBrec, E. H., Palmer, A., and Falkow, S., 1965c, Protection of monkeys against experimental shigellosis with attenuated vaccines, *J. Bacteriol.* **90**:63–68.

Formal, S. B., Maenza, R. M., Austin, S., and LaBrec, E. H., 1967, Failure of parenteral vaccines to protect monkeys against experimental shigellosis, *Proc. Soc. Exp. Biol. Med.* **125**:347–349.

Formal, S. B., Gemski, P., Jr., Baron, L. S., and LaBrec, E. H., 1970, Genetic transfer of *Shigella flexneri* antigens to *Escherichia coli* K-12, *Infect. Immun.* **1**:279–287.

Formal, S. B., Gemski, P., Jr., Baron, L. S., and LaBrec, E. H., 1971a, A chromosomal locus which controls the ability of *Shigella flexneri* to evoke keratoconjunctivitis, *Infect. Immun.* **3**:73–79.

Formal, S. B., DuPont, H. L., Hornick, R. B., Snyder, M. J., Libonati, J. P., and LaBrec, E. H., 1971b, Experimental models in the investigation of the virulence of dysentery bacilli and *Escherichia coli*, *Ann. N.Y. Acad. Sci.* **176**:190–196.

Formal, S. B., LaBrec, E. H., Hornick, R. B., and Snyder, M. J., 1971c, Atenuation of strains of dysentery bacilli, presented at the International Symposium on Enterobacterial Vaccines, Berne, 1968, *Symp. Ser. Immunobiol. Standard.* **15**:73–78.

Fowler, J. E., Jr., and Stamey, T. A., 1977, Studies of introital colonization in women with recurrent urinary infections. VII. The role of bacterial adherence, *J. Urol.* **117**:472.

French, G. L., 1976, Enteropathogenic *E. coli*, *Lancet* **1**:1411–1412.

Freter, R., 1956, Experimental enteric shigella and vibrio infections in mice and guinea pigs, *J. Exp. Med.* **104**:411–418.

Freter, R., and Gangarosa, E. J., 1963, Oral Immunization and production of coproantibody in human volunteers, *J. Immunol.* **91**:724–729.

Fubara, E. S., and Freter, R., 1972, Availability of locally synthesized and systemic antibodies in the intestine, *Infect. Immun.* **6**:965–981.

Fubara, E. S., and Freter, R., 1973, Protection against enteric bacterial infection by secretory IgA antibodies, *J. Immunol.* **111**:395–403.

Gangarosa, E. J., and Merson, M. H., 1977, Epidemiologic assessment of the relevance of the so-called enteropathogenic serogroups of *Escherichia coli* in diarrhea, *N. Engl. J. Med.* **296**:1210–1213.

Gangarosa, E. J., Beisel, W. R., Benyajati, C., Spring, H., and Piyaratn, P., 1960, The nature of the gastrointestinal lesion in Asiatic cholera and its relation to pathogenesis, *Am. J. Trop. Med. Hyg.* **9**:125–135.

Gangarosa, E. J., Perera, D. R., Mata, L. J., Mendizabal-Morris, C. A., Guzman, G., and Reller, L. B., 1970, Epidemic Shiga bacillus dysentery in Central America. II. Epidemiologic studies in 1969, *J. Infect. Dis.* **122**:181–190.

Gemski, P., Jr., Takeuchi, A., Washington, O., and Formal, S. B., 1972, Shigellosis due to *Shigella dysenteriae*. I. Relative importance of mucosal invasion versus toxin production in pathogenesis, *J. Infect. Dis.* **126**:523–530.

Germanier, R., and Furer, E., 1975, Isolation and characterization of Gal E mutant Ty21a of *Salmonella typhi*: A candidate strain for a live, oral typhoid vaccine, *J. Infect. Dis.* **131**:553–558.

Giannella, R. A., Broitman, S. A., and Zamcheck, N., 1970, Salmonellosis: Relevance of reduced gastric acid secretion to severity of diarrhea and effects on the small bowel, *Gastroenterology* **60**:666.

Giannella, R. A., Broitman, S. A., and Zamcheck, N., 1971a, Salmonella enteritis. I. Role of reduced gastric secretion in pathogenesis, *Am. J. Digest. Dis.* **16**:1000–1006.

Giannella, R. A., Broitman, S. A., and Zamcheck, N., 1971b, Salmonella enteritis. II. Fulminant diarrhea in and effects on the small intestine, *Am. J. Digest. Dis.* **16**:1007–1013.

Giannella, R. A., Formal, S. B., Dammin, G. J., and Collins, H., 1973a, Pathogenesis of salmonellosis: Studies of fluid secretion, mucosal invasion, and morphologic reaction in the rabbit ileum, *J. Clin. Invest.* 52:441–453.

Giannella, R. A., Broitman, S. A., and Zamcheck, N., 1973b, Influence of gastric acidity on bacterial and parasitic enteric infections, *Ann. Intern. Med.* 78:271–276.

Giglioli, G., 1933a, Agglutinins for the typhoid-paratyphoid group in random sample of the population of British Guiana, *J. Hyg.* 33:379–386.

Giglioli, G., 1933b, Agglutinins found in the serum of subjects inoculated with typhoid-paratyphoid vaccine, *J. Hyg.* 33:387–395.

Giles, C., and Sangster, G., 1948, An outbreak of infantile gastroenteritis in Aberdeen: The association of a special type of *Bact. coli* with infection, *J. Hyg.* 46:1–9.

Gilman, R. H., Terminel, M., Levine, M. M., Hernandez-Mendoza, P., and Hornick, R. B., 1975, Comparison of the relative efficacy of blood, urine, rectal swab, bone marrow and rose spot cultures for recovery of *Salmonella typhi* in typhoid fever, *Lancet* 1:1211–1215.

Gilman, R. H., Hornick, R. B., Woodward, W. E., DuPont, H. L., Snyder, M. J., Levine, M. M., and Libonati, J. P., 1977, Immunity in typhoid fever: Evaluation of Ty21a—an epimeraseless mutant of *S. typhi* as a live oral vaccine, *J. Infect. Dis.* 136:717–723.

Gindrat, J.-J., Gothefors, L., Hanson, L., and Winberg, J., 1972, Antibodies in human milk against *E. coli* of the serogroups most commonly found in neonatal infections, *Acta Paediatr. Scand.* 61:587–590.

Girard, J. P., and de Kalbermatten, A., 1970, Antibody activity in human duodenal fluid, *Eur. J. Clin. Invest.* 1:188–195.

Gitelson, S., 1971, Gastrectomy, achlorhydria and cholera, *Israel J. Med. Sci.* 7:663–667.

Goldblum, R. M., Ahlstedt, S., Carlsson, B., Hanson, L. A., Jodal, U., Lidin-Janson, G., and Sohl-Akerlurd, A., 1975, Antibody-forming cells in human colostrum after oral immunisation, *Nature (London)* 257:797–798.

Goldschmidt, M. C., and DuPont, H. L., 1976, Enteropathogenic *Escherichia coli*: Lack of correlation of serotype with pathogenicity, *J. Infect. Dis.* 133:153–156.

Gorbach, S. L., 1971, Intestinal microflora, *Gastroenterology* 60:1110–1129.

Gorbach, S. L., and Khurana, C. M., 1972, Toxigenic *Escherichia coli.* A cause of infantile diarrhea in Chicago, *N. Engl. J. Med.* 287:791–795.

Gorbach, S. L., Banwell, J. G., Chatterjee, B. D., Jacobs, B., and Sack, R. B., 1971, Acute undifferentiated human diarrhea in the tropics. I. Alterations in the intestinal microflora, *J. Clin. Invest.* 50:881–889.

Gorbach, S. L., Kean, B. H., Evans, D. G., Evans, D. J., Jr., and Bessudo, D., 1975, Travelers' diarrhea and toxigenic *Escherichia coli, N. Eng. J. Med.* 292:933–936.

Gotoff, S. P., Lepper, M. H., and Fielder, M. A., 1963, Antibody response as an adjunct in the investigation of an outbreak of shigellosis, *Am. J. Hyg.* 78:261–268.

Gotze, O., and Muller-Eberhard, H. J., 1971, The C3-activator system: An alternative pathway of complement activation, *J. Exp. Med.* 134:90S–108S.

Gray, J. A., and Trueman, A. M., 1971, Severe salmonella gastroenteritis associated with hypochlorhydria, *Scot. Med. J.* 16:255–258.

Greisman, S., and Hornick, R. B., 1972, Cellular inflammatory responses of man to bacterial endotoxin: A comparison with PPD and other bacterial antigens, *J. Immunol.* 109:1210–1222.

Gross, R. J., Scotland, S. M., and Rowe, B., 1976, Enterotoxin testing of *Escherichia coli* causing epidemic infantile enteritis in the U.K., *Lancet,* 1:629–631.

Gross, R. J., Cravioto, A., Scotland, S. M., Cheasty, T., and Rowe, B., 1978, The occurrence of colonisation factor (CF) in enterotoxigenic *Escherichia coli, FEMS Microbiol. Lett.* 3:231–233.

Grunbaum, A. S., 1896a, Preliminary note on the use of the agglutinative action of human serum for the diagnosis of enteric fever, *Lancet* 2:806–807.

Grunbaum, A. S., 1896b, On the agglutinative action of human serum in its relation to the sero-diagnosis of enteric fever, *Lancet* 2:1747–1748.

Guerrant, R. L., Brunton, L. L., Schnaitman, T. C., Rebhun, L. I., and Gilman, A. G., 1974, Cyclic adenosine monophosphate and alteration of Chinese hamster ovary cell morphology: A rapid, sensitive *in vitro* assay for the enterotoxins of *Vibrio cholerae* and *Escherichia coli, Infect. Immun.* 10:320–327.

Guerrant, R. L., Moore, R. A., and Sande, M. A., 1975, Role of toxigenic and invasive bacteria in acute diarrhea of childhood, *N. Engl. J. Med.* 293:567–573.

Gurwith, M. J., Wiseman, D. A., and Chow, P., 1977, Clinical and laboratory assessment of the pathogenicity of serotyped enteropathogenic *Escherichia coli, J. Infect. Dis.* 135:736–743.

Gyles, C. L., 1971, Heat-labile and heat-stable forms of the enterotoxin from *E. coli* strains enteropathogenic for pig, *Ann. N.Y. Acad. Sci.* 176:314–322.

Gyles, C. L., 1974a, Immunological study of the heat-labile enterotoxins of *Escherichia coli* and *Vibrio cholerae, Infect. Immun.* 9:564–570.

Gyles, C., 1974b, Relationships among heat-labile enterotoxins of *Escherichia coli* and *Vibrio cholerae, J. Infect. Dis.* 129:277–283.

Gyles, C., So, M., and Falkow, S., 1974, The enterotoxin plasmids of *Escherichia coli, J. Infect. Dis.* 130:40–49.

Hardy, A. V., DeCapito, T., and Halbert, S. P., 1948, Studies of the acute diarrheal diseases. XIX. Immunization in shigellosis, *Publ. Health Rep.* 63:685–688.

Harris, J. C., DuPont, H. L., and Hornick, R. B., 1972, Fecal leukocytes in diarrheal illness, *Ann. Intern. Med.* 76:697–703.

Harrison, P., and Banvard, J., 1947, Coproantibody excretion during enteric infection, *Science* 106:188–189.

Hejfec, L. B., Salmin, L. V., Lehtman, M. Z., Kuzminova, M. L., Vasileva, A. V., Levina, L. A., Bencianova, T. G., Pavlova, E. A., and Antonova, A. A., 1966, A controlled field trial and laboratory study of five typhoid vaccines in the USSR, *Bull WHO* 34:321–329.

Hejfec, L. B., Levina, L. A., Kuzminova, M. L., Salmin,

L. V., Slavina, A. M., and Vasileva, A. V., 1968, Controlled field trials of paratyphoid B vaccine and the evaluation of the effectiveness of a single administration of typhoid vaccines, *Bull. WHO* **38**:907–915.

Hentges, D. J., 1967a, Inhibitor of *Shigella flexneri* by the normal intestinal flora. I. Mechanisms of inhibition by *Klebsiella, J. Bacteriol.* **93**:1369–1373.

Hentges, D. J., 1967b, Influence of pH on the inhibitory activity of formic and acetic acids for shigella, *J. Bacteriol.* **93**:2029–2030.

Hentges, D. J., 1969, Inhibition of *Shigella flexneri* by the normal intestinal flora. II. Mechanisms of inhibition by coliform organisms, *J. Bacteriol.* **97**:513–517.

Hentges, D. J., and Freter, R., 1962, *In vivo* and *in vitro* antagonism in intestinal bacteria against *Shigella flexneri.* I. Correlation between various tests, *J. Infect. Dis.* **110**:30–37.

Hentges, D., and Maier, B. R., 1970, Inhibition of Shigella flexneri by the normal intestinal flora. III. Interactions with *Bacteroides fragilis* strains *in vitro, Infect. Immun.* **2**:364–370.

Herzberg, M., Nash, P., and Hino, S., 1972, Degree of immunity induced by killed vaccines to experimental salmonellosis in mice, *Infect. Immun.* **5**:83–90.

Higgins, A. R., Floyd, T. M., and Kader, M. A., 1955, Studies in shigellosis. III. A controlled evaluation of a monovalent *Shigella* vaccine in a highly endemic environment, *Am. J. Trop. Med. Hyg.* **4**:281–288.

Hill, I. R., and Porter, P., 1974, Studies of bactericidal activity to *Escherichia coli* of porcine serum and colostral immunoglobulins and the role of lysozyme with secretory IgA, *Immunology* **26**:1239–1250.

Hohmann, A., and Wilson, M. R., 1975, Adherence of enteropathogenic *Escherichia coli* to intestinal epithelium *in vivo, Infect. Immun.* **12**:886–880.

Holmgren, J., 1973, Comparison of the tissue receptors for *Vibrio cholerae* and *Escherichia coli* enterotoxins by means of gangliosides and natural cholera toxoid, *Infect. Immun.* **8**:851–859.

Hone, R., Fitzpatrick, S., Keane, C., Gross, R. J., and Rowe, B., 1973, Infantile enteritis in Dublin caused by *Escherichia coli* O142, *J. Med. Microbiol.* **6**:505–510.

Horgan, E. S., 1932, Qualitative or quantitative methods in the serological diagnosis of enteric infections, *J. Hyg.* **32**:523–528.

Hornick, R. B., Greisman, S. E., Woodward, T. E., DuPont, H. L., Dawkins, A. T., and Snyder, M. J., 1970, Typhoid fever: Pathogenesis and immunologic control, *N. Engl. J. Med.* **283**:686–691, 739–746.

Hsu, H. S., and Mayo, D. R., 1973, Interactions between macrophages of guinea pigs and salmonellae. III. Bactericidal action and cytophilic antibodies of macrophages of infected guinea pigs, *Infect. Immun.* **8**:165–172.

Huckstep, R. L., 1962, *Typhoid Fever and Other Salmonella Infections,* E. and S. Livingstone, Edinburgh.

Hughes, J. M., Murad, F., Chang, B., and Guerrant, R. L., 1978, Role of cyclic GMP in the action of heat-stable enterotoxin of *Escherichia coli, Nature (London)* **271**:755–756.

Iida, K., Fujita, T., Inai, S., Sasaki, M., Kato, T., and Kobayashi, K., 1976, Complement fixing abilities of IgA myeloma proteins and their fragments: The activation of complement through the classical pathway, *Immunochemistry* **13**:747–752.

Isaacson, R. E., Nagy, B., and Moon, H. W., 1977, Colonization of porcine small intestine by *Escherichia coli*: Colonization and adhesion factors of pig enteropathogens that lack K88, *J. Infect. Dis.* **135**:531–539.

Isaacson, R. E., Fusco, P. C., Brinton, C. C., and Moon, H. W., 1978, *In vitro* adhesion of *Escherichia coli* to porcine small intestinal cells: Pili as adhesive factors, *Infect. Immun.* **21**:392–397.

Ishizaka, T., Ishizaka, K., Borsos, T., and Rapp, H., 1966, C′1 fixations by human isoagglutinins: Fixation of C′1 by gamma G and gamma M but not by gamma A antibody, *J. Immunol.* **97**:716–726.

Istrati, G., 1961, Recherches sur l'immunité active de l'homme dans la dysenterie bacillaire, *Arch. Roum. Pathol. Exp.* **20**:53–62.

Istrati, G., and Istrati, M., 1964, Vaccination antidysenterique, *Arch. Roum. Pathol. Exp. Microbiol.* **23**:289–298.

Istrati, G., Istrati, M., Meitert, T., and Ciufeco, C., 1963, Vaccination anti-dysenterique. Recherches experimentales sur l'homme et les animaux, *Arch. Roum. Pathol. Exp. Microbiol.* **22**:531–536.

Istrati, G., Meitert, T., and Ciufeco, C., 1965, Recherches sur l'immunité active de l'homme dans la dysenterie bacillaire, *Arch. Roum. Pathol. Exp. Microbiol.* **24**:677–686.

Istrati, G., Meitert, T., and Ciufecu, C., 1967a, Transformation von Shigellen in Stamme, die fuer den Menschen und fuer das meerschweinschenauge Apothogen sind, *Zbl. Bakteriol Abt. Orig.* **203**:295–299.

Istrati, G., Meitert, T., Ciufecu, C., Popescu, P., Antonescu, O., Georgescu, G., Grumberg, A., Mitroin, C., and Epure, G., 1967b, Beobachtungen Anlasslich der Verabreichung von Impfstoff aus lebender apathogener *Shigella flexneri* 2a an Kindern einer Schulergruppe, *Zbl. Bakteriol. Abt. Orig.* **204**:555–563.

Jenkin, C. R., and Rowley, D., 1963, Basis for immunity to typhoid in mice and the question of "cellular immunity," *Bacteriol. Rev.* **27**:391–404.

Jenkin, C. R., Rowley, D., and Auzins, L., 1964, The basis for immunity to mouse typhoid. 1. The carrier state, *Aust. J. Exp. Biol. Med.* **42**:215–228.

Jones, G. W., and Rutter, J. M., 1972, Role of the K88 antigen in the pathogenesis of neonatal diarrhea caused by *Escherichia coli* in piglets, *Infect. Immun.* **6**:918–927.

Jones, G. W., and Rutter, J. M., 1974a, Contribution of the K88 antigen of *Escherichia coli* to enteropathogenicity; protection against disease by neutralizing the adhesive properties of K88 antigen, *Am. J. Clin. Nutr.* **27**:1441–1449.

Jones, G. W., and Rutter, J. M. 1974b, The association

of K88 antigen with haemagglutinating activity in porcine strains of *Escherichia coli, J. Gen. Microbiol.* **84:**135–144.

Jóo, L., 1971, Present status and perspectives of vaccination against typhoid fever, from International Conference on the Application of Vaccines against Viral, Rickettsial, and Bacterial Diseases of Man, in: *PAHO Scientific Publication No. 226,* pp. 329–341, Washington, D.C.

June, R. C., Ferguson, W. W., and Worfer, M. T., 1953, Experiments in Feeding adult volunteers with *Escherichia coli* 55, B5, a coliform organism associated with infant diarrhea, *Am. J. Hyg.* **57:**222–236.

Kantor, H. S., Tao, P., and Wisdom, C., 1974a, Action of *Escherichia coli* enterotoxin: Adenylate cyclase behaviour of intestinal epithelial cells in culture, *Infect. Immun.* **9:**1003–1010.

Kantor, H. S., Tao, P., and Gorbach, S. L., 1974b, Stimulation of intestinal adenyl cyclase by *Escherichia coli* enterotoxin: Comparison of strains from an infant and an adult with diarrhea, *J. Infect. Dis.* **129:**1–9.

Kaplan, M. E., Dalmasso, A. P., and Woodson, M., 1972, Complement-dependent opsonization of incompatible erythrocytes of human secretory IgA, *J. Immunol.* **108:**275–278.

Kauffmann, F., 1947, The serology of the coli group, *J. Immunol.* **57:**71–100.

Kauffmann, F., Orskov, F., and Ewing, W. H., 1956, Designations for the K antigens of *Escherichia coli* serotypes, *Int. Bull. Bacteriol. Nomencl.* **6:**63–64.

Kent, T. H., Formal, S. B., and LaBrec, E. H., 1966a, Acute enteritis due to *Salmonella typhimurium* in opium-treated guinea pigs, *Arch. Pathol.* **81:**501–508.

Kent, T. H., Formal, S. B., and LaBrec, E. H., 1966b, Salmonella gastroenteritis in rhesus monkeys, *Arch. Pathol.* **82:**272–279.

Keusch, G. T., 1973, Pathogenesis of shigella diarrhea. III. Effects of shigella enterotoxin in cell culture, *Tr. N.Y. Acad. Sci.* **35:**51–58.

Keusch, G. T., and Donta, S. T., 1975, Classification of enterotoxins on the basis of activity in cell culture, *J. Infect. Dis.* **131:**58–63.

Keusch, G. T., and Jacewicz, M., 1973, Serum enterotoxin-neutralizing antibody in human shigellosis, *Nature (London), New Biol.* **241:**31–32.

Keusch, G. T., and Jacewicz, M., 1975, The pathogenesis of shigella diarrhea. V. Relationship of shiga enterotoxin, neurotoxin and cytotoxin, *J. Infect. Dis. Suppl.* **131:**522–540.

Keusch, G. T., Grady, G. F., Mata, L. J., and McIver, J., 1972a, The pathogenesis of shigella diarrhea. 1. Enterotoxin production by *Shigella dysenteriae* 1, *J. Clin. Invest.* **51:**1212–1218.

Keusch, G. T., Grady, G. F., Takeuchi, A., and Sprinz, H., 1972b, The pathogenesis of shigella diarrhea. II. Enterotoxin-induced acute enteritis in the rabbit ileum, *J. Infect. Dis.* **126:**92–95.

Keusch, G. T., Jacewicz, M., and Hirschman, S. Z., 1972c, Quantitative microassay in cell culture for enterotoxin of *Shigella dysenteriae* 1, *J. Infect. Dis.* **125:**539–541.

Keusch, G. T., Jacewicz, M., Levine, M. M., Hornick, R. B., and Kochwa, S., 1976, Pathogenesis of shigella diarrhea: Serum anticytotoxin antibody response produced by toxigenic and nontoxigenic *Shigella dysenteriae* 1, *J. Clin. Invest.* **57:**194–202.

Kirby, A. C., Hall, E. G., and Coackley, W., 1950, Neonatal diarrhoea and vomiting. Outbreaks in the same maternity unit, *Lancet* **2:**201–207.

Koupal, L. R., and Deibel, R. H., 1975, Assay, characterization and localization of an enterotoxin produced by salmonella, *Infect. Immun.* **11:**14–22.

Koya, G., Kosakai, N., Kono, M., Mori, M., and Fukasawa, Y., 1954, Observations on the multiplication of *Escherichia coli* O111:B4 in the intestinal tract of adult volunteers in feeding experiments, *Jpn. J. Med. Sci. Biol.* **7:**197–201.

Kubinyi, L., Kiss, I., and Lendvai, K. G., 1972, Epidemiological evaluation of the efficiency of oral vaccination against enteropathogenic *Escherichia coli, Acta Microbiol. Acad. Sci. Hung.* **19:**175–186.

Kubinyi, L., Kiss, I., and Lendvai, K. G., 1974, Epidemiological-statistical evaluation of oral vaccination against infantile *Escherichia coli* enteritis, *Acta Microbiol. Acad. Sci. Hung.* **21:**187–191.

LaBrec, E. H., and Formal, S. B., 1961, Experimental shigella infections. IV. Fluorescent antibody studies of an infection in guinea pigs, *J. Immunol.* **87:**562–572.

LaBrec, E. H., Schneider, H., Magnani, T. J., and Formal, S. B., 1964, Epithelial cell penetration as an essential step in the pathogenesis of bacillary dysentery, *J. Bacteriol.* **88:**1503–1518.

Landy, M., 1954, Studies on Vi antigen. VI. Immunization of human beings with purified Vi antigen, *Am. J. Hyg.* **60:**52–62.

Landy, M., and Lamb, E., 1953, Estimation of Vi antibody employing erythrocytes treated with purified Vi antigen, *Proc. Soc. Exp. Biol. Med.* **82:**593–598.

Landy, M., Trapani, R. J., Webster, M. E., and Jarvis, F. G., 1963, Immunological properties of Vi antigen isolated by chemical fractionation and by electrophosesis, *Tex. Rep. Biol. Med.* **21:**214–229.

Lariviere, S., Gyles, C. L., and Barnum, D. A., 1973, Preliminary characterization of the heat-labile enterotoxin of *Escherichia coli* FII (P155), *J. Infect. Dis.* **128:**312–320.

Lee, M. R., Ikari, N. S., Branche, W. C., Jr., and Young, V. M., 1966, Microtiter bacterial hemagglutination technique for detection of shigella antibodies, *J. Bacteriol.* **91:**463.

Levin, D. M., Wong, K. H., Reynolds, H. V., Sutton, A., and Northrup, R. S., 1975, Vi antigen From *Salmonella typhosa* and immunity against typhoid fever. II. Safety and immunogenicity in humans, *Infect. Immun.* **12:**1290–1294.

Levine, M. M., 1974, Epidemiologic and sero-epidemiologic methods in evaluation of the endemicity of typhoid fever in Peru, D.T.P.H. thesis, University of London.

Levine, M. M., and Daya, V., 1978, Hemagglutination, pili, and diarrheagenic potential of *Escherichia coli* strains in man, 18th Interscience Conference on Antimicrobial Agents and Chemotherapy, Atlanta, October.

Levine, M. M., and Hornick, R. B., 1975, Lactulose therapy in shigella carrier state and acute dysentery, *Antimicrob. Agents Chemother.* 8:581–584.

Levine, M. M., DuPont, H. L., Gangarosa, E. J., Hornick, R. B., Snyder, M. J., Libonati, J. P., Glaser, K., and Formal, S. B., 1972, Shigellosis in custodial institutions. II. Clinical, immunologic and bacteriologic response of institutionalized children to oral attenuated shigella vaccines, *Am. J. Epidemiol.* 96:40–49.

Levine, M. M., DuPont, H. L., Formal, S. B., Hornick, R. B., Takeuchi, A., Gangarosa, E. J., Snyder, M. J., and Libonati, J. P., 1973a, Pathogenesis of *Shigella dysenteriae* 1 (Shiga) dysentery, *J. Infect. Dis.* 127:261–270.

Levine, M. M., DuPont, H. L., Khodabandelou, M., and Hornick, R. B., 1973b, Long-term shigella carrier state, *N. Engl. J. Med.* 288:1169–1171.

Levine, M. M., Rice, P. A., Gangarosa, E. J., Morris, G. K., Snyder, M. J., Formal, S. B., Wells, J. G., Gemski, P., Jr., and Hammond, J., 1973c, An outbreak of sonne shigellosis in a population receiving oral attenuated shigella vaccines, *Am. J. Epidemiol.* 99:30–36.

Levine, M. M., Gangarosa, E. J., Werner, M., and Morris, G. K., 1974a, Shigellosis in custodial institutions. III. Prospective clinical and bacteriologic surveillance of children vaccinated with oral attenuated shigella vaccines, *J. Pediatr.* 84:803–806.

Levine, M. M., DuPont, H. L., Formal, S. B., Hornick, R. B., Gangarosa, E. J., Snyder, M. J., and Libonati, J. P., 1974b, Vacuna de *Shigella dysenteriae*-1 (Shiga): Simposio sobre Disenteria Shiga en Centro America, in: *PAHO Scientific Publication No. 283,* pp. 142–145, Washington, D.C.

Levine, M. M., Gangarosa, E. J., Barrow, W. B., Morris, G. K., Wells, J. G., and Weiss, C. F., 1975, Shigellosis in custodial institutions. IV. *In vivo* stability and transmissibility of oral attenuated streptomycin-dependent shigella vaccines, *J. Infect. Dis.* 131:704–707.

Levine, M. M., DuPont, H. L. Hornick, R. B., Snyder, M. J., Woodward, W., Gilman, R. H., and Libonati, J. P., 1976a, Attenuated streptomycin-dependent *Salmonella typhi* oral vaccine: Potential deleterious effects of lyophilization, *J. Infect. Dis.* 133:424–428.

Levine, M. M., Gangarosa, E. J., Barrow, W. B., and Weiss, C. F., 1976b, Shigellosis in custodial institutions. V. Effect of intervention with streptomycin-dependent *Shigella sonnei* vaccine in an institution with endemic disease, *Am. J. Epidemiol.* 104:88–92.

Levine, M. M., Woodward, W. E., Formal, S. B., Gemski, P., Jr., DuPont, H. L., Hornick, R. B., and Snyder, M. J., 1977a, Studies with a new generation of oral attenuated shigella vaccine: *Escherichia coli* bearing surface antigens of *Shigella flexneri, J. Infect. Dis.* 136:577–582.

Levine, M. M., Caplan, E. S., Waterman, D., Cash, R. A., Hornick, R. B., and Snyder, M. M., 1977b, Diarrhea caused by *Escherichia coli* that produce only heat-stable enterotoxin, *Infect. Immun.* 17:78–82.

Levine, M. M., Bergquist, E. J., Nalin, D. R., Waterman, D. H., Hornick, R. B., Young, C. R., and Sotman, S., 1978a, *Escherichia coli* strains that cause diarrhea but do not produce heat-labile or heat-stable enterotoxins and are non-invasive, *Lancet* 1:1119–1122.

Levine, M. M., Grados, O., Gilman, R. H., Woodward, W. E., Solis-Plaza, R., and Waldman, W., 1978b, Diagnostic value of the widal test in areas endemic for typhoid fever, *Am. J. Trop. Med. Hyg.* 27:795–800.

Levine, M. M., Nalin, D. R., Hoover, D. L., Bergquist, E. J., Hornick, R. B., and Young, C. R., 1979, Immunity to enterotoxigenic *Escherichia coli, Infect. Immun.* 23:729–736.

McClelland, D. B. L., Samson, R. R., Parkin, D. M., and Shearman, D. J. C., 1972, Bacterial agglutination studies with secretory IgA prepared from human gastrointestinal secretions and colostrum, *Gut* 13:450–458.

MacKaness, G. B., Blanden, R. V., and Collins, F. M., 1966, Host–parasite relations in mouse typhoid, *J. Exp. Med.* 124:573–583.

Mackel, D. C., Langley, L. F., and Venice, L. A., 1961, The use of the guinea pig conjunctivae as an experimental model for the study of virulence of shigella organisms, *Am. J. Hyg.* 73:219–223.

Mackenzie, E. F. W., and Windle Tayler, E., 1945, A study of the Vi agglutination test for the detection of typhoid carriers, *J. Hyg.* 44:31–36

McIver, J., Grady, G., and Keusch, G. T., 1975, Production and characterization of exotoxins(s) of *Shigella dysenteriae* type I, *J. Infect. Dis.* 131:559–566.

McIver, J., Grady, G. F., and Formal, S. B., 1977, Immunization with *Shigella dysenteriae* type I: Evaluation of antitoxic immunity in prevention of experimental disease in rhesus monkeys *(Macaca mulatta), J. Infect. Dis.* 136:416–421.

Mata, L. J., Gangarosa, E. J., Caceres, A., Perera, D. R., and Mejicanos, M. L., 1970, Epidemic Shiga bacillus dysentery in Central America. 1. Etiologic investigations in Guatemala, 1969, *J. Infect. Dis.* 122:170–180.

Meitert, T., Istrati, G., Sulea, I. T., Baron, E., Andronescu, C., Gogulescu, L., Templea, C., Ianopol, L., Galan, L., Fleseriu, M., Onciu, C., Bogos, L., Lupovici, R., Boghitoiu, A., Ohmt, E., Popescu, G., Mihailiuc, I., Maffei, S., Tapu, T., and Zebreniuc, D., 1973, Prophylaxie de la dysenterie bacillaire par le vaccin vivant antidysenterique dans une collectivité d'enfants neuropsychiques, *Arch. Roum. Pathol. Exp. Microbiol.* 32:35–44.

Mel, D. M., Papo, R. G., Terzin, A. L., and Vuksic, L., 1965a, Studies on vaccination against bacillary dysentery. II. Safety tests and reactogenicity studies on a live dysentery vaccine intended for use in field trials, *Bull. WHO* 32:637–645.

Mel, D. M., Terzin, A. L., and Vuksic, L., 1965b, Studies on vaccination against bacillary dysentery. III. Effective oral immunization against *Shigella flexneri* 2a in a field trial, *Bull. WHO* 32:647–655.

Mel, D. M., Arsic, B. L., Nikolic, B. D., and Radovanovic, M. L., 1968, Studies on vaccination against bacillary dysentery. IV. Oral immunization with live mon-
otypic and combined vaccines, *Bull. WHO* 39:375–380.

Mel, D. M., Gangarosa, E. J., and Radovanovic, M. D.,
1971, Studies on vaccination against bacillary dysentery. VI. Protection of children by oral immunization
with streptomycin-dependent shigella strains, *Bull. WHO*
45:457–464.

Mel, D. M., Arsic, B. L., Radovanovic, M. L., and Litvinjenko, S. A., 1974a, Live oral shigella vaccine: Vaccination schedule and the effect of booster dose, *Acta
Microbiol. Acad. Sci. Hung.* 21:109–114.

Mel, D. M., Arsic, B. L., Radovanovic, M. L., Kaljolovic,
R., and Litvinjenko, S., 1974b, Safety tests in adults
and children with live oral typhoid vaccine, *Acta Microbiol. Acad. Sci. Hung.* 21:161–166.

Mendizabal-Morris, C. A., Mata, L. J., Gangarosa, E. J.,
and Guzman, G., 1971, Epidemic Shiga bacillus dysentery in Central America: Derivation of the epidemic
and its progression in Guatemala, 1968–69, *Am. J. Med.
Hyg.* 20:927–933.

Merson, M. H., Goldman, D. A., Boyer, K. M., Peterson,
N. J., Patton, C., Everett, L. G., Downs, H., Steckler,
A., and Barker, W. H., Jr., 1974, An outbreak of *Shi-
gella sonnei* gastroenteritis on Colorado River raft trips,
Am. J. Epidemiol. 100:186–196.

Merson, M. H., Morris, G. K., Sack, D. A., Wells, J. G.,
Feeley, J. C., Sack, R. B., Creech, W. B., Kapikian,
A. Z., and Gangarosa, E. J., 1976, Travelers diarrhea
in Mexico: A prospective study of physicans and family
members attending a congress, *N. Engl. J. Med.*
294:1299–1305.

Miller, R. M., Garbus, J., and Hornick, R. B., 1972, Lack
of enhanced oxygen consumption by polymorphonuclear leukocytes on phagocytosis of virulent *Salmonella
typhi, Science* 175:1010–1011.

Mochmann, H., Ocklitz, H. W., Weh, L., and Heinrich,
H., 1974, Oral Immunization with an extract of *Esch-
erichia coli* enteritidis, *Acta. Microbiol. Acad. Sci.
Hung.* 21:193–196.

Moon, H. W., Nagy, B., and Isaccson, R. E., 1977, Intestinal colonization and adhesion by enterotoxigenic
Escherichia coli: Ultrastructural observations on adherence of ileal epithelium of the pig, *J. Infect. Dis.
Suppl.* 136:S124–129.

Morgan, R. L., Isaacson, R. E., Brinton, C. C., and Moon,
H. W., 1978, Immunization of suckling pigs against enteric enterotoxigenic *Escherichia coli* infection by vaccinating dams with purified pili, *Infect. Immun.*

Mujibur Rahaman, M., Moslemuddin Khan, M., Aziz, K.
M. S., Shafiqul Islam, M., and Golam Kibriya, K. M.,
1975, An outbreak of dysentery caused by *Shigella dysenteriae* type I on a Coral Island in the Bay of Bengal,
J. Infect. Dis. 132:15–19.

Mullan, N. A., Burgess, M. N., and Newsome, P. M.,
1978, Characterization of a partially purified, methanol-
soluble heat-stable *Escherichia coli* enterotoxin in infant
mice, *Infect. Immun.* 19:779–784.

Nagy, B., Moon, H. W., and Isaacson, R. E., 1977, Colonization of porcine intestine by enterotoxigenic *Escherichia coli*: Selection of piliated forms *in vivo*, adhesion
of piliated forms to epithelial cells *in vitro*, and incidence
of a pilus antigen among porcine enteropathogenic *E.
coli, Infect. Immun.* 16:344–352.

Nagy, B., Moon, H. W., Isaacson, R. E., To, C. C., and
Brinton, C. C., 1978, Immunization of suckling pigs
against enteric enterotoxigenic *Escherichia coli* infection by vaccinating dams with purified pili, *Infect.
Immun.* 21:269–274.

Nakamura, M., 1972, Alteration of shigella pathogenicity
by other bacteria, *Am. J. Clin. Nutr.* 25:1441–1451.

Nalin, D. R., Al-Mahmud, A., Curlin, G., Ahmed, A., and
Peterson, J., 1974a, Cholera toxoid boosts serum *Escherichia coli* antitoxin in humans, *Infect. Immun.*
10:747–749.

Nalin, D. R., Bhattacharjee, A. K., and Richardson, S.
H., 1974b, Cholera-like toxic effect of culture filtrates
of *Escherichia coli, J. Infect. Dis.* 130:595–601.

Neter, E., 1959, Enteritis due to enteropathogenic *Escherichia coli, J. Pediatr.* 55:223–239.

Neter, E., 1962, Epidemiologic and immunologic studies
of *Shigella sonnei* dysentery, *Am. J. Publ. Hlth.*
52:61–67.

Neter, E., and Dunphy, D., 1957, The duration of the
hemagglutination response in the serum of children with
shigellosis and salmonellosis, *Pediatrics* 20:78–86.

Neter, E., and Shumway, C. N., 1950, *E. coli* serotype
D433: Occurrence in intestinal and respiratory tracts,
cultural characteristics, pathogenicity, sensitivity to antibiotics, *Proc. Soc. Exp. Biol. Med.* 75:504–507.

Neter, E., and Walker, J., 1954, Hemagglutination test for
specific antibodies in dysentery caused by *Shigella sonnei, Am. J. Clin. Pathol.* 24:1424–1429.

Neter, E., Korns, R. F., and Trussell, R. E., 1953, Association of *Escherichia coli* serogroup O III with two
hospital outbreaks of epidemic diarrhea of the newborn
infant in New York during 1947, *Pediatrics* 12:377–383.

Neter, E., Westphal, O., Luderitz, O., Gino, R. M., and
Gorzynski, E. A., 1955, Demonstration of antibodies
against enteropathogenic *Escherichia coli* in sera of children of various ages, *Pediatrics* 16:801–808.

North, R. J., 1975, Nature of "memory" in T-cell-mediated antibacterial immunity: Anamnestic production
of mediator T Cells, *Infect. Immun.* 12:754–760.

North, R. J., and Deissler, J. F., 1975, Nature of "memory" in T-cell-mediated antibacterial immunity: Cellular
parameters that distinguish between the active immune
response and a state of "memory," *Infect. Immun.*
12:761–767.

O'Brien, A. D., Thompson, M. R., Cantey, J. R., and
Formal, S. B., 1977a, Production of a *Shigella dysen-
teriae*-like toxin by pathogenic *Escherichia coli*, Pro-
gram and Abstracts of the 77th Annual Meeting of the
American Society of Microbiology, May 1977, New
Orleans, Abstr. No. B103.

O'Brien, A. D., Thompson, M. R., Gemski, P., Doctor,
B. P., and Formal, S. B., 1977b, Biological properties

of *Shigella flexneri* 2a toxin and its serological relationship to *Shigella dysenteriae* 1 toxin, *Infect. Immun.* 15:796–798.

Ofek, I., Mirelman, D., and Sharon, N., 1977, Adherence of *Escherichia coli* to human mucosal cells mediated by mannose receptors, *Nature (London)* 265:623–625.

Ogawa, H., Nakamura, A., and Sakazaki, R., 1968, Pathogenic properties of "enteropathogenic" *Escherichia coli* from diarrheal children and adults, *Jpn. J. Med. Sci. Biol.* 21:333–349.

Ogra, P. L., and Karzon, D. J., 1969, Distribution of poliovirus antibody in serum, nasopharynx, and alimentary tract following segmental immunization of lower alimentary tract with poliovaccine, *J. Immunol.* 102:1423–1430.

Ogra, P. L., Karzon, D. T., Righthand, F., and MacGillivray, M., 1968, Immunoglobulin response in serum and secretions after immunization with live and inactivated poliovaccine and natural infection, *N. Engl. J. Med.* 279:893–900.

Olarte, J., and Ramos-Alvarez, M., 1965, Epidemic diarrhea in premature infants: Etiological significance of a newly recognized type of *Escherichia coli* (O142:K86 [B]:H6), *Am. J. Dis. Child.* 109:436–438.

Olitsky, P. K., and Kligler, I. J., 1920, Toxins and antitoxins of *Bacillus dysenteriae shiga*, *J. Exp. Med.* 31:19–33.

Olitzki, A., 1972, *Enteric Fevers—Causing Organisms and Host's Reactions*, Karger, Basel.

Ornellas, E. P., Roantree, R. J., and Steward, J. P., 1970, The specificity and importance of humoral antibody in the protection of mice against intraperitoneal challenge with complement-sensitive and complement-resistant salmonella, *J. Infect. Dis.* 121:113–123.

Orskov, F., Orskov, I., Rees, T. A., and Sahab, K., 1960, Two New *E. coli* O antigens: 0141 and 0142 and two new coli K-antigens: K85 and K86. *Acta Pathol. Microbiol. Scand.* 48:48–50.

Orskov, F., Orskov, I., Jann, B., and Jann, K., 1971, Immunoelectrophoretic patterns of extracts from all *Escherichia coli* O and K antigen test strains: Correlation with pathogenicity, *Acta Pathol. Microbiol. Scand.* 79B:142–152.

Orskov, F., Orskov, I., and Furowicz, A. J., 1972, Four new *Escherichia coli* O antigens, 0148, 0151, 0152, 0153 and one new H antigen, H50, found in strains isolated from enteric diseases in man, *Acta Path. Microbiol. Scand.* 80B:435–440.

Orskov, F., Orskov, I., Evans, D. J., Jr., Sack, R. B., Sack, D. A., and Waldstrom, T., 1976, Special *Escherichia coli* serotypes among enterotoxigenic strains from diarrhoea in adults and children, *Med. Microbiol. Immunol.* 162:73–80.

Orskov, I., and Orskov, F., 1966, Episome carried K88 surface antigen of *Escherichia coli*. I. Transmission of the determinent of the K88 antigen and the influences on the transfer of chromosomal markers, *J. Bacteriol.* 91:69–75.

Orskov, I., and Orskov, F., 1977, Special O:K:H serotypes among enterotoxigenic *E. coli* strains from diarrhea in adults and children: Occurrence of the CF (colonization factor antigen and of haemagglutinating abilities), *Med. Microbiol. Immunol.* 163:99–110.

Orskov, I., Orskov, F., Sojka, W. J., and Wittig, W., 1964, K antigens K88ab (L) and K88ac (L) in *E. coli*. A new O antigen: 0141 and a new K antigen: K88 (B), *Acta Pathol. Microbiol. Scand.* 62:439–447.

Orskov, I., Orskov, F., Smith, H. W., and Sojka, W. J., 1975, The establishment of K99, a thermolabile, transmissible *Escherichia coli* K antigen, previously called "Kco," possessed by calf and lamb enteropathogenic strains, *Acta Path. Microbiol. Scand. Sect. B* 83:31–36.

Peller, S., 1928, Typhoid fever in Palestine, *J. Hyg.* 28:318–323.

Pierce, N. F., 1973, Differential inhibitory effects of cholera toxoids and ganglioside on the enterotoxins of *Vibrio cholerae* and *Escherichia coli*, *J. Exp. Med.* 137:1009–1023.

Plaut, A. G., and Keonil, P., 1969, Immunoglobulins in human small intestinal fluid, *Gastroenterology* 56:522–530.

Polish Typhoid Committee, 1965, evaluation of typhoid vaccines in the laboratory and in a controlled field trial in Poland, *Bull. WHO* 32:15–27.

Porter, P., Kenworthy, R., Noakes, D. E., and Allen, W. D., 1974, Intestinal antibody secretion in the young pig in response to oral immunization with *Escherichia coli*, *Immunology* 27:841–853.

Powell, D. W., Plotkin, G. R., and Maenza, R. M., 1971, Experimental diarrhea. I. Intestinal water and electrolyte transport in rat salmonella enterocolitis, *Gastroenterology* 60:1053–1064.

Public Health Laboratory Service Working Party, 1961, The detection of the typhoid carrier state, *J. Hyg.* 59:231–247.

Quie, P. G., Messner, R. P., and Williams, R. C., 1968, Phagocytosis in subacute bacterial endocarditis: Localization of the primary opsonic site to Fc fragment, *J. Exp. Med.* 128:553–570.

Raska, K., and Raskova, H., 1976, Recognizing epidemic strains of *E. coli*, *Lancet* 1:1300.

Rauss, K., Ketyi, I., Matusovits, E., Szendrai, L., Vertenyi, A., and Varbiro, B., 1972, Specific oral prevention of infantile enteritis. III. Experiments with corpuscular vaccine, *Acta Microbiol. Acad. Sci. Hung.* 19:19–28.

Rauss, K., Ketyi, I., Szendrei, L., and Vertenyi, A., 1974, Immunization of infants against *Escherichia coli* enteritis, *Acta Microbiol. Acad Sci. Hung.* 21:181–185.

Reed, W. P., and Cushing, A. H., 1975, Role of immunoglobulins in protection against shigella-induced keratoconjunctivitis, *Infect. Immun.* 2:1265–1268.

Reed, W. P., and Williams, R. C., Jr., 1971, Intestinal immunoglobulins in shigellosis, *Gastroenterology* 61:35–45.

Reitman, M., 1967, Infectivity and antigenicity at streptomycin-dependent salmonella typhosa, *J. Infect. Dis.* 117:101–107.

Reitman, M., and Iverson, W. P., 1953, The immunizing properties of dihydrostreptomycin-dependent *Salmonella typhosa*, *Antibiot. Ann.*, pp. 604–608.

Reller, L. B., Navarro Rivas, E., Masferrer, R., Bloch, M., and Gangarosa, E. J., 1971, Epidemic Shiga-bacillus dysentery in Central America: Evaluation of the outbreak in El Salvador, 1969–70, *Am. J. Trop. Med. Hyg.* **20**:934–940.

Reynolds, D. W., Carpenter, L., and Simon, W. H., 1970, Diagnostic specificity of Widal's reaction for typhoid fever, *JAMA* **214**:2192–2193.

Rhame, F. S., Root, R. K., MacLowry, J. D., Dadisman, T. A., and Bennett, J. V., 1973, Salmonella septicemia from platelet transfusions: Study of an outbreak traced to a hematogenous carrier of *Salmonella cholerasuis*, *Ann. Intern. Med.* **78**:633–641.

Robbins, J. B., McCracken, G. H., Jr., Gotschlich, E. C., Orskov, F., Oskov, I., and Hanson, L. A., 1974, *Escherichia coli* KI capsular polysaccharide associated with neonatal meningitis, *N. Engl. J. Med.* **290**:1216–1220.

Rout, W. R., Formal, S. B., Dammin, G. J., and Giannella, R. A., 1974, Pathophysiology of salmonella diarrhea in the rhesus monkey: Intestinal transport, morphological and bacteriological studies, *Gastroenterology* **67**:59–70.

Rowe, B., Taylor, J., and Bettelheim, K. A., 1970, An investigation of travellers' diarrhea, *Lancet* **1**:1–5.

Rowe, B., Gross, R. J., and Scotland, S. M., 1976, Serotypeing of *E. coli*, *Lancet* **2**:37–38.

Rowe, B., Scotland, S. M., and Gross, R. J., 1977, Enterotoxigenic *Escherichia coli* causing infantile enteritis in Britain, *Lancet* **1**:90–91.

Rowley, D., Turner, K. J., and Jenkin, C. R., 1964, The basis for immunity to mouse typhoid. III. Cell-bound antibody, *Austr. J. Exp. Biol. Med.* **42**:237–248.

Rutter, J. M., and Jones, G. W., 1973, Protection against enteric disease caused by *Escherichia coli*—A model for vaccination with a virulence determinant, *Nature (London)* **242**:531–532.

Rutter, J. M., Burrows, M. R., Sellwood, R., and Gibbons, R. A., 1975, A genetic basis for resistance to enteric disease caused by *E. coli*, *Nature (London)* **257**:135–136.

Ryder, R. W., Wachsmuth, I. K., Buxton, A. E., Evans, D. G., DuPont, H. L., Mason, E., and Barrett, F. F., 1976, Infantile diarrhea produced by heat-stable enterotoxigenic *Escherichia coli*, *N. Engl. J. Med.* **295**:849–853.

Sack, D. A., and Sack, R. B., 1975, Test for enterotoxigenic *Escherichia coli* using Yl adrenal cells in miniculture, *Infect. Immun.* **2**:334–336.

Sack, D. A., Merson, M. H., Wells, J. G., Sack, R. B., and Morris, G. K., 1975, Diarrhea associated with heat-stable enterotoxin-producing strains of *Escherichia coli*, *Lancet* **2**:239–241.

Sack, D. A., McLaughlin, J. C., Sack, R. B., Orskov, F., and Orskov, I., 1977, Enterotoxigenic *Escherichia coli* isolated from patients at a hospital in Dacca, *J. Infect. Dis.* **135**:275–280.

Sack, G. H., Jr., Pierce, N. F., Hennessey, K. N., Mitra, R. C., Sack, R. B., and Guha Mazumler, D. N., 1972, Gastric acidity in cholera and non-cholera diarrhea, *Bull. WHO* **47**:31–36.

Sack, R. B., 1973, Immunization with *Escherichia coli* enterotoxin protects against homologous enterotoxin challenge, *Infect. Immun.* **8**:641–644.

Sack, R. B., 1975, Human diarrheal disease caused by enterotoxigenic *Escherichia coli*, *Ann. Rev. Microbiol.* **29**:333–353.

Sack, R. B., 1976a, Serotyping of *E. coli*, *Lancet* **1**:1132.

Sack, R. B., 1976b, Enterotoxigenic *Escherichia coli*—An emerging pathogen, *N. Engl. J. Med.* **295**:893–895.

Sack, R. B., Gorbach, S. L., Banwell, J. G., Jacobs, B., Chatterjee, B. D., and Mitra, R. C., 1971, Enterotoxigenic *Escherichia coli* isolated from patients with severe cholera-like disease, *J. Infect. Dis.* **123**:378–385.

Sack, R. B., Jacobs, B., and Mitra, R., 1974, Antitoxin responses to infections with enterotoxigenic *Escherichia coli*, *J. Infect. Dis.*, **129**:330–335.

Sack, R. B., Hirschhorn, N., Brownlee, I., Cash, R. A., Woodward, W. E., and Sack, D. A., 1975a, Enterotoxigenic *Escherichia coli*-associated diarrheal disease in Apache children, *N. Engl. J. Med.* **292**:1041–1045.

Sack, R. B., Hirschhorn, N., Brownlee, I., Cash, R. A., Woodward, W. E., Sack, D. A., and Cash, R. A., 1975b, Antibodies to heat-labile *Escherichia coli* enterotoxin in Apaches in Whiteriver, Arizona, *Infect. Immun.* **12**:1475–1477.

Sakazaki, R., Tamura, K., and Saito, M., 1967, Enteropathogenic *Escherichia coli* associated with diarrhea in children and adults, *Jpn. J. Med. Sci. Biol.* **20**:387–399.

Salit, I. E., and Gotschlich, E. C., 1977, Type 1 *Escherichia coli* pili: Characterization of binding to monkey kidney cells, *J. Exp. Med.* **146**:1182–1194.

Sandefur, P. D., and Peterson, J. W., 1976, Isolation of skin permeability factors from culture filtrate of *Salmonella typhimurium*, *Infect. Immun.* **14**:671–679.

Sandefur, P. D., and Peterson, J. W., 1977, Neutralization of salmonella toxin-induced elongation of chinese hamster ovary cells by cholera antitoxin, *Infect. Immun.* **15**:988–992.

Sansone, P., Saslaw, M. S., and Hennekens, C. H., Jr., 1972, High titer Widal reaction, *JAMA* **220**:1615–1616.

Schneider, H., and Formal, S. B., 1963, Spontaneous loss of guinea pig virulence in a strain of *Shigella flexneri* 2a, *Bacteriol. Proc.*, p. 66.

Schubert, J. H., Edwards, P. R., and Ramsey, C. H., 1959, Detection of typhoid carriers by agglutination tests, *J. Bacteriol.* **77**:648–654.

Sellwood, R., Gibbons, R. A., Jones, G. W., and Rutter, J. M., 1975, Adhesion of enteropathogenic *Escherichia coli* to pig intestinal brush borders: The existence of two Pig phenotypes, *J. Med. Microbiol.* **8**:405–411.

Sereny, B., 1957, Experimental keratoconjunctivitis shigellosa, *Acta Microbiol. Hung.* **4**:368–376.

Shaughnessy, H. J., Olsson, R. C., Bass, K., Friewer, F., and Levinson, S. O., 1946, Experimental human baccillary dysentery: Polyvalent dysentery vaccine in its prevention, *JAMA* **132:**352–368.

Shedlofsky, S., and Freter, R., 1974, Synergism between ecologic and immunologic control mechanisms of intestinal flora, *J. Infect. Dis.* **129:**296–303.

Shiga, K., 1898, Ueber den Erreger der Dysenterie in Japan, *Zentrabl. Bakteriol. Abt. I* **23:**599–600.

Shiga, K., 1906, Observations on the epidemiology of dysentery in Japan, *Phil. J. Sci.* **1:**485–500.

Shiga, K., 1936, The trend of prevention, therapy and epidemiology of dysentery since the discovery of its causative organism, *N. Engl. J. Med.* **215:**1205–1211.

Shore, E. G., Dean, A. G., Holik, K. J., and Davis, B. R., 1974, Enterotoxin-producing *Escherichia coli* and diarrheal disease in adult travelers: A prospective study, *J. Infect. Dis.* **129:**577–582.

Skerman, F. J., Formal, S. B., and Falkow, S., 1972, Plasmid-associated enterotoxin production in a strain of *Escherichia coli* isolated from humans, *Infect. Immun.* **5:**622–624.

Smith, H. W., 1974, A search for transmissible pathogenic characters in invasive strains of *Escherichia coli*: The discovery of a plasmid controlled lethal character closely associated, or identical, with colicine V, *J. Gen. Microbiol.* **83:**95–111.

Smith, H. W., and Halls, S., 1967, Studies on *Escherichia coli* enterotoxin, *J. Pathol. Bacteriol.* **93:**531–543.

Smith, H. W., and Linggood, M. A., 1971a, The transmissible nature of enterotoxin production in a human enteropathogenic strain of *Escherichia coli, J. Med. Microbiol.* **4:**301–305.

Smith, H. W., and Linggood, M. A., 1971b, Observation on the pathogenic properties of the K88, Hly, and Ent plasmids of *Escherichia coli* with particular reference to porcine diarrhea, *Med. Microbiol.* **4:**467–485.

Smith, H. W., and Linggood, M. A., 1972, Further observations on *Escherichia coli* enterotoxins with particular regard to those produced by atypical piglet strains and by calf and lamb strains: The transmissible nature of these enterotoxins and of a K antigen possessed by calf and lamb strains, *J. Med. Microbiol.* **5:**243–250.

Smith, H. W., and Sack, R. B., 1973, Immunologic cross-reactions of enterotoxins from *Escherichia coli* and *Vibrio cholerae, J. Infect. Dis.* **127:**164–170.

Soni, S. D., and Rajapaksa, T. J., 1973, Cholera-like illness in salmonellosis, *Lancet* **1:**1006.

South, M. A., 1971, Enteropathogenic *Escherichia coli* disease: New developments and perspectives, *J. Pediatr.* **79:**I–II.

South, M. A., Cooper, M. D., Wollheim, F. A., Hong, R., and Good, R. A., 1966, The IgA system. I. Studies of the transport and immunochemistry of IgA in the saliva, *J. Exp. Med.* **123:**615–627.

Speirs, J. I., Stavric, S., and Konowalchuk, J., 1977, Assay of *Escherichia coli* heat-labile enterotoxin with Vero cells, *Infect. Immun.* **16:**617–622.

Sprinz, H., 1969, Pathogenesis of intestinal infections, *Arch. Pathol.* **87:**556–562.

Staack, H. H., and Spaun, J., 1953, Serological diagnosis of chronic typhoid carriers by Vi hemagglutination, *Acta Pathol. Microbiol. Scand.* **32:**420–423.

Standfast, A. F. B., 1960, A report on the laboratory assays carried out at the Lister Institute of Preventive Medicine on the typhoid vaccines used in the field study in Yugoslavia, *Bull. WHO* **23:**37–45.

Stirm, S., Orskov, F., Orskov, I., and Birch-Anderson, A., 1967a, Episome-carried surface antigen K88 of *Escherichia coli*. III. Morphology, *J. Bacteriol.* **93:**740–748.

Stirm, S., Orskov, F., Orskov, I., and Mansa, B., 1967b, Episome-carried surface antigen K88 of *Escherichia coli*. II. Isolation and chemical analysis, *J. Bacteriol.* **93:**731–739.

Stuart, G., and Krikorian, K. S., 1928, Serologic diagnosis of the enterica by the method of qualitative receptor analysis, *J. Hyg.* **28:**105–126.

Swaney, L. M., Ying-Ping, L., Chuen-Mo, T., Cheng-Chin, T., Ippen-Ihler, K., and Brinton, C. C., Jr., 1977, Isolation and characterization of *Escherichia coli* phase variants and mutants deficient in type 1 pilus production, *J. Bacteriol.* **130:**495–505.

Takeda, Y., Okamoto, K., and Miwatani, T., 1977, Toxin from the culture filtrate of *Shigella dysenteriae* that causes morphological changes in Chinese hamster ovary cells and is distinct from the neurotoxin, *Infect. Immun.* **18:**546–548.

Takeuchi, A., 1967, Electron microscope studies of experimental salmonella infection. I. Penetration into the intestinal epithelium by *Salmonella typhimurium, Am. J. Pathol.* **50:**109–136.

Takeuchi, A., 1971, Penetration of the intestinal epithelium by various micro-organisms, *Curr. Top. Pathol.* **54:**1–27.

Takeuchi, A., and Sprinz, H., 1967, Electron microscope studies of experimental salmonella infection in the preconditional guinea pig. II. Response of the intestinal mucosa to the invasion by *Salmonella typhimurium, Am. J. Pathol.* **51:**137–161.

Takeuchi, A., Sprinz, H., LaBrec, E. H., and Formal, S. B., 1965, Experimental bacillary dysentery: An electron microscopic study of the response of the intestinal mucosa to bacterial invasion, *Am. J. Pathol.* **47:**1011–1044.

Takeuchi, A., Formal, S. B., and Sprinz, H., 1968, Experimental acute colitis in the rhesus monkey following peroral infection with *Shigella flexneri, Am. J. Pathol.* **52:**503–529.

Taylor, J., Powell, B. W., and Wright, J., 1949, Infantile diarrhoea and vomiting: A clinical and bacteriological investigation, *Br. Med. J.* **2:**117–125.

Tomasi, T. B., Jr., 1972, Secretory immunoglobulins, *N. Engl. J. Med.* **287:**500–506.

Tomasi, T. B., Jr., and Zigelbaum, S. D., 1963, The selective occurrence of gamma A globulins in certain body fluids, *J. Clin. Invest.* **42:**1552–1560.

Tulloch, E. F., Jr., Ryan, K. J., Formal, S. B., and Franklin, F. A., 1973, Invasive enteropathic *Escherichia coli* dysentery: An acute outbreak in 28 adults, *Ann. Intern. Med.* **79**:13–17.

Tully, J. G., and Gaines, S., 1961, H antigen of *Salmonella typhosa, J. Bacteriol.* **81**:924–932.

Tully, J. G., Gaines, S., and Tigertt, W. D., 1963, Studies on infection and immunity in experimental typhoid fever. IV. Role of H antigen in protection, *J. Infect. Dis.* **112**:118–124.

Van Heynigan, W. E., 1971, The exotoxin of *Shigella dysenteriae,* in: *Microbial Toxins,* Vol. IIA: *Bacterial Protein Toxins.* (S. Kadis, T. C. Monte, and S. Ajl., eds.), pp. 255–269, Academic Press, New York.

Vicari, G., Olitzki, A. L., and Olitzki, A., 1960, The action of the thermolabile toxin of *Shigella dysenteriae* on cells cultivated *in vitro, Br. J. Exp. Pathol.* **41**:179–189.

Wallace, R. B., and Donta, S. T., 1975, Paper presented at American Public Health Association Meeting, Nov. 18, Abstr. No. 345C.

Watson, K. C., 1957, The relapse state in typhoid fever treated with chloramphenicol, *Am. J. Trop. Med. Hyg.* **6**:72–80.

Webster, M. E., Landy, M., and Freeman, M. E., 1952, Studies on Vi antigen II. Purification of Vi antigen from *Escherichia coli* 5396/38, *J. Immunol.* **69**:135–142.

Wells, P. S., and Hsu, H. S., 1970, Interactions between macrophages of guinea pigs and salmonellae. II. Phagocytosis of macrophages of normal guinea pigs, *Infect. Immun.* **2**:145–149.

Wentworth, F. H., Brock, D. W., Stulberg, C. S., and Page, R. H., 1955, Clinical and serological observations of two human volunteers following the ingestion of *Escherichia coli* O127:B8, *Proc. Soc. Exp. Biol. Med.* **91**:586–588.

Wernet, P., Breu, H., Knop, J., and Rowley, D., 1971, Antibacterial action of specific IgA and transport, IgM, IgA and IgG from serum into the small intestine, *J. Infect. Dis.* **124**:223–226.

Whipp, S. C., Moon, H. W., and Lyon, N. C., 1975, Heat-stable *Escherichia coli* enterotoxin production *in vivo, Infect. Immun.* **12**:240–244.

Widal, G. F. I., and Sicard, A., 1896, Recherches de la reaction agglutinate de le sang et le serum desséchés des typhiques et dans la serosité des vesications, *Bull*

Mem Soc. Med. Hop. Paris 3rd Ser.* **12**:681–682.

Wilson, G. S., and Miles, A. A., 1964, *Topley and Wilson's Principles of Bacteriology and Immunity,* 5th ed., pp. 1833–1842, E. Arnold, London.

Wilson, M. R., and Hohmann, A. W., 1974, Immunity to *Escherichia coli* in pigs: Adhesion of enteropathogenic *Escherichia coli* to isolated intestinal epithelial cells, *Infect. Immun.* **10**:776–782.

Wong, K. H., Feeley, J. C., Northrup, R. S., and Forlines, M. E., 1974a, Vi antigen from *Salmonella typhosa* and immunity against typhoid fever. I. Isolation and immunologic properties in animals, *Infect. Immun.* **9**:348–353.

Wong, K. H., Feeley, J. C., Pittman, M., and Forlines, M. E., 1974b, Adhesion of Vi antigen inactivated by acetone or by heat and phenol, *J. Infect. Dis.* **129**:501–506.

Woodward, T. E., Smadel, J. E., and Parker, R. T., 1954, The therapy of typhoid fever, *Med. Clin. N. Am.* **38**:577–590.

Yee, R. B., and Buffenmyer, B. L., 1970, Infection of cultured mouse macrophages with *Shigella flexneri, Infect Immun.* **1**:459–463.

Young, V. M., Gillem, H. C., Massey, E. D., and Baker, H. J., 1960, A study on the detection and specificity of antibodies to *Shigella flexneri* types using preserved polysaccharide-sensitized human erythrocytes, *Am. J. Publ. Health* **50**:1866–1872.

Young, V. M., Lee, M. R., Branche, W. C., Jr., and Kenton, D. M., 1967, *Shigella flexneri* antibody levels in healthy subjects from various regions of the United States, *Am. J. Publ. Health* **57**:2104–2110.

Yugoslav Typhoid Commission, 1957, Field and laboratory studies with typhoid vaccines, *Bull WHO* **16**:897–910.

Yugoslav Typhoid Commission, 1964, A controlled field trial of the effectiveness of acetone-dried and inactivated and heat-phenol-inactivated typhoid vaccines in Yugoslavia, *Bull WHO* **30**:623–630.

Zenser, T. V., and Metzger, J. F., 1974, Comparison of the action of *Escherichia coli* enterotoxin on the thymocyte adenylate cyclase–cyclic adenosine monophosphate system to that of cholera toxin and prostaglandin E_1, *Infect. Immun.* **10**:503–509.

12

Immunology of *Vibrio cholerae*

RICHARD A. FINKELSTEIN

1. Introduction

The problems of immunization against the cholera vibrios and the disease cholera, for which they are responsible, can best be appreciated using Fig. 1 as a frame of reference. The figure, kindly provided by Dr. Edward T. Nelson (Nelson *et al.*, 1976), is a scanning electron micrograph of *Vibrio cholerae* organisms, magnified approximately 5000 times, adhering to the intestinal mucosal epithelium about 5 hr after their introduction into the lumen of an isolated ileal loop in an adult rabbit. [The adult rabbit ileal loop model, reintroduced by S. N. De (De and Chatterje, 1953), is widely used as an experimental system for the controlled investigation of aspects of pathogenicity and immunology of cholera and other enterotoxic enteropathies.] The tissue was extensively washed prior to its preparation for electron microscopy, so it is evident that the vibrios are adherent with a degree of firmness that resists detachment. The small bowel, in health, is normally relatively free of bacteria because of the efficiency of the normal clearance mechanisms, the mucus layer (Florey, 1933), and peristalsis (Dixon, 1960). Thus it also becomes evident that the cholera vibrios can, by their specific adhesive properties, circumvent the normal defensive barriers to colonize the small bowel in huge numbers in close association with the intestinal epithelium, the target tissue for their enterotoxin. Unlike shigellae and salmonellae, chol-

era vibrios have never been shown to penetrate the intestinal epithelial cells, although they do occasionally insert themselves between the microvilli (Nelson *et al.*, 1976). Accumulating evidence (Jones, 1975) permits one to state, axiomatically, that the ability to adhere to the intestinal mucosa is an important attribute of virulence of any nonpenetrating bacterial pathogen of the small bowel.

The figure reveals no particular surface structure (pili, fimbriae, or capsular material) on the cholera vibrios that is associated with their ability to adhere, except perhaps for a slight fuzziness of the cell envelope visible at higher magnification (Nelson *et al.*, 1976). Thus in the case of the cholera vibrios (or at least with this particular strain) adhesion appears to depend on a specific interaction between the surface of the vibrio and the surface of the microvilli. In this regard there may be some heterogeneity in distribution of receptors on the intestinal surface, since some areas are clearly free of vibrios whereas the bacteria are densely packed in others. In infant rabbit tissue, in contrast, the distribution of vibrios is more uniform and adhesion is more rapid (Nelson *et al.*, 1976). Attachment of vibrio to vibrio is also evident in the photograph; whether the mechanism of this interaction is the same as that involved in the vibrio–intestine association is not yet clear.

The figure also reveals the single polar flagellum of the cholera vibrios, their organ of locomotion. Other micrographs, taken early in the course of infection (Nelson *et al.*, 1976), show the vibrios primarily in an end-on attachment to the epithelium with their flagella free in the lumen, thus dispelling any possible

RICHARD A. FINKELSTEIN • Department of Microbiology, University of Missouri School of Medicine, Columbia, Missouri 65212.

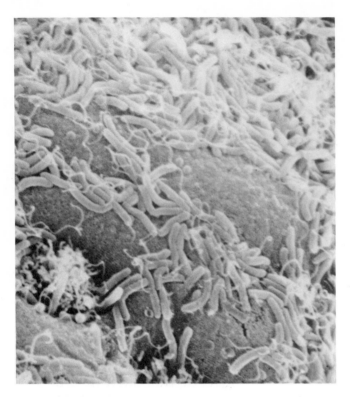

Figure 1. Scanning electron micrograph (SEM) (5000×) of *V. cholerae* on the surface of the intestinal mucosa in an adult rabbit ileal loop approximately 5 hr after intraluminal inoculation. The tissue was washed extensively prior to preparation for SEM. Courtesy of Dr. Edward T. Nelson (Nelson *et al.*, 1976).

notion that the flagellum is itself an organ of attachment. However, the motility of the vibrios is increasingly being recognized as an attribute of virulence (Guentzel and Berry, 1975), perhaps by enabling the vibrios to penetrate the "mucous zone" (Schrank and Verwey, 1976), although it cannot be ignored that other intestinal pathogens such as shigellae and some strains of enterotoxic *Escherichia coli* (Finkelstein *et al.*, 1976) are nonmotile.

Not shown in the figure are various other potential weapons in the armamentarium of the cholera vibrios which must be considered in the total picture—the enzymes (mucinases, sialidase, proteases, etc.), the lipopolysaccharide endotoxin, their mechanism(s) for acquiring essential nutrients, and the now well-characterized protein exoenterotoxin (choleragen),* which is totally responsible for the

cardinal clinical manifestation of cholera, the copious isotonic diarrhea. The toxin has been demonstrated also to bind rapidly and firmly to the surface of the intestinal mucosa (Peterson *et al.*, 1972: Walker *et al.*, 1974). Following this interaction, the biological effects of the enterotoxin are no longer prevented or reversed by specific antibodies (Mosley and Ahmed, 1969).

The (anatomically) superficial nature of the insult induced by the cholera vibrios and their enterotoxin is contrasted to the marked physiological disturbances induced in the cholera patient. A patient with cholera may present in shock with practically no vital signs, as a consequence of the acute loss of fluid and electrolytes in the voluminous choleraic stool. Solely with adequate intravenous rehydration such a patient can be restored to "health" within a couple of hours, although he may continue to pass stools at a rate of 20 liters or so a day for 3 or 4 more days. There are no systemic manifestations other than those associated with fluid loss and electrolyte imbalances.

Since the disease is so easily treated—after correction of the initial losses, patients can be maintained by fluids administered *per os* (Hir-

*The term "exoenterotoxin" was coined (Finkelstein, 1969) to connote that this toxin is (1) elaborated by growing vibrios into the surrounding menstruum and (2) produced in and is active at the level of the intestines during the natural disease. "Choleragen" is a laboratory epithet which was given to the active principle found in *V. cholerae* cultures before it was clear that it was indeed *the* cholera enterotoxin (Finkelstein *et al.*, 1964). It has since been legitimized (Dorland, 1974).

schhorn *et al.*, 1974; Nalin and Cash, 1974)—mortality in cholera reflects a failure in health care delivery. Appropriate antibiotic therapy (Hirschhorn *et al.*, 1974) plays an adjunctive role by reducing the infective period, the amount of fluids required, and the duration of hospitalization, but does not replace physiological treatment. Although cholera patients respond with antibodies to the cholera vibrios and their enterotoxin (as will be detailed below), it is not yet clear whether the immune response plays a significant role in recovery. The facts that the effects of the toxin are long lived and that the toxin, once fixed to tissue receptors, is no longer neutralizable by antibody suggest rather that, following the clearance of the vibrios as a continuing source of enterotoxin, recovery may be more dependent on replacement, by regeneration, of the poisoned epithelial cells.

That effective immunity to cholera is feasible was convincingly demonstrated by volunteer studies which showed that convalescents from induced cholera were solidly resistant to homologous rechallenge for (at least) 1 year (Cash *et al.*, 1974a). However, scientifically controlled field studies, conducted over the past decade, have also demonstrated convincingly the inadequacy of available conventional and experimental cholera vaccines, administered parenterally, in controlling cholera, although some protective effect is elicited in some population groups (Section 3, Cholera Vaccines: Historical Aspects).

Cholera is one of only relatively few infectious diseases in which immune mechanisms must be operative essentially outside the body, i.e., at the surface (or in the lumen) of the intestine. Dental caries, pertussis, and other enterotoxic enteropathies are the only other examples that come quickly to mind. Pathogens such as *Neisseria gonorrhoeae*, nontoxigenic *Corynebacterium diphtheriae*, and shigellae have a limited invasiveness that could render them susceptible to humoral and cell-mediated immune mechanisms, and thus they cannot be considered strictly "surface pathogens." *V. cholerae*, which has the additional merit of possessing relatively well-defined antigens that do generate resistance to infection and/or its effects, should be an interesting and relevant tool to immunologists concerned with aspects of local immunity but not necessarily

in cholera itself. As will be noted later, the cholera enterotoxin—itself a potent protein antigen subject to all the classical and neoclassical methods of assay for antigens and antibodies—also has significant and powerful modulating effects on immunological responsiveness to other antigens under experimental conditions.

Additionally, it should be emphasized that cholera is the prototype for an emerging group of newly recognized enterotoxic enteropathies that as a whole are probably much more significant than cholera in terms of worldwide morbidity and mortality. Thus information and principles developed from studies of the cholera model should be applicable to the other enterotoxic enteropathies. In some cases the applicability may be quite direct, since some of the causative agents elaborate enterotoxins which are immunologically related to the cholera enterotoxin. The list of enterotoxigenic bacteria is expanding rapidly. It currently includes strains of *Escherichia coli*, nonagglutinable (NAG) vibrios [or noncholera vibrios (NCV), or "*Vibrio enteritidis*" (Finkelstein, 1973)], *Vibrio parahaemolyticus*, *Shigella* spp., *Salmonella* spp., *Clostridium perfringens*, *Bacillus cereus*, *Pseudomonas* spp., *Enterobacter* spp., *Aerobacter* spp., *Klebsiella* spp., and *Aeromonas* spp. (and even blue-green algae). In at least some instances, e.g., *E. coli* heat-labile enterotoxin and NAG vibrio toxin, an immunological relationship with choleragen has been established. Likewise, the heat-labile *E. coli* toxin has been shown to have a mode of action similar to that of choleragen in activating host cell adenylate cyclase (Evans *et al.*, 1972).

2. Cholera: Historical Aspects

Prior to the 1900s cholera swept the world in what have been regarded as six major pandemic waves (Pollitzer, 1959) with almost incalculable numbers of cases and a mortality ranging as high as 60–70%. In the first half of the present century, with only occasional exceptions, such as the Egyptian outbreak in 1947 with 20,000 deaths among some 33,000 reported cases, cholera tended to recede into its ancestral home in the Bengal region of the Indo-Pakistani subcontinent. Concurrently, interest in cholera outside the endemic region generally waned, and in the 1950s only a handful of laboratories were engaged in experimental studies on cholera.

The outbreak of classical cholera in Thailand in 1958 and the subsequent emergence of the present seventh great pandemic of El Tor cholera, which first erupted in Hong Kong in 1961 and then spread practically worldwide (see Kamal, 1974), renewed interest in the unresolved problems of this infectious disease and led to a decade and a half of remarkable progress in understanding the pathophysiology, pathogenesis, therapy, and immunology of cholera.

El Tor vibrios were differentiated from classical *V. cholerae* because they were first isolated, in 1905, at the El Tor Quarantine Station in the Sinai peninsula, from people (pilgrims to Mecca) who did not have cholera. The isolates were further distinguished by their ability to hemolyze sheep or goat erythrocytes—a property not shared by classical strains. A number of additional tests have since been introduced to differentiate these two groups of choleragenic vibrios, including, among others, the ability of agar-grown fresh isolates to agglutinate chicken erythrocytes in a slide test (Finkelstein and Mukerjee, 1963), sensitivity to polymyxin B (Gan and Tjia, 1963), and sensitivity to particular cholera phages (Mukerjee and Takeya, 1974). For some time after their initial isolation the hemolytic El Tor vibrios were considered to be incapable of causing epidemic cholera and were excluded from the International Sanitary Regulations even though they had been associated periodically with isolated outbreaks of choleralike diarrheal disease ("paracholera"), especially in Indonesia. Although strains isolated early in the present pandemic were markedly hemolytic, this property was lost as the epidemic spread. Most current isolates are either nonhemolytic or only weakly hemolytic, while retaining other distinctive characteristics of El Tor vibrios. However, by the vast majority of taxonomic and immunological criteria, the two groups of choleragenic vibrios are similar (See Finkelstein, 1973). With the present inescapable evidence of the ability of El Tor vibrios to cause epidemic cholera clinically identical with that caused by classical *V. cholerae*, El Tor vibrios are now universally accepted as a biotype of *Vibrio cholerae*

and are so recognized by the World Health Organization. Nevertheless, there are significant epidemiological differences between the two biotypes, El Tor and classical *V. cholerae*. The El Tor vibrios generally appear to produce less toxin than classical *V. cholerae* strains (Vasil *et al.*, 1974) and are better able to survive adverse environmental conditions (Felsenfeld, 1974). Perhaps for these reasons they have significantly higher infection-to-case ratios than classical *V. cholerae* (Bart *et al.*, 1970) and thus are more likely to become endemic. However, both groups of vibrios share the same somatic antigens, operationally designated AB and AC, representing the Ogawa and Inaba serotypes, respectively (see Finkelstein, 1975), and the enterotoxins produced by both biotypes are immunologically closely related, although not invariably completely identical (Finkelstein *et al.*, 1974b; Vasil *et al.*, 1974).

An additional large and heterogenous group of vibrios which are serologically unrelated to the cholera vibrios have, on occasion, been incriminated in outbreaks of diarrheal disease (see Aldova *et al.*, 1968). These organisms, because they are not agglutinated by diagnostic antisera which recognize the true cholera vibrios (i.e., Inaba or Ogawa serotype El Tor and classical biotypes of *V. cholerae*), have come to be known as nonagglutinable (NAG) vibrios or noncholera vibrios (NCV). Some genetic relatedness to the true cholera vibrios has been demonstrated (Colwell, 1970; Citarella and Colwell, 1970; Bhaskaran, 1974); enterotoxin from some strains appears to be immunologically related to the cholera enterotoxin (Zinnaka and Carpenter, 1972; Ohashi *et al.*, 1972). It has therefore been recommended (Sakazaki *et al.*, 1970; International Committee on Nomenclature of Bacteria, 1972) that the NAG vibrios be included in the species *V. cholerae*, which would then distinguish the true immunologically related cholera vibrios as *V. cholerae* serotype I and the NAG vibrios as *V. cholerae* followed by other serotype designations. This recommendation, if accepted, would necessitate a change in the present International Health Regulations. Otherwise, any country experiencing a case of noncholera vibrio diarrhea would be obliged to report it and be subject to quarantine regulations. Alternatively, the author has previously suggested (1973) that they be classified in a new species, "*Vibrio enteritidis.*" Although the taxonomic considerations cited above have some validity, these organisms have never been incriminated in widespread epidemic diarrhea characteristic of cholera vibrios and thus have neither their historic nor their epidemiological significance. The claim that NAG vibrios share flagellar antigens with cholera vibrios (Sakazaki *et al.*, 1970) has been disputed by Smith (1974). Other than the need to recognize that effective antitoxic immunity against the cholera vibrio enterotoxin may also offer some degree of protection against diarrheal disease due to these organisms, they will not be considered further in this chapter.

3. Cholera Vaccines: Historical Aspects

Cholera vaccines were introduced in the late 1800s shortly after the first isolation of the cholera vibrios by Koch in 1882 and some time before the recognition, by Nobechi and Kabeshima in the 1920s, that there were two major serotypes of cholera vibrios, Inaba and Ogawa. Vaccines composed of "attenuated" living vibrios and administered parenterally were developed by Ferran in 1885 and, later, by Haffkine in 1893, whereas the killed vibrio vaccine which, with only slight modification, is still in use was introduced by Kolle in 1896. Cvjetanović (1965) summarized earlier experiences with cholera vaccines in the field and concluded that "these early studies give circumstantial evidence, although no proof, that some types of cholera vaccine were perhaps moderately effective."

The reasons why the earlier field trials failed to yield conclusive evidence regarding the efficacy of cholera vaccine were (1) that the studies were largely improperly designed, i.e., the control and vaccinated groups were not strictly comparable—sometimes volunteer vaccinees were used or on occasion inhabitants of some villages or regions were vaccinated and other populations were used as controls; (2) there was lack of uniformity in surveillance and definitions of what constitutes a case of cholera; and (3) that the vaccines used were poorly standardized and differed from study to study.

The Pakistan-SEATO Cholera Research Laboratory in Dacca, East Pakistan (now the Cholera Research Laboratory in Bangladesh), initiated the first of the series of modern double-blind, scientifically controlled field studies of the prophylactic efficacy of cholera vaccines and antigens in appropriate placebo-treated control and vaccinated groups. The results of the first study, with a divalent (Inaba and Ogawa) killed vibrio vaccine of exceptionally high potency in the mouse protection test and some degree of reactogenicity, indicated that a single dose of vaccine effectively reduced the incidence of diarrhea associated with *V. cholerae* from 6.1 cases per 1000 among controls to 1.7 per 1000 among vaccinees (Oseasohn *et al.*, 1965) in the heavily endemic region of East Bengal.

Subsequent studies (summarized by Joó, 1974, and Finkelstein, 1975) extended these observations into different population groups and included evaluations of cell-free somatic antigen preparations, different dose regimens, and, in one instance, the incorporation of an oil adjuvant in a killed whole cell vaccine.

As a result of these studies it is now possible to restate, with confidence, Cvjetanović's earlier conclusion (1965) as follows: *It has now been demonstrated unequivocally that some parenterally administered cholera vaccines offer a limited but significant degree of protection against cholera for a limited period of time in some population groups.*

In general, the best results, in terms of degree and duration of protection (about 70% for a year), were obtained in adults in the heavily endemic region of Bangladesh. Vaccine, administered in a single dose, was almost completely ineffective in younger children in the same area, where it should be recognized that cholera is largely a pediatric disease. Adults in the endemic region have a much lower incidence of cholera than children (Mosley, 1969). Significant protection of 3 months' duration was obtained in the pediatric population given two doses of vaccine.

In trials conducted in Calcutta and in the Philippines, a neoepidemic area, the protective effect hardly approached significance and lasted less than 6 months. Inclusion of an oil adjuvant, in the Philippine study, increased the protection significantly but caused severe local reactions which precluded further use of that particular material.

From the experience gained from the field studies it is evident that some protection can be attained in the gut from parenterally administered killed cellular vaccines, although it is equally clear that this time-honored conventional approach to cholera immunization is relatively inefficient. Isolated somatic antigen preparations (Watanabe, 1974) offered no significant advantages over killed whole cellular vaccines. It is also clear that the results are partially dependent on the nature of the population at risk. In a heavily endemic region vaccine appears to "boost" preexistent levels of immunity which were probably acquired as a consequence of repeated natural exposure to cholera antigens. In neoepidemic areas, in children, and in other "immunological virgins" the beneficial effects of vaccine are probably not worth the expense and trouble of administering it (see Cvjetanović, 1974).

In recognition of the facts that cholera is not likely to pose a significant problem in a sanitarily developed country like the United States, that it is almost perfectly treatable should it occur here, and that the vaccine has only limited effectiveness, the United States has dropped the requirement for evidence of cholera vaccination even among travelers from epidemic areas. Other nations have followed suit, although cholera vaccination is still required by some.

Other useful information also emerged from the field trials. Since none of the vaccines tested induced significant levels of antitoxic antibodies, clearly it is possible to obtain some degree of protection dependent solely on antibacterial mechanisms. Vaccinees respond with the production of circulating antibacterial antibodies readily demonstrable either by the complement-dependent vibriocidal test (Finkelstein, 1962) (and later less sensitive modifications) or by agglutination tests. According to Mosley (1969) the circulating antibody level has predictive value—a doubling of the antibody titer in a population (with age or as result of vaccine) is associated with a 50% reduction in the case rate. However, it should not be inferred from this that there is a cause-and-effect relationship, i.e., it should not be concluded that serum antibody is directly protective—the serum antibody level could be indicative of an immune response which results in protection at the gut level, or it could be related to or reflective of the coproantibody level.

The field trials also revealed that the serotype of the vibrios rather than the biotype was the more important consideration. Inaba somatic antigen prepared from an El Tor biotype strain protected against classical Inaba vibrios in Bangladesh equally as well as a classical monovalent whole cell Inaba vaccine, and classical vaccine protected practically as well as El Tor vaccine against El Tor disease in the Philippines. It seems evident that the cell-wall-associated somatic antigens play the major role in antibacterial immunity to cholera and that these antigens do not differ significantly among El Tor and classical biotypes of the same serotype. Although an El Tor vaccine was slightly superior to a classical vaccine against El Tor cholera in the Philippines, the results might also reflect quantitative differences in antigen content among the strains used. Surprisingly, this aspect has hardly ever been investigated, although Finkelstein and Pongpairojana (1968) reported significant differences in antigenicity of vaccines composed of different strains of *V. cholerae* when tested in rabbits.

The issues of the protective roles of the type specific antigens, B and C, and of the shared antigen, A, were not completely settled by the field studies, largely because the epidemic strains failed to cooperate by providing sufficient numbers of cases of both serotypes to permit a critical examination. Purified Ogawa antigen was found to provide some protection against Inaba serotype cholera in older subjects in Bangladesh. There were insufficient numbers of Ogawa cases for evaluation of homologous immunity (Benenson *et al.*, 1968b). Although monovalent Inaba cells and purified antigen were protective, monovalent Ogawa whole cell vaccine was ineffective in protecting children against Inaba cholera even though vibriocidal antibody was induced. On this basis Mosley *et al.* (1970) concluded that vaccine-induced protection was type specific. However, in the Philippines, Inaba vaccine provided some protection against Ogawa infection (Azurin, 1973). Again the situation may be complicated by the previous antigenic experience (original antigenic sin) and by competition between antigenic determinants. Pike and Chandler (1974) found that some, but not all, rabbits immunized with Ogawa antigen produced precipitins against Inaba antigen and *vice versa*. Watanabe (1974) claimed that the common antigen of Ogawa vibrios is a weaker antigen than that in Inaba vibrios.

4. Antigens of *V. cholerae*

4.1. Somatic Antigen(s)

Surprisingly little is known about the basic nature and structure of *V. cholerae* antigens, especially in comparison with the definitive studies that have been performed with other microorganisms such as *Salmonella*.

The heat-stable somatic antigen responsible for the major serologic activity in vibriocidal and agglutination tests is extractable from the cholera vibrios by conventional procedures used for isolation of endotoxic lipopolysaccharide (LPS) of other gram-negative species (Finkelstein, 1962), and it shares many of their biological properties. Cholera vibrios have long been known to be exquisitely sensitive to the cidal effects of antibody and complement and, in fact, were the first organisms used experimentally for this purpose (the Pfeiffer phenomenon). Isolated endotoxin, in nanogram amounts, inhibits the predominant vibriocidal antibodies in a type-specific manner corresponding with the ABC operational concept elaborated by Burrows *et al.* (1946). This assay, designated the "vibriocidal antibody inhibition test" (VAIT) (Finkelstein, 1962), can be used to characterize the predominant vibriocidal antibodies in serum from either cholera convalescents or vaccinees or to identify the immunological specificity of antigen using known antisera. A number of less sensitive, but equally useful, modifications of the vibriocidal test have been introduced subsequently (Feeley, 1965; Benenson *et al.*, 1968a; Deb *et al.*, 1969; Holmgren *et al.*, 1971; Joó, 1973).

Depending on the sensitivity of the test, vibriocidal antibody may be found more or less frequently in the serum of normal people who have never had contact with antigens of *V. cholerae* (Finkelstein *et al.*, 1965). Titers are more prevalent and higher in Southeast Asians (Basaca-Sevilla *et al.*, 1964) than in North Americans. Cross-reactions with *Brucella*, *Citrobacter*, and *Yersinia* (Feeley, 1969; Gan-garosa *et al.*, 1970; Barua and Watanabe, 1972) may account, in part, for this "natural" antibody activity, but there must be other occult cross-reactive antigens. Ahmed *et al.* (1970) reported that the natural antibody activity was sensitive to 2-mercaptoethanol, implying that it is largely of the IgM class of immunoglobulins. In general, there is a strong correlation between vibriocidal and agglutinating antibody titers in immune sera and in sera from cholera convalescents (Finkelstein *et al.*, 1965; Feeley, 1965; Sack *et al.*, 1966), although exceptions occur.

Interestingly, although the isolated cholera LPS has properties similar to endotoxin from other gram-negative bacteria (Finkelstein, 1964; Milner and Finkelstein, 1966), it appears to be lacking in 2-keto-3-deoxyoctonate (KDO) (Jackson and Redmond, 1971; Redmond *et al.*, 1973; Jann *et al.*, 1973), which is a component of the core region of LPS from most Enterobacteriaceae (Westphal, 1975). Although the carbohydrate determinants responsible for the immunological specificity of the cholera vibrios have not yet been identified, glucose, heptose (believed to be L-glycero-D-manno-heptose), mannose, glucosamine, glycerol, ethanolamine, and fructose have been found in Inaba LPS (Jackson and Redmond, 1971; Redmond *et al.*, 1973; Jann *et al.*, 1973). In addition, an unusual amino sugar, D-quino-vosamine (2-amino-2, 6-dideoxyglucose), has been found in both serotypes (Jann *et al.*, 1973). The lipid A region, the biologically active portion of the endotoxin (Westphal, 1975), is generally similar to that of other species, although there appears to be a higher content of odd-numbered fatty acids (Armstrong and Redmond, 1974; Hisatsune *et al.*, 1975). The peptidoglycan, lysozyme-sensitive, inner, "rigid" or R-layer of the vibrios, which consists of a polymer of *N*-acetyl glucosamine, *N*-acetyl muramic acid, diamino pimelic acid, L- and D-alanine, and D-glutamic acid, does not participate in serological reactions of whole cells (Hisatsune *et al.*, 1974).

Biologically and immunologically reactive LPS is found in significant amounts in supernatant fluids of broth cultures of *V. cholerae* in the absence of significant lysis of the bacterial cells (Finkelstein *et al.*, 1964, 1966; Finkelstein and LoSpalluto, 1970; Pike and Chandler, 1975).

4.2. Protein Antigens

The possibility that "outer membrane *proteins*" of the cholera vibrios participate in their serological reactions has not been examined, although this aspect is coming into prominence with other gram-negative organisms, such as the gonococci (Johnston *et al.*, 1976). Some suggestion that a protein surface component may be responsible for a small proportion, perhaps 10%, of the vibriocidal activity of antisera against live vibrios may be derived from the work of Neoh and Rowley (1970, 1971, 1972). The "protein" antigen was reported to be heat stable and was shared by both Inaba and Ogawa serotypes. In partial support of these observations Pike and Chandler observed (1975) that extensive adsorption with phenol-water-extracted antigen left a residuum of 1.5–2% of the vibriocidal activity of antisera raised against live vibrios, although partially purified somatic antigen from cell-free culture supernates could totally adsorb the antibody from the same sera.

4.3. Ribosomal Preparations

As has been shown with a number of other bacteria, crude ribosomal preparations from both serotypes of cholera vibrios induce protection (Pitkin and Actor, 1972; Jensen *et al.*, 1972; Guentzel and Berry, 1974). It is not unlikely that the protection is dependent on small amounts of contaminating somatic antigen in an effective adjuvant (see also Eisenstein, 1975).

4.4. Flagellar Antigens and "Adhesins"

V. cholerae possesses only one polar flagellum, which confers on the vibrios a rather exceptional motility. According to Sanarelli (1919, as quoted by Pollitzer, 1959), "*V. cholerae* is endowed with a speed three times greater than that of *Bacillus prodigiosis*, five times that of *Salmonella typhosa*, ten times that of *Escherichia coli*, and twelve times that of *B. megatherium*." Koch (in Pollitzer, 1959) described the movement of vibrios as akin to that of a host of gnats.

Although earlier reports (see Pollitzer, 1959) suggested some serological differences among flagellar "H" antigens in cholera vibrios, this was not substantiated by Kauffman (1950). Aside from the studies of Sakazaki and of Smith cited earlier, little work has been done on flagellar antigens *per se* in recent years. According to Follett and Gordon (1963), vibrio flagella have a sheath and a core of different composition: "the core consists of the protein 'flagellin,' whereas the sheath is probably of cell-wall origin." This may explain why antibody against somatic antigen preparations, boiled cells, and purified somatic antigen can inhibit the motility of cholera vibrios (Williams *et al.*, 1974). *Vibrio parahaemolyticus*, a halophilic vibrio which is increasingly being recognized as a cause of enteritis associated with eating raw fish and seafood, also has a sheathed single polar flagellum but, in addition, produces lateral (peritrichous) flagella on solid medium (Yabuuchi *et al.*, 1974). Isolated polar flagellin from *V. parahaemolyticus* shares a common antigen with *V. cholerae*, other vibrios, and related genera according to work of Shinoda *et al.* (1976), but the lateral flagellin is more antigenically specific; *V. cholerae* does not produce lateral flagella.

The ability of specific diagnostic antisera to inhibit vibrio motility has been exploited by Benenson *et al.* (1964; Greenough *et al.*, 1965) and others (Barua *et al.*, 1967) to facilitate rapid diagnosis of cholera patients and carriers.

The motility of cholera vibrios is becoming recognized as an attribute of virulence, perhaps in enabling the vibrios to penetrate the mucus layer of the small bowel to adhere to the intestinal epithelium (Guentzel and Berry, 1975). Interestingly, however, nonmotile mutants were also less virulent for mice inoculated intraperitoneally with vibrios in hog gastric mucin (Eubanks *et al.*, 1976). It is therefore possible that other unrecognized alterations in the cell envelope may affect both motility and virulence. Jones (1975) has suggested that *V. cholerae* may have two kinds of hemagglutinin/adhesins: one, described by Lankford and Legsomburana (Lexomboon) (1965), associated with a surface "slime layer," and the other expressed only by motile cultures. The flagellum itself is not a hemagglutinin, according to Jones, since it is possible to find motile cultures which are hemagglutinin negative. That the flagellum is not an organ of adhesion to epithelial cells was demonstrated clearly by Nelson *et al.* (1976). Vibrios visualized, by scanning electron microscopy, early in the infection were primarily in an end-on attachment mode with their flagella free in the lumen (Figure 1). There was a lag period of approximately 1 hr before intralumenal vibrios adhered in large numbers to the intestinal epithelium of adult rabbits. This could be the time needed to penetrate the mucus layer, since adherence was much more rapid with washed intestinal sections *in vitro*. Adherence was also much more rapid and uniform in infant rabbits, suggesting that there is greater availability of receptors in the more susceptible infant animal.

Although a subculture of *V. cholerae* strain 569B Inaba (the strain most widely used for enterotoxin production) was found to be only weakly motile and of reduced virulence in mice by Guentzel and by Eubanks (1975, 1976), this strain has been demonstrated to have equivalent virulence to other strains tested in human beings (Cash *et al.*, 1974a). Forty-seven of 58 volunteers given 10^6 live vibrios of strain 569B orally with bicarbonate developed diarrheal disease. It must be recalled that many enteric pathogens are nonmotile, e.g., the shigellae. Most recently, an exceptionally diarrheagenic strain of toxigenic *E. coli* (Throop D) associated with a truly choleraic diarrheal disease was also found to be nonmotile (Finkelstein *et al.*, 1976). It is possible that highly toxinogenic strains can compensate for lower motility by producing disease "at a distance" through greater toxin production. E. T. Nelson (personal communication) has observed that strain 569B adheres less well than the strain, 3083, he used in most of his studies, although there is no doubt concerning its pathogenicity and virulence in rabbits and human beings. The role of motility in virulence of cholera vibrios is, at least to this observer, still to be settled.

That antibodies which inhibit motility are also protective does not *prove* the point—they could be operative by preventing attachment either directly by interaction with the putative adhesin(s), indirectly by steric mechanisms, or by other means to be discussed further below. Isolation of the actual adhesin(s) and the demonstration that antibodies against the purified material (if it is antigenic) are protective would help resolve the problem.

4.5. Mucinase(s)

The mucinases of the cholera vibrios were postulated to play a role in virulence of cholera vibrios by Burnet and Stone (1947) and subsequent investigators in the "pre-cholera enterotoxin era." This work ceased when it was shown by Gangarosa *et al.* (1960) that there was no histological evidence of epithelial desquamation, *assumed* from the earlier work to be *the* host response to mucinase. A further blow was dealt by the observation that partially purified choleragen, with low mucinase activity, was fully capable of evoking the characteristic fluid response, whereas preparations with high mucinase activity were not enterotoxic (Finkelstein *et al.*, 1966). Nevertheless, cholera mucinase (sialidase) may (1) help the vibrios penetrate the mucus layer and (2) enhance responsiveness to the cholera enterotoxin by converting other sialidase-sensitive membrane gangliosides to the sialidase-resistant G_{M1} (GGnSLC) ganglioside, which appears to be the receptor for the binding (B) region of the cholera enterotoxin. However, hard evidence that mucinase plays a role in virulence or is susceptible to immunological intervention is not yet available.

Cuatrecasas (1973) has reported that incubation of isolated fat cells with the G_{M1} ganglioside increases their ability to bind cholera toxin and increases their sensitivity to its biological effects. Hollenberg *et al.* (1974) have also shown that the responsiveness of transformed mouse cell lines to cholera enterotoxin is related to the G_{M1} ganglioside content of their membranes. The addition of exogenous G_{M1} to G_{M1}-deficient cells results in a functional incorporation, such that the cells previously unresponsive to choleragen become responsive (Moss *et al.*, 1976). Thus it seems clear that the sialidase-resistant monosialosyl ganglioside, G_{M1}, is at least a portion of the receptor or receptor complex (King and Van Heyningen, 1975). King and Van Heyningen (1973) found that the ability of di- and trisialosyl gangliosides and intestinal scrapings to deactivate (bind) cholera toxin was enhanced by treatment with sialidase from *Corynebac-*

terium diphtheriae or by *V. cholerae* sialidase, found as a contaminant in impure preparations of cholera enterotoxin. However, it is not clear that G_{M1} produced in an intestinal (or other) cell membrane by such treatment would be a functional receptor for cholera toxin. In contrast, Holmgren *et al.* (1975a) found that *V. cholerae* sialidase did not accomplish the conversion of di- and trisialosylgangliosides of intestinal mucosa to G_{M1}, nor did it markedly increase binding of or sensitivity to cholera toxin *in vitro* or *in vivo*. These workers suggested that the contradictions between their results and those of King and Van Heyningen may be due to the inclusion of muscular layer tissue in the study done by the latter group, although the latter indicated that they were careful not to include muscle.

4.6. Cholera Enterotoxin (Choleragen)

The remaining major antigen to consider in the immunology of cholera is the cholera enterotoxin or choleragen. The toxin is an oligomeric protein of 84,000 daltons, which consists of a number of noncovalently associated subunits representing functionally and immunologically distinct regions of the holotoxin. The two major regions of the toxin, A and B, have been separated from each other and recombined, thus reconstituting the physicochemical, biological, and immunological characteristics of the holotoxin (Finkelstein *et al.*, 1974a). The A region, 28,000 daltons (Klapper *et al.*, 1976), is responsible for the biological activity of the toxin (see Gill, 1975; Gill and King, 1975), whereas the B region, 56,000 daltons (LoSpalluto and Finkelstein, 1972), is responsible for binding of the toxin to its receptor(s), presumably containing G_{M1} ganglioside, on the host cell membrane. The B region is entirely equivalent to *choleragenoid*, the spontaneously formed "natural toxoid" (Finkelstein and LoSpalluto, 1969; Finkelstein *et al.*, 1971a,b). The A region consists of two peptides, A_1 and A_2, joined by a disulfide bond at position 5 of the A_2 chain. B (choleragenoid) is a polymer of noncovalently associated B chains. Choleragenoid binds to the same receptors as the holotoxin (Peterson *et al.*, 1972) and can prevent the binding and effects of toxin added subsequently (Pierce, 1973). Partial amino acid sequences have been deter-

mined for each of the three kinds of peptide chains which comprise the toxin, A_1, A_2, and B (Kurosky *et al.*, 1976; Klapper *et al.*, 1976; Ohtomo *et al.*, 1976; Mendez *et al.*, 1975; Lai *et al.*, 1976; Sattler *et al.*, 1975; S. van Heyningen, 1976). There is some disagreement as to the precise number and size of the peptide components. We (Klapper *et al.*, 1976) tend to agree with a model suggested by Lai *et al.* (1976), which proposes that the choleragen formed by the cholera vibrios contains six 10,000-dalton B chains per single A region (A_1–A_2). In the course of its isolation and purification, some of the B chains dissociate and recombine, yielding choleragenoid demonstrated to be somewhat heterogeneous (Finkelstein and LoSpalluto, 1970) and an average population of toxin molecules containing somewhat more than five B chains per A region. On the other hand, Gill (1976), who has been using toxin prepared exclusively in our laboratory, claims there are only five B chains per A region.

Figure 2 illustrates the serological reactivity of the major components of the cholera enterotoxin with their respective antisera. Rabbit antiserum prepared against the A region (wells 3 and 6) precipitates with the A region (well 1) and with the holotoxin (well 5), but does not precipitate with separated B region (well 2) or choleragenoid (well 4). Equine anticholeragenoid (Finkelstein, 1970b) (well 7) precipi-

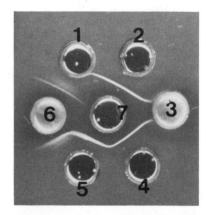

Figure 2. Ouchterlony double immunodiffusion precipitation reactions of cholera enterotoxin and its components. Contents of wells are as follows: 1, A region, 15 μg; 2, B region, 15 μg; 3, anti-A immunoglobulin, rabbit, 50 μl; 4, choleragenoid, 15 μg; 5, choleragen, 15 μg; 6, same as 3; 7, anticholeragenoid, equine, 50 μl.

tates with choleragen (well 5), choleragenoid (well 4), and separated B region (well 2) but does not recognize the immunologically distinct A region (well 1). The cholera enterotoxin is most widely standardized by the so-called Lb (limit of bluing) test introduced by Craig (1971). An Lb dose is defined as that amount of toxin which overcomes the neutralizing activity of one arbitrarily defined unit of antitoxin to produce a characteristic skin reaction in rabbits under standardized conditions. The test is analogous to the Lr test used previously with diphtheria toxin. One Lb dose is approximately 0.038 µg of highly purified cholera toxin.

It has been known for more than a decade that antiserum against choleragen is both neutralizing and protective (Finkelstein, 1965; Finkelstein and Atthasampunna, 1967). In the early studies, however, the enterotoxin preparations were contaminated with significant amounts of vibrio somatic antigen which induced respectable levels of vibriocidal antibodies. Thus immunity to experimental challenge with live vibrios could not be attributed exclusively to antitoxic mechanisms. Following the isolation of the toxin to homogeneity, it was found that protection against live vibrio challenge could be obtained in the absence of a rise in vibriocidal antibody (Finkelstein, 1970a). Parenterally induced purely antitoxic immunity can be protective against intestinal challenge, at least experimentally. The immunity induced with toxin antigen prepared from strain 569B was protective against challenge with cholera vibrios of both serotypes and biotypes and from diverse sources. Thus there is only a single major immunological type of cholera enterotoxin, although enterotoxin isolated from an El Tor vibrio strain has been found to lack an antigenic determinant found in toxin from strain 569B (Finkelstein *et al.*, 1974b; Vasil *et al.*, 1974).

The findings that antitoxic immunity was protective in a variety of experimental animal systems (Feeley, 1974; see Finkelstein, 1975) stimulated interest in their possible application to control of cholera in man.

Based on the precedents established by the obvious successes of immunity elicited by parenterally administered tetanus and diphtheria formalinized toxoids, under the auspices of the U.S. National Institutes of Health and the Cholera Research Laboratory in Dacca, an effort was initiated to evaluate the efficacy of purely antitoxic immunity elicited by parenterally administered formalinized cholera enterotoxoid in a scientifically controlled field study. However, experimental lots of formalinized toxoid prepared under contract by Wyeth laboratories were found to revert partially to toxicity and to cause delayed painful local reactions at the site of inoculation in volunteers and in laboratory animals (Hornick *et al.*, 1972; Verwey *et al.*, 1972; Northrup and Chisari, 1972). That particular lot of formalinized toxoid also elicited substantial vibriocidal antibody. Thus it was not clear from the preliminary studies in volunteers (Hornick *et al.*, 1972), which suggested that some protection had been achieved, whether the protection was antibacterial, antitoxic, or both.

Subsequently, the residual somatic antigen content was reduced to insignificant levels (Rappaport *et al.*, 1974a) and a stable, nonreverting toxoid was prepared by treatment of the toxin with glutaraldehyde (Rappaport *et al.*, 1974b). This, however, resulted in loss of antigenicity of the product (Peterson *et al.*, 1975) which appeared to be partially restored by adjuvant in experimental animals (Rappaport *et al.*, 1974b) but not in volunteers (Peterson *et al.*, 1975).

A similar glutaraldehyde-treated protamine-alum adjuvanted toxoid was evaluated in Bangladesh in 66,000 individuals who were given two injections of 100 µg each or a placebo 6 weeks apart (Curlin, 1975b). Statistically significant protection was obtained against Inaba serotype cholera during the first 24 weeks of the field trial, but the cumulative protection was only of the order of 35%. The protection was more marked with hospitalized patients than with outpatients, suggesting that antitoxic immunity may reduce the severity of the disease. Interestingly and inexplicably, no protection was observed against Ogawa serotype cholera, although in an earlier preliminary report (Curlin, 1975a) equal protection was observed against both serotypes. The conclusion was that "these results suggest that antitoxic immunity may play a role in resistance to cholera, but it will be necessary to markedly enhance the duration and level of protection."

Ohtomo *et al.* (1974) have prepared a stable

302 RICHARD A. FINKELSTEIN

toxoid by treating purified toxin with formaldehyde in the presence of glycine. This product, with an alum adjuvant, is currently being evaluated in the Philippines (Ohtomo et al., 1975).

Saletti and Ricci (1974a,b) have also prepared stable toxoids, although they still contain appreciable amounts of somatic antigen. More recently, Germanier et al. (1976) have prepared a stable, antigenic toxoid by heating purified toxin to form "procholeragenoid" (Finkelstein et al., 1971b), a relatively nontoxic, high molecular weight polymer, and then treating with formaldehyde to inactivate the slight residual toxicity. Procholeragenoid was earlier found to produce better gut immunity than monomeric forms of the toxin antigen after parenteral administration in mice (Fujita and Finkelstein, 1972) and rabbits (Holmgren, 1973), but whether similar effects would result in man remains to be established. The glutaraldehyde toxoid described by Rappaport et al. (1974b) contained polymeric forms of the toxin antigen but was rather ineffective in eliciting protection in humans. Polymers of staphylococcal enterotoxin were found by Warren et al. (1975) to be more immunogenic in monkeys than monomeric forms. They suggested that the highly polymerized derivatives may elicit a thymus-independent humoral response, as has been demonstrated with other high molecular weight bacterial antigens.

5. Host Responses to *V. cholerae* Antigens

Despite the anatomically superficial nature of *V. cholerae* infection, the host generally exhibits a vigorous antibody response to both somatic antigen(s) and the cholera enterotoxin. It is not, however, as yet clear whether, or how much, the serological response contributes to recovery or resistance to reinfection.

In all systems studied the effects of cholera enterotoxin are long lasting—perhaps even for the life span of the affected cells. In the study in which cholera enterotoxin was instilled into the small bowel of volunteers (Benyajati, 1966), the subject who received a sufficient dose manifested diarrhea over a period of 2 days—too short a period for an effective im-

munological response but, perhaps fortuitously, a period of time coincident with that needed for almost total regeneration of the intestinal epithelium (see Isselbacher, 1975). Similarly, cholera patients appropriately treated with antibiotics, which effectively eliminate the vibrios as a continuing source of enterotoxin, continue to have diarrhea for 48 hr or more (Hirschhorn et al., 1974). Nevertheless, the duration and volume, relative to those of patients not treated with antibiotics, are approximately halved. Early antibiotic treatment reduces the serum antitoxic antibody response but does not affect the vibriocidal antibody response (Pierce et al., 1970). Thus the antivibrio immune response may be significant in the ultimate elimination of the vibrios from the non-antibiotic-treated patient but the antitoxic response may not play any role in recovery, although it may be significant (with antibacterial antibody) in resistance to reinfection. The gut of cholera patients generally becomes cleared of cholera vibrios during convalescence. Exceptions, in the form of chronic gallbladder carriers, occur rarely (Azurin et al., 1967; Wallace et al., 1967) and through unknown mechanisms. The antitoxic titer, in naturally acquired cholera, remains elevated for at least 12–18 months according to Pierce et al. (1970). However, in volunteers convalescent from induced cholera, both circulating antitoxic and antibacterial antibody levels had practically returned to baseline within a year, although the volunteers were still resistant to cholera (Cash et al., 1974a). It should be recalled, however, that the patients studied by Pierce were in the heavily endemic region, whereas the volunteers were from an immunologically virgin population. Nevertheless, the volunteer study suggests that immunological memory in the gut may be more long lived than is generally assumed.

It was also shown, in the volunteer study, that some degree of protection was elicited by parenterally administered killed whole cell vaccine, by orally administered whole cell vaccine, and by parenterally administered toxoid. However, the levels of immunity were not as high as those achieved by convalescence from induced cholera. Since the toxoid vaccine used contained some somatic antigen and induced vibriocidal antibody, it is not clear that the protection elicited by toxoid was purely antitoxic in nature. Results of serological tests, antibacterial or antitoxic, on the vaccinees and convalescents were not predictive of their response to challenge. Ganguly *et al.* (1975) have shown that a small proportion of volunteers immunized orally with two doses of killed or live whole cell vaccines responded with intestinal antibody predominantly of the IgA class. The killed vaccine was more effective than the live attenuated vaccine strain used which failed to colonize the gut in this as well as in previous studies (Sanyal and Mukerjee, 1969; Cash *et al.*, 1974b).

The observation that some immunity was generated by orally administered killed vibrio cells supports the contention, long championed by Freter (Freter and Gangarosa, 1963; Freter, 1974), that effective immunity can be generated by the oral route, but it is still not clear whether immunity could be induced by a regimen which is likely to prove feasible in the field.

Oral administration of various forms of toxin antigen (formol toxoid, choleragenoid, and procholeragenoid), even in a single dose, was found by Fujita and Finkelstein (1972) to generate effective intestinal immunity (as well as a humoral antibody response) in mice, although the amounts of antigen required were somewhat larger than those which produced immunity following parenteral aministration. More recently, however, Pierce and Gowans (1975) have found that, in rats, the most effective response was elicited by parenteral priming followed by peroral boosting: perorally administered antigen by itself was relatively ineffective. These investigators concluded that the antitoxin-containing cells (ACC), predominantly containing IgA, arise in Peyer's patches or mesenteric lymph nodes and drain into thoracic duct lymph. Subsequent homing of the ACC to the lamina propria was not totally antigen dependent but was significantly influenced by antigen applied in the lumen of the gut.

In rabbits Holmgren *et al.* (1975b) have confirmed the earlier observations of Fujita and Finkelstein (1972) that aggregated forms of toxin antigen produced better immunity than monomeric forms after parenteral administration. These workers showed, in addition, that primary enteral administration of toxin antigen did result in immunity, although multiple doses were needed. Protection following enteral antigen was mediated by locally synthesized antibodies, whereas both serum-derived and locally produced antibodies appeared to be involved after parenteral immunization. The potential protective effect of serum IgG antitoxin was confirmed by Pierce and Reynolds (1974) in passive protection studies in dogs.

Most of the reported experimental studies on immunization with cholera antigens have dealt with responses to isolated antigens, i.e., either somatic antigen preparations of one kind or another or with toxin antigen in various forms, although it is widely recognized that ultimately effective immunity to cholera may best be attained using combinations of the two. Evidence that this may well be the case has been provided most recently by Svennerholm and Holmgren (1976), who showed that subcutaneous immunization of rabbits with a combination of LPS and enterotoxin induced a hundredfold higher degree of protection against intestinal challenge with live cholera vibrios than that attained with either antigen separately. The synergistic effect was apparently not attributable to the adjuvant action of either antigen but rather to the interference, by immunization, with two separate events in the pathogenesis of cholera, i.e., colonization and the action of the enterotoxin.

Immune response kinetics at the cellular level, using vibriolytic and hemolytic plaque assays, were studied by Kateley *et al.* (1974). These workers found that specific antitoxin-producing plaque cells, synthesizing immunoglobulin of the IgM, IgG1, IgG2a, IgG2b, and IgA classes, were produced following parenteral administrations of antigen in mice. The absence of a background of antibody-producing cells in normal mice indicates that the system should be particularly useful in further studies of the cellular aspects of the immune response.

6. Mechanisms of Immunity against Cholera

The observations reviewed in the previous section strongly suggest that immunity against cholera is mediated by antibacterial or by antitoxic antibodies (or by both). In both instances, circulating antibodies, as well as locally produced antibodies appear to be able to result in protection. It is, however, not yet clear which route of immunization and what kind of antigen preparation are most desirable to protect humans against cholera. The most effective immunity is that generated by the actual disease itself in which all components can be involved, i.e., both humoral and local antibodies against both the bacteria and their toxin. The question then arises as to the means with which these antibodies exert their protective effect at the surface of the intestinal epithelium.

Antibodies of the major immunoglobulin classes against both the bacteria and the toxin have been found in the gut contents by Northrup and Hossain (1970), Waldman et al. (1972), Waldman and Ganguly (1974), and Pierce and Reynolds (1975). Waldman and Ganguly (1974) concluded that local cell-mediated immunity (CMI) could play a role in protection and immunity on mucosal surfaces. This, immune effector system, especially with regard to the gut, has not been sufficiently studied to permit firm conclusions, although it seems quite unlikely that CMI could play a major role.

With regard to the mode of action of the protective effect in antitoxic immunity, it has been demonstrated that, once bound to host cells, the toxin is no longer neutralizable by antibody (Mosley and Ahmed, 1969). It would thus appear that the primary protective effect of antitoxic antibody must be to prevent the toxin from interacting with the epithelial cell surface. Secretory immunoglobulin (sIgA), the major immunoglobulin in intestinal secretions, has been shown to function in prevention of entry of antigen (Stokes et al., 1975). The inability of sIgA to fix complement by the conventional pathway would not be a deterrent to toxin neutralization by binding and prevention of interaction with host membrane receptors. Although its quantity and relative resistance to proteolytic digestion would suggest the primary importance of sIgA, antibody of other subclasses, when present, could also function in the same way. Anti-vibrio sIgA could also function in preventing attachment and promoting clearance of the vibrios, as will be discussed below. It is interesting to note that antitoxic immunity in the gut appears to be more effective against challenges with live vibrios than it is against the toxin itself (Finkelstein,

1970a). This is probably because, in the more natural challenges with live vibrios, the immune mechanisms have to deal with only small amounts of toxin released gradually by the growing vibrios, whereas a bolus of toxin may be more difficult to handle.

The mechanisms involved in antibacterial immunity are apparently more complex. Freter and his associates (Freter, 1969, 1970, 1972, 1974; Fubara and Freter, 1972a) performed the pioneer work on the protective role of "coproantibody," defined as "antibody present on the mucosal surface, or in the lumen of the intestine, regardless of immunoglobulin class, origin or function of such antibody." Initially (see Freter, 1969) it was found that in rabbits which were protected by antibacterial immunization (passive or active) against intraintestinal challenge with living vibrios, multiplication of the vibrios occurred to the same degree in protected and in control ileal loops—the major difference being in the distribution of the vibrios. In immunized loops the vibrios occurred predominantly in the lumen, whereas in control loops a substantial proportion of the vibrio population was associated with the mucosal surface with a degree of firmness that resisted washings.

Subsequent studies provided evidence (1) that there was a direct effect of coproantibody on adsorption of the vibrios to the mucosa and (2) that there is a complement-independent, antibody-dependent antibacterial mechanism on the mucosal surface, apparently dependent on actively metabolizing mucosal cells. Fubara and Freter (1972b) and Steele et al. (1974) have shown that anti-vibrio IgA, containing insignificant amounts of complement-mediated vibriocidal or opsonic activity, had good protective activity in mice and rabbits. Based on further studies on the mechanism of protection, the conclusion was reached that antibody cross-linking was essential to protection and that prevention of adherence and agglutination was probably causally associated with protection (Steele et al., 1975; Bellamy et al., 1975). Whether agglutination per se is involved in resistance to natural cholera in man is somewhat problematical, since it is unlikely that the density of the infecting dose would be such that vibrio–antibody–vibrio interaction would occur. In the experimental systems, larger, more dense inocula were employed. Agglutination of the inoculum, which was mixed with antibody, was observed and could, in effect, have reduced the challenge dose.

7. Cholera Toxin as an Immune Modulator: Effects on Leukocytes, Lymphocytes, and Leukemic cells

In addition to its role as the causative agent of the diarrhea of cholera and its potential role in protective immunity, the cholera enterotoxin has profound experimental effects on a variety of other metabolic events (unrelated to the disease, cholera). This is a result of its unique, specific, and promiscuous ability to interact with the practically ubiquitous G_{M1} ganglioside-containing receptors on the surface of eukaryotic cells and to activate adenylate cyclase leading to increased levels of cyclic $3',5'$-adenosine monophosphate (cAMP). The number of such observations of the effects of cholera enterotoxin in extraintestinal tissues is growing (Finkelstein, 1973, 1976). It has become almost axiomatic that if a certain observed experimental effect is stimulated by cholera toxin then it is a cyclase/cAMP-mediated effect and *vice versa*. Of particular interest are the experimental effects of the cholera toxin on the immunological and inflammatory functions of leukocytes and, consequently, on immunological responsiveness.

Northrup and Fauci (1972) were the first to observe that cholera enterotoxin was a potent immunological adjuvant. Submicrogram to microgram amounts, administered intravenously in mice in conjunction with 10^8 sheep RBCs, increased by more than tenfold (over controls) the number of splenic plaque-forming cells. Subsequently, the toxin was found to have both adjuvant and immunosuppressive effects, dependent on both the time of administration and the dose of toxin employed (Chisari *et al.*, 1974; Kateley *et al.*, 1975). Treatment with toxin before administration of an antigen was immunosuppressive. The secondary immune response to sheep RBC was also affected by cholera toxin. In large doses, however, the toxin can produce severe depletion of lymphoid cells from splenic red pulp, thymic cortical atrophy, and hypercalcemia (Chisari

and Northrup, 1974). Dependent on the amount of antigen, the time sequence, and the dose employed, the *in vitro* anamnestic response to keyhole limpet hemocyanin could be either enhanced or inhibited by cholera toxin or dibutyryl cAMP (Cook *et al.*, 1975). These findings are in agreement with pharmacological evidence suggesting that increased intracellular cAMP triggers differentiation of lymphoid functions and inhibits proliferation. Thus, cholera toxin administered before antigen challenge would be expected to restrict clonal expansion, but toxin given after a proliferation response to antigen challenge would indicate antibody production.

The observed modulations of the immune response appear to depend on the ability of the toxin to interact with both T and B lymphocytes and to increase the production of cAMP. Sultzer and Craig (1973) concluded that the toxin affected both T and B lymphocytes, since it inhibited the mitogenic response (i.e., depressed DNA synthesis) in lymphocytes stimulated with optimal concentrations of either T- or B-cell mitogens. These findings were extended by Hart and Finkelstein (1975), who showed that choleragenoid did not inhibit mitogen stimulation but could block the inhibition caused by choleragen. Thus binding alone is insufficient: the inhibition of the mitogenic effect is dependent on the subsequent activation of adenylate cyclase. Somewhat similar results were reported by Vischer and LoSpalluto (1975), although they observed a greater sensitivity of the phytohemaglutinin (PHA) response to inhibition by choleragen. In the doses employed by the investigators cited above, the cholera toxin did not affect the viability of the cells used, as determined by morphological criteria and Trypan Blue exclusion. Hart (1975a) presented evidence that the lymphocyte receptor is a glycolipid and, further, employed the toxin as a marker to evaluate detergent-induced dissociation of thymocyte and splenocyte plasma membranes (Hart, 1975b). Holmgren *et al.* (1974) also showed that the toxin and choleragenoid inhibited the mitogenic responses of mouse thymocytes and splenocytes to Con A (note: it is not unlikely that the responses observed to high doses of choleragenoid in this and other studies may be due to residual traces of toxin present as a contaminant, although the pos sibility that choleragenoid may be active directly cannot be excluded). These workers also showed that "capping" of toxin-treated thymocytes could be induced, in a small proportion of the cells, by subsequent treatment with antitoxin and fluorescein-labeled antiimmunoglobulin. Specific cap formation of immunoglobulin-bearing cells was, however, not blocked by treatment with choleragen, thus providing additional evidence for the fluid membrane theory. Only the B region of the toxin (called by them the L, or light, subunits) could be demonstrated to bind to thymocytes. Approximately 4×10^4 molecules of toxin or choleragenoid were bound per cell. G_{M1} ganglioside, and to a markedly lesser degree G_{D1a} and G_{A1}, decreased the inhibitory effect of cholera toxin on Con-A-induced thymocyte stimulation.

Révész and Greaves (1975a) have also demonstrated capping of choleragen-treated human and mouse lymphocytes. Human lymphocytes responded over a wide range of concentrations of toxin, but mouse lymphocytes showed capping only at lower choleragen concentrations. This was interpreted to be due to a higher concentration of G_{M1} on mouse lymphocytes. Neuraminidase treatment or G_{M1} insertion (both methods would produce more receptors) decreased the toxin-induced redistribution of the membrane. Capping was also inhibited by colchicine and cytochalasin, suggesting that microfilaments and microtubules play a significant role in membrane molecular mobility. Cells deficient in G_{M1}, such as human acute leukemia cells, become responsive to choleragen after treatment with neuraminidase or by G_{M1} insertion. In contrast, transformed rodent cell lines (BHK and NIL), which are deficient in all gangliosides, bind choleragen only after G_{M1} insertion. These observations have been extended (Révész and Greaves, 1975b; Greaves et al., 1976) as a means of cell surface phenotyping of human leukemias. Generally, malignant transformation is associated with a simplification of membrane glycolipids. The ability to bind cholera toxin, before and after G_{M1} insertion and neuraminidase treatment, can therefore be used to classify leukemic cells. Almost all normal human cells tested, with the exception of normoblasts from cord blood and erythrocytes, have been found to bind cholera toxin. On the other hand, none of the leukemic cells from 17 cases of acute lymphoblastic leukemia bound cholera toxin; all chronic myeloid leukemic cells tested had toxin receptors, except in blast crisis. Other types of leukemias had varied abilities to bind cholera toxin. The results have important implications on the mechanisms of malignant transformation and expression. It is of some interest to mention that choleragenoid has been demonstrated to sensitize transformed cells to "targeted immune lysis" mediated by anticholeragenoid and complement (Forman and Finkelstein, 1977).

In part based on observations on the effects of cholera toxin on the immune response, Bourne et al. (1974) have hypothesized that "certain vasoactive hormones, mediators of inflammation and cyclic AMP serve to protect the host from the dangerous consequences of an unregulated immune response. This regulation is mediated by a general inhibitory action of cyclic AMP on immunologic and inflammatory functions of leukocytes." The parallel inhibitory effects of histamine, β-catecholamines, prostaglandins, cAMP, and cholera toxin on effector cell functions, such as histamine release from basophils and mast cells, release of lysosomal hydrolases, immune cytolysis, and sheep erythrocyte plaque formation, were summarized by these workers. Additionally, it has been observed that cholera toxin inhibits the cell-mediated responses involved in the pathogenesis of experimental schistosomiasis, prolongs allograft survival in mice, and eliminates foreign body granuloma formation around plastic beads (Warren et al., 1974). The cholera toxin thus appears to be the most potent and long-acting inhibitor of cell-mediated immunity yet described.

Cholera toxin has been recently observed to depress in vitro production of IgE by peripheral blood lymphocytes of two human donors with elevated serum IgE concentrations (Patterson et al., 1976). It has also been found to inhibit the chemotactic responsiveness of rabbit peritoneal neutrophils to a chemotactic factor from Escherichia coli (Rivkin et al., 1975). The latter effect was blocked by choleragenoid. The toxin apparently inhibited the expression of Fc receptor activity, as manifested by decreased rosette formation following the addition of sensitized erythrocytes to murine myeloma cells. However, thousand-fold larger doses of toxin were required for this effect than were required to increase cAMP levels (Zuckerman and Douglas, 1975). In the absence of a control with choleragenoid (the authors used glutaraldehyde toxoid, which does not bind), it is not clear whether the observed inhibition was related to activation of cyclase or simply to a steric hindrance caused by the toxin bound to the surface of the lymphocytes.

Although it is clear that the cholera enterotoxin is a potent modulator of immune responsiveness under defined experimental conditions, there is no information as to whether any of these effects occur in cholera patients. As discussed above, cholera patients exhibit conventional responses to cholera antigens during the disease process and into recovery. In view of the absence of systemic metabolic effects, other than those attributable to the dehydration and electrolyte imbalance, it seems clear that little, if any, active toxin is absorbed. Thus, if the toxin serves as an immune modulator during the disease, it must be at the local level. Judging from the respectable antibody responses observed during cholera, the immune modulating effects, if any, must be more to the adjuvant than to the immunosuppressive side. It might be of some interest to compare the responsiveness of cholera patients and appropriate controls to exogenous antigen(s) administered *per os* and systemically.

8. Prospects for the Future

It is apparent from much of the information cited above that conventional approaches to immunization against cholera have fallen short of their goals of providing effective and durable immunity. The most promising observations are those generated by the experimental study of Svennerholm and Holmgren (1976), which demonstrated that a combination of antitoxic and antibacterial immunity exerted a significant synergistic protective effect in rabbits, and the study of Cash *et al.* (1974a) in volunteers, which demonstrated that recovery from an attack of induced cholera resulted in immunity against homologous challenge for at least a year. The latter illustrates the effectiveness of what is essentially a locally stimulated immune response combining antitoxic and antibacterial elements. To these should be added the widely documented observations that antibody to the choleragenoid or B region of the toxin molecule effectively neutralizes the toxin and protects against experimental cholera and that anticholeragenoid also effectively neutralizes the heat-labile enterotoxins of *E. coli* and the so-called nonagglutinable vibrios, as well as an enterotoxinlike factor of *Salmonella* (Sandefur and Peterson, 1977).

The message which appears to emerge from these considerations is that the most effective means of stimulating immunity against cholera will be a form of local immunization, simulating that induced by the disease itself, and combining both antibacterial and antitoxic effects. This can best be obtained (as experience with poliovirus vaccine suggests) by the use of a living attenuated mutant, one which will replicate and colonize the small bowel and which, at the same time, will secrete a nontoxic antigen sufficiently similar to the cholera enterotoxin to generate an effective local antitoxic response as well as a local antibacterial response. Theoretically, a mutant cholera vibrio, which produces choleragenoid without the A region of the cholera toxin or choleragenoid with a functionally altered A region (preferably a genetically stable deletion or missense mutant), such that it can no longer activate cyclase and hence is no longer toxic, would be ideal. Such a mutant might also be expected to generate some degree of resistance to the other enterotoxic enteropathies which depend on enterotoxins immunologically related to the cholera enterotoxin and which are far more important than cholera as causes of morbidity and mortality in the world. Unfortunately, such a mutant has not yet been generated, although some encouraging progress has been made.

Following nitrosoguanidine mutagenesis of the highly toxinogenic, virulent parent strain *V. cholerae* 569B Inaba, a mutant, M13, was isolated. This mutant failed to produce cholera toxin in amounts detectable by the usual biological and immunological tests and was completely avirulent after repeated serial passages in experimental animal models (Finkelstein *et al.*, 1974b; Vasil *et al.*, 1974; Holmes *et al.*, 1975). Unlike previously described adventitiously isolated avirulent forms (Sanyal and Mukerjee, 1969), M13 was prototrophic like the wild-type parent and extensively colonized adult rabbit ileal loops and the intestinal tract of infant rabbits. This mutant was fed to volunteers, in doses of 10^{10} viable organisms after appropriate alkalinization of the stomach, and failed to cause symptoms of cholera in any individual (Woodward *et al.*, 1975, 1976). The volunteers who had been infected with M13 were found to be significantly resistant to subsequent challenge with the virulent parent strain. Unfortunately, however, even though none of the volunteers manifested any symptoms of cholera or other untoward effects following infection with M13, an isolate from one of the subjects appeared, in subsequent laboratory tests, to have regained the capacity to elaborate enterotoxin in significant amounts. Although, at that time, no additional genetic markers had been introduced in M13 to establish unequivocally that reversion had occurred, it must be presumed that M13 is unstable and therefore is unsuitable for larger scale studies in human beings. Nevertheless, the study established that it is feasible to induce effective immunity in man through infection with an avirulent mutant. This mutant, it should be recalled, was short of the theoretical ideal in that it did not elaborate significant amounts of toxin antigen. Attempts to generate a mutant that will produce nontoxic cross-reactive material (CRM) are currently in progress in our laboratory.*

* Honda and Finkelstein (1979) have isolated a mutant, Texas Star-SR, from a hypertoxinogenic strain of *V. cholerae*, serotype Ogawa, biotype El Tor, which fails to produce any detectable A (*active*, ADP-ribosylating) portion of the cholera enterotoxin but which produces the highly immunogenic B (*binding*, or choleragenoid) region in amounts similar to those of the wild-type parent. As predicted, this mutant was avirulent in laboratory animal models, in which it was shown to colonize from relatively small inocula. Chinchillas infected enterally with Texas Star-SR were shown to develop resistance to subsequent intraintestinal challenge with virulent wild-type cholera vibrios. It is not yet clear whether the immunity is antibacterial, anticolonizing, or antitoxic, or results from a combination of these factors. However, antiserum prepared from the toxin-related protein isolated from cultures of the mutant was found to neutralize both cholera and *E. coli* enterotoxins to similar high titers. Because of previous information indicating that the disease cholera is itself an immunizing process, and that an avirulent hypotoxinogenic mutant, M13, elicited immunity in volunteers, it may be expected

Inasmuch as some studies cited above have suggested that antivibrio immunity may be predominantly serotype specific, it may be necessary to generate CRM mutants of both Inaba and Ogawa serotypes (or a CRM mutant of one serotype and a stable *tox⁻* mutant of the other) for the highest degree of protection against cholera. Such mutants could have advantages in addition to their ability to stimulate directly immunity against cholera (and related enteropathies). Conceivably, by occupying the ecological niche of the small bowel, they could prevent superinfection by virulent strains. By virtue of the poor sanitation in the cholera-receptive areas of the world, such mutants could also disseminate from person to person and might therefore be able to induce some degree of "communicable herd immunity." It is hoped that such a mutant will be available for preliminary studies in man in the near future.

ACKNOWLEDGMENTS

Studies in the author's laboratory cited herein were supported in large measure by Grant AI-08877 from the U.S. Public Health Service under the United States–Japan Cooperative Medical Science Program administered by the National Institute of Allergy and Infectious Diseases. The author is also grateful for the participation of his collaborators and associates and is especially grateful to Mrs. Sara Leary for her superb secretarial contributions.

The literature survey for this chapter was completed, and the chapter submitted, in September 1976.

References

Ahmed, A., Bhattacharjee, A. K., and Mosley, W. H., 1970, Characteristics of the serum vibriocidal and ag-

that Texas Star-SR will also generate effective immunity against cholera. If a substantial local antitoxic response is generated, the mutant may also stimulate resistance to immunologically related enterotoxic enteropathies, such as diarrhea due to LT-producing *E. coli*. The structural and immunological relatedness of *E. coli* LT to choleragen has recently been demonstrated (Clements and Finkelstein, 1979).

glutinating antibodies in cholera cases and in normal residents of the endemic and non-endemic cholera areas, *J. Immunol.* 105:431–441.

Aldova, E., Laznickova, K., Stepankova, E., and Lietava, J., 1968, Isolation of nonagglutinable vibrios from an enteritis outbreak in Czechoslovakia, *J. Infect. Dis.* 118:25–31.

Armstrong, I. L., and Redmond, J. W., 1974, The fatty acids present in the lipopolysaccharide of *Vibrio cholerae* 569B (Inaba), *Biochim. Biophys. Acta* 348:302–305.

Azurin, J. C., 1973, Different aspects of cholera in the Philippines, in: *Proceedings of the 8th Joint Conference, U.S.–Japan Cooperative Medical Science Program, Cholera Panel: Advances in Research on Cholera and Related Diseases, Tokyo, August 22–23, 1972, and Round Table Discussions on International Quarantine Against Cholera, Kumamoto, August 20, 1972,* pp. 230–234, Japanese Cholera Panel, National Institute of Health, Tokyo.

Azurin, J. C., Kobari, K., Barua, D., Alvero, M., Gomez, C. Z., Dizon, J. J., Nakano, E., Suplido, R., and Ledesma, L., 1967, Long-term carrier of cholera: Cholera Dolores, *Bull. WHO* 37:745–749.

Bart, K. J., Huq, Z., Khan, M., and Mosley, W. H., 1970, Seroepidemiologic studies during a simultaneous epidemic of infection with El Tor Ogawa and classical Inaba *Vibrio cholerae, J. Infect. Dis.* 121(Suppl.): S17–S24.

Barua, D., and Watanabe, Y., 1972, Vibriocidal antibodies induced by *Yersinia enterocolitica* serotype IX, *J. Hyg. (Camb.)* 70:161–169.

Barua, D., Wake, A., Gomez, C. Z., Paguio, A., Azurin, J. C., Dizon, J. J., Ramos, R., and Cordova, V., 1967, Some observations on the detection of cholera carriers, *Bull. WHO* 37:804–806.

Basaca-Sevilla, V., Pesigan, T. P., and Finkelstein, R. A., 1964, Observations on serological responses to cholera immunizations, *Am. J. Trop. Med. Hyg.* 13:100–107.

Bellamy, J. E. C., Knop, J., Steele, E. J., Chaicumpa, W., and Rowley, D., 1975, Antibody cross-linking as a factor in immunity to cholera in infant mice, *J. Infect. Dis.* 132:181–188.

Benenson, A. S., Islam, M. R., and Greenough, W. B., III, 1964, Rapid identification of *Vibrio cholerae* by darkfield microscopy, *Bull. WHO* 30:827–831.

Benenson, A. S., Saad, A., and Mosley, W. H., 1968a, Serological studies in cholera. 2. The vibriocidal antibody response of cholera patients determined by a microtechnique, *Bull. WHO* 38:277–285.

Benenson, A. S., Mosley, W. H., Fahimuddin, M., and Oseasohn, R. O., 1968b, Cholera vaccine field trials in East Pakistan. 2. Effectiveness in the field, *Bull. WHO* 38:359–372.

Benyajati, C., 1966, Experimental cholera in humans, *Br. Med. J.* 1966(1):140–142.

Bhaskaran, K., 1974, Vibrio genetics, in: *Cholera* (D. Barua and W. Burrows, eds.), pp. 41–59, Saunders, Philadelphia.

Bourne, H. R., Lichtenstein, L. M., Melmon, K. L., Henney, C. S., Weinstein, Y., and Shearer, G. M., 1974, Modulation of inflammation and immunity by cyclic AMP, *Science* 184:19–28.

Burnet, F. M., and Stone, J. D., 1947, Desquamation of intestinal epithelium in vitro by *V. cholerae* filtrates: Characterization of mucinase and tissue disintegrating enzymes, *Aust. J. Exp. Biol. Med. Sci.* 25:219–226.

Burrows, W., Mather, A. N., McGann, V. G., and Wagner, S. M., 1946, Studies on immunity to Asiatic cholera. II. The O and H antigenic structure of the cholera and related vibrios, *J. Infect. Dis.* 79:168–197.

Cash, R. A., Music, S. I., Libonati, J. P., Craig, J. P., Pierce, N. F., and Hornick, R. B., 1974a, Response of man to infection with *Vibrio cholerae*. II. Protection from illness afforded by previous disease and vaccine, *J. Infect. Dis.* 130:325–333.

Cash, R. A., Music, S. I., Libonati, J. P., Schwartz, A. R., and Hornick, R. B., 1974b, Live oral cholera vaccine: Evaluation of the clinical effectiveness of two strains in humans, *Infect. Immun.* 10:762–764.

Chisari, F. V., and Northrup, R. S., 1974, Pathophysiologic effects of lethal and immunoregulatory doses of cholera enterotoxin in the mouse, *J. Immunol.* 113:740–749.

Chisari, F. V., Northrup, R. S., and Chen, L. C., 1974, The modulating effect of cholera enterotoxin on the immune response, *J. Immunol.* 113:729–739.

Citarella, R. V., and Colwell, R. R., 1970, Polyphasic taxonomy of the genus *Vibrio*: Polynucleotide sequence relationships among selected *Vibrio* species, *J. Bacteriol.* 104:434–442.

Clements, J. D., and Finkelstein, R. A., 1979, Isolation and characterization of homogenous heat-labile enterotoxins with high specific activity from *Escherichia coli* cultures, *Infect. Immun.* 24:760–769.

Colwell, R. R., 1970, Polyphasic taxonomy of the genus *Vibrio*: Numerical taxonomy of *Vibrio cholerae, Vibrio parahaemolyticus*, and related *Vibrio* species, *J. Bacteriol.* 104:410–433.

Cook, R. G., Stavitsky, A. B., and Schoenberg, M. D., 1975, Regulation of the *in vitro* early anamnestic antibody response by exogenous cholera enterotoxin and cyclic AMP, *J. Immunol.* 114:426–434.

Craig, J. P., 1971, Cholera toxins, in: *Microbial Toxins*, Vol. IIA (S. Kadis, T. C. Montie, and S. J. Ajl, eds.), pp. 189–254. Academic Press, New York.

Cuatrecasas, P., 1973, Gangliosides and membrane receptors for cholera toxin, *Biochemistry* 12:3558–3566.

Curlin, G., 1975a, Current progress in the cholera toxoid field trial in Bangladesh, in: *Proceedings of the 10th Joint Conference, U.S.–Japan Cooperative Medical Science Program, Cholera Panel: Symposium on Cholera, Kyoto, 1974* (H. Fukumi and M. Ohashi, eds.), pp. 98–102, Japanese Cholera Panel, National Institute of Health, Tokyo.

Curlin, G., 1975b, Cholera toxoid field trial, in: *Abstracts [of the] 11th Joint Conference on Cholera, The*

U.S.–Japan Cooperative Medical Science Program, New Orleans, La., Nov. 4, 5, 6, 1975, pp. 41–42, US DHEW, Public Health Service, NIH, Washington, D.C.

Cvjetanović, B., 1965, Earlier field studies of the effectiveness of cholera vaccines, in: *Proceedings of the Cholera Research Symposium, Jan. 24–29, 1965, Honolulu, Hawaii* (U.S. Public Health Service Publ. No. 1328), pp. 355–361, U.S. Government Printing Office, Washington, D.C.

Cvjetanović, B., 1974, Economic considerations in cholera control, in: *Cholera* (D. Barua and W. Burrows, eds.), pp. 435–445, Saunders, Philadelphia.

De, S. N., and Chatterje, D. N., 1953, An experimental study of the mechanism of action of *Vibrio cholerae* on the intestinal mucous membrane, *J. Pathol. Bacteriol.* **66:**559–562.

Deb, B. C., Sinha, R., and Shrivastava, D. L., 1969, Vibriocidal antibody titrations: A comparison of three methods, *Indian J. Med. Res.* **57:**167–174.

Dixon, J. M. S., 1960, The fate of bacteria in the small intestine, *J. Pathol. Bacteriol.* **79:**131–140.

Dorland, W. A. N., 1974, Choleragen, in: *Illustrated Medical Dictionary* (25th ed.), p. 308, Saunders, Philadelphia.

Eisenstein, T. K., 1975, Evidence for O antigens as the antigenic determinants in "ribosomal" vaccines prepared from *Salmonella, Infect. Immun.* **12:**364–377.

Eubanks, E. R., Guentzel, M. N., and Berry, L. J., 1976, Virulence factors involved in the intraperitoneal infection of adult mice with *Vibrio cholerae, Infect. Immun.* **13:**457–463.

Evans, D. J., Jr., Chen, L. C., Curlin, G. T., and Evans, D. G., 1972, Stimulation of adenyl cyclase by *Escherichia coli* enterotoxin, *Nature (London), New Biol.* **236:**137–138.

Feeley, J. C., 1965, Comparison of vibriocidal and agglutinating antibody responses in cholera patients, in: *Proceedings of the Cholera Research Symposium, Jan. 24–29, 1965, Honolulu, Hawaii* (U.S. Public Health Service Publ. No. 1328), pp. 220–222, U.S. Government Printing Office, Washington, D.C.

Feeley, J. C., 1969, Somatic O antigen relationship of *Brucella* and *Vibrio cholerae, J. Bacteriol.* **99:**645–649.

Feeley, J. C., 1974, Antitoxic immunity in cholera, in: *Cholera* (D. Barua and W. Burrows, eds.), pp. 307–314, Saunders, Philadelphia.

Felsenfeld, O., 1974, The survival of cholera vibrios, in: *Cholera* (D. Barua and W. Burrows, eds.), pp. 359–366, Saunders, Philadelphia.

Finkelstein, R. A., 1962, Vibriocidal antibody inhibition (VAI) analysis: A technique for the identification of the predominant vibriocidal antibodies in serum and for the recognition and identification of *Vibrio cholerae* antigens, *J. Immunol.* **89:**264–271.

Finkelstein, R. A., 1964, Observations on mode of action of endotoxin in chick embryos, *Proc. Soc. Exp. Biol. Med.* **115:**702–707.

Finkelstein, R. A., 1965, Observations on the nature and mode of action of the choleragenic product(s) of cholera vibrios, in: *Proceedings of the Cholera Research Symposium, Jan. 24–29, 1965, Honolulu, Hawaii* (U.S. Public Health Service Publ. No. 1328), pp. 264–270, U.S. Government Printing Office, Washington, D.C.

Finkelstein, R. A., 1969, The role of choleragen in the pathogenesis and immunology of cholera, *Tex. Rep. Biol. Med.* **27:**181–201 (Suppl. 1).

Finkelstein, R. A., 1970a, Antitoxic immunity in experimental cholera: Observations with purified antigens and the ligated ileal loop model, *Infect. Immun.* **1:**464–467.

Finkelstein, R. A., 1970b, Monospecific equine antiserum against cholera exo-enterotoxin, *Infect. Immun.* **2:**691–697.

Finkelstein, R. A., 1973, Cholera, *CRC Crit. Rev. Microbiol.* **2:**553–623.

Finkelstein, R. A., 1975, Immunology of cholera, *Curr. Top. Microbiol. Immunol.* **69:**137–196.

Finkelstein, R. A., 1976, Progress in the study of cholera and related enterotoxins, in: *Selected Topics in Bacterial Toxinology* (A. Bernheimer, ed.), pp. 53–84, Wiley, New York.

Finkelstein, R. A., and Atthasampunna, P., 1967, Immunity against experimental cholera, *Proc. Soc. Exp. Biol. Med.* **125:**465–469.

Finkelstein, R. A., and LoSpalluto, J. J., 1969, Pathogenesis of experimental cholera: Preparation and isolation of choleragen and choleragenoid, *J. Exp. Med.* **130:**185–202.

Finkelstein, R. A., and LoSpalluto, J. J., 1970, Preparation of highly purified choleragen and choleragenoid, *J. Infect. Dis. Suppl.* **121:**S63–S72.

Finkelstein, R. A., and Mukerjee, S., 1963, Hemagglutination: A rapid method for differentiating *Vibrio cholerae* and El Tor vibrios, *Proc. Soc. Exp. Biol. Med.* **112:**355–359.

Finkelstein, R. A., and Pongpairojana, S., 1968, A test of antigenicity for the selection of strains for inclusion in cholera vaccines, *Bull. WHO* **39:**247–259.

Finkelstein, R. A., Norris, H. T., and Dutta, N. K., 1964, Pathogenesis of experimental cholera in infant rabbits. I. Observations on the intraintestinal infection and experimental cholera produced with cell-free products, *J. Infect. Dis.* **114:**203–216.

Finkelstein, R. A., Powell, C. J., Jr., Woodrow, J. C., and Krevans, J. R., 1965, Serological responses in man to a single small dose of cholera vaccine with special reference to the lack of influence of ABO blood group on natural antibody or immunological responsiveness, *Bull. Johns Hopkins Hosp.* **116:**152–160.

Finkelstein, R. A., Atthasampunna, P., Chulasamaya, M., and Charunmethee, P., 1966, Pathogenesis of experimental cholera: Biologic activities of purified procholeragen A, *J. Immunol.* **96:**440–449.

Finkelstein, R. A., Peterson, J. W., and LoSpalluto, J. J., 1971a, Conversion of cholera exo-enterotoxin (choleragen) to natural toxoid (choleragenoid), *J. Immunol.* **106:**868–871.

Finkelstein, R. A., Fujita, K., and LoSpalluto, J. J., 1971b, Procholeragenoid: An aggregated intermediate in the formation of choleragenoid, *J. Immunol.* 107:1043–1051.

Finkelstein, R. A., Boesman, M., Neoh, S. H., LaRue, M. K., and Delaney, R., 1974a, Dissociation and recombination of the subunits of the cholera enterotoxin (choleragen), *J. Immunol.* 113:145–150.

Finkelstein, R. A., Vasil, M. L., and Holmes, R. K., 1974b, Studies on toxinogenesis in *Vibrio cholerae*. I. Isolation of mutants with altered toxinogenicity, *J. Infect. Dis.* 129:117–123.

Finkelstein, R. A., Vasil, M. L., Jones, J. R., Anderson, R. A., and Barnard, T., 1976, "Clinical cholera" caused by enterotoxigenic *Escherichia coli, J. Clin. Microbiol.* 3:382–384.

Florey, H. W., 1933, Observations on the functions of mucus and the early stages of bacterial invasion of the intestinal mucosa, *J. Pathol. Bacteriol.* 37:283–298.

Follett, E. A. C., and Gordon, J., 1963, An electron microscope study of vibrio flagella, *J. Gen. Microbiol.* 32:235–239.

Forman, J., and Finkelstein, R. A., 1977, Inability of choleragenoid-sensitized cells to induce T-cell-mediated cytolysis, *J. Immunol.* 118:1655–1658.

Freter, R., 1969, Studies of the mechanism of action of intestinal antibody in experimental cholera, *Tex. Rep. Biol. Med.* 27(Suppl. 1):299–316.

Freter, R., 1970, Mechanism of action of intestinal antibody in experimental cholera. II. Antibody-mediated antibacterial reaction at the mucosal surface, *Infect. Immun.* 2:556–562.

Freter, R., 1972, Parameters affecting the association of vibrios with the intestinal surface in experimental cholera, *Infect. Immun.* 6:134–141.

Freter, R., 1974, Gut-associated immunity to cholera, in: *Cholera* (D. Barua and W. Burrows, eds.), pp. 315–331, Saunders, Philadelphia.

Freter, R., and Gangarosa, E. J., 1963, Oral immunization and production of coproantibody in human volunteers, *J. Immunol.* 91:724–729.

Fubara, E. S., and Freter, R., 1972a, Availability of locally synthesized and systemic antibodies in the intestine, *Infect. Immun.* 6:965–981.

Fubara, E. S., and Freter, R., 1972b, Source and protective function of coproantibodies in intestinal disease, *Am. J. Clin. Nutr.* 25:1357–1363.

Fujita, K., and Finkelstein, R. A., 1972, Antitoxic immunity in experimental cholera: Comparison of immunity induced perorally and parenterally in mice, *J. Infect. Dis.* 125:647–655.

Gan, K. H., and Tjia, S. K., 1963, A new method for the differentiation of *Vibrio comma* and *Vibrio* El Tor, *Am. J. Hyg.* 77:184–186.

Gangarosa, E. J., Beisel, W. R., Benyajati, C., Sprinz, H., and Piyaratn, P., 1960, The nature of gastrointestinal lesion in Asiatic cholera and its relation to pathogenesis: A biopsy study, *Am. J. Trop. Med. Hyg.* 9:125–135.

Gangarosa, E. J., DeWitt, W. E., Feeley, J. C., and Adams, M. R., 1970, Significance of vibriocidal antibodies with regard to immunity in cholera, *J. Infect. Dis. Suppl.* 121:S36–S43.

Ganguly, R., Clem, L. W., Benčič, Z., Sinha, R., Sakazaki, R., and Waldman, R. H., 1975, Antibody response in the intestinal secretions of volunteers immunized with various cholera vaccines, *Bull. WHO* 52:323–330.

Germanier, R., Fürer, E., Varallyay, S., and Inderbitzen, T. M., 1976, Preparation of a purified antigenic cholera toxoid, *Infect. Immun.* 13:1692–1698.

Gill, D. M., 1975, Involvement of nicotinamide adenine dinucleotide in the action of cholera toxin *in vitro, Proc. Natl. Acad. Sci. USA* 72:2064–2068.

Gill, D. M., 1976, The arrangement of subunits in cholera toxin, *Biochemistry* 15:1242–1248.

Gill, D. M., and King, C. A., 1975, The mechanism of action of cholera toxin in pigeon erythrocyte lysates, *J. Biol. Chem.* 250:6424–6432.

Greaves, M., Capellaro, D., Brown, G., Révész, T., Janossy, G., Lister, Beard, M., Rapson, N., and Catovsky, D., 1976, Analysis of human leukaemic cells using cell surface binding probes and the fluorescence activated cell sorter, in: *Modern Trends in Human Leukaemia II* (R. Neth, R. C. Gallo, K. Mannweiler, and W. C. Moloney, eds.), pp. 243–260, Suppl. *Hämatologie und Bluttransfusion,* Vol. 19, J. F. Lehmanns Verlag, München.

Greenough, W. B., III, Benenson, A. S., and Islam, M. R., 1965, Experience in darkfield examination of stools from diarrheal patients, in: *Proceedings of the Cholera Research Symposium, Jan. 24–29, 1965, Honolulu, Hawaii* (U.S. Public Health Service Publ. No. 1328), pp. 56–58, U.S. Government Printing Office, Washington, D.C.

Guentzel, M. N., and Berry, L. J., 1974, Protection of suckling mice from experimental cholera by maternal immunization: Comparison of the efficacy of whole-cell, ribosomal-derived, and enterotoxin immunogens, *Infect. Immun.* 10:167–172.

Guentzel, M. N., and Berry, L. J., 1975, Motility as a virulence factor for *Vibrio cholerae, Infect. Immunity* 11:890–897.

Hart, D. A., 1975a, Evidence for the non-protein nature of the receptor for the enterotoxin of *Vibrio cholerae* on murine lymphoid cells, *Infect. Immun.* 11:742–747.

Hart, D. A., 1975b, Studies on nonidet P_{40} lysis of murine lymphoid cells. I. Use of cholera toxin and cell surface Ig to determine degree of dissociation of the plasma membrane, *J. Immunol.* 115:871–875.

Hart, D. A., and Finkelstein, R. A., 1975, Inhibition of mitogen stimulation of human peripheral blood leukocytes by *Vibrio cholerae* enterotoxin, *J. Immunol.* 114:476–480.

Hirschhorn, N., Pierce, N. F., Kobari, K., and Carpenter, C. C. J., Jr., 1974, The treatment of cholera, in: *Cholera* (D. Barua and W. Burrows, eds.), pp. 235–252, Saunders, Philadelphia.

Hisatsune, K., Kondo, S., Kawata, T., Zinnaka, Y., Fu-koyoshi, S., and Takeya, K., 1974, Studies on the cell walls of *Vibrio cholerae*: Isolation and characterization of the outer membranes and lipopolysaccharide of NAG vibrio 4715, in: *Proceedings of the Ninth Joint Cholera Research Conference, U.S.–Japan Cooperative Med. Sci. Program, Geographic Med. Branch, NIAID, NIH, Grand Canyon, Arizona, Oct. 1–3, 1973* (Department of State Publ. 8762, East Asian and Pacific Series 211), pp. 111–123, U.S. Department of State, Washington, D.C.

Hisatsune, K., Kondo, S., Kawata, T., Takeya, K., and Kishimoto, Y., 1975, Studies on the cell walls of *Vibrio cholerae*: Fatty acid composition of the lipopolysac-charides, in: *Proceedings of the 10th Joint Conference, U.S.–Japan Cooperative Medical Science Program, Cholera Panel: Symposium on Cholera, Kyoto, 1974* (H. Fukumi and M. Ohashi, eds.), pp. 45–51, Japanese Cholera Panel, National Institute of Health, Tokyo.

Hollenberg, M. D., Fishman, P. H., Bennett, V., and Cuatrecasas, P., 1974, Cholera toxin and cell growth: Role of membrane gangliosides, *Proc. Natl. Acad. Sci. USA* **71:**4224–4228.

Holmes, R. K., Vasil, M. L., and Finkelstein, R. A., 1975, Studies on toxinogenesis in *Vibrio cholerae*. III. Characterization of nontoxinogenic mutants in vitro and in experimental models, *J. Clin. Invest.* **55:**551–560.

Holmgren, J., 1973, Experimental studies on cholera immunisation: The protective immunogenicity in rabbits of monomeric and polymeric crude exotoxin, *J. Med. Microbiol.* **6:**363–370.

Holmgren, J., Svennerholm, A.-M., and Ouchterlony, Ö., 1971, Quantitation of vibriocidal antibodies using agar plaque techniques, *Acta Pathol. Microbiol. Scan. Sect. B.* **79:**708–714.

Holmgren, J., Lindholm, L., and Lönnroth, I., 1974, Interaction of cholera toxin and toxin derivatives with lymphocytes. I. Binding properties and interference with lectin-induced cellular stimulation, *J. Exp. Med.* **139:**801–819.

Holmgren, J., Lönnroth, I., Månsson, J.-E., and Svennerholm, L., 1975a, Interaction of cholera toxin and membrane G_{M1} ganglioside of small intestine, *Proc. Natl. Acad. Sci. USA* **72:**2520–2524.

Holmgren, J., Svennerholm, A.-M., Ouchterlony, Ö., Andersson, Å., Wallerström, G., and Westerberg-Berndtsson, U., 1975b, Antitoxic immunity in experimental cholera: Protection, and serum and local antibody responses in rabbits after enteral and parenteral immunization, *Infect. Immun.* **12:**1331–1340.

Honda, T., and Finkelstein, R. A., 1979, Selection and characterization of a *Vibrio cholerae* mutant lacking the A (ADP-ribosylating) portion of the cholera enterotoxin, *Proc. Natl. Acad. Sci. USA* **76:**2052–2056.

Hornick, R. B., Music, S. I., Libonati, J. P., Snyder, M. J., Woodward, T. E., 1972, Cholera in volunteers, in: *Proceedings of the 7th Joint Conference, U.S.–Japan Cooperative Medical Science Program, Cholera Panel:*

Symposium on Cholera, Woods Hole, Mass., Aug. 9–11, 1971, pp. 37–38, National Institute of Health, Tokyo.

International Committee on Nomenclature of Bacteria, Subcommittee on Taxonomy of Vibrios, 1972, Report (1966–1970) of the Subcommittee on Taxonomy of Vibrios to the International Committee on Nomenclature of Bacteria, *Int. J. Syst. Bacteriol.* **22:**123.

Isselbacher, K. J., 1975, The intestinal cell surface: Properties of normal, undifferentiated, and malignant cells, in: *The Harvey Lectures, Delivered under the Auspices of the Harvey Society of New York, 1973–1974* (Series 69), pp. 197–221, Academic Press, New York.

Jackson, G. D. F., and Redmond, J. W., 1971, Immunochemical studies of the O-antigens of *Vibrio cholerae*: The constitution of a lipopolysaccharide from *V. cholerae* 569B (Inaba), *FEBS Lett.* **13:**117–120.

Jann, B., Jann, K., and Beyaert, G. O., 1973, 2-Amino-2,6-dideoxy-D-glucose (D-quinovosamine): A constituent of the lipopolysaccharides of *Vibrio cholerae*, *Eur. J. Biochem.* **37:**531–534.

Jensen, R., Gregory, B., Naylor, J., and Actor, P., 1972, Isolation of protective somatic antigen from *Vibrio cholerae* (Ogawa) ribosomal preparations, *Infect. Immun.* **6:**156–161.

Johnston, K. H., Holmes, K. K., and Gotschlich, E. C., 1976, The serological classification of *Neisseria gonorrhoeae*. I. Isolation of the outer membrane complex responsible for serotypic specificity, *J. Exp. Med.* **143:**741–758.

Jones, G. W., 1975, The adhesive properties of enteropathogenic bacteria, in: *Microbiology—1975* (D. Schlessinger, ed.), pp. 137–142, American Society for Microbiology, Washington, D.C.

Joó, I., 1973, Occurrence of "natural" vibriocidal antibodies in the population of a non-endemic area, *Boll. Ist. Sieroter. Milan.* **52:**224–229.

Joó, I., 1974, Cholera vaccines, in: *Cholera* (D. Barua and W. Burrows, eds.), pp. 333–355, Saunders, Philadelphia.

Kamal, A. M., 1974, The seventh pandemic of cholera, in: *Cholera* (D. Barua and W. Burrows, eds.), pp. 1–14, Saunders, Philadelphia.

Kateley, J. R., Lyons, S. F., and Friedman, H., 1974, Immunocyte response to a purified bacterial toxin (choleragen) and toxoid: Cytokinetics, immunoglobulin class, and specificity, *J. Immunol.* **112:**1452–1460.

Kateley, J. R., Kasarov, L., and Friedman, H., 1975, Modulation of in vivo antibody responses by cholera toxin, *J. Immunol.* **114:**81–86.

Kauffmann, F., 1950, On the serology of the *Vibrio cholerae, Acta Pathol. Microbiol. Scand.* **27:**283–299.

King, C. A., and Van Heyningen, W. E., 1973, Deactivation of cholera toxin by a sialidase-resistant monosialosylganglioside, *J. Infect. Dis.* **127:**639–647.

King, C. A., and Van Heyningen, W. E., 1975, Evidence for the complex nature of the ganglioside receptor for cholera toxin, *J. Infect. Dis.* **131:**643–648.

Klapper, D. G., Finkelstein, R. A., and Capra, J. D., 1976, Subunit structure and *N*-terminal amino acid sequence of the three chains of cholera enterotoxin, *Immunochemistry* 13:605–611.

Kurosky, A., Markel, D. E., Touchstone, B., and Peterson, J. W., 1976, Chemical characterization of the structure of cholera toxin and its natural toxoid, *J. Infect. Dis. Suppl.* 133:S14–S22.

Lai, C. Y., Mendez, E., and Chang, D., 1976, Chemistry of cholera toxin: The subunit structure, *J. Infect. Dis. Suppl.* 133:S23–S30.

Lankford, C. E., and Legsomburana, U., 1965, Virulence factors of choleragenic vibrios, in: *Proceedings of the Cholera Research Symposium, January 24–29, 1965, Honolulu, Hawaii* (U.S. Public Health Service Publ. No. 1328), pp. 109–120, U.S. Government Printing Office, Washington, D.C.

LoSpalluto, J. J., and Finkelstein, R. A., 1972, Chemical and physical properties of cholera exo-enterotoxin (choleragen) and its spontaneously formed toxoid (choleragenoid), *Biochim. Biophys. Acta* 257:158–166.

Mendez, E., Lai, C. Y., and Wodnar-Filipowicz, A., 1975, Location and the primary structure around the disulfide bonds in cholera toxin, *Biochem. Biophys. Res. Commun.* 67:1435–1444.

Milner, K. C., and Finkelstein, R. A., 1966, Bioassay of endotoxin: Correlation between pyrogenicity for rabbits and lethality for chick embryos, *J. Infect. Dis.* 116:529–536.

Mosley, W. H., 1969, The role of immunity in cholera: A review of epidemiological and serological studies, *Tex. Rep. Biol. Med.* 27:227–241 (Suppl. 1).

Mosley, W. H., and Ahmed, A., 1969, Active and passive immunization in the adult rabbit ileal loop model as an assay for production of antitoxin immunity by cholera vaccines, *J. Bacteriol.* 100:547–549.

Mosley, W. H., Woodward, W. E., Aziz, K. M. A., Rahman, A. S. M. Mizanur, Chowdhury, A. K. M. Alauddin, Ahmed, A., and Feeley, J. C., 1970, The 1968–1969 cholera-vaccine field trial in rural East Pakistan: Effectiveness of monovalent Ogawa and Inaba vaccines and a purified Inaba antigen, with comparative results of serological and animal protection tests, *J. Infect. Dis. Suppl.* 121:S1–S9.

Moss, J., Fishman, P. H., Manganiello, V. C., Vaughan, M., and Brady, R. O., 1976, Functional incorporation of ganglioside into intact cells: Induction of choleragen responsiveness, *Proc. Natl. Acad. Sci. USA* 73:1034–1037.

Mukerjee, S., and Takeya, K., 1974, Vibrio-phages and viobriocins, in: *Cholera* (D. Barua and W. Burrows, eds.), pp. 61–83, Saunders, Philadelphia.

Nalin, D. R., and Cash, R. A., 1974, Oral therapy for cholera, in: *Cholera* (D. Barua and W. Burrows, eds.), pp. 253–261, Saunders, Philadelphia.

Nelson, E. T., Clements, J. D., and Finkelstein, R. A., 1976, *Vibrio cholerae* adherence and colonization in experimental cholera: Electron microscopic studies, *Infect. Immun.* 14:527–547.

Neoh, S. H., and Rowley, D., 1970, The antigens of *Vibrio cholerae* involved in the vibriocidal action of antibody and complement, *J. Infect. Dis.* 121:505–513.

Neoh, S. H., and Rowley, D., 1971, Quantitative assay of a protein antigen of *Vibrio cholerae* involved in the vibriocidal action of antibody and complement, *Aust. J. Exp. Biol. Med. Sci.* 49:605–612.

Neoh, S. H., and Rowley, D., 1972, Protection of infant mice against cholera by antibodies to three antigens of *Vibrio cholerae, J. Infect. Dis.* 126:41–47.

Northrup, R. S., and Chisari, F. V., 1972, Response of monkeys to immunization with cholera toxoid, toxin, and vaccine: Reversion of cholera toxoid, *J. Infect. Dis.* 125:471–479.

Northrup, R. S., and Fauci, A. S., 1972, Adjuvant effect of cholera enterotoxin on the immune response of the mouse to sheep red blood cells, *J. Infect. Dis.* 125:672–673.

Northrup, R. S., and Hossain, S. A., 1970, Immunoglobulins and antibody activity in the intestine and serum in cholera. II. Measurement of antibody activity in jejunal aspirates and sera of cholera patients by radioimmunodiffusion, *J. Infect. Dis. Suppl.* 121:S142–S146.

Ohashi, M., Shimada, T., and Fukumi, H., 1972, *In vitro* production of enterotoxin and hemorrhagic principle by *Vibrio cholerae*, NAG, *Jpn. J. Med. Sci. Biol.* 25:179–194.

Ohtomo, N., Muraoka, T., Inoue, H., Sasaoka, H., and Takahashi, H., 1974, Preparation of cholera toxin and immunization studies with cholera toxid, in: *Proceedings of the Ninth Joint Cholera Research Conference, U.S.–Japan Cooperative Medical Science Program, Geographic Med. Branch, NIAID, NIH, Grand Canyon, Arizona, Oct. 1–3, 1973* (Department of State Publ. 8762, East Asian and Pacific Series 211), pp. 132–142, U.S. Department of State, Washington, D.C.

Ohtomo, N., Muraoka, T., and Ogonuki, H., 1975, General properties of a preparation of cholera toxid, in: *Abstracts, Eleventh Joint Conference on Cholera, The U.S.–Japan Medical Science Program, New Orleans, La., Nov. 4, 5, 6, 1975*, p. 44, U.S. Department of HEW, Publ. Health Serv., NIH, Washington, D.C.

Ohtomo, N., Muraoka, T., Tashiro, A., Zinnaka, Y., and Amako, K., 1976, Size and structure of the cholera toxin molecule and its subunits, *J. Infect. Dis. Suppl.* 133:S31–S40.

Oseasohn, R. O., Benenson, A. S., and Fahimuddin, Md., 1965, Field trial of cholera vaccine in rural East Pakistan, *Lancet* 1:450–453.

Patterson, R., Suszko, I. M., Metzger, W. J., and Roberts, M., 1976, In vitro production of IgE by human peripheral blood lymphocytes: Effect of cholera toxin and β adrenergic stimulation, *J. Immunol.* 117:97–101.

Peterson, J. W., LoSpalluto, J. J., and Finkelstein, R. A., 1972, Localization of cholera toxin *in vivo, J. Infect. Dis.* 126:617–628.

Peterson, J. W., Verwey, W. F., Craig, J. P., Guckian,

J. C., Williams, H. R., and Pierce, N. F., 1975, The response to glutaraldehyde toxoid in human volunteers—A progress report, in: *Proceedings of the 10th Joint Conference, U.S.–Japan Cooperative Medical Science Program, Cholera Panel: Symposium on Cholera, Kyoto, 1974* (H. Fukumi and M. Ohashi, eds.), pp. 89–97, Japanese Cholera Panel, National Institute of Health, Tokyo.

Pierce, N. F., 1973, Differential inhibitory effects of cholera toxoids and ganglioside on the enterotoxins of *Vibrio cholerae* and *Escherichia coli, J. Exp. Med.* **137:**1009–1023.

Pierce, N. F., and Gowans, J. L., 1975, Cellular kinetics of the intestinal immune response to cholera toxoid in rats, *J. Exp. Med.* **142:**1550–1563.

Pierce, N. F., and Reynolds, H. Y., 1974, Immunity to experimental cholera. I. Protective effect of humoral IgG antitoxin demonstrated by passive immunization, *J. Immunol.* **113:**1017–1023.

Pierce, N. F., and Reynolds, H. Y., 1975, Immunity to experimental cholera. II. Secretory and humoral antitoxin response to local and systemic toxoid administration, *J. Infect. Dis.* **131:**383–389.

Pierce, N. F., Banwell, J. G., Sack, R. B., Mitra, R. C., and Mondal, A., 1970, Magnitude and duration of antitoxic response to human infection with *Vibrio cholerae, J. Infect. Dis. Suppl.* **121:**S31–S35.

Pike, R. M., and Chandler, C. H., 1974, The spontaneous release of somatic antigen from *Vibrio cholerae, J. Gen. Microbiol.* **81:**59–67.

Pike, R. M., and Chandler, C. H., 1975, Partial purification and properties of somatic antigen spontaneously released from *Vibrio cholerae, Infect. Immun.* **12:**187–192.

Pitkin, D., and Actor, P., 1972, Immunity to *Vibrio cholerae* in the mouse, *Infect. Immun.* **5:**428–432.

Pollitzer, R., 1959, *Cholera,* World Health Organization, Geneva.

Rappaport, R. S., Rubin, B. A., and Tint, H., 1974a, Development of a purified cholera toxoid. I. Purification of toxin, *Infect. Immun.* **9:**294–303.

Rappaport, R. S., Bonde, G., McCann, T., Rubin, B. A., and Tint, H., 1974b, Development of a purified cholera toxoid. II. Preparation of a stable, antigenic toxoid by reaction of purified toxin with glutaraldehyde, *Infect. Immun.* **9:**304–317.

Redmond, J. W., Korsch, M. J., and Jackson, G. D. F., 1973, Immunochemical studies of the O-antigens of *Vibrio cholerae:* Partial characterization of an acid-labile antigenic determinant, *Aust. J. Exp. Biol. Med. Sci.* **51:**229–235.

Révész, T., and Greaves, M., 1975a, Ligand-induced redistribution of lymphocyte membrane ganglioside GMl, *Nature (London)* **257:**103–106.

Révész, T., and Greaves, M. F., 1975b, Interaction of cholera toxin with lymphocyte membrane gangliosides, in: *International Symposium on Membrane Receptors of Lymphocytes* (M. Seligmann, J.-L. Preud'homme,

and I. Kourilsky, eds.), pp. 403–414, ASP Biological and Medical Press, Amsterdam.

Rivkin, I., Rosenblatt, J., and Becker, E. L., 1975, The role of cyclic AMP in the chemotactic responsiveness and spontaneous motility of rabbit peritoneal neutrophils: The inhibition of neutrophil movement and the elevation of cyclic AMP levels by catecholamines, prostaglandins, theophylline and cholera toxin, *J. Immunol.* **115:**1126–1134.

Sack, R. B., Barua, D., Saxena, R., and Carpenter, C. C. J., 1966, Vibriocidal and agglutinating antibody patterns in cholera patients, *J. Infect. Dis.* **116:**630–640.

Sakazaki, R., Tamura, K., Gomez, C. Z., and Sen., R., 1970, Serological studies on the cholera group of vibrios, *Jpn. J. Med. Sci. Biol.* **23:**13–20.

Saletti, M., and Ricci, A., 1974a, Experiments with cholera toxin detoxified with glutaraldehyde, *Bull. WHO* **51:**633–639.

Saletti, M., and Ricci, A., 1974b, Experiments on monkeys with cholera toxin partially purified and detoxified with formol and glycine, *Bull. WHO* **51:**641–645.

Sandefur, P. D., and Peterson, J. W., 1977, Neutralization of *Salmonella* toxin-induced elongation of Chinese hamster ovary cells by cholera antitoxin, *Infect. Immun.* **15:**988–992.

Sanyal, S. C., and Mukerjee, S., 1969, Live oral cholera vaccine: Report of a trial on human volunteer subjects, *Bull. WHO* **40:**503–511.

Sattler, J., Wiegandt, H., Staerk, J., Kranz, T., Ronneberger, H. J., Schmidtberger, R., and Zilig, H., 1975, Studies of the subunit structure of choleragen, *Eur. J. Biochem.* **57:**309–316.

Schrank, G. D., and Verwey, W. F., 1976, Distribution of cholera organisms in experimental *Vibrio cholerae* infections: Proposed mechanisms of pathogenesis and antibacterial immunity, *Infect. Immun.* **13:**195–203.

Shinoda, S., Kariyama, R., Ogawa, M., Takeda, Y., and Miwatani, T., 1976, Flagellar antigens of various species of the genus *Vibrio* and related genera, *International J. Systematic Bacteriol.* **26:**97–101.

Smith, H. L., Jr., 1974, Antibody responses in rabbits to injections of whole cell, flagella, and flagellin preparations of cholera and noncholera vibrios, *Appl. Microbiol.* **27:**375–378.

Steele, E. J., Chaicumpa, W., and Rowley, D., 1974, Isolation and biological properties of three classes of rabbit antibody to *Vibrio cholerae, J. Infect. Dis.* **130:**93–103.

Steele, E. J., Chaicumpa, W., and Rowley, D., 1975, Further evidence for cross-linking as a protective factor in experimental cholera: Properties of antibody fragements, *J. Infect. Dis.* **132:**175–180.

Stokes, C. R., Soothill, J. F., and Turner, M. W., 1975, Immune exclusion is a function of IgA, *Nature (London)* **255:**745–746.

Sultzer, B. M., and Craig, J. P., 1973, Cholera toxin inhibits macromolecular synthesis in mouse spleen cells, *Nature (London), New Biol.* **244:**178–180.

Svennerholm, A.-M., and Holmgren, J., 1976, Synergistic protective effect in rabbits of immunization with *Vibrio cholerae* lipopolysaccharide and toxin/toxoid, *Infect. Immun.* **13**:735–740.

Van Heyningen, S., 1976, The subunits of cholera toxin: Structure, stoichiometry, and function, *J. Infect. Dis. Suppl.* **133**:S5–S13.

Vasil, M. L., Holmes, R. K., and Finkelstein, R. A., 1974, Studies on toxinogenesis in *Vibrio cholerae*. II. An *in vitro* test for enterotoxin production, *Infect. Immun.* **9**:195–197.

Verwey, W., Craig, J. P., Feeley, J. C., Greenough, W. B., III, Guckian, J. C., and Pierce, N. F., 1972, Response of human volunteers to the parenteral injection of partially purified cholera toxoid: Clinical and serological observations, in: *Proceedings of the 7th Joint Conference, U.S.–Japan Cooperative Medical Science Program Cholera Panel, Symposium on Cholera, Woods Hole, Mass., Aug. 9–11, 1971* (H. Fukumi and M. Ohashi, eds.), pp. 99–100, Japanese Cholera Panel, National Institute of Health, Tokyo.

Vischer, T. L., and LoSpalluto, J. J., 1975, The differential effect of cholera toxin on the lymphocyte stimulation induced by various mitogens, *Immunology* **29**:275–282.

Waldman, R. H., and Ganguly, R., 1974, Immunity to infections on secretory surfaces, *J. Infect. Dis.* **130**:419–440.

Waldman, R. H., Benčič, Z., Sinha, R., Deb, B. C., Sakazaki, R., Tamura, K., Mukerjee, S., and Ganguly, R., 1972, Cholera immunology. II. Serum and intestinal secretion antibody response after naturally occurring cholera, *J. Infect. Dis.* **126**:401–407.

Walker, W. A., Field, M., and Isselbacher, K. J., 1974, Specific binding of cholera toxin to isolated intestinal microvillous membranes, *Proc. Natl. Acad. Sci. USA* **71**:320–324.

Wallace, C. K., Pierce, N. F., Anderson, P. N., Brown, T. C., Lewis, G. W., Sanyal, S. N., Segre, G. V., and Waldman, R. H., 1967, Probable gallbladder infection in convalescent cholera patients, *Lancet* **1**:865–868.

Warren, J. R., Spero, L., Metzger, J. F., and McGann, V. G., 1975, Immunogenicity of formaldehyde-inactivated enterotoxins A and C₁ of *Staphylococcus aureus*, *J. Infect. Dis.* **131**:535–542.

Warren, K. S., Mahmoud, A. A. F., Boros, D. L., Rall, T. W., Mandel, M. A., and Carpenter, C. C. J., Jr., 1974, *In vivo* suppression by cholera toxin of cell-mediated and foreign body inflammatory responses, *J. Immunol.* **112**:996–1007.

Watanabe, Y., 1974, Antibacterial immunity in cholera, in: *Cholera* (D. Barua and W. Burrows, eds.), pp. 283–306, Saunders, Philadelphia.

Westphal, O., 1975, Bacterial endotoxins, *Int. Arch. Allergy Appl. Immunol.* **49**:1–43.

Williams, H. R., Jr., Verwey, W. F., Schrank, G. D., and Hurry, E. K., 1974, An *in vitro* antigen–antibody reaction in relation to an hypothesis of intestinal immunity to cholera, in: *Proceedings of the Ninth Joint Cholera Research Conference, U.S.–Japan Cooperative Medical Science Program, Geographic Medicine Branch, NIAID, NIH, Grand Canyon, Arizona, Oct. 1–3, 1973* (Department of State Publ. 8762, East Asian and Pacific Series 211), pp. 161–173, U.S. Department of State, Washington, D.C.

Woodward, W. E., Gilman, R. H., Hornick, R. B., Libonati, J. P., and Cash, R. A., 1975, Efficacy of a live oral cholera vaccine in human volunteers, in: *Proceedings of the Eleventh Joint Conference on Cholera Sponsored by the U.S.–Japan Cooperative Medical Science Program, Geographic Medicine Branch, National Institute of Allergy and Infectious Diseases, NIH, New Orleans, La., Nov. 4–6, 1975*, pp. 330–335, U.S. Department of HEW, Public Health Service, NIH, Washington, D.C.

Wooward, W. E., Gilman, R. H., Hornick, R. B., Libonati, J. P., and Cash, R. A., 1976, Efficacy of a live oral cholera vaccine in human volunteers, in: *Developments in Biological Standardization*, Vol. 33: *International Symposium on Vaccination of Man and Animals by the Nonparenteral Route* (R. H. Regamey, W. Hennessen, E. C. Hulse, and F. T. Perkins, acting eds.), pp. 108–112, Karger, Basel.

Yabuuchi, E., Miwatani, T., Takeda, Y., and Arita, M., 1974, Flagellar morphology of *Vibrio parahaemolyticus* (Fujino *et al.*) Sakazaki, Iwanami and Fukumi 1963, *Jpn. J. Microbiol.* **18**:295–305.

Zinnaka, Y., and Carpenter, C. C. J., Jr., 1972, An enterotoxin produced by noncholera vibrios, *Johns Hopkins Med. J.* **131**:403–411.

Zuckerman, S. H., and Douglas, S. D., 1975, Inhibition of Fc receptors on a murine lymphoid cell line by cholera exotoxin, *Nature (London)* **255**:410–412.

13

Immunology of Anaerobic Bacterial Infections

DAN DANIELSSON and DWIGHT W. LAMBE, Jr.

1. Introduction

It is well known that oxygen and oxidizing free radicals can be very toxic for any form of life not equipped to utilize oxygen. What we call anaerobes have not developed the ability to withstand these substances. Since it is beyond the scope of this chapter to discuss all the possible mechanisms by which oxygen proves toxic to anaerobic bacteria, the reader is referred to Smith (1975) on the effects of oxygen on anaerobes.

Anaerobic bacteria compose the majority of the indigenous flora of our skin and mucous membranes and can cause significant human diseases. Examination of host interactions with anaerobes will be concerned with three areas of interest:

1. The specific and nonspecific immune defense mechanisms which determine the relation of anaerobes to the host under normal conditions, as well as during and after anaerobic bacterial infections.
2. Specific immunity against anaerobic bacterial infections or, more specifically, against highly potent toxins of some anaerobes, e.g., *Clostridium tetani, C. bo-*

tulinum, and *C. perfringens,* which can be effectively achieved by active or passive immunization.
3. The application of immunodiagnostic techniques to some anaerobic bacterial infections which can be utilized for (a) the demonstration of the organisms, or of toxins, in clinical specimens; (b) the immunological identification of organisms isolated by culture; and (c) the demonstration of a specific immune response.

We will mainly follow this outline in describing the immunology of anaerobic bacterial infections, but first we will briefly discuss evolutionary, historical, and ecological aspects of the anaerobes.

2. Evolutionary and Historical Aspects

Anaerobic bacteria are of great interest from an evolutionary viewpoint, since they most likely represent the first forms of life of this planet. The first anaerobic bacteria probably appeared 2 billion years ago. They most likely preceded the aerobes that became tolerant to oxygen produced by the efficient photosynthesizers, i.e., first the algae, and later the multicellular plants. In order to survive this new situation the anaerobes had to restrict their life to environments with low oxidation–reduction potentials, which became their nat-

DAN DANIELSSON • Department of Clinical Bacteriology and Immunology, Central County Hospital, Orebro, Sweden. DWIGHT W. LAMBE, Jr. • Department of Microbiology, College of Medicine, East Tennessee State University, Johnson City, Tennessee 37601.

317

ural ecological niches. Some anaerobes, i.e., clostridia, developed the ability to form spores that enabled them to survive high concentrations of oxygen or highly oxidized environments (Smith, 1975).

The well-recognized clinical entities tetanus and gas gangrene, each caused by specific clostridial species, have been known since ancient times and were described by Hippocrates and Celcus. Botulism, a disease also caused by a *Clostridium,* was described in Germany a little more than 200 years ago as *Wurstvergiftung,* i.e., sausage poisoning. However, it was not until the late nineteenth century that clostridia were discovered and isolated as the first pathogenic anaerobic bacteria with the use of rather primitive anaerobic culture techniques. As methodology subsequently improved, anaerobic organisms such as *Peptococcus, Peptostreptococcus, Veillonella, Actinomyces, Bacteroides,* and *Fusobacterium* were isolated and described.

The last two decades witnessed the introduction and refinement of the Hungate technique (1950), the use of prereduced anaerobically sterilized (PRAS) culture media, and sophisticated technical equipment for the handling and inoculating of specimens and cultivation of the anaerobic organisms (Aranki *et al.,* 1969; Holdeman and Moore, 1972). As a consequence of these technical improvements, anaerobic bacteria in health and disease have been subjected to a reappraisal during the last decade.

Anaerobic bacterial infections are of historical interest from an immunological standpoint in that many of the principles for immunotherapy and immunoprevention of infectious diseases originated from the experiments by Behring and Kitasato (1890) with the toxins of the anaerobic *Clostridium tetani* and the aerobic *Corynebacterium diphtheriae* and their discoveries of the preventive effect of serum from immunized animals.

3. The Anaerobic Flora and the Host

The presence of anaerobic bacteria in soil and on our skin and mucous membranes is well known. However, improved culture and isolation techniques for anaerobes have demonstrated their ecological importance. Anaerobic bacteria outnumber aerobes by factors of 2–10 : 1 in skin, oral cavity, and upper respiratory and genital tracts, and by as much as 1000:1 in the large intestine (Gibbons, 1974; Smith, 1975). Viable anaerobes occur at a concentration of $2–4 \times 10^{11}$ organisms per gram dry weight of feces (Atterbery *et al.,* 1974). This means that approximately 20–30% of the wet weight of fecal material makes up a solid mass of living bacteria, and nearly all of these are anaerobes. Several hundred species have been described and characterized; several others await description.

Colonization with both aerobic and anaerobic bacteria occurs immediately after birth. Many host factors influence colonization, e.g., age, diet, and the hormonal status (Rosebury, 1962; Atterbery *et al.,* 1974; Smith, 1975). We must also recognize that the skin, oral cavity, and upper respiratory, genital, and gastrointestinal tracts make up their own ecologies in their different sites. Both aerobes and anaerobes will thus find their own ecological niches; as a result, the microbes in any part of the body may differ from one individual to another because differences in the microenvironment promote the growth of one group of microbes and inhibit that of others. Even in parts of the body like the oral cavity, where one would think the microflora would be fairly uniform, there are several microenvironmental areas, each with its own particular microflora, e.g., the buccal folds, the tongue, the teeth, and the gingival sulci (Gibbons, 1974).

To a very great extent, we still do not know the factors governing the ecology of these microenvironments. We can only recognize that they do exist. This also means that the indigenous microbial flora of the different parts of our body can only be described in general terms. However, the great majority tend to be members of a few major groups. The macroorganism and its microflora form a balanced ecological system in which the anaerobes make up a considerable part. Under normal conditions this ecological system is very tenaciously held and can be changed only by rather drastic measures. For further details and references on these subjects, see Rosebury (1962) and Smith (1975).

4. Spectrum of and Host Factors Contributing to Anaerobic Bacterial Infections

Not too long ago, tetanus, botulism, and gas gangrene were among the few distinct and well-recognized anaerobic bacterial infectious diseases of importance. Through the years we have learned how to cope with these diseases by application of immunoprophylaxis and immunotherapy, prevention by surgical revision of necrotic tissues in wounds, or prevention by food hygiene.

Diseases associated with other anaerobes were overlooked for a long time, but with the use of improved culture and isolation techniques anaerobic bacteria have been recognized with increased frequency. Infectious diseases caused by one or more of the endogenous anaerobes are much more common than those due to anaerobic bacteria of exogenous origin. These anaerobes of endogenous origin are often isolated in combination with aerobes; the isolation of five, ten, or even more species has been noted. This also means that the old concept of Koch and Ehrlich ''one microbe, one disease, and one antimicrobial substance'' can no longer be used generally, since in many situations we have to deal with polymicrobial infections.

Intact host barriers, especially the mucous membranes of the oropharyngeal cavity and the intestinal and urogenital tracts, where endogenous anaerobes occur abundantly, are of utmost importance for the protection of invasion. Humoral and cellular nonspecific defense factors as well as specific humoral and cellular immune mechanisms are certainly also of importance but at present badly understood as related to infection with these organisms.

The susceptibility of the compromised host to anaerobic infections was analyzed by Finegold *et al.* (1970) in a series of 224 patients with such infections; they also made a literature review of 306 patients. They found that the conditions predisposing to infection in the compromised host may also predispose to anaerobic infection. However, certain conditions seemed particularly important, e.g., carcinoma of the colon, uterus, and the lung, because of the prevalence of anaerobic organisms as normal flora in these or adjacent sites and a milieu favorable for anaerobic growth by obstruction and stasis and/or by tissue necrosis with lowering of local E_h. Finegold *et al.* (1970) noted a high incidence of septicemia with anaerobes, especially with clostridia, in patients with hematopoietic and lymphoreticular malignancies; such patients who are treated with radiation and/or antimetabolites are predisposed to infection in general.

There are no reports of an increased frequency of anaerobic infections in patients with agamma- or hypogammaglobulinemia, T-cell defects, or complement deficiencies. Finegold *et al.* (1970) found no conclusive evidence that corticosteroid therapy, leukopenia, antineoplastic therapy (except in hematological and lymphoreticular malignancies), splenectomy, collagen disease, or organ transplantation predisposed to anaerobic infection to any greater extent than to infection in general. Since most organ transplantation patients are treated with azathioprine as an immunosuppressive agent, it is worth mentioning that the unsplit molecule of this antimetabolite has a pronounced antibacterial activity against intestinal anaerobes but not against intestinal aerobes. Concentrations exceeding 10 times the MIC of azathioprine against these bacteria were demonstrated in jejunal secretion (Danielsson and Persson, 1977).

Finegold *et al.* (1970) found diabetes mellitus to be particularly associated with anaerobic cholecystitis and anaerobic osteomyelitis. Intestinal antisepsis with oral aminoglycosides (to which anaerobes are very resistant) predisposed to infections with anaerobes as well as other resistant organisms. However, bowel sterilization with antimicrobials having high activity against anaerobes will significantly reduce postoperative *Bacteroides* infections in patients undergoing elective colon surgery (Willis *et al.*, 1977). The rare disease acatalasemia (genetic lack of catalase in blood) predisposes to putrid progressive oral gangrene with anaerobes due to local tissue necrosis because accumulated peroxide turns hemoglobin to methemoglobin lacking normal oxygen-carrying ability (Finegold *et al.*, 1970; Takahara, 1952).

Some indigenous anaerobic bacteria appear to be frequently associated with human disease, whereas others, although present in large numbers in the normal microflora, seldom if ever are involved in disease. Table 1 shows the genera of anaerobic bacteria that are frequently associated with human disease and those that are seldom, if ever, disease producing. In the following sections we will emphasize the virulence, pathogenic, and immunological aspects as related specifically to the most frequently disease-related anaerobes.

5. Clostridial Infections

5.1. General Characteristics

The clostridia are anaerobic, spore-forming rods. They compose a large, widespread, and important group of bacteria with several well-defined pathogenic and nonpathogenic species. The habitat in nature for most of them is the intestinal tract of humans, animals, and fish; the soil; and water. Under normal conditions, clostridial organisms seem to have no obvious capacity to penetrate intact skin or mucous membranes.

Pathogenic clostridia are known for their production of biologically potent toxins and enzymes that are responsible for their local and systemic histotoxic effects. However, the mere isolation of clostridia from a wound does not necessarily mean a clinically significant clostridial infection. Necrotic tissue with a low oxidation–reduction potential must be present for the establishment of a clinically significant clostridial infection with unrestrained growth of these organisms resulting in toxin production and tissue invasion.

5.2. Immunology of Tetanus

5.2.1. Introduction

Tetanus has been recognized as a disease entity since ancient times and was described by Hippocrates. Little more than 100 years ago it was proposed by Wells to be due to a nerve poison, a hypothesis that was proved in 1884 by Carlo and Rattone. The same year, Nicolaier showed that the causative agent was present in a mixed culture of soil, but he did not succeed in isolating it. In 1889 Kitasato managed to culture and isolate the tetanus bacillus and showed it to be a spore-forming rod. One year later, Behring and Kitasato (1890) demonstrated the presence of neurotoxin in culture filtrates and showed that immunization of laboratory animals with small doses of the toxin created protection. Specific antibodies were present in serum of these animals. Protection could be passively transferred with serum to other animals.

The tetanus bacillus can be found in most places of our environment, although its natural habitat seems to be high productivity soil (Smith, 1975). The cultural and biochemical characteristics are motility, production of indol, and lack of acid production from glucose; final identification is based on its production of tetanospasmin. The details for isolation and identification were recently reviewed by Smith (1975). Several serotypes of the tetanus bacillus have been described by Mandia (1955). This serotyping has been found to be of little or no practical value, since tetanospasmin with similar antigenic properties is produced by toxigenic strains of all serotypes.

5.2.2. Biochemistry and Biological Properties of Tetanospasmin

Toxigenic strains of the tetanus bacillus grown in appropriate fluid media produce three exotoxins: the tetanolysin, the nonspasmogenic toxin, and the highly neurotoxic tetanospasmin, which is responsible for clinical tetanus. Tetanospasmin was one of the first toxins to be obtained in a highly purified, crys-

---

TABLE 1. Genera of Anaerobes Associated with Human Disease

Frequently associated with human disease	Seldom, if ever, associated with human disease
Actinomyces	Acidaminococcus
Anaerobic cocci (Peptococcus, Peptostreptococcus, Streptococcus)	Veillonella
	Borrelia
	Butyrivibrio
Bacteroides	Lachnospira
Clostridium	Lactobacillus
Fusobacterium	Leptotrichia
Treponema	Succinimonas
	Succinivibrio
	Propionibacterium
	Arachnia
	Desulfovibrio
	Bifidobacterium

talline state (Pillemer *et al.*, 1946, 1948). The usual ways to determine the amount of purified toxin, or toxin in culture filtrates, are by (1) LD_{50} determinations in mice, (2) neutralization of the toxic activity by standard antitoxin, and (3) the Ramon flocculation test with standard flocculating antitoxin to determine Lf/mg N (Lf = flocculating unit). One Lf corresponds to the quantity of antigen bound by one international unit (IU) of standard tetanus antitoxin, a reaction visible *in vitro* by flocculation. One IU tetanus antitoxin is the neutralizing power, specific for tetanus toxin. equal to 0.03384 mg of an international standard preparation (WHO Expert Committee on Biological Standardization, 1970).

Purified tetanospasmin has an LD_{50}/mg N of $1–5 \times 10^8$ mice and an Lf of 3000–3200/mg N. Its molecular weight is 150,000, and it has a sedimentation value of 6.8–7.0 S (Dawson and Mauritzen, 1968; Dowdle *et al.*, 1970). The amino acid composition of tetanospasmin and its chemical configuration have been analyzed by several investigators with fairly consistent results (Dawson and Mauritzen, 1968; Dowdle *et al.*, 1970; Bizzini *et al.*, 1970; Holmes and Ryan, 1971).

The receptor sites of tetanospasmin were studied by van Heyningen and Mellanby (1971). They showed that the gangliosides in nerve tissue, when complexed with cerebroside, will fix tetanus spasmogenic toxin in a ratio of two molecules of ganglioside with one molecule of toxin. It thus appears that gangliosides determine the site of attachment but are not directly involved in the action of the toxin. The specific neurotoxic action of tetanospasmin seems to be primarily the inhibition of the release of the amino acids glycine and γ-aminobutyric acid (GABA), which are major inhibitory transmitters in the spinal cord synapses (Osborne and Bradford, 1973). This leaders to spasmodic contraction of the muscles because of ungoverned propagation of impulses through the ramifying connections of the motor neurons in the central nervous system. This view is consistent with the findings of Choudbury *et al.* (1972), who showed, with the use of fluorescein-labeled antitoxin, that the toxin was primarily in the synaptosomes, i.e., that part of the nerve cell that contains appreciable amounts of gangliosides.

5.2.3. Pathogenic Mechanisms

The tetanus bacillus has no invasive or histotoxic properties in itself, clinical tetanus being the result of the neurotoxic action of tetanospasmin locally produced by the tetanus bacillus growing in a contaminated wound, usually of traumatic origin. The toxin can reach the central nervous system by two routes, humorally through the lymph and the blood and neurally by way of the tissue spaces of the peripheral nerves. So-called descending tetanus is produced by toxin reaching the central nervous system humorally and is usually seen in men and horses; ascending tetanus, sometimes called local tetanus, is produced by toxin reaching the central nervous system neurally.

Clinical tetanus seems to occur only under exceptional circumstances. During World War I tetanus bacilli were found in nearly 20% of wounded soldiers. Yet the disease developed in less than 1% of the wounded who were not immunized or did not receive antitoxin (van Heyningen, 1955). Necrotic tissue with an E_h potential less than -100 mV is essential to promote growth of the tetanus bacillus and the strain must be toxigenic for production of tetanospasmin (Smith, 1975). Most cases of tetanus result from small, localized wound infections, the majority of them in the lower extremities. The incubation period in man varies from a few days to several weeks. Once clinical tetanus is established, it is a grave disease with mortality rates between 30% and 70%. The mortality is inversely related to the length of incubation period, being approximately 70% in those cases with an incubation period of less than 5 days, around 30% in cases with incubation periods of 1 week to 10 days and 3–12% in those few cases with incubation periods of two weeks or more (CDC Tetanus Surveillance Report No. 3, 1968–1969).

5.2.4. Natural Acquired Immunity

It has been generally considered that natural immunity is not acquired against tetanus and that no immunity is produced by the disease itself (Eckmann, 1963; Adams *et al.*, 1969; Furste and Wheeler, 1972). The small amount of toxin produced, much of it immediately fixed by nerve cells, does not appear to be sufficient to induce antibody production. However, there are several observations suggesting the possibility of some acquired natural immunity against tetanus. Veronesi *et al.* (1973) point out that nonvaccinated individuals, such as gardeners and persons in similar professions, working for many years in contact with high-productivity soil, do not contract the disease any more frequently than others. Serological surveys of such persons have demonstrated blood levels of 0.01 unit/ml or higher of tetanus antitoxin. These workers also note that some nonvaccinated individuals without detectable titers of humoral antibodies (≤ 0.001 unit/ml) react very promptly to the first dose of toxoid ("good responders"), while others need two or three doses of toxoid ("normal responders" or "bad responders"). The "good responders" might well be individuals sensitized naturally. A third observation supporting the hypothesis of some natural acquired immunity is that tetanus does occur more frequently among newborns, children, and young people, at least in the countries where tetanus is prevalent (Eckmann, 1963; Adams *et al.,* 1969). A fourth relevant observation is the great variation in intensity and extension of clinical tetanus, with the exception of umbilical tetanus, which is always fatal. In practice, it is not possible to rely on these observations suggesting that some natural immunity is acquired against tetanus. Experience has taught us that active or passive immunization is of extreme importance for the prevention of the disease.

5.2.5. Immunoprophylaxis and Immunotherapy

The immunogenicity of tetanospasmin was beautifully demonstrated by Behring's and Kitasato's experimental animal studies in 1890. To begin with, the high toxicity of tetanospasmin was a drawback for use in active immunization, until it was found that treatment with formaldehyde transformed it to a toxoid. The antigenic properties of the toxin were retained, and the toxoid has proved to be one of the most reliable vaccines in man when it is adsorbed to alum (Eckmann, 1963, 1967; Adams *et al.,* 1969).

The prevention of clinical tetanus by passive or active immunization was overwhelmingly shown during World Wars I and II. Prophylactic passive immunization was introduced toward the end of 1914, with a tenfold drop in the incidence of cases. Active immunization with toxoid was instituted before World War II, which resulted in another tenfold drop as compared with prophylactic passive immunication (van Heyningen, 1955). The success of immunoprophylaxis of soldiers suggested the desirability of immunizing civilians. In 1943 active immunization of young children against both tetanus and diphtheria was made compulsory in Lyons; since then, the practice has become almost universal.

In most countries of the Western hemisphere, the incidence of clinical tetanus is as low as 0.08–0.20 per 100,000 (Smith, 1975). In the United States 97% of clinical tetanus occurred among those who had not been vaccinated (CDC Tetanus Surveillance Report No. 3, 1968–1969). The mean age of mortality cases has doubled since World War II because of lower vaccination rates among older people. The incidence of tetanus in vaccinated children is estimated to be approximately 4 in 100 million, i.e., practically immeasurable (CDC Tetanus Surveillance Report No. 3, 1968–1969; The Tetanus Report of the Swedish Medical Board for Public Health, No. 2, March, 1976). While diseases like smallpox and poliomyelitis have been almost totally eradicated by achieving high levels of immunity through massive vaccination programs, tetanus as a disease is not eradicable because *Clostridium tetani* will always be in our environment.

a. Active Immunization. According to common practice, active immunization against tetanus is developed with two injections of adsorbed tetanus toxoid, spaced 4–6 weeks apart, and a third dose after at least 6 months but preferably after 1 year (Edsall, 1959; Eckmann, 1967). In many industrialized countries this type of complete vaccination against tetanus is performed during the first year of life. Without all three injections it is not complete.

From a practical point of view it is important to know how long immunity from complete vaccination will last, as well as what happens to people who have received only one or two injections earlier. Edsall (1959) as well as Fischlewitz and Sturm (1967) showed that persons will respond to a booster injection even if 15–20 years have passed after the last dose of a complete vaccination. Antibody responses, well above the limit of protection (≥ 0.01 IU antitetanus antitoxin/ml), were recorded. Recently Ullberg-Olsson and Eriksson (1975) showed that individuals who had previously received only one dose of tetanus vaccine and who were revaccinated 8–13 years later responded 8 days after the booster dose with an antitoxin content of 0.01 IU/ml or more, levels generally considered protective. A control group who had received two or three earlier vaccine injections was treated in the same way and responded with an antitoxin content of ≥ 1 IU/ml. The advantage of a complete basic immunization is obvious, but the investigation of Ullberg-Olsson and Eriksson (1975) highlights the antigenicity of this vaccine.

b. Passive and Combined Passive–Active Immunization. If every individual had a complete vaccination with tetanus toxoid, passive immunization with antitetanus immune globulin would not be necessary. However, in unvaccinated patients with contaminated wounds not amenable to complete surgical excision, passive immunization with hyperimmune antitetanus immune globulin becomes necessary.

Heterologous antitetanus antitoxin is usually no longer used. Human antitetanus immune globulin has been available since the early 1960s (Ellis, 1963; Levine *et al.*, 1966; Eckmann, 1970). In contrast to heterologous antitoxin, homologous tetanus immune globulin is less subject to immune elimination and is unlikely to provoke type 1 and/or type 3 hypersensitivity reactions. It is thus safer and protective for longer intervals.

The recommended dose of human antitetanus immunoglobulin is 3000–6000 IU (Furste and Wheeler, 1972). The antibodies will not neutralize or dissociate tetanus toxin already fixed by the nervous tissue. Therefore, once clinical tetanus is already established, immunotherapy will not influence greatly the fatality rate, if the interval between onset and antitoxin is more than 24 hr (CDC Tetanus Surveillance Report No. 3, 1968–1969). Nevertheless, antitetanus immune globulin is administered to neutralize toxin not yet fixed by nervous tissue.

Whether active immunization should be started at the same time as passive immunization has been debated lately (Eckmann, 1967). Ullberg-Olsson (1975a,b) studied the possible effect of passive vaccination with as much as 6000–45,000 IU human antitetanus immune globulin on the simultaneous active vaccination with alum-adsorbed tetanus toxoid. She showed that the rise in titer after the third injection with toxoid was of the same magnitude as in patients receiving active immunization only. A typical response to the second injection of toxoid might be masked by the passively administered antibodies. Although the number of patients in this investigation was rather small, the studies indicate that large doses of human immune globulin do not appear to affect the response obtained by complete vaccination with three doses of tetanus toxoid. Simultaneous active immunization is now the current recommended procedure in Sweden when unvaccinated patients at risk for tetanus are prophylactically given human antitetanus immune globulin. Toxoid adsorbing passively administered antibody, thereby reducing neutralization of the quantitatively smaller amount of toxin being generated, does not seem to be a problem.

5.2.6. Immunodiagnosis of Tetanus Infection

Isolation of *C. tetani* is not difficult with the use of current anaerobic techniques (Smith, 1975). The production of neurotoxin must be specifically tested with experimental animals (mice) and their controls protected with specific antitoxin. A tentative diagnosis can be made by homogenizing a small amount of excised necrotic tissue in a small volume of saline. The material is then centrifuged and mice are injected with 0.2-ml amounts intramuscularly alongside their tail or intravenously. Control mice are given antitoxin. If the unprotected mice show spasm of the tail within 2 or 3 days or die overnight, it can be assumed that the specimen contained tetanus toxin.

5.3. Immunology of Botulism

5.3.1. Introduction

Although a few cases of botulism due to wound infection have been reported (Davis *et al.*, 1951; Merson and Dowell, 1973), botulism is primarily not an infectious disease but a poisoning caused by eating food in which *Clostridium botulinum* has grown and produced toxin. The very word "botulism" (Latin for sausage) was coined in 1870 by Mueller. The causative organism was isolated and described as *Clostridium* by van Ermengen in 1897 in the course of an outbreak of this disease, and hence the organism was labeled *C. botulinum*.

Symptoms of clinical botulism in man appear after periods varying from less than a day to several days after ingestion of toxin-containing food. They include double vision, thirst, vomiting, constipation, difficulty in swallowing and speaking, and, worst of all, respiratory paralysis, which can be fatal.

There are several strains of *C. botulinum* with the ability to produce a potent neurotoxin having similar pharmacological action. The organisms are today divided into eight toxigenic types on the basis of the antigenic characteristics of the neurotoxins produced. These toxigenic strains and toxins are labeled A, B, C1, C2, D, E, F, and G. Only A, B, and E strains have been implicated in human disease. The toxigenic strains of these botulinum bacteria are found in soil and in sediments of coastal and sea water. They are, like other *C. botulinum* strains, restricted to the Northern Hemisphere, mostly between the latitudes of 35 N and 55 N (Smith, 1975).

5.3.2. Biochemical and Biological Properties of Botulinum Toxin

Botulinum toxin is one of the most biologically potent toxins known. It is a neurotoxin, acting peripherally at the neuromuscular junction, apparently by preventing release of acetylcholine from the demyelinated ends of the cholinergic motor nerves (Wright, 1955). It is one of the few toxins that not only is not destroyed but also actually may be activated by acids and proteolytic enzymes in the gut. The disease is entirely toxemic and can be exactly simulated by parenteral or oral administration of the isolated toxin.

Most but not all of the botulinum neurotoxins are synthesized as nontoxic prototoxins, or as slightly active progenitor toxins. Some of them are activated to full toxicity by the proteolytic enzymes produced by these organisms (Smith, 1975). Procedures for production of botulinum toxin are relatively simple and have been described by several investigators (Sterne and Wentzel, 1950; Duff *et al.*, 1957; Gordon *et al.*, 1957; Skulberg, 1964). Toxin preparations are easy to crystallize, but it has been shown that these are toxin-hem-

agglutinating complexes with a molecular weight of 900,000–1,000,000. The molecular weight of the toxin itself is 140,000–150,000 and has an LD_{50}/mg N of $1–5 \times 10^8$ in mice. The molecular weight seems to have the ability to depolymerize and repolymerize.

All of the eight types of botulinum toxin are heat labile at 100°C for a few minutes. They are also destroyed by protein denaturants. Treatment with formaldehyde changes the toxin to toxoid with good antigenic properties.

Almost all botulinum strains carry bacteriophage. The production of C1, C2, and D toxins is mediated by bacteriophage (Eklund *et al.*, 1971; Eklund and Poysky, 1974). In this respect they resemble pathogenic corynebacteria producing diphtheria toxin. When such strains are cured of their phages by physical or chemical means, toxigenicity is lost. For further information on botulinum toxin, the reader is referred to the review by Boroff and Das Gupta (1971).

5.3.3. Immunoprophylaxis and Immunotherapy

Botulism in man is a rare disease today. However, it is a serious disease, with fatality rates from 5–50% (Gangarosa *et al.*, 1971; Smith, 1975). There is no naturally acquired immunity. Treatment is directed to neutralization of circulating toxin by the administration of specific heterologous antitoxin in a total dose of 100,000 units by the intravenous route. The antitoxin will not reverse the effects of toxin which has already damaged the myoneural junction, but it will neutralize that which has not yet been fixed by the receptor cells. Early administration is therefore important. Efforts are also made to remove unabsorbed toxin from the gastrointestinal canal by stomach lavage and high enemas. Patients with botulism often require ventilatory support and intensive nursing care under close medical supervision because of the possibility of rapidly developing respiratory paralysis. Prophylactic antitoxin, gastric lavage, and high enemas are also recommended to other individuals who have eaten the contaminated food.

Immunotherapy was reported by Smith (1975) to be highly effective in cases of type E botulism, being less effective in cases of type B and type A botulism. The reason for this difference is not clearly understood, but the latter two toxins have been demonstrated for several days in serum after contaminated food has been eaten (Smith, 1975).

Immunization against botulism is not practiced routinely. It has been suggested for Eskimos and the Indians of the coast of Alaska and British Columbia in whom the incidence of botulism, particularly type E, is higher than in any other people in the world because of their food habits (Smith, 1975). Otherwise, the best way of preventing botulism is proper handling and preservation of food.

5.3.4. Diagnosis

Clinically suspected botulism can be diagnosed by the demonstration of toxin in serum or feces of the patient. Mice are used as test animals, and 0.3–0.5 ml serum or fecal extract is injected intraperitoneally. Corresponding tests are done with suspected toxin-containing food that is also subjected to bacteriological culture procedures. Identification of the immunotype of an isolated strain is done by neutralization with specific antitoxin.

5.4. Immunology of Gas Gangrene

5.4.1. Introduction

Gas gangrene is associated with infection or invasion of pathogenic proteolytic clostridia, of which the four most important species are *C. perfringens (welchii), C. novyi, C. septicum,* and *C. sordellii* (MacLennan, 1962; Brummelkamp, 1974). These clostridia are found in soil, in sediments of coastal water, and, in large numbers, as members of the indigenous flora of the large bowel in man and animals, where they seem to live in harmony with the host. They produce a variety of potent toxins with enzymatic action which play a major role in the initiation of gas gangrene. An excellent review of the biological properties of these toxins was recently given by Smith (1975).

Gas gangrene is a serious disease with high mortality, hence the general view that clostridial infections should be considered with apprehension. However, if all types of such infections are regarded they are neither grave nor very rare. Unrestrained growth of these organisms resulting in an invasive infection occurs only under exceptional circumstances. As with *C. tetani,* necrotic tissue with a low oxidation–reduction potential must be present for the establishment of an invasive clostridial infection. These prerequisites are usually present in accidental traumatic injuries of muscles, and sometimes after surgical trauma, e.g., after large bowel operations.

5.4.2. Pathogenic Mechanisms

Gas gangrene comprises the clinical entities of a rapidly spreading myonecrosis of healthy muscle, necrotic cellulitis, and postabortal uterine infection (MacLennan, 1962; Brummelkamp, 1974). These follow infection by pathogenic clostridia of severely injured muscle or other tissues which develop when the blood supply to the muscle has been interrupted. The anoxia and the consequent anaerobic glycolysis result in a fall of the E_h to levels permitting multiplication and toxin production of the clostridia. Those species, i.e., *C. perfringens, C. novyi, C. septicum,* and *C. sordellii,* associated with gas gangrene produce a variety of biologically potent toxins that are labeled α, β, δ, ε, κ, etc. The α toxin is a phospholipase-C-splitting lecithin to phosphorylcholine and a diglyceride (Smith, 1975). It is the most important of the toxins and appears to be essential for the initiation of the pathological process. Other toxins seem to be of minor importance but may contribute to the development of the pathological process once this has started. For more extensive information on clostridial toxins, their mode of action, and their toxicological typing, see MacLennan (1962), Willis (1969), and Smith (1975).

5.4.3. Immunoprophylaxis and Immunotherapy

The α toxins, converted to toxoids by formaldehyde, are potent antigens. From our knowledge of their major importance in gas gangrene it therefore seems logical to attempt immunoprophylaxis and immunotherapy directed against these toxins. This has in fact been practiced since the early 1940s with potent antitoxins prepared by hyperimmunization of horses with detoxified toxin filtrates or detoxified toxin preparations of *C. perfringens, C. novyi,* and *C. septicum.* In experimental animal studies these antitoxins were shown to have a high degree of protection when given prior to induction of gas gangrene.

However, the results in established clinical gas gangrene were more disappointing, since it was found that administration of antitoxin did not stop the disease unless extensive surgical removal of necrotic tissue and muscles was also done (Macfarlane, 1943; MacLennan and Macfarlane, 1944). Despite this, serum therapy is generally considered valuable in neutralizing toxins detrimental to the patient. Recommended doses vary from 10,000 to 27,000 IU of *C. perfringens* and *C. novyi* antitoxins and from 5000 to 13,000 IU of *C. septicum* antitoxin given intravenously before surgery and every 4 hr for 1–2 days after the operation (MacLennan and Macfarlane, 1944; Brummelkamp, 1974).

Active immunization of domestic animals with α toxoid of *C. perfringens*, *C. novyi*, and *C. septicum* is of demonstrable value against diseases caused by these organisms (Thomson *et al.*, 1969; Macheak *et al.*, 1972). Studies along these lines were also initiated during World War II by British and American workers, and it was found that an appreciable antibody response could be elicited in animals, as well as in man (Robertson and Keppie, 1943; Altemeier and Tytell, 1952). There are, however, no data on the effects of such active immunization on the subsequent exposure of man to gas gangrene. In this connection, the experimental work by Boyd *et al.* (1972) is of interest. Experimental gas gangrene with *C. perfringens* and *C. novyi* was induced in sheep that suffered muscle injuries by high-velocity missiles. Control sheep were vaccinated with α toxoids of *C. perfringens*, *C. novyi*, and *C. septicum*. These toxoids were adsorbed to alum, and two 2-ml doses spaced 1 month apart were given subcutaneously. Immunization was found to be almost completely effective in preventing gas gangrene on challenge even 1 year after immunization. It was of interest to note that antitoxin levels in serum increased significantly after challenge, but Boyd *et al.* (1972) did not state what Ig class(es) protective antibodies belonged to. Since sheep and man have similar muscle masses, these authors state that it is not unreasonable to assume that the protective level required in man may be comparable to that in sheep.

Despite these promising results, there is at present little interest in active immunization against gas gangrene, because this disease is rare today, because penicillin can be used prophylactically (Owen-Smith and Matheson, 1968), and because with hyperbaric oxygen in combination with antibiotics is an effective treatment (Brummelkamp, 1974).

5.5. Other Immune Phenomena Related to *Clostridium perfringens*

We have pointed out earlier that *C. perfringens* is found in large numbers in the large intestine of both humans and animals, which seems to be its natural habitat (Atterbery *et al.*, 1974; Smith, 1975). Despite its potential to produce highly fatal toxins, *C. perfringens* seems to dwell well with its host, as long as it is confined to the large intestine. This also seems to be relevant for other pathogenic as well as apathogenic clostridia. The factors that protect the host from invasion with these organisms and control the organisms' production of their highly fatal toxins are poorly understood. There is certainly a complex cooperation between specific and nonspecific cellular as well as humoral mechanisms governing this host–parasite relationship. Doubtless this is an open field for future research for a better understanding of these interrelationships. A few interesting observations should be mentioned.

Månsson and Olhagen (1967) and Månsson *et al.* (1971) observed in swine fed a high-protein diet the development of arthritis, parakeratosis, and proliferative glomerulonephritis. The symptoms were correlated with a change of the intestinal microflora and a significant increase in the number of *C. perfringens*, particularly strains showing increased α toxin production, increased proteolytic activity, and immediate and active fermentation of salicin. It is not clear if the pathological conditions in the swine were due to some sort of hypersensitivity reactions to *C. perfringens*, α toxin, or other substances produced by the organisms. It is of interest to note, however, that the hypersensitivity was transferred to normal animals by lymphocytes from an experimental animal which had *C. perfringens* in the gut flora. Whether these observations have any implication for rheumatoid arthritis or other autoimmune disease in humans remain speculative at present.

Danielsson *et al.* (1974b), in a study of patients with Crohn's disease and healthy controls, demonstrated with the indirect immunofluorescent technique the occurrence of moderate to high serum titers (1 : 40–1 : 320) of IgG, IgA, and IgM antibodies in both groups to one strain of *C. perfringens* but no or very low titers (≤1 : 20) against other strains. It is not clear whether these represent cross-reacting antibodies, naturally occurring antibodies, or the result of a specific immune response against *C. perfringens,* or whether these antibodies had any protective role.

6. Infections Due to Nonsporing Anaerobic Gram-Positive Rods

The genera *Bifidobacterium, Lactobacillus, Eubacterium, Actinomyces,* and *Propionibacterium* comprise the non-spore-forming anaerobic gram-positive rods. They all form part of the indigenous flora of the upper respiratory tract, the oral cavity, or the intestinal or urogenital tract (Rosebury, 1962; Smith, 1975). Many species of these genera, except bifidobacteria, have been implicated in human as well as animal infections, but they are of relatively minor importance. Actinomycosis and infections with propionibacteria are, however, of some interest from immunological points of view, and will therefore be briefly discussed.

6.1. Immunology of Actinomycosis

6.1.1. Introduction

Actinomycosis, a disease of both man and animals, has been recognized since the late nineteenth century. Cervicofacial, pulmonary, and abdominal involvement can occur. The agents of human actinomycosis in the order of their importance are *Actinomyces israellii, Arachnia propionica, Actinomyces naeslundii, A. viscosus,* and *A. odontolyticus.* Of these, *A. naeslundii* and *A. viscosus* grow aerobically but grow better under anaerobic conditions, They are all members of the normal flora of the oral cavity and upper respiratory tract but have pathogenic properties when introduced into tissue below the mucous membranes. There has been much confusion about these organisms because of the difficulties of differentiating one from the other accomplished only in the past 10–15 years. For de-

tailed descriptions of isolation of *Actinomyces* and related organisms, the reader is referred to Georg (1970, 1974) and Holdeman and Moore (1972).

6.1.2. Pathogenesis

Actinomycosis is a disease that usually runs a chronic course. In this respect it can be considered as a slow bacterial infection like leprosy and brucellosis. Histopathology of actinomycotic lesions is characterized by a heavy infiltration of inflammatory cells, fibroblasts, giant cells, and granulomas, i.e., the picture of a chronic inflammatory reaction. When it runs a course of acute inflammation, suppuration ensues. The "sulfur granules" so often found in actinomycosis are a mycelial mass of cells held together by a polysaccharide–protein complex secreted by the organisms, probably as a capsular material. The whole complex is cemented together by calcium phosphate as a result of the phosphatase activity of the organisms and possibly of the host (Frazier and Fowler, 1967; Crawford, 1971).

6.1.3. Diagnosis

The demonstration or identification of the causative agents in human actinomycosis is frequently hampered by antecedent and ongoing antibiotic treatment of this chronic infection. Humoral immune responses can be used as an aid in the diagnosis of this disease.

Since *A. israelii* and *A. propionica* are the most common etiological agents of actinomycosis, most immunological and serological studies have concentrated on these two species. There are two serotypes recognized within both *A. israelii* and *A. propionica,* with minor antigenic relationships between each serotype (Brock and Georg, 1969a; Slack *et al.,* 1969; Slack and Gerencser, 1970). Antibodies against these organisms have been produced in rabbits; gel diffusion, agglutination, and immunofluorescent techniques have been employed to aid in this identification. Direct immunofluorescent techniques are now the accepted method for the identification of isolated organisms or for their demonstration in exudates, as well as for differentiating them from other related bacteria (Brock and Georg, 1969b; Holmberg and Forsum, 1973).

Various immunological techniques, including complement fixation, hemagglutination, and agar gel diffusion, have been used as tools for the serodiagnosis of actinomycosis. The results obtained and reported are somewhat conflicting with regard to sensitivity and specificity since positive results have been obtained in individuals with no clinical evidence of actinomycosis (Georg *et al.,* 1968; Holm and Kwapinski, 1959; Lerner, 1974). These results are most likely due to differences in the antigenic preparations used and their lack of purity. In this respect, the results recently reported by Holmberg *et al.* (1975a) are of interest. A standard reference antigen of the two *A. israelii* serotypes was characterized with the crossed immunoelectrophoresis technique. A sonic lysate of *A. israelii* was chosen and tested against heterologous rabbit antisera for related as well as unrelated organisms. None of these heterologous antisera had antibodies against the standard antigen of the sonic lysate of *A. israelii.* Holmberg *et al.* (1975a,b) therefore chose the sonic lysate of *A. israelii* as reference antigen for examining human sera in crossed immunoelectrophoresis tests. In sera from nine patients with proven actinomycosis, precipitating antibodies were detected against this reference standard antigen. These human sera contained one to four precipitins, most of which disappeared during the following year after successful treatment. One patient maintained the initial precipitin pattern during follow-up studies, and even increased the number of precipitating antibodies during exacerbations. Sera from blood donors, from patients with tuberculosis, nocardiosis, candidosis, chronic acne vulgaris, or chronic periodontal disease contained no precipitins at all against the reference antigen. These thus show that crossed immunoelectrophoresis with a standard reference antigen is a specific and valuable diagnostic tool in patients with actinomycosis. More work is needed, however, to test the sensitivity of the method.

6.1.4. Immunopathology of Actinomycosis

Precipitating, complement-fixing, and agglutinating antibodies appearing during the course of clinical actinomycosis might well have implications for the development of the histopathological picture. The continuous presence of antigenic material and the appearance of complement-fixing and precipitating antibodies might form the basis for the formation of local immune complexes with the ability to initiate a hypersensitivity reaction. Immunohistopathological investigations of actinomycotic lesions with the use of the immunofluorescence technique would be of great interest in this respect.

6.2. Immunology of Propionibacteria Infections

There has been much confusion in literature regarding the taxonomy of propionibacteria. They have been considered in the past as anaerobic corynebacteria or anaerobic diphtheroids. They are now called *Propionibacterium* because of this distinguished ability to produce propionic acid. The three most often encountered species, as part of the human microflora or in clinical specimens, are *Propionibacterium acnes, P. avidum,* and *P. granulosum* (Johnson and Cummins, 1972).

6.2.1. Significance of *P. acnes* in Clinical Specimens

P. acnes is the most common *Propionibacterium* encountered in clinical specimens. Two serotypes are recognized, and immunofluorescent techniques have been found quite helpful to differentiate between the two as well as other related bacteria (Holmberg and Forsum, 1973). When strains of this species are isolated from clinical specimens, it is not always clear whether they have etiological significance or represent mere contamination. However, Felner (1974) reported the isolation of *P. acnes* in 15 patients with endocarditis, five of whom had cardiovascular surgery. Levin (1966) and Johnson *et al.* (1968) reported similar findings. Kamme *et al.* (1974) used an immunodiagnostic approach to prove the clinical significance of *P. acnes* isolated in material from late chronic infections after total hip arthroplasty. In serum from such patients these workers demonstrated high agglutination titers against these organisms. The titers were significantly reduced 6 months after reoperation, i.e., the findings of *P. acnes* in these clinical specimens were associated with an active immune response.

6.2.2. Adjuvant Effect of Propionibacteria

O'Neill *et al.* (1973) and Wilkinson *et al.* (1973) have reported an increased phagocytic activity of polymorphonuclear leukocytes, stimulation of lysosomal hydrolases, increase in the weight of the spleen, and enhancement of humoral and cellular immunity when strains of anaerobic propionibacteria are injected into some animal species. The adjuvant effectiveness in humans is under current investigation.

7. Infections Due to Anaerobic Gram-Negative Rods

7.1. General Characteristics

The anaerobic, gram-negative non-spore-forming rods compose a large and important group of bacteria of both man and animals. They are part of the indigenous microflora of the mouth, upper respiratory tract, and intestinal and genital tracts. The six genera recognized are *Bacteroides, Fusobacterium, Leptotrichia, Butyrivibrio, Succinivibrio,* and *Selenomonas.* The last four are very seldom encountered in clinical specimens and appear to have no pathogenic significance (Smith, 1975). Some species of the genus *Bacteroides,* e.g., *B. fragilis* and *B. melaninogenicus,* and of *Fusobacterium* are, however, encountered in clinical specimens from soft tissue infections that often originate from lesions or traumatic injuries of the mucous membranes in the mouth, or the respiratory, gastrointestinal, or genital tract.

7.2. Immunology of *Bacteroides fragilis* Infections

7.2.1. Introduction

Bacteroides fragilis used to be subdivided into five subspecies according to their biochemical characteristics: ssp. *fragilis,* ssp. *thetaiotaomicron,* ssp. *vulgatus,* ssp. *ovatus,* and ssp. *distasonis* (Holdeman and Moore, 1972). Recently, Cato *et al.* (1976) assigned species status to each of the five subspecies.

B. fragilis is the most frequent anaerobic gram-negative nonsporing bacillus found in clinical specimens (Lambe and Moroz, 1976). Its role in bacteremia and septicemia is well documented (Gleb and Seligman, 1970; Felner and Dowell, 1971; Wilson *et al.,* 1972; Danielsson *et al.,* 1974a; Lambe *et al.,* 1975). It has been implicated in endocarditis (Masri and Grieco, 1972; Felner, 1974), pleuropulmonary infections (Bartlett and Finegold, 1972), anaerobic empyema (Sullivan *et al.,* 1973), abdominal wound infections following surgical or other mechanical trauma (Thadepalli *et al.,* 1973), septic abortion (Rotherman and Schick, 1969), and joint infections (Ziment *et al.,* 1969). It is of interest to note that *B. vulgatus* is one of the most common anaerobes isolated from normal fecal specimens, whereas *B. fragilis* is more commonly encountered than *B. vulgatus* in significant clinical infections.

7.2.2. Virulence Factors

A number of workers have studied the lipopolysaaccharide (LPS) O antigen of *B. fragilis* (Hofstad and Kristoffersen, 1970; Ushijima *et al.,* 1971; Sonnenwirth *et al.,* 1972; Hofstad *et al.,* 1972; Meisel-Mikolajczyk and Dworczynski, 1973). Most of these studies dealt with the biochemical composition of LPS. It was similar in many respects to that of other aerobic gram-negative bacteria (Lüderitz *et al.,* 1966). However, Hofstad and Kristoffersen (1970) and Ushijima *et al.* (1971) could not detect 2-ketodeoxyoctonate (KDO). Sonnenwirth *et al.* (1972) reported the presence of KDO in *B. fragilis* using the method described by Warren (1959). Hofstad and Kristoffersen (1970) used the Shwartzman reaction in rabbits to demonstrate that LPS of *B. fragilis* had endotoxic activity. However, compared to endotoxin of aerobic gram-negative bacteria, the activity was low.

The role of a number of other factors potentially contributing to pathogenicity elaborated by the various subspecies of *B. fragilis* has been investigated by several authors. Müller and Werner (1970a,b) have demonstrated the production of neuraminidase. They found that strains isolated from specimens of clinical infections had a higher neuraminidase activity than those isolated from stool specimens. Moreover, the neuraminidase activity of *B. fragilis* was higher than the activity of the neuraminidase formed by other *Bacteroides* strains. The neuraminic-acid-containing glycoprotein of human plasma was altered by the neuraminidase of *B. fragilis* and the activity of this enzyme was demonstrated *in vivo* as well as *in vitro.* Certain strains of *B. fragilis* produce a fibrinolysin (Werner and Müller, 1971). Werner and Rintelen (1968) demonstrated the production of extracellular deoxyribonuclease by various species of *Bacteroides*. However, the role of these enzymes in determining the pathogenicity of *Bacteroides* species is unclear and has not been investigated experimentally.

Kasper (1976) demonstrated a capsule on *B. fragilis* ssp. *fragilis* by electron microscopy; this capsule was absent in other subspecies of *B. fragilis*. Kasper *et al.* (1977) used several techniques to show that only *B. fragilis* ssp. *fragilis* was encapsulated. Onderdonk *et al.* (1977) showed in a rat model of intraabdominal sepsis that implantation of encapsulated *B. fragilis* strains alone resulted in abscess formation whereas unencapsulated strains seldom produced this effect. The ability to form abscesses was related to purified capsular polysaccharide alone, which may represent a virulence factor for *B. fragilis*.

7.2.3. Serological Classification

The first serological studies of *B. fragilis*, carried out with the agglutination technique, provided little evidence that serological classification would be possible (Eggerth and Gagnon, 1933; Henthorne *et al.*, 1936). Four *Bacteroides* serogroups were described by Weiss and Rettger (1937), but these findings were not extended to serotype *Bacteroides* strains isolated from specimens of clinically significant infections.

Recently, more detailed serological studies on the antigenic characteristics of certain species of the *B. fragilis* group were reported by Beerens *et al.* (1971), Shinjo *et al.* (1971), and Romond *et al.* (1972). These workers described six serotypes based on agglutination tests with antiserum prepared in rabbits against six strains of the *B. fragilis* group. By assigning species status to subspecies, they referred to *B. thetaiotaomicron* as serotype A, *B. ovatus* as serotype B, *B. vulgatus* as serotype C, *B. distasonis* a serotype D, and to *B. fragilis* as serotypes E_1 E_2. In a study by Shinjo *et al.* (1971) on 131 strains of the *B. fragilis* group, 93% of the strains possessed the E antigen. The presence of the E antigen was equated to pathogenicity, although criteria to relate the E antigen to pathogenesis, such as animal studies of the presence of virulence factors, were lacking. Heterogeneity in serotype E was also noted; furthermore, cross-reactions with *B. thetaiotaomicron* and *B. fragilis* occurred

with their unadsorbed antisera, and 15 strains of *B. fragilis* failed to react with the six antisera. No attempts were made by these authors to characterize the antigens involved.

A new approach to the serological classification of *B. fragilis* by agglutination was taken by Lambe and Moroz (1976). A detailed classification scheme was elaborated, and the two unique features of this scheme were the use of adsorbed antisera which were monospecific with respect to the immunizing antigens and the use of a larger number of antisera (seven) than that employed by other workers. This study included 98 strains of *B. fragilis* isolated from human clinical specimens and normal feces. The strains tested represented the following geographical areas: Georgia, California, Arizona, New York, and North Carolina of the United States, Sweden, England, and France. The serological classification scheme was composed of 21 serogroups and 24 subserogroups, with a total of 45 serological patterns (Table 2). Each of the seven absorbed antisera failed to cross-react with the other subspecies of the *B. fragilis* group and also with the seven other *Bacteroides* species.

Strains isolated from various human sources were serogrouped with the absorbed antisera. Certain serogroups were rarely encountered, whereas other serogroups were common. Seventy-three percent of all strains isolated from clinical specimens belonged to one of eight serogroups. Twenty-five isolates from blood specimens of bacteremic patients occurred in 14 different serogroups (Moroz, 1975).

The serological studies by Lambe's group look promising for future immunological classification of this large and heterogeneous group of bacteria. These investigations show, however, that the antigenic composition of any particular strain may be rather complicated. These antigens resisted treatment at 100°C for 60 min, but further immunochemical characterizations are needed.

Lambe (1979) developed a polyvalent conjugate (fluorescein isothiocyanate-labeled antibody reagent) for *B. fragilis* which contained conjugates against three strains of *B. fragilis*. This polyvalent conjugate stained 93% of the 111 *B. fragilis* strains tested; the other 7% of *B. fragilis* strains stained some times but not others. The conjugate was specific for *B. fragilis* since 91 strains of anaerobes other than

TABLE 2. Agglutination Results of 98 Strains of *Bacteroides fragilis* ssp. *fragilis* Using Seven Adsorbed *B. fragilis* ssp. *fragilis* Antisera[a]

Serogroup	Subsero-group	Strain No.	Adsorbed antisera (strain No.)						
			1 (289-71)	2 (322-72A)	3 (586-71)	4 (531-71A)	5 (988-72B)	6 (270-72A)	7 (898-72)
I	—	289-71	320	—[b]	—[b]	—[b]	—[b]	—[b]	—[b]
		413-72	40	—	—	—	—	—	—
		411-72A	20	—	—	—	—	—	—
		662-71	40	—	—	—	—	—	—
II	—	322-72A	—	320	—	—	—	—	—
		950-70A	—	20	—	—	—	—	—
		565-71	—	20	—	—	—	—	—
		566-71	—	20	—	—	—	—	—
		442-72B	—	40	—	—	—	—	—
		1586-74	—	80	—	—	—	—	—
		1271-74	—	20	—	—	—	—	—
III	—	586-71	—	—	320	—	—	—	—
		946-72A	—	—	20	—	—	—	—
		863-72	—	—	20	—	—	—	—
		80-72B	—	—	20	—	—	—	—
		850-72A	—	—	40	—	—	—	—
IV	—	531-71A	—	—	—	160	—	—	—
		3-72A	—	—	—	80	—	—	—
V	—	988-72B	—	—	—	—	80	—	—
		380-72	—	—	—	—	20	—	—
VI	—	270-72A	—	—	—	—	—	1280	—
		800-72B	—	—	—	—	—	40	—
		357-72	—	—	—	—	—	160	—
		186-76	—	—	—	—	—	20	—
VII	—	898-72	—	—	—	—	—	—	80
		1227-72	—	—	—	—	—	—	80
		449-71C	—	—	—	—	—	—	40
		1280-73A	—	—	—	—	—	—	40
		1361-73C	—	—	—	—	—	—	40
		1361-73A	—	—	—	—	—	—	40
		1162-74	—	—	—	—	—	—	20
		190-76	—	—	—	—	—	—	40
VIII	a	513-72	20	—	20	20	—	—	—
	b	414-72	20	—	40	—	40	—	—
	c	168-72	40	—	40	—	80	160	—
	d	488-72F	20	—	40	—	—	20	20
	e	694-71B	40	—	20	40	—	20	80
IX	a	141-74	40	—	—	40	—	—	—
X	a	1279-73B	20	—	—	—	—	—	80
		1589-74	20	—	—	—	—	—	40
XI	a	424-72	—	20	—	—	—	—	40
		1270-74	—	40	—	—	—	—	20
	b	1269-74	—	20	40	—	—	—	40
XII	a	76-72	—	—	20	—	40	—	—
		473-72A	—	—	20	—	20	—	—
	b	974-72	—	—	40	20	40	—	—
	c	375-72	—	20	40	40	20	—	—
		185-76	—	80	40	20	20	—	—
	d	189-76	—	—	80	—	20	—	80

(Continued)

TABLE 2. (Continued)

Serogroup	Subsero-group	Strain No.	1 (289-71)	2 (322-72A)	3 (586-71)	4 (531-71A)	5 (988-72B)	6 (270-72A)	7 (898-72)
					Adsorbed antisera (strain No.)				
XIII	a	50-72F	40	—	—	40	20	—	—
		423-72C	20	—	—	40	20	—	—
	b	958-72A	20	—	—	20	20	40	—
	c	786-72	—	—	—	80	80	20	40
XIV	a	337-75	—	—	—	20	—	—	40
		338-75	—	—	—	20	—	—	40
XV	a	1587-74	—	—	—	—	40	—	20
XVI	a	1588-74	—	—	—	—	—	20	40
	b	275-72	—	20	—	—	—	20	40
	c	191-76	—	20	—	—	40	40	40
XVII	a	1226-72	20	80	—	—	—	20	—
	b	1344-72	20	40	40	80	—	80	—
		184-76	20	40	20	40	—	20	—
	c	196-72C	160	20	—	40	—	320	20
	d	658-71A	40	20	—	80	20	20	40
		559-71C	80	20	—	40	40	20	80
		188-76	20	20	—	20	80	80	80
XVIII	a	625-71A	80	—	20	20	20	40	—
		447-71A	40	—	20	20	80	40	—
		1179-72A	40	—	40	40	80	20	—
		515-72	40	—	20	20	40	20	—
	b	1-74	40	—	40	40	160	—	40
		2-74	40	—	20	40	160	—	40
		580-71	20	—	20	20	20	—	160
	c	593-71	80	—	20	40	80	160	20
		183-72	80	—	80	20	40	160	80
		1215-72A	320	—	40	160	40	20	40
XIX	a	1598-74	—	20	—	20	40	—	40
		23-74A	—	40	—	40	80	—	40
		23-74B	—	80	—	40	80	—	80
		913-70	—	20	—	40	40	—	40
		207-72A	—	20	—	80	40	—	40
	b	295-72D	—	20	20	20	20	—	80
	c	34-74B	—	80	—	80	80	40	80
		664-71D	—	20	—	40	20	40	160
XX	a	445-71	—	—	160	—	20	20	20
	b	164-72	—	40	20	—	20	20	20
	c	824-73	20	40	20	—	40	40	80
XXI	a	371-74	80	40	20	40	40	—	—
		514-72	20	20	40	20	40	—	—
	b	507-72A	80	40	40	20	20	20	—
		609-72B	160	20	80	80	20	80	—
		101-72B	20	40	80	40	40	80	—
	c	136-72	40	20	80	20	20	—	20
	d	814-72A	80	40	80	80	80	160	160
		700-72A	80	20	40	40	20	20	20
		109-72	80	40	40	40	40	80	160
		187-76	20	40	20	80	40	40	80
		192-76	40	40	40	20	20	40	40

[a] Reprinted from Lambe and Moroz (1976).
[b] —, ≤10.

B. fragilis, and aerobes, failed to give positive fluorescence.

The *B. fragilis* conjugate was used successfully on a limited number of smears from clinical specimens to detect *B. fragilis* in clinical specimens. Further evaluation of this conjugate needs to be performed on a large number of clinical specimens, although this conjugate shows promise of alerting the clinician to the presence of *B. fragilis* the same day the clinical material is submitted to the laboratory.

7.2.4. Immune Responses

Little information regarding the humoral immune status against anaerobic gram-negative rods was available until a few years ago. Laporte and Brochard (1939) failed to detect flocculating antibody to *Bacteroides funduliformis* (now *Fusobacterium necrophorum*) in normal adults, but antibody to this organism was detected in six patients with septicemia. Monteiro *et al.* (1971) showed the absence of serum antibody to indigenous *Bacteroides* flora (not speciated) in normal subjects, but antibody that reacted with fecal anaerobic bacteria was demonstrated in the washings of the intestinal mucosa of patients with colitis by the indirect immunofluorescent (IF) technique.

Danielsson *et al.* (1972) demonstrated an active immune response against *B. fragilis* ssp. *fragilis* isolated from the perirectal abscess of a patient with Crohn's disease. Antibodies against this strain, but not against a heterologous *Bacteroides* strain, were demonstrated by tube agglutination, the agar gel diffusion (AGD) technique, and indirect IF. A significant fourfold decrease of agglutination and IF titers and a disappearance of precipitating antibodies occurred during an observation period of 5 months after the perirectal abscess had healed. Serum specimens from a limited number of blood donors showed no reactivity with the test antigens.

Later, Danielsson *et al.* (1974a) reported studies of the immune response with agglutination, indirect IF, AGD, and passive hemagglutination tests in a group of patients with septicemia and wound infections. Five patients with *B. fragilis* septicemia showed, as compared with healthy blood donors, elevated agglutination titers against their homologous as well as certain heterologous strains; one to four precipitin bands were detected by AGD

with test antigens of the patient's homologous strains, and occasionally also with heterologous test antigens. Serum from ten blood donors gave agglutination titers of less than 1 : 10 and no precipitin bands by AGD.

The antibody response against *B. fragilis* strains of the patients with abscesses or wound infections was also studied (Danielsson *et al.,* 1974a). Two patients were infected with *B. fragilis* and a third with *B. thetaiotaomicron.* Significant increases of the antibody titers to antigens of homologous but not heterologous strains were demonstrated by agglutination and indirect IF in all three patients.

Rissing *et al.* (1974) used the AGD technique to detect precipitins in 12 patients with bacteremia and eight patients with lung abscess due to *B. fragilis.* In half of the patients, precipitin lines were formed with one or more extracts of *B. fragilis.* In contrast to these findings, Lambe *et al.* (1975), in a study of eight patients with septicemia or pyothorax from whom *B. fragilis* was isolated, demonstrated precipitins by the AGD in the sera of all the patients. The discrepancy between the two studies may be related to the method used for detection of precipitins. Lambe *et al.* (1975) also detected antibodies in the sera of the eight patients by agglutination and indirect IF tests, in titers up to 1 : 160 and 1 : 320. Some of the patient sera reacted with homologous, as well as heterologous, test antigens. These findings suggested two possibilities: an antigenic relationship between certain strains of *B. fragilis* or evidence of past or present infection with strains of a similar serotype. In support of the first hypothesis is the antigenic relationship of 98 strains of *B. fragilis* discussed earlier and the findings of Lambe and Moroz (1976) that 79% of the *B. fragilis* strains possessed a common antigen when tested with unadsorbed antisera.

Lambe and Coleman (unpublished data) developed antigen–antibody reference systems for two strains of *B. fragilis* by use of crossed immunoelectrophoresis (CIE) which showed up to seven precipitates. The two *B. fragilis* strains studied were isolated from a patient with a diagnosis of tumor of the colon; the patient developed peritonitis and septicemia following removal of the tumor. Blood and an abdominal wound yielded pure cultures of *B. fragilis.* Comparison of the two *B. fragilis* strains and their antisera produced in rabbits with tandem-CIE and CIE with intermediate gel showed that the blood strain of *B. fragilis* was more complex antigenically than the abdominal wound isolate.

Sera were collected from the patient at 2 days after onset of fever (acute) and at 8 and 25 days after onset of fever (convalescent). The acute serum and the 8-day serum showed up to three precipitates, whereas the 25-day convalescent serum showed four precipitates. Although further work is needed, it appears likely that CIE may be useful as a rapid diagnostic test to detect antibody in patients with septicemia due to *B. fragilis.*

The above-cited studies have shown the occurrence of an active humoral immune response in patients having clinically significant infections with *B. fragilis,* implying that the demonstration of such an immune response would signify a clinical infection. In contrast, we have not been able to demonstrate precipitins or agglutinins with the standard tube agglutination test in serum from blood donors or other healthy individuals. With the more sensitive passive hemagglutination technique, using untreated sheep erythrocytes sensitized with heat extract antigens from *B. fragilis,* Quick *et al.,* (1972) demonstrated titers of $\geq 1 : 4$ in normal adults. We have reported similar findings in blood donors and healthy individuals, but the titers were usually low and within the range of $1 : 10$–$1 : 40$ (Danielsson *et al.,* 1974a; Persson and Danielsson, 1974). We also showed (Danielsson *et al.,* 1974a) that these antibodies are sensitive to treatment with β-mercaptoethanol, in contrast to those found in sera from patients with significant clinical *B. fragilis* infections. It is of interest to mention the regular findings of significantly higher titers of agglutinins and hemagglutinins in patients with Crohn's disease of the chronic type (Danielsson *et al.,* 1974b; Persson and Danielsson, 1974). The immunological implications of these findings in relation to the histopathological picture of the diseased intestinal mucosa of these patients are still unclear. However, since these antibodies have complement-fixing capacity and are elicited most likely by the continuous presence of antigens in the intestinal lumen, they might well be responsible for the inflammatory reaction typical for the Crohn lesions. We have no information regarding the effect of antibodies detected serologically in serum and the duration of colonization of a given *Bacteroides,* e.g., if immune elimination from the intestinal lesion occurs. We are also lacking knowledge to what extent secretory antibodies are operating at the mucosal level against these organisms in healthy individuals and in patients with acute or chronic bowel disease, nor do we know whether other non-specific factors protect the intestinal mucosa against the attachment of these microorganisms to epithelial cells.

7.3. Immunology of *Bacteroides melaninogenicus* Infections

7.3.1. Introduction

Bacteroides melaninogenicus is an anaerobic, non-spore-forming, gram-negative bacillus that produces a brown-black to black pigmented colony. The three subspecies are *B. melaninogenicus* ssp. *melaniogenicus, B. melaninogenicus* ssp. *asaccharolyticus,* and *B. melaninogenicus* ssp. *intermedius* (Moore and Holdeman, 1973). *B. melaninogenicus* is found as a normal inhabitant in the human intestine (Burdon, 1928), on male and female external genitalia (Burdon, 1928), in the throat (Burdon, 1928; Oliver and Wherry, 1921), and in the gingival crevices of man (Gibbons *et al.,* 1963; Socransky *et al.,* 1963; Burdon, 1928).

B. melaninogenicus has been isolated in mixed culture from many types of infections: tooth abscesses (Kerébel and Sedallian, 1972; Burdon, 1928), periodontal diseases (Macdonald, 1962; Weiss, 1937), gingival infections (Courant and Bader, 1966), orofacial infections (Dormer and Babett, 1972), soft tissue infections (Nobles, 1973), liver abscesses (Sabbaj *et al.,* 1972), lung abscesses (Shevky *et al.,* 1934; Burdon, 1932; Cohen, 1932; Burdon, 1928), pleuropneumonia infections (Bartlett and Finegold, 1972), infected surgical wounds, and urine from a patient with a suspected kidney infection (Oliver and Wherry, 1921), appendicitis and peritonitis (Altemeier, 1938), surgical infections (Weiss, 1943), the uterus and blood from patients with puerperal infection (Schwarz and Dierkmann, 1927), and other infections (Smith and Holdeman, 1968; Shevky *et al.,* 1934).

B. melaninogenicus was implicated as a key

agent in certain mixed anaerobic infections (Gibbons *et al.*, 1963). Experiments were designed to compare the infectivity of mixtures of indigenous bacteria containing *B. melaninogenicus* with that of mixtures in which *B. melaninogenicus* was not present (Socransky and Gibbons, 1965). Several methods were used to delete *B. melaninogenicus* from naturally occurring mixtures of indigenous bacteria of the oral cavity and intestinal tract. Inoculation of these mixtures lacking *B. melaninogenicus* into the groin of guinea pigs failed to produce infections. However, if a strain of *B. melaninogenicus* was added to these mixtures, infection accompanied by inflammatory reaction occurred. When the *B. melaninogenicus* strain alone was injected into guinea pigs, infection did not occur, thus indicating the synergistic nature of the infectious mixture.

7.3.2. Virulence Factors

The mechanism responsible for the pathogenicity of *B. melaninogenicus* is not clear (Socransky and Gibbons, 1965), although *B. melaninogenicus* has been shown to produce a number of possible virulence factors. Gibbons and Macdonald (1961) demonstrated that *B. melaninogenicus* produced an enzyme capable of hydrolyzing collagen; Hausman and Kaufman (1969) found that, unlike the collagenase of clostridia which is released into the growth medium (Seifter *et al.*, 1959), the collagenase of *B. melaninogenicus* is tightly bound to a particulate fraction of the bacterial cell. Since the destruction of collagen is probably necessary for establishing localized infections, and since *B. melaninogenicus* is the only member of the oral flora that appears to produce collagenase, Smith (1975) postulated that collagenase is probably the principal virulence factor of this organism. Furthermore, the production of collagenase is probably the key factor which establishes *B. melaninogenicus* as an essential agent in a mixed anaerobic infection (Smith, 1975). Kaufman *et al.* (1972) found that more severe lesions were produced in rabbits by combining a strain of a fusiform bacterium with a cell-free extract of *B. melaninogenicus* which possessed collagenolytic activity than when either agent alone was injected into rabbits. The end-products of the breakdown of collagen are probably peptides and amino acids which serve as feedback repressors of collagenase. The utilization of these substances by bacteria accompanying *B. melaninogenicus* would result in the continued production of this enzyme (Smith, 1975).

Strains of *B. melaninogenicus* contain endotoxic lipopolysaccharide (Hofstad, 1968, 1969, 1970; Mergenhagen *et al.*, 1961; Sonnenwirth *et al.*, 1972). Hofstad and Kristoffersen (1971) demonstrated that the sugar components of the LPS of *B. melaninogenicus* were galactose, glucose, mannose, rhamnose and traces of fucose, galactosamine, and glucosamine. Heptose and 2-keto-3-deoxy-octonate (KDO) were not demonstrated (Hofstad, 1968). In contrast, Sonnenwirth *et al.* (1972) demonstrated low levels of KDO in a strain of *B. melaninogenicus*. The role of LPS of *B. melaninogenicus* in infections is not known (Smith, 1975), although Hofstad (1970) demonstrated its endotoxic properties with the local Shwartzman reaction and lethality in mice. Other potential pathogenic factors produced by *B. melaninogenicus* include fibrinolysin (Weiss, 1943), and deoxyribonuclease and ribonuclease (Macdonald and Gibbons, 1962).

7.3.3. Serology

Preliminary serological investigations of *B. melaninogenicus*, utilizing the IF staining technique, were performed by Griffin (1970). Lambe (1974) and Lambe and Jerris (1976) described four specific serogroups of *B. melaninogenicus* by IF studies: nine strains of serogroup A, *B. melaninogenicus* ssp. *melaninogenicus;* 82 strains of serogroup B, *B. melaninogenicus* ssp. *asaccharolyticus;* and 38 strains of serogroup C and nine strains of serogroup C1, *B. melaninogenicus* ssp. *intermedius*. The most common serogroup isolated from clinical specimens was serogroup B. A few strains (two of 11) of *B. melaninogenicus* ssp. *melaninogenicus* failed to react with the serogroup A conjugate, and two of 84 strains of *B. melaninogenicus* ssp. *asaccharolyticus* failed to react with serogroup B conjugate. These strains probably represent new rarely occurring serogroups. The four conjugates failed to react with 192 strains of other anaerobic or aerobic bacteria tested.

Serological homogeneity of *B. melaninogenicus* by some workers, of heterogeneity by others, was based on the agglutination technique (Werner and Sebald, 1968; Courant and Gibbons, 1967; Pulverer, 1958; Shevky *et al.*, 1934). The study which closely corroborated Lambe's serogrouping by IF was the agglutination study of Pulverer (1958), who described four serogroups with the agglutination test. He noted the biochemical and serological relationships of the four groups; the four groups were confirmed by the precipitation test.

Lambe and Jerris (1976) developed polyvalent and serogroup-specific IF conjugates that reacted with 158 strains of the four serogroups described previously. The polyvalent conjugate may be used to detect *B. melaninogenicus* isolates; the four specific serogroup IF conjugates may be used to identify the specific serogroup. This identification by IF as soon as a colony is visible on the isolation plate is useful for a rapid identification of *Bacteroides melaninogenicus* from clinical specimens. By contrast, isolation in pure culture, development of characteristic pigmentation, and biochemical identification of *B. melaninogenicus* may require several days to 2 weeks.

7.3.4. Immune Responses

Circulating antibodies to *B. melaninogenicus* have been detected in normal human sera (Hofstad, 1974; Quick *et al.*, 1972; Courant and Gibbons, 1967). Courant and Gibbons (1967) demonstrated the presence of low levels of circulating antibodies in normal human sera with the hemagglutination test. Erythrocytes were sensitized with crude LPS derived from strains isolated from a variety of sources. Hofstad (1974) prepared erythrocytes sensitized with purified LPS from *B. melaninogenicus;* hemagglutinating antibody titers in the sera of healthy human subjects ranged from 1 : 10 to 1 : 320.

An active immune response against *B. melaninogenicus* in humans infected with this organism has not been reported.

7.4. Immunology of *Fusobacterium* Infections

7.4.1. Introduction

Fusobacteria are anaerobic, gram-negative, non-spore-forming rods which produce butyric acid as a major end-product of carbohydrate fermentation. The normal habitat of the fusobacteria is the mouth, and many of the diseases caused by this organism are associated with the respiratory tract (Smith, 1975). *F. nucleatum* is the most common of the fusobacteria isolated from clinical specimens, although *F. necrophorum, F. mortiferum, F. naviforme, F. gonidiaformans,* and *F. varium* may also be isolated from clinical specimens (Holdeman *et al.*, 1974).

Fusobacteria have been isolated from pleuropulmonary infections (Bartlett and Finegold, 1972), bacteremia and septicemia (Felner and Dowell, 1971; Danielsson *et al.*, 1974a), intestinal fistulas (Danielsson *et al.*, 1974a), and soft tissue infections such as wounds and abscesses (Zabransky, 1970). Species of this organism have also been isolated from lesions of endocarditis and sinus infection (Smith, 1975).

7.4.2. Virulence Factors

The presence of endotoxic LPS in fusobacteria has been demonstrated by several workers (Kristoffersen, 1969a,b; Mergenhagen *et al.*, 1961). Electron microscopic studies indicated that the LPS of *Fusobacterium* was morphologically similar to the LPS of other anaerobic and aerobic gram-negative bacteria (Hofstad *et al.*, 1972). Kristoffersen and Hofstad (1970) studied the LPS extracted by the phenol–water procedure from three different strains of oral fusobacteria. In contrast to the LPS extracted from *B. melaninogenicus* (Hofstad, 1968) and *B. fragilis* (Hofstad and Kristoffersen, 1970), the LPS of the fusobacteria contained heptose and KDO. In addition, the LPS from the three different strains contained glucosamine. There were certain differences in the sugar components of the LPS of the three strains: LPS of one of the strains contained glucose and rhamnose, LPS from another contained glucose and mannose, and LPS from the third contained galactose and mannose. This may be of significance, since the specificity of the O antigen in *Salmonella* and related Enterobacteriaceae is determined by the differences in the sugar components of the polysaccharide side chains (Kristoffersen and Hofstad, 1970).

7.4.3. Serology

Kristoffersen (1969a,c,d) described a group-reactive precipitinogen found in strains of oral fusobacteria. This group-specific antigen contained protein, a carbohydrate component, and small amounts of lipid (Kristoffersen, 1969d).

7.4.4. Immune Responses

IgG antibodies in human sera against the purified group-specific antigen were detected by the indirect hemagglutination technique (Kristoffersen, 1969e). Hofstad (1974) detected antibodies in healthy children and blood donors to purified lipopolysaccharide from *F. nucleatum* using the indirect hemagglutination technique.

Danielsson *et al.* (1974a) demonstrated an active immune response against *Fusobacterium* in patients infected with this organism, which indicates the significance of these organisms as pathogenic agents. These authors used the tube agglutination test, passive HA test, indirect IF test, and AGD to study serum specimens from a patient with *F. necrophorum* septicemia. The five sera collected from this patient over a 21-week period showed significant titers by HA and indirect FA tests to his *F. necrophorum* isolate, as well as to a stock strain of *F. necrophorum*, but not to a stock strain of *F. varium*. Two precipitins were detected by AGD. Negative or low titers were obtained in sera from ten blood donors by HA and indirect FA tests. The tube agglutination test was unsuitable, since *F. necrophorum* spontaneously agglutinated.

8. Infections Due to Anaerobic Gram-Positive Cocci

8.1. General Characteristics

Certain anaerobic and microaerophilic gram-positive cocci, e.g., *Peptostreptococcus anaerobius*, *Peptostreptococcus productus*, *Streptococcus intermedius*, *Streptococcus constellatus*, *Peptococcus prevotii*, *Peptococcus asaccharolyticus*, and *Peptococcus saccharolyticus*, are part of the normal human flora of either the upper respiratory tract (Thomas and Hare, 1954), gastrointestinal tract (Moore *et al.*, 1969), or genitourinary tract (Gibbons, 1972). Anaerobic cocci have been isolated in pure culture and/or in association with other anaerobic and aerobic or-

ganisms from a variety of pathological processes (Finegold *et al.*, 1968; Lambe *et al.*, 1972; Pien *et al.*, 1972).

8.2. Serology

Serological studies of various *Peptococcus* species, *Peptostreptococcus* species, and *Streptococcus* species have included whole cell agglutination (McDonald *et al.*, 1937; Weiss and Mercado, 1938), precipitin tests (Weiss and Mercado, 1938), and fluorescent antibody tests (Porschen and Spaulding, 1974).

Coleman and Lambe (1979) studied strains of *S. intermedius*, *S. constellatus*, and *S. morbillorum* by crossed immunoelectrophoresis (CIE). The *S. intermedius* strains studied were isolated from blood, abscesses (brain, liver, back), wounds (occipital, jaw, dorsal), pleural fluid, ascitic fluid, kidney pus, sphenoid sinus, vagina, and cervix; *S. constellatus* strains were isolated from blood, wounds (abdominal, buccal), pleural fluid, maxillary sinus, and scrotum pus; and *S. morbillorum* was isolated from neck and mouth drainage, cornea, buccal mucosa, abdominal fluid, and arm wound. These streptococci were biochemically similar to, but were differentiated from, certain other streptococci such as *S. sanguis*, *S. mitis*, *S. mutans*, and *S. bovis*. Since these streptococci were biochemically similar, CIE was used to study the antigenic structure of *S. intermedius*, *S. constellatus*, and *S. morbillorum* and to compare the cytoplasmic antigens of these organisms with those of certain other species of streptococci. CIE with intermediate gel showed up to six common antigens between *S. intermedius* and *S. constellatus*. Biochemically, *S. intermedius* and *S. constellatus* were also similar. DNA homology studies are needed to determine the taxonomic relationship of these two species. CIE studies showed that the two *S. morbillorum* strains were antigenically more distinct than *S. constellatus* and *S. intermedius*. One *S. morbillorum* strain had one common antigen with *S. intermedius;* the second *S. morbillorum* strain showed no common antigens with *S. intermedius*. No common antigens were observed between *S. morbillorum* and *S. constellatus*. The strain of *S. morbillorum* which was antigenically distinct from the other streptococci species was isolated as the predominant organism from a corneal

ulcer. In the original isolation plate it grew as
tiny, clear satelliting colonies only around colonies of *Staphylococcus epidermidis*. After
repeated subcultures for 3 weeks, *S. morbillorum* grew in pure culture. Tandem-CIE,
which was used to compare the cytoplasmic
antigens of *S. sanguis* and *S. mitis* with those
of *S. constellatus*, *S. intermedius*, and *S. morbillorum*, showed common antigens between
S. sanguis and *S. constellatus*. *S. mitis* shared
a common antigen with *S. constellatus* and one
strain of *S. morbillorum*.

References

Adams, E. B., Laurence, D. R., and Smith, J. W. G.,
1969, *Tetanus*, Blackwell Scientific Publications, Oxford.

Altemeier, W. A., 1938, The bacterial flora of acute per-
forated appendicitis with peritonitis, *Ann. Surg.*
107:517–528.

Altemeier, W. A., and Tytell, A., 1952, Toxoid immunization of experimental gas gangrene; further studies,
AMA Arch. Surg. **65:**633–640.

Anderson, J. D., and Sykes, R. B., 1973, Characterization
of a β-lactamase obtained from a strain of *Bacteroides
fragilis* resistant to β-lactam antibiotics, *J. Med. Microbiol.* **6:**201–206.

Aranki, A., Syed, S. A., Kenney, E. B., and Freter, R.,
1969, Isolation of anaerobic bacteria from human gingiva and mouse cecum by means of simplified glove box
procedure, *Appl. Microbiol.* **17:**568–576.

Atterbery, H. R., Sutter, V. L., and Finegold, S. M., 1974,
Normal human intestinal flora, in: *Anaerobic Bacteria:
Role in Disease* (A. Balows, R. M. DeHaan, L. B. Guze,
and V. R. Dowell, eds.), pp. 81–98, Thomas, Springfield, Ill.

Bartlett, J. G., and Finegold, S. M., 1972, Anaerobic pleuropulmonary infections, *Medicine* **51:**413–450.

Beerens, H., Wattre, P., Shinjo, T., and Romond, C.,
1971, Premiers résultats d'un essai de classification
sérologique de 131 souches de *Bacteroides* du groupe
fragilis (Eggerthella), *Ann. Inst. Pasteur* **121:**187–198.

Behring, Dr., and Kitasato, Dr., 1890, Ueber das Zustan-
denkommen der Diptherie-Immunitat und der Tetanus-
Immunitat bei Thieren *Deutsch. Med. Wehnschr.*
49:1113–1114.

Bizzini, B., Blass, J., Turpin, A., and Raynand, M., 1970,
Chemical characterization of tetanus toxin and toxoid:
Amino acid composition, number of SH and S-S groups
and *N*-terminal amino acid, *Eur. J. Biochem.* **17:**100–105.

Boroff, D. A., and Das Gupta, B. R., 1971, Botulinum
toxin, in: *Microbial Toxins*, Vol. 2 (A. S. Kadis, T. C.
Montio, and S. J. Ajl, eds.), Academic Press, New
York.

Boyd, N. A., Thomason, R. O., and Walker, P. D., 1972,
The prevention of experimental *Clostridium novyi* and
Cl. perfringens gas gangrene in high velocity missiles
wounds by active immunization, *J. Med. Microbiol.*
5:467–472.

Brock, D. W., and Georg, L. K., 1969a, Characterization
of *Actinomyces israelii*, serotypes 1 and 2, *J. Bacteriol.*
97:589–593.

Brock, D. W., and Georg, L. K., 1969b, Determination
and analysis of *Actinomyces israelii* serotypes by fluorescent antibody procedures, *J. Bacteriol.* **97:**581–588.

Brummelkamp, W. H., 1974, Treatment of clostridial infections, in: *Anaerobic Bacteria: Role in Disease* (A.
Balows, R. M. DeHaan, L. B. Guze, and V. R. Dowell,
eds.), pp. 521–552, Thomas, Springfield, Ill.

Burdon, K. L., 1928, *Bacterium melaninogenicum* from
normal and pathogenic tissues, *J. Infect. Dis.* **42:**161–171.

Burdon, K. L., 1932, Isolation and cultivation of *Bacterium melaninogenicum*, *Proc. Soc. Exp. Biol. Med.*
29:1144–1145.

Cato, E. P., and Johnson, J. L., 1976, Reinstatement of
species rank for *Bacteroides fragilis*, *B. ovatus*, *B. distasonis*, *B. thetaiotaomicron*, and *B. vulgatus:* Designation of neotype strains for *Bacteroides fragilis* (Veil-
lon and Zuber) Castellani and Chalmers and *Bacteroides
thetaiotaomicron* (Distaso) Castellani and Chalmers,
Int. J. Syst. Bacteriol. **26:**230–237.

Choudbury, R. P., Mandal, S., Chatterjee, R., and Na-
rayanaswami, A., 1972, Site of action of tetanus toxin
in the central nervous system—Subcellular site of binding of tetanus toxin in the cerebrum, *Ind. J. Med. Res.*
60:1175–1180.

Cohen, J., 1932, The bacteriology of abscess of the lung
and methods for its study, *Arch. Surg.* **24:**171–188.

Coleman, R. M., and Lambe, D. W., Jr., 1979, Serologic
studies of *Streptococcus intermedius*, *Streptococcus
constellatus*, and *Streptococcus morbillorum* by crossed
immunoelectrophoresis, *Am. J. Clin. Path.* **72:**12–20.

Courant, P. R., and Bader, H., 1966, *Bacteroides melaninogenicus* and its products in the gingiva of man, *Per-
iodontics* **4:**131–136.

Courant, P. R., and Gibbons, R. J., 1967, Biochemical and
immunological heterogeneity of *Bacteroides melaninogenicus*, *Arch. Oral Biol.* **12:**1605–1613.

Crawford, J. J., 1971, Interaction of *Actinomyces* organisms with cationic polypeptides. I. Histochemical studies of infected human and animal tissues, *Infect. Immun.*
4:632–641.

Danielsson, D., and Persson, S., 1977, Antibacterial activity of azathioprine (Imuran[R]) against anaerobic intestinal bacteria—Implications in Crohn's disease, in:
*Proceedings from the Xth International Congress of
Chemotherapy*, pp. 295–298, Zurich.

Danielsson, D., Lambe, D. W., Jr., and Persson, S., 1972,
The immune response in a patient to an infection with
Bacteroides fragilis ss. *fragilis* and *Clostridium difficile*,
Acta Pathol. Microbiol. Scand. Ser. B. **80:**709–712.

Danielsson, D., Lambe, D. W., Jr., and Persson, S., 1974a, Immune response to anaerobic infections, in: *Anaerobic bacteria: Role in Disease* (A. Balows, R. M. DeHaan, B. Guze, and V. R. Dowell, eds.), pp. 173–191, Thomas, Springfield, Ill.

Danielsson, D., Kjellander, J., Persson, S., and Wallensten, J., 1974b, Studies on Crohn's disease. IV. Investigation of the immune response to aerobic and anaerobic intestinal bacteria in a patient with Crohn's disease, in: S. Persson, Dissertation, *Acta Universitatis Upsaliensis*, Vol. 188, pp. 1–20, Faculty of Medicine, Uppsala.

Davis, J. B., Mattman, L. H., and Wiley, M., 1951, *Clostridium botulinum* in a fatal wound infection, *JAMA* 146:646–648.

Dawson, D. J., and Mauritzen, C. M., 1968, Studies on tetanus toxin and toxoid. II. Isolation and characterization of the tetanus toxin and toxoid, *Aust. J. Biol. Sci.* 21:559–568.

Del Bene, V. E., and Farrar, W. E., Jr., 1973, Cephalosporinase activity in *Bacteroides fragilis, Antimicrob. Agents, Chemother.* 3(3):369–372.

Dormer, B. J., Jr., and Babett, J. A., 1972, Orofacial infection due to bacteroides a neglected pathogen, *J. Oral Surg.* 30:658–660.

Dowdle, F. B., Koper, G., and Schaafsma, A. W., 1970, Studies on the immunotherapy of tetanus. I. Purification and characterization of tetanus toxin, *S. Afr. J. Med. Sci.* 35:75–80.

Duff, J. T., Wright, G. C., Klerer, J., Moore, D. E., and Bibler, R. H., 1957, Studies on immunity to toxins of *Clostridium botulinum*. I. A simplified procedure for isolation of type A toxin, *J. Bacteriol.* 73:42–47.

Eckmann, L., 1963, *Tetanus, Prophylaxis and Therapy,* Grune, New York.

Eckmann, L., 1967, Principles on tetanus, in: *International Conference on Tetanus, Berne 1966,* pp. 576–577, Huber, Bern.

Eckmann, L., 1970, Zur Anwendung von menschlichem Antitetanus-hyperimmunglobulin, *Schweiz. Med. Wochenschr.* 100:1656–1657.

Edsall, G., 1959, Specific prophylaxis of tetanus, *JAMA* 171:417–427.

Eggerth, A. H., and Gagnon, B. H., 1933, The bacteroides of human feces, *J. Bacteriol.* 25:389–413.

Eklund, M. W., and Poysky, F. T., 1974, Interconversion of type C and D strains of *Clostridium botulinum* by specific bacteriophages, *Appl. Microbiol.* 27:251–258.

Eklund, M. W., Poysky, F. T., Reed, S. M., and Smith, C. A., 1971, Bacteriophage and the toxigenicity of *Clostridium botulinum* type C, *Science* 172:480–482.

Ellis, M., 1963, Human antitetanus serum in the treatment of tetanus, *Br. Med. J.* 1:1123–1126.

Felner, J. M., 1974, Infective endocarditis caused by anaerobic bacteria, in: *Anaerobic Bacteria: Role in Disease* (A. Balows, R. M. DeHaan, B. Guze, and V. R. Dowell, eds.), pp. 345–352, Thomas, Springfield, Ill.

Felner, J. M., and Dowell, V. R., Jr., 1971, "Bacteroides" bacteremia, *Am. J. Med.* 50:787–796.

Finegold, S. M., Miller, A. B., and Sutter, V. L., 1968, Anaerobic cocci in human infection, *Bacteriol. Proc.* 68:94.

Finegold, S. M., Marsh, V. H., and Bartlett, J. G., 1970, Anaerobic infections in the compromised host, in: *Proceedings of the International Conference on Nosocomial Infections,* pp. 123–234, Center for Disease Control, August 3–6, 1970, Waverly Press, Baltimore.

Fischlewitz, J., and Sturm, W., 1967, Booster effect in persons vaccinated in the army against tetanus 10–25 years ago, in: *Principles on Tetanus* (D. Eckmann, ed.), pp. 317–319, Huber, Bern.

Frazier, P. D., and Fowler, B. O., 1967, X-ray diffraction and infrared study of the "sulphur granules" of *Actinomyces bovis, J. Gen. Microbiol.* 46:445–450.

Furste, W., and Wheeler, W. L., 1972, Tetanus: A team disease, in: *Current Problems in Surgery,* Year Book Medical Publishers, Chicago.

Gangarosa, E. J., Donadio, J. A., Armstrong, R. W., Meyer, K. F., Brachman, P. S., and Dowell, V. R., 1971, Botulism in the United States, 1899–1969, *Am. J. Epidemiol.* 93:92–101.

Georg, L. K., 1970, Diagnostic procedures for the isolation and identification of the etiologic agents of actinomycosis, in: *Proceedings of the International Symposium on Mycoses,* pp. 71–81, World Health Organization, Washington, D. C.

Georg, L. K., 1974, The agents of human actinomycosis, in: *Anaerobic Bacteria: Role in Disease* (A. Balows, R. M. DeHaan, L. B. Guze, and V. R. Dowell, eds.), pp. 237–256, Thomas, Springfield, Ill.

Georg, L. K., Coleman, R. M., and Brown, J. M., 1968, Evaluation of an agar gel precipitin test for the serodiagnosis of actinomycosis, *J. Immunol.* 100:1288–1292.

Gibbons, R. J., 1972, Ecology and cariogenic potential of oral streptococci, in: *Streptococci and Streptococcal Disease* (L. W. Wannamaker and J. M. Matsen, eds.), pp. 371–385, Academic Press, New York.

Gibbons, R. J., 1974, Aspects of the pathogenicity and ecology of the indigenous flora of man, in: *Anaerobic Bacteria: Role in Disease* (A. Balows, R. M. DeHaan, L. B. Guze, and V. R. Dowell, eds.), pp. 267–286, Thomas, Springfield, Ill.

Gibbons, R. J., and Macdonald, J. B., 1961, Degradation of collagenous substrates by *Bacteroides melaninogenicus, J. Bacteriol.* 81:614–621.

Gibbons, R. J., Socransky, S. S., Sawyer, S., Kapsimalis, B., and Macdonald, J. B., 1963, The microbiota of the gingival crevice area of man. II. The predominant cultivable organisms, *Arch. Oral Biol.* 8:281–289.

Gleb, A. F., and Seligman, S. J., 1970, *Bacteroidaceae* bacteremia: Effect of age and focus of infection upon clinical course, *JAMA* 212:1038–1041.

Gordon, M., Fiock, M. A., Yarinsky, A., and Duff, J. T., 1957, Studies on immunity to toxins of *Clostridium bo-*

tulinum. III. Preparation, purification and detoxification of type E toxin, *J. Bacteriol.* **74**:533–538.

Griffin, M. H., 1970, Fluorescent antibody techniques in the identification of the gram-negative nonsporeforming anaerobes, *Health Lab. Sci.* **7**:78–83.

Hausman, E., and Kaufman, E., 1969, Collagenase activity in a particulate fraction from *Bacteroides melaninogenicus*, *Biochem. Biophys. Acta* **194**:612–615.

Henthorne, J. C., Thompson, L., and Beaver, D., 1936, Gram-negative bacilli of the genus *Bacteroides*, *J. Bacteriol.* **31**:255–274.

Hofstad, T., 1968, Chemical characteristics of *Bacteroides melaninogenicus* endotoxin, *Arch. Oral Biol.* **13**:1149–1155.

Hofstad, T., 1969, Serological properties of lipopolysaccharide from oral strains of *Bacteroides melaninogenicus*, *J. Bacteriol.* **97**:1078–1082.

Hofstad, T., 1970, Biological activities of endotoxins from *Bacteroides melaninogenicus*, *Arch. Oral Biol.* **15**:343–348.

Hofstad, T., 1974, Antibodies reacting with lipopolysaccharides from *Bacteroides melaninogenicus*, *Bacteroides fragilis*, and *Fusobacterium nucleatum* in serum from normal human subjects, *J. Infect. Dis.* **129**:349–352.

Hofstad, T., and Kristoffersen, T., 1970, Chemical characteristics of endotoxin from *Bacteroides fragilis* NCTC 9343, *J. Gen. Microbiol.* **61**:15–19.

Hofstad, T., and Kristoffersen, T., 1971, Lipopolysaccharide from *Bacteroides melaninogenicus* isolated from the supernatant fluid after ultracentrifugation of the water phase following phenol–water extraction, *Acta Pathol. Microbiol. Scand.* **79**:12–18.

Hofstad, T., Kristoffersen, T., and Selvig, K. A., 1972, Electron microscopy of endotoxic lipopolysaccharide from *Bacteroides*, *Fusobacterium*, and *Sphaerophorus*, *Acta Pathol. Microbiol. Scand.* **80**:413–419.

Holdeman, L. V., and Moore, W. E. C. (eds.), 1972, *Anaerobe Laboratory Manual*, Virginia Polytechnic Institute and State University, Blacksburg, Va.

Holdeman, L. V., Cato, E. P., and Moore, W. E. C., 1974, Current classification of clinically important anaerobes, in: *Anaerobic Bacteria: Role in Disease* (A. Balows, R. M. DeHaan, B. Guze, and V. R. Dowell, eds.), pp. 67–74, Thomas, Springfield, Ill.

Holm, P., and Kwapinski, J. B. 1959, Studies on the detection of *Actinomyces* antibodies in human sera by using pure antigenic fractions of *Actinomyces israelli*, *Acta Pathol. Microbiol. Scand.* **45**:107–112.

Holmberg, K., 1975, Studies on the *Actinomycetaceae* by means of numerical taxonomy, immunofluorescence, and crossed immunoelectrophoresis, Ph.D. thesis, Karolinska Institutet, Stockholm, Sweden.

Holmberg, K., and Forsum, U., 1973, Identification of *Actinomyces*, *Rothia*, and *Propionibacterium* species by defined immunofluorescence, *Appl. Microbiol.* **25**:834–843.

Holmberg, K., Nord, C.-E., and Wadstrom, T., 1975a, Serological studies of *Actinomyces israelii* by crossed

immunoelectrophoresis: Standard antigen–antibody system for *A. israelii, Infect. Immun.* **12**:387–397.

Holmberg, K., Nord, C.-E., and Wadstrom, T., 1975b, Serological studies of *Actinomyces israelii* by crossed immunoelectrophoresis: Taxonomic and diagnostic applications, *Infect. Immun.* **12**:398–403.

Holmes, M. J., and Ryan, W. L., 1971, Amino acid analysis and molecular weight determination of tetanus toxin, *Infect. Immun.* **3**:133–140.

Hungate, R. E., 1950, The anaerobic mesophilic cellulolytic bacteria, *Bacteriol. Rev.* **14**:1–49.

Johnson, J. L., 1973, Use of nucleic-acid homologies in taxonomy of anaerobic bacteria, *Int. J. Syst. Bacteriol.* **23**:308–315.

Johnson, J. L., and Cummins, C. S., 1972, Cell wall composition and deoxyribonucleic acid similarities among the anaerobic coryneforms, classic propionibacteria, and strains of *Arachnia propionica*, *J. Bacteriol.* **109**:1047–1066.

Johnson, W. D., Cobbs, C. G., and Arditi, L. I., 1968, Diphtheroid endocariditis after insertion of a prosthetic heart valve, *JAMA* **203**:919–921.

Kamme, C., Lidgren, L., Lindberg, L., and Mårdh, P-A., 1974, *Scand. J. Infect. Dis.* **6**:161–165.

Kasper, D. L., 1976, The polysaccharide capsule of *Bacteroides fragilis* ss. *fragilis*: Immunochemical and morphologic definition, *J. Infect. Dis.* **133**:79–87.

Kasper, D. L., and Seiler, M. W., 1975, Immunochemical characterization of the outer membrane complex of *Bacteroides fragilis* ss. *fragilis*, *J. Infect. Dis.* **132**:440–450.

Kasper, D. L., Hayes, M. E., Reinop, B. G., Croft, F. D., Onderdonk, A. B., and Polk, B. F., 1977, Isolation and identification of encapsulated strains of *Bacteroides fragilis*, *J. Infect. Dis.* **136**:75–81.

Kaufman, E. J., Mashimo, P. A., Hausman, E., Hanks, C. T., and Ellison, S. A., 1972, Fusobacterial infection: Enhancement by cell free extracts of *Bacteroides melaninogenicus* possessing collagenolytic activity, *Arch. Oral Biol.* **17**:577–578.

Kerébel, B., and Sedallian, A., 1972, Action de *Bacteroides melaninogenicus* sur la dentine *in vitro*, *Schweiz. Monatsschr. Zahnheilk.* **82**:731–734.

Kristoffersen, T., 1969a, Immunochemical studies of oral fusobacteria. I. Major precipitinogens, *Acta Pathol. Microbiol. Scand.* **77**:235–246.

Kristoffersen, T., 1969b, Immunochemical studies of oral fusobacteria. II. Some properties of undigested cell wall preparations, *Acta Pathol. Microbiol. Scand.* **77**:247–257.

Kristoffersen, T., 1969c, Immunochemical studies of oral fusobacteria. III. Purification of a group reactive precipitinogen, *Acta Pathol. Microbiol. Scand.* **77**:446–456.

Kristoffersen, T., 1969d, Immunochemical studies of oral fusobacteria. IV. Some chemical properties of a group reactive precipitinogen, *Acta Pathol. Microbiol. Scand.* **77**:457–464.

Kristoffersen, T., 1969e, Immunochemical studies of oral fusobacteria. VI. Distribution of a group reactive antigen among some bacteria and occurrence of antibodies in human sera to this antigen, *Acta Pathol. Microbiol. Scand.* **77:**717–726.

Kristoffersen, T., and Hofstad, T., 1970, Chemical composition of lipopolysaccharide endotoxins from human oral fusobacteria, *Arch. Oral Biol.* **15:**909–916.

Lambe, D. W., Jr., 1974, Determination of *Bacteroides melaninogenicus* serogroups by fluorescent antibody staining, *Appl. Microbiol.* **28:**561–567.

Lambe, D. W., Jr., 1979, Characterization of a polyvalent conjugate of *Bacteroides fragilis* by fluorescent antibody staining, *Am. J. Clin. Path.* **71:**97–101.

Lambe, D. W., Jr., and Jerris, R. C., 1976, Description of a polyvalent conjugate and a new serogroup of *Bacteroides melaninogenicus* by fluorescent antibody staining, *J. Clin. Microbiol.* **3:**506–512.

Lambe, D. W., Jr., and Moroz, D. M., 1976, Serogrouping of *Bacteroides fragilis* subsp. *fragilis* by the agglutination test, *J. Clin. Microbiol.* **3:**586–592.

Lambe, D. W., Jr., Vroon, D. H., and Rietz, C. W., 1972, Infections due to anaerobic cocci, in: *Anaerobic Bacteria: Role in Disease* (A. Balows, R. M. DeHaan, L. B. Guze, and V. R. Dowell, eds.), pp. 585–599, Thomas, Springfield, Ill.

Lambe, D. W., Jr., Danielsson, D., Vroon, D. H., and Carver, R. K., 1975, Immune response in eight patients infected with *Bacteroides fragilis, J. Infect. Dis.* **131:**499–508.

Laporte, A., and Brochard, H., 1939, La réaction de floculation du sérum en présence d'un estrait alcoolique microbein dans les infections a *Bacillus funduliformis, C. R. Soc. Biol. (Paris)* **131:**4–7.

Latham, W. C., Bent, D. F., and Levine, L., 1962, Tetanus toxin production in the absence of protein, *Appl. Microbiol.* **10:**146–152.

Levin, J., 1966, Diphtheroid bacterial endocarditis after insertion of a Starr valve, *Ann. Intern. Med.* **64:**396–399.

Levine, L., McCombe, J. A., Roderick, D. E. M., Dwyer, C., and Latham, W. C., 1966, Active–passive tetanus immunization. Choice of toxoid, dose of tetanus immunoglobulin and timing of injections, *N. Engl. J. Med.* **274:**186–190.

Lerner, P. I., 1974, Serologic screening for actinomycosis, in: *Anaerobic Bacteria: Role in Disease* (A. Balows, R. H. DeHaan, L. B. Guze, and V. R. Dowell, Jr. eds.), pp. 571–584, Thomas, Springfield, Ill.

Lüderitz, O., Staub, A. M., and Westphal, O., 1966, Immunochemistry of O and R antigens of *Salmonella* and related Enterobacteriaceae, *Bacteriol. Rev.* **30:**192–255.

Macdonald, J. B., 1962, On the pathogenesis of mixed anaerobic infections of mucous membranes, *Ann. R. Coll. Surg. Engl.* **31:**361–378.

Macdonald, J. B., and Gibbons, R. J., 1962, The relationship of indigenous bacteria to periodontal disease, *J. Dent. Res.* **41:**320–326.

Macfarlane, M. G., 1943, The therapeutic value of gas gangrene antitoxin, *Br. Med. J.* **2:**636–640.

Macheak, M. E., Claus, K. D., and Maloy, S. E., 1972, Potency testing *Clostridium novyi*-containing bacterins:

Comparison of immunologic response in guinea pigs and sheep, *Am. J. Vet. Res.* **33:**1201–1208.

MacLennan, J. D., 1962, The histotoxic clostridial infections of man, *Bacteriol. Rev.* **26:**177–276.

MacLennan, J. D., and Macfarlane, M. G., 1944, Treatment of gas gangrene, *Br. Med. J.* **1:**683–685.

Mandia, J. W., 1955, The position of *Clostridium tetani* within the serological schema for proteolytic clostridia, *J. Infect. Dis.* **97:**66–72.

Månsson, I., and Olhagen, B., 1967, Intestinal *Clostridium perfringens* in arthritis and parakeratosis induced by dietary factors: Experimental studies in pigs, *Bull. Off. Int. Epiz.* **67:**1319–1327.

Månsson, I., Norberg, R., Olhagen, B., and Björklund, N. E., 1971, Arthritis in pigs induced by dietary factors: Microbiologic, clinical and histologic studies, *Clin. Exp. Immunol.* **9:**677–693.

Masri, A. F., and Grieco, M. H., 1972, Bacteroides endocarditis: Report of a case, *Am. J. Med. Sci.* **263:**357–367.

McDonald, J. R., Henthorne, J. C., and Thompson, L., 1937, Role of anaerobic streptococci in human infections, *Arch. Pathol.* **23:**230–240.

Meisel-Mikolajczyk, F., and Dworczynski, A., 1973, Chemical composition of endotoxins of *Eggerthella convexa* (*Bacteroides fragilis*) strain, *Bull. Acad. Pol. Sci. Ser. Sci. Biol.* **6:**193–197.

Mergenhagen, S. E., Hampp, E. G., and Scherp, H. W., 1961, Preparation and biological activities of endotoxins from oral bacteria, *J. Infect. Dis.* **108:**304–310.

Merson, M. H., and Dowell, V. R., Jr., 1973, Epidemiologic, clinical and laboratory aspects of wound botulism, *N. Engl. J. Med.* **289:**1005–1010.

Monteiro, E., Fossey, J., Shiner, M., Draser, B. S., and Allison, A. C., 1971, Antibacterial antibodies in rectal and colonic mucosa in ulcerative colitis, *Lancet* **1:**249–251.

Moore, W. E. C., and Holdeman, L. V., 1973, New names and combinations in the genera *Bacteroides* Castellani and Chambers, *Fusobacterium* Knorr, *Eubacterium* Prévot, *Propionibacterium* Delwich, and *Lactobacillus* Orla-Jensen, *Int. Syst. Bacteriol.* **23:**69–74.

Moore, W. E. C., and Holdeman, L. V., 1974, Human fecal flora: The normal flora of 20 Japanese-Hawaiians, *Appl. Microbiol.* **27:**961–979.

Moore, W. E. C., Cato, E. P., and Holdeman, L. V., 1969, Anaerobic bacteria of the gastrointestinal flora and their occurrence in clinical infections, *J. Infect. Dis.* **119:**641–649.

Moroz, D. A., 1975, A serological study of *Bacteroides fragilis* subsp. *fragilis* by the tube agglutination technique, Master's thesis, Emory University, Atlanta, Ga.

Müller, H. E., and Werner, H., 1970a, Die Neuraminidase als pathogenetischer Fator bei eivem durch *Bacteroides fragilis* bedingten Abscess, *Z. Med. Mikrobiol. Immunol.* **156:**98–106.

Müller, H. E., and Werner, H., 1970b, *In vitro* Untersuchungen über das Vorkommen von Neuraminidase bei Bacteroides arten, *Pathol. Microbiol.* **36**:135–152.

Nobles, E. R., 1973, Bacteroides infections, *Ann. Surg.* **177**:601–606.

Oliver, W. W., and Wherry, W. B., 1921, Notes on some bacterial parasites of the human mucous membranes, *J. Infect. Dis.* **28**:341–344.

Onderdonk, A. B., Kasper, D. L., Cisneros, R. L., and Bartlett, J. G., 1977, The capsular polysaccharide of *Bacteroides fragilis* as a virulence factor: Comparison of the pathogenic potential of encapsulated and unencapsulated strains, *J. Infect. Dis.* **136**:82–89.

O'Neill, G. J., Henderson, D. C., and White, R. G., 1973, The role of anaerobic coryneforms on specific and nonspecific immunological reactions. I. Effect on particle clearance and humoral and cell mediated immune responses, *Immunology* **24**:977–995.

Osborne, R. H., and Bradford, H. F., 1973, Tetanus toxin inhibits amino acid release from nerve endings *in vitro*, *Nature (London)* **244**:157–158.

Owen-Smith, M. S., and Matheson, J. M., 1968, Successful prophylaxis of gas gangrene of the high-velocity missile wound in sheep, *Br. J. Surg.* **55**:36–39.

Pearson, H. E., and Smiley, D. F., 1968, *Bacteroides* in pilonidal sinuses, *Am. J. Surg.* **113**:336–338.

Persson, S., and Danielsson, D., 1974, Studies on Crohn's disease. V. On the occurrence of serum antibodies to *Bacteroides fragilis* and serogroups of *E. coli* in patients with Crohn's disease, in: S. Persson, Dissertation, *Acta Universitatis Upsaliensis*, Vol. 188, pp. 1–20, Faculty of Medicine, Uppsala.

Pien, F. D., Thompson, R. L., and Martin, W. J., 1972, Clinical and bacteriologic studies of anaerobic gram positive cocci, *Mayo Clin. Proc.* **47**:251–257.

Pillemer, L., Wittler, R., and Grossberg, D. B., 1946, The isolation and crystallization of tetanal toxin, *Science* **103**:615–616.

Pillemer, L., Wittler, R. G., Burrell, J. I., and Grossberg, D. B., 1948, The immunochemistry of toxins and toxoids. VI. The crystallization and characterization of tetanal toxin, *J. Exp. Med.* **88**:205–221.

Pinkus, G., Veto, G., and Braude, A. I., 1968, *Bacteroides* penicillinase, *J. Bacteriol.* **96**:1437–1438.

Porschen, R. K., and Spaulding, E. H., 1974, Fluorescent antibody study of the gram-positive anaerobic cocci, *Appl. Microbiol.* **28**:851–855.

Pulverer, G., 1958, Zur Morphologie, Biochemie, und Serologie des *Bacteroides melaninogenicus*, *Z. Hyg. Infektionskr. Med. Mikrobiol. Immunol. Virol.* **145**:293–303.

Quick, J. D., Goldberg, H. S., and Sonnenwirth, A., 1972, Human antibody to Bacteroidaceae, *Abstr. Annu. Meet. Am. Soc. Microbiol.*, p. 94.

Regamey, R. H., 1965, Gammaglobuline antitétanique humaine et séroprophylaxis du tétanos, in: *Progress in Immunobiological Standardization* (Regamey, Hennesen, Ikic, and Ungar, eds.), pp. 93–116, Karger, Basel.

Rissing, J. P., Crowder, J. G., Smith, J. W., and White,

A., 1974, Detection of *Bacteroides fragilis* infection by precipitin antibody, *J. Infect. Dis.* **130**:70–73.

Robertson, M., and Keppie, J., 1943, Gas gangrene; active immunization by means of concentrated toxoids, *Lancet* **2**:311–314.

Romond, C., Beerens, H., and Wattre, P., 1972, Identification sérologique des *Bactéroides* en relation avec leur pouvoir pathogene, *Arch. Roum. Pathol. Exp. Microbiol.* **31**:351–355.

Rosebury, T., 1962, *Microorgranisms Indigenous to Man*, McGraw-Hill, New York.

Rotherman, E. G., and Schick, S. F., 1969, Nonclostridial anaerobic bacteria in septic abortion, *Am. J. Med.* **46**:80–89.

Sabbaj, J., Sutter, V. L., and Finegold, S. M., 1972, Anaerobic pyogenic liver abscess, *Ann. Intern. Med.* **77**:629–638.

Schwarz, O. H., and Dierkmann, W. J., 1927, Puerperal infection due to anaerobic streptococci, *Am. J. Obstet. Gynecol.* **13**:467–485.

Sedallian, A., Frocrain, C., and Rouxel, A., 1972, Bactéroides du groupe fragilis identification biochemique et sérologique, *Quest Med.* **24**:2563–2568.

Seifter, S., Gallop, P. M., Klein, L., and Meilman, E., 1959, Studies on collagen. II. Properties of purified collagenase and its inhibition, *J. Biol. Chem.* **234**:285–293.

Shevky, M., Kohl, C., and Marshall, M. S., 1934, *Bacterium melaninogenicum*, *J. Lab. Clin. Med.* **19**:689–694.

Shinjo, T., Beerens, H., and Romond, C. H., 1971, Classification sérologique de 131 souches de *Bactéroides* du groupe *fragilis* (Eggerthella), *Ann. Inst. Pasteur* **22**:85–100.

Skulberg, A., 1964, Studies on the formation of toxin by *Clostridium botulinum*, Doctoral thesis, Norges Veterinaerhögskole, Oslo.

Slack, J. M., Lanfried, S., and Gerencser, M. A., 1969, Morphological, biochemical and serological studies of 64 strains of *Actinomyces israelii*, *J. Bacteriol.* **97**:873–884.

Slack, J. M., and Gerencser, M. A., 1970, Two new serological groups of *Actinomyces*, *J. Bacteriol.* **103**:266–267.

Smith, L. Ds., 1975, *The Pathogenic Anaerobic Bacteria*, Thomas, Springfield, Ill.

Smith, L. Ds., and Holdeman, L. V., 1968, *The Pathogenic Anaerobic Bacteria*, Thomas, Springfield, Ill.

Socransky, S. S., and Gibbons, R. J., 1965, Required role of *Bacteroides melaninogenicus* in mixed anaerobic infections, *J. Infect. Dis.* **115**:247–253.

Socransky, S. S., Gibbons, R. J., Dale, H. C., Bortnick, L., Rosenthal, E., and Macdonald, J. B., 1963, The microbiota of the gingival crevice area of man. I. Total microscopic and viable counts and counts of specific organisms, *Arch. Oral Biol.* **8**:275–280.

Sonnenwirth, A. C., Yin, E. T., Sarmiento, E. M., and Wessler, S., 1972, Bacteroidaceae endotoxin detection by *Limulus* assay, *Am. J. Clin. Nutr.* **25**:1452–1454.

Sterne, M., and Wentzel, L. M., 1950, A new method for

the large scale production of high-titer botulinum formol-toxoid types C and D, *J. Immunol.* **65:**175–183.

Sullivan, K. M., O'Toole, R. D., Fischer, R. H., and Sullivan, K. N., 1973, Anaerobic empyema thoracis: The role of anaerobes in 226 cases of culture-proven empyemas, *Arch. Intern. Med.* **13:**521–527.

Swenson, R. M., Michaelson, T. C., Daly, M. J., and Spaulding, E. H., 1973, Anaerobic bacterial infections of the female genital tract, *Obstet. Gynecol.* **42:**538–541.

Takahara, S., 1952, Progressive oral gangrene probably due to lack of catalase in the blood (acatalasemia), *Lancet* **2:**1101–1104.

Thadepalli, H., Gorbach, S. L., Broido, P. W., Norsen, J., and Hyhus, L., 1973, Abdominal trauma, anaerobes, and antibiotics, *Surg. Gynecol. Obstet.* **137:**270–276.

Thomas, C. G. A., and Hare, R., 1954, The classification of anaerobic cocci and their isolation in normal human beings and pathological processes, *J. Clin. Pathol.* **7:**300–304.

Thomson, R. O., Batty, I., Thomson, A., Kerry, J. B., Epps, B. H. G., and Foster, W. H., 1969, The immunogenicity of a multicomponent clostridial oil emulsion vaccine in sheep, *Vet. Res.* **85:**81–85.

Ullberg-Olsson, K., 1975a, Active immunization against tetanus in man. III. Antibody response to vaccine injections in the presence of therapeutic doses of human tetanus immune globulin. A record of five cases, *Eur. Surg. Res.* **7:**305–314.

Ullberg-Olsson, K., 1975b, Active immunization against tetanus in man and guinea pigs. An experimental and clinical study, Doctoral thesis, Karolinska Institutet, Stockholm.

Ullberg-Olsson, K., and Eriksson, E., 1975, Active immunization against tetanus in man. I. Duration of anamnestic reaction after one dose of vaccine, *Eur. Surg. Res.* **7:**249–258.

Ushijima, T., Ueno, K., Suzuki, S., and Kurimoto, U., 1971, Morphology and chemistry of the bacterial cell wall. II. Sugar composition and location of O-antigen in the cell wall of *Bacteroides convexus. J. Electron Microsc.* **20:**32–39.

Van Ermengen, E., 1897, Ueber einen neuen anaeroben Bacillus und seine Beziehung zum Botulismus, *Z. Hyg.* **26:**1–56.

van Heyningen, W. E., 1955, The role of toxins in pathology, in: *Society of General Microbiology, Symposium No. 5,* pp. 17–39, Cambridge University Press, Cambridge.

van Heyningen, W. E., and Mellanby, J., 1971, Tetanus toxin, in: *Microbial Toxins,* Vol. II (A. S. Kadis, T. C. Montie, and S. J. Ajl, eds.), Academic Press, New York.

Veronesi, R., Cecin, H., Corréa, A., Tavares, J., Moraes, C., and Nascimento, O. J., 1973, New concepts on tetanus immunization: Naturally acquired immunity. Preliminary report, *Rev. Hosp. Clin. Fac. Med. Univ. Sao. Paulo* **28:**313–318.

Warren, L., 1959, The thiobarbituric acid assay of sialic acids, *J. Biol. Chem.* **234:**1971–1975.

Weiss, C., 1937, Observations on *Bacterium melaninogenicum:* Demonstration of fibrinolysin, pathogenicity, and serological types, *Proc. Soc. Exp. Biol. Med.* **37:**473–476.

Weiss, C., 1943, The pathogenicity of *Bacteroides melaninogenicus* and its importance in surgical infections, *Surgery* **13:**683–691.

Weiss, C., and Mercado, D. G., 1938, Studies of anaerobic streptococci from pulmonary abscesses, *J. Infect. Dis.* **62:**181–185.

Weiss, J. E., and Rettger, L. F., 1937, The gram-negative bacteroides of the intestine, *J. Bacteriol.* **33:**423–434.

Werner, H., and Sebald, M., 1968, Etude sérologique d'anaerobies Gram-négatif asporulés, et particulièrement de *Bacteroides convexus* et *Bacteroides melaninogenicus, Ann. Inst. Pasteur* **115:**350–366.

Werner, H., and Rintelen, G., 1968, Untersuchungen über die Konstanz der Kohlenhydratspaltung bei intestinal Bacteroides (Eggerthella)—Arten, *Zen. Bakteriol. Orig.* **208:**521–528.

Werner, H., and Müller, H. E., 1971, Immunelektrophoretishe Untersuchungen über die Einwirkung von Bacteroides-, Fusobacterium-, Leptotrichia- and Sphaerophorus-Aten auf menschliche Plasmaproteine, *Zbl. Bakteriol. I. Abt. Orig.* **216:**96–113.

Wilkinson, P. C., O'Neill, G. J., and Wapshaw, K. G., 1973, Role of anaerobic coryneforms in specific and non-specific immunological reactions. II. Production of a chemotactic factor specific for macrophages, *Immunology* **24:**997–1006.

Willis, A. T., 1969, *Clostridia of Wound Infection,* Butterworth, London.

Willis, A. T., Ferguson, I. R., Jones, P. H., Phillips, K. D., and Edwards, D., 1977, Metronidazole in prevention and treatment of bacteroides infections in elective colonic surgery, *Br. Med. J.* **1:**607–610.

Wilson, W. R., Martin, W. F., Wilkowske, C. J., and Washington, J. A., 1972, Anaerobic bacteremia, *Mayo Clin. Proc.* **47:**639–646.

Wright, G. P., 1955, The neurotoxins of *Clostridium botulinum* and *Clostridium tetani, Pharmacol. Rev.* **7:**413–465.

Zabransky, R. J., 1970, Isolation of anaerobic bacteria from clinical specimens, *Mayo Clin. Proc.* **45:**256–264.

Ziment, I., Davis, A., and Finegold, S. M., 1969, Joint infection by anaerobic bacteria: A case report and review of the literature, *Arthritis Rheum.* **12:**627–634.

14

Immunology of *Mycobacterium tuberculosis*

MAURICE J. LEFFORD

1. Introduction

Tuberculosis is an infectious disease caused predominantly by *Mycobacterium tuberculosis,* but other mycobacterial species may produce an indistinguishable or closely similar disease in man. Tuberculosis was recognized by early physicians such as Hippocrates, and archeological studies indicate that man has been afflicted by this disease for many thousands of years. Although almost any organ may be affected, pulmonary tuberculosis is the most common manifestation of clinical disease.

There is indirect evidence that tuberculosis has been prevalent for thousands of years in Europe. The peak incidence of the disease probably occurred in the nineteenth century, as a result of the rapid urbanization and poor living conditions that followed the industrial revolution. The paramount importance of the disease during the naissance of microbiology and post-Laennnec clinical medicine, in the latter part of the nineteenth century and early twentieth century, is reflected by the extensive literature on tuberculosis. During the past 80 years the prevalence of tuberculosis in technologically advanced countries has dropped steadily (Styblo *et al.,* 1969). Much as one might wish otherwise, this improvement is probably not attributable to the undoubted scientific contributions to the control of tuberculosis, such as pasteurization of milk, im-

munization, and effective chemotherapy. The initial decline in tuberculosis incidence predates these innovations and was a consequence of improved socioeconomic conditions (Styblo, 1968). It has been predicted that if the incidence of tuberculosis in the United States and Western Europe continues to decline at its present rate, the disease should become virtually extinct in these countries within 100 years. However, in the United States today, there are still approximately 30,000 new cases of tuberculosis a year, which are mainly concentrated where poverty is worst: the decayed inner cities, Indian reservations, and the area north of the border with Mexico (Tuberculosis in the United States, 1976). Tuberculosis continues to be prevalent in the poorer countries of the world, in which it remains the most important communicable disease.

Tuberculosis is a peculiarly interesting example of host–parasite relationships in chronic diseases. Although the causative organism will, under favorable conditions, infect almost the entire population, only a relatively small proportion of hosts develop clinical disease. In most patients with overt tuberculosis the disease progresses with variable rapidity, but in some it regresses spontaneously for no apparent reason. Tuberculosis is also the archetype of diseases which induce cell-mediated immunity in relatively "pure" form: a material role for humoral immunity has never been substantiated in this disease. Finally, tuberculosis is unique in that the causative organisms have most potent immunological adjuvants incorporated within their cell walls (Lederer, 1976). These not only play a role in the immune re-

MAURICE J. LEFFORD ● Department of Immunology and Microbiology, Wayne State University of Medicine, Detroit, Michigan 48201.

sponse to tubercle bacilli but also can modulate the immune response in unrelated host–parasite systems and in neoplasia (Yashphe, 1971).

2. Bacteriology

Mycobacteria are nonmotile, nonsporing, aerobic rods belonging to the family Mycobacteriaceae, order Actinomycetales. They do not stain easily but are stainable by carbol fuchsin, particularly when heated. Once stained, they are resistant to decolorization by mineral acids and are hence termed acid-fast bacilli (AFB).

The genus *Mycobacterium* includes a wide variety of species that differ widely with respect to their pathogenicity to man. The spectrum of pathogenicity ranges from harmless saprophytes like *M. phlei* to highly virulent organisms such as *M. tuberculosis* and *M. bovis*. These last two species, especially *M. tuberculosis,* are largely responsible for clinical tuberculosis in man, in whom both produce an essentially similar disease. There are other mycobacterial species that are potentially pathogenic to man: *M. africanum, M. avium, M. chelonei, M. fortuitum, M. intracellulare, M. kansasii, M. leprae, M. marinum, M. scrofulaceum, M. simiae, M. szulgai, M. ulcerans,* and *M. xenopi* (Runyon, 1974). With the exception of leprosy, which is described elsewhere in this volume, the immunological characteristics of diseases produced by all the pathogenic mycobacteria are similar and will be considered as one.
as one.

3. Natural History of Tuberculosis

The common portals of entry of *M. tuberculosis* and *M. bovis* are the respiratory and alimentary tracts, respectively. There is no conspicuous lesion at the site of entry, but the organism reaches the draining lymph nodes where multiplication and pathological changes occur. During this period it is probable that a bacteremia occurs and bacilli are seeded through the body in locations such as the lungs, brain, kidneys, and bones. The host develops delayed hypersensitivity (DTH) to

tuberculin, but the infection is usually self-limiting and even inapparent. This type of infection is termed "primary tuberculosis." Occasionally, primary tuberculosis is progressive and may be expressed as mediastinal lymph node, peritoneal, renal, skeletal, miliary, or meningeal disease. Such progressive primary disease has a brisk tempo and may be rapidly fatal.

The common outcome of primary tuberculosis is that the host remains well but the state of tuberculin hypersensitivity persists. However, a small proportion of such subjects subsequently develop clinical tuberculosis, often after many years of health. Such disease is called postprimary, reinfection, or "secondary tuberculosis." The term "reinfection tuberculosis" implies that it is caused by organisms that have been contracted from an exogenous source, but there is contrary evidence that such disease is caused by recrudescence of endogenous primary infection that was acquired many years before.

The reinfection theory draws its support from the observation that secondary tuberculosis differs from primary tuberculosis with respect to its anatomical location and pathology. More direct evidence has recently been obtained through the use of mycobacteriophage typing. *M. tuberculosis* cultures of different phage types were isolated sequentially from patients before and after antituberculosis chemotherapy. The implication of this finding is that these patients contracted an exogenous reinfection (Raleigh *et al.,* 1975). The evidence for reactivation of endogenous disease is drawn from animal experiments and epidemiological studies (Stead, 1967). Animals which have been infected with mycobacteria are extremely resistant to reinfection, which can be established only with large challenge inocula. By analogy, it would be equally difficult to reinfect man. This conjecture is corroborated by the observation that, in heavy exposure situations, the incidence of tuberculosis is higher among previously tuberculin-negative than tuberculin-positive subjects. The converse is also true, namely, that where exposure to exogenous tubercle bacilli is light, the incidence of tuberculosis is higher in tuberculin-positive subjects. This paradox is explicable only in terms of reactivation of endogenous latent disease, and it is this theory that is more widely accepted. There remains the problem of why a host who can resist a large inoculum of reinfecting organisms cannot with equal ease prevent the growth of a small number of endogenous bacilli. Since the vast majority of such patients reveal no evidence of immunodeficiency, other explanations have been sought.

In low-prevalence situations, such as apply in the United States, the incidence of tuberculosis is higher in that part of the population more than 40 years old and the case rate continues to rise with advancing years. The low incidence of tuberculosis in the younger population is due to the low prevalence of tubercle bacilli, as a consequence of which the risk of primary tuberculosis and its sequelae is diminishing. The older part of the population is the remnant of a cohort which was at greater risk to primary tuberculosis during childhood and is therefore subject to recrudescence of latent infection. The risk of reactivation of infection in any individual is very small but cumulative. Hence the longer a person lives, the more likely he is to suffer the "accident" of secondary tuberculosis (Comstock, 1975).

In the present era of chemotherapy, when the natural history of tuberculosis is rarely observed, it is appropriate to note that untreated secondary tuberculosis is not necessarily progressive and fatal. There are many living testimonials to this fact, survivors of the era preceding the advent of antituberculosis chemotherapy.

4. Bacterial Factors in Pathogenicity

M. tuberculosis and *M. bovis* are obligate parasites and can be isolated in the wild only from tuberculous hosts and their fomites. Hence any freshly isolated or wild strain of *M. tuberculosis* is, by definition, virulent to man. The quantitative assessment of degree of virulence is measured in experimental animals, of which the most commonly used are guinea pigs and mice.

Most wild strains of *M. tuberculosis* are of remarkably uniform virulence to guinea pigs, but it is common for laboratory strains to become attenuated, either by accident or design. A classical example of the latter is the vaccine strain of BCG, which was derived by atten-

uation of virulent strain of *M. bovis*. In the past 25 years two groups of wild strains of *M. tuberculosis* have been identified that are of reduced virulence to guinea pigs. The first group comprises strains of *M. tuberculosis* which have become resistant either *in vivo* or *in vitro* to the antibacterial drug isoniazid (Barnett *et al.*, 1953; Karlson, 1954). The second group of strains has been isolated most frequently from untreated patients in South India (Mitchison *et al.*, 1960). It should be emphasized that neither group of strains is of reduced virulence in mice and there is no clear evidence that they are less virulent in man (Mitchison, 1964).

Theoretically, there are three components of virulence. The first, which may be termed "intrinsic" virulence, is the ability of the organism to multiply within tissues of the non-immune host. For example, *M. tuberculosis* H37Rv grows more rapidly than BCG, both in mouse tissues *in vivo* prior to the induction of immunity and in normal mouse macrophages *in vitro* (Pierce *et al.*, 1953; Mackaness *et al.*, 1954). The second component of virulence is the ability of the organism to survive the immune mechanisms of the host. The parasite may induce an immune response in the host yet resist the established effector mechanism, namely, the microbicidal action of activated macrophages. Other possibilities are that the parasite may be poorly immunogenic or may engender an inappropriate immune response, so that the host is unable to muster an effective antibacterial reaction. Finally, virulence may be a reflection of the ability of the parasite to elaborate toxic materials. More than one of these factors may be involved in the host–parasite interaction at any given time.

In some bacterial genera virulence has been clearly associated with a secretory product or structural constituent of the organism, e.g., the polysaccharide capsule of pneumococci. No such clear-cut explanation of mycobacterial virulence has been elucidated, although two cell wall components have been suspected: cord factor (Bloch, 1950) and strongly acidic lipids (Middlebrook *et al.*, 1959). Cord factor is a dimycolate of trehalose and is probably identical (Goren, 1975) with the cell wall component P3, which has been independently isolated by another group of workers (Azuma *et al.*, 1974). Cord factor suspended in mineral oil kills normal mice when injected intraperitoneally. This action is thought to be effected through damage inflicted on the mitochondria of the hepatic parenchyma (Kato, 1968). Cord factor in an oil-in-water emulsion can also produce tuberculoid granulomata in mice (Bekierkunst et al., 1969; Meyer et al., 1975). The relationship between cord factor and virulence is somewhat ambiguous, since cord factor can be isolated from attenuated strains of virulent mycobacteria and from nonpathogenic species. Another reservation concerning cord factor is that the mitochondrial pathology that is produced in liver cells has not been reported in macrophages parasitized with virulent M. tuberculosis, so it is a moot point whether cord factor is responsible for the death of infected macrophages.

There is a strong correlation between the presence of highly acidic lipids, particularly the sulfatides, and virulence of strains of M. tuberculosis in guinea pigs (Goren et al., 1974a). Mycobacterial sulfatides are not by themselves toxic but potentiate the toxicity of cord factor. Recently, the sulfatides have been shown to affect macrophages, as will be described in a subsequent section. In related studies it was found that phthiocerol dimycoserate (DIM) was found in cell walls of the more virulent organisms, while a specific phenolic phthiocerol diester was present in the less virulent strains (Goren et al., 1974b). Mycobacteria do not secrete exotoxins, neither can the lipopolysaccharides of the mycobacterial cell wall be considered toxic in the same sense as those of the enterobacteriaceae.

Pathogenic mycobacteria are high immunogenic, except when administered in such high doses that the host is overwhelmed before an immune response can be generated. The nature of the immune response in tuberculosis will be discussed in detail in a later section.

5. Host Factors in Pathogenicity

5.1. Genetic Factors in Tuberculosis

M. tuberculosis and M. bovis are each highly pathogenic to man, and other mycobacterial species are much less so. The natural reservoir of M. tuberculosis is man; cattle are the primary host of M. bovis; and M. avium causes disease in birds and to a lesser extent in man. Other mycobacteria (excepting M. leprae and M. lepraemurium) are not so dependent on a primary host, since they occur in such habitats as soil and water.

A number of experimental animal species permit the growth of M. tuberculosis in their tissues. These include nonhuman primates, guinea pigs, rabbits, hamsters, mice, and rats. Guinea pigs and nonhuman primates are highly susceptible to both M. tuberculosis and M. bovis. Rabbits are resistant to M. tuberculosis but readily succumb to M. bovis. Mice die following large intravenous inocula of virulent tubercle bacilli; rats are not similarly killed, despite the fact that they do support tuberculous infection (Ratcliffe, 1952; Lefford et al., 1973a). Hamsters have been little studied (Ratcliffe, 1952) but are unusual in that they can be killed by strains as attenuated as BCG (Jespersen and Bentzon, 1964).

A host species may be resistant to a parasite because either innate, unacquired resistance or specific, required resistance is high. Studies of tuberculosis in guinea pigs, rats, mice, and hamsters indicate that all species are innately susceptible but that they vary with respect to their acquired immunity (Ratcliffe, 1952; Ratcliffe and Palladino, 1953). It had been argued that rats are innately unsusceptible to tuberculosis (Ornstein and Steinbach, 1925), but this host supports the multiplication of M. tuberculosis and rapidly develops a high level of acquired immunity (Lefford et al., 1973a). Tuberculosis in monkeys, guinea pigs, and rabbits differs from that in mice and rats in that in the former the lesions undergo a coagulative necrosis (caseation), a characteristic feature of human disease. Of all these animal species, the guinea pig develops a state of tuberculin hypersensitivity which most closely resembles that observed in man.

Pertinent to the question of species susceptibility is the appropriateness of animal models to human disease. Guinea pigs have been the species most used in experimental tuberculosis because they develop high levels of tuberculin hypersensitivity and their lesions undergo caseous necrosis. More recently, mice have been more widely used because they are less expensive and inbred strains are easily maintained and facilitate cell transfer experiments. No experimental animal species exhibits one important feature of human disease: the ability of the majority of hosts to survive primary infection, linked with the predisposition of a minority to succumb much later to a recrudescence of latent infection.

Genetic variation within a species has been most carefully documented in rabbits, in which low- and high-resistance lines have been bred (Lurie, 1964). There is less convincing evidence of significant variation between guinea pig strains (Mitchison, 1964), but there is unanimity that the C57BL is the most susceptible strain of mice (Pierce *et al.*, 1947; Gray *et al.*, 1960; Youmans and Youmans, 1972). It has been suggested that intraspecies susceptibility is determined by the facility with which a given strain responds immunologically to the infection (Plant and Glynn, 1976).

Genetically determined variation in susceptibility is difficult to establish in man because of the importance of environmental influences. The primary determinants of any infectious disease are related to duration and intensity of exposure to the pathogenic agent. These determinants are invariably associated with concomitants of poverty, such as overcrowding, inadequate hygiene, and malnutrition. Consequently it is often impossible to differentiate genetic from environmental factors. This problem has been discussed at length by Rich (1951), who concludes that among human racial/ethnic groups good evidence exists only for the high resistance of Jews and the high susceptibility of Blacks to tuberculosis. American Indians appear to have an increased susceptibility to tuberculosis compared to the white population, but this difference is not as well documented as it is for the black population (Rich, 1951).

5.2. Nongenetic Factors in Tuberculosis

Since immunity to tuberculosis is of the cell-mediated type, anything that depresses such immunity will predispose the subject to tuberculosis. Diseases of the lymphoid system and immunodepressive agents, including cancer chemotherapy drugs and corticosteroids, exert such an effect. Endocrine disorders, such as hypothyroidism, adrenal cortical insufficiency, and diabetes also increase suscepti-

bility to diverse infections, including tuberculosis.

The incidence of tuberculosis varies with age and sex depending on whether the disease occurs in high- or low-prevalence populations. In high-prevalence populations there is a high incidence in infancy and early childhood with a second peak affecting young adults. The first peak has been attributed to the immunological immaturity of infants. However, since the risk of clinical tuberculosis is greatest during the first year following exposure to infection, regardless of age, the high incidence of tuberculosis in young children may simply reflect their close contact with family members who are excreting tubercle bacilli. Tuberculosis of adolescence and early adult life is more common in females. This phenomenon has been attributed to the "stress" of menstruation and pregnancy, but the evidence is inconclusive (Rich, 1951).

In low-prevalence populations there is an increasing incidence of tuberculosis with advancing age, and it is tempting to attribute this to a progressive loss of immunological responsiveness. There is some evidence for this general hypothesis in man and experimental animals (Walford, 1969). The effect of age on humoral immune responses has been studied extensively in mice, and there is good evidence that both primary and secondary immune responses are depressed in old age (Heidrick and Makinodan, 1972). The CMI responses of aged mice and humans are also depressed as evidenced by less vigorous reactivity of their T lymphocytes to polyclonal mitogens and alloantigens (Rodey *et al.*, 1971; Weksler and Hutteroth, 1974). Tuberculosis immunity and hypersensitivity have not been studied expressly in aged animals, but it appears that immunological memory to tuberculosis persists in aged guinea pigs (Baldwin and Gardner, 1921). In man it has been shown that primary sensitization with dinitrochlorobenzene (DNCB) was less successful in those aged 70 years or more. Some of those subjects who could not be sensitized to DNCB were nonetheless sensitive to tuberculin PPD, suggesting that cell-mediated immunological memory remained intact during ageing (Waldorf *et al.*, 1968). In light of these observations it is presumptuous to attribute the relatively high incidence of tuberculosis in the aged to loss of immunological competence until better evidence is forthcoming.

5.3. Local and Systemic Responses of Tuberculosis

5.3.1. Initial Interaction between Macrophages and Mycobacteria

In the early literature much was made of the acute inflammation which ensues on infection with tubercle bacilli (Vorwald, 1933). It seems probable that such observations were artifactual. If care is taken to inoculate mycobacteria atraumatically, e.g., intravenously or by inhalation into the lungs, no such acute reaction is seen. On the contrary, the infecting organisms are soon found within mononuclear phagocytes, in which they multiply without at first exciting any tissue reaction. The proclivity of pathogenic mycobacteria to enter and multiply within macrophages *in vivo* extends to *in vitro* situations. Neither specific antibody nor nonspecific serum factors are necessary for macrophages to ingest tubercle bacilli in tissue culture.

Following the *in vitro* ingestion of mycobacteria by macrophages, the organisms lie within cytoplasmic vacuoles, termed phagosomes. In the case of living, virulent *M. tuberculosis,* the bacteria are surrounded by an electron-translucent "clear substance" that extends to the unit membrane of the phagosome. The clear substance is elaborated by living bacilli, since it is not present if dead organisms are ingested (Armstrong and Hart, 1971). Furthermore, elaboration of clear substance may be a correlate of virulence because it is a much less conspicuous feature of phagocytosed BCG. Another correlate of clear substance formation is failure of the secondary lysosomes to fuse with the phagosome to produce a phagolysosome. The inhibition of lysosome–phagosome fusion may be instrumental in permitting the replication of the bacilli, unhindered by the potentially microbicidal contents of the lysosomes. Inhibition of phagolysosome formation is not shared by all pathogenic mycobacteria. Live *M. lepraemurium* bacilli do not inhibit fusion of lysosomes with phagosomes (Hart *et al.,* 1972). Two possible mechanisms by which lyso-

some–phagosome fusion is inhibited have been proposed. There is evidence that secretion of cyclic AMP by the ingested bacilli stabilizes the lysosomal membranes (Lowrie *et al.,* 1975). Alternatively, the sulfatides normally present in the cell walls of *M. tuberculosis* may inhibit the formation of phagolysosomes. Such effects may not be restricted to mycobacterial sulfatides but may be common to a range of extensively ionized polyanionic substances (Goren *et al.,* 1976). The degree of inhibition of phagolysosome formation appears to be proportional to the bacterial content of sulfatide (Goren *et al.,* 1976). Since virulent strains of *M. tuberculosis* have a higher content of sulfatide than less virulent strains, it is conceivable that inhibition of phagolysosome formation may be one of the factors that determine mycobacterial virulence. The above studies have been performed with normal mouse peritoneal macrophages maintained *in vitro*. Of even greater interest would be information on the interaction between tubercle bacilli and macrophages from immunized mice.

The interaction between isolated macrophages and attenuated mycobacteria, such as BCG, is almost symbiotic. The parasite undergoes limited growth in the host cell, which remains essentially unharmed. The same is true of the early stages of parasitization with virulent organisms, but eventually the host cell dies and disintegrates following extensive intracellular replication of the parasite. The exact cause of cell death is unknown, and it may be unnecessary to invoke an agent peculiar to mycobacteria. The unrestricted replication of most intracellular parasites will eventually cause cell death, presumably by the release of metabolites which damage the phagolysosomal membrane, permitting the escape of noxious material directly into the cytoplasm of the host cell. Nonetheless, components of the tubercle bacillus have been closely examined for evidence of "specific" toxicity, as described previously.

5.3.2. Lymphoproliferative Response

Following infection the tubercle bacilli multiply at the site of implantation and travel to the regional lymph node. In the node a proliferative response ensues involving the T lymphocytes of the paracortical zone. The interval between infection and lymphoproliferation and the magnitude of the latter are functions of the inoculum size (Lefford *et al.*, 1973b). With larger inocula the latent period is abbreviated and lymphoproliferation is increased. At the time when lymphocyte replication reaches its peak, histological tubercles make their first appearance in the lymph node, the animal exhibits delayed hypersensitivity to tuberculin and becomes immune to challenge with tubercle bacilli, and nonspecific resistance in maximal (North *et al.*, 1972). During these events the draining lymph node becomes substantially enlarged. Although this sequence of events has been discerned through animal studies, it is probable that similar changes occur in man. Thus, in primary tuberculosis the parenchymatous tissue lesion at the site of infection may be inconspicuous or invisible, while the draining lymph nodes are grossly enlarged.

The lymphoproliferative response is not simply some nonspecific reaction to the presence of tubercle bacilli in the lymph node, because the dividing cells can transfer both tuberculin hypersensitivity and antituberculosis immunity to normal recipients (Lefford *et al.*, 1973b; Lefford and McGregor, 1978). The properties of the sensitized lymphocytes change with time. Initially they are actively dividing large lymphocytes, or immunoblasts. The immunoblasts leave the lymph node in the efferent lymph, drain into the thoracic duct and thence into the circulating blood. They are relatively radioresistant, are sensitive to antimitotic agents (such as vinblastine) but do not recirculate from blood to lymph, are short-lived, and disappear within a few days. Subsequently a population of long-lived, nondividing, recirculating, small lymphocytes is found in the thoracic duct and elsewhere which mediates antituberculosis immunity (Lefford *et al.*, 1973b). These cells persist in immunized animals for an indefinite period, even after viable bacilli have been entirely eliminated (Lefford and McGregor, 1974).

There is compelling evidence that the sensitized lymphocytes are T cells: they are sensitive to anti-Thy 1 serum and complement, and immunity is not induced or is defective in T-lymphocyte-deprived mice (North, 1973). Furthermore, since immunity and DTH are transferrable with lymphocytes, but not serum, the T lymphocytes do not function merely as antibody helper cells (Lefford, 1975a).

5.3.3. Tubercle Formation

At the time when lymphocyte proliferation achieves its peak in the draining lymph nodes, histological "tubercles" make their first appearance at sites where tubercle bacilli are located. The histological tubercle consists of a focus of mononuclear cells comprising lymphocytes, macrophages, and epithelioid cells. The lymphocytes and macrophages are derived from blood-borne cells that have migrated into the lesions, and tubercle bacilli are frequently found within the macrophages. Epithelioid cells are probably derived from macrophages, from which they are distinguishable by both light and electron microscopy, but their function is unclear (Epstein, 1967). Multinucleate giant cells, which are also derived from macrophages, are a prominent feature of the tubercles of man but are inconspicuous in some other species. In man there is often coalescence of adjacent tubercles whose centers undergo coagulative necrosis or caseation. Such larger lesions become visible as macroscopic tubercles from which tuberculosis derives its name. However, closely similar granulomas are found in sarcoidosis, zirconium sensitivity, and berylliosis, and less commonly in other chronic inflammations. Such lesions are termed "hypersensitivity granulomas" because they arise as a consequence of a cell-mediated immune response (Epstein, 1967).

The macrophages that make up tuberculous granulomas differ morphologically and histochemically from normal tissue macrophages. The former have a better-developed Golgi apparatus, more numerous secondary lysosomes, increased mitochondria, and an increase in lysosomal enzymes (Grogg and Pearce, 1952; Epstein, 1967). Such changes are thought to denote an increased activity of the cells, and hence the term "activated macrophages" has been coined. This subject will be discussed further in the next section, but it should be stressed here that even within a tuberculous lesion there is substantial heterogeneity with respect to activation (Dannenberg *et al.*, 1968). A given lesion may include macrophages which have presumably arrived only recently and are not yet activated, activated macrophages, and previously activated, effete cells.

5.3.4. Macrophage Activation

The macrophages in tuberculous lesions are difficult to isolate and study. However, analogous changes may take place in the free macrophages of the peritoneal cavity of experimental animals, and these cells can be obtained without difficulty and studied in detail. Activated macrophages differ from normal macrophages with respect to increases in cell size, spreading on glass, activity of the surface membrane which appears ruffled, pinocytosis, phagocytosis, cytoplasmic content of phase- and electron-dense bodies (secondary lysosomes), Golgi vesicles, lysosomal acid hydrolases, respiratory enzymes, and microbicidal activity (Grogg and Pearce, 1952; Cohn and Wiener, 1963; Blanden, 1968; Blanden et al., 1969; Turk and Poulter, 1974).

It is presumed that during a CMI response, there is an interaction between specifically sensitized T lymphocytes and the corresponding antigen as a result of which lymphokines are produced, which in turn cause macrophage activation. This hypothesis is supported by experiments in which normal macrophages have been activated in vitro by lymphokines (Nathan et al., 1971; Simon and Sheagren, 1971; Poulter and Turk, 1976).

The induction of macrophage activation by the putative mediators of an immunologically specific reaction is highly satisfying. Unfortunately, similar morphological changes can also be induced in macrophages by a variety of nonimmunological stimulants (Cohn and Parks, 1967a,b). From the point of view of host–parasite relations, the most important criterion of macrophage activation is increased microbicidal activity (Blanden, 1968; Blanden et al., 1969; Krahenbuhl and Remington, 1971; Simon and Sheagren 1971). One should beware of a common but unsubstantiated assumption that any macrophage which is activated by some other criterion is also a more effective microbicidal cell. The weakness of this assumption lies in our ignorance of how macrophages kill bacteria. A number of possible microbicidal mechanisms will now be considered.

Activated macrophages have a greatly increased content of acid hydrolases, and it seems plausible that these might act as bactericidal agents. However, the enzymes themselves are relatively innocuous to most facultative intracellular parasites, although acid conditions alone may be deleterious (Looke and Rowley, 1962).

Lysozyme is a major secretory product of macrophages and is involved in the killing of gram negative organisms. However, lysozyme production is not increased by activation of macrophages, whose increased microbicidal activity cannot be ascribed to this enzyme (Gordon et al., 1974).

Intermediate products of oxidative phosphorylation have been implicated in the killing of bacteria. One such product is hydrogen peroxide, which may kill microorganisms either by direct action or through the peroxidase or catalase enzyme systems. It was formerly believed that macrophages did not possess a peroxidase (Cohn and Wiener, 1963), but recently this enzyme has been detected (Romeo et al., 1973). Another possible bactericidal product of cell metabolism is singlet oxygen (Maugh, 1973). The attractiveness of these bactericidal mechanisms is that oxidative phosphorylation by macrophages is markedly increased following exposure to lymphokines (Nathan et al., 1971; Poulter and Turk, 1976). It may be that the bactericidal mechanism depends on a combination of acidity, lysozyme, and hydrogen peroxide (Klebannof and Hamon, 1975).

Before leaving this subject, two further points require emphasis. First, normal unactivated macrophages have considerable bactericidal activity against a wide range of pathogens. The survivors of this initial kill subsequently multiply and cause progressive infection. Hence increased microbicidal activity may be a quantitative rather than a qualitative change. Second, although the ability of macrophages to kill many pathogens is beyond dispute, there is no evidence that even activated cells can kill pathogenic mycobacteria. The best that macrophages can do is prevent the intracellular multiplication of tubercle bacilli, which may eventually die of attrition (Patterson and Youmans, 1970; Godal et al., 1971). The possibility also exists that it is not the parasitized macrophages that limit the infection but the granulomatous lesions in which the microorganisms are trapped. Granuloma formation in turn may be dependent on lymphokines which act on macrophages, such as migration inhibitory factor (David *et al.*, 1964), macrophage chemotactic factor (Ward *et al.*, 1970), and macrophage aggregation factor (Gotoff and Vizral, 1972). Conditions within the granulomas with respect to pH and the supply of oxygen and nutrients may be highly unfavorable to tubercle bacilli, which are obligatory aerobes.

The activated macrophages in tuberculosis granulomas not only inhibit the growth of tubercle bacilli but also inhibit or kill other microorganisms that are ingested (Mackaness, 1964a,b; Blanden *et al.*, 1966, 1969; Ruskin and Remington, 1968). Such killing of immunologically unrelated bacteria is termed nonspecific immunity or nonspecific resistance. This phenomenon has created some confusion concerning the relative importance of immunologically specific and nonspecific factors in tuberculosis and other situations in which CMI is involved (Coppel and Youmans, 1969).

Essentially, the activation or "arming" of macrophages is a process which depends on an immunologically specific cell-mediated response to an appropriate antigen, in this case living mycobacteria. The specific component of the response resides within clone(s) of sensitized lymphocytes. Following exposure to the homologous antigen these lymphocytes are stimulated to release soluble mediators, or lymphokines, which mediate a number of phenomena including the attraction (or chemotaxis) of macrophages into the reaction site and the subsequent activation of these macrophages (Granger, 1972). The nonspecific component of the immune response concerns the killing of the parasites. Once activated, the macrophage does not discriminate between ingested parasites on an immunological basis. Hence the phagocyte's antimicrobial mechanism is directed equally against ingested mycobacteria, listeriae, brucellae, salmonellae, or toxoplasmas. Activated macrophages also exhibit a capacity to kill a limited range of extracellular targets, such as *Listeria monocytogenes* and tumor cells (Bast *et al.*, 1974; Middlebrook *et al.*, 1974; Hibbs *et al.*, 1972). The activated macrophage is analogous to a bullet that has been fired. Regardless of the target to which the bullet has been directed, it will damage anything that lies in its path. In summary, the process by which macrophages are activated during infection involves an immunologically specific event, but the antibacterial effector mechanism of the cells is nondiscriminatory.

Under certain experimental conditions, macrophages remote from the site of primary infection may become activated (Mackaness, 1962; Blanden *et al.*, 1969). This is likely to occur when infection is heavy and/or widely disseminated. Such an eventuality is unlikely in human tuberculosis but might conceivably occur in miliary tuberculosis, tuberculous bronchopneumonia, or extensive pulmonary tuberculosis.

5.3.5. Delayed Hypersensitivity

Infection with tubercle bacilli, whether virulent or attenuated, is invariably accompanied by tuberculin hypersensitivity of the delayed type (DTH) (Zinsser, 1921). So close is the association between DTH and tuberculosis infection that lack of hypersensitivity is notable for its rarity. DTH implies a general state of tissue hypersensitivity, but, since the usual method of detection is a tuberculin skin test, it is too easily assumed that a negative test necessarily denotes absence of DTH. It has long been known that this is not so. For example, animals that do not exhibit dermal sensitivity may be as susceptible to systemic tuberculin shock as skin-reactive hosts (Freund, 1929), and tuberculin skin hypersensitivity can be transferred with lymphoid cells from donors with negative skin tests (Collins and Mackaness, 1970; Dwyer and Kantor, 1973).

It should now be apparent that although a positive tuberculin skin test is unambiguous evidence of past or present mycobacterial infection, a negative skin test is not nearly so easy to interpret. This situation is further complicated by the discovery of lymphokines and antigen-specific lymphocyte transformation (LT). Lymphokines are released following the interaction of specifically sensitized lymphocytes and the homologous antigen. A number of functions have been ascribed to lymphokines (Granger, 1972), and each function has its own assay. The most widely applied assay is inhibition of macrophage migration, which is mediated by a lymphokine designated migration inhibitory factor (MIF) (David *et al.*, 1964). When an animal is infected with *M. tu-*

berculosis, it develops DTH as well as MIF and LT reactivity to tuberculin (Mills, 1966; Oppenheim *et al.,* 1967; Thor and Dray, 1968). The association among DTH, MIF, and LT, is common, but not invariable, and the *in vitro* assays may be used to detect specific sensitization in the absence of skin hypersensitivity. Thus it has been shown that lymph node cells of desensitized animals can still react in MIF assays (Schlossman *et al.,* 1971) and skin-test-negative human subjects may yield positive MIF or LT tests (Rocklin *et al.,* 1970; Thomas *et al.,* 1971).

The association between tuberculin skin hypersensitivity and tuberculosis infection has been repeatedly confirmed since the beginning of this century (von Pirquet, 1909). This relationship has generated a longstanding controversy concerning the relevance of delayed hypersensitivity (DTH) to cell-mediated antibacterial immunity, in general, and the argument has concentrated on tuberculin hypersensitivity and antituberculosis immunity in particular. One contention is that DTH is an essential part of the CMI response to *M. tuberculosis.* The skin reaction is regarded as a peripheral manifestation of the cellular events that control the infection in tuberculosis lesions (Mackaness, 1967; Mackaness and Blanden, 1967). The opposing hypothesis is that hypersensitivity is the cause of focal tissue damage which impairs the host's antibacterial response (Rich, 1951). This wearisome controversy refuses to die, but recent contributions portend a more conciliatory attitude on the part of the protagonists (Youmans, 1975; Lefford, 1975b; Salvin and Neta, 1975). Much of the evidence in support of the opposing contentions is indirect and will not be reviewed here. Instead, consideration will be given to the type of evidence that would contribute substantially to the resolution of this issue.

The hypothesis that DTH and immunity are integral components of a single CMI response implies that these functions are mediated by the same or closely linked populations of lymphocytes. This hypothesis becomes untenable if DTH and immunity can be completely dissociated. Earlier claims of successful dissociation of DTH and immunity have been severely criticized (Mackaness, 1967). In recent years methods of segregating lymphocyte subpopulations have become available and have

shed light on the present problem. The major classes of lymphocytes are bone marrow derived (B) and thymus-dependent (T) cells. It has been shown that all CMI functions (DTH, cellular immunity, LT, and MIF) are mediated by T lymphocytes (Arnason *et al.,* 1962; North, 1973; Jaffer *et al.,* 1973; Clinton *et al.,* 1974; Chess *et al.,* 1974), although B lymphocytes may also produce MIF (Rocklin *et al.,* 1974). This evidence supports the close relationship among MIF, LT, DTH, and immunity. Murine T-lymphocyte (Lyt) subclasses are now identifiable on the basis of antigenic markers on the cell surface (Kisielow *et al.,* 1975; Boyse *et al.,* 1977). So far, three functionally separate subpopulations have been identified: Lyt 1^+, 2^-, 3^-; Lyt 1^-, 2^+, 3^+; and Lyt 1^+, 2^+, 3^+. Some T-lymphocyte functions have been shown to be restricted to a particular subpopulation. Thus DTH and helper cell function are mediated by lymphocytes with the Lyt 1^+ surface marker whereas cytotoxic and suppressor cells possess the Lyt 2, Lyt 3 antigens (Cantor *et al.,* 1976; Huber *et al.,* 1976). Further experiments along these lines should determine whether or not immunity and DTH are mediated by a single Lyt population, and this controversy will finally be laid to rest. Meanwhile, the practical consequences of the relationship between DTH and immunity will be examined.

If DTH and immunity are mediated by the same or closely related cell populations, then the tuberculin test signifies not only that tuberculous infection has occurred but also that specific immunity has been induced. Furthermore, maneuvers which engender or sustain DTH will be of putative benefit to the patient, desensitization will be contraindicated, and the value of antituberculosis vaccines can be judged by the facility with which they induce DTH.

If, on the other hand, DTH and immunity are entirely separate functions of different cell populations, then, at best, tuberculin sensitivity is irrelevant to tuberculoimmunity (Nieburger *et al.,* 1973; Reggiardo and Middlebrook, 1974). Espousal of the notion that DTH is deleterious to immunity has two logical consequences: the practice of therapeutic desensitization and the development of nonsensitizing or nonallergenic vaccines (Youmans, 1975). It is virtually impossible to completely desensitize a tuberculous guinea pig without killing it (Rothschild *et al.*, 1934). Less heroic doses of tuberculin have been used in man, but there is no good evidence that they have any therapeutic effect. The quest for a nonallergenic vaccine still survives despite unremittingly disappointing results, which will be discussed later.

Hypersensitivity and immunity to tuberculosis are long lived. There is ample evidence in the older literature that tuberculin-positive subjects maintain their state of hypersensitivity indefinitely, and, through the association of DTH and immunity, it is presumed that the latter is also persistent. The long duration of CMI in tuberculosis is often attributed to the residence within the host of small numbers of living tubercle bacilli which provide continuous antigenic stimulation. Although the persistence of viable tubercle bacilli in man is undisputed, it seems implausible that so few organisms could constitute a measurable antigenic stimulus, particularly since the bacilli are often imprisoned within calcareous lymph nodes. It is equally possible that in high-prevalence populations, booster doses of tubercle bacilli might be acquired on a recurrent basis from exogenous sources. Recent studies indicate that immunity to tuberculosis is mediated by long-lived lymphocytes obviate the necessity to invoke a continuous or recurrent source of antigenic stimulation (Lefford *et al.*, 1973b), particularly since DTH and immunity were also sustained in animals from whom no viable organisms could be recovered (Lefford and McGregor, 1974).

Even in the prechemotherapy era it was noted that some tuberculin-positive subjects lost their hypersensitivity without apparent cause or ill effects (Gelien and Hamman, 1913). The phenomenon can be reproduced in animals that have been infected with attenuated *M. tuberculosis* (Baldwin and Gardner, 1921; Willis, 1928). Despite loss of hypersensitivity, immunity was still present in such hosts and hypersensitivity reappeared at an accelerated rate after reinfection with virulent tubercle bacilli. Spontaneous loss of tuberculin hypersensitivity has been reported more frequently in recent years (Adams *et al.*, 1959), and there are indications that the development and decay of DTH over a period of a few years is now the rule rather than the exception

(Katz *et al.*, 1972). A related phenomenon is the loss of tuberculin hypersensitivity following the chemotherapy or chemoprophylaxis of tuberculosis (Robinson *et al.*, 1955; Houk *et al.*, 1968; Atuk and Hunt, 1971). The evidence from experimental animal studies is conflicting: sometimes chemotherapy influences hypersensitivity (Steenken and Wolinsky, 1952; Brosbe *et al.*, 1965), and sometimes not (Bretey and Canetti, 1957; Narain *et al.*, 1970). The study of Lefford and McGregor (1974) is critical in this regard because they took care to eradicate living BCG from the immunized hosts, yet hypersensitivity and immunity remained unimpaired. It should be noted that these results are consistent with the general experience in man, in whom DTH is unaffected by chemotherapy.

How are these contradictory results to be explained? A critical analysis of the data reveals that tuberculin hypersensitivity is unstable when it is either of recent onset, of low degree, or of both. In the prechemotherapy era, exposure to tubercle bacilli was heavy and recurrent, and the incidence of clinical tuberculosis was high. These circumstances favor the induction of a high degree of tuberculin hypersensitivity which is stable. Currently, the opportunities for heavy exposure and recurrent infection are few, and early infection is often aborted by chemotherapy. Experience with BCG vaccination also indicates that immunity decays substantially over a 15-year period (Medical Research Council, 1972). The evidence suggests that, as the prevalence of tuberculosis in the United States continues to fall, it will be unwise to assume that tuberculin-positive subjects have acquired a lifelong immunity to that disease.

5.3.6. Antibody Response

Tuberculosis induces an antibody response to mycobacterial antigens in addition to CMI. The relevance of the humoral response to resistance to infection is problematic. Efforts to transfer either DTH or immunity with serum from tuberculous and/or hypersensitivity animals have usually failed. The few successful experiments have been discounted on technical grounds (Bloom and Chase, 1967). The lack of biological activity of serum from tuberculous animals confirms the preeminent role of CMI in this infection.

The possibility exists that humoral antibodies in tuberculosis might play an ancillary role in the response of the host. Florid DTH reactions with necrosis and polymorphonuclear cell infiltration, suggestive on an Arthus reaction, are sometimes seen in man and guinea pigs, but antibodies have not been convincingly implicated. Similarly, the involvement of antibodies in granuloma formation and the tissue necrosis of caseation is unconvincing (Chapman, 1972). Finally, there is no evidence that antibodies can enhance tuberculous infection through inhibition of CMI, in the way that antibodies can enhance tumors (Heppner, 1972). Some investigators have found an association among advanced disease, high antibody titers, and depressed DTH (Bhatnagar et al., 1977). Such an association might be expected on theoretical grounds but is uncommon in practice (Takahashi et al., 1961; Daniel and Baum, 1969).

5.3.7. The Problem of Active Tuberculosis

It has been estimated that less than 5% of those infected with tubercle bacilli subsequently develop clinically significant disease (Rees and Meade, 1974). Thus over 95% of putatively susceptible hosts mount an immune response that completely controls the primary infection. It remains unclear why a small proportion of infected hosts ever develop active disease. A plethora of intangibles have been invoked as contributory factors: unfavorable socioeconomic conditions, heredity, hormonal influences, and physical and psychological stress. It is relevant in the present context to consider the possible role of an inadequate or inappropriate specific immune response.

Except for the very small number of patients with diseases of the lymphoid system and other immunodepressive states, there is little evidence of primary failure of the specific immune response in patients with tuberculosis. With few exceptions, these patients display DTH to tuberculin and many also have circulating antibodies to one or more components of the tubercle bacillus. The question of an inappropriate CMI (hypersensitivity) response has already been raised in the discussion of the role of DTH in tuberculosis. The evidence for the adverse effects of DTH derive from observations that in normal subjects a very large (> 15 mm diameter) tuberculin reaction is a poor prognostic sign (Medical Research Council, 1972) and that patients with extensive progressive disease also exhibit high degrees of hypersensitivity (Rich, 1951). Unfortunately, there is evidence to support the diametrically opposite hypothesis, namely, that absolute tuberculin anergy is also associated with severe disease, e.g., miliary tuberculosis and tuberculous bronchopneumonia (British Medical Journal, 1970; Bhatnagar et al., 1977).

In recent years there has been an increasing awareness of another type of inappropriate immune response, namely, an antibody response that inhibits the development and/or expression of CMI (Lagrange et al., 1974). This concept postdates the heyday of tuberculosis research and is not considered in the monographs of Rich (1951) and Lurie (1964). If this hypothesis is correct, one would predict that patients with active tuberculosis would have high antibody levels in the blood and diminished CMI, as in lepromatous leprosy (Godal et al., 1974). A recent study has shown that, among subjects infected with tubercle bacilli, there is an inverse relation between the levels of DTH to tuberculin and humoral antibodies reactive with the same material (Bhatnagar et al., 1977). Those who were tuberculin positive but without active disease had high levels of DTH and low antibody titers, whereas the converse was true in those with miliary tuberculosis. The latter situation was rectified by antituberculosis chemotherapy, from which it was deduced that the suppression of DTH and enhancement of antibody production were an effect rather than a cause of progressive disease.

The notion that tuberculosis subjects suffer from some generalized immunodepression has already been rejected. However, the possibility of a slow decay of immunological memory deserves serious consideration. It has been noted that the lymphocytes in which immunity is vested are long lived (Lefford et al., 1973b), but this should not imply that they are immortal. Specific loss of immunological memory to tuberculosis in the elderly derives some support from observations that they do not exhibit tuberculin sensitivity as frequently as expected. These individuals might well be predisposed to reactivation of endogenous disease.

6. Immunodiagnosis of Tuberculosis

6.1. Serological Tests

Diagnostic tests have been developed which depend on humoral and cellular immunity, respectively. A wide variety of serological tests have been described that measure antibodies directed against one or more components of the tubercle bacillus: carbohydrate, protein, or phosphatide (Middlebrook and Dubos, 1948; Boyden, 1951; Takahashi and Ono, 1958). In recent years more sensitive tests such as antigen-binding capacity, indirect fluorescent antibody, and immunodiffusion assays have been used (Janicki et al., 1973). The present view is that none of these methods is suitable for use in the routine clinical laboratory because the diagnostic power of these tests is not adequately sensitive or specific (David and Selin, 1976). Although the protagonists of a particular antibody test have vindicated its use (Takahashi et al., 1961), the general experience is that these assays do not discriminate efficiently between tuberculin-negative healthy subjects, tuberculin-positive healthy subjects and patients with active tuberculosis (Daniel and Baum, 1969).

6.2. Tuberculin Test

Three tests of cellular immunity are available: the delayed hypersensitivity skin test (the tuberculin test), the antigen-specific inhibition of macrophage migration *in vitro* (David et al., 1964), and lymphocyte blast transformation (Pearmain et al., 1963). All these tests depend on the use of an antigen preparation derived from mycobacteria, of which there are two types: old tuberculin (OT) and purified protein derivative (PPD). OT is a crude concentrate of a culture filtrate of human tubercle bacilli. PPD is prepared from a culture filtrate of *M. tuberculosis* that has been precipitated with either ammonium sulfate (as in the United States) or trichloroacetic acid (as in Britain). From a chemical and antigenic point of view, PPD is still a crude product, but it contains less carbohydrate and nu-

cleic acid than OT and relatively more protein. Tuberculins are standardized by biological assay, rather than total mass or protein content, and are quantitated in tuberculin units (TU). One TU is equivalent to 0.00002 mg protein of PPD-S, the human tuberculin preparation against which all new batches of PPD are standardized. It must be realized that PPD is a highly heterogeneous material from the chemical and, more importantly, the antigenic point of view (Janicki et al., 1971; Chase and Kawata, 1974). No two lots of PPD are antigenically identical; neither is it known which antigens are specific to *M. tuberculosis*. Finally, there is substantial cross-reactivity between tuberculins prepared from different mycobacterial species (Landi and Held, 1970).

There are several methods for performing tuberculin tests. The standard diagnostic method is the Mantoux test, in which tuberculin is injected intradermally into the volar surface of the forearm with a needle and syringe. A number of other tests are extant which should not be used in diagnostic practice but are suitable for large-scale screening, e.g., of school children. These tests include the tine, Heaf, and jet injector (MacLean, 1975). The jet injector test is superior to the tine and Heaf tests in that a precisely known quantity of tuberculin is injected and the size of the wheal provides an indication of whether the injection procedure has been performed correctly. The tests are read not earlier than 24 hr after injection of tuberculin, and the optimum time is 72 hr. It is odd that reactions often develop more slowly in man than in the usual experimental animals. The results are expressed in terms of diameter of induration or vesiculation (Table 1). Erythema is disregarded.

The dose of tuberculin is critical only for the Mantoux and jet injector methods, in which

TABLE 1. Evaluation of Tuberculin Tests

Test	Usage	Diameter of induration (mm)		
		Negative	Doubtful	Positive
Mantoux[a]	Diagnostic	0–4	5–9	10
Jet injector[a]	Screening			
Tine	Screening	0–1	2–5	6 or vesiculation
Heaf	Screening			

[a] 5TU test.

an attempt is made to introduce a precise quantity of antigen. Formerly, a range of tuberculin doses was commonly used, commencing with a low dose that was increased in a stepwise fashion in patients with negative reactions. This approach is now discouraged in favor of a standard dose of 5 TU (Comstock *et al.,* 1971). In the event that this dose yields a doubtfully positive result (Table 1) the test should be repeated with the same dose. High doses of tuberculin may indeed produce positive results in otherwise negative reactors, but it is felt that such results are indicative of cross-reactivity to environmental mycobacteria rather than infection with *M. tuberculosis* or *M. bovis.* In this connection it should be understood that no diagnostic test is free of error. The 5 TU test may fail to detect some tuberculous patients who are low reactors, but it minimizes the misdiagnosis of normal subjects as tuberculous. Since the incidence of tuberculosis in the United States is low, it is preferable to err in the direction of false-negative than false-positive results, so that the total number of incorrect results is minimized.

The reading of tuberculin tests also presents some difficulties. There may be substantial reading variations between observers, and even the same observer may have difficulty in reproducing his own measurements. This problem becomes significant for reactions that are close to the critical size for "doubtful" or "positive" classification (Carruthers, 1970).

6.3. MIF and LT Tests

Assays of antigen-induced lymphocyte transformation (LT) and migration inhibitory factor (MIF) have also been used as diagnostic tests for tuberculosis. However, these tests are as vulnerable as the skin test to variation between lots of PPD and dosage problems. Furthermore, they cannot be applied routinely to large populations and hence the incidence of the false-negative and false-positive results is difficult to evaluate. In general, there is a close association among dermal sensitivity, MIF, and LT tests, but examples of dissociation have been recorded (Rocklin *et al.,* 1970; Thomas *et al.,* 1971). In certain studies the *in vitro* tests have been shown to be more sensitive than the skin test, but there is no evidence for thinking that the former are intrins-

ically more sensitive (David, 1973). The skin test is preferable on account of its practicality.

6.4. Diagnosis of Nontuberculous Mycobacterioses

Tuberculins have been prepared from mycobacterial species, other than *M. tuberculosis,* in the expectation that through their use specific diagnosis of nontuberculous mycobacterioses might be possible. The cross-reactivity that exists between mycobacterial species and their tuberculins has vitiated these hopes. When patients with a mycobacteriosis are tested with numerous tuberculins, the outcome is often a nonsense pattern of sensitivity. Consequently, the use of such tuberculins has been discouraged and their distribution by the Center for Disease Control, Atlanta, has been curtailed. These materials are still available through commercial sources and may prove useful under the following conditions. If a specific pathogen is suspected, then the appropriate tuberculin should be chosen. The patient should be tested concomitantly with the "specific" tuberculin and human tuberculin PPD. The "specific" tuberculin test should be regarded as positive only if the diameter of induration is at least 5 mm greater than that obtained with human PPD.

6.5. Positive Tuberculin Test

A positive tuberculin test denotes either current or past infection with *M. tuberculosis* or *M. bovis,* vaccination with BCG, or active infection with some other mycobacterial pathogen. The use of the 5TU test has effectively precluded positive results arising from environmental contact with saprophytic or poorly pathogenic mycobacteria. Thus, to all intents and purposes, there is no such thing as a false-positive tuberculin test to 5TU. False positives may be obtained if a 250 TU dose is employed.

6.6. Negative Tuberculin Test

As a corollary of the preceding section, nontuberculous subjects will have negative tuberculin tests. However, false-negative tests may be obtained either because of technical failure of the test or because a tuberculous patient fails to respond (Wijsmuller, 1971).

6.6.1. Technical Failure of the Tuberculin Test

Some of the reasons for technical failure have already been alluded to: faulty injection of tuberculin and incorrect reading. Other factors include inactive tuberculin due to either aging, storage at room temperature, inappropriate dilution, or contamination.

6.6.2. Failure of the Subject to Respond

The minimal requirements for a positive tuberculin test are a population of sensitized lymphocytes, blood monocytes, and a normally functioning capillary bed which permits the egress of these cells into the tissues. Failure of a sensitized subject to respond represents a lack of one or more of these requirements. However, in many cases it is not possible to determine what the cause of nonreactivity, or anergy, is. Tuberculin anergy may be either transient or persistent.

6.6.3. Transient Anergy

Newborn infants are unable to express DTH during the first few weeks of life. This is true of human infants who are exposed to virulent tubercle of BCG vaccination, and newborn experimental animals (Janicki and Aron, 1968). Such anergy is not due to primary failure of the immune response because newborn subjects fail to express DTH after receiving specifically sensitized lymphocytes (Waksman and Matoltsy, 1958; Warrick *et al.*, 1960). Hence anergy appears to result from an inability to generate inflammatory reactions. However, despite the lack of tuberculin hypersensitivity following BCG vaccination, neonates are effectively immunized against tuberculosis.

Acute infections, particularly acute viral exanthems, notably measles, may be associated with loss of tuberculin sensitivity. Recent studies have revealed that myxo- and paramyxoviruses can bind to lymphocytes and alter their surface properties, presumably through the action of viral neuraminidase. Lymphocytes so affected lose their ability to circulate normally and consequently cannot function properly. Such effects are transient, but antigen-reactive proliferating lymphocytes may be killed by virus infection (Woodruff and Woodruff, 1975), an event which might delete an entire clone of cells (Romano *et al.*, 1977).

Similar anergy may occur following vaccination with living attenuated viruses, e.g., yellow fever, poliomyelitis, and measles.

There is a latent period of several weeks between infection with tubercle bacilli and the development of hypersensitivity. A tuberculin test that is performed in this interval will give a negative result, even though the patient is infected.

Cytotoxic drugs, such as cancer chemotherapy agents, produce transient immunosuppression due to damage inflicted on lymphocytes and bone marrow precursors of monocytes. Total body irradiation has similar effects. Corticosteroids are both lympholytic and antiinflammatory and thereby inhibit DTH reactions.

Desensitization with tuberculin causes temporary loss of dermal hypersensitivity in experimental animals. This has been shown to be due not to destruction of sensitized lymphocytes but rather to their absence from the circulation due to sequestration in the lymph nodes. Lymphocytes recovered from the nodes function normally in MIF assays (Schlossman *et al.*, 1971). Spontaneous desensitization in man may occur as a result of antigen overload as in miliary tuberculosis or extensive caseous tuberculosis.

A miscellany of unrelated disorders are sometimes associated with loss of sensitivity. These include overexposure to sunlight, hypnosis, acute alcoholism, and scurvy. The last example is of interest because similar loss of sensitivity is present in scorbutic guinea pigs, in which it has been shown that the essential defect is vascular (Zweiman *et al.*, 1966).

6.6.4. Persistent Anergy

Chronic destructive diseases of the bone marrow and lymphoid system deprives the host of lymphocytes and macrophages with a consequent inability to generate DTH reactions. Such diseases include lymphomas and amyloidosis.

Advanced disseminated tuberculosis produces a chronic desensitization (see Section 6.6.3., fifth paragraph).

Chronic debilitating diseases, such as carcinomatosis and syphilis, are associated with loss of sensitivity for no known reason.

A normal immune response to tuberculosis depends on normal thyroid function (Lurie,

1964), so it not surprising that hypothyroidism is associated with anergy.

Loss of hypersensitivity in tuberculosis subjects, occurring either spontaneously or following antituberculosis chemotherapy, has been discussed previously.

There is a relatively low incidence of tuberculin sensitivity in the aged, despite the fact that this cohort of the population was at one time heavily exposed to tuberculosis and bears stigmata of earlier infection, such as calcified Ghon foci or mediastinal lymph nodes. A number of explanations have been offered to explain this anomaly. It has already been argued that there may be a gradual reduction of immunological capacity with age which accounts for the loss of tuberculin hypersensitivity and increased incidence of tuberculosis. Others have suggested that such lack of hypersensitivity is more apparent than real, in that the thin skin of the elderly does not support a good DTH reaction. Wijsmuller (1971), however, argues that the skin of the aged will support a DTH reaction provided the test is performed properly but admits that it may be difficult to perform a good intradermal injection in these subjects.

Some patients with active tuberculosis of modest severity are anergic for no known reason. These subjects show no increased susceptibility to the infection, and their anergy is ascribed to genetic nonresponsiveness (*British Medical Journal*, 1970).

A most interesting cause of unresponsiveness to tuberculin is sarcoidosis. Lack of reactivity in this disease may persist despite BCG vaccination. Sarcoidosis is characterized by granulomas which are indistinguishable from noncaseous tubercles. This histological similarity has prompted the search for an etiological relationship between the two diseases. The general view is that the two diseases are entirely unrelated, but a minority hold that sarcoidosis is an atypical form of tuberculosis (Scadding, 1960).

The significance of anergy in relation to antituberculosis immunity will depend on the underlying causes, some of which are more serious diseases than tuberculosis.

6.6.5. Repeated Tuberculin Tests

It may be necessary to repeat tuberculin skin tests on patients, either because the orig-

inal test gave a doubtful result or as part of a surveillance program, e.g., population surveys or regular examination of subjects who are exposed to tuberculosis infection. In either case one needs to know whether or not a given test result may have been influenced by the preceding tests. There is ample evidence that repeat tests may increase the tuberculin sensitivity of certain subjects, particularly if the same site is used for injection of antigen (O'Grady, 1967). A given site is apt to be retested because the central portion of the volar surface of the forearm is habitually used. Consequently, the left arm may be used for the first test, the right arm for the second test, and the left arm for the third test. There is a good chance that the first and third test sites will overlap.

The problem of retesting is a small one, in practice, because only a small group of subjects are effectively influenced. Normal, tuberculin-negative people are not converted to positivity by retesting. Subjects whose initial test gave a small reaction in the "doubtful" range may react more vigorously following repeated tests (Narain *et al.*, 1966). Another situation in which testing alters the tuberculin status is in BCG-vaccinated subjects, in whom repeated tests serve to sustain tuberculin sensitivity at a higher level than untested controls (Olakowski and Mardon, 1971).

7. Antituberculosis Immunization

7.1. Living BCG Vaccine

Only one type of antituberculosis vaccine has been widely used in man, namely, BCG (Bacille de Calmette et Guérin). BCG is a laboratory-attenuated strain of *M. bovis* that was originally prepared at the Pasteur Institute in Lille, France. Since then, the organism has been distributed to many other laboratories and has suffered the vicissitudes of serial subcultivation on a variety of artificial media for decades. Consequently, although all BCG strains are derived from the original Pasteur strain, many of the substrains differ substantially from the parental strain and from each other (Ladefoged *et al.*, 1976). BCG is used as a living vaccine. For many years it was available only in a liquid menstruum, in which form it had a short effective life span, did not travel well, and could not be assayed fully prior to distribution. Nowadays, all commercial vaccines are lyophilized, in which state viability, effectiveness, and lack of toxicity of these vaccines can also be assayed prior to distribution. There is no question that BCG vaccines are efficacious in a wide variety of experimental animal models (Frappier *et al.,* 1971), but there is continuing debate over their usefulness in man.

This disagreement arises from the relative failure of BCG in three controlled studies sponsored by the USPHS (Palmer *et al.,* 1958; Comstock and Palmer, 1966; Comstock and Webster, 1969). On the other hand, BCG was found to be highly efficacious in other controlled trials, notably that organized by the British Medical Research Council (Medical Research Council, 1972). The cause of this discrepancy will never be known for certain, but the general view is that the vaccine used in the American studies was inadequate (Hart, 1967; Sutherland, 1971; Guld, 1971). Comstock and Palmer (1966) have ascribed the ineffectiveness of BCG in their study to "natural" immunization with environmental mycobacteria, but this analysis has been disputed (ten Dam *et al.,* 1976). The general consensus is that BCG vaccine is effective, occasional contrary views notwithstanding (Naganna, 1974). The standard dose of vaccine is 0.075 mg wet weight, which contains approximately 10^6 viable organisms, but lower doses are recommended for infants in whom severe regional lymphadenopathy may occur (ten Dam *et al.,* 1976). At one time it was standard procedure to tuberculin-test prospective vaccinees and then immunize only those who were tuberculin negative. This approach presents no problems in technically advanced countries, but in developing countries, particularly in rural areas, the populace has to be brought together twice: first to tuberculin-test and then to read the tests and vaccinate the tuberculin-negative subjects. Present practice is to vaccinate the entire population (or subpopulation) regardless of its tuberculin status, since BCG is not harmful to tuberculin-positive subjects, although they may react more vigorously to the vaccine.

Following vaccination there is usually conversion of tuberculin-negative subjects to tuberculin positivity within 2 months. The question arises as to whether an individual who falls to convert to tuberculin positivity should be revaccinated. Provided that the lot of vaccine has sensitized most of the subjects, nonconverters are as well protected as converters (Hart *et al.,* 1967). In the Medical Research Council (1972) study, BCG vaccination conferred 87%, 70%, and 59% protection at 2½, 5, and 10–15 years, respectively, following vaccination. The progressive loss of protection with time is disappointing but may equally apply to the immunity acquired accidentally through primary infection with virulent tubercle bacilli. The duration of hypersensitivity following vaccination is variable but may be sustained for as long as 5 years (Horwitz and Bunch-Christensen, 1972).

7.2. Vaccines Other Than Living BCG

The only other antituberculosis vaccine that has been used in man is a living vole bacillus (*M. microti*) vaccine, which was as effective as living BCG (Medical Research Council, 1972). However, during the past 50 years numerous nonviable immunizing agents have been tested in experimental animals. The search for an alternative to living BCG vaccine has been prompted by three considerations. The first is that an inanimate product is intrinsically safer and more reliable than a living vaccine. Second, some believe that a nonsensitizing vaccine is preferable to living BCG because of the supposed harmful effects of hypersensitivity. Finally, a nonsensitizing vaccine has been sought because the tuberculin conversion produced by living BCG precludes the use of the tuberculin test in the diagnosis of tuberculosis. Of the numerous vaccines that have been studied, three have received attention in recent years. One is the preparation of Ribi *et al.* (1966), which consists of BCG cell walls in an oil-in-water emulsion. This vaccine is effective only when injected intravenously, as a result of which the oil-associated cell wall fragments form pulmonary microemboli. The subsequent pulmonary granulomatosis, though protective, renders the vaccine unacceptable in man. This vaccine was at first thought to be nonsensitizing, but subsequent investigations proved otherwise (Anacker *et al.,* 1969).

Crowle (1972) has devised a vaccine based on a trypsin extract of mycobacteria. This material is most effective when incorporated in mineral oil and does not sensitize to tuberculin but sensitizes towards itself. Finally, the mycobacterial RNA vaccine of Youmans and Youmans (1967) also requires incorporation in mineral oil and is nonsensitizing.

The requirement for a mineral oil vehicle precludes the use of any of these vaccines in man. Furthermore, although each is effective when tested according to the method of its originator, none is more effective than living BCG. Additionally, the protective capacity of the Youmans and Crowle vaccines has not been confirmed independently. It is concluded that, in the foreseeable future, only living BCG vaccine will be used as an antituberculosis vaccine in man.

8. Immunotherapy

8.1. Tuberculin

Koch introduced tuberculin as a therapeutic agent in 1900, and it was widely used for several decades. However, its efficacy was never proven, and it had fallen out of fashion long before the availability of effective chemotherapy. Even in the postchemotherapy era, tuberculin therapy was used in a few specific instances. Some clinicians used intrathecal tuberculin as an adjunct to chemotherapy in the treatment of tuberculous meningitis in the hope of preventing the formation of adhesions in the subarachnoid space. At present, there are no indications for a rational therapeutic use of tuberculin.

8.2. Transfer Factor

It has been noted that transfer of DTH in experimental animals and man can be achieved with living lymphoid cells but not serum. In experimental rodent systems, disrupted cells and subcellular fractions fail to transfer hypersensitivity. Surprisingly, this is not true for man, in whom disrupted blood leukocytes were found to transfer hypersensitivity (Lawrence, 1955). Similar results have since been obtained in subhuman primates. Subsequently, a purified subcellular product that transferred DTH was isolated and has been named "transfer factor" (Lawrence, 1974).

This material has a molecular weight of less than 10,000, is dialyzable, and is resistant to DNase, RNase, and trypsin. A given sample of transfer factor may confer sensitivity to multiple antigens, and the specificity of the agent is in doubt. Another property of transfer factor is that it can be serially transferred through man without loss of activity. The implication of this observation is that donor transfer factor induces the cells of the recipient to produce more transfer factor.

Transfer factor can confer reactivity to patients with defects of CMI, but the response varies with the nature of the defect. Patients with Hodgkin's disease, sarcoidosis, and thymic aplasia usually fail to respond, whereas those with mucocutaneous candidiasis and the Wiskott–Aldrich syndrome may be converted to hypersensitivity. It has been suggested that postthymic lymphocytes are a prerequisite for a favorable response to transfer factor (Kirkpatrick, 1975). Transfer factor is not used in the management of tuberculosis but is being tested in lepromatous leprosy.

References

Adams, J. M., Kalajan, V. A., Mork, B. O., Rosenblatt, M., Rothrock, W. J., and O'Loughlin, B. J., 1959, Reversal of tuberculin reaction in early tuberculosis, Chest Dis. 35:348–356.

Anacker, R. L., Ribi, E., Tarmina, D. F., Fadness, L., and Mann, R. E., 1969, Relationship of footpad sensitivity to purified protein derivatives and resistance to airborne infection with Mycobacterium tuberculosis of mice vaccinated with mycobacterial cell walls, J. Bacteriol. 100:51–57.

Armstrong, J. A., and Hart, P. D., 1971, Response of cultured macrophages to Mycobacterium tuberculosis, with observations on fusion of lysosomes with phagosomes, J. Exp. Med. 134:713–740.

Arnason, B. G., Jankovic, B. D., Waksman, B. H., and Wennersten, C., 1962, Role of the thymus in immune reactions in rats. I. Suppressive effect of thymectomy at birth on reactions of delayed (cellular) hypersensitivity and the circulating small lymphocyte, J. Exp. Med. 116:177–188.

Atuk, N. O., and Hunt, E. H., 1971, Serial tuberculin testing and isoniazid therapy in general hospital employees, JAMA 218:1795–1798.

Azuma, I., Ribi, E., Meyer, T. J., and Zbar, B., 1974, Biologically active components from mycobacterial cell walls. I. Isolation and composition of cell wall skeleton and component P3, J. Natl. Cancer Inst. 52:95–101.

Baldwin, E. R., and Gardner, L. U., 1921, Reinfection in tuberculosis. Experimental arrested tuberculosis and subsequent infections, *Am. Rev. Tuberc.* **5**:429–517.

Barnett, M., Bushby, S. R. M., and Mitchison, D. A., 1953, Tubercle bacilli resistant to isoniazid: Virulence and response to treatment with isoniazid in guinea pigs and mice, *Br. J. Exp. Pathol.* **34**:568–581.

Bast, R. C., Cleveland, R. P., Littman, B. H., Zbar, B., and Rapp, H. J., 1974, Acquired cellular immunity: Extracellular killing of *Listeria monocytogenes* by a product of immunologically activated macrophages, *Cell. Immunol.* **10**:248–259.

Bekierkunst, A., Levij, I. S., Yarkoni, E., Vilkas, E., Adam, A., and Lederer, E., 1969, Granuloma formation induced in mice by chemically defined mycobacterial fractions, *J. Bacteriol.* **100**:95–102.

Bhatnagar, R., Malaviya, A. N., Narayanan, S., Rajgopalan, P., Kumar, R., and Bharadwaj, O. P., 1977, Spectrum of immune response abnormalities in different clinical forms of tuberculosis, *Am. Rev. Resp. Dis.* **115**:207–212.

Blanden, R. V., 1968, Modification of macrophage function, *J. Reticuloendothel. Soc.* **5**:179–202.

Blanden, R. V., Mackaness, G. B., and Collins, F. M., 1966, Mechanisms of acquired resistance in mouse typhoid, *J. Exp. Med.* **124**:585–600.

Blanden, R. V., Lefford, M. J., and Mackaness, G. B., 1969, The host response to Calmette-Guérin bacillus infection in mice, *J. Exp. Med.* **129**:1079–1107.

Bloch, H., 1950, Studies on the virulence of tubercle bacilli. Isolation and biological properties of a constituent of virulent organisms, *J. Exp. Med.* **91**:197–218.

Bloom, B. R., and Chase, M. W., 1967, Transfer of delayed-type hypersensitivity. A critical review and experimental study in the guinea pig, *Prog. Allergy.* **10**:151–255.

Boyden, S. V., 1951, The absorption of proteins on erythrocytes treated with tannic acid and subsequent haemagglutination by antiprotein sera, *J. Exp. Med.* **93**:107–120.

Boyse, E. A., Cantor, H., and Shen, F. W., 1977, Nomenclature for antigens demonstrable on lymphocytes, *Immunogenetics* **5**:189.

Bretey, J., and Canetti, G., 1957, Effect of early administration of isoniazid on the immunizing activity of normal BCG and isoniazid-resistant BCG in guinea pigs, *Am. Rev. Tuberc.* **75**:650–655.

British Medical Journal, 1970, Tuberculin anergy, **4**:573.

Brosbe, E. A., Sugihari, P. T., and Adams, J. M., 1965, Prevention of tuberculosis and reversal of tuberculin reaction in guinea pigs, *Proc. Soc. Exp. Biol. Med.* **119**:46–49.

Cantor, H., Shen, F. W., and Boyse, E. A., 1976, Separation of helper T cells from suppressor T cells expressing different Ly components. II. Activation by antigen: After immunization, antigen-specific suppressor and helper activities are mediated by distinct T-cell subclasses, *J. Exp. Med.* **143**:1391–1401.

Carruthers, K. J. M., 1970, Observer and experimental variation in tuberculin testing, *Tubercle* **51**:48–67.

Chapman, J. S., 1972, A review of early events in tubercle formation, *Acta Pathol. Microbiol. Scand. Sect. A* **80**:189–194 (Suppl. 233).

Chase, M. W., and Kawata, H., 1974, Multiple mycobacterial antigens in diagnostic tuberculins, *Dev. Biol. Stand.* **29**:308–330.

Chess, L., MacDermott, R. P., and Schlossman, S. F., 1974, Immunologic functions of isolated human lymphocyte subpopulations. II. Antigen triggering of T and B cells *in vitro, J. Immunol.* **113**:1122–1127.

Clinton, B. A., Magoc, T. J., and Aspinall, R. L., 1974, The abrogation of macrophage migration inhibition by pretreatment of immune exudate cells with anti-θ antibody and complement, *J. Immunol.* **112**:1741–1746.

Cohn, Z. A., and Parks, E., 1967a, The regulation of pinocytosis in mouse macrophages. II. Factors inducing vesicle formation, *J. Exp. Med.* **125**:213–232.

Cohn, Z. A., and Parks, E., 1967b, The regulation of pinocytosis in mouse macrophages. III. The induction of vesicle formation by nucleosides and nucleotides, *J. Exp. Med.* **125**:457–466.

Cohn, Z. A., and Wiener, E., 1963, The particulate hydrolases of macrophages. I. Comparative enzymology, isolation and properties, *J. Exp. Med.* **118**:991–1008.

Collins, F. M., and Mackaness, G. B., 1970, The relationship of delayed hypersensitivity to acquired antituberculous immunity. I. Tuberculin sensitivity and resistance to reinfection in BCG-vaccinated mice, *Cell. Immunol.* **1**:253–265.

Comstock, G. W., 1975, Frost revisited: The modern epidemiology of tuberculosis, *Am. J. Epidemiol.* **101**:363–382.

Comstock, G. W., and Palmer, C. E., 1966, Long-term results of BCG vaccination in the southern United States, *Am. Rev. Resp. Dis.* **93**:171–183.

Comstock, G. W., and Webster, R. G., 1969, Tuberculosis studies in Muscogee County, Georgia. VII. A twenty-year evaluation of BCG vaccination in a school population, *Am. Rev. Resp. Dis.* **100**:839–845.

Comstock, G. W., Furculow, M. L., Greenberg, R. A., Grzybowski, S., MacLean, R. A., Baer, H., and Edwards, P. Q., 1971, The tuberculin skin test, *Am. Rev. Resp. Dis.* **104**:769–775.

Coppel, S., and Youmans, G. P., 1969, Specificity of acquired resistance produced by immunization with mycobacterial cells and mycobacterial fractions, *J. Bacteriol.* **97**:114–120.

Crowle, A. J., 1972, Trypsin-extracted immunizing antigen of the tubercle bacillus: A practical vaccine? *Adv. Tuberc. Res.* **18**:31–102.

Daniel, T. M., and Baum, G. L., 1969, The immunoglobulin response to tuberculosis. II. Molecular characterization of hemagglutinating antibody to tuberculoprotein in serum from patients with tuberculosis, *Am. Rev. Resp. Dis.* **99**:249–254.

Dannenberg, A. M., Meyer, O. T., Esterly, J. R., and

Kambara, T., 1968, The local nature of immunity in tuberculosis, illustrated histochemically in dermal BCG lesions, *J. Immunol.* **100**:931–941.

David, H. L., and Selin, M. J., 1976, Immune response to mycobacteria, in: *Manual of Clinical Immunology* (N. R. Rose and H. Friedman, eds.), pp. 324–331, American Society for Microbiology, Washington, D.C.

David, J. R., 1973, Lymphocyte mediators and cellular hypersensitivity, *N. Engl. J. Med.* **288**:143–149.

David, J. R., Al-Askari, S., Lawrence, H. S., and Thomas, L., 1964, Delayed hypersensitivity *in vitro*. I. The specificity of inhibition of cell migration by antigens, *J. Immunol.* **93**:264–273.

Dwyer, J., and Kantor, F. S., 1973, Regulation of delayed hypersensitivity. Failure to transfer delayed hypersensitivity to desensitized guinea pigs, *J. Exp. Med.* **137**:32–41.

Epstein, W. L., 1967, Granulomatous hypersensitivity, *Prog. Allergy* **11**:36–88.

Frappier, A., Portelance, V., St. Pierre, J., and Panisset, M., 1971, BCG Strains: Characteristics and relative efficacy, in: *Status of Immunization in Tuberculosis,* pp. 157–178, U.S. Department of Health, Education and Welfare, Washington, D.C.

Freund, J., 1929, The sensitiveness of tuberculous guinea pigs one month old to the toxicity of tuberculin, *J. Immunol.* **17**:465–471.

Gelien, J., and Hamman, L., 1913, The subsequent history of 1000 patients who received tuberculin tests, *Bull. Johns Hopkins Hosp.* **24**:180–186.

Godal, T., Rees, R. J. W., and Lamvik, J. P., 1971, Lymphocyte-mediated modification of blood-derived macrophage function *in vitro*; inhibition of growth of intracellular mycobacteria with lymphokines, *Clin. Exp. Immunol.* **8**:625–637.

Godal, T., Myrvang, B., Stanford, J. L., and Samuel, D. R., 1974, Recent advances in the immunology of leprosy with special reference to new approaches in immunoprophylaxis, *Bull. Inst. Pasteur* **72**:273–310.

Gordon, S., Todd, J., and Cohn, Z. A., 1974, *In vitro* synthesis and secretion of lysozyme by mononuclear phagocytes, *J. Exp. Med.* **139**:1228–1248.

Goren, M. B., 1975, Cord factor revisited: A tribute to the late Dr. Hubert Bloch, *Tubercle* **56**:65–71.

Goren, M. B., Brokl, O., and Schaefer, W. B., 1974a, Lipids of putative relevance to virulence in *Mycobacterium tuberculosis*: Correlation of virulence with elaboration of sulfatides and strongly acidic lipids, *Infect. Immun.* **9**:142–149.

Goren, M. B., Brokl, O., and Schaefer, W. B., 1974b, Lipids of putative relevance to virulence in *Mycobacterium tuberculosis*: Phthiocerol dimycoserate and the attenuation indicator, *Infect. Immun.* **9**:150–158.

Goren, M. B., Hart, P. D., Young, M. R., and Armstrong, J. A., 1976, Prevention of phagosome-lysosome fusion in cultured macrophages by sulfatides of *Mycobacterium tuberculosis*, *Proc. Natl. Acad. Sci. USA* **73**:2510–2514.

Gotoff, S. P., and Vizral, I. F., 1972, The macrophage aggregation assay for delayed hypersensitivity: Development of the response, role of the macrophage, and the independence of humoral antibody, *Cell. Immunol.* **3**:53–61.

Granger, G. A., 1972, Lymphokines—The mediators of cellular immunity, *Ser. Haematol.* **5**:8–40.

Gray, D. F., Graham-Smith, H., and Noble, J. L., 1960, Variations in natural resistance to tuberculosis, *J. Hyg.* **58**:215–227.

Grogg, E., and Pearce, A. G. E., 1952, The enzymic and lipid histochemistry of experimental tuberculosis, *Br. J. Exp. Pathol.* **33**:567–576.

Guld, J., 1971, BCG as an immunizing agent, in: *Status of Immunization in Tuberculosis,* pp. 149–156, U.S. Department of Health, Education, and Welfare, Washington, D.C.

Hart, P. D., 1967, Efficacy and applicability of mass BCG vaccination in tuberculosis control, *Br. Med. J.* **1**:587–592.

Hart, P. D., Sutherland, I., and Thomas, J., 1967, The immunity conferred by effective BCG and vole bacillus vaccines, in relation to individual variations in induced tuberculin sensitivity and to technical variations in the vaccines, *Tubercle* **48**:201–210.

Hart, P. D., Armstrong, J. A., Brown, C. A., and Draper, P., 1972, Ultrastructural study of the behavior of macrophages toward parasitic mycobacteria, *Infect. Immun.* **5**:803–807.

Heidrick, M. L., and Makinodan, T., 1972, Nature of cellular deficiencies in age-related decline of the immune system, *Gerontologia* **18**:305–320.

Heppner, G. H., 1972, Blocking antibodies and enhancement, *Ser. Haematol.* **5**:41–66.

Hibbs, J. B., Lambert, L. H., and Remington, J. S., 1972, Possible role of macrophage mediated nonspecific cytotoxicity in tumor resistance, *Nature (London), New Biol.* **235**:48–50.

Horwitz, O., and Bunch-Christensen, K., 1972, Correlation between tuberculin sensitivity after 2 months and 5 years among BCG vaccinated subjects, *Bull. WHO* **47**:49–58.

Houk, V. N., Kent, D. C., Sorensen, K., and Baker, J. H., 1968, The eradication of tuberculosis infection by isoniazid chemoprophylaxis, *Arch. Environ. Health* **16**:46–50.

Huber, B., Devinsky, O., Gershon, R. K., and Cantor, H., 1976, Cell-mediated immunity: Delayed-type hypersensitivity and cytotoxic responses are mediated by different T-cell subclasses, *J. Exp. Med.* **143**:1534–1539.

Jaffer, A. M., Jones, G., Kasdon, E. J., and Schlossman, S. F., 1973, Local transfer of delayed hypersensitivity by T lymphocytes, *J. Immunol.* **111**:1268–1269.

Janicki, B. W., and Aron, S. A., 1968, Induction of tuberculin hypersensitivity and serologic unresponsiveness to tubercle bacilli in newborn and young guinea pigs, *J. Immunol.* **101**:121–127.

Janicki, B. W., Chaparas, S. D., Daniel, T. M., Kubica,

G. P., Wright, G. L., and Yee, G. S., 1971, A reference system for antigens of *Mycobacterium tuberculosis*, *Am. Rev. Resp. Dis.* **104**:602–604.

Janicki, B. W., Good, R. C., Minden, P., Affronti, L. F., and Hymes, W. F., 1973, Immune responses in Rhesus monkeys after Bacillus Calmette-Guerin vaccination and aerosol challenge with *Mycobacterium tuberculosis*, *Am. Rev. Resp. Dis.* **107**:359–366.

Jespersen, A., and Bentzon, M. W., 1964, The virulence of various strains of BCG determined in the golden hamster, *Acta Tuberc. Scand.* **44**:222–249.

Karlson, A. G., 1954, Regression of tuberculous lesions in guinea pigs infected with isoniazid-resistant tubercle bacilli, *Am. Rev. Tuberc.* **70**:531–532.

Kato, M., 1968, Studies of the biochemical lesion in experimental tuberculosis in mice. VII. Effect of derivatives and chemical analogs of cord factor on structure and function of mouse liver mitochondria, *Am. Rev. Resp. Dis.* **98**:668–676.

Katz, J., Kunofsky, S., and Krasnitz, A., 1972, Variation in sensitivity to tuberculin, *Am. Rev. Resp. Dis.* **106**:202–212.

Kirkpatrick, C. H., 1975, Properties and activities of transfer factor, *J. Allergy Clin. Immunol.* **55**:411–421.

Kisielow, P., Hirst, J. A., Shiku, H., Beverly, P. C. L., Hoffman, M. K., Boyse, E. A., and Oettgen, H. F., 1975, Ly antigens as markers for functionally distinct sub-populations of thymus-derived lymphocytes of the mouse, *Nature (London)* **253**:219–220.

Klebanoff, S. J., and Hamon, C. B., 1975, Antimicrobial systems of mononuclear phagocytes, in: *Mononuclear Phagocytes in Immunity, Infection and Pathology* (R. van Furth, ed.), pp. 507–528, Blackwell Scientific Publications, Oxford.

Krahenbuhl, J. L., and Remington, J. S., 1971, *In vitro* induction of non-specific resistance in macrophages by specifically sensitized lymphocytes, *Infect. Immun.* **4**:337–343.

Ladefoged, A., Bunch-Christensen, J., and Guld, J., 1976, Tuberculin sensitivity in guinea pigs after vaccination with varying doses of BCG of 12 different strains, *Bull. WHO* **53**:435–444.

Lagrange, P. H., Mackaness, G. B., and Miller, T. E., 1974, Influence of dose and route of antigen injection on the immunological induction of T cells, *J. Exp. Med.* **139**:528–542.

Landi, S., and Held, H. R., 1970, Comparative study of ^{14}C-labeled purified protein derivative from various mycobacteria, *Appl. Microbiol.* **20**:704–709.

Lawrence, H. S., 1955, The transfer in humans of delayed skin sensitivity to streptococcal M-substance and to tuberculin with disrupted leucocytes, *J. Clin. Invest.* **34**:219–230.

Lawrence, H. S., 1974, Transfer factor in cellular immunity, *Harvey Lect.* **68**:239–350.

Lederer, E., 1976, Natural and synthetic immunostimulants related to the mycobacterial cell wall, in: *Proceedings of the Fifth International Symposium on Medicinal Chemistry*, Elsevier Scientific Publishing Company, Amsterdam.

Lefford, M. J., 1975a, Transfer of adoptive immunity to tuberculosis in mice, *Infect. Immun.* **11**:1174–1181.

Lefford, M. J., 1975b, Delayed hypersensitivity and immunity in tuberculosis, *Am. Rev. Resp. Dis.* **111**:243–246.

Lefford, M. J., and McGregor, D. D., 1974, Immunological memory in tuberculosis. I. Influence of persisting viable organisms, *Cell. Immunol.* **14**:417–428.

Lefford, M. J., and McGregor, D. D., 1978, The lymphocyte mediators of delayed hypersensitivity: The early phase cells, *Immunology* **34**:581–590.

Lefford, M. J., McGregor, D. D., and Mackaness, G. B., 1973a, Immune response to *Mycobacterium tuberculosis* in rats, *Infect. Immun.* **8**:182–189.

Lefford, M. J., McGregor, D. D., and Mackaness, G. B., 1973b, Properties of lymphocytes which confer adoptive immunity to tuberculosis in rats, *Immunology* **25**:703–715.

Looke, E., and Rowley, D., 1962, The lack of correlation between sensitivity of bacteria to killing by macrophages or acidic conditions, *Aust. J. Exp. Biol. Med. Sci.* **40**:315–320.

Lowrie, D. B., Jacket, P. S., and Ratcliffe, N. A., 1975, *Mycobacterium microti* may protect itself from intracellular destruction by releasing cyclic AMP into phagosomes, *Nature (London)* **254**:600–602.

Lurie, M. B., 1964, *Resistance to Tuberculosis: Experimental Studies in Native and Acquired Defense Mechanisms*, Harvard University Press, Cambridge, Mass.

Mackaness, G. B., 1962, Cellular resistance to infection, *J. Exp. Med.* **116**:381–406.

Mackaness, G. B., 1964a, The behaviour of microbial parasites in relation to phagocytic cells *in vitro* and *in vivo*, *Symp. Soc. Gen. Microbiol.* **14**:213–240.

Mackaness, G. B., 1964b, The immunological basis of acquired cellular resistance, *J. Exp. Med.* **120**:105–120.

Mackaness, G. B., 1967, The relationship of delayed hypersensitivity to acquired cellular resistance, *Br. Med. Bull.* **23**:52–54.

Mackaness, G. B., and Blanden, R. V., 1967, Cellular immunity, *Prog. Allergy* **11**:89–140.

Mackaness, G. B., Smith, N., and Wells, A. Q., 1954, The growth of intracellular tubercle bacilli in relation to their virulence, *Am. Rev. Tuberc.* **69**:479–494.

MacLean, R. A., 1975, Tuberculin testing antigens and techniques, *Chest* **68**:455–459.

Maugh, T. H., 1973, Singlet oxygen: A unique microbicidal agent in cells, *Science* **182**:44–45.

Medical Research Council, 1972, BCG and vole bacillus vaccines in the prevention of tuberculosis in adolescence and early adult life, *Bull. WHO* **46**:371–385.

Meyer, T. J., Ribi, E., and Azuma, I., 1975, Biologically active components from mycobacterial cell walls. V. Granuloma formation in mouse lungs and guinea pig skin, *Cell. Immunol.* **16**:11–24.

Middlebrook, G., and Dubos, R. J., 1948, Specific serum agglutination of erythrocytes sensitized with extracts of tubercle bacilli, *J. Exp. Med.* **88**:521–528.

Middlebrook, G., Coleman, C. M., and Schaefer, W. B., 1959, Sulfolipid from virulent tubercle bacilli, *Proc. Natl. Acad. Sci. USA* **45**:1801–1804.

Middlebrook, G., Salmon, B. J., and Kreisberg, J. I., 1974, Sterilization of *Listeria monocytogenes* by guinea pig peritoneal exudate cell cultures, *Cell. Immunol.* **14**:270–283.

Mills, J. A., 1966, The immunologic significance of antigen induced lymphocyte transformation *in vitro, J. Immunol.* **97**:239–247.

Mitchison, D. A., 1964, The virulence of tubercle bacilli from patients with pulmonary tuberculosis in India and other countries, *Bull. Int. Union Tuberc.* **35**:287–306.

Mitchison, D. A., Wallace, J. G., Bhatia, A. L., Selkon, J. B., Subbaiah, T. V., and Lancaster, M. C., 1960, A comparison of the virulence in guinea-pigs of South Indian and British tubercle bacilli, *Tubercle* **41**:1–22.

Naganna, K., 1974, Some of the BCG trials and certain aspects involved in them, *Am. Rev. Resp. Dis.* **109**:497–499.

Narain, R., Nair, S. S., Rao, G. R., Chandrasekhar, P., and Lal, P., 1966, Enhancing of tuberculin allergy by previous tuberculin testing, *Bull. WHO* **34**:623–628.

Narain, R., Bagga, A. S., Naganna, K., and Mayurnath, S., 1970, Influence of isoniazid on naturally acquired tuberculin allergy and on induction of allergy by BCG vaccination, *Bull. WHO* **43**:56–64.

Nathan, C., Karnovsky, M. L., and David, J. R., 1971, Alterations of macrophage functions by mediators from lymphocytes, *J. Exp. Med.* **133**:1356–1376.

Nieburger, R. G., Youmans, G. P., and Youmans, A. S., 1973, Relationship between tuberculin hypersensitivity and cellular immunity to infection in mice vaccinated with viable attenuated mycobacterial ribonucleic acid preparation, *Infect. Immun.* **8**:42–47.

North, R. J., 1973, Importance of thymus-derived lymphocytes in cell-mediated immunity to infection, *Cell. Immunol.* **7**:166–176.

North, R. J., Mackaness, G. B., and Elliott, R. W., 1972, The histogenesis of immunologically committed lymphocytes, *Cell. Immunol.* **3**:680–694.

O'Grady, F., 1967, Tuberculin reaction in tuberculosis, *Br. Med. Bull.* **23**:76–80.

Olakowski, T., and Mardon, K., 1971, The restorative influence of repeated tuberculin testing on tuberculin sensitivity in BCG-vaccinated schoolchildren, *Bull. WHO* **45**:649–655.

Oppenheim, J. J., Wolstencroft, R. A., and Gell, P. G. H., 1967, Delayed hypersensitivity in the guinea-pig to a protein-hapten conjugate and its relationship to *in vitro* transformation of lymph node, spleen, thymus and peripheral blood lymphocytes, *Immunology* **12**:89–102.

Ornstein, G. G., and Steinbach, M. M., 1925, The resistance of the albino rat to infection with tubercle bacilli, *Am. Rev. Tuberc.* **12**:77–86.

Palmer, C. E., Shaw, L. W., and Comstock, G. W., 1958, Community trials of BCG vaccination, *Am. Rev. Tuberc.* **77**:877–907.

Patterson, R. J., and Youmans, G. P., 1970, Demonstration in tissue culture of lymphocyte-mediated immunity to tuberculosis, *Infect. Immun.* **1**:600–603.

Pearmain, G. E., Lycette, R. R., and Fitzgerald, P. H., 1963, Tuberculin-induced mitosis in peripheral blood leucocytes, *Lancet* **1**:637–638.

Pierce, C., Dubos, R. J., and Middlebrook, G., 1947, Infection of mice with mammalian tubercle bacilli grown in Tween-albumin liquid medium, *J. Exp. Med.* **86**:159–174.

Pierce, C. H., Dubos, R. J., and Schaefer, W. B., 1953, Multiplication and survival of tubercle bacilli in the organs of mice, *J. Exp. Med.* **97**:189–205.

Plant, J., and Glynn, A. A., 1976, Genetics of resistance to infection with *Salmonella typhimurium* in mice, *J. Infect. Dis.* **133**:72–78.

Poulter, L. W., and Turk, J. L., 1976, Mediation of macrophage effector function by lymphokine, in: *Future Trends in Inflammation II* (G. P. Velo, D. A. Willoughby, and J. P. Giroud, eds.), Birkhauser Verlag, Basel.

Raleigh, J. W., Wichelhausen, R. H., Rado, T. M., and Bates, J. H., 1975, Evidence for infection by two distinct strains of *Mycobacterium tuberculosis* in pulmonary tuberculosis: Report of 9 cases, *Am. Rev. Resp. Dis.* **112**:497–503.

Ratcliffe, H. L., 1952, Tuberculosis induced by droplet nuclei infection; pulmonary tuberculosis of pre-determined initial intensity in mammals, *Am. J. Hyg.* **55**:36–48.

Ratcliffe, H. L., and Palladino, V. F., 1953, Tuberculosis induced by droplet nuclei infection: Initial homogeneous response of small mammals (rats, mice, guinea pigs, and hamsters) to human and to bovine bacilli, and the rate and pattern of tubercle development, *J. Exp. Med.* **97**:61–68.

Rees, R. J. W., and Meade, T. W., 1974, Comparison of the modes of spread and the incidence of tuberculosis and leprosy, *Lancet* **1**:47–48.

Reggiardo, Z., and Middlebrook, G., 1974, Delayed-type hypersensitivity and immunity against aerogenic tuberculosis in guinea pigs, *Infect. Immun.* **9**:815–820.

Ribi, E., Larson, C., Wicht, W., List, R., and Goode, G., 1966, Effective non-living vaccine against experimental tuberculosis in mice, *J. Bacteriol.* **91**:975–983.

Rich, A. R., 1951, *The Pathogenesis of Tuberculosis*, 2nd ed., Thomas, Springfield, Ill.

Robinson, A., Meyer, M., and Middlebrook, G., 1955, Tuberculin hypersensitivity in tuberculous infants treated with isoniazid, *N. Engl. J. Med.* **252**:983–985.

Rocklin, R. E., MacDermott, R. P., Chess, L., Schlossman, S. F., and David, J. R., 1974, Studies on mediator production by highly purified human T and B lymphocytes, *J. Exp. Med.* **140**:1303–1316.

Rocklin, R. E., Reardon, G., Sheffer, A., Churchill, W. H., and David, J. R., 1970, Dissociation between two *in vitro* correlates of delayed hypersensitivity; Absence of migration inhibitory factor (MIF) in the presence of antigen-induced incorporation of ³H-thymidine, in: *Pro-*

ceedings of the Fifth Leukocyte Culture Conference (J. E. Harris, ed.), pp. 639–648, Academic Press, New York.

Rodey, G. E., Good, R. A., and Yunis, E. J., 1971, Progressive loss *in vitro* of cellular immunity with aging in strains of mice susceptible to autoimmune disease, *Clin. Exp. Immunol.* **9:**305–311.

Romano, T. J., Nowakowski, M., Bloom, B. R., and Thorbecke, G. J., 1977, Selective viral immunosuppression of the graft-versus-host reaction, *J. Exp. Med.* **145:** 666–675.

Romeo, D., Cramer, R., Marzi, M., Soranzo, M. R., Zabucchi, G., and Rossi, F., 1973, Peroxidase activity of alveolar and peritoneal macrophages, *J. Reticuloendothel. Soc.* **13:**399–409.

Rothschild, H., Friedenwald, J. S., and Bernstein, C., 1934, The relation of allergy to immunity in tuberculosis, *Bull. Johns Hopkins Hosp.* **54:**232–276.

Runyon, E. H., 1974, Ten mycobacterial pathogens, *Tubercle* **55:**235–240.

Ruskin, J., and Remington, J. S., 1968, Immunity and intracellular infection: Resistance to bacteria in mice infected with a protozoan, *Science* **160:**72–74.

Salvin, S. B., and Neta, R., 1975, A possible relationship between delayed hypersensitivity and cell-mediated immunity, *Am. Rev. Resp. Dis.* **111:**373–377.

Scadding, J. G., 1960, *Mycobacterium tuberculosis* in the aetiology of sarcoidosis, *Br. Med. J.* **2:**1617–1623.

Schlossman, S. F., Levin, H. A., Rocklin, R. E., and David, J. R., 1971, The compartmentalization of antigen-reactive lymphocytes in desensitized guinea pigs, *J. Exp. Med.* **134:**741–750.

Simon, H. B., and Sheagren, J. N., 1971, Cellular immunity *in vitro*. I. Immunologically mediated enhancement of macrophage bactericidal activity, *J. Exp. Med.* **133:**1377–1389.

Stead, W. W., 1967, Pathogenesis of a first episode of chronic tuberculosis in man: Recrudescence of residuals of the primary infection or exogenous reinfection, *Am. Rev. Resp. Dis.* **95:**729–745.

Steenken, W., and Wolinsky, E., 1952, Antituberculous properties of hydrazines of isonicotinic acid (Rimifon, Marsilid), *Am. Rev. Tuberc.* **65:**365–375.

Styblo, K., 1968, Progress report from the Tuberculosis Surveillance Research Unit, *Bull. Int. Union Tuberc.* **41:**255–264.

Styblo, K., Meijer, J., and Sutherland, I., 1969, Tuberculosis Surveillance Research Unit Report No. 1: The transmission of tubercle bacilli. Its trend in a human population, *Bull. Int. Union Tuberc.* **52:**1–104.

Sutherland, I., 1971, State of the art in immunoprophylaxis in tuberculosis, in: *Status of Immunization in Tuberculosis*, pp. 113–125, U.S. Department of Health, Education, and Welfare, Washington, D.C.

Takahashi, Y., and Ono, K., 1958, Hemagglutination reaction by the phosphatide of the tubercle bacillus, *Science* **127:**1053–1054.

Takahashi, Y., Mochizuki, K., and Nagayama, Y., 1961,

The behavior of three different kinds of antibodies in tuberculosis: Antiprotein, antipolysaccharide and antiphosphatide, *J. Exp. Med.* **114:**569–579.

ten Dam, H. G., Toman, K., Hitze, K. L., and Guld, J., 1976, Present knowledge of immunization against tuberculosis, *Bull. WHO* **54:**255–269.

Thomas, J. W., Clements, D., and Grzybowski, S., 1971, *In vitro* lymphocyte responses and skin test reactivity following BCG vaccination, *Clin. Exp. Immunol.* **9:**611–623.

Thor, D. E., and Dray, S., 1968, A correlate of human delayed hypersensitivity: Specific inhibition of capillary tube migration of sensitized human lymph node cells by tuberculin and histoplasmin, *J. Immunol.* **101:** 51–61.

Tuberculosis in the United States, 1976, U.S. Department of Health, Education, and Welfare, Washington, D.C.

Turk, J. L., and Poulter, L. W., 1974, Macrophage activation in delayed hypersensitivity, in: *Future Trends in Inflammation* (G. P. Velo, D. A. Willoughby, and J. P. Giroud, eds.), pp. 343–360, Piccin Medical Books, Padua, Italy.

von Pirquet, C. F., 1909, Quantitative experiments with the cutaneous tuberculin reaction, *J. Pharmacol. Exp. Ther.* **1:**151–174.

Vorwald, A. J., 1933, A comparison of tissue reactions to pulmonary infection with tubercle bacilli in animals of varying resistance, *Am. Rev. Tuberc.* **27:**270–290.

Waksman, B. H., and Matoltsy, M., 1958, Quantitative study of local passive transfer of tuberculin sensitivity with peritoneal exudate cells in the guinea pig, *J. Immunol.* **81:**235–241.

Waldorf, D. S., Willkens, R. F., and Decker, J. L., 1968, Impaired delayed hypersensitivity in an aging population, *JAMA* **203:**831–834.

Walford, R. L., 1969, *The Immunologic Theory of Aging*, Williams and Wilkins, Baltimore.

Ward, P. A., Remold, H. G., and David, J. R., 1970, The production by antigen-stimulated lymphocytes of a leukotactic factor distinct from migration inhibitory factor, *Cell. Immunol.* **1:**162–174.

Warrick, W. J., Good, R. A., and Smith, R. T., 1960, Failure of passive transfer of delayed hypersensitivity in the newborn human infant, *J. Lab. Clin. Med.* **56:**139–147.

Weksler, M. E., and Hutteroth, T. H., 1974, Impaired lymphocyte function in aged humans, *J. Clin. Invest.* **53:**99–104.

Wijsmuller, G., 1971, The negative tuberculin test, *J. Med. Assoc. State Ala.* **41:**353–357.

Willis, H. S., 1928, Studies on immunity to tuberculosis: The waning of cutaneous hypersensitiveness to tuberculin and the relation of tuberculoimmunity to tuberculoallergy, *Am. Rev. Tuberc.* **17:**240–252.

Woodruff, J. F., and Woodruff, J. J., 1975, T lymphocyte interaction with viruses and virus infected tissues, *Prog. Med. Virol.* **19:**120–160.

Yashphe, D. J., 1971, Immunological factors in nonspecific stimulation of host resistance to syngeneic tumors, *Israel J. Med. Sci.* **7**:90–107.

Youmans, A. S., and Youmans, G. P., 1967, Preparation and effect of different adjuvants on the immunogenic activity of mycobacterial ribosomal fraction, *J. Bacteriol.* **94**:836–843.

Youmans, G. P., 1975, Relation between delayed hypersensitivity and immunity in tuberculosis, *Am. Rev. Resp. Dis.* **111**:109–118.

Youmans, G. P., and Youmans, A. S., 1972, Response of vaccinated and non-vaccinated syngeneic C57Bl/6 mice to infection with *Mycobacterium tuberculosis, Infect. Immun.* **6**:748–754.

Zinsser, H., 1921, Studies on the tuberculin reaction and on specific hypersensitiveness in bacterial infection, *J. Exp. Med.* **34**:495–524.

Zweiman, B., Schoenwetter, W. F., and Hildreth, E. A., 1966, The effect of the scorbutic state on tuberculin hypersensitivity in the guinea pig. I. Passive transfer of tuberculin hypersensitivity, *J. Immunol.* **96**:296–300.

15

Immunobiology of Leprosy

WARD E. BULLOCK

1. Introduction

Leprosy continues to be one of the major unconquered diseases of the world as witnessed by the fact that the total number of cases probably exceeds 12 million (WHO, 1977). Furthermore, this infection produces some form of physical disability in more than 25% of cases (Bechelli and Mártinéz Dominquez, 1966). Until recently, the staggering medical, social, and economic consequences of leprosy have received insufficient attention from the governments and medical research communities of more affluent nations. Within the past decade, however, the need for a global attack on leprosy has become widely recognized and tangible progress has been made.

Fortunately, important advances have been made in the pharmacology of antileprosy drugs at a time when the incidence of primary resistance to dapsone by *Mycobacterium leprae* is increasing (Pearson *et al.*, 1977). The successful cultivation of the "noncultivatable" species, *Mycobacterium lepraemurium*, in a synthetic medium represents a major step toward the ultimate goal of propagating *M. leprae in vitro* (Nakamura, 1972). In addition, the successful transmission of *M. leprae* from man to armadillo is expected to be a great boon to progress in leprosy since infected animals provide enormous numbers of organisms, the yield from livers being as high as 1×10^8 bacilli per gram of tissue (Kirchheimer and Sanchez, 1976). Indeed, the increased availability of *M. leprae* has provided considerable impetus to a massive program for development of an

antileprosy vaccine under the auspices of the World Health Organization.

Application of the newer knowledge in immunology to the problems of leprosy during the past few years has led to significant advances in our understanding of the mechanisms of this complex infection. It is the purpose of this chapter to review these advances in order to bring the fundamental immunobiological problems inherent in the paradigm of leprosy to the attention of a larger number of clinical investigators.

2. The Bacillus, *Mycobacterium leprae*

Human leprosy is caused by an acid-fast staining bacillus first discovered in 1873 (Hansen, 1874). Unfortunately, little information has become available in the ensuing century concerning the antigenic makeup and taxonomic status of this pathogen. The dearth of information stems from the fact that all efforts to cultivate the organism *in vitro* have failed.* Nevertheless, numerous studies of leprosy bacilli extracted from infected tissues have provided sufficient information to permit assignment of these organisms to the genus *Mycobacterium*. Although *M. leprae* appears to differ from other members of the genus in certain cytochemical properties, particularly in its phenoloxidase activity (Prabhakaran *et al.*, 1968) and in the extractability of its acid-fast property by pyridine (Fisher and Barksdale, 1973), three major lines of evidence support its generic status as a *Mycobacterium*. First,

WARD E. BULLOCK • Department of Medicine, University of Kentucky Medical Center, Lexington, Kentucky 40506.

---

* The recent claim by Skinsnes *et al.* (1978) of successful *M. leprae* cultivation on hyaluronic-acid-based medium has not been confirmed at the time of writing.

M. leprae contains mycolic acids characteristic of the mycobacteria. These are most closely related to the types present in *Mycobacterium tuberculosis* and *Mycobacterium kansasii* (Etemadi and Convit, 1974). Second, it possesses a superficial network of ropelike peptidoglycolipid filaments that resembles in morphology and structure the surface filaments characteristic of other mycobacteria (Sata and Makoto, 1968; Gordon and White, 1971). Third, extracts of *M. leprae* contain multiple antigens common to other mycobacteria (Navalkar *et al.*, 1964; Abe, 1970; Closs *et al.*, 1979).

The long replication time of *M. leprae*, estimated to be 10–20 days in the logarithmic phase of growth (Shepard and McRae, 1965), suggests that it is a member of the "slow-growing" subgroup of mycobacteria. However, preliminary toxonomic studies indicate that it might be more closely related to certain "fast-growing" groups of mycobacteria (Paul *et al.*, 1975; Stanford *et al.*, 1975). These findings raise the interesting possibility that *M. leprae* may not have evolved from a slow-growing progenitor but rather may have had as its ancestor an environmental saprophyte.

The microbial factors responsible for pathogenesis of the granulomatous infection produced by *M. leprae* are poorly understood. It is known that killed *M. leprae* produce an adjuvant effect in experimental animals when injected in a water-and-oil emulsion (Carter *et al.*, 1969; Stewart-Tull and Davies, 1972). Furthermore, the distribution of organisms to local or distant lymphoid organs and the associated histological reactions are indistinguishable from those observed after injection of killed *M. tuberculosis*. In comparative studies, Stewart-Tull and Davies (1972) observed that *M. leprae* isolated from human tissue contains 4–5 times less adjuvant activity than do equal numbers of *M. tuberculosis* grown *in vitro*. One possible explanation for this difference is the fact that the surface network of peptidoglycolipid filaments on *M. leprae* harvested from tissues is less dense than the network on *M. tuberculosis* grown *in vitro* (Gordon and White, 1971). Since these filaments are adjuvant active (White *et al.*, 1964), the lesser adjuvant effect of *M. leprae* might be explained on this basis. Whether the quantity of peptidoglycolipid surface structure on *M.* *leprae* may be altered under various conditions is unknown.

Shepard and McCrae (1971) observed that during continuous passage of *M. leprae* in mouse footpads, certain isolates could be differentiated into "fast" and "slow" growers, as determined by the average rate of growth between inoculation and harvest and by the number of bacilli in the harvest. The property of "fastness" was stable on repeated mouse passage. In addition, histological studies showed that "fast" strains grew to a higher level of organisms without inducing a tissue infiltrate of lymphocytes and macrophages. Conversely, an inflammatory cell infiltrate did appear in footpads infected by "slow" growers that was associated with termination of the logarithmic growth phase. This inverse relationship between the numbers of bacilli and degree of lymphocyte infiltration in response to "fast" and "slow" organisms, respectively, raises a critical question to which there is no answer at present: are there inherent differences among strains of *M. leprae* that may explain, at least in part, the different types of inflammatory responses observed in various forms of leprosy?

3. Epidemiology and Host Factors in Leprosy

Traditionally, it has been assumed that leprosy is transmitted by direct skin-to-skin contact because dermatological manifestations are the most frequent presenting sign, and infection rates are high among young children of parents with lepromatous leprosy. This assumption may be incorrect as suggested by the fact that the numbers of acid-fast bacilli shed from the intact skin of lepromatous patients are very small (Pedley, 1970). Many bacilli may be shed from ulcerating lesions, but these do not occur with high frequency. Conversely, the nasal mucus contains approximately 1×10^8/ml of acid-fast bacilli (Shepard, 1962). This number of equivalent to the quantity of *M. tuberculosis* in the sputum of patients with cavitary pulmonary tuberculosis (Rees and Meade, 1974). Furthermore, the leprosy bacilli in dried nasal mucus may remain viable for several days (Rees, 1976). These observations have stimulated a reexamination of the hypothesis that primary leprosy can be acquired via the respiratory tract, despite the fact that no cases have been reported of primary nasal infection in the absence of skin lesions (Brinckerhoff and Moore, 1909; Solis and Wade, 1925). The gastrointestinal tract may provide another route of infection, since large numbers of *M. leprae* are shed in breast milk (Pedley, 1968). And finally, leprosy may be transmitted by biting insects; viable acid-fast bacilli can be isolated from the midgut of laboratory-bred mosquitoes and bed bugs for at least 48 hr after they have fed on lepromatous patients (Narayanan *et al.*, 1972).

Little is known of the host factors that determine susceptibility to actual disease once an individual has been infected by *M. leprae*, whatever the route. Doull *et al.* (1942) estimated that the risk of acquiring leprosy among household contacts of lepromatous patients was 8 times the risk in households free of leprosy within an endemic area. Nevertheless, calculation of the cumulative age-specific attack rates for household contacts to the age of 25 years gave an expected prevalence for all types of leprosy no greater than 293 per 1000 for males and 140 per 1000 for females. Lara and Nolasco (1956) demonstrated that two-thirds of the children reared by parents with lepromatous leprosy who contracted clinical leprosy actually healed completely without therapy as judged by clinical follow-up for as long as 20 years.

More recently, Godal and Negassi (1973) and Myrvang (1974) studied the immune response to *M. leprae* among groups of healthy individuals whose job assignments placed them in various degrees of contact with leprosy patients. The percentage of positive responses to *M. leprae* by skin test and lymphocyte transformation was far higher (about 50%) among those with occupational or household contact than among personnel from nonendemic areas (< 1%). Thus human resistance to *M. leprae* appears to be high overall, with a far greater prevalence of infection than of disease. A major question still to be answered is whether apparently healthy individuals who are skin test negative to *M. leprae* are at a greater risk of contracting leprosy, especially the lepromatous type. A 15- to 20-year follow-up of 156 lepromin-negative "normals" in India by Dharmendra and Chatterjee (1955)

revealed that 22 (14%) subsequently acquired leprosy, whereas only 17 (3.2%) of 524 lepromin-positive subjects did so. These results are interesting, but it is impossible to draw definitive conclusions because of several uncontrolled variables within the study.

Many workers believe that genetic factors must play some role in susceptibility to leprosy, especially among those "destined" to develop lepromatous disease. As yet, no conclusive evidence in support of this hypothesis has been forthcoming. The concordance of lepromatous leprosy in monozygotic twins is not sufficiently high to implicate clearly a genetic predisposition (WHO Memorandum, 1973). Tests of genetic polymorphic systems, including eight red blood cell antigens, have detected no differences between tuberculoid and lepromatous patients (Salzano, 1967; Blumberg *et al.*, 1967). More than ten studies of HLA phenotype frequencies among patients with leprosy have failed to demonstrate consistent differences between patients and controls (Rea *et al.*, 1976b). However, in studies of families, De Vries *et al.* (1976) and Fine *et al.*, (1979) demonstrated a significant, nonrandom segregation of parental HLA haplotypes in siblings with tuberculoid leprosy. Thus the importance of HLA-linked genes in determining susceptibility to leprosy remains undecided.

Notwithstanding the current paucity of evidence for a role of genetic factors in leprosy, it is quite possible that HLA-linked genes are present in man which are important in determining susceptibility to leprosy but are not necessarily the same as those determining the HLA SD antigens. Studies of HLA LD phenotype frequencies among leprosy patients will be of interest, since putative immune response genes in man may be located in the same region of the HLA complex as genes that determine the LD alleles recognized in the mixed leukocyte culture (MLC) reaction.

4. Immunopathological Spectrum of Leprosy

Infection by *M. leprae* evokes a chronic inflammatory cell response that varies greatly in histological appearance and in the associated clinical manifestations. Nevertheless, polar forms of leprosy have been defined with sufficient clarity to serve as reference points for the clinical spectrum of disease that extends between them. The classification of Ridley and Jopling (1966; Ridley, 1974) is used most commonly to refract the spectrum of leprosy. At one pole is tuberculoid leprosy, designated as TT. Borderline forms of tuberculoid leprosy are defined as BT, and cases with features of both tuberculoid and lepromatous disease are BB. Within the lepromatous portion of the spectrum are described borderline lepromatous leprosy (BL), intermediate lepromatous leprosy (LI), and polar lepromatous leprosy (LL). Histologically, the lesions of TT and BT leprosy are characterized by foci of granulomas containing epithelioid cells, giant cells, and a dense infiltration of lymphocytes. Acid-fast staining bacilli are observed infrequently. Systemic distribution of granulomas within various organs of the reticuloendothelial system does occur; however, the prevalence of such lesions is unknown (Okada, 1954; Desikan and Job, 1966).

In lepromatous leprosy, granulomas are composed of histiocytic cells that are "foamy" in appearance and contain many *M. leprae*. Lymphocytes are scanty and, if present, are diffusely distributed. Epithelioid cells and giant cells are absent. Less severe forms of lepromatous disease are classified histologically by the relative numbers of lymphocytes, foamy macrophages, giant cells, and bacilli present within granulomas. Granulomatous pathology is common within the lymph nodes, spleen, and liver (Sharma and Shrivastav, 1958; Desikan and Job, 1968; Karat *et al.*, 1971). Within lymph nodes the paracortical region is infiltrated by masses of undifferentiated cells belonging to the histiocyte–macrophage series that are laden with acid-fast bacilli (Turk and Waters, 1971). Lymphocytes appear to be displaced from this area, whereas the germinal centers are usually increased in size and number. As lepromatous patients improve clinically under long-term antimicrobial therapy, the histiocytic infiltrate in lymph nodes tends to regress with a concomitant "return" of lymphocytes to the paracortical areas. Nevertheless, residual clusters of foamy histiocytes have been observed even after 10 years of therapy. Detailed information as to the nature of splenic pathology

in lepromatous leprosy is limited. Although sinusoids of the red pulp are infiltrated by foamy macrophages containing acid-fast bacilli, the white pulp appears to be involved by granulomas more consistently (Bernard and Vazquez, 1973). Lymphocytes normally present within the periarteriolar lymphocyte sheaths of the Malpighian corpuscles may be extensively replaced by masses of histiocytes. In the liver, focal granulomata containing acid-fast bacilli are observed most frequently around the portal tracts and scattered within the lobules (Karat *et al.*, 1971). Hypertrophy of the Kupffer cells is common.

5. Inflammatory Response in Leprosy

Studies of the inflammatory response in leprosy patients by the skin window technique indicate that the local exudative cellular response is qualitatively normal throughout the clinical spectrum of leprosy (Bullock *et al.*, 1974b). On the other hand, if quantitative collection chambers are applied to sites of skin abrasion, the number of leukocytes migrating into these chambers from lepromatous patients over a 24-hr period is approximately one-half the number from normal controls and patients with tuberculoid leprosy. Support for the possibility of a nonspecific defect in the expression of inflammatory reactions by lepromatous patients is provided by the fact that sera from these patients often contain high levels of a chemotactic factor inactivator that irreversibly inactivates the leukotactic factors of *Escherichia coli*, as well as the C3a and C5a fragments of complement (Ward *et al.*, 1976). In general, the presence of this factor correlates with skin test anergy to a series of antigens. Thus in active lepromatous disease, as in sarcoidosis (Maderazo *et al.*, 1976) and Hodgkin's disease (Ward and Berenberg, 1974), it is possible that elevated levels of chemotactic factor inactivator may suppress the chemotactic attraction of polymorphonuclear (PMN) and mononuclear leukocytes to sites of acute and chronic inflammatory stimuli.

It has been suggested that an inherited digestive defect of macrophages specific for *M. leprae* might explain the occurrence of disseminated disease in lepromatous leprosy (Barbieri and Correa, 1967). However, recent studies indicate that macrophages from patients with lepromatous and tuberculoid leprosy and from normal donors do not differ in their ability to digest heat-killed *M. leprae in vitro* or in their ability to sustain the viability of *M. leprae* in tissue culture (Godal and Rees, 1970; Drutz *et al.*, 1974). Furthermore, macrophages and PMN cells from lepromatous donors possess normal or supernormal phagocytic and microbicidal activity against a variety of gram-positive and gram-negative organisms, as well as *Candida albicans*; iodination of ingested bacteria by phagocytic leukocytes of lepromatous patients also appears to be qualitatively normal (Drutz *et al.*, 1974). There are no significant differences between lepromatous patients without complications and normals in the capacity of their PMN leukocytes to reduce nitroblue tetrazolium (NBT) dye, a measure of oxidative function in these cells during infectious processes (Goihman-Yahr *et al.*, 1975). Conversely, NBT reduction by peripheral blood mononuclear cells may be markedly increased (Lim *et al.*, 1974). This finding suggests an intense stimulation of metabolic oxidative pathways in blood cells observed to contain bacilli during the chronic bacteremia associated with more than 70% of untreated cases of lepromatous leprosy (Mostert, 1936; Drutz *et al.*, 1972). No abnormalities of lysosomal activity in the macrophages of lepromatous patients have been detected by routine histochemical techniques (Job, 1970); however, detailed studies have not been performed.

Much needed are ultrastructural studies of macrophage behavior with specific reference to the fusion of lysosomes with phagosomes containing *M. leprae*. Certain mycobacterial species are known to interfere with fusion of lysosomes to phagosomes containing viable organisms. Thus lysosomes fail to fuse with phagosomes containing living *M. tuberculosis* and related species but do appear to fuse with phagosomes containing viable *M. lepraemurium* and all species of dead mycobacteria tested to date (Armstrong and Hart, 1971, 1975). If phagosome–lysosome fusion can be demonstrated in monocyte-derived macrophages from normal and lepromatous individuals after ingestion of *M. leprae* judged to be viable, then studies on the susceptibility of *M. leprae* to destruction by lysosomal enzymes

would be of value. Indeed, the elimination of dead *M. leprae* by macrophages in lepromatous patients appears to be accomplished poorly, since approximately 90% of the organisms within infected tissues appear to be nonviable by microscopic techniques. (Rees and Valentine, 1962; Shepard and McRae, 1965; Levy *et al.*, 1969).

M. leprae produces a capsulelike substance of lipid composition that contributes to the extensive intracellular inclusions (globi) seen in the foamy macrophages of lepromatous leprosy (Imaeda, 1965). Some intriguing questions are raised by the persistence of this lipid material *in vivo*, as contrasted with the successful degradation of *M. leprae in vitro* when killed organisms are presented to lepromatous macrophages in a low ratio. It would be of interest to know if these lipids are directly inhibitory to macrophage digestive function or if they act indirectly by inducing humoral or cellular mechanisms of macrophage inhibition, thereby perpetuating the depression of cell mediated immunity (CMI) so characteristic of lepromatous infection.

It is also possible that *M. leprae* may survive in the macrophages of lepromatous patients by escaping from phagocytic vacuoles into the cytoplasm where there are no specifically developed mechanisms for microbial killing. Supportive evidence for this hypothesis is very limited (Evans *et al.*, 1973), although another intracellular pathogen, *Trypanosoma cruzi*, does appear to survive in experimentally infected macrophages by escaping from phagocytic vacuoles into the cytoplasm (Kress *et al.*, 1975). Conversely, the epimastigotes *are* contained and effectively degraded within phagolysosomes of macrophages obtained from donors who have been preimmunized with BCG.

Finally, it is possible that the macrophages of lepromatous patients are unresponsive to lymphokines. That this is not the case for at least one lymphokine, migratory inhibitory factor (MIF), is suggested by a study of Han *et al.* (1974), in which monocyte-derived macrophages from lepromatous and normal donors were exposed to MIF produced by incubating *M. leprae* with lymphocytes from tuberculoid patients. The migration of macrophages from both normal and lepromatous donors was inhibited equally by MIF.

6. Lymphocyte Function in Leprosy

6.1. *M. leprae*—Specific Responses

6.1.1. Cell-Mediated Immunity

Patients with lepromatous leprosy are universally anergic to the antigens of *M. leprae* by skin testing. This is true whether tests are performed with integral lepromin (a heat-killed suspension of *M. leprae* plus tissue components prepared from lepromatous nodules) or with bacillary antigens separated from tissues (Dharmendra preparation). Patients with tuberculoid leprosy respond to both test preparations; to integral lepromin, they respond with transient induration at 48–72 hr (Fernandez reaction) followed by nodule formation, sometimes with ulceration, that peaks at 21–28 days (Mitsuda reaction). The nodule is formed by granulomatous inflammation composed of epithelioid cells, giant cells, and lymphocytes. Conversely, biopsy of the test site in lepromatous patients reveals a minimal reaction in which these cell types are conspicuously absent (Rees, 1964). The Dharmendra preparation evokes erythema and induration at 24–78 hr in the skin of tuberculoid patients but not in lepromatous patients (Dharmendra and Lowe, 1942). Patients with tuberculoid leprosy tend to lose skin reactivity to *M. leprae* if their disease advances toward the lepromatous form. In contrast, it is unusual for lepromatous patients to recover skin reactivity, even though successful therapy may have eradicated *identifiable* acid-fast bacilli from biopsy specimens.

Diminution of the delayed-type hypersensitivity (DTH) response to skin testing with antigens of *M. leprae* in more bacilliferous patients is closely paralleled by *in vitro* tests of lymphocyte response to these antigens. Thus when lymphocytes are tested from donors with TT, BB, and LL leprosy, respectively, the blastogenic responses to *M. leprae* can be shown to diminish progressively with each group tested until background levels are reached in LL leprosy (Myrvang *et al.*, 1973). Furthermore, incubation of *M. leprae* with lymphocytes from lepromatous donors fails to elicit a factor capable of inhibiting the migration of macrophages from normals or lepromatous patients (Han *et al.*, 1974). Similar failure of MIF production by lymphocytes from

lepromatous donors has been reported by Katz *et al.* (1971) and Godal *et al.*, (1972).

6.1.2. Antibodies

Antibodies to *M. leprae* that cross-react with other mycobacteria can be demonstrated in the serum of 75–95% of the lepromatous patients by the passive hemagglutination test, by complement fixation (CT), and by agar gel precipitin tests (Levine, 1951; Almeida, 1962; Navalkar *et al.*, 1964; Myrvang *et al.*, 1974; Harboe *et al.*, 1978). Titers of antibody assayed by these methods decrease slowly during treatment (Ross, 1954; Rees *et al.*, 1965). However, no long-term studies have been performed to determine whether titers are actually reduced to the levels that may be present in healthy controls of similar socioeconomic background. Low titers of antibodies to mycobacteria have been detected in 30–70% of sera from patients with tuberculoid leprosy by passive hemagglutination and CF tests. In polar tuberculoid cases (TT) the frequency of precipitating antibodies is very low (< 10%) (Myrvang *et al.*, 1974). Immunochemical characterization of the antimycobacterial antibodies has not been performed.

6.2. Nonspecific Responses

6.2.1. Cell-Mediated Immunity

In addition to having profound and specific anergy to *M. leprae*, many patients with lepromatous leprosy also have a generalized, nonspecific impairment of CMI. *In vivo*, this deficiency is manifested by depression of DTH responses to skin tests with microbial antigens (Guinto and Mabalay, 1962; Buck and Hasenclever, 1963; Bullock, 1968) and by impaired responses to sensitizing haptens (Waldorf *et al.*, 1966; Bullock, 1968; Turk and Waters, 1969). Significant prolongation of skin homograft survival and diminished lymphocyte transfer reactions in these patients also have been reported (Han *et al.*, 1971a,b).

In vitro studies of lymphocytes from lepromatous patients have demonstrated poor blastogenic responses to phytohemagglutinin (PHA) (Dierks and Shepard, 1968; Bullock and Fasal, 1971; Mehra *et al.*, 1972; Lim *et al.*, 1975) and to the antigens of purified protein derivative (PPD) (Bullock and Fasal, 1971; Myrvang *et al.*, 1973), bacillus Calmette-Guérin (BCG) (Godal *et al.*, 1972; Myrvang *et al.*, 1973), and *Streptococcus* (Sheagren *et al.*, 1969; Bullock and Fasal, 1971), respectively. In one study of the two-way MLC reaction between pairs of lepromatous patients, the blastogenic response did not differ significantly from the mean response in MLC between lymphocytes from tuberculoid patients; however, control studies of MLC reactions between normal lymphocyte donors were not performed (Godal *et al.*, 1971).

The normal ratio of T : B lymphocytes in peripheral blood may be altered severely among patients with lepromatous leprosy. T lymphocytes or subpopulations thereof, measured by nonspecific rosette formation with sheep red blood cells, may be sharply reduced from normal levels in both percentage and absolute count (Dwyer *et al.*, 1973; Lim *et al.*, 1974; Nath *et al.*, 1974; Mendes *et al.*, 1974). Conversely, B-cell numbers may be elevated as counted in autoradiographs after exposure of lymphocytes to radiolabeled anti-human IgM serum (Dwyer *et al.*, 1973) or as enumerated by surface labeling with fluoresceinated antiserum to human immunoglobulins (Gajl-Peczalska *et al.*, 1973; Mendes *et al.*, 1974). The population of B lymphocytes bearing complement receptor sites (EAC rosette-forming cells) has been quantitated by two groups. Both found the absolute numbers of these cells to be below normal in lepromatous patients (Mendes *et al.*, 1974; Sher *et al.*, 1976). In one study blood levels of EAC-binding lymphocytes returned to normal after patients had received more than 6 months of therapy (Sher *et al.*, 1976). These findings suggest that C3 receptor sites on the surfaces of lymphocytes from some lepromatous patients may be blocked by circulating immune complexes that are complement binding. Further studies attempting to elute complexes from lymphocytes are needed. In most cases of tuberculoid leprosy the blood levels of T and B cells have been normal.

Several points are worth emphasizing regarding the nonspecific depression of CMI observed in lepromatous leprosy:

1. The nonspecific impairment of CMI is not restricted to lepromatous leprosy; it has been well documented in tuberculoid leprosy (BT type), although the depression generally is less severe and can be detected less consistently (Guinto and Mabalay, 1962; Buck and Hasenclever, 1963; Bullock, 1968).

2. The nonspecific depression is less severe than the specific impairment of CMI to *M. leprae*. Current information suggests that the nonspecific depression of CMI is of approximately the same magnitude as observed in active sarcoidosis but less severe than that associated with Hodgkin's disease. In neither sarcoidosis nor leprosy does the nonspecific depression appear to be severe enough to block the DTH response to PPD in patients who have or recently have had active tuberculosis (Godal *et al.*, 1971).

3. Several investigators have found that effective antimicrobial therapy can reverse the nonspecific component of anergy in leprosy (Bullock, 1968; Sheagren *et al.*, 1969; Lim *et al.*, 1975; Nath *et al.*, 1977). Abnormalities of T : B cell ratios also appear to be corrected by therapy (Lim *et al.*, 1974b; Nath *et al.*, 1974; Sher *et al.*, 1976).

4. Some studies indicate that there is less nonspecific depression of CMI among lepromatous patients who experience concomitant erythema nodosum leprosum (ENL) (Waldorf *et al.*, 1966; Sheagren *et al.*, 1969; Lim *et al.*, 1975).

5. The nonspecific component of anergy apparently does not predispose to secondary infection by other pathogens that challenge the cell-mediated immune defenses. A very high prevalence of active tuberculosis has been reported in lepromatous patients at autopsy (Mitsuda and Ogawa, 1937; Desikan and Job, 1968), but uncontrolled epidemiological factors could explain these findings. Of interest is one report of five volunteers with lepromatous leprosy who submitted themselves to intracutaneous inoculation with 1.45×10^7 viable *Leishmania braziliensis* organisms (Convit *et al.*, 1971). Serial biopsies of the inoculation sites revealed that all five responded with granuloma formation of a tuberculoid type in which leishmanial forms could not be detected 4 months after inoculation. Studies of the mortality experience in leprosy are lim-

ited, but the available evidence does not point to an increased frequency of malignancy (Oleinick, 1969; Purtilo and Pangi, 1975).

Although current evidence is against a marked increase in susceptibility to secondary infection in leprosy, a number of clinical reports have kept open the question. A high prevalence of necrosis and retarded resolution at the sites of smallpox vaccination have been observed (Denney, 1922; Ramanujam and Ramu, 1966; Saha et al., 1973). Several investigators have detected a significantly higher prevalence of hepatitis B surface antigenemia among lepromatous patients than among tuberculoid patients or normal controls of similar socioethnic background (Blumberg et al., 1970; Francis and Smith, 1972; Dutta and Saha, 1973). Few of these studies were controlled for the fact that lepromatous cases are more often confined to institutions. Hence it is unresolved whether the higher prevalence of hepatitis B surface antigenemia among lepromatous patients is indeed secondary to the nonspecific depression of CMI. The issue of host defense against chronic viral infections is further complicated by the fact that Papageorgiou et al. (1973) detected high titers of Epstein–Barr virus in a group of lepromatous patients. The high titers may have resulted from an impaired ability to restrict replication of a latent virus. However, nonspecific enhancement of B-cell function with antibody responses disproportionate to the antigenic stimulus is also a distinct possibility in these patients, as suggested later in this section and in Section 7.4.

6. The sera of lepromatous patients often contain factor(s) that nonspecifically depress the lymphoblastic response *in vitro*. These factor(s) can depress PHA and antigen-induced transformation of lymphocytes from normal controls and leprosy patients (Bullock and Fasal, 1971; Nelson *et al.*, 1971; Mehra *et al.*, 1972; Fliess *et al.*, 1975). In addition, sera from untreated patients may severely depress the MLC reaction between cell populations

from normal donors (Nelson *et al.*, 1975). The factors have not been characterized, but preliminary work has shown that those capable of depressing blastogenic responses to antigens are heat stable, nondialyzable, and present in serum at low concentrations (Bullock and Fasal, 1971) see Section 7.4.3 for discussion of C-reactive protein and its putative immunosuppressor activity).

7. The severity of nonspecific immune depression may vary considerably within the population of lepromatous patients. Among the variables that may modulate the degree of depression are race, sex, duration of disease, nutritional status, the presence of ENL, depressor factors in serum, and duration of therapy. Consequently, it is not unexpected that two groups of investigators have been unable to detect nonspecific suppression of CMI among these patients (Convit *et al.*, 1971; Rea *et al.*, 1976a). In the latter study the patients were quite young and presented with a short disease history. Most did not have polar (LL) lepromatous leprosy by histological criteria, and 80% were experiencing ENL at the time of testing (see item 4).

6.2.2. Alterations in Immunoglobulin Levels

Hypergammaglobulinema is characteristic of lepromatous leprosy. Bullock *et al.* (1970) quantitated the levels of IgG, IgA, and IgM classes in sera from 158 lepromatous and 35 tuberculoid patients and compared them with controls of similar racial and sociogeographic background. Mean levels of IgG, IgA, and IgM all were significantly elevated in lepromatous sera, as compared with controls, whereas the serum levels in tuberculoid patients did not differ from normal. Linear regression equations relating levels of Ig classes to length of therapy with DDS revealed that IgG and IgA levels did not decline significantly in association with prolonged therapy over several months or years. However, there was a significant negative correlation between IgM levels and treatment; that is, IgM levels decreased as duration of therapy increased. Other workers have reported variable increases in the IgG, IgA, and IgM classes in lepromatous leprosy, but hyperglobulinema is uncommon in tuberculoid leprosy (Lim and Fusaro, 1968; Jha *et al.*, 1971). There is little information on IgD levels in leprosy; in most reports of IgE levels it has been difficult to exclude the presence of parasites.

7. Immunopathological Correlates of Disease Activity

The pathogenesis of primary leprosy and its subsequent evolution to a form that is clinically recognizable or histologically classifiable is poorly understood. The granulomas of leprosy rarely caseate unless they are within a confined space, such as the neural sheath, and healing proceeds without dense scar formation or subsequent calcification (Enna and Brand, 1970). Thus no stigmata equivalent to the calcified scars of a healed Ghon complex remain to mark the site of "primary" infection in leprosy. Whether truly primary or not, the earliest lesions that can be recognized as leprosy appear in the skin. The histopathology is essentially "indeterminant," i.e., characterized by nonspecific inflammation and a rare acid-fast bacillus within small dermal nerves or, less commonly, in the subepidermal zone and arrectores pilorum muscles (Büngeler, 1943; Ridley, 1972). Histological classification of a leprous lesion is not possible until granuloma formation has progressed over a period of weeks or months. Thereafter, the cellular infiltrate may be of tuberculoid type involving nerves or the subepidermal zone. More suggestive of lepromatous pathology, however, are infiltrates situated in a perineural or perivascular location that contain foamy macrophages and many bacilli. Clear evidence for a perivascular distribution of lesions can be found quite early in many cases. Given the perivascular distribution of lesions and the proclivity of *M. leprae* to invade vascular channels (Fite, 1941), it seems probable that bacteremia is a feature of many primary leprosy infections, as it is in tuberculosis (Rich, 1951). The course of leprosy subsequent to the putative bacteremia may then be characterized by a tendency toward self-healing as in tuberculoid leprosy or by progression to lepromatous forms.

7.1. Reversal Reactions

The histopathology of polar tuberculoid (TT) or lepromatous leprosy (LL) is relatively stable, with little tendency for "downgrading" (deterioration) of the CMI response in the former or for "upgrading" in the latter. In borderline cases, however, marked changes may occur in the cellular composition of granulomatous infiltrates that can be of considerable clinical importance. Most notable is an acute inflammatory reaction within the dermis, the so-called reversal reaction (Tajiri, 1955; Ridley, 1969). This reaction is observed in 10–15% of patients with borderline lepromatous leprosy (BL) after the bacterial load has been reduced by treatment for several months. Occasionally, "reversal" reactions occur spontaneously without treatment (Fernandez *et al.*, 1962). Clinically, leprous infiltrates within the dermis become quite erythematous and indurated. Histologically, there is edema within reactional sites plus an influx of lymphocytes, epithelioid cells, and giant cells, whereas the number of bacilli is reduced relative to surrounding areas. Reversal reactions persist for several weeks or months, and the lepromin reaction frequently converts to positive, although it may revert to negative at a later date. Among untreated or drug-resistant patients, deterioration of CMI may be signaled by a "downgrading" type of inflammatory reaction, in which the numbers of lymphocytes within granulomas actually decrease concomitantly with an increase in bacilli.

Reversal reactions may signal improvement in the patient's immunological status but, unfortunately, the neurological consequences of "immunological improvement" may be severe. Peripheral nerves are consistently involved in all forms of leprosy, most probably via the endoneurial blood vessels. Schwann cells are selectively colonized by *M. leprae*, and as bacilli proliferate within these cells, the latter degenerate with release of mycobacterial antigens (Weddell *et al.*, 1964). In tuberculoid patients with relatively high resistance to *M. leprae*, the nerve is invaded by mononuclear inflammatory cells that infiltrate the interfascicular spaces, the perineurium, and the nerve bundles. The intense granulomatous response with epithelioid cell formation leads to focal demyelination, axonal degeneration, and ultimate fibrosis (Dastur *et al.*, 1970; Pearson and Ross, 1975).

In lepromatous cases there is extensive proliferation of bacilli within Schwann cells and perineurial cells. Infiltration of the epineurium and perineurium by macrophages but not by lymphocytes or epithelioid cells leads to progressive increase in fibrous connective tissue with adhesion formation between the endoneurium and perineurium (Job, 1971). Because CMI in lepromatous leprosy is deficient, structural and functional preservation of nerves is much greater than in tuberculoid disease. Axonal destruction does occur in lepromatous leprosy but it proceeds more slowly, primarily as a result of irreversible damage to Schwann cells by *M. leprae*. During a reversal reaction there is increased edema within the rather rigid inflammatory tissue surrounding nerve fascicles. As a result, surviving strands of Schwann cells are liable to sudden compression with rapid loss of nerve function. Furthermore, the augmented mononuclear cell response within nerves contributes to destruction of Schwann cells and their axons. Presumably, the neurological damage incurred during a reversal reaction arises nonspecifically as the consequence of a CMI reaction, from either mediators produced by sensitized lymphocytes or activated macrophages influenced by lymphocytes (Wisniewski and Bloom, 1975).

7.2. Erythema Nodosum Leprosum (ENL)

ENL is a common and often serious reactional syndrome that is encountered almost exclusively in lepromatous leprosy. Although it is not uncommon for untreated patients to present with ENL, there has been an unequivocal increase in the prevalence of ENL during the era of effective antileprosy therapy inaugurated by introduction of the sulfones in 1948 (Petit and Waters, 1967). ENL is usually of sudden onset over 24–48 hr, and, unlike the erythema nodosum associated with other conditions, nodules are not confined to the lower extremities. Instead they are widely distributed especially on the face, trunk, and upper extremities. Nodules may proceed to frank

suppuration requiring several weeks to heal, usually without scarring. Occasionally, ENL may be chronic, lasting for several months. A variant form of ENL-like reaction (the Lucio phenomenon) occurs most frequently among Latin Americans with diffuse lepromatous leprosy (Moschella, 1967). This form presents as crops of small macules that undergo necrosis often with antecedent hemorrhagic blistering. The eschar heals with scar formation.

Histopathological changes of ENL are most pronounced in the dermis. In early nodules, large collections of PMN leukocytes infiltrate the lepromatous granulomas, and frequently there is panniculitis (Mabalay *et al.*, 1965). A proliferative vasculitis may involve both arteries and veins in which the entire wall is invaded by PMN cells and eosinophils. The vascular lumina may be obliterated by endarteritis or endophlebitis, and occasionally there is frank necrosis of the vessel wall (Job *et al.*, 1964). In healing lesions the PMN cell infiltrate is replaced by lymphocytes, plasma cells, histiocytes, and scar formation. Typically, ENL triggered by sulfones does not appear until the third or fourth month of therapy, at which time the numbers of viable *M. leprae* within ENL reactions are reduced. Diaminodiphenylsulfone (DDS) itself does not possess ENL-stimulating activity, and both the frequency and severity of ENL decline as the bacterial load is reduced through years of therapy (Waters and Helmy, 1974).

Histologically, ENL lesions closely resemble Arthus-type reactions. Consequently, it is widely held that ENL is triggered by lysis of *M. leprae* secondary to drug treatment or spontaneous changes in host CMI. The release of antigens that diffuse into dermal blood vessels might then lead to local antigen–antibody complex formation and subsequent inflammatory reactions. Despite its appeal, this hypothesis has been difficult to substantiate. In fact, only one group has succeeded in demonstrating deposits of immunoglobulin (Ig), complement, and antigen in the lesions of ENL by immunofluorescence microscopy (Wemambu *et al.*, 1969). The difficulty in detecting components of antigen–antibody complexes within tissues may stem from the fact that many of the lesions biopsied for examination are too mature for successful detection of immunoreactive material. Indeed, it is known that both the triggering antigen (Cochrane *et al.*, 1959) and the Ig-complement components of complexes are lost from the site of an experimentally induced Arthus reaction within several hours (Cream *et al.*, 1971). Therefore, an intensive search for complex deposition in very early lesions of ENL may prove more successful. In addition, specialized techniques, such as histamine-induced wheal formation, may yield fluid specimens that contain crystalloid or amorphous deposits suggestive of immune complexes by electron microscopic examination (Braverman and Yen, 1975).

7.3. Complications Attributed to Circulating Immune Complexes

Severe ENL is frequently associated with distressing constitutional disturbances. Among these are pyrexia, acute iridocyclitis (Choyce, 1964), neuritis, orchitis, lymphadenitis (Karat *et al.*, 1968), and polyarthritis (Karat *et al.*, 1967). Although *M. leprae* does not invade the renal parenchyma, many reports have stressed the high prevalence of glomerulonephritis among patients with ENL (Drutz and Gutman, 1973; Johny *et al.*, 1975). The most frequent pathological findings described by light microscopy are acute proliferative glomerulonephritis and focal mesangial hypercellularity with thickening of the glomerular capillary loops. Using immunofluorescence microscopy, two groups have detected diffuse discontinuous linear deposits of IgG, IgM, and C3 along the walls of glomerular capillary membranes of patients with leprosy-associated nephritis (Tin Shwe, 1972b; Iveson *et al.*, 1975). In some cases, immunofluorescent studies have been negative; however, electron microscopy revealed considerable regional thickening of basement membranes with foci of rarefaction, or reduplication. In addition, there were subendothelial or subepithelial deposits of electron-dense material (Bullock *et al.*, 1974a; Date *et al.*, 1977).

It is reasonable to presume that many of the clinical disorders associated with ENL are secondary to the phlogistic effects of circulating antigen–antibody complex deposition in tissues. However, much remains to be done to clarify the role of putative circulating complexes in the clinical pathology of leprosy.

Total serum hemolytic complement activity (CH_{50}) and individual components of complement are normal in uncomplicated leprosy (Saitz *et al.*, 1968; Tin Shwe and Petty, 1971; Petchclai *et al.*, 1973). In patients with ENL, most workers have found complement levels to be markedly elevated and only rarely has hypocomplementemia been observed (Saitz *et al.*, 1968; Sheagren *et al.*, 1969; Gelber *et al.*, 1974).

One method for detection of circulating immune complexes relies on the reaction of these complexes with the C1q component of complement to form a precipitate in an agarose gell diffusion assay (Agnello *et al.*, 1970). By this method C1q-precipitating substances have been detected in the sera of patients with leprosy, and among those with ENL the incidence of positive reactions exceeds 50% (Moran *et al.*, 1972; Rojas-Espinosa *et al.*, 1972; Gelber *et al.*, 1974). Nevertheless, it has not been established that these C1q-precipitating substances are actually leprosy-related antigen–antibody complexes. For example, the sera of patients with the extensive inflammatory reactions of ENL may contain small amounts of DNA that will readily precipitate C1q in the assay. Furthermore, C1q will precipitate with aggregated γ-globulin, mycobacterial antigens, and bacterial endotoxins. Additional studies therefore are needed in which leprosy sera are screened for endotoxin activity, freed of possible γ-globulin aggregates by ultracentrifugation, and pretreated with DNase to reduce the frequency of false-positive reactions (Agnello *et al.*, 1970).

Recently, the C1q deviation test, a more sensitive variation of the C1q-precipitin assay (Sobel *et al.*, 1975) and the Raji cell assay (Theofilopoulos *et al.*, 1976), have been developed to detect circulating immune complexes. The Raji cell assay detects complexes of immunoglobulin plus complement by allowing the C3b and C3d fragments of complement already fixed to antigen–antibody complexes to react with receptors for complement on the surfaces of cells from a human lymphoblastoid line of B cells. Thus the Raji cell test appears to be more specific for detection of immune complexes, particularly those formed by antibody of the IgM class. Using both assays, Tung *et al.* (1977) obtained a positive C1q deviation test in 30 of 46 (67%) patients with leprosy; only two of the 30 sera (7%) were also positive by the Raji cell test. Furthermore, no complexes were detected by Raji cell assay in the sera of 14 patients with ENL that had tested positive by the C1q assay. It should be noted that actual fixation of complement by circulating immune complexes is a prerequisite for their detection by Raji cells. Therefore, small complexes that fix complement less well may be underestimated by this assay (Theofilopoulos et al., 1976), whereas C1q tests may overestimate complexes for the reasons cited above. In any event, these preliminary studies suggest that the C1q-reactive material in the serum of leprosy patients may not be antigen–antibody complexes in some cases.

In some lepromatous patients, with or without ENL, deposits of IgM localized to the dermal–epidermal basement membrane have been demonstrated by direct immunofluorescence microscopy. The immunofluorescent banding appears as a continuous linear staining pattern of the basement membrane that is finely granular at high magnification (Bullock et al., 1974a). It is morphologically indistinguishable from the banding observed in the skin of patients with systemic lupus erythematosus (SLE), and ignorance of this fact has lead to serious diagnostic errors. Unlike in SLE, however, basement membrane deposits of other Ig classes and of C3 have been detected infrequently in leprosy. Preliminary attempts to elute anti-basement membrane antibody from skin biopsies have been unsuccessful (Quismorio et al., 1975). At present, the significance of these Ig collections is unknown. They may simply be nonspecific deposits of IgM; alternatively, they may be autoantibodies to basement membrane or antibodies to mycobacterial glycoproteins that cross-react with components of the basement membrane. It is also possible that the basement membrane of skin may act as a trap for IgM-containing antigen–antibody complexes that diffuse upward from antigen-containing infiltrates deeper within the dermis.

7.4. Serological Disturbances

7.4.1. Biological False-Positive Reactions

The reported prevalence of biological false-positive (BFP) reactions in serological tests for syphilis is high among patients with lepromatous leprosy, ranging from approximately 8% to more than 65% (Nelson, 1952; Garner et al., 1969). In fact, the frequency with which BFP reactions are observed in agglutination and flocculation tests employing cardiolipin-type antigens is related to the lecithin content of cardiolipin. As the relative concentration of lecithin in cardiolipin is increased, the percentage and intensity of BFP reactions decrease in sera from leprosy patients, whereas the intensity of reactions in syphilitic sera is increased (Kent et al., 1957; Almeida, 1962). Efforts to eliminate BFP reactions in the sera of leprosy patients have been unsuccessful, and confirmatory treponemal tests are essential. Of these, the fluorescent treponemal antibody adsorption test (FTA-ADS) and the Treponema pallidum immobilization test (TPI) have proved most useful, although the latter is technically more difficult. The results obtained by these two techniques generally are in close agreement, with the prevalence of serological reactivity among lepromatous patients ranging from 5% to 15% (Cannefax et al., 1959; Scotti et al., 1970). The latter figure is unusually high and suggests that even in "specific" treponemal tests BFP reactions do occur in leprosy. In fact, Ruge (1967) selected 16 untreated leprosy patients whose sera were TPI test positive and demonstrated a progressive decline in titer over a 2-year period, during which time the patients received antileprosy therapy but no antitreponemal therapy. It is also possible that sera from some lepromatous patients can induce discontinuous treponemal fluorescence in the FTA-ADS test of the type occasionally observed in tests of sera from patients with SLE. These false-positive tests are caused by antibodies reactive to DNA in the treponemal nuclei (Kraus et al., 1971). Thus, in difficult cases, preadsorption of leprous serum with DNA or pretreatment of the Treponema substrate with DNase may be indicated (Wright, 1973).

7.4.2. Autoantibodies

Additional serological abnormalities that may be detected in patients with lepromatous leprosy include rheumatoid factor (RF) activity, cryoproteinemia, elevated titers of antistreptolysin O(ASO) activity, thyroglobulin antibodies, antinuclear factors, and antibodies to testicular germinal cells (Wall and Wright, 1974).

Most, but not all, investigators have reported elevated serum titers of RF among lepromatous patients (Rea *et al.*, 1976a). The highest reported prevalence of seropositivity by latex fixation testing is 58% (Cathcart *et al.*, 1961). The antiglobulin activity of RF positive sera is present chiefly in the 19 S macroglobulin fraction; however, low molecular weight (7 S) RF has been detected by chromatographic and density gradient preparative techniques (Bonomo and Dammacco, 1971).

Cryoglobulinemia is present in more than 30% of patients with lepromatous leprosy (Matthews and Trautman, 1965). Usually the cryoglobulins are a mixed polyclonal type composed of IgG and IgM, respectively. In most instances the IgM component exhibits anti-IgG activity (Bonomo and Dammacco, 1971). Elevation of the ASO titer has been observed in many lepromatous patients and has been attributed either to a high frequency of streptococcal infections or to general "hyperactivity" of the antibody-mediated immune system (Abe *et al.*, 1967; Tin Shwe, 1972a). Actually, the elevated ASO titer in some leprous sera is specious and is caused by a nonspecific inhibitor of ASO activity that is bound to serum β-lipoproteins. The "false" elevation of ASO titer can be reduced in many cases by precipitating the nonspecific inhibitor of ASO activity with dextran sulfate (W. E. Bullock, unpublished observations; Baylet *et al.*, 1973). On occasion, this simple technique may be of value in establishing more precisely the etiology of glomerulonephritis in patients with ENL.

Low titers of thyroglobulin antibodies have been detected in the sera of up to 48% of lepromatous patients (Bonoma *et al.*, 1963). In most cases antibodies are of the 19 S macroglobulin class (Bonomo and Dammacco, 1967), in contrast to the typical 7 S character of thyroglobulin antibodies in patients with Hashimoto's thyroiditis. Bonomo *et al.* (1965) also detected antinuclear factor in 16 of 55 lepromatous sera by means of a fluorescent antibody test; lupus cell preparations were positive in four of ten patients whose sera were positive for antinuclear factor. Azoury and

Gum (1967) detected antinuclear factor in sera from two of ten patients. The pattern of nuclear staining was homogeneous (associated with antibodies to nuclear protein), and both patients were affected by multiple joint swellings or polyarthralgias. In neither report was the possibility excluded of a drug-induced lupus syndrome, a matter of potential importance because of the structural similarity of DDS to drugs (procainamide and sulfonamides) that may induce the clinical and laboratory abnormalities of SLE.

7.4.3. C-Reactive Protein

Elevation of serum orosomucoid, an acid glycoprotein, has been reported in up to 63% of lepromatous cases (Ross, 1960). Likewise, serum levels of C-reactive protein (CRP) may be very high, especially in patients with ENL (Bush, 1958). Of interest is the fact that CRP, a γ-migrating protein, is known to bind to human T lymphocytes. Associated with this binding there is a reduction in the capacity of T cells to respond to allogeneic cells in MLC; T-cell responses to antigen stimulation and the production of lymphokines are also impaired (Mortensen *et al.*, 1977). Hokama *et al.* (1974) have suppressed lymphocyte responses to PHA by adding high concentrations of CRP to cultures. However, Mortensen *et al.* (1975) have been unable to suppress the response of T lymphocytes to PHA by high concentrations of CRP. Although the studies with PHA are contradictory, the recent evidence for immunosuppressive activity by CRP suggests that it may have an immunoregulatory function and that the elevated levels in lepromatous patients may contribute to the suppression of CMI.

7.4.4. Amyloid-Related Factors

Lepromatous leprosy may be complicated by secondary amyloidosis, although the prevalence thereof may vary considerably in different locales. Gingival biopsies were positive for amyloid in 31% of patients hospitalized at one hospital in the United States (Williams *et al.*, 1965). Among natives of New Guinea, amyloid was present in rectal biopsies from 14 of 86 (16%) lepromatous patients (McAdam *et al.*, 1975). The prevalence of amyloid among patients in South India may be lower, as suggested by one study in which gingival biopsies were positive in only two of 79 (2.5%) patients (Satyanarayana et al., 1972). Amyloidosis is rare in patients with tuberculoid leprosy; those cases in which amyloid has been documented are frequently complicated by chronic neurotrophic ulcers that could predispose to amyloid deposition.

Elevated levels of a nonimmunoglobulin, amyloid-related serum protein component (ARSC), have been detected in lepromatous sera; this protein is antigenically related to the fibrillar protein found in tissue deposits of secondary amyloid (Levin et al., 1973). Levels of ARSC are elevated in 29–64% of patients with lepromatous infections but only in 12–14% of patients with tuberculoid leprosy (Kronvall et al., 1975; McAdam et al., 1975). The concentration of ARSC may rise to very high levels during the acute inflammatory response of ENL before declining over a period of several days or weeks. Of note is the fact that ARSC is not elevated in all leprosy patients with proved amyloidosis. These observations suggest that leprosy may be a valuable model for studying the metabolism of ARSC and the relationship of fluctuating levels to amyloid deposition. It would also be of interest to study the capacity of antiinflammatory drugs such as colchicine, thalidomide, and sterioids to inhibit rises in ARSC during episodes of ENL and their effectiveness in preventing the ultimate development of amyloidosis.

8. Immunotherapy

The introduction of DDS as a cheap and effective drug for treatment of leprosy has done much to dispel the therapeutic gloom that prevailed prior to 1948. Unfortunately, relapse rates are high, ranging from 1% to 6% per year, even among patients whose skin biopsies have become negative for recognizable bacilli after years of therapy (Noordeen, 1971). In some cases viable drug-sensitive bacilli have been recovered by inoculation of immunodepressed mice with biopsy material from patients treated with DDS for as long as 10 years (Waters et al., 1974). Furthermore, the prevalence of proved resistance to DDS by M. leprae has been increasing; a recent estimate Malaysia indicates that at least 2.2% of lepromatous

patients treated with DDS habor organisms resistant to this drug (Pearson et al., 1975). Rifampin has excellent bactericidal activity against M. leprae and may provide an improved therapeutic regimen in combination with DDS (U.S. Leprosy Panel, 1975). Unfortunately, there is already disturbing information that drug-sensitive M. leprae organisms capable of multiplying in mice have been recovered from patients treated for 2–5 years with combination therapy including daily rifampin (Rees, 1975).

Since the fundamental problem in lepromatous leprosy is failure of the CMI response against M. leprae, correction of this deficiency has been attempted by several methods. Efforts to induce positive skin test reactivity to lepromin by administering BCG vaccine to lepromatous patients have succeeded in approximately 50% of cases (Schujman, 1956). The histological appearance is reported to differ between lepromin tests performed before and after BCG vaccination; after BCG there is frequently an increase in lymphocyte infiltration at the lepromin test site, often in association with giant cell formation (Kuper, 1958). Regretably, skin reactivity to lepromin does not persist and reverts to negative in less than 6 months. Intensive immunotherapy with repeated BCG stimulation is worthy of further investigation and conceivably could prove to be of value, especially as an adjunct to antibiotic therapy (Convit et al., 1974). It should be mentioned at this point that the immunoprophylactic use of BCG vaccination for protection of children exposed to leprosy in the home has met with variable success. In Uganda, where the predominant form of leprosy is tuberculoid, BCG vaccination appears to afford a highly significant degree of protection, as compared with results in a control population (Brown et al., 1968). However, in Burma, where the incidence of lepromatous leprosy is higher, the degree of protection afforded by BCG is not significant (Bechelli et al., 1974).

The discovery of transfer factor (TF) by Lawrence et al. (1963), and demonstration that it is an initiator of DTH, has spurred efforts to benefit the lepromatous patient by injections of TF or injection of homologous lymphocytes. Paradisi et al. (1969) reported successful transfer of DTH to antigens of M. leprae in four of 12 lepromatous patients given

1.8 × 10⁶ blood leukocytes from lepromin positive donors. Subsequently, Bullock *et al.* (1972) observed conversion from anergy to weak skin positivity to *M. leprae* in six of nine patients given 4.1 × 10⁸ lymphocytes or TF from equivalent cell numbers donated by individuals reactive to *M. leprae*. In six patients the positive skin reactions were induced at test sites remote from the injection of TF or cells. In a seventh patient a positive test reaction was induced only locally at the TF injection site. No long-term clinical benefit resulted from the TF or cell injections. Nevertheless, five patients experienced significant inflammatory changes within their skin lesions that were characterized by increased erythema and induration. In two of three patients in whom skin biopsies were obtained before and after administration of TF there was an influx of lymphocytes in the post TF specimen. These "flare" reactions were of short duration (7–12 days). Nevertheless, they were very similar to the more chronic reversal reactions that may arise spontaneously after prolonged antibiotic therapy and regarded by some clinicians as a harbinger of clinical improvement.

Silva *et al.* (1973) failed to transfer sensitivity to *M. leprae* with TF or RNA from lyphocytes of skin-test-positive donors, although reactivity to other antigens was transferred successfully in some cases. Conversely, Mendes *et al.* (1974a) were successful in transferring lepromin sensitivity to three of eight lepromatous patients. More recently, Hastings *et al.* (1976) have employed multiple doses of TF given three times weekly for 12 weeks (one dose equivalent of 2 × 10⁸ lymphocytes). Each patient developed the "flare" reactions described by Bullock *et al.* (1972). These reactions persisted throughout the course of TF therapy and waned after treatment was discontinued. Biopsies of the reactional skin areas revealed an influx of lymphocytes within the granulomas, and during TF therapy the rate of fall in the bacterial index was accelerated (Hastings and Job, 1978). Unfortunately, the accelerated decline in the bacterial index was not maintained after discontinuing TF, and TF did not significantly decrease the percentage of dermis involved by granulomas. While intriguing, these findings are too limited to permit meaningful judgment as to the possible value of TF in leprosy. On the other hand,

they do provide strong impetus for the conduct of well-controlled, double-blind studies on the value of TF in leprosy and other serious intracellular infections as, for example, coccidiodomycosis.

Recently, massive numbers of allogeneic cells (2 × 10¹⁰) have been given to patients with lepromatous leprosy in an effort to increase their CMI response to *M. leprae* (Lim *et al.*, 1972). Theoretically, such a large number of cells might exert a salutary effect either by release of TF in considerable amounts or by stimulation of host T-cell macrophage function, as a consequence of a graft-vs.-host reaction known as the "allogeneic effect" (Katz, 1972). It has been reported that such therapy will result in rapid destruction of bacilli, partial healing of lesions, and restitution of lymphocytes to the thymus-dependent areas of lymph nodes—all within a period of several weeks (Lim *et al.*, 1972). As attractive as this unconfirmed claim of dramatic reversal in the clinical course of lepromatous leprosy may be, the administration of massive allogeneic cell infusions to leprosy patients is fraught with serious ethical and practical considerations. Unlike TF therapy, massive infusions of leukocytes from several different donors is likely to result in transmission of type B hepatitis to some cases despite screening of donors for HB$_s$ antigenemia. The risk of infecting lepromatous patients with type B hepatitis virus or others such as cytomegalovirus is of special concern in view of the nonspecific depression of CMI often associated with lepromatous disease. In addition, there is a risk of inducing harmful graft-vs.-host reactions in lepromatous patients by massive allogeneic cell infusion. Although Lim *et al.* (1972) did not report such reactions among their patients, it is mandatory that the therapeutic use of allogeneic cells in large numbers be approached with great caution.

It is clear that immunological responses can be suppressed or even abrogated by both lymphocytes and macophages in a number of experimental models and in clinical disease (Waldman and Broder, 1977). For example, potent suppressor cell activity has been demonstrated in mice experimentally infected with *Mycobacterium lepraemurium* (Bullock *et al.*, 1978). These studies suggest that similar augmentation of suppressor cell activity may exist in patients with lepromatous leprosy. Whether significant suppressor cell activity actually is present and whether it may be responsible in part for the poor cell-mediated immune response to *M. leprae* remains to be determined.

A major objective of WHO is to increase the effectiveness of leprosy control by development of a vaccine. Hope that pilot vaccine field trials can be conducted in the near future has been engendered by increased supplies of *M. leprae* from infected armadillos and by improved methods of purifying bacilli free from armadillo tissue. *M. leprae* purified from armadillo tissues can induce high levels of DTH in guinea pigs in the absence of oil adjuvants and without inducing sensitization to armadillo tissues (Mehra and Bloom, 1979). Positive skin reactions to sonicates of *M. leprae* can be elicited as long as one year after sensitization. Several groups are studying the effect of different procedures for purifying *M. leprae* on the capacity of the antigen preparations to induce skin sensitivity and lymphocyte transformation to *M. leprae*.

ACKNOWLEDGMENTS

The author expresses appreciation to Mrs. Jill Van Veen and Ms. Sandra Page for excellent typing assistance. This work was supported by NIH Grant AI-10094 of the U.S. Public Research Service.

References

Abe, M., 1970, Studies on the antigenic specificity of *Mycobacterium leprae*. I. Demonstration of soluble antigens in leprosy nodules by immunodiffusion, *Int. J. Lepr.* 38:113–125.

Abe, M., Chinone, S., and Hirako, T., 1967, Rheumatoid-factor-like substance and antistreptolysin O antibody in leprosy serum: Significance in erythema nodosum leprosum, *Int. J. Lepr.* 35:336–344.

Agnello, V., Winchester, R. J., and Kunkel, H. G., 1970, Precipitin reactions of the C1q component of complement with aggregated γ-globulin and immune complexes in gel diffusion, *Immunology* 19:909–919.

Almeida, J. O., 1962, Serological studies on leprosy: A comparison of complement-fixation tests using antigens prepared from tubercle bacilli and beef-heart lipids with other serological reactions, *Bull. WHO* 26:233–240.

Armstrong, J. A., and Hart, P. D., 1971, Response of cultured macrophages *Mycobacterium tuberculosis*, with observations on fusion of lysosomes with phagosomes, *J. Exp. Med.* 134:713–740.

Armstrong, J. A., and Hart, P. D., 1975, Phagosome-lysosome interactions in cultured macrophages infected with virulent tubercle bacilli, *J. Exp. Med.* 142:1–16.

Azoury, F. J., and Gum, O. B., 1967, Antinuclear factors in nephrotic syndrome secondary to systemic lupus erythematosus and in leprosy, *Am. J. Med. Sci.* 253:661–666.

Barbieri, T. A., and Correa, W. M., 1967, Human macrophage culture: The leprosy prognostic test (LPT) *Int. J. Lepr.* 35:377–381.

Baylet, R., Gouatter, P., and Yven, J., 1973, Sur l'existence de fausses antistreptolysines dans la lèpre, *Sem. Hop. Paris* 49:1093–1096.

Bechelli, L. M., and Martínez Domínguez, V., 1966, The leprosy problem in the world, *Bull. WHO* 34:811–826.

Bechelli, L. M., Kyaw Lwin, Gallego Garbajosa, P., Gyi, M. M., Uemura, K., Sundaresan, T., Tamondong, C., Matejka, M., Sansarricq, H., and Walter, J., 1974, B. C. G. vaccination of children against leprosy: Nine-year findings of the controlled WHO trial in Burma, *Bull. WHO* 51:93–99.

Bernard, J. C., and Vazquez, C. A. J., 1973, Visceral lesions in lepromatous leprosy, *Int. J. Lepr.* 41:94–101.

Blumberg, B. S., Melartin, L., Lechat, M., and Guinto, R. S., 1967, Association between lepromatous leprosy and Australia antigen, *Lancet* 2:173–175.

Blumberg, B. S., Melartin, L., Guinto, R., and Lechat, M., 1970, Lepromatous leprosy and Australia antigen with comments on the genetics of leprosy, *J. Chron. Dis.* 23:507–516.

Bonomo, L., and Dammacco, F., 1967, Characterization of thyroglobulin antibodies in leprosy, *Immunology* 13:565–576.

Bonomo, L., and Dammacco, F., 1971, Immune complex cryoglobulinemia in lepromatous leprosy, *Clin. Exp. Immunol.* 9:175–181.

Bonomo, L., Dammacco, F., Pinto, L., and Barbieri, G., 1963, Thyroglobulin antibodies in leprosy, *Lancet* 2:807–809.

Bonomo, L., Tursi, A., Trimigliozzi, G., and Dammacco, F., 1965, L. E. Cells and antinuclear factors in leprosy, *Br. Med. J.* 2:689–690.

Braverman, I. M., and Yen, A., 1975, Demonstration of immune complexes in spontaneous and histamine-induced lesions and in normal skin of parents with leukocytoclastic angiitis, *J. Invest. Dermatol.* 64:105–112.

Brinckerhoff, W. R., and Moore, W. L., 1909, Studies upon leprosy. IV. Upon the utility of the examination of the nose and the nasal secretions for the detection of incipient cases of leprosy, *Public Health Bull.* 27:3–29.

Brown, J. A. K., Stone, M. D., and Sutherland, I., 1968,

B. C. G. vaccination of children against leprosy in Uganda: Results at end of second follow-up, *Br. Med. J.* **1**:24–27.

Buck, A. A., and Hasenclever, H. F., 1963, Influence of leprosy on delayed-type skin reactions and serum agglutination titers to *Candida albicans, Am. J. Hyg.* **77**:305–316.

Bullock, W. E., 1968, Studies on immune mechanisms in leprosy. I. Depression of delayed allergic response to skin test antigens, *N. Engl. J. Med.* **278**:298–304.

Bullock, W. E., and Fasal, P., 1971, Studies of immune mechanisms in leprosy. III. The role of cellular and humoral factors in impairment of the *in vitro* immune response, *J. Immunol.* **106**:888–889.

Bullock, W. E., Jr., Ho, M. F., and Chen, M. J., 1970, Studies of immune mechanisms in leprosy. II. Quantitative relationships of IgG, IgA, and IgM immunoglobulins, *J. Lab. Clin. Med.* **75**:863–870.

Bullock, W. E., Fields, J. P., and Brandriss, M., 1972, An evaluation of transfer factor therapy in lepromatous leprosy, *N. Engl. J. Med.* **287**:1053–1059.

Bullock, W. E., Callerame, M. L., and Panner, B. J., 1974a, Immunohistologic alteration of skin and ultrastructural changes of glomerular basement membranes in leprosy, *Am. J. Trop. Med. Hyg.* **23**:78–83.

Bullock, W. E., Ho, M. F., and Chen, M. J., 1974b, Quantitative and qualitative studies of the local cellular exudative response in leprosy, *J. Reticuloendothel. Soc.* **16**:259–268.

Bullock, W. E., Carlson, E. M., and Gershon, R. K., 1978, The evolution of immunosuppressive cell populations in experimental mycobacterial infection, *J. Immunol.* **120**:1709–1716.

Büngeler, W., 1943, Die pathologische Anatomie der Lepra. II. *Arch. Pathol. Anat. Physiol. (Virchow's)* **310**:493–565.

Bush, O. B., Jr., 1958, C-reactive protein in leprosy, *Int. J. Lepr.* **26**:123–136.

Cannefax, G. R., Ross, H., and Bancroft, H., 1959, Reactivity of the RPCF test in leprosy compared with other syphilis tests, *Public Health Rep.* **74**:45–48.

Carter, R. L., Jamison, D. G., and Vollum, R. L., 1969, Histological changes evoked in mice by Freund's complete adjuvant, *J. Pathol.* **96**:503–512.

Cathgart, E. S., Williams, R. C., Ross H., and Calkins, E., 1961, The relationship of the latex fixation test to the clinical and serologic manifestations of leprosy, *Am. J. Med.* **31**:758–765.

Choyce, D. P., 1964, The eyes in leprosy, in: *Leprosy in Theory and Practice*, 2nd ed. (R. G. Cochrane and T. F. Davey, eds.), pp. 310–321, Williams and Wilkins, Baltimore.

Closs, O., Mshana, R. N., and Harboe, M., 1979, Antigenic analysis of *Mycobacterium leprae, Scand. J. Immunol.* **9**:297–302.

Cochrane, C. G., Weigle, W. O., and Dixon, F. J., 1959, The role of polymorphonuclear leukocytes in the initi-

ation and cessation of the Arthus vasculitis, *J. Exp. Med.* **110**:481–494.

Convit, J., Pinardi, M. E., and Rojas, F. A., 1971, Some considerations regarding the immunology of leprosy, *Int. J. Lepr.* **39**:556–564.

Convit, J., Pinardi, M., Rodriguez-Ocha, G., Ulrich, M., Avila, J. L., and Goihman-Yahr, M., 1974, Elimination of *Mycobacterium leprae* subsequent to local *in vivo* activation of macrophages in lepromatous leprosy by other mycobacteria, *Clin. Exp. Immunol.* **17**:261–265.

Cream, J. J., Bryceson, A. D. M., and Ryder, G., 1971, Disappearance of immunoglobulin and complement from the Arthus reaction and its relevance to studies of vasculitis in man, *Br. J. Dermatol.* **84**:106–109.

Dastur, D. K., Pandya, S. S., and Antia, N. H., 1970, Nerves in the arm in leprosy. 2. Pathology, pathogenesis and clinical correlations, *Int. J. Lepr.* **38**:30–48.

Date, A., Thomas, A., Mathai, R., and Johny, K. V., 1977, Glomerular pathology in leprosy, *Am. J. Trop. Med. Hyg.* **26**:266–272.

Denney, O. E., 1922, Specific leprous reactions and abnormal vaccinia induced in lepers by small pox vaccination, *Public Health Rep.* **37**:3141–3149.

Desikan, K. V., and Job, C. K., 1966, Leprous lymphadenitis: Demonstration of tuberculoid lesions, *Int. J. Lepr.* **34**:147–154.

Desikan, K. V., and Job, C. K., 1968, A review of postmortem findings in 37 cases of leprosy, *Int. J. Lepr.* **36**:32–44.

De Vries, R. R. P., Nijenhuis, L. E., Lai, A., Fat, R. F. M., and Van Rood, J. J., 1976, HLA-linked genetic control of host response to *Mycobacterium leprae, Lancet* **2**:1328–1330.

Dharmendra and Chatterjee, K. R., 1955, Prognostic value of the lepromin test in contacts of leprosy cases, *Lepr. India* **27**:149–152.

Dharmendra and Lowe, J., 1942, The immunological skin tests in leprosy. II. The isolated protein antigen in relation to the classical mitsuda reaction and the early reaction to lepromin, *Indian J. Med. Res.* **30**:9–15.

Dierks, R. E., and Shepard, C. C., 1968, Effect of phytohemagglutinin and various mycobacterial antigens on lymphocyte cultures from leprosy patients, *Proc. Soc. Exp. Biol. Med.* **127**:391–395.

Doull, J. A., Guinto, R. S., Rodriguez, J. N., and Bancroft, H., 1942, The incidence of leprosy in Cordova and Talisay, Sebu, P. I., *Int. J. Lepr.* **10**:107–131.

Drutz, D. J., and Gutman, R. A., 1973, Renal manifestations of leprosy: Glomerulonephritis, a complication of erythema nodosum leprosum, *Am. J. Trop. Med. Hyg.* **22**:496–502.

Drutz, D. J., Chen, T. S. N., and Lu, W. H., 1972, The continuous bacteremia of lepromatous leprosy, *N. Engl. J. Med.* **287**:159–164.

Drutz, D. J., Cline, M. J., and Levy, L., 1974, Leukocyte antimicrobial function in patients with leprosy, *J. Clin. Invest.* **53**:380–386.

Dutta, R. N., and Saha, K., 1973, Australia antigen and lepromatous leprosy: Its incidence, persistence and relation to cell mediated immunity, *Indian J. Med. Res.* **61**:1–8.

Dwyer, J. M., Bullock, W. E., and Fields, J. P., 1973, Disturbance of the blood T : B lymphocyte ratio in lepromatous leprosy, *N. Engl. J. Med.* **228**:1036–1039.

Enna, C. D., and Brand, P. W., 1970, Peripheral nerve abscess in leprosy: Report of three cases encountered in dimorphous and lepromatous leprosy, *Lepr. Rev.* **41**:175–180.

Etemadi, A. H., and Convit, J., 1974, Mycólic acids from "noncultivable" mycobacteria, *Infect. Immun.* **10**:236–239.

Evans, M. J., Newton, H. E., and Levy, L., 1973, Early response of mouse foot pads to *Mycobacterium leprae*, *Infect. Immun.* **7**:76–85.

Fernandez, J. M. M., Carboni, E. A., Mercau, R. A., and Serial, A., 1962, Transformation of two borderline-lepromatous leprosy cases to tuberculoid with healing, *Int. J. Lepr.* **30**:254–265.

Fine, P. E. M., Wolf, E., Pritchard, J., Watson, B., Bradley, D. J., Festenstein, H., and Chacko, C. J. G., 1979, HLA-linked genes and leprosy: A family study in Karigiri, South India, *J. Infect. Dis.* **140**:152–161

Fisher, C. A., and Barksdale, L., 1973, Cytochemical reactions of human leprosy bacilli and mycobacteria: Ultrastructural implications, *J. Bacteriol.* **113**:1389–1399.

Fite, G. L., 1941, Vascular lesions of leprosy, *Int. J. Lepr.* **9**:193–202.

Fliess, E. L., Ruibal-Ares, B., and Braun, A., 1975, Serum factors affecting the cell migration inhibition response to lepromin, *Int. J. Lepr.* **43**:320–325.

Francis, T. I., and Smith, J. A., 1972, Australia [Au(1)] antigen in Nigerian patients with leprosy, *Int. J. Lepr.* **40**:68–72.

Gajl-Peczalska, K. J., Soo Duk Lim, Jacobson, R. R., and Good, R. A., 1973, B lymphocytes in lepromatous leprosy, *N. Engl. J. Med.* **288**:1033–1035.

Garner, M. F., Backhouse, J. L., Collins, C. A., and Roeder, P. J., 1969, Serological tests for treponemal infection in leprosy patients, *Br. J. Vener. Dis.* **45**:19–22.

Gelber, R. H., Drutz, D. J., Epstein, W. V., and Fasal, P., 1974, Clinical correlates of C1q-precipitating substances in the sera of patients with leprosy, *Am. J. Trop. Med. Hyg.* **23**:471–475.

Godal, T., and Negassi, K., 1973, Subclinical infections in leprosy, *Br. Med. J.* **2**:557–559.

Godal, T., and Rees, R. J. W., 1970, Fate of *Mycobacterium leprae* in macrophages of patients with lepromatous or tuberculoid leprosy, *Int. J. Lepr.* **38**:439–442.

Godal, T., Myklestad, B., Samuel, D. R., and Myrvang, B., 1971, Characterization of the cellular immune defect in lepromatous leprosy: A specific lack of circulating *Mycobacterium leprae*-reactive lymphocytes, *Clin. Exp. Immunol.* **9**:821–831.

Godal, T. Myrvang, B., Froland, S. S., Shao, J., and Melaku, G., 1972, Evidence that the mechanism of immunological tolerance ("central failure") is operative in the lack of host resistance in lepromatous leprosy, *Scand. J. Immunol.* **1**:311–321.

Goihman-Yahr, M., Rodriguez-Ochoa, G., Aranzazu, N., and Convit, J., 1975, Polymorphonuclear activation in leprosy, *Clin. Exp. Immunol.* **20**:257–264.

Gordon, J., and White, R. G., 1971, Surface peptido-glycolipid filaments on Mycobacterium leprae, *Clin. Exp. Immunol.* **9**:539–547.

Guinto, R. S., and Mabalay, M. A., 1962, Note on tuberculin reaction in leprosy, *Int. J. Lepr.* **30**:278–283.

Han, S. H., Weiser, R. S., and Kau, S. T., 1971a, Prolonged survival of skin allografts in leprosy patients, *Int. J. Lepr.* **39**:1–6.

Han, S. H., Weiser, R. S., Tseng, J. J., and Kau, S. T., 1971b, Lymphocyte transfer reactions in leprosy patients, *Int. J. Lepr.* **39**:715–718.

Han, S. H., Weiser, R. S., Wang, J. J., Tsai, L. C., and Lin, P. R., 1974, The behavior of leprous lymphocytes and macrophages in the macrophage migration-inhibition test, *Int. J. Lepr.* **42**:186–192.

Hansen, G. A., 1874, Causes of leprosy, *Nor. Mag. Laegevidensk.* **4**:76–79.

Harboe, M., Closs, O., Bjune G., Kronvall, G., and Axelsen, N. H., 1978, Mycobacterium leprae specific antibodies detected by radioimmunoassay, *Scand. J. Immunol.* **7**:111–120.

Hastings, R. C., and Job, C. J., 1978, Reversal reaction in lepromatous leprosy following transfer factor therapy, *Am. J. Trop. Med. Hyg.* **27**:995–1004.

Hastings, R. C., Morales, M. J., Shannon, E. J., and Jacobson, R. R., 1976, Preliminary results on the safety and efficacy of transfer factor in leprosy, *Int. J. Lepr.* **44**:275.

Hokama, Y., Su, D. W. P., Skinsenes, O. K., Kim, R., Kimura, L., and Yanagihara, E., 1974, Effect of C-reactive protein, PHA, PWM and choline phosphate in ^{3}H-thymidine uptake of leukocytes of leprosy patients and normal individuals, *Int. J. Lepr.* **42**:19–27.

Imaeda, T., 1965, Electron microscopy: Approach to leprosy research, *Int. J. Lepr.* **33**:669–683.

Iveson, J. M. I., McDougall, A. C., Leathem, A. J., and Harris, H. J., 1975, Lepromatous leprosy presenting with polarthritis, myositis and immune-complex glomerulonephritis, *Br. Med. J.* **2**:619–621.

Jha, P., Balakrishnan, K., Talwar, G. P., and Bhutani, L. K., 1971, Status of humoral immune responses in leprosy, *Int. J. Lepr.* **39**:14–19.

Job, C. K., 1970, Lysosomal activity of macrophages in leprosy, *Arch. Pathol.* **90**:547–552.

Job, C. K., 1971, Pathology of peripheral nerve lesions in lepromatous leprosy—A light and electron microscopic study, *Int. J. Lepr.* **39**:251–268.

Job, C. K., Gude, S., and Macaden, V. P., 1964, Erythema nodosum leprosum, *Int. J. Lepr.* **32**:177–184.

Johny, K. V., Karat, A. B. A., Rao, P. S. S., and Date, A., 1975, Glomerulonephritis in leprosy—A percutaneous renal biopsy study, *Lepr. Rev.* **46**:29–37.

Karat, A. B. A., Karat, S., Job, C. K., and Furness, M. A., 1967, Acute exudative arthritis in leprosy: Rheumatoid-arthritis-like syndrome in association with erythema nodosum leprosum, *Br. Med. J.* **3**:770–772.

Karat, A. B. A., Karat, S., Job, C., and Sudarsanam, D., 1968, Acute necrotizing lepromatous lymphadenitis: An erythema-nodosum-leprosum like reaction in lymph nodes, *Br. Med. J.* **2**:223–224.

Karat, A. B. A., Job, C. K., and Rao, R. S. S., 1971, Liver in leprosy: Histological and biochemical findings, *Br. Med. J.* **1**:307–310.

Katz, D. H., 1972, The allogeneic effect on immune responses: Model for regulatory influence of T lymphocytes on the immune system, *Transplant. Rev.* **12**: 141–179.

Katz, S. I., DeBetz, B. H., and Zaias, N., 1971, Production of macrophage inhibitory factor by patients with leprosy, *Arch. Dermatol.* **103**:358–361.

Kent, J. F., Otero, A. B., and Harrigan, R. E., 1957, Relative specificity of serologic tests for syphilis in *Mycobacterium leprae* infections, *Am. J. Clin. Pathol.* **27**:539–545.

Kirchheimer, W. F., and Sanchez, R. M., 1976, Quantitative aspects of leprosy in armadillos, *Int. J. Lepr.* **44**:84–87.

Kraus, S. J., Haserick, J. R., Logan, L. C., and Bullard, J. C., 1971, Atypical fluorescence in the fluorescent treponemal antibody absorption (FIA-ABS) test related to deoxyribonucleic acid (DNA) antibodies, *J. Immunol.* **106**:1665–1669.

Kress, Y., Bloom, B. R., Wittner, M., Rowen, A., and Tanowitz, H., 1975, Resistance of *Trypansoma cruzi* to killing by macrophages, *Nature (London)* **257**:394–396.

Kronvall, G., Husby, G., Samuel, D., Bjune, G., and Wheate, H., 1975, Amyloid-related serum component (protein ASC) in leprosy patients, *Infect. Immun.* **11**:969–972.

Kuper, S. W. A., 1958, Histological changes in the lepromin reaction induced by BCG in leprosy patients, in: *Transactions of Chest and Heart Disease Conference*, p. 67–71, London.

Lara, C. B., and Nolasco, J. O., 1956, Self-healing or abortive and residual forms of childhood leprosy and their probable significance, *Int. J. Lepr.* **24**:245–263.

Lawrence, H. S., Al-Askari, S., David, J., Franklin, E. C., and Zweiman, B., 1963, Tranfer of immunological information in humans with dialysates of leukocyte extracts, *Tr. Assoc. Am. Physicians* **76**:84–91.

Levin, M., Pras, M., and Franklin, E. C., 1973, Immunologic studies of the major non-immunoglobulin protein of amyloid, *J. Exp. Med.* **138**:373–380.

Levine, M., 1951, Hemagglutination of tuberculin sensitized sheep cells in Hansen's disease, *Proc. Soc. Exp. Biol. Med.* **76**:171–173.

Levy, L., Fasal, P., and Murray, L. P., 1969, Morphology of *Mycobacterium leprae* in tissue sections, *Arch. Dermatol.* **100**:618–620.

Lim, S. D., and Fusaro, R. M., 1968, Leprosy. IV. Quantitation of immune globulins (IgG, IgA, and IgM) in leprosy sera, *Int. J. Lepr.* **36**:144–153.

Lim, S. D., Fusaro, R., and Good, R. A., 1972, Leprosy. VI. The treatment of leprosy patients with intravenous infusions of leukocytes from normal persons, *Clin. Immunol. Immunopathol.* **1**:122–139.

Lim, S. D., Kim, W. S., Kim, L. S., Good, R. A., and Park, B. H., 1974a, NBT responses of neutrophils and monocytes in leprosy, *Int. J. Lepr.* **42**:150–153.

Lim, S. D., Kiszkiss, D. F., Jacobson, R. R., Choi, Y. S., and Good, R. A., 1974b, Thymus-dependent lymphocytes of peripheral blood in leprosy patients, *Infect. Immun.* **9**:394–399.

Lim, S. D., Jacobson, R. R., Park, B. H., and Good, R. A., 1975, Leprosy. XII. Quantitative analysis of thymus-derived lymphocyte response to phytohaemagglutinin in leprosy, *Int. J. Lepr.* **43**:95–100.

Mabalay, M. D., Helwig, E. B., Tolentino, J. G., and Binford, C. H., 1965, The histopathology and histochemistry of erythema nodosum leprosum, *Int. J. Lepr.* **33**:28–49.

McAdam, K. P. W. J., Anders, R. F., Smith, S. R., Russell, D. A., and Price, M. A., 1975, Association of amyloidosis with erythema nodosum leprosum reactions and recurrent neutrophil leukocytosis in leprosy, *Lancet* **2**:572–575.

Maderazo, E. G., Ward, P. A., Woronick, C. L., Kubik, J., and DeGraff, A. C., Jr., 1976, Leukotactic dysfunction in sarcoidosis, *Ann. Intern. Med.* **84**:414–419.

Matthews, L. J., and Trautman, J. F., 1965, Clinical and serological profiles in leprosy, *Lancet* **2**:915–918.

Mehra, V., and Bloom, B. R., 1979, The induction of cell-mediated immunity to human *M. leprae* in the guinea pig, *Infect. Immun.* **23**:787–794.

Mehra, V. L., Talwar, G. P., Balakrishnan, K., and Bhutani, L. K., 1972, Influence of chemotherapy and serum factors on the mitogenic response of peripheral leukocytes of leprosy patients to phytohaemagglutinin, *Clin. Exp. Immunol.* **12**:205–213.

Mendes, E., Raphael, A., Mota, N. G. S., and Mendes, N. F., 1974a, Cell-mediated immunity in leprosy and transfer of delayed hypersensitivity reactions, *J. Allergy Clin. Immunol.* **53**:223–229.

Mendes, N. F., Kopersztych, S., and Mota, N. G. S., 1974b, T and B lymphocytes in patients with lepromatous leprosy, *Clin. Exp. Immunol.* **16**:23–30.

Mitsuda, K., and Ogawa, M. A., 1937, Study of one hundred and fifty autopsies on cases of leprosy, *Int. J. Lepr.* **5**:53–60.

Moran, C. J., Ryder, G., Turk, J. L., and Waters, M. F. R., 1972, Evidence for circulating immune complexes in lepromatous leprosy, *Lancet* **2**:572–573.

Mortensen, R. F., Osmand, A. P., and Gewurz, H., 1975, Effects of C-reactive protein on the lymphoid system. I. Binding to thymus-dependent lymphocytes and alteration of their functions, *J. Exp. Med.* **141**:821–839.

Mortensen, R. F., Braun, D., and Gewurz, H., 1977, Effects of C-reactive protein on the lymphoid system. III.

Inhibition of antigen-induced lymphocyte stimulation and lymphokine production, *Cell. Immunol.* **28**:59–68.

Moschella, S. L., 1967, The lepra reaction with necrotizing skin lesions, *Arch. Dermatol.* **95**:565–575.

Mostert, H. V. R., 1936, Bacillaemia in leprosy, *Lepr. Rev.* **7**:6–10.

Myrvang, B., 1974, Immune responsiveness to *Mycobacterium leprae* of healthy humans: Application of the leukocyte migration inhibition test, *Acta Pathol. Microbiol. Scand. Sect. B* **82**:707–714.

Myrvang, B., Godal, T., Ridley, D. S., Froland, S. S., and Song, Y. K., 1973, Immune responsiveness to *Mycobacterium leprae* and other mycobacterial antigens throughout the clinical and histopathological spectrum of leprosy, *Clin. Exp. Immunol.* **14**:541–553.

Mryvang, B., Feek, C. M., and Godal, T., 1974, Antimycobacterial antibodies in sera from patients throughout clinico-pathological disease spectrum of leprosy, *Acta Pathol. Microbiol. Scand.* **82B**:701–706.

Nakamura, M., 1972, Multiplication of *M. lepraemurium* in cell-free medium containing α-ketoglutaric acid and cytochrome c, *J. Gen. Microbiol.* **73**:193–195.

Narayanan, E., Shankara Manja, K., Bedi, B. M. S., Kirchheimer, W. F., and Balasurbrahmanyan, M., 1972, Arthropod feeding experiments in lepromatous leprosy, *Lepr. Rev.* **43**:188–193.

Nath, I., Curtis, J., Bhutani, L. K., and Talwar, G. P., 1974, Reduction of a subpopulation ot T lymphocytes in lepromatous leprosy, *Clin. Exp. Immunol.* **18**:81–87.

Nath, I., Curtiss, J., Sharma, A. K., and Talwar, G. P., 1977, Circulating T-cell numbers and their mitogenic potential in leprosy—Correlation with mycobacterial load, *Clin. Exp. Immunol.* **29**:393–400.

Navalkar, R. G., Norlin, M., and Ouchterlony, O., 1964, Characterization of leprosy sera with various mycobacterial antigens using double diffusion-in-gel analysis. II, *Int. Arch. Allergy* **8**:250–260.

Nelson, D. S., Nelson, M., Thurston, J. M., Waters, M. F. R., and Pearson, J. M. H., 1971, Phytohaemagglutinin-induced lymphocyte transformation in leprosy, *Clin. Exp. Immunol.* **9**:33–43.

Nelson, D. S., Penrose, J. M., Waters, M. F. R., Pearson, J. M. H., and Nelson, M., 1975, Depressive effect of serum from patients with leprosy on mixed lymphocyte reactions, *Clin. Exp. Immunol.* **22**:388–392.

Nelson, R. A., Jr., 1952, Changing concepts in the serodiagnosis of syphilis: Specific treponemal antibody versus Wasserman Reagin, *Br. J. Vener. Dis.* **28**:160–168.

Noordeen, S. K., 1971, Relapse in lepromatous leprosy, *Lepr. Rev.* **42**:43–48.

Okada, S., 1954, Studies on tuberculoid visceral leprosy: Tuberculoid granuloma in the liver, revealed by puncture biopsy, *Int. J. Lepr.* **22**:41–46.

Oleinick, A., 1969, Altered immunity and cancer risk: A review of the problem and analysis of the cancer mortality experience of leprosy patients, *J. Natl. Cancer Inst.* **43**:775–781.

Papageorgiou, P. S., Sorokin, C. F., Kouzoutzakoglou,

K., Bonforte, R. J., Workman, P. L., and Glade, P. R., 1973, Host responses to Epstein-Barr virus and cytomegolovirus infection in leprosy, *Infec. Immun.* **7**:620–624.

Paradisi, E. R., de Bonaparte, Y. P., and Morgenfeld, M. C., 1969, Response in two groups of anergic patients to the transfer of leukocytes from sensitive donors, *N. Engl. J. Med.* **280**:859–861.

Paul, R. C., Stanford, J. L., and Carswell, J. W., 1975, Multiple skin testing in leprosy, *J. Hyg.* **75**:57–68.

Pearson, J. M. H., and Ross, W. F., 1975, Nerve involvement in leprosy—Pathology, differential diagnosis and principles of management, *Lepr. Rev.* **46**:199–212.

Pearson, J. M. H., Rees, R. J. W., and Waters, M. F. R., 1975, Sulphone resistance in leprosy: A review of one hundred proven clinical cases, *Lancet* **2**:69–72.

Pearson, J. F. H., Cap, J. A., Haile, G. S., and Rees, R. J. W., 1977, Dapsone-resistant leprosy and its implications for leprosy control programs, *Lepr. Rev.* **48**:83–94.

Pedley, J. C., 1968, The presence of *M. leprae* in the lumina of the female mammary gland, *Lepr. Rev.* **39**:201–202.

Pedley, J. C., 1970, Summary of results of a search of the skin surface for *Mycobacterium leprae, Lepr. Rev.* **41**:167–168.

Petchclai, B., Chutanondh, R., Prasongsom, S., Hiranras, S., and Ramasoota, T., 1973, Complement profile in leprosy, *Am. J. Trop. Med. Hyg.* **22**:761–764.

Petit, J. H. S., and Waters, M. F. R., 1967, The etiology of erythema nodosum leprosum, *Int. J. Lepr.* **35**:1–10.

Prabhakaran, K., Kirchheimer, W. F., and Harris, E. B., 1968, Oxidation of phenolic compounds by *Mycobacterium leprae* and inhibition of phenolase by substrate analogues and copper chelators, *J. Bacteriol.* **95**:2051–2053.

Purtilo, D. T., and Pangi, C., 1975, Incidence of cancer in patients with leprosy, *Cancer* **35**:1259–1261.

Quismorio, F. P., Rea, T. H., Levan, N. E., and Friou, G. J., 1975, Immunoglobulin deposits in lepromatous leprosy skin, *Arch. Dermatol.* **111**:331–334.

Ramanujam, K., and Ramu, G., 1966, Small pox vaccination and acute exacerbation of leprosy, *Lepr. India* **38**:3–9.

Rea, T. H., Quismorio, F. P., Harding, B., Nies, K. M., Di Saia, P. J., Levan, N. E., and Friou, G. J., 1976a, Immunologic responses in patients with lepromatous leprosy, *Arch. Dermatol.* **112**:791–800.

Rea, T. H., Levan, N. E., and Terasaki, P., 1976b, Histocompatibility antigens in patients with leprosy, *J. Infect. Dis.* **134**:615–618.

Rees, R. J. W., 1964, The significance of the lepromin reaction in man, *Prog. Allergy* **8**:224–258.

Rees, R. J. W., 1975, in: *Proceedings of the U.S.–Japan Cooperative Medical Science Program, Workshop on Chemotherapy*, Bethesda, Md., October 26, p. 3.

Rees, R. J. W., 1976, personal communication.

Rees, R. J. W., and Meade, T. W., 1974, Comparison of

the modes of spread and the incidence of tuberculosis and leprosy, *Lancet* **1**:47–48.

Rees, R. J. W., and Valentine, R. C., 1962, The appearance of dead leprosy bacilli by light and electron microscopy, *Int. J. Lepr.* **30**:1–9.

Rees, R. J. W., Chatterjee, K. R., Pepys, J., and Tee, R. D., 1965, Some immunologic aspects of leprosy, *Am. Rev. Resp. Dis.* **92**(2):139–149.

Rich, A. R., 1951, *The Pathogenesis of Tuberculosis*, 2nd ed., pp. 797, 827, Thomas, Springfield, Ill.

Ridley, D. S., 1969, Reactions in leprosy, *Lepr. Rev.* **40**:77–81.

Ridley, D. S., 1972, The pathogenesis of the early skin lesion in leprosy, *J. Pathol.* **111**:191–206.

Ridley, D. S., 1974, Histological classification and the immunological spectrum of leprosy, *Bull. WHO* **51**:451–465.

Ridley, D. S., and Jopling, W. H., 1966, Classification of leprosy according to immunity, *Int. J. Lepr.* **34**:255–273.

Rojas-Espinosa, O., Mendez-Navarrete, I., and Estrada-Parra, S., 1972, Presence of C1q-reactive immune complexes in patients with leprosy, *Clin. Exp. Immunol.* **12**:215–223.

Ross, H., 1954, The results of a modified Middlebrook Dubos hemagglutination test in leprosy, *Int. J. Lepr.* **22**:174–180.

Ross, H., 1960, Immunochemical determination of orosomucoid in the blood serum of leprosy patients, *Int. J. Lepr.* **28**:267–270.

Ruge, H. G. C., 1967, Treponemal immobilization tests in leprosy, *Br. J. Vener. Dis.* **43**:191–196.

Saha, K., Mittal, M. M., and Ray, L. S. N., 1973, Consequences of small pox vaccination in leprosy patients, *Infec. Immun.* **8**:301–308.

Saitz, E. W., Dierks, R. E., and Shepard, C. C., 1968, Complement and the second component of complement in leprosy, *Int. J. Lepr.* **36**:400–404.

Salzano, F. M., 1967, Blood groups and leprosy, *J. Med. Genet.* **4**:102–106.

Sato, S., and Makoto, I., 1968, The surface structure of *M. leprae*, *Int. J. Lepr.* **36**:303–308.

Satyanarayana, B. V., Raju, P. S., Raja Kumari, K., and Reddy, C. R. R. M., 1972, Amyloidosis in leprosy, *Int. J. Lepr.* **40**:278–280.

Schujman, S., 1956, Subsequent evolution of the induced Mitsuda reaction in clinically and bacteriologically negative lepromatous cases, *Int. J. Lepr.* **24**:51–56.

Scotti, A. T., Mackey, D. M., and Trautman, J. R., 1970, Syphilis and biologic false positive reactors among leprosy patients, *Arch. Dermatol.* **101**:328–330.

Sharma, K. D., and Shrivastav, J. B., 1958, Lymph nodes in leprosy, *Int. J. Lepr.* **26**:41–50.

Sheagren, J. N., Block, J. B., Trautman, J. R., and Wolff, S. M., 1969, Immunologic reactivity in patients with leprosy, *Ann. Intern. Med.* **70**:295–302.

Shepard, C. C., 1962, The nasal excretion of *Mycobacterium laprae* in leprosy, *Int. J. Lepr.* **30**:10–18.

Shepard, C. C., and McRae, D. H., 1965, *Mycobacterium leprae* in mice: Minimal infectious dose, relationship

between staining quality and infectivity, and effect of cortisone, *J. Bacteriol.* **89**:365–372.

Shepard, C. C., and McRae, D., 1971, Hereditary characteristic that varies among isolates of *Mycobacterium leprae, Infec. Immun.* **3**:121–126.

Sher, R., Holm, G., Kok, S. H., Koornhof, H. J., and Glover, A., 1976, T and CR and lymphocyte profile in leprosy and the effect of treatment, *Infec. Immun.* **13**:31–35.

Silva, C., Lima, A. O., Andrade, L. M. C., and Mattos, O., 1973, Attempts to convert lepromatous into tuberculoid-type leprosy with blood lymphocyte extracts from sensitized donors, *Clin. Exp. Immunol.* **15**:87–92.

Skinsnes, 1978, *Int. J. Lepr.* **46**:394–413

Sobel, A. T., Bokish, V. A., and Müller-Eberhard, H. J., 1975, C1q deviation test for the detection of immune complexes, aggregates of IgG and bacterial products in human sera, *J. Exp. Med.* **142**:139–151.

Solis, F., and Wade, H. W., 1925, Bacteriologic findings in children of lepers with special reference to nasal lesions, *J. Philipp. Isl. Med. Assoc.* **5**:365–369.

Stanford, J. L., Rook, G. A. W., Convit, J., Godal, T., Kronvall, G., Rees, R. J. W., and Walsh, G. P., 1975, Preliminary taxonomic studies on the leprosy bacillus, *Br. J. Exp. Pathol.* **56**:579–585.

Stewart-Tull, D. E. S., and Davies, M., 1972, Adjuvant activity of *Mycobacterium* leprae, *Infec. Immun.* **6**:909–912.

Tajiri, I., 1955, The "acute infiltration" reaction of lepromatous leprosy, *Int. J. Lepr.* **23**:370–384.

Theofilopoulos, A. N., Wilson, C. B., and Dixon, F. J., 1976, The Raji cell radioimmune assay for detecting immune complexes in human sera, *J. Clin. Invest.* **57**:169–182.

Tin Shwe, 1972a, Antistreptolysin O titer in leprosy, *Int. J. Lepr.* **40**:389–391.

Tin Shwe, 1972b, Immune complexes in glomeruli of patients with leprosy, *Lepr. Rev.* **52**:282–289.

Tin Shwe, and Petty, R. E., 1971, Activation of complement (C3) in patients with leprosy, *Lepr. Rev.* **42**:277–281.

Tung, K. S. K., Kim, B., Bjorvatn, B., Kronvall, G., McLaren, L. C., and Williams, R. C., Jr., 1977, Discrepancy between C1q deviation and Raji cell tests in detection of circulating immune complexes in patients with leprosy, *J. Infect. Dis.* **136**:216–221.

Turk, J. L., and Waters, M. F. R., 1969, Cell-mediated immunity in patients with leprosy, *Lancet* **2**:243–246.

Turk, J. L., and Waters, M. F. R., 1971, Immunological significance of changes in lymph nodes across the leprosy spectrum, *Clin. Exp. Immunol.* **8**:363–376.

U.S. Leprosy Panel, 1975, Rifampin therapy of lepromatous leprosy, *Am. J. Trop. Med. Hyg.* **24**:475–484.

Waldman, T. A., and Broder, S., 1977, Suppressor cells in the regulation of the immune response, *Prog. Clin. Immunol.* **3**:155–199.

Waldorf, D. S., Sheagren, J. N., Trautman, J. R., and Block, J. B., 1966, Impaired delayed hypersensitivity in patients with lepromatous leprosy, *Lancet* **2**:773–775.

Wall, J. R., and Wright, D. J. M., 1974, Antibodies against testicular germinal cells in lepromatous leprosy, *Clin. Exp. Immunol.* **17**:51–59.

Ward, P. A., and Berenberg, J. L., 1974, Defective regulation of inflammatory mediators in Hodgkin's disease: Supernormal levels of chemotactic factor inactivator, *N. Engl. J. Med.* **290**:76–80.

Ward, P. A., Goralnick, S. J., and Bullock, W. E., 1976, Defective leukotaxis in patients with lepromatous leprosy, *J. Lab. Clin. Med.* **87**:1025–1032.

Waters, M. F. R., and Helmy, H. S., 1974, The relationship of Dapsone (DDS) therapy to erythema nodosum leprosum, *Lepr. Rev.* **45**:299–307.

Waters, M. F. R., Rees, R. J. W., McDougall, A. C., and Wedell, A. G. M., 1974, Ten years of dapsone in lepromatous leprosy: Clinical, bacteriological and histological assessment and the finding of viable leprosy bacilli, *Lepr. Rev.* **45**:288–298.

Weddell, A. G. M., Jamison, D. G., and Palmer, E., 1964, Recent investigations into the sensory and neurohistological changes in leprosy, in: *Leprosy in Theory and Practice* (R. G. Cochrane and T. F. Davey, eds.), pp. 205–220, Williams and Wilkins, Baltimore.

Wemambu, S. M. G., Turk, J. L., Waters, M. F. R., and Rees, R. J. W., 1969, Erythema nodosum leprosum: A clinical manifestation of the Arthus phenomenon, *Lancet* **2**:933–935.

White, R. G., Jolles, P., Samour, D., and Lederer, R., 1964, Correlation of adjuvant activity and chemical structure of wax D fractions of mycobacteria, *Immunology* **7**:158–171.

Williams, R. C., Jr., Cathcart, E. S., Calkins, E., Fite, G. L., Tubio, J. B., and Cohen, A. S., 1965, Secondary amyloidosis in lepromatous leprosy: Possible relationships of diet and environment, *Ann. Intern. Med.* **62**:1000–1007.

Wisniewski, H. M., and Bloom, B. R., 1975, Primary demyelination as a nonspecific consequence of a cell-mediated immune reaction, *J. Exp. Med.* **141**:346–359.

WHO Memorandum, 1973, Immunological problems in leprosy research. 2, *Bull. WHO* **48**:483–491.

WHO, 1977, *Technical Report Series No. 607,* World Health Organization, Geneva, Switzerland.

Wright, D. J. M., 1973, The significance of the fluorescent treponemal antibody (FTA-ABS) test in collagen disorders and leprosy, *J. Clin. Pathol.* **26**:968–972.

16

Immunology of Syphilis

PETER L. PERINE

1. Introduction

Syphilis has been a controversial disease since it was first recognized in Europe in the late fifteenth century. Historians debate its origins; physicians, its manifestations; epidemiologists, methods for its control; microbiologists, the metabolism and structure of its etiological agent, *Treponema pallidum*; and immunologists, the comparative roles of humoral and cellular immunity in protection against or the pathogenesis of this disease. As a result, the volume of writing on syphilis is enormous. That reviewed in this chapter deals primarily with the biology and immunology of *T. pallidum* published since the monograph by Turner and Hollander (1957) and the bibliographical review by Willcox and Guthe (1966). A recent symposium on the biology of parasitic spirochetes (Johnson, 1976) describes many of the recent advances in the immunobiology of syphilis.

2. Treponematoses

2.1. Evolutionary Aspects

Syphilis is one of the treponematoses, a group of chronic granulomatous diseases caused by spirochetes belonging to the genus *Treponema* (Table 1). These diseases comprise venereal and endemic syphilis, yaws, pinta, and cuniculosis, which are differentiated by their clinical manifestations, their ability to produce

disease in experimental animal hosts and certain epidemiological features. None of the pathogenic treponemes can be grown *in vitro*, and superinfection experiments in animals (Turner and Hollander, 1957) and man (*WHO Technical Report,* 1970) demonstrate various degrees of cross-immunity between the treponemes causing syphilis (*T. pallidum*), yaws (*T. pertenue*), pinta (*T. careteum*), and rabbit cuniculosis (*T. cuniculi*).

The most notable feature of the treponematoses is the progression of disease by stages separated by periods of quiescence, each stage presenting different clinical manifestations and lesion morphology. Together with a common morphology and immunology, this reflects a common ancestor. It has been postulated that pinta was the first treponematosis to evolve within the Afro–Asian land mass, followed by yaws and then syphilis (Hackett, 1963). This is also the order of increasing virulence of the respective, causative treponemes.

Syphilis is considered to be a relatively recent disease. Its recognition in Europe coincided with the return of Columbus from the New World in the late fifteenth century, and it is a commonly held belief that members of his crew acquired and imported syphilis from America. However, there is considerable evidence that endemic syphilis, if not venereal syphilis, was prevalent in the Middle East and Europe centuries before Columbus, masquerading as a form of "leprosy" (Hackett, 1963). Whatever its origin, syphilis spread throughout Europe as the "great pox" with the amazing rapidity usually characteristic of a new

PETER L. PERINE ● Center for Disease Control, Venereal Disease Control Division, Atlanta, Georgia 30333.

TABLE 1. Classification of the Treponematoses

Disease (synonyms)	Organisms	Mode of transmission	Natural host	Experimental host	Geographic distribution
Venereal syphilis (lues)	*T. pallidum*	Venereal	Man	Rabbits, hamsters, primates, guinea pigs	Worldwide
Endemic syphilis (bejel, dichuchwa)	*T. pallidum* subspecies	Intimate nonvenereal contact	Man		Arid areas of Middle East, Africa, Asia, Australia
Yaws (frambesia tropica, pian)	*T. pertenue, T. friborg-blanc*	Intimate nonvenereal contact	Man, subhuman primates	Hamsters, rabbits, guinea pigs	Intertropical Zone of Africa, America, Southeast Asia, Oceania
Pinta (mal del pinto, carete)	*T. careteum*	Intimate nonvenereal contact	Man	Rabbits, primates	Tropical forests of Central and South America
Cuniculosis	*T. paraleus-cuniculi*	Venereal	Rabbit	Hamsters, guinea pigs	Worldwide

pathogen in a nonimmune population (Fleming, 1964).

2.2. Host and Environmental Factors

The type of disease produced by a given treponeme is conditioned by the host and environmental factors (Willcox, 1974). For example, in the preantibiotic era, there were striking racial differences to syphilitic infection in whites and blacks. In early syphilis, lymphoid involvement was much more extensive in blacks, and ocular and bone lesions were from 2 to 4 times as common. In late syphilis, bone lesions and cardiovascular syphilis were 2 times as frequent in blacks, whereas, conversely, neurosyphilis of any kind was 3 times more common in whites (Moore, 1939). Whether or not these racial differences reflect a genetic predisposition to certain manifestations and complications of syphilis has yet to be determined. One way to look at this would be to study the distribution frequency of HLA antigens in patients with different types of syphilitic lesions. Studies of the racial differences in syphilis would be more difficult, since these are not as obvious today, perhaps because antibiotic treatment aborts disease progression, dramatically reducing the number of patients who develop tertiary syphilis.

Climate and age play a major role in the epidemiology of yaws and pinta (Willcox, 1960).

These treponematoses are found in warm, humid areas located between the Tropics of Cancer and Capricorn. Pinta occurs only in South and Central America, and yaws occurs primarily in Africa and Oceania. Yaws and pinta are acquired during childhood by nonvenereal contract with infectious lesions and are facilitated by poor sanitation, overcrowding, and fomites. There is recent evidence that some species of nonhuman primates in West Africa are infected with a yawslike treponeme (Fribourg-Blanc and Mollaret, 1969), raising the intriguing possibility of a zoonotic reservoir for this disease.

2.3. Nonvenereal Treponematoses

The progression of disease by stages is not as well delineated in pinta and yaws as it is in syphilis. Since neither *T. careteum* nor *T. pertenue* can penetrate intact skin or mucosa, transmission of infection requires intimate contact between an infectious lesion and minor skin abrasions caused by insect bites or injury. The primary lesions appear on the skin of the site of invasion. In pinta the primary, pigmented papule heals after a period of several months, and adjacent secondary maculopapular lesions develop. These slowly depigment, leaving white areas of atrophic skin characteristic of "tertiary" or late pinta.

In contrast to pinta, yaws involves the osseous tissue as well as the skin. The primary "mother yaw" is a relatively large granulomatous lesion, usually found on the extremities, which lasts 1–3 months. Secondary papillomas erupt 3–6 months after the mother yaw heals and are accompanied by swelling of the bones of the extremities and nose. Tertiary yaws occurs 5–10 years after infection and is characterized by destructive gummatous lesions of the extremities and face, which often ulcerate.

Endemic syphilis or bejel is similar to yaws and pinta by its nonvenereal transmission and its predilection to infect the young. It is caused by a treponeme identical to *T. pallidum* and is found today mainly among nomadic populations living in arid areas of North Africa and the Middle East. The mucous membranes are usually involved, and, in contrast to yaws and pinta, systemic spread of infection with cardiovascular and nervous system involvement has been reported (Grin and Guthe, 1973).

2.4. Treatment

A number of antimicrobial drugs are proven efficacy for all stages of the treponematoses except the destructive lesions of cardiovascular and neurosyphilis. Penicillin is the most widely used antibiotic. Although there is no evidence that *T. pallidum* has developed any degree of resistance to penicillin, there have been several reports of treponemelike forms persisting in tissues of man and experimental animals after adequate and repeated courses of penicillin therapy (Yobs *et al.*, 1968; Rein, 1976). As noted by Turner *et al.* (1969) only rarely have these treponemelike forms been proven to be *T. pallidum* by animal inoculation and in many instances the organism was isolated from cerebrospinal fluid (Hardy *et al.*, 1970, Tremont, 1976), aqueous humor (Smith and Israel, 1968), or other infected tissue that is largely impervious to penicillin.

Penicillin in appropriate doses sterilizes syphilis infection, but if treatment is delayed until the early latent stage the treponemal antigen tests usually remain reactive for life. This suggests that *T. pallidum* or its antigens persist in the host or that periodic anamnestic stimulation is provided by the avirulent treponemes of the normal intestinal flora.

Treatment of syphilis or yaws may induce a Jarisch–Herxheimer reaction, which is characterized by the onset of fever, chills, leukocytosis, and an aggravation of syphilitic lesions lasting for several hours. The etiology of this reaction is obscure, but recent evidence indicates that it may be caused by an endotoxinlike substance released by the dying spirochetes (Gelfand *et al.*, 1976).

3. The Organism

3.1. Classification of Treponemes

The treponemes are classified into two separate groups: pathogens which cannot be grown *in vitro* and the avirulent, cultivated strains (Smibert, 1976). There are more than 60 species of avirulent treponemes, many of which are present in the microflora of the gastrointestinal and genitourinary tracts of man and animals. They may at times be opportunistic pathogens and are a frequent cause of diagnostic confusion in syphilis because of their similar morphology and motility. Moreover, some avirulent treponemes share common antigens with the pathogenic treponemes and give rise to cross-reacting antibodies in the host. Several were initially isolated in culture from syphilitic lesions and were falsely assumed to be the cause of syphilis (Noguchi, 1911). These treponemes continue to be a source of taxonomic confusion. For example, the Nichols nonpathogenic strain of *T. pallidum* cultured by Kast and Kolmer in 1933 was isolated from rabbits infected with the pathogenic Nichols strain of *T. pallidum*, which, in turn, was originally isolated from the cerebrospinal fluid of a neurosyphilitic by Nichols and Hough in 1913!

The major importance of the avirulent treponemes has been their use as antigens in serodiagnostic tests for syphilis, the study of their metabolism in attempts to develop a culture medium suitable for pathogenic treponemes, and their potential value as a syphilis vaccine. The most widely used are *T. phagedenis*, which includes the Reiter, English Reiter, and Kazan strains; *T. refringens*, which includes avirulent Nichols and Noguchi strains; and *T. denticola*, which has more than 40 strains including *T. macrodentium* and *T. vencentii* (Smibert, 1976).

Although there is only one species of pathogenic *T. pallidum*, there is considerable experimental evidence, based on superinfection studies in rabbits, for strains of *T. pallidum* which differ in virulence and/or immunogenicity. To demonstrate this phenomenon, rabbits were first inoculated intratesticularly with the Nichols strain and challenged 3–4 months later with 500 virulent treponemes obtained from patients residing in different geographic areas. Four of 11 strains so tested produced cutaneous lesions in rabbits that were immune to challenge with the Nichols strain (Turner and Hollander, 1957). Similar differences may exist between the Nichols strain(s) used to study experimental syphilis in different parts of the world, since they were often obtained from different sources at different times and their serial passage in rabbits over the past 65 years provided ideal conditions for genetic mutation. Serial passage of the Nichols strain in rabbits; however, has not affected its virulence for rabbits or man. The minimum infective dose of *T. pallidum* in rabbits is approximately the same as in man and ranges between one organism and 50 organisms (Magnuson *et al.*, 1956).

3.2. Morphology

T. pallidum organisms are slender, motile, gram-negative, helical-shaped, and cylindrical; they belong to the order Spirochaetales, which also includes the genera *Cristispira*, *Borrelia*, *Spirochaeta*, and *Leptospira*. Pathogenic treponemes are about 0.2 μm in diameter and range in length from 5 μm to 20 μm (Wiegand *et al.*, 1972). The coils are about 0.3 μm deep and have a constant interval or wavelength of about 1.0 μm (Hovind-Hougen, 1976). Because of their small mass and low refractive index, treponemes are not easily visualized by ordinary light microscopy unless dark-field illumination, phase contrast, and negative stain techniques are used.

The most distinguishing feature of the pathogenic treponemes is their unique motility, a rapid spinning, corkscrewlike rotation, often interrupted by marked flexing around its long axis. Slow-moving *T. pallidum* organisms appear as flat sine waves when photographed under high magnification, but avirulent treponemes and other members of the order Spirochaetales are irregularly coiled and helical (Cox, 1972). Despite their morphological similarities, an experienced microscopist can usually differentiate pathogenic from nonpathogenic treponemes.

The electron microscope has been used by a number of investigators to study the ultrastructure of *T. pallidum* (Ovcinnikov and Delektorskij, 1971; Wiegand *et al.*, 1972; Hovind-Hougen, 1976; Holt, 1978). The basic structural elements (Fig. 1) are an outer envelope covering the cell; a protoplasmic cylinder with tapered ends consisting of the cell wall, cell membrane, and the enclosed cytoplasm; and the axial fibrils (Holt, 1978).

The outer envelope or sheath is a triple-layered membrane of unknown chemical composition and function. Its position suggests that it may be analogous to the typical prokaryotic capsule and is the probable site of attachment for complement-dependent immobilizing antibody (Holt, 1978). The outer envelope of freshly isolated *T. pallidum* may be coated by an acid mucopolysaccharide slime layer (Zeigler *et al.*, 1976). The origin of the slime layer is uncertain; it may be an important virulence factor since it is not found on avirulent treponemes. Christiansen (1963) proposed that the slime layer is derived from the host and its function is to protect the organism from immune destruction by antibod-

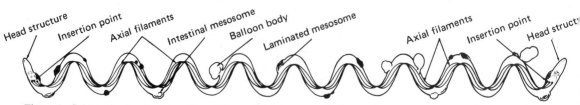

Figure 1. Schematic drawing of a *T. pallidum* without a mucoid layer, illustrating various anatomical structures. From Wiegand *et al.* (1972).

ies and phagocytosis. The slime layer may also play a role in adhesion phenomena, such as the attachment of treponemes to cell membranes (Holt, 1978).

Directly beneath the outer envelope is the cell wall–cell membrane complex, which encloses the protoplasmic cylinder. This complex contains peptidoglycan and is sensitive to lysozyme and osmotic stress (Jackson and Black, 1971; Hardy and Nell, 1961). The axial filaments, presumed to be responsible for motility, lie in a bundle between the outer envelope and cell wall. These originate near the terminus of the organism from basal bodies and traverse the cell in a helical arrangement. The protein subunits of the axial filaments are antigenic; those of the avirulent Reiter treponeme stimulate antibodies that cross-react with the axial filament subunits of pathogenic treponemes, which is the basis for the Reiter protein complement-fixation test for syphilis antibody (Hardy et al., 1975).

The cytoplasm of treponemes contains ribosomes for protein synthesis and a number of other organelles of unknown function, such as fibrils, multilaminated bodies resembling bacterial mesosomes, and granular cysts (Wiegand et al., 1972). The last are contiguous with the outer envelope and may contain some of the structural elements of the organism. Ovcinnikov and Delektorskij (1971) suggest that granular cysts are formed in the presence of antimicrobial drugs and/or host immune forces to protect the organism.

Only minor morphological changes occur in tissue infected with treponemes. In biopsies of primary and secondary syphilitic lesions the majority of treponemes are found in the extracellular, peripheral areas surrounding small blood vessels and lymphatics. A few are also found within the cytoplasm of a variety of cells, including plasma cells (Azar et al., 1970; Ovcinnikov and Delektorskij, 1970), phagocytes, fibroblasts, epithelial and endothelial cells (Sykes et al., 1974). The intracellular localization of T. pallidum may be a requirement for their multiplication (Fitzgerald et al., 1975) or may protect the organism from treponemicidal drugs or immune factors (Ovcinnikov and Delektorskij, 1971). It is not known whether viable treponemes enter nonphagocytic cells by phagocytosis or by direct invasion.

3.3. Multiplication and Metabolism

T. pallida organisms multiply slowly by transverse division, with a generation time in vivo estimated at 30–33 hr (Magnuson et al., 1948; Turner and Hollander, 1957). Despite a tremendous effort by many able investigators, none of the pathogenic treponemes has been successfully cultivated in vitro, at least in a reproducible manner (reviewed by Willcox and Guthe, 1966; Fitzgerald et al., 1976). Most of these efforts have been devoted to defining the factors which influence the survival of T. pallidum in vitro, or the study of the metabolic potential of freshly isolated treponemes, in the hope that this information would lead to the development of media that would support the growth and multiplication of the organism.

Nelson (1948) formulated a cell-free medium that maintained T. pallidum motility for as long as 16 days and used it to measure treponemal immobilizing (TPI) antibodies in syphilitic serum (Nelson and Mayer, 1949). The primary function of the medium appeared to be the creation of a state of anaerobiosis by addition of sulfhydryl reducing compounds and by incubation in an atmosphere of 95% nitrogen and 5% carbon dioxide. No significant multiplication of the organism occurred in TPI medium, and virulence for rabbits was lost long before motility ceased (Weber, 1960).

Although anaerobiosis is an essential requirement for survival of T. pallidum in Nelson's medium, there is recent evidence that the organism requires small concentrations of oxygen for its metabolism and multiplication (Baseman, 1977). Cox and Barber (1974) found that T. pallidum utilizes oxygen in vitro at a rate comparable to that of aerobic Leptospira to metabolize pyruvate and glucose by oxidative phosphorylation (Schiller and Cox, 1977). That virulent treponemes derive their metabolic energy from oxidative phosphorylation but are readily killed when exposed to atmospheric oxygen seems paradoxical. However, the oxygen requirement may be narrowly defined in terms of redox potential and oxygen tension, and may be difficult to establish and maintain in vitro for the period of time required for several generations of growth (Fieldsteel et al., 1977; Sandok et al., 1978). Moreover, the organism may lack a mechanism for neutralizing toxic metabolites accumulating *in vitro* that are detoxified by the host *in vivo* (Fitzgerald *et al.*, 1975).

Recent experiments designed to meet the nutritional, redox potential, and detoxifying requirements for growth of *T. pallidum* by co-incubation in a variety of tissue culture systems have been unsuccessful, with one possible exception. Although motility and virulence were enhanced (Fitzgerald *et al.*, 1975; Fieldsteel *et al.*, 1977), multiplication did not occur. Jones *et al.* (1976) succeeded in cultivating *T. pallidum* for two generations in tissue culture, but their results have not been confirmed (Foster *et al.*, 1977; Sandok *et al.*, 1978).

The *T. pallidum*–cell interaction in tissue cultures has other interesting characteristics (Fitzgerald *et al.*, 1977). Treponemes are usually attached to cells by their pointed ends, and the rapid, initial attachment is followed by a cycle of detachment and reattachment for several hours. Attachment is temperature dependent and is prevented by previous incubation of the organism with syphilis immune rabbit serum. Avirulent or heat-killed virulent treponemes' not attaching to cells indicates that attachment is an active phenomenon and a virulence characteristic of pathogenic treponemes. Attachment and even penetration of the treponeme into the cell do not destroy the cell, which may explain the occasional intracellular location of *T. pallidum* in cells of syphilitic lesions. These findings may partially explain some aspects of the pathogenesis of syphilis.

4. The Infection

4.1. Experimental Animals

Man is the only natural host for *T. pallidum*. Nonhuman primates and most warm-blooded animals are easily infected and occasionally harbor other treponemes. However, higher primates, rabbits, hamsters, and guinea pigs are the only animals which regularly develop syphilitic lesions and only primates manifest some of the lesions of tertiary syphilis (Turner and Hollander, 1957; Kuhn, 1970; Elsas *et al.*, 1968). Many animal species that fail to develop syphilitic lesions after infection may be naturally resistant to *T. pallidum*, although in oth-

ers such as the mouse the treponemes remain dormant, but infectious, for the lifetime of the host. In the last case conventional tests for reagin antibody are usually negative but treponemal antibody tests may become reactive (Ohta, 1972).

Elevated body temperatures are prejudicial to the survival of treponemes within the host. Syphilitic lesions heal quickly or fail to develop at body temperatures above 40°C (Turner and Hollander, 1957). Conversely, experimental syphilis in some animal species may be enhanced by housing the animal in environments between 4°C and 18°C. This phenomenon may explain the predilection of *T. pallidum* to cause syphilitic lesions on exposed body surfaces or on the extremities.

4.2. Acquired Syphilis

4.2.1. Venereal Infection

Syphilis is almost always transmitted by sexual intercourse. Drying and air are prejudicial to the survival of *T. pallidum*. The risk of transmission depends on the duration of contact and the number of virulent organisms present in the contact lesion(s). The organism can penetrate normal mucous membrane in the rabbit (Mahoney and Bryant, 1933), but infection probably occurs more commonly by its invasion through small breaks in the skin or mucosa. After breaching the skin barrier, the majority of the organisms invade the local perivascular lymphatics and reach the bloodstream within minutes or hours (Raiziss and Severac, 1937); intermittent spirochetemia continues throughout the course of untreated natural and experimental infection (Frazier *et al.*, 1952). The organisms are carried to virtually every organ and tissue of the body, where, perhaps aided by an active process of cellular attachment, they lodge and begin multiplication. After an interval of 9–90 days the first macroscopic lesion, the chancre, appears at the site of invasion. The chancre is commonly painless and in women is frequently in a concealed position, such as the cervix or vagina, and the patient is often unaware or unmindful of its presence. The organisms evoke an inflammatory response composed primarily of lymphocytes, plasma cells, and macrophages. This results in a local obstructive endarteritis and lymphadenitis, leading to necrosis and ulceration of the chancre. The serous exudate of the chancre is rich in treponemes and is therefore highly infectious. The ulcerated chancre heals without scar formation within a few weeks.

Due: 3/17/20

Sumant Puri

sumantpuri@Temple.edu

in one of three ways: one-third of patients develop symptoms and signs of tertiary syphilis, one-third remain seropositive for syphilis but do not develop symptoms or lesions of tertiary syphilis, and the remaining one-third presumably progress to "spontaneous" cure with no

clinical or laboratory evidence of infection (Clark and Danbolt, 1964). The lesions of tertiary syphilis are noninfectious and are of two types (Kampmeier, 1964). The most common are destructive lesions produced by obliterative small vessel endarteritis. In the nervous system this produces general paresis or tabes dorsalis. If it involves the vasa vasorum of the aortic arch, an aneurysm and aortic valve incompetence result. These lesions are the result of immune factors directed against T. pallidum persisting in the perivascular tissue of the affected vessels, and are irreversible with treatment. In many cases the tissue damage is devastating and often fatal. The second type of tertiary lesion is the gumma, an allergic lesion resembling the tubercle which may occur in any organ or tissue (Fig. 2). Gummas are usually "benign" since they seldom cause physical incapacity or death. They have become rare since the advent of penicillin, probably because they are remarkably sensitive to small doses of penicillin and other antibiotics (Kampmeier, 1964).

An important and unexplained observation is that all patients infected with T. pallidum pass through the successive stages of syphilis. Clark (1939) thought that as many as one in every five men and one in every three infected women acquire syphilis without developing primary lesions, and that the proportion of patients with late syphilis who have no history of early infection is so high, "even among the most intelligent, as to rouse the suspicion that

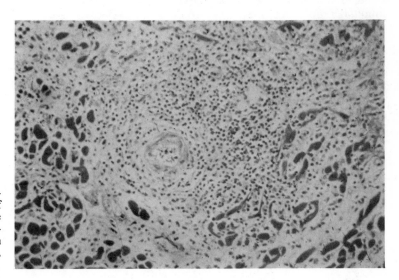

Figure 2. Gumma seen in myocardium with a central zone of necrosis surrounded by large numbers of plasma cells and lymphocytes. Vascular proliferation is present on the periphery (950 ×, H & E stain).

infection may have occurred in the complete absence of primary and secondary syphilis.''

4.2.2. Congenital Infection

Congenital syphilis is caused by the transmission of *T. pallidum* from the mother to the fetus across the placenta. Transmission is influenced by the duration of untreated maternal infection and the gestational age of the fetus. It is most likely to occur during the early stages of syphilis in the mother (Kaufman *et al.*, 1977), which corresponds to the time when high levels of spirochetemia are likely to be present.

There is considerable evidence based on the pathological study of fetuses aborted from women with untreated syphilis that infection seldom occurs before 18 weeks' gestation (McCord, 1929; Dippel, 1944). Beck and Daily (1938) proposed that the trophoblast of the developing placenta destroys treponemes by its erosive action on maternal tissue and that the cytotrophoblast or Langhans' layer acts as a barrier to the invasion of the organism before 18 weeks' gestation. The slow involution of the cytotrophoblast after this time would explain the increasing incidence of congenital infection after the fifth month of gestation. Silverstein (1962) challenged this widely accepted theory. He observed that large numbers of mature plasma cells were characteristic of fetal syphilitic lesions. He postulated that these lesions were due to a specific inflammatory response directed against *T. pallidum*. Fetal infection before the gestational age of immunocompetence, therefore, would seldom be recognized because of the absence of inflammation and pathological lesions.* Harter and Benirschke (1976) confirmed the presence of *T. pallidum* in tissues from two of five abortuses of five women with recent untreated syphilis. The fetuses' gestational ages were 9 and 10 weeks. The spirochetes were detected by specific fluorescent antibody and silver stains; they were few in number and did not cause surrounding necrotic lesions or incite an inflammatory response. These authors conclude that *T. pallidum* rarely, if ever, overwhelms the early fetus, leading to intrauterine

*Silverstein's work reversed a widely held belief that the fetus was incapable throughout gestation of responding specifically to an antigenic stimulus.

death and expulsion, which is so common in the last trimester.

The fate of the fetus infected with *T. pallidum* early in gestation is unknown. It is conceivable that a state of immunological tolerance ensues so that the infant at birth has no clinical, pathological, or laboratory evidence of syphilis except for reactive reagin and treponemal antigen tests resulting from passive transfer of maternal IgG antibody. In a recently completed but unpublished study of congenital syphilis in a high-prevalence Ethiopian population, Perine *et al.* (1978) found that three of 14 neonates born of mothers with untreated latent syphilis had virulent *T. pallidum* in their cerebrospinal fluid (CSF). This was demonstrated by producing syphilitic orchitis in rabbits after injection of 1.0 ml of CSF obtained during the first 48 hr of life. None of the three infected neonates had clinical, radiological, or laboratory evidence of syphilis; the CSF cell count and protein concentration were normal for this age group and the CSF VDRL and FTA ABS serological tests were negative. Their serum reagin antibody titers ranged from 1 : 2 to 1 : 8, and in each instance the titer lower than that of the mother. Each of the neonates' FTA treponemal antigen test was reactive at a serum dilution of 1 : 50 and 1 : 200 when an anti-IgG conjugate was used, but not with an anti-IgM conjugate, indicating that there was no production of specific IgM antibody by the neonates. Finally, lymphocytes from peripheral blood of these neonates did not undergo significant blastogenesis when exposed to *T. pallidum* (Nichols strain) in an *in vitro* lymphocyte transformation test (Friedmann, 1977). Because the duration of maternal infection was unknown (none had symptoms or signs of primary or secondary syphilis during their pregnancy), the gestational age at the time of fetal infection could not be determined. It is possible that the fetuses were infected in the third trimester and were incubating syphilis at the time of birth. All of the infected infants were treated with penicillin within 3 weeks of age or as soon as they were proven to be infected with syphilis; their clinical and immunological status was unchanged from birth at the time of treatment.

Chesney and Kemp (1924) demonstrated *T. pallidum* by rabbit inoculation of CSF from five of 34 patients with secondary syphilis, when the CSF was normal according to routine laboratory and serological tests. It is not surprising, therefore, that "normal" CSF of congenital syphilitics contains virulent treponemes, since congenital syphilis is analogous to the disseminated disease of secondary syphilis. What is surprising in congenital syphilis is that the patient may be seronegative and not develop manifestations of congenital syphilis until much later in life, as has been reported in congenital syphilitic labyrinthitis (Kerr, 1970).

Approximately 30% of infected fetuses die *in utero* from syphilis and are miscarried or stillborn. The remainder are born live, but only a very small percentage have manifestations of congenital syphilis at birth or develop them within the first few days of life (Peterson, 1944). Thus the majority of infants appear to be healthy, and, although most will show definite clinical manifestations of syphilis within 6–12 months, the manifestations of the infection may be so minimal as to be unnoticed (Benirschke, 1974). These children then enter latency, which may be followed by the onset of tertiary lesions between the third and fifteenth years.

The lesions of fetal and early congenital syphilis are remarkable for their content of treponemes and plasma cells. Those of late congenital syphilis have a morphology similar to the of lesions of acquired tertiary syphilis. Among the lesions that are unique for late congenital syphilis are interstitial keratitis, Clutton's joints (a painless hydrarthrosis usually of the knee), malformation of the permanent molar teeth ("mulberry" molars), and hypertrophic osteitis of the tibia producing the well-known saber-shin deformity of the tibia.

4.2.3. Infection in Compromised Hosts

There is virtually no published information about syphilis infection in patients with congenital immunodeficiency or in those immunosuppressed by chemotherapeutic drugs. Turner and Hollander (1954) found that the administration of cortisone in moderate to large doses to rabbits with skin chancres changed the character of the syphilitic lesions from a cartilaginous consistency to ones which were soft and filled with a mucoid material identified as hyaluronic acid. In contrast to lesions in untreated rabbits, which have a marked mononuclear inflammatory reaction, the chancres of cortisone-treated rabbits were relatively acellular and the numbers of *T. pallidum* present were greatly increased. On withdrawal of cortisone, the chancres reverted to their precortisone characteristics but became much larger than those of control animals similarly inoculated, and a high proportion of animals developed signs of extensive disease. These changes were attributed to the immunosuppressive effect of cortisone. The mode of action of cortisone at the cellular level is poorly understood, but studies in cortisone-treated mice suggest that the drug induces functional defects in accessory and T-helper cells (Lee *et al.*, 1975). Advantage has been taken of the effect of cortisone in syphilitic rabbits to produce testicular lesions that contain large numbers of *T. pallidum* for experimental use that are relatively free of contamination by rabbit tissue (Hardy and Nell, 1975).

Smolin *et al.* (1970) also found that treatment of rabbits with antilymphocyte serum alone or in combination with cortisone acetate before inoculation of *T. pallidum* significantly shortened the time of onset and the appearance of syphilitic lesions, which were larger and more necrotic.

5. Immune Response to Infection

5.1. Immunopathological Phenomena

The cause of tissue damage in syphilis is not known. Most believe that it is caused primarily by the immune response of the host to the treponeme, its metabolic products, or soluble antigens rather than by direct tissue destruction. Much of the evidence in support of this concept is derived from the histopathological appearance of syphilitic lesions and the observation that those of congenital syphilis do not develop unless infection occurs after the age of fetal immunocompetence. Also, the gumma of tertiary syphilis closely resembles the cellular immune response to the tubercle bacillus in a tuberculin-sensitive host. The deposition of soluble treponemal antigen–antibody complexes causes glomerulonephritis and nephrotic syndrome in secondary (Gamble and Reardan, 1975) and congenital (Wiggelinkhuizen *et al.* 1973) syphilis. Finally, autoimmune phenomena are not uncommon in syphilis, as evidenced by the host response to cardiolipin antigen and the paroxysmal cold hemoglobinuria associated with tertiary and congenital syphilis. The cold hemoglobinuria is mediated by autoantibody, first described by Donath and Landsteiner in 1904, that reacts with the P blood group antigen at temperatures below 20°C and causes hemolysis when the antibody-coated cell is warmed to 37°C (Leddy and Swisher, 1971).

5.2. Natural Resistance

Man has no natural immunity to syphilis, and the likelihood of acquiring syphilis after exposure is related to the degree and duration of contact and the number and virulence of organisms at the contact site. Nonspecific host factors probably account for the natural resistance of some experimental animals to syphilis, but their contribution to acquired immunity is largely unknown. As mentioned previously, elevated body temperatures are prejudicial to treponeme survival. Fever therapy produced by inoculation of malaria parasites was routinely used with some success to treat neurosyphilis before the penicillin era.

The immune immobilization of *T. pallidum* *in vitro* by treponemal antibodies requires complement and lysozyme. One of the characteristic features of this reaction is a lag phase of several hours' duration before treponemes are immobilized. Turner and Hollander (1957) postulated that the mucoid slime layer prevents the fixation of antibodies to treponemal cell wall antigens and that the lag phase in the immobilization of treponemes reflects the destruction of this protective coating by lysozyme. Müller *et al.* (1973) showed that, in a lysozyme-free medium, damage to the cell wall by treponemal antibodies and complement could be repaired by the organism. Lysozyme acts on the mucopeptide layer of the cell wall only when it is damaged by a preceding complement-dependent immune reaction. This observation suggests that animals which are genetically complement or lysozyme deficient might be expected to develop severe syphilis infections. Titus (1977) found this to be the case in lysozyme-deficient rabbits but not in others lacking the sixth component of complement.

The sex of experimental animals influences the rate of lesion development and severity of syphilis. Female rabbits usually have milder infections, as is usually the case in human syphilis. The reasons for this are unknown, but it has been suggested that it may be associated with hormonal regulation, a greater ability of macrophages to process antigen in the female, or enhanced B- or T-lymphocyte stimulation in the female (Miller, 1976).

5.3. Acquired Resistance

Many of the experimental studies center on investigations of the immune response in syphilis, particularly under what circumstances and for how long immunity remains once established, the differing degrees of immunity at different stages of the disease, the mechanism of immune development, and the part played by humoral antibody and cell-mediated immunity.

Once infected with *T. pallidum*, both man (Magnuson *et al.* 1956) and experimental animals (Turner and Hollander, 1957; Magnuson and Rosenau, 1948) acquire a resistance to superinfection that is directly related to the duration of the primary or "immunizing" infection and inversely related to the number of treponemes in the challenge inoculum. Magnuson and Rosenau (1948) observed that challenge with homologous *T. pallidum* after syphilis infection in rabbits had one of three results: (1) symptoms were produced without evidence of resistance; (2) a symptomless infection resulted, detectable only by lymph node transfer; or (3) the host was not reinfected, as evidenced by the absence of local lesions and negative lymph node transfer. In a later, classical study, Magnuson *et al.* (1956) challenged 52 human volunteers who had had previous syphilis with 100,000 virulent *T. pallidum*, Nichols strain, given intracutaneously at a single site. Of 11 patients previously treated for early syphilis, nine developed dark-field-positive lesions, while two developed dark-field-negative lesions. All of these patients responded with increased reagin antibody titers and were considered to be reinfected. None of the five patients with untreated latent syphilis showed clinical or serological response to virulent challenge and were "resistant" to reinfection. Only ten of 26 patients previously treated for proved or presumed late latent syphilis were reinfected; one developed a dark-field-positive lesion and nine had dark-field-negative lesions. One of the latter lesions was a gumma. These workers concluded that resistance to syphilis develops first to a stage where infection is symptomless and later to the point where no infection is established.

Turner and Nelson (1950) found the rate of development of resistance to reinfection to be directly related to the degree of antigenic stimulus stemming from the multiplication of treponemes in the host: the larger the inoculum, the shorter the incubation period, the larger the lesions, the greater the degree of resistance. The relatively small contribution of duration of infection to resistance was demonstrated by producing subclinical infections in rabbits by judicious administration of penicillin (Hollander *et al.*, 1952). If sublethal amounts of penicillin were given after the appearance of primary lesions, the rate of lesion development was only one-sixth of that of untreated infections.

Hunter in 1810 showed that patients with primary syphilis could often not be reinoculated successfully with material from their primary lesion ("chancre immunity"). He also observed the same phenomenon in secondary syphilis and wrongly concluded that the lesions of secondary syphilis were noninfectious. The reinoculation experiments of Magnuson *et al.* (1956) on human volunteers showed that resistance to reinfection is not complete until the lesions of secondary syphilis have healed and that once established this resistance tends to persist for life. Resistance to reinfection is considered to be solid evidence of acquired immunity, but knowledge of the effector mechanisms is meager.

5.3.1. Humoral Antibody Response

The search to identify the resistance or immune factors in syphilis historically focused on treponemal antibodies. The Wassermann or reagin antibody was initially thought to be specific for syphilis, but the ubiquitous nature of the cardiolipin antigen in mammalian tissue and the lack of any correlation between the presence of large amounts of reagin and resistance to reinfection proved that it did not contribute to syphilis immunity (Eagle and Fleischman, 1948).

Reagin antibodies should not be confused with IgE. In syphilis they refer to IgM and IgG immunoglobulins that are of considerable diagnostic value. The reagin antibody is often the first to be produced after infection, and its titer correlates with the amount of tissue injury caused by syphilis (Schipper and Chesney, 1950). Serial measurements of reagin titer, most commonly by the VDRL test, are used to assess therapeutic response in early syphilis; adequate treatment is followed by a decline in titer, and reinfection in the absence of clinical lesions is indicated by a rise in titer.

A number of antibodies specific for treponemal antigens are also produced during syphilis. These include antibodies that react *in vitro* with *T. pallidum* to cause its immobilization and lysis in the presence of complement (the TPI antibody of Nelson and Mayer, 1949), agglutination (Hardy and Nell, 1955), hemagglutination of erythrocytes coated with treponemes (Tomizawa *et al.*, 1969), and opsonization (Metzger and Michalska, 1974).

The demonstration of "protective" antibodies in the serum of rabbits by Eberson (1921) and the rough correlation between high TPI titers in syphilitic rabbits and resistance to reinfection by Turner and Nelson (1950) supported the concept that antibodies alone accounted for immunity to syphilis. This concept has been challenged by the observation that passively transferred maternal antibody provided little or no protection to the fetus (Kemp and Fitzgerald, 1938) and the failure by many investigators to establish any correlation between the presence of TPI antibody and host resistance (McLeod and Magnuson, 1951; Magnuson *et al.*, 1951; Miller, 1973).

Other experimental evidence, however, supports the concept that humoral antibody contributes to syphilis immunity. Perine *et al.* (1973) showed that large amounts (80 ml/kg) of syphilis-immune rabbit serum given by intraperitoneal injection arrested the progression of early syphilomas in rabbits and delayed the appearance of syphilitic lesions if given to nonimmune rabbits before intradermal challenge with virulent *T. pallidum*. These authors and others (Septijian *et al.*, 1973; Turner *et al.*, 1973) also noted that the syphilitic lesions in immune serum-treated rabbits were smaller, did not ulcerate, and were often dark-field negative. Weiser *et al.* (1976) and Bishop and

Miller (1976a) demonstrated that the development of lesions was completely suppressed as long as immune serum was given. Titus (1977) showed that the protective factors in immune serum were contained in the IgG fraction, and Bishop and Miller (1976b) established a close correlation between the neutralizing or protective activity of immune serum and its TPI antibody titer.

Although the manner by which treponemal antibodies act is unknown, they probably serve to immobilize the organisms, prevent their attachment to cells, and destroy them when conbined with complement. There is no convincing evidence that viable, pathogenic treponemes are actively phagocytized (Turner, 1970). Reynolds (1941) observed that treponemes inoculated into the subcutaneous tissues of immune rabbits did not disseminate from the site of inoculation, whereas in nonimmune rabbits the organisms entered the regional lymphatics within minutes and were rapidly disseminated by the draining lymphatics and bloodstream. The promptness of this localizing effect in the immune animal suggests that the immune forces involved were humoral rather than cellular. This suggestion is supported by the findings of Turner et al. (1973), who noted that passively transferred immune serum decreased the number of metastatic syphilitic lesions in recipient rabbits. One protective effect of immune serum, therefore, is probably to limit multiplication and dissemination of treponemes. That immune factors other than antibody operate in syphilis is indicated by the experiments of Magnuson and Rosenau (1948) in which rabbits treated with penicillin 24 weeks after an immunizing infection were completely immune to challenge with 10^5 virulent treponemes. A comparable level of protection cannot be achieved by passive transfer of immune serum.

5.3.2. Cell-Mediated Response

A great deal of experimental evidence indicates that cell-mediated immune responses play an important role in both the immunopathology of and acquired immunity to syphilis. This includes an impairment of cellular immunity in the early stages of acquired and congenital syphilis, progressive development of strong delayed hypersensitivity during the course of the infection, and enhancement of the experimental infection in rabbits with antilymphocyte serum and corticosteroids.

The most convincing evidence for the participation of cell-mediated immunity (CMI) in syphilis is derived from the histopathological appearance of the gummatous lesions and the delayed skin reactions produced by syphilitic tissue extracts (luetins) in the late stages of infection. Gummas are destructive allergic granulomas containing surprisingly few treponemes and can be produced in the skin of some patients with tertiary syphilis by inoculation of virulent T. pallidum (Magnuson et al., 1956). Luetin skin tests were introduced by Neisser in 1908 as a diagnostic aid but were soon abandoned because they were almost uniformly negative in early syphilis and because they lacked specificity, no doubt because of contamination of luetin preparations with autologous tissue. Later studies with relatively pure formalin- or heat-killed T. pallidum as antigen improved the specificity of the "luotest" and confirmed earlier observations that delayed skin reactions were usually negative in primary and early secondary syphilis but positive thereafter, except in general paresis (Marshak and Rothman, 1951; Turner and Hollander, 1957). Wright and Grimble (1974) proposed that a specific anergy to T. pallidum occurred during early syphilis, since the response to other common skin test antigens (candida, mumps, etc.) was not impaired.

The response of lymphocytes from syphilitic patients to both treponemal antigens and nonspecific mitogens has been investigated by several groups. Levene et al. (1969) found that transformation of lymphocytes in response to phytohemagglutinin (PHA) was impaired in patients with secondary syphilis. They attributed this phenomenon to a factor present in the plasma of patients with secondary syphilis, since lymphocytes from these patients responded normally to PHA in nonsyphilitic plasma. The nonspecific activity of the plasma factor was shown by its ability to impair PHA transformation of lymphocytes from normal patients. The nature of the plasma factor has not been defined. It may be present in serum of patients with primary and secondary syphilis (Kantor, 1975), but it has different physical properties than does antibody (Wright and

Grimble, 1974), being inactivated on freezing at −70°C (Friedmann and Turk, 1978). Musher *et al.* (1975) showed that lymphocytes from patients with primary and secondary syphilis were not transformed *in vitro* when exposed to *T. pallidum, T. refringens, T. reiteri,* trichophytin, and monilia antigens. Suppression was unrelated to serum factors, and lymphocyte response to mitogens (PHA, pokeweed mitogen, and streptolysin) was identical to that of normal control lymphocytes. Friedmann and Turk (1978) also reported suppression of lymphocyte transformation in Ethiopian patients with primary and secondary syphilis. Autologous plasma from these patients inhibited the response of their own lymphocytes and those from a single healthy European control subject to PPD and PHA. These findings contrast with the results from an earlier study in England in which impaired lymphocyte transformation was found only in patients with early secondary syphilis (Friedmann and Turk, 1975). In both of these studies lymphocyte transformation by *T. pallidum* was restored 7–10 days after treatment, perhaps as the result of the generation of increased sensitized T lymphocytes by the release of spirochetal antigens by the abrogation of immunological paralysis by reduction of antigen load, or by the appearance in the peripheral circulation of lymphocytes that had been trapped in syphilitic lesions. The differences in lymphocyte transformation between Ethiopian and English patients may reflect unknown genetic differences in their response to *T. pallidum.* Impaired lymphocyte transformation during secondary syphilis in both populations may be related to depletion of the thymus-dependent lymphocytes from the paracortical areas of lymph nodes as a direct response to the presence of large numbers of spirochetes (Turner and Wright, 1972).

Since congenital syphilis corresponds to the secondary stage of acquired infection, it is not surprising that Friedmann (1977) found that peripheral lymphocytes from neonates born of mothers with untreated latent syphilis and some older infants with active congenital syphilis were unresponsive to PPD and *T. pallidum,* even when lymphocytes from their mothers were reactive to both antigens. This phenomenon may also be related to a depletion of thymus-dependent lymphocytes from lymphoid tissue, which has been described in the spleens of infants dying with congenital syphilis (Levene *et al.,* 1971). Skin sensitization by dinitrochlorobenzene is also impaired in infants with congenital syphilis (Parent and Smythe, 1973).

Other *in vitro* parameters of lymphocyte function have not been so well investigated as lymphocyte transformation. Fulford and Brostoff (1972) performed an assay of leukocyte migration inhibitory factor production on a total of 47 patients with syphilis at various stages, using commercially prepared Reiter protein as antigen. Stimulation of leukocyte migration was observed in primary syphilis and inhibition of migration in active tertiary syphilis. These were interpreted as evidence for weak and strong delayed hypersensitivity, respectively. Neither stimulation nor inhibition of leukocyte migration was seen in patients with secondary syphilis, indicating either failure or suppression of CMI in secondary syphilis.

Cell-mediated immune responses in experimental rabbit syphilis are somewhat different from those of man. The intradermal injection of treponemal antigens or virulent or attenuated *T. pallidum* in repeated doses does not evoke an allergic reaction in syphilitic rabbits, regardless of the duration of the infection (Rich *et al.,* 1933; Magnuson *et al.,* 1956; Miller, 1973). Whereas the production of leukocyte inhibitory factor is stimulated in primary syphilis of man, migration of rabbit peritoneal exudate cells from syphilitic rabbits is not inhibited in the presence of Reiter protein during the first 4 weeks of rabbit syphilis, which corresponds to the primary stage of the human infection. However, the migration of these peritoneal exudate cells is inhibited later in rabbit syphilis as the syphilitic lesions begin to heal (Pavia *et al.,* 1977a). These results indicate that macrophage inhibitory factor (MIF) is not produced in the early stages of syphilis but is present later in infection.

In other experiments Pavia *et al.* (1977b) demonstrated suppressed lymphocyte transformation to T-cell mitogens (Con A, PHA, and pokeweed mitogen) during the first 4 weeks of experimental rabbit syphilis but a normal level of transformation to B-cell mitogen (antirabbit immunoglobulin) and to Reiter protein. They also found that rabbit serum obtained during the first 4 weeks of infection significantly reduced the blastic response of autologous lymphocytes to Con A. They concluded that T-cell reactivity is markedly reduced during early infection, although B-cell reactivity (humoral immunity) was normal throughout infection.

Pavia *et al.* (1977c) further assessed the apparent selectivity of the lymphocyte response during experimental rabbit syphilis by separating peripheral lymphocytes into T- and B-cell populations and monitoring their response to different mitogens and to *T. pallidum*. It was clear that Con A- and PHA-induced transformation of purified T cells was markedly reduced during early infections, although the response to B-cell mitogens (antiimmunoglobulin G and lypopolysaccharide) was normal. A surprising finding was the transformation of lymphocytes in the T-cell population by *T. pallidum* which was diminished by autologous syphilitic serum. The authors concluded that the poor blastogenic response of T lymphocytes to Con A and PHA is due to the presence of regulatory factors, such as soluble inhibitory substances and/or suppressor T cells.

Although evidence indicates that CMI is activated in syphilis, attempts to increase host resistance to *T. pallidum* by activating the mononuclear phagocyte system before infection have been unsuccessful. Rabbits injected with BCG strain of *Mycobacterium bovis* before challenge with *T. pallidum* developed syphilitic lesions at the same time and of the same magnitude as did non-BCG-treated controls (Graves and Johnson, 1975; Schell *et al.*, 1975). Furthermore, the administration of two doses of BCG before infection enhanced syphilitic lesion development. Using a different approach, Schell and Musher (1974) showed that syphilitic rabbits have an enhanced ability to suppress challenge infection by *Listeria monocytogenes*. They attributed this enhanced listericidal activity to nonspecific sensitized T lymphocytes and *T. pallidum*, although there was no evidence that the activated macrophages were phagocytosing treponemes.

The demonstration of impaired T-cell function in early syphilis and of delayed hypersensitivity to treponemal antigens in the late stages of disease does not necessarily establish a protective role for CMI in syphilis. Attempts to measure protection by passive transfer of immune lymphocytes in experimental animals, as was done with immune serum, have been hampered by the lack of syngeneic rabbits, which would ensure survival of donor cells in the recipient. Metzger and Smogor (1975) transferred lymphocytes obtained from the popliteal lymph nodes of syphilis-immune, outbred female rabbits to nonimmune rabbits of the same breed and sex. The donor rabbits were made immune to syphilis either by immunization with *T. pallidum* rendered noninfectious by storage at 4°C (Metzger and Smogor, 1969) or by infection with virulent organisms. The infections in the latter group were terminated by penicillin treatment 3 months after infection. Nonimmune rabbits given a total of 7×10^6 immune lymphocytes intravenously showed evidence of protection when challenged with 10^4 virulent *T. pallidum* 24 hr after lymphocyte transfer, as measured by an absence of syphilitic lesions at the challenge sites or by a reduced number and delayed incubation period of chancres in the recipient rabbits (mean 18.6 days) compared to normal controls (mean 11.6 days). There was no difference in protection between rabbits given lymphocytes from immunized or penicillin-treated rabbits. Recipients given lymphocytes from normal rabbits developed syphilis lesions after the same period of incubation as did control rabbits (11–13 days).

By contrast, Baughn *et al.* (1977) could not transfer protection to virulent challenge with 10^3 *T. pallidum* by passive transfer of 10^9 spleen lymphocytes from chancre-immune rabbits. The adoptive transfer experiments were performed in both outbred and inbred rabbits. The latter were shown to be syngeneic by maintaining skin grafts for more than 19 months and by exhibiting no histocompatibility differences in one-way, mixed lymphocyte reactions. The failure to transfer protection with immune lymphocytes, therefore, did not result from decreased survival of donor lymphocytes. Furthermore, transfer of tuberculin hypersensitivity was readily accomplished in syngeneic rabbits with the same number of sensitized splenic lymphocytes that were used in the syphilis experiments. It is possible that had Baughn *et al.* (1977) used lymphocytes from lymph nodes draining syphilitic lesions instead of splenic lymphocytes in their adoptive transfer experiments, protection would have been observed. Hardy *et al.* (1978) found that lymph node lymphocytes respond earlier in the course of experimental infection and more intensely to T-cell mitogens and treponemal antigens than do sensitized splenic lymphocytes.

In any consideration of acquired resistance to syphilis, the relative efficiency of local, as well as systemic, factors in immunity should be kept in mind (Weiser *et al.*, 1976). It is possible that effective specific immunity, cellular and/or humoral, can be mounted locally in the primary lesion and initiate healing before strong systemic immunity develops. Local cellular immunity may be mediated by activated macrophages or by lymphokines secreted by sensitized lymphocytes.

6. Immunodiagnosis

Serological tests play a major role in the diagnosis of syphilis, especially during latent infection. There are two general categories of serological tests: nontreponemal tests, which detect antibodies of the IgG or IgM class historically termed "reagin," and treponemal tests, which detect antibodies specific for treponemal antigens (Table 2).

The prototype of the nontreponemal tests was introduced by Wasserman *et al.* in 1906. They used an aqueous extract of syphilitic fetal liver as antigen in a complement-fixation test to detect what they thought was specific syphilis antibody. Shortly thereafter, it was shown that alcoholic extracts of nonsyphilitic organs contained the same lipoidal antigen, and that the Wasserman antibody was therefore an autoantibody directed against a constituent of normal tissue. Presumably the in-

TABLE 2. Serological Tests for Syphilis

Test system	Reporting system	Antigen	Antibody	Sensitivity	Specificity	Prototype[a]
Flocculation	Nonreactive, weakly reactive, or reactive, titer in dilutions (dils)	Cardiolipin	"Reagin," IgM (early), IgG	Good	Good but false positives; common in low-syphilis-prevalence populations	VDRL, RPR
Complement fixation	As above, or reactive 1+ to 4+	Cardiolipin	As above	Good but less than flocculation tests	As above	Wassermann
Complement fixation	As above	Reiter treponeme protein	IgG, IgM	Decreased in latent syphilis	Good, but detects treponemal group antigen	RPCF
Immobilization	As above	Viable *T. pallidum*, Nichols strain	IgG	Decreased in early and late syphilis	Very good	TPI
Indirect fluorescent antibody	Nonreactive, borderline, or reactive 1+ to 4+	Killed *T. pallidum*, Nichols strain	IgG and IgM, in a ratio of 3:1	Very good	Very good	FTA ABS
Hemagglutination	Nonreactive or reactive	*T. pallidum* attached to sheep or turkey erythrocytes	As above	Very good but less sensitive than FTA ABS in primary syphilis	Very good	TPHA

[a] See text for explanation of abbreviations.

flammatory response in syphilis damages cells, causing the release of the phospholipid antigen. The nontreponemal tests are, therefore, not specific for syphilis, and are often reactive in certain chronic infections and connective tissue disorders (Garner, 1970).

A large number of nontreponemal tests have been described (Table 2). All use cardiolipin antigen (commercially prepared from beef heart) mixed with measured amounts of lecithin and cholesterol to detect reagin antibody by either flocculation or complement fixation. These tests have enormous value in syphilis since they are sensitive, inexpensive, and simple to perform. The titer of reagin antibody correlates well with the rate of tissue destruction and is the sole guide for assessing the effectiveness of therapy in the absence of syphilitic lesions. Reagin is present in about 70% of patients with primary syphilis and in high titer in all secondary syphilitics (Figure 3). Reagin is variably present in patients with tertiary syphilis, and may be absent in the cerebrospinal fluid of neurosyphilitics, especially those with tabes dorsalis.

The reagin titer should decrease within a few months after effective therapy for syphilis. The antibody may not disappear altogether in patients treated during the secondary stage or later in the course of syphilis. Patients who have received adequate treatment for these stages of syphilis usually remain seropositive ("serofast") in low titer for life. This phenomenon presumably reflects persisting tissue injury with release of lipoidal antigens.

The prototype of the treponemal antigen tests was the *Treponema pallidum* immobilization (TPI) test developed by Nelson and Mayer in 1949. Viable *T. pallidum*, Nichols strain, organisms were used to detect immo-

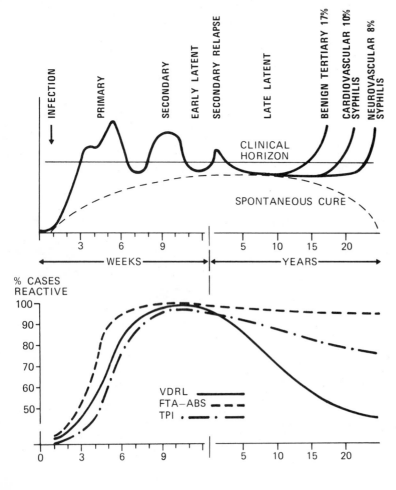

Figure 3. Clinical and serological course of syphilis. Approximately one-third of untreated patients develop tertiary syphilis, one-third remain seroreactive but do not develop tertiary lesions, and the remaining one-third become seronegative or "spontaneously" cured. The fluorescent treponemal antibody adsorption (FTA ABS) and the *Treponema pallidum* immobilization (TPI) tests are not quantitated. The titer of the Venereal Disease Research Laboratory (VDRL) reagin antibody test usually falls to low levels after the secondary stage unless tertiary syphilis ensues.

bilizing antibodies in syphilitic serum in the presence of complement (see Section 5.2). The TPI remains the most specific tests for syphilis antibody, but because of its technical complexity and expense it has been all but replaced by the fluorescent treponemal antibody (FTA) or *T. pallidum* hemagglutination (TPHA) assays.

The FTA test is an indirect fluorescent antibody test and uses as antigen a suspension of dead *T. pallidum* extracted from rabbit testicular tissue. To improve specificity, test serum is adsorbed with lyophilized supernatant from cultures of the Reiter biotype of *T. phagedenis* (commercially available as "Sorbent") before testing; this process presumably removes from the test serum cross-reacting treponemal antibodies produced against the avirulent treponemes of the gastrointestinal tract. The FTA adsorption (FTA ABS) test is more sensitive than the TPI test and has comparable specificity.

The hemagglutination tests for syphilis antibody were developed in the past decade. The antigen is a suspension of formalized, tanned sheep or turkey erythrocytes which have been sensitized with sonicated *T. pallidum*, Nichols strain. These tests are comparable to the FTA ABS in sensitivity and specificity.

The treponemal antibody tests are used to confirm reactive nontreponemal reagin tests. They are occasionally positive in diseases other than syphilis, such as sytemic lupus erythematosus. This reactivity may be due to the production of anti-DNA antibodies which attach to the DNA of *T. pallidum* used in the FTA ABS test (Wright *et al.*, 1975). Neither the FTA ABS nor TPHA test is quantitated since the antibody is usually present in very high titer so as to make quantitation meaningless. These tests, moreover, seldom revert to negative status during the course of treated or untreated syphilis.

The IgM FTA test was introduced to facilitate the diagnosis of early congenital syphilis in the absence of dark-field-positive lesions (Scotti and Logan, 1968). The test procedure is exactly like the FTA ABS except that fluorescein-labeled antihuman IgM is used as conjugate to detect only IgM antitreponemal antibody produced by the infant and not IgG of maternal origin. The test has not been widely used because the false-negative rate is consid-

erable in delayed-onset disease (Kaufman *et al.*, 1974). Reimer *et al.* (1975) questioned the specificity of the IgM FTA test for syphilis because syphilitic infants make relatively large amounts of IgM antibodies (rheumatoid factor) to maternal IgG allotypes (Gm factors).

7. Immunoprevention

7.1. Passive Immunization

The protection against virulent challenge afforded a normal rabbit given syphilis-immune serum is an example of passive immunization. The therapeutic potential of syphilis-immune serum was demonstrated in monkeys by Metchnikoff and Roux in 1905, but Ehrlich's "magic bullet," arsphenamine, introduced as a singularly effective treponenicidal drug for treatment of syphilis in 1910, obviated the therapeutic value of syphilis-immune serum. Furthermore, the experiments of Metchnikoff and Roux (1905), as well as those of Finger and Landsteiner (1906), showed that small amounts of syphilis-immune serum given prophylactically only modified the appearance of challenge syphilitic lesions, and did not afford complete protection.

7.2. Active Immunization

The feasibility of a syphilis vaccine is based on the development of specific immunity to *T. pallidum* during the course of syphilis. Unfortunately, most attempts have failed to induce artificial immunity in experimental animals by vaccination with *T. pallidum* inactivated by a variety of chemical and physical methods, nonpathogenic treponemes, and treponemal fractions or by-products (Miller, 1976). The primary reason for failure is lack of knowledge about the immunogenic antigens of *T. pallidum*.

Metzger *et al.* (1969) noted that syphilitic serum contains antibodies that differ in their ability to agglutinate *T. pallidum*, one of which was directed against a heat-labile treponemal protein. They showed that this protein antigen was present in freshly extracted treponemes stored at 4°C in phosphate-buffered saline (PBS), pH 7.4, for as long as 10 days. Thereafter, the organisms were not agglutinated by syphilitic serum, and the preparation did not stimulate the production of antibody to the heat-labile antigen. They demonstrated that the heat-labile antigen was destroyed by proteolytic enzymes, formalin, and phenol. To test the immunogenicity of the heat-labile antigen, treponemes were first rendered noninfectious by storage at 4°C and then given to nonimmune female rabbits in 28 divided doses over 7 weeks, for a total of 8×10^9 organisms. When immunized rabbits were challenged with 10^5 virulent *T. pallida* 5 weeks after completion of the immunization schedule, none of the 16 immunized rabbits developed lesions. However, ten of the 16 immunized rabbits were asymptomatically infected, as measured by positive lymph node transfer experiments.

Miller (1973) produced complete protection, lasting for at least 1 year, to virulent challenge with 10^3 and 10^5 homologous *T. pallidum* by immunizing male rabbits with a total of 3.71×10^9 γ-irradiated (620,000 R) treponemes, in 60 divided doses over a 37-week period. He had previously shown that treponemes irradiated with 520,000 R remained viable, did not multiply, and were noninfectious (Miller, 1967). Immunized rabbits, however, were not protected against virulent challenge with 10^3 *T. pertenue*.

These studies prove that a syphilis vaccine is possible, although hardly practical. The large number of organisms and the prolonged immunization schedules required to produce transient, limited protection mimic the natural course of infection. Although it may be possible to isolate and concentrate the treponemal immunogens so that only a few vaccine doses need to be given, the utility of such a vaccine in human populations is questionable. It is even difficult to determine who would be immunized. For example, if the syphilis vaccine prevents only symptomatic infection, the vaccinated individual runs the risk of not being diagnosed and treated before tertiary complications ensue. Moreover, the vaccine is likely to induce the production of both reagin and treponemal antibodies, with the result that diagnostic serological tests would be useless. Finally, as demonstrated by Miller (1973), immunization with only one species of treponemes does not provide protection from infection with other pathogenic species, and the differences in protection afforded by different strains of *T. pallidum* in rabbits (Turner and

Hollander, 1957) indicate that a multivalent vaccine would probably be necessary.

Unfortunately, vaccine experiments have not shed much light on the respective roles of humoral and cellular immunity in syphilis. Miller (1973) observed that although TPI antibody developed during the course of immunization and was present at the time of the first challenge with virulent treponemes, it was not present in rabbits rechallenged 1 year after immunization was completed, nor did the challenge organisms provoke an anamnestic rise in TPI antibody. In future vaccine experiments it would be of great interest to know whether or not serum and/or lymphocytes from immunized animals adoptively transferred to normal animals protect the recipient against virulent challenge.

8. Conclusion

Clearly, our knowledge of the biological properties of *T. pallidum* and the pathogenesis of syphilis is limited. The evidence is incontrovertible that both man and experimental animals acquire a resistance to reinfection by *T. pallidum* during the course of untreated infection. The relative contribution of humoral and cell-mediated immunity to acquired resistance has yet to be determined.

The bulk of experimental evidence indicates that acquired immunity in syphilis does not necessarily eliminate *T. pallidum* from the host. The presence of treponemes in the lesions of tertiary syphilis occurs in the face of strong immunity to reinfection. These organisms may survive and escape immune destruction by residing within host cells or by acquiring a mucoid slime layer that protects it against treponemicidal antibodies, phagocytic cells, or other cells potentiated by lymphokines. It is possible that the strong systemic immunity at this stage of infection depends more on memory B cells and possibly T-helper cells than it does on circulating antibody levels (Weiser *et al.*, 1976). Such cells could be quickly mobilized to sites of infection and set up intense local production of treponemicidal antibody. If this amnestic response is the major determinant of protective immunity, it would explain the need for frequent and large doses of immune serum to convey passive immunity in experimental rabbits. In the actively immunized animal it could account for the reported lack of correlation between the serum levels of treponemal antibody and resistance to superinfection (Magnuson *et al.*, 1951; Metzger *et al.*, 1969; Miller, 1973).

The contribution of cell-mediated responses to acquired immunity in syphilis remains controversial. A major problem has been the lack of a suitable culture system for *T. pallidum* that would provide large numbers of organisms free of tissue contamination for use in *in vitro* tests of lymphocyte function and vaccine studies. There is solid evidence in both man and experimental rabbits that cellular hypersensitivity to *T. pallidum* is impaired in the early stages of syphilis. This apparent defect in cell-mediated immunity may be due to a decrease in the number of T cells in the peripheral blood, as has been reported in viral infections (Niklasson and Williams, 1974), the destruction and depletion of thymus-dependent lymphocytes by *T. pallidum* (Turner and Wright, 1972), the presence of T-suppressor cells (Pavia *et al.*, 1977c), or the presence of a plasma or serum inhibitory substance (Levene *et al.*, 1969). The last may be a lymphocytotoxic treponemal factor (Friedmann and Turk, 1975), a blocking antibody, or treponemal antigen–antibody immune complexes which are known to cause suppression of T-cell blastogenesis (Hellstrom and Hellstrom, 1970; Ryan *et al.*, 1975). Wright and Grimble (1974) proposed that this period of transient immunosuppression could be due to competition between treponemal antigens, where one antigen selectively competes and interferes with the response to other antigens, thereby creating a state of partial or split tolerance. This phenomenon may also explain the suppression of lymphocyte transformation in neonates infected with *T. pallidum* who have no signs of congenital syphilis.

The failure by Baughn *et al.* (1977) to adoptively transfer syphilis immunity in syngeneic rabbits with spleen lymphocytes calls into question the contribution of cellular immunity to acquired immunity in syphilis. It is well known that there is no relationship between delayed hypersensitivity to tuberculin and acquired immunity to tuberculosis (Youmans, 1975), and this may be the case in syphilis. Delayed hypersensitivity to treponemal anti-

gens, however, is the cause of the destructive lesions of tertiary syphilis.

The complexity of the immune response in syphilis, particularly the delicate balance eventually achieved between the host and parasite in latent syphilis, is, in the view of Turner (1970), "one of the most interesting and challenging unknowns in the realm of infectious diseases. The more one seeks the whole, the more parts one discovers, yet at rare intervals great synthesizing flashes bring simplicity from complexity."

References

Azar, H. A., Pham, T. D., and Kurban, A. T., 1970, An electron microscopic study of a syphilitic chancre, *Arch. Pathol.* **90:**143–150.

Baseman, J. B., 1977, Summary of the workshop of the biology of *Treponema pallidum*: Cultivation and vaccine development, *J. Infect. Dis.* **136:**308–311.

Baughn, R. E., Musher, D. M., and Simmons, C. B., 1977, Inability of spleen cells from chancre-immune rabbits to confer immunity to challenge with *Treponema pallidum*, *Infect. Immun.* **17:**535–540.

Beck, A. C., and Daily, W. T., 1938, Syphilis in pregnancy, in: *Syphilis* (F. R. Moulton, ed.), pp. 101–114, American Association for the Advancement of Science Publication No. G, Washington, D.C.

Benirschke, K., 1974, Syphilis—the placenta and the fetus, *Am. J. Dis. Child.* **128:**142–143.

Bishop, N. N., and Miller, J. N., 1976a, Humoral immunity in experimental syphilis I. The demonstration of resistance conferred by passive immunization, *J. Immunol.* **117:**191–196.

Bishop, N. N., and Miller, J. N., 1976b, Humoral immunity in experimental syphilis. II. The relationship of neutralizing factors in immune serum to acquired resistance, *J. Immunol.* **117:**197–207.

Chesney, A. M., and Kemp, J. E., 1924, Incidence of *Spirochaeta pallida* in cerobrospinal fluid during the early stages of syphilis, *J. Am. Med. Assoc.* **83:**1725–1728.

Christiansen, S., 1963, Protective layer covering pathogenic treponemata, *Lancet* **1:**423–425.

Clark, E. G., and Danbolt, N., 1964, The Oslo study of the natural course of untreated syphilis, *Med. Clin. N. Am.* **48:**613–623.

Cox, C. D., 1972, Shape of *Treponema pallidum*, *J. Bacteriol.* **109:**943–944.

Cox, C. D., and Barber, M. K., 1974, Oxygen uptake by *Treponema pallidum*, *Infect. Immun.* **10:**123–127.

Dippel, A. L., 1944, The relationship of congenital syphilis to abortion and miscarriage, and the mechanisms of intrauterine protection, *Am. J. Obstet. Gynecol.* **47:**369–379.

Eagle, H., and Fleischman, R., 1948, The antibody response in rabbits to killed suspensions of pathogenic *T. pallidum, J. Exp. Med.* **87**:369–384.

Eberson, F., 1921, Immunity studies in experimental syphilis, *Arch. Derm. Syph.* **4**:490–511.

Elsas, F. J., Smith, J. L., Israel, C. W., and Gager, W. E., 1968, Late syphilis in the primate, *Br. J. Vener. Dis.* **44**:267–273.

Fieldsteel, A. H., Becker, F. A., and Stout, J. G., 1977, Prolonged survival of virulent *Treponema pallidum* in cell-free and tissue culture systems, *Infect. Immun.* **18**:173–182.

Finger, E., and Landsteiner, K., 1906, Untersuchungen über Syphilis an Affen, *Arch. Derm. Syph.* **78**:335–367.

Fitzgerald, T. J., Miller, J. N., and Sykes, J. A., 1975, *Treponema pallidum* (Nichols strain) in tissue cultures: Cellular attachment, entry and survival, *Infect. Immun.* **11**:1133–1140.

Fitzgerald, T. J., Miller, J. N., Sykes, J. A., and Johnson, R. C., 1976, Tissue culture and *Treponema pallidum*, in: *The Biology of Parasitic Spirochetes* (R. Johnson, ed.), pp. 57–64, Academic Press, New York.

Fitzgerald, T. J., Johnson, R. C., Sykes, J. A., and Miller, J. N., 1977, Interaction of *Treponema pallidum* (Nichols strain) with cultured mamalian cells: Effects of oxygen, reducing agents, serum supplements, and different cell types, *Infect. Immun.* **15**:444–452.

Fleming, W. L., 1964, Syphilis through the ages, *Med. Clin. N. Am.* **48**:587–612.

Foster, J. W., Kellogg, D. S., Clark, J. W., and Ballows, A., 1977, The *in vitro* culture of *Treponema pallidum*: Corroborative studies, *Br. J. Vener. Dis.* **53**:338–339.

Frazier, C. N., Bensel, A., and Keuper, C. S., 1952, Further observation on the duration of spirochetemia in rabbits with asymptomatic syphilis, *Am. J. Syph.* **36**:167–173.

Fribourg-Blanc, A., and Mollaret H. H., 1969, Natural treponematosis of the African primate, *Primates Med.* **3**:113–121.

Friedmann, P. S., 1977, Cell-mediated immunological reactivity in neonates and infants with congenital syphilis, *Clin. Exp. Immunol.* **30**:271–276.

Friedmann, P. S., and Turk, J. L., 1975, A spectrum of lymphocyte responsiveness in human syphilis, *Clin. Exp. Immunol.* **21**:59–64.

Friedmann, P. S., and Turk, J. L., 1978, The role of cell-mediated immune mechanisms in syphilis in Ethiopia, *Clin. Exp. Immunol.* **31**:59–65.

Fulford, K. W. M., and Brostoff, J., 1972, Leucocyte migration and cell-mediated immunity in syphilis, *Br. J. Vener. Dis.* **48**:483–488.

Gamble, C. N., and Reardan, J. B., 1975, Immunopathogenesis of syphilitic glomerulonephritis, *N. Engl. J. Med.* **292**:449–454.

Garner, M. F., 1970, The biological false-positive reaction to serologic tests for syphilis, *J. Clin. Pathol.* **23**:31–34.

Gelfand, J. A., Elin, R. J., Berry, F. W., and Frank, M. M., 1976, Endotoxemia associated with the Jarisch–Herxheimer reaction, *N. Engl. J. Med.* **295**:211–213.

Graves, S., and Johnson, R., 1975, Effect of pretreatment with *Mycobacterium bovis* (strain BCG) and immune syphilitic serum on rabbit resistance to *Treponema pallidum, Infect. Immun.* **12**:1029–1036.

Grin, E. I., and Guthe, T., 1973, Evaluation of a previous mass campaign against endemic syphilis in Bosnia and Herzegovina, *Br. J. Vener. Dis.* **49**:1–19.

Hackett, C. J., 1963, On the origin of the human treponematoses, *Bull. WHO* **29**:7–41.

Hardy, J. B., Hardy, P. H., Oppenheimer, E. H., Ryan, S. J., Jr., and Sheff, R. N., 1970, Failure of penicillin in a newborn infant with congenital syphilis, *J. Am. Med. Assoc.* **212**:1345–1349.

Hardy, P. H., Jr., 1976, Pathogenic treponemes, in: *The Biology of Parasitic Spirochetes* (R. Johnson, ed.), pp. 107–119, Academic Press, New York.

Hardy, P. H., and Nell, E. E., 1955, Specific agglutination of *Treponema pallidum* by sera from rabbits and human beings with treponemal infections, *J. Exp. Med.* **101**:367–382.

Hardy, P. H., and Nell, E. E., 1961, Influence of osmotic pressure on the morphology of the Reiter treponeme, *J. Bacteriol.* **82**:967–978.

Hardy, P. H., and Nell, E. E., 1975, Isolation and purification of *Treponema pallidum* from syphilitic lesions in rabbits, *Infect. Immun.* **11**:1296–1299.

Hardy, P. H., Fredericks, W. R., and Nell, E. E., 1975, Isolation and antigenic characteristics of axial filament from the Reiter treponeme, *Infect. Immun.* **11**:380–386.

Hardy, P. H., Nell, E. E., Klein, J. R., and Prendergast, J. H. U., 1978, Specific stimulation of cells from various lymphoid tissues of rabbits with early syphilitic infection, *Abst. 18th Interscience Conference on Antibiotic Agents and Chemotherapy*, p. 197, American Society Microbiology, Washington, D.C.

Harter, C. A., and Benirschke, K., 1976, Fetal syphilis in the first trimester, *Am. J. Obstet. Gynecol.* **124**:705–711.

Hellstrom, K. E., and Hellstrom, I., 1970, Immunological enhancement as studied by cell culture techniques, *Annu. Rev. Microbiol.* **24**:373–398.

Hollander, D. H., Turner, T. B., and Nell, E. E., 1952, Effect of long-continued subcurative doses of penicillin during the incubation period of experimental syphilis, *Bull. Johns Hopkins Hosp.* **90**:105–120.

Holt, S. C., 1978, Anatomy and chemistry of spirochetes, *Microbiol. Rev.* **42**:114–160.

Hovind-Hougen, K., 1976, Determination by means of electron microscopy of morphological criteria of value for classification of some spirochetes, in particular treponemes, *Acta. Path. Microbiol. Scand. B Suppl.* **255**:1–41.

Jackson, S., and Black, S. H., 1971, Ultrastructure of *Treponema pallidum* Nichols following lysis by physical and chemical methods. 1. Envelope, wall, membrane and fibrils, *Arch. Mikrobiol.* **76**:308–324.

Johnson, R. C. (ed.), 1976, *The Biology of Parasitic Spirochetes,* Academic Press, New York.

Jones, R. H., Finn, M. A., Thomas, J. J., and Folger, C., 1976, Growth and subculture of pathogenic *T. pallidum* (Nichols strain) in BHK-21 cultured tissue cells, *Br. J. Vener. Dis.* **52**:18–23.

Kampmeier, R. H., 1964, The late manifestations of syphilis: Skeletal, visceral and cardiovascular, *Med. Clin. N. Am.* **18**:667–697.

Kantor, F. S., 1975, Infection, anergy and cell-mediated immunity, *N. Engl. J. Med.* **292**:629–634.

Kast, C. C., and Kolmer, J. A., 1933, On the cultivation of *Spirochaeta pallida* in living tissue media, *Am. J. Syph.* **17**:529–532.

Kaufman, R. E., Jones, O. G., Blount, J. H., and Wiesner, P. J., 1977, Questionnaire survey of reported early congenital syphilis, *Sex. Transm. Dis.* **4**:135–139.

Kaufman, R. E., Olansky, D. C., and Wiesner, P. J., 1974, The FTA-ABS (IgM) test for neonatal congenital syphilis: A critical review, *J. Am. Vener. Dis. Assoc.* **1**:79–84.

Kemp, J. E., and Fitzgerald, E. M., 1938, Studies in experimental congenital syphilis and the transference of immunity from immune syphilitic female rabbits to their offspring, *J. Invest. Dermatol.* **1**:353–365.

Kerr, A. G., 1970, Congenital syphilitic labyrinthitis, *Arch. Otolaryngol.* **91**:474–478.

Kuhn, U. S. G., 1970, The treponematoses, in: *The Chimpanzee,* Vol. 3 (G. H. Bourne, ed.), pp. 71–81, Karger, New York.

Lee, K., Langman, R. E., Paetkan, V. H., and Diener, E., 1975, The cellular basis of cortisone-induced immunosuppression of the antibody response studied by its reversal *in vitro, Cell. Immunol.* **17**:405–417.

Leddy, J. P., and Swisher, S. N., 1971, Acquired immune hemolytic disorders, in: *Immunological Diseases* (M. Santer, D. W. Talmage, B. Rose, W. B. Sherman, and J. H. Vaughan, eds.), pp. 1083–1110, Little, Brown, Boston.

Levene, G. M., Turk, J. L., Wright, D. J. M., and Grimble, G. S., 1969, Reduced lymphocyte transformation due to a plasma factor in patients with active syphilis, *Lancet* **2**:246–247.

Levene, G. M., Wright, D. J. M., and Turk, J. L., 1971, Cell-mediated immunity and lymphocyte transformation in syphilis, *Proc. R. Soc. Med.* **64**:426–428.

McCord, J. R., 1929, Study of 200 autopsies made on syphilitic fetuses, *Am. J. Obstet. Gynecol.* **18**:597–601.

McLeod, C. P., and Magnuson, H. J., 1951, Development of treponemal immobilizing antibodies in mice following injection of killed *Treponema pallidum, J. Vener. Dis. Inform.* **32**:274–279.

Magnuson, H. J., and Rosenau, B. J., 1948, The rate of development and degree of acquired immunity in experimental syphilis, *Am. J. Syph.* **32**:418–436.

Magnuson, H. J., Eagle, H., and Fleischman, R., 1948, The minimal infectious inoculum of *Spriochaeta pallida* (Nichols strain) and a consideration of its rate of multiplication *in vivo, Am. J. Syph.* **32**:1–18.

Magnuson, H. J., Thompson, F. A., and McLeod, C. P., 1951, Relationship between treponemal immobilizing antibodies and acquired immunity of experimental syphilis, *J. Immunol.* **67**:41–48.

Magnuson, H. J., Thomas, E. W., Olansky, S., Kaplan, B. T., De Mello, L., and Cutler, J. C., 1956, Inoculation of syphilis human volunteers, *Medicine* **35**:33–82.

Mahoney, J. F., and Bryant, K. K., 1933, Contact infection of rabbits in experimental syphilis, *Am. J. Syph.* **17**:188–193.

Marshak, L. C., and Rothman, S., 1951, Skin testing with a purified suspension of *Treponema pallidum, Am. J. Syph.* **35**:35–41.

Metchnikoff, E., and Roux, E., 1905, Etudes experimentales sur la syphilis, *Ann. Inst. Pasteur* **19**:673–698.

Metzger, M., and Michalska, E., 1974, *Treponema pallidum* opsonophagocytic test, *Arch. Immunol. Ther. Exp. (Warsz)* **22**:745–758.

Metzger, M., Michalska, E., Podwinska, J., and Smogor, W., 1969, Immunogenic properties of the protein component of *Treponema pallidum, Br. J. Vener. Dis.* **45**:299–304.

Metzger, M., and Smogór, W., 1969, Artificial immunization of rabbits against syphilis, *Br. J. Vener. Dis.* **45**:308–312.

Metzger, M., and Smogór, W., 1975, Passive transfer of immunity to experimental syphilis in rabbits by immune cells, *Arch. Immun. Ther. Exp.* **23**:625–630.

Miller, J. N., 1967, Immunity in experimental syphilis. IV. The immunogenicity of *Treponema pallidum* attenuated by γ-irradiation, *J. Immunol.* **99**:1012–1016.

Miller, J. N., 1973, Immunity in experimental syphilis. VI. Successful vaccination of rabbits with *Treponema pallidum,* Nichols strain, attenuated by γ-irradiation, *J. Immunol.* **110**:1206–1215.

Miller, J. N., 1976, Potential for vaccines for venereal diseases, *Bull. N.Y. Acad. Med.* **52**:986–1003.

Moore, J. E., 1939, Unsolved clinical problems of syphilogy, *Am. J. Syph.* **23**:701–711.

Müller, F., Feddersen, H., and Segerling, M., 1973, Studies on the action of lysozyme in immune immobilization of *Treponema pallidum* (Nichols strain), *Immunology* **24**:711–719.

Musher, D. M., Schell, R. F., Jones, R. H., and Jones, A. M., 1975, Lymphocyte transformation in syphilis: An *in vitro* correlate of immune suppression *in vivo? Infect. Immun.* **11**:1261–1264.

Nelson, R. A., Jr., 1948, Factors affecting the survival of *Treponema pallidum in vitro, Am. J. Hyg.* **48**:120–132.

Nelson, R. A., and Mayer, M. M., 1949, Immobilization of *Treponema pallidum in vitro* by antibody produced in syphilitic infection, *J. Exp. Med.* **89**:369–393.

Nichols, H. J., and Hough, W. H., 1913, Demonstration

of *Spirochaeta pallida* in the cerebrospinal fluid from a patient with nervous relapse following use of salvarsan, *J. Am. Med. Assoc.* **60**:108–110.

Niklasson, P. M., and Williams, R. C., Jr., 1974, Studies of peripheral blood T- and B-lymphocytes in acute infections, *Infect. Immun.* **9**:1–7.

Noguchi, H., 1911, A method for the pure cultivation of pathogenic *Treponema pallidum (Spirochaeta pallida)*, *J. Exp. Med.* **14**:99–108.

Ohta, Y., 1972, *Treponema pallidum* antibodies in syphilitic mice as determined by immunofluorescence and passive hemagglutination techniques, *J. Immunol.* **108**:921–926.

Ovcinnikov, N. M., and Delektorskij, V. V., 1970, Ultrafine structure of the cell elements in hard chancres of the rabbit and their interrelationship with *Treponema pallidum, Bull. WHO* **42**:437–444.

Ovcinnikov, N. M., and Delektorskij, V. V., 1971, Current concepts of the morphology and biology of *Treponema pallidum* based on electron microscopy, *Br. J. Vener. Dis.* **47**:315–328.

Parent, M. A., and Smythe, P. M., 1973, Dinitrochlorobenzene sensitization in congenital syphilis, *Lancet* **2**:1273.

Pavia, C. S., Folds, J. D., and Baseman, J. B., 1977a, Development of macrophage migration inhibition in rabbits infected with virulent *Treponema pallidum, Infect. Immun.* **17**:651–654.

Pavia, C. S., Baseman, J. B., and Folds, J. D., 1977b, Selective response of lymphocytes from *Treponema pallidum* infected rabbits to mitogens and *Treponema reiteri, Infect. Immun.* **15**:417–422.

Pavia, C. S., Folds, J. D., and Baseman, J. B., 1977c, Selective *in vitro* response of thymus-derived lymphocytes from *Treponema pallidum*-infected rabbits, *Infect. Immun.* **18**:603–611.

Perine, P. L., Weiser, R. S., and Klebanoff, S. J., 1973, Immunity to syphilis I. Passive transfer in rabbits with hyperimmune serum, *Infect. Immun.* **8**:787–790.

Perine, P. L., Krause, D. W., Awoke, S., and Duncan, M. E., 1978, Congenital syphilis in Ethiopia, unpublished manuscript.

Peterson, J. C., 1944, Congenital syphilis, in: *Essentials of Syphilogy* (R. H. Kampmeier, ed.), pp. 412–445, Lippincott, Philadelphia.

Purtilo, D. T., Hallgren, H. M., and Yunis, E. J., 1972, Depressed maternal lymphocyte response to phytohaemagglutinin in human pregnancy, *Lancet* **1**:769–771.

Raiziss, G. W., and Severac, M., 1937, Rapidity with which *Spirochaeta pallida* invades the blood stream, *Arch. Derm. Syph. (Chicago)* **35**:1101–1109.

Reimer, C. B., Black, C. M., Phillips, D. J., Logan, L. C., Hunter, E. F., Pender, B. J., and McGrew, B. E., 1975, The specificity of fetal IgM: Antibody or anti-antibody? *Ann. N.Y. Acad. Sci.* **254**:77–93.

Rein, M. F., 1976, Biopharmacology of syphilotherapy, *J. Am. Vener. Dis. Assoc.* **3**:109–127.

Reynolds, F. W., 1941, The fate of *Treponema pallidum*

inoculated subcutaneously into immune rabbits, *Bull. Johns Hopkins Hosp.* **69**:53–60.

Rich, A. R., Chesney, A. M., and Turner, T. B., 1933, Experiments demonstrating that acquired immunity in syphilis is not dependent upon allergic inflammation, *Bull. Johns Hopkins Hosp.* **52**:179–202.

Ryan, J. L., Arbeit, R. O., Dickler, H. B., and Henkart, P. A., 1975, Inhibition of lymphocyte mitogenesis by immobilized antigen–antibody complexes, *J. Exp. Med.* **142**:814–826.

Sandok, P. L., Jenkin, H. M., Matthews, H. M., and Roberts, M. S., 1978, Unsustained multiplication of *Treponema pallidum* (Nichols virulent strain) *in vitro* in the presence of oxygen, *Infect. Immun.* **19**:421–429.

Schell, R. F., and Musher, D. M., 1974, Detection of nonspecific resistance to *Listeria monocytogenes* in rabbits infected with *Treponema pallidum, Infect. Immun.* **9**:658–662.

Schell, R., Musher, D., Jacobson, K., Schwethelm, P., and Simmons, C., 1975, Effect of macrophage activitation on infection with *Treponema pallidum, Infect. Immun.* **12**:505–511.

Schiller, N. L., and Cox, C. D., 1977, Catabolism of glucose and fatty acids by virulent *Treponema pallidum, Infect. Immun.* **16**:60–68.

Schipper, G. J., and Chesney, A. M., 1950, The effect of the method of inoculation on the behavior of the serologic test for syphilis in experimental syphilis of the rabbit, *Am. J. Syph.* **34**:25–33.

Scotti, A. T., and Logan, L., 1968, A specific IgM antibody test in neonatal congenital syphilis, *J. Pediatr.* **73**:242–243.

Septijian, M. D., Salussalo, D., and Thivolet, J., 1973, Attempt to protect rabbits against experimental syphilis by passive immunization, *Br. J. Vener. Dis.* **49**:335–337.

Silverstein, A. M., 1962, Congenital syphilis and the timing of immunogenesis in the human fetus, *Nature (London)* **194**:196–197.

Smibert, R. M., 1976, Classification of nonpathogenic treponemes, borrelia, and spirochaeta, in: *The Biology of Parasitic Spirochetes* (R. Johnson, ed.), pp. 121–131, Academic Press, New York.

Smith, J. L., and Israel, C. W., 1968, Recovery of spirochaetes in the monkey by passive transfer from human late seronegative syphilis, *Br. J. Vener. Dis.* **44**:109–115.

Smolin, G., Nozik, R. A., and Okumoto, M. S., 1970, Growth of *Treponema pallidum* in rabbits, *Am. J. Ophthalmol.* **70**:273–276.

Sykes, J. A., Miller, J. N., and Kalan, A. J., 1974, Treponema pallidum within cells of a primary chancre from a human female, *Br. J. Vener. Dis.* **50**:40–44.

Titus, R. G., 1977, Studies on immunity in experimental syphilis, Ph.D. thesis, University of Washington, Seattle.

Tomizawa, T., Kasamatsu, S., and Yamaya, S., 1969, Usefulness of the hemagglutination test using *Treponema pallidum* (TPHA) for the serodiagnosis of syphilis, *Jpn. J. Med. Sci. Biol.* **22**:341–350.

Tremont, E. C., 1976, Persistence of *Treponema pallidum* following penicillin G therapy: Report of two cases, *J. Am. Med. Assoc.* **236**:2206–2207.

Turner, D. H., and Wright, D. J. M., 1972, Lymphadenopathy in early syphilis, *J. Pathol.* **110**:305–308.

Turner, T. B., 1970, Syphilis and the treponematosis, in: *Infectious Agents and Host Reaction* (S. Mudd, ed.), pp. 346–389, Saunders, Philadelphia.

Turner, T. B., Hardy, P. H., and Newman, B., 1969, Infectivity tests in syphilis, *Br. J. Vener. Dis.* **45**:183–196.

Turner, T. B., Hardy, P. H., Jr., Newman, B., and Nell, E. E., 1973, Effects of passive immunization on experimental syphilis in the rabbit, *Johns Hopkins Med. J.* **133**:241–251.

Turner, T. B., and Hollander, D. H., 1954, Studies on the mechanism of action of cortisone in experimental syphilis, *Am. J. Syph.* **38**:371–387.

Turner, T. B., and Hollander, D. H., 1957, *Biology of the Treponematoses,* World Health Organization, Monograph Series 35, Geneva.

Turner, T. B., and Nelson, R. A., 1950, The relationship of treponemal immobilizing antibody to immunity in syphilis, *Tr. Assoc. Am. Physicians* **63**:112–117.

Wassermann, A., Neisser, A., and Brück, C., 1906, Eine serodiagnostische Reaktion bei Syphilis, *Dtsch. Med. Wochenschr.* **32**:745–746.

Weber, M. W., 1960, Factors influencing the *in vitro* survival of *Treponema pallidum, Am. J. Hyg.* **71**:401–417.

Weiser, R. S., Erickson, D., Perine, P. L., and Pearsall, N. N., 1976, Immunity to syphilis: Passive transfer in rabbits using serial doses of immune serum, *Infec. Immun.* **13**:1402–1407.

Wiegand, S. E., Strobel, P. L., and Glassman, L. H., 1972, Electron miscroscopic anatomy of pathogenic *Treponema pallidum, J. Invest. Dermatol.* **58**:186–204.

Wiggelinkhuizen, J., Kaschula, R. O. C., Uys, C. J., Kuijten, R. H., and Dale, J., 1973, Congenital syphilis and glomerulonephritis with evidence for immune pathogenesis, *Arch. Dis. Child.* **48**:375–381.

Willcox, R. R., 1960, Evolutionary cycle of the Treponematoses, *Br. J. Vener. Dis.* **36**:78–90.

Willcox, R. R., 1974, Changing patterns of treponemal disease, *Br. J. Vener. Dis.* **50**:169–178.

Willcox, R. R., and Guthe, T., 1966, *Treponema pallidum: A Biographical Review of the Morphology, Culture, and Survival of T. pallidum and Associated Organisms,* World Health Organization, Geneva, World Health Organization Technical Report No. 455, 1970, Geneva.

Wright, D. J. M., and Grimble, A. S., 1974, Why is the infectious stage of syphilis prolonged? *Br. J. Vener. Dis.* **50**:45–49.

Wright, J. T., Cremer, A. W., and Ridgway, G. L., 1975, False positive FTA-ABS results in patients with genital herpes, *Br. J. Vener. Dis.* **51**:329:330.

Yobs, A. R., Clark, J. W., Mothershed, S. E., Bullard, J. C., and Artley, C. W., 1968, Further observations on the persistence of *Treponema pallidum* after treatment in rabbits and humans, *Br. J. Vener. Dis.* **44**:116–130.

Youmans, G. P., 1975, Relation between delayed hypersensitivity and immunity in tuberculosis, *Am. Rev. Resp. Dis.* **111**:109–118.

Zeigler, J. A., Jones, A. M., Jones, R. H., and Kubica, K. M., 1976, Demonstration of extracellular material at the surface of pathogenic *T. pallidum* cells, *Br. J. Vener. Dis.* **52**:1–8.

17

Immunology of Mycoplasma Infection

GERALD W. FERNALD, WALLACE A. CLYDE, Jr., and
FLOYD W. DENNY

1. Introduction

"Mycoplasma(s)" is the trivial name for organisms in class Mollicutes, which contains two families and five genera (Freundt, 1974a; Edward, 1974). These organisms are distinguished from bacteria by the absence of cell wall and small size, with a genome mass of $4–8 \times 10^8$ daltons (Bak *et al.*, 1969). Although they resemble large viruses in size and filterability, unlike viruses they are able to grow on cell-free media. The lack of a cell wall also accounts for the resistance to penicillins which characterizes all mycoplasmas. This class of microorganisms is thus unique in that it includes the smallest free-living forms to be found in nature.

Mycoplasma infections have quite recently been recognized by medical scientists, although veterinarians have contended with a variety of species since the early 1900s. There are over 40 mycoplasma species which infect a variety of animals and plants (Table 1). The list includes exotic organisms, such as *Thermoplasma* and insect mycoplasmas. The economic importance of certain of the plant organisms has been appreciated only recently. As mycoplasma infections become more generally recognized, the role of host immunity

in the pathogenesis of disease is demanding increased attention. This chapter is intended to provide a view of the field of mycoplasmology as it relates to the science of immunology. The immunology of *Mycoplasma pneumoniae* infection will be emphasized because this entity is the only human disease clearly known to be caused by mycoplasmas.

Mycoplasma species tend to be host, organ, and tissue specific (Freundt, 1974b). This specificity is reflected in some instances by taxonomic nomenclature, such as in the human species—*M. buccale, M. orale, M. faucium,* and *M. pneumoniae*. Exceptions to this generality are found in closely related animal hosts, i.e., *M. pulmonis* is a common respiratory pathogen of both rats and mice, and *M. gallisepticum* infects chickens as well as turkeys. There are nine mycoplasma species found in man (Table 2). Some of the human mycoplasmas may be found in one or more nonhuman primates. *M. pneumoniae* is clearly recognized as a human respiratory tract pathogen. *M. orale* and *M. salivarium* are part of the normal respiratory flora, and *M. hominis* and *Ureaplasma urealyticum* (T strains) commonly inhabit the genital tract. These organisms are not found normally in other nonprimate hosts. *Acholeplasma laidlawii* is ubiquitous and may be cultured from a large variety of animals, culture materials, and sewage. The widespread use of animal sera or cells in culture systems appears to explain many reported isolations of various nonhuman

GERALD W. FERNALD, WALLACE A. CLYDE, Jr., and FLOYD W. DENNY • Department of Pediatrics, University of North Carolina School of Medicine, Chapel Hill, North Carolina 27514.

TABLE 1.   Ecology of the Mycoplasmatales

Habitat	Genera	Characteristic features	Species
Mammals	*Mycoplasma*	Pleuropneumonia in cattle	*mycoides*
		Bronchiectasis in rats	*pulmonis*
		Polyarthritis in rats	*arthritidis*
		Agalactia in goats	*agalactiae*
		"Rolling disease" in mice	*neurolyticum*
		Pneumonia in man	*pneumoniae*
	Acholeplasma	Nasal parasite in swine	*granularum*
	Ureaplasma	Urogenital parasite in man	*urealyticum*
	Spiroplasma	Suckling mouse cataract agent	—
Birds	*Mycoplasma*	Synovitis in poultry	*synoviae*
		Sinusitis in turkeys	*gallisepticum*
Insects	*Spiroplasma*	Plant disease vectors	*citri*
Plants	*Spiroplasma*	Citrus stubborn disease	*citri*
Hot springs	*Thermoplasma*	60°C optimum, pH 2.0	*acidophillum*
Soil and wastes	*Acholeplasma*	Ubiquitous; infected with mycoplasma virus	*laidlawaii*

strains from clinical specimens (Freundt, 1974c). Unless strict microbiological controls are employed, such contaminating organisms may be misinterpreted as etiological agents (Edward, 1974; Jansson *et al.*, 1971).

In addition to the unique features of mycoplasmas discussed above, the nature of the mycoplasma–host cell relationship is of special interest to the immunologist. In most instances these organisms parasitize surface membranes. A large number of species seem to be nonpathogenic commensals and exhibit little or no direct effect on the tissue to which they attach. In several instances, to be discussed in detail later, the pathogenicity of the organism seems to relate to the host immune response rather than toxicity of the infecting agent *per se*. These facts suggest that mycoplasmas are old and well-adapted parasites. Not only is study of the host reaction to human

mycoplasmas important, but also the variety of disease models to be found in animals may provide clues to the etiology of certain idiopathic human diseases (Edward, 1974).

Mycoplasmas provide interesting models for experimental immunology. Techniques of membrane lysis and reaggregation provide a specialized means for presenting selected antigens, including haptens, to a host. The organisms also are susceptible to complement injury and complement-mediated immune lysis (Brunner *et al.*, 1971, 1973d, 1976). The simplicity of mycoplasmas relative to bacteria—and complexity relative to erythrocytes—makes them useful tools for study of cell membrane lytic phenomena.

2.   Microbial Aspects of Mycoplasma Infection

2.1.   Antigenicity

2.1.1.   Antigenic Components of Mycoplasmas

Since mycoplasmas lack a cell wall, their antigenic constituents reside within the triple-layered membrane and intracellular substance. Membrane structural components are glycolipids analogous to the lipopolysaccharides of gram-negative bacteria (Smith *et al.*, 1973). These glycolipid haptens are capable of stimulating antibody synthesis when attached to proteins (Sobeslavsky *et al.*, 1966). In the case of *M. pneumoniae*, galactosyl and glycosyl diglycerides in the surface membrane

TABLE 2.   Mycoplasmas Indigenous to Man

Site	Species	Pathobiology
Respiratory tract	*M. pneumoniae*	Bronchitis, pneumonia
Oropharynx	*M. orale*	Normal flora
	M. buccale	Normal flora
	M. faucium	Normal flora
	M. salivarium	Normal flora
	M. lipophilum	Normal flora
	M. fermentans	Normal flora
	M. hominis	?Pharyngitis
Urogenital tract	*U. urealyticum*	Congenital pneumonia
		Amnionitis
		?Nonspecific urethritis
	M. hominis	Postpartum sepsis
	M. fermentans	Normal flora

appear to be the antigens responsible for stimulation of humoral immunity. Using lectins, Schiefer *et al.* (1974) studied the carbohydrate structures on the surface membranes of a variety of mycoplasmas. Both glucose and galactose were detected on untreated *M. pneumoniae, M. mycoides, M. pulmonis, M. gallinarum,* and *M. gallisepticum.* Pronase treatment had no effect, indicating that there were no glycoproteins. No carbohydrate structures were detected on *M. fermentans* and *A. laidlawii* until they were treated with pronase, suggesting that the glycolipids were hidden under a protein layer. *M. hominis* had no lectin activity, even after pronase treatment. Further analysis of *M. hominis* by Schiefer *et al.* (1975) has shown 87% of the membrane is phosphatidylglcerol; although this is a biologically active antigen, it is masked by surface proteins. Thus the antigenically active components of intact mycoplasmas are glycolipids contained in the cell membrane; exposed sugars on the membrane surface account for only a limited variety of specificities. Glycoproteins have not been found in most mycoplasmas.

A variety of proteins are demonstrable in mycoplasma membranes, accounting for 40–60% of the membrane components (Kahane and Marchesi, 1973). Of the 15 polypeptides identified in delipidated *M. pneumoniae* membranes by polyacrylamide gel electrophoresis, six were located on the external surface of the membrane by ^{125}I labeling. Only one of these surface proteins was a glycoprotein. Analysis of soluble proteins in sonically disrupted *M. pneumoniae* preparations yielded 25 bands on polyacrylamide gels, five of which were found in the culture medium (Lipman and Clyde, 1969). These proteins apparently are contained in the cell sap or are loosely attached to the interior cell membrane, since the membrane proteins are not soluble unless lysed with detergents (Hollingdale and Lemke, 1969).

2.1.2. Immune Response to Mycoplasma Components

Parenteral injection of whole mycoplasmas stimulates both humoral and cellular immune responses. If complete adjuvant is employed, a variety of antibodies are generated to membrane antigens and soluble proteins (Lemke,

1973). However, infection or intravenous inoculation of organisms without adjuvant generates only antibodies to cell membrane surface antigens (i.e., growth inhibiting, metabolic inhibiting, and indirect hemagglutinating reactivity). Similar antibodies are produced in rabbits by glycolipid haptens reaggregated with *M. laidlawii* membranes (Razin *et al.,* 1971). The activity of these antibodies can be blocked with the purified glycolipid haptens (Sobeslavsky *et al.,* 1966).

Soluble, lipid-depleted proteins of *M. pneumoniae* react weakly with CF antibodies from infected or immunized animals, as compared to the chloroform–methanol extracted lipid antigen, which reacts strongly (Kenny and Grayston, 1965). There is evidence, however, that mycoplasma protein antigens react with T lymphocytes. Mizutani and Mizutani (1975) have reported experiments comparing a lipid-depleted *M. pneumoniae* preparation with its acetone-soluble fraction in a macrophage migration-inhibition system. Whole, untreated organisms and the acetone-insoluble fraction were equally active inhibitors of the migration of peritoneal exudate cells from immunized guinea pigs. The lipid fraction was inactive. When tested for complement-fixing activity the reverse was found; the lipid antigen titered 1 : 512, while the lipid-depleted antigen titered 1 : 8. Mizutani (1975) has also reported that activity for delayed-typed skin reactions is retained in the lipid-depleted fraction of *M. pneumoniae.* These experiments suggest that the protein antigens of *M. pneumoniae* induce primarily cell-mediated immune responses while humoral immune responses are directed against the glycolipid haptens. Further experiments designed to characterize these apparently distinct components of *M. pneumoniae* should serve to clarify which antigens stimulate biologically important immunity in mycoplasma infections.

2.2. Pathogenicity

2.2.1. Attachment Mechanisms and Mobility

Three mycoplasma species have been found to have specific means of attaching to surfaces, as illustrated schematically in Fig. 1 (Clyde, 1975). These organisms, *M. pulmonis, M. gallisepticum,* and *M. pneumoniae,* also have a characteristic mobility which seems to

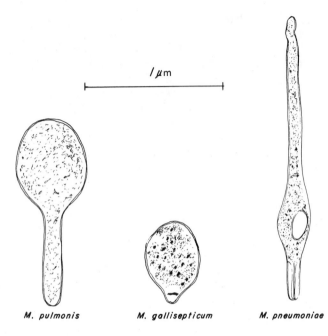

*1 μ*m

M. pulmonis   M. gallisepticum   M. pneumoniae

Figure 1. Schematic representation of three pathogenic mycoplasma species. Reproduced with permission of ASM publications (Clyde, 1975).

relate to the special attachment organelle. Bredt (1974) has shown that these mycoplasmas maintain contact with the surface of culture vessels by special structures and that movement across the surface proceeds from this lead point. The bleb of *M. gallisepticum* has been shown to be the point of attachment to animal cells (Zucker-Franklin *et al.*, 1966). *M. pulmonis* appears also to attach to ciliated epithelial cells by a specialized structure (Richter, 1970).

The most completely studied mycoplasma attachment system is that of *M. pneumoniae*. It attaches to a variety of surfaces, including plastic and glass (Somerson *et al.*, 1967; Taylor-Robinson and Manchee, 1967a), erythrocyte membranes (Sobeslavsky *et al.*, 1968), tissue culture cells (Manchee and Taylor-Robinson, 1969), spermatozoa (Taylor-Robinson and Manchee, 1967b), and tracheal epithelium of hamster and man (Collier *et al.*, 1971). Neuraminic acid receptors appear to be important for attachment of *M. pneumoniae* to erythrocytes and ciliated epithelium, since the interaction is blocked by either neuraminidase treatment of the target cell or treatment of the mycoplasma with sialic acid (Sobeslavski *et al.*, 1968).

The specialized structure of *M. pneumoniae* was discovered by Biberfeld and Biberfeld

(1970). Collier and Clyde (1974) determined that this specialized structure was the point of attachment to hamster and human bronchial epithelium *in vivo* and to human ciliated epithelium in sputum, thereby demonstrating that the specialized tip is functional in human disease (Fig. 2). The characteristic location of *M. pneumoniae* between the microvilli of ciliated respiratory epithelial cells with the tip, identified by its electron-dense central core, in contact with but not fused to the host cell membrane, suggests that this association of organism and host cell is the biologically effective form. Presumably mycoplasmas which do not penetrate the mucus blanket and attach to the mucosal cells are cleared from the respiratory tract by mechanical and phagocytic action.

The interaction of *M. pneumoniae* and pulmonary macrophages is influenced by the organism's cytadsorbing properties. Both *M. pneumoniae* and *M. pulmonis* attach to macrophages *in vitro*. However, they resist endocytosis until antimycoplasma antibody is added to the medium (Powell and Clyde, 1975; Jones and Hirsch, 1971). It is tempting to speculate that this antiphagocytic feature of *M. pneumoniae* and *M. pulmonis* may contribute to their ability to maintain prolonged colonization of the host tissues. Other phenomena

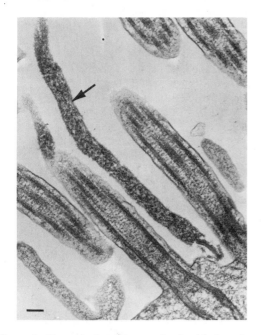

Figure 2. Electron photomicrograph of epithelium from hamster bronchus showing filamentous *Mycoplasma pneumoniae* organism (arrow) attached between cilia. The bar represents 0.1 μm. Reproduced with permission of CIBA Foundation (Collier, 1972).

appear to be involved, since *M. salivarium,* which colonizes the gingival sulci, does not cytadsorb and is phagocytosed by both polymorphonuclear and mononuclear phagocytes in the absence of serum or antibody (Parkinson and Carter, 1975). *M. hominis,* which colonizes the genital mucosa, appears to resist phagocytosis, whether or not antibody is present (Simberkoff and Elsbach, 1971).

2.2.2. Systemic Invasiveness of Mycoplasmas

Mycoplasmas colonize the human oral respiratory and genital mucosal surfaces but rarely penetrate systemically. *M. hominis* septicemia has been reported following gynecological surgery (Tully and Smith, 1968) and normal vaginal delivery (McCormack *et al.,* 1973). There is recent evidence that human ureaplasmas can penetrate the gravid uterus, based on reports of the isolation of these strains from internal organs of abortuses (Jones, 1967) and amniotic membranes (Brunell *et al.,* 1969). Recovery of *M. pneumoniae* from the bullae of Stevens-Johnson syndrome has been reported (Lyell *et al.,* 1967), but most large

series give no indication of systemic spread. In the hamster model *M. pneumoniae* is restricted to an extracellular location external to the basement membrane (Collier *et al.,* 1971). While immunosuppression promotes systemic invasion by *M. pulmonis* in mice (Denny *et al.,* 1972), antithymocyte serum treatment does not alter the virulence of *M. pneumoniae* for the hamster (Taylor and Taylor-Robinson, 1975; Taylor *et al.,* 1974). Although a few well-designed studies have been directed to this question, more work needs to be done to define the invasiveness of human mycoplasmas under ordinary conditions.

2.3. Toxicity

2.3.1. Specific Mycoplasma Toxins

Specific toxins are produced by some mycoplasmas. *M. neurolyticum* produces a neurotoxin which causes a specific encephalopathy in mice (but not in rats) called "rolling disease." The exotoxin is specific for receptors in the cerebellum of mice and physiologically disrupts the blood–brain barrier through endothelial cell cytoplasmic swelling leading to capillary occlusion (Sabin, 1941). *M. gallisepticum* strain S6 produces a cerebral arteritis in turkeys and pathophysiological changes similar to those of *M. neurolyticum,* although a specific exotoxin has not been demonstrated (Thomas *et al.,* 1966). This lesion does not appear in turkeys infected with nontoxic strains, which are nevertheless fully virulent, or in chickens inoculated with strain S6.

M. pneumoniae produces hydrogen peroxide, which is responsible for the hemolytic property of *M. pneumoniae* colonies (Clyde, 1963). Peroxide has been postulated to be a virulence factor responsible for the pathogenic effects of *M. pneumoniae* on respiratory epithelium (Cohen and Somerson, 1967). There is little direct evidence that this is so *in vivo.* Rather, direct cell-to-cell interaction is probably the critical factor, since a noncytadsorbing *M. pneumoniae* strain which produces H_2O_2 is avirulent for tracheal organ cultures and hamsters (Lipman and Clyde, 1969).

While the specific toxic factors of *M. pneumoniae* are not known, it is clear that the organism alters the metabolism and physiology of the host cell. Hu *et al.* (1975) have shown decreased uptake of galactose, orotic acid, and amino acids within 24 hr of infection of tracheal rings. Related inhibition of host cell ribonucleic acid and protein synthesis was also noted. No inhibitory effects were produced by a noncytadsorbing, avirulent *M. pneumoniae* strain. Host cell injury required continued protein synthesis by the attached mycoplasmas, since erythromycin treatment within 24 hr of infection reversed the injurious effects.

2.3.2. Immunosuppressive Effects of Mycoplasmas

Toxicity of mycoplasmas for lymphocytes has also been recognized. Copperman and Morton (1966) described reversible inhibition of mitosis in cultured lymphocytes by nonviable suspensions of *M. hominis*. The inhibitor was shown to be arginine deaminase, and the effect was common to all arginine-utilizing mycoplasmas (Simberkoff *et al.*, 1969). This phenomenon becomes important when an arginine-utilizing mycoplasma, such as *M. arthritidis*, is employed to stimulate lymphocytes from an immunized host. Controlling for both nonspecific inhibition and specific stimulation of mitosis is then critical (Cole *et al.*, 1975a).

An *in vivo* immunosuppressive effect of *M. arthritidis* on antibody responses to phage φ5 has been reported in rats (Kaklamanis and Pavlatos, 1972). Lymphocyte responses to PHA were also suppressed in these animals. *M. arthritidis* membranes produce a similar immunosuppressive effect on antibody responses to bacterial antigens in rabbits (Bergquist *et al.*, 1974). A possible explanation for the immunosuppressive effect of *M. arthritidis* extracts on the *in vivo* immune response has been offered by Eckner *et al.* (1974), who found that thymus cellularity was markedly decreased in young mice inoculated with this material. Histologically T-dependent cortical areas of the thymus and paracortical areas in lymph nodes were depleted by this treatment. Phytohemagglutinin and concanavalin A responses were suppressed, but the antibody response to sheep erythrocytes remained intact, suggesting a selective suppression of a T-lymphocyte subpopulation. A similar involutionary effect on mouse tissues by *M. fermentans* has been reported by Gabridge and Schneider (1975), although evaluation of immune mechanisms was not carried out.

Biberfeld and Sterner (1976a) have documented anergy to tuberculin skin testing in patients with *M. pneumoniae* pneumonia. In light of the universal use of BCG in Sweden, negative PPD skin tests early after onset of disease were notable in 22 of 36 patients. Repeated skin testing yielded a return of delayed hypersensitivity to tuberculin within 3–6 weeks, but prolonged tuberculin anergy was observed for more than 5 months in two patients. Control skin tests with *Candida* or other frequently positive antigens were not studied.

In a subsequent report Biberfeld and Sterner (1976b) extended these observations to include 47 recently infected subjects with the same results. In addition, lymphocyte activation *in vitro* by PPD and *M. pneumoniae* antigens was studied in 13 patients. In eight cases thymidine uptake stimulated by PPD was threefold lower during the *M. pneumoniae* illness than after recovery. This documentation of tuberculin nonreactivity, both *in vivo* and *in vitro*, strongly suggests that mycoplasma infections exert direct effects on the immune response of the host as do certain viruses such as measles. The implications of this phenomenon, if confirmed, are far-reaching both for experimental studies on the pathogenesis of mycoplasma diseases and for vaccine immunoprophylaxis.

2.3.3. Immunostimulatory Effects of Mycoplasmas

An apparently nonspecific stimulation of rat lymphocytes by *M. pulmonis in vitro* has been reported by Ginsburg and Nicolet (1973). Extensive blastogenesis was observed after 2 days of culture, resembling the mitogenic effect of lectins. Heating to 60°C or filtration (0.22 nm) removed the agent, suggesting that live organisms were involved. The mitogenicity of *M. pulmonis* has been confirmed by Cole *et al.* (1975b) in studies on mouse lymphocytes. In neither study was there evidence of prior sensitization of the lymphocytes; rather, the evidence favors a direct nonspecific effect of the viable mycoplasma on lymphocytes.

In a second paper Ginsburg's experiments have been reconfirmed in germ-free animals and the effect of other mycoplasmas on rat lymphocytes is reported (Naot *et al.*, 1977). In these experiments *M. pneumoniae*, *M. fermentans*, *M. hominis*, *M. orale*, and *A. laid-*

lowii did not activate rat lymphocytes but *M. pulmonis*, *M. arthritidis*, and *M. neurolyticum* did.

Biberfeld and Gronowicz (1976) reported that *M. pneumoniae* is a polyclonal activator for B lymphocytes in pathogen-free mice. The phenomenon has also been observed with human B cells (Biberfeld, 1977). They proposed that such direct stimulation of antibody-forming cells could account for the early production of nonspecific IgM antibodies in natural infection. Further evidence of mycoplasma-mediated activation of lymphocytes *in vitro* was presented by Cole and co-workers, who reported that interferon is induced by several mycoplasma species in sheep and human lymphocyte cultures (Cole *et al.*, 1976).

Cole *et al.* (1977) reported studies on the mitogenic potential of a large number of mycoplasma strains. Both arginine-utilizing and glucose-fermenting species, including *A. laidlawii* and *S. citri*, were mitogenic for mouse lymphocytes. In the case of the arginine deaminase-containing mycoplasmas, heat inactivation removed the inhibitory effect and allowed expression of a heat stable mitogenic factor. The mitogenic factor in *M. pneumoniae* reported by Biberfeld and Gronowicz (1976) was also heat stable, but in Ginsburg and Nicolet's experiments with *M. pulmonis* it was not. Further characterization of this factor (or factors) should be forthcoming now that its existence is established.

2.4. Interactions of Mycoplasmas and Other Microbial Flora in Man

The normal flora of the oral cavity, upper respiratory tract, and genital tracts includes a variety of bacteria, fungi, viruses and mycoplasmas. The intimate association of these organisms suggests the possibility of synergistic or antagonistic interactions between the various microorganisms. Microbial interaction involving mycoplasmas exists in animals (Fabricant, 1968) and in several experimental models (Reed, 1972). Type I pneumococcus, normally avirulent for hamsters, produces fatal sepsis if the animals are initially infected with *M. pneumoniae* (Liu et al., 1972). The demonstration that mycoplasmas stimulate interferon in leukocyte cultures raises the possibility that they could modify intercurrent viral infections (Cole *et al.*, 1976).

In man certain complications of *M. pneumoniae* infection—especially sinusitis (Griffin and Klein, 1971) and otitis media (Sobeslavsky *et al.*, 1965)—may depend on related bacterial infection, although the exact nature of these events has not been established. The frequent association of ureaplasmas (Shepard, 1970), as well as chlamydiae (Dunlop *et al.*, 1972), with nonspecific urethritis suggests the possibility of an interaction between these organisms. Although *M. salivarium* is intimately associated with gingival and dental plaque bacteria, there is no evidence that this is a pathogenic interaction (Kumagai *et al.*, 1971).

3. Host Factors in Human Mycoplasma Infections

With the exception of *M. pneumoniae*, the human mycoplasma species may generally be categorized as common parasitic inhabitants of the oropharynx or genital tract. The colonization rate seems to vary in different populations. Oropharyngeal mycoplasmas are found less frequently in young children and edentulous adults than in others (Razin *et al.*, 1964). Ureaplasmas occur in the genitourinary tracts of sexually active males and females more frequently than in children or sexually inactive adults. Such variables have been difficult to control in studies of the possible etiological role of these organisms in nonspecific urethritis and complications of pregnancy (McCormack, 1974).

Genetic factors generally do not appear to dictate expression of *M. pneumoniae* disease, since the problem is worldwide in distribution and occurs equally in males and females. However, more severe disease has been reported in patients with sickle cell disease (Shulman *et al.*, 1972) and B-lymphocyte immunodeficiency (Foy *et al.*, 1973). Although these are genetic disorders, the pathogenetic defects related to *M. pneumoniae* have not been studied.

The age-related pattern of *M. pneumoniae* disease suggests that host factors are important in mediating clinical expressions (Fernald *et al.*, 1975). While infection occurs as early as the first few months of life, it tends to be asymptomatic; pneumonia is diagnosed infrequently in infants and preschool children. After age 5, lower respiratory symptoms become increasingly apparent. The peak incidence of *M. pneumoniae* pneumonia is reached around 10 years of age, and this infection remains the most common cause of pneumonia in the adolescent and young adult. Thus in contrast to the common viral respiratory infections, which are most severe early in life, *M. pneumoniae* infections become increasingly manifest as the host matures.

Studies of the pathogenesis of *M. pneumoniae* disease indicate that much of the pathology detectable clinically and histologically is a manifestation of the host immune response to the organism (Fernald and Clyde, 1976). Epidemiological data indicate that reinfections with *M. pneumoniae* are quite common and that the severity of disease expression may relate directly to multiple encounters of host and organism (Fernald *et al.*, 1975). This phenomenon will be considered in detail in a subsequent section.

4. Microbe–Host Interactions

4.1. Host Response to Infection

With the exception of *M. pneumoniae,* there is little or no information on the immunology and immunopathology of human mycoplasma infections. For this reason, the remaining sections of this chapter will be concerned chiefly with this organism.

To understand the nature of the relationship between *M. pneumoniae* and the respiratory epithelium, one must be aware of the full spectrum of this infection. Characteristically several weeks pass from the period of acquisition and incubation to the termination of the carriage state. Symptoms, ranging from mild upper respiratory illness to bronchitis and pneumonia, appear 2–3 weeks after exposure, reach maximum espression in the next 2 weeks, and then gradually decline. Pathogenesis of the disease depends on attachment of the *M. pneumoniae* organisms to ciliated epithelial cells of the respiratory tract. Direct toxic effects of organism products on host cells have been demonstrated in tracheal organ cultures (Collier, 1972; Hu *et al.*, 1975). Indirectly, organisms and their products resulting from death and phagocytic degradation are responsible for stimulating the local immune-inflammatory response which constitutes the pneumonia characteristic of this infection. A review of *M. pneumoniae* disease pathogenesis has been published elsewhere (Fernald and Clyde, 1976). The following discussion deals with those features concerned with the immunological response of the host.

4.1.1. Pulmonary Histopathology

Because of the generally benign nature of *M. pneumoniae* pneumonia and its consequent low mortality, very few descriptions of human lung pathology are available (Maisel *et al.*, 1967). The lesions include peribronchiolar lymphocyte and plasma cell infiltration and edema of bronchiolar walls, interstitial infiltrates, some evidence of vasculitis, and a striking endobronchial exudate composed of both polymorphonuclear and mononuclear phagocytes. Such cases are the extreme, and the usual histopathology of *M. pneumoniae* disease can only be surmised. The sputum in nonfatal cases mirrors the endobronchial exudates described above, and the mycoplasmas can be seen attached to desquamated epithelial cells (Collier and Clyde, 1974). Fortunately, animal models have been developed for study of the evolution of the infection, its pathology and both humoral and cellular immune responses.

The most successfully exploited animal model of *M. pneumoniae* disease has been the Syrian hamster (Eaton *et al.*, 1944; Dajani *et al.*, 1965; Fernald and Clyde, 1976). The guinea pig can also be infected with *M. pneumoniae* (Brunner *et al.*, 1973c) and promises to be useful, particularly for studies on cell-mediated immune mechanisms. Tracheal rings from hamsters and human fetuses have been employed by Collier *et al.* (1972) for a series of *in vitro* experiments concerning the host cell–parasite relationship. These experimental models will be alluded to frequently in the following sections concerning the pathogenesis and immunology of mycoplasma infection in man.

Of the several laboratory animals which can be infected with *M. pneumoniae,* the hamster has been most popular. As described by Dajani *et al.* (1965), hamsters inoculated intranasally remain infected for a period of several weeks. Peak organism titers are reached in the nasal turbinates within 7 days and in the trachea and lungs by 10 days. Thereafter, the quantity of organisms decreases gradually, reaching low levels by 6–8 weeks; cultures often remain positive for several months. When previously infected animals receive an intranasal challenge with live organisms, resistance to infection is seen in the form of lower numbers of organisms colonizing the lung and no pneumonia when the lungs are examined at 10–14 days after infection (Fernald and Clyde, 1970).

As in man, the pneumonia in hamsters reaches its peak by 14 days. The lesions are not detectable grossly or radiologically; therefore, direct temporal correlations with human disease are not possible. Nevertheless, the pulmonary histopathology is similar to human pneumonia, characteristically consisting of a peribronchial round cell infiltrate and a polymorphonuclear and mononuclear endobronchial exudate. The alveoli and terminal bronchioles are usually not involved, suggesting a tropism of the organisms for ciliated epithelium. In severely infected lungs perivascular infiltrates are often seen, but interstitial mononuclear infiltrates are uncommon. The lesions evolve slowly over a period of 2–3 weeks and often persist for 8–12 weeks. Thus in terms of histological characteristics and timing of the pneumonic cellular response, the hamster provides a good model of human *M. pneumoniae* pneumonia.

4.1.2. Humoral Immunity in the Lung

One approach to characterization of local immunity in *M. pneumoniae* infection has been to search for specific secretory antibodies. Biberfeld and Sterner (1971) detected IgA, IgM, and IgG specific for *M. pneumoniae* in sputum of infected patients with a sensitive immunofluorescence technique. Brunner and Chanock (1973) developed a very sensitive radioimmunoprecipitation (RIP) technique to detect IgA-specific antibody in nasal secretions. Utilizing this assay in human volunteers, it was shown not only that secretory IgA was generated during *M. pneumoniae* infection but also that its presence correlated directly with resistance to challenge infection (Brunner *et al.*, 1973b). In some of Brunner's subjects it was clear that the presence or absence of serum antibody had no influence on local resistance to reinfection.

Examination of sputum cytology in patients infected with *M. pneumoniae* gives further evidence that local antibody is actively involved in the disease process. In some sputa with purulent characteristics, rosette formations consisting of infected epithelial cells surrounded by polymorphonuclear leukocytes were observed (Collier and Clyde, 1974). These cellular formations have also been seen in hamsters, as mentioned below, in which case the rosettes have been shown to depend on the presence of antibody and complement (Clyde, 1971).

Experiments with the hamster model have also shown that circulating antibody does not assure local immunity to *M. pneumoniae* (Fernald and Clyde, 1970). Thus, although systemic immune responses accompanying *M. pneumoniae* infection are certain evidence of past experience, mild infection can occur without generating detectable serum antibody. Presumably reinfection occurs after local antibody has disappeared since persisting levels of serum antibody do not guarantee resistance to reinfection of the respiratory tract. While this concept seems to hold true in general, there is recent evidence in *M. pulmonis* infection in mice that passively adminstered serum antibody does provide resistance to small numbers of organisms inoculated intranasally (Taylor and Taylor-Robinson, 1976). Thus, response to reinfection with *M. pneumoniae* in hamsters, and in man, is dependent on size of infectious inoculum and the existing state of both local and systemic immunity in the host.

The lymphoid cellular infiltrates seen in infected hamster lungs resemble the lesions of delayed hypersensitivity. It was presumed that this mononuclear infiltrate was composed of thymic-dependent (T) lymphocytes and monocytes, and that cell-mediated immunity might play a major role in the pathogenesis of this pulmonary disease. This presumption seems to be in conflict with the generally held concept that the secretory antibody system was preeminent in controlling surface respiratory infection (Fernald, 1969). Accordingly, experiments were performed to characterize the nature of lymphoid cells infiltrating the bronchial lamina propria in *M. pneumoniae* infected lungs (Fernald *et al.*, 1972). Frozen sections of hamster lungs at various stages of infection were stained with rabbit antihamster immunoglobulins by the indirect immunofluorescence technique. Contrary to expectations, the majority of cells stained for IgM and IgG. Although IgA-containing plasmacytes were demonstrable, they increased only a few-fold over normal uninfected controls. IgM-stainable cells were not present in uninfected lungs and appeared to be derived from outside the lamina propria. A further peculiarity observed was that IgM production continued to predominate during the 21-day period of observation, never being surpassed—although perhaps at some points equaled—by IgG-containing cells.

These data were obtained in the hamster and do not necessarily apply to *M. pneumoniae* pneumonia in man. However, there is evidence that while IgA production predominates in areas of the body where continuous microbial stimulation prevails (i.e., upper respiratory tract and gut), the immune response of the lower respiratory tract may be less restricted (Kaltreider, 1976; Kaltreider and Chan, 1976). Also, Martinez-Tello *et al.* (1968) have found IgA-, IgG-, and IgM-containing plasma cells in a ratio of 5 : 5 : 1 in uninfected bronchial mucosa at autopsy. In patients with cystic fibrosis IgA and IgG cells were increased with IgA predominating. Thus the findings of IgG, IgA, and IgM antibodies in sputum of *M. pneumoniae* patients by Biberfeld and Sterner (1971) are not at odds with the selective IgA response in nasal washings (Brunner *et al.,* 1973b). Furthermore, local IgM and IgG production has been described in other infectious disease models (Miller and North, 1973). Thus the possibility remains that the localization of IgM and IgG plasmacytes in the pulmonary lamina propria is characteristic of human *M. pneumoniae* infection. Corroboration of this concept must await studies of freshly obtained autopsy material or possibly lung biopsy tissue.

Indirect evidence of antibody activity in bronchial washings of hamsters experiencing both primary and challenge infections has been described by Clyde (1971). In these experiments rosette forms consisting of sloughed epithelial cells surrounded by polymorphonuclear phagocytes were seen in smears of bronchial exudate during the second week of infection. They appeared to decline in number as the degree of infection and pneumonia decreased during the third week. On reinfection the same figures reappeared within 3 days,

coincident with the accelerated pneumonic response characteristic of reinfection in the hamster. Reconstruction of rosette formation was accomplished *in vitro* and revealed that a combination of organisms attached to ciliated epithelial cells, immune serum, and complement were required to attract leukocytes to form rosettes. Although the antibody in the bronchial washings was not characterized immunologically, its opsonizing and complement-activating capacities suggest that it was IgG, rather than IgA.

In experiments reviewed above there is strong suggestion that local antibody production is an important component of the immune response to *M. pneumoniae* infection. The predominance of peribronchial plasmacytes in the hamster implicates B lymphocytes as the source of the local immune response. However, the synthesis of secretory antibodies in response to *M. pneumoniae* infection says nothing of their function or origin. A variety of antibodies composed of IgM, IgG, and IgA are probably secreted into the bronchial lumen during the course of the disease. Opsonic antibodies are likely to be of biological significance for both polymorphonuclear and mononuclear phagocytosis of *M. pneumoniae* organisms. One may speculate that the sheltered position of *M. pneumoniae* attached between cilia and microvillae of respiratory epithelial cells precludes efficient removal by phagocytic activity. This could explain the prolonged carriage of organisms following resolution of clinical disease. The mechanism by which antibody may eradicate organisms is suggested by the experiments of Williams and Gibbons (1972) and Fubara and Freter (1973) concerning the action of antibodies which block attachment of oral and intestinal bacteria.

4.1.3. Cell-Mediated Immunity in the Lung

Experimental studies in other systems have demonstrated that production of macrophage migration-inhibitory factor is elicited from lymphocytes in bronchial washings by chemical haptens (Waldman and Henny, 1971), foreign erythrocytes (Kaltreider and Salmon, 1973), and infectious agents (Jurgenson *et al.,* 1973). Similar experiments have not been reported following mycoplasma infections, although production of MIF in response to *M.*

pneumoniae has been described in hamster peritoneal exudates (Arai *et al.,* 1971; Biberfeld, 1973). An alternative and more direct approach to evaluation of cell-mediated immunity in mycoplasma infections would be to study the influence of T lymphocytes on the phagocytosis of mycoplasmas. Techniques for studying mycoplasmas and macrophages have reached a stage of development conducive to the success of such a study, and data soon should be available.

An alternative approach to study of cell-mediated immunity in *Mycoplasma pneumoniae* infection has been to employ immunosuppression of the T-lymphocyte population with antithymocyte serum (ATS). In ATS-immunosuppressed animals, *M. pneumoniae* organisms proliferate within the respiratory tract, but only slightly more than in the infected controls treated with normal rabbit serum. No evidence of epithelial cell destruction or systemic escape of organisms has been detected. Histologically, minimal or no peribronchial lymphoid infiltrates develop in ATS-treated animals, indicating rather complete suppression of the local immune infiltrate (Taylor *et al.,* 1974). Clinically, hamsters do not express disease symptoms when infected with *M. pneumoniae* so no comparison of the clinical ATS treatment can be made.

Decreased serum antibody production in the immunosuppressed animals was an accompanying feature of ATS treatment. Both specific *M. pneumoniae* antibody (Fernald, unpublished data) and antibodies to control antigens were suppressed (Fernald and Clyde, 1976). The serum antibody response to intraperitoneal injection of sheep erythrocytes was markedly reduced, but serum agglutinins to whole *Brucella* organisms were normal compared to those of controls. Since the latter system is known to be T-cell independent, at least in chickens (Rouse and Warner, 1972), it would appear that only T-lymphocyte-mediated antibody production is blocked by ATS. This suggests the necessity of an intact T-lymphocyte system in the production of àntibodies to *M. pneumoniae.*

The endobronchial exudate characteristic of *M. pneumoniae* disease in hamsters is not similarly suppressed by ATS (Fernald and Clyde, 1976). Quantitatively, PMN phagocytes are significantly reduced in number, but mononuclear cells are unaffected. These experiments raise the possibility that T lymphocytes are essential for effective mobilization of the phagocytic response to *M. pneumoniae* in the respiratory tract, both by mediating synthesis of opsonizing antibodies and via the effect of lymphokines on mononuclear and polymorphonuclear phagocyte function.

M. pneumoniae infection has been described in immunodeficient children by Foy *et al.* (1973), providing an experiment of nature for comparison with the animal data discussed above. Four patients, ages 12–19 years, were all severely B-cell deficient, as evidenced by low or absent immunoglobulins, absent isohemagglutinins, positive Schick test, and absent plasma cells in lymph node and/or rectal biopsies. The subjects were not apparently suffering from defective cell-mediated immunity by clinical history, and three out of four demonstrated normal allograft rejection. *M. pneumoniae* infection was diagnosed by recovery of organisms from the respiratory tract on one or more occasions from each patient, but, as predicted, no serological response was detectable. Although physical findings of pneumonia and bronchitis were recorded, none of the three patients who were X-rayed had pulmonary infiltrates. The absence of radiological lesions and the prolonged course and severity of the illness were felt to be uncharacteristic of *M. pneumoniae* pneumonia. In spite of the lack of an immune response, all four patients did respond to tetracycline and erythromycin and suffered no apparent sequellae.

Comparison of Foy's aggammaglobulinemic patients and the ATS-hamster model reveals many similarities; the relative lack of pathogenicity of *M. pneumoniae* and the lack of pneumonic lesions in the absence of B-cell function are most notable. Foy *et al.* suggested that their data supported the idea that cell-mediated immunity is important in resistance to *M. pneumoniae,* since this system was apparently intact in their patients. Although studies in normal hamsters support this view (Fernald and Clyde, 1970), the evidence from ATS-suppressed hamster experiments suggests that T lymphocytes are only indirectly responsible. That is, suppression of the immune response with ATS prevents the expression of localized immune infiltrates and prolongs the carriage of organisms, but there is no evidence of systemic invasion or extension of the infection locally (Taylor *et al.*, 1974). Thus we are led to conclude that most of the disease associated with *M. pneumoniae* infection relates to the host immune response. This concept becomes more important in considering the feasibility of immunoprophylaxis. This subject will be discussed in a subsequent section.

4.1.4. Systemic Humoral and Cellular Immunity

A variety of techniques have been employed for titration of serum antibodies arising from *M. pneumoniae* infection. These range from nonspecific streptococcus MG agglutinins and cold hemagglutinins to complement fixation, indirect (passive) hemagglutination, and various growth-inhibiting antibody assays, the last being the most specific. When analyzed in terms of immunoglobulin class and time elapsed since onset of infection, the antibody response to *M. pneumoniae* infection behaves predictably (Fernald *et al.*, 1967b). In the first few weeks of illness IgM production is prominent and accounts for all of the cold hemagglutinin and indirect hemagglutinating activity. Complement-fixing and growth-inhibiting antibodies derive from both IgM and IgG, but the non-complement-fixing character of IgA is reflected as a gap in the CF antibody profile; later in convalescence, IgG composes most of the antibody activity in serum. Similar studies have been reported by Biberfeld (1968, 1971a), who emphasized the variability of individual immunoglobulin responses when large numbers of individuals are examined.

Cell-mediated immunity to *M. pneumoniae* was first demonstrated by Leventhal *et al.* (1969) as antigen-specific lymphocyte blast transformation *in vitro,* following experimental infection in human volunteers. Later studies revealed that antigen-stimulable lymphocytes are detectable in all but very acute bleedings, usually preceding the appearance of CF and GI antibody (Fernald, 1972, and unpublished data). Biberfeld *et al.* (1974) have documented peripheral lymphocyte stimulability as long as 10 years after documented clinical disease. Since subclinical infections are known to occur, this finding may be subject to reinterpretation.

Other parameters of systemic cell-mediated immunity to *M. pneumoniae* which have been assessed are lymphocyte production of leukocyte migration-inhibition factor and delayed cutaneous hypersensitivity in man, macrophage migration inhibitory production in hamsters, and cutaneous delayed hypersensitivity in guinea pigs. Biberfeld (1974) found homologous antigen-specific inhibition of peripheral leukocyte migration in seven out of ten patients with *M. pneumoniae* pneumonia 3–6 weeks after onset of illness. The reaction was short lived as compared to *in vitro* lymphocyte reactivity in the same patient; lymphocytes from only one of four patients tested after 6 months generated migration-inhibitory activity response to antigenic stimulation. Mizutani *et al.* (1971) have demonstrated delayed-type skin reactions to *M. pneumoniae* in patients diagnosed by serological and X-ray findings, and have observed similar skin responses in guinea pigs infected with *M. pneumoniae* (Mizutani and Mizutani, 1975). While these studies confirm that cell-mediated immunity is stimulated during infection, such systemic manifestations shed no light on the pathogenicity of local disease in the lung or on the ability of the host to resist infection.

4.2. Immunopathological Aspects of *M. pneumoniae* Infection

A variety of systemic expressions of immunological reactivity have been described in *M. pneumoniae* disease. In addition to cold hemagglutinins and antibodies to streptococcus MG, antibodies to brain, liver, heart, and lung are detectable in some patients (Biberfeld, 1971b). These antibodies are composed of IgM and have been shown to react with specific antigens: the I antigens of the erythrocyte membrane (Costea *et al.*, 1972) and cellular antigens from several organs. In the case of streptoccus MG it has been shown that this organism and *M. pneumoniae* share a glycosyl diglyceride antigen (Plackett *et al.*, 1969). Except for cold hemagglutinins, which may cause hemolytic anemia or thromboembolic phenomena (Purcell and Chanock, 1967), the role of these antibodies in *M. pneumoniae* disease is unknown. The finding by Biberfeld (1971b) of antibrain antibodies in patients with encephalitis, as well as those without neurological symptoms, illustrates this point.

Clinical findings associated with *M. pneumoniae* infection are myriad and include skin rashes, Stevens–Johnson syndrome, encephalopathy, Guillain–Barré syndrome, myocarditis, and arthritis (Couch, 1973). Pancreatitis and hepatitis have been added to this list (Mardh and Ursing, 1973), although the evidence of a causal relationship has been questioned (Leinikki *et al.*, 1973). The evidence for a causal association in most of these reports consists of elevated serum antibody titers and in some cases a positive throat culture. The failure to culture organisms from tissues peripheral to the lung is not surprising, since all evidence indicates that *M. pneumoniae* does not penetrate the mucosal basement membrane. Biberfeld and Norberg (1974) have reported detection of circulating immune complexes in convalescent sera by means of a platelet aggregation technique. The antigenic component of these complexes is unknown. If the antigen is derived from *M. pneumoniae*, its identification would confirm that soluble products from the organism do reach systemic circulation.

It is difficult to prove the alleged association of *M. pneumoniae* with the clinical syndromes listed above, because of the frequency of infection and reinfection with this organism. Serological evidence alone, particularly if not clearly denoting a fourfold or greater titer rise, does not prove recent *M. pneumoniae* infection; CF antibodies may persist for 2 or more years. Furthermore, since nonspecific rashes and erythema multiforme are commonly associated with a wide variety of infectious agents, one must be skeptical of a direct association, even when there is evidence of recent *M. pneumoniae* infection.

4.3. Immunological Implications of Reinfection with *M. pneumoniae*

It is now clearly established that *M. pneumoniae* infection can be acquired as early as the first year of life and that it recurs at intervals of approximately 2–4 years through childhood to the young adult years. It has long been recognized that *M. pneumoniae* pneumonia is less common in small children than in older family members. Serological surveys suggest that many childhood infections went unnoticed, or at least were not medically diagnosed

(Chanock *et al.*, 1960). The frequency of *M. pneumoniae* disease in military recruits who entered training with serological evidence of previous infection also suggested that reinfection was common (Steinberg *et al.*, 1969). Recurrent *M. pneumoniae* pneumonia was documented by Foy *et al.* (1971) in an adult, and Biberfeld *et al.* (1974) reported second infections in a Swedish father and son.

A prospective study of respiratory infections in children attending a day-care center in Chapel Hill, North Carolina, provided a unique opportunity to study *M. pneumoniae* infections (Fernald *et al.*, 1975). In this group of approximately 50 children, age 6 weeks to 9 years, 27 *M. pneumoniae* infections were documented in 22 subjects. The five reinfections occurred after 1½–3 year intervals. Most of these episodes were not recognized clinically in spite of daily medical attention provided at the facility. Complement-fixing and growth-inhibiting antibody responses were significant even in the youngest infants but tended to fall to undetectable levels within a few months. The brevity of the systemic antibody response in these generally asymptomatic children contrasted with observations in adult pneumonia cases, in whom CF and GI antibodies persist at least several years.

The cellular immune response in these children was assessed by performing peripheral lymphocyte cultures on each subject during the sixth year of study. Although it was not possible to test for *M. pneumoniae* stimulability before and after each infection, the tendency for antigen-sensitive lymphocytes to remain detectable for up to 10 years following *M. pneumoniae* pneumonia suggested that this retrospective approach was feasible. The results are displayed in Fig. 3. Maximum CF and GI antibody titers obtained following each infection are also displayed in this figure. In spite of the mildness of these childhood infections, antibody rises detected in early infancy were as high those in older children. In contrast to the early expression of humoral immunity, peripheral lymphocyte stimulability did not rise to significant levels until age 5. Thereafter antigen-responsive lymphocytes became detectable, although not to the degree seen in adults.

These data suggest that asymptomatic *M. pneumoniae* infections in infancy generate

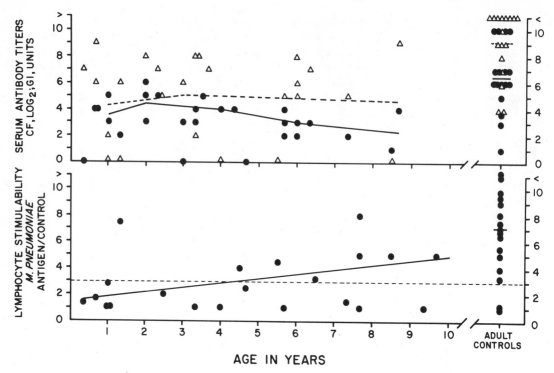

Figure 3. Immune response to *M. pneumoniae* in infants and children with upper respiratory infection. ●, Maximum complement-fixation titer in each individual case in upper portion of figure; solid line indicates mean. △, Growth inhibition levels in same sera; dashed line indicates mean by age. Dotted line in lower panel indicates level of significance for peripheral lymphocyte culture response to *M. pneumoniae*; each ● represents one case with proven infection. Reproduced by permission of Institut National de la Sante et de la Recherche Medicale, Paris (Fernald and Clyde, 1974).

only a restricted immune response, since antigen-reactive lymphocytes do not reach detectable numbers in circulating blood. An analogous situation has been described by Goldberg *et al.* (1971) in rabbits immunized orally with bovine serum albumin. Antigen-reactive cells were present in the lamina propria, and serum antibodies were detectable, but only when the antigen dose was increased were sensitized lymphocytes found in the peripheral blood. These data are compatible with the concept that local immune systems within the lung are compartmentalized and are functionally separate from systemic immunity. Thus it is possible to stimulate effective local immunity without a significant systemic response or to stimulate circulating antibody and lymphocytes without generating effective local immunity. The former is a natural consequence of mild natural infection; the latter appears to be common following parenteral inoculation

with killed *M. pneumoniae* vaccines (Fernald and Clyde, 1974).

Inferences can be drawn from the data that have been summarized concerning the key role played by immune experience relative to *M. pneumoniae* disease. In Table 3 are listed several points which provide evidence that immune mechanisms may be responsible for the disease caused by this organism. First, there is a dissociation between infection and illness, with illness occurring after there has been ample opportunity for prior infection. Second, in experimental animals pulmonary lesions occur that resemble natural human disease and consist of antibody-producing cells and phagocytes. Repeat inoculation of experienced animals results in more rapid and intense production of these pulmonary changes. Third, these pathological changes are obliterated if the animals receive antithymocyte serum. Fourth, although the organism localizes on the

TABLE 3. Evidence for Immune Mediation of *Mycoplasma pneumoniae* Disease

1. Repeated infections without disease occur during 1st decade of life; disease is more common in 2nd decade.
2. In experimental animals, repeated infection produces accelerated and exaggerated pulmonary histopathology.
3. Immunosuppressed animals and patients with immune deficiencies may be infected without occurrence of pulmonary histopathology.
4. Some patients develop sterile nonrespiratory tract complications: skin, blood, central nervous system, and joints.
5. Many patients develop "autoantibodies": cold agglutinins (anti-I), antibrain, antilung, and antiheart.

The foregoing epidemiological, clinical, and experimental observations—some apparently contradictory to others—can be assimilated into a unified concept, shown diagramatically in Fig. 4. Depicted are the first four decades in the life of a hypothetical individual, indicating opportunities for exposure to *M. pneumoniae* and the outcome in terms of both infection and illness. The vertical dimension of the figure shows the relative degree of protective immunity possessed by the individual, as well as the presumed mediators of this immunity. The occurrence of silent infections during early childhood is indicated by the first two exposures, which probably generate transient immunity that is only partially protective. It has been shown that circulating antigen-reactive cells reflecting immune experience may not develop early but do appear later in childhood, as indicated above exposure 3. The presence of serum and local antibody appears to correlate with, and may mediate resistance to, reinfection in the respiratory tract. If this parameter wanes with time, surface reinfection would become possible again, as in exposure 4. Immunological memory residing in the systemic cellular component then could

respiratory mucosa, distant complications are being recognized. These include manifestations such as Stevens–Johnson syndrome, hemolytic anemia and thromboembolic processes, several neurological syndromes, and arthritis. Fifth, it is being recognized that many patients develop antibodies of the IgM class that react with various tissues. Similarities between lipids in host tissues and those of mycoplasma may explain these "autoantibodies."

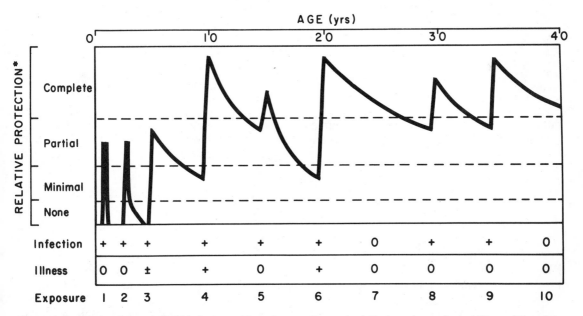

Figure 4. A concept of the relationship between *Mycoplasma pneumoniae* infections, immunity and illness. *Complete protection suggests both local and systemic humoral and cellular immunity. Partial protection prevails when local immunity has waned but systemic immunity persists. Minimal protection may be present in the absence of all but barely detectable systemic cellular immunity.

initiate an anamnestic response, including appearance of systemic and local antibody and local cellular responses in the lungs. These changes constitute the clinical and radiographic findings of "atypical" pneumonia occurring at 10 years, the age of peak incidence. With the loss of local immunity, but presence of adequate systemic immune mechanisms, exposure 5 could produce a surface infection leading to a booster effect, but no disease. The possibility for recurrent pneumonia is illustrated by exposure 6 at age 20, by which time the immune parameters have diminished back to the level of cellular memory. Exposure 7 occurs with full protective immunity, and neither infection nor illness is seen. Beyond this point, infection may recur and restimulate the protected state, or be prevented as shown by exposures 8–10. This hypothesis centers on the proposition that the disease produced by *M. pneumoniae* could represent host response to infection in consequence of minimal immunity from prior experience. This is not "hypersensitivity" of either the immediate or the delayed type, but rather what could be termed "anamnestic pneumonia."

5. Immunodiagnosis of Mycoplasma Infection

5.1. Serological Reactions to Mycoplasmas

Serological tests have been employed to study the immune response to several of the human mycoplasmas (Sethi, 1973). Serum antibodies have been interpreted as evidence that the organisms were stimulating a host response. Such data are important in defining the ecology of mycoplasmas in the human oral and genital tract and suggesting their role in disease processes. In man, *M. pneumoniae* is the only mycoplasma definitely associated with clinical disease. As discussed above, the pathogenicity of other human species is equivocal, but *M. hominis* and the ureaplasmas are implicated in diseases of the perinatal period. Since the serology of *M. pneumoniae* has been developed extensively while that of other human mycoplasmas remains experimental, only the former will be considered in this section.

A variety of serological methods have been developed to study *M. pneumoniae* infections. The cold hemagglutination reaction is the most commonly employed. It depends on the development of an IgM antibody to an I-antigen-like glycolipid of *M. pneumoniae* (Costea *et al.*, 1972). While this test is simple and can be applied during the acute stage of the disease, it is found in only 50% of patients with pneumonia and is limited by its nonspecificity, especially in young children (Sussman *et al.*, 1966). Specific serological tests for *M. pneumoniae* include indirect immunofluorescence, complement fixation, indirect hemagglutination, metabolic-inhibiting, growth inhibition, complement-mediated lysis and radioimmunoprecipitation. Immunofluorescent antibody was the first to be assayed (Liu *et al.*, 1959) and remains a sensitive and reliable method. Its specificity relates to the antiglobulin reagent employed, making this one of the preferred methods of assaying immunoglobulin specific antibody in serum (Umetsu *et al.*, 1975), and respiratory secretions (Biberfeld and Sterner, 1971).

The complement-fixation (CF) test, performed in a microtiter system with chloroform–methanol extracted lipid antigen (Kenny and Grayston, 1965) and guinea pig complement, is the most reliable and commonly used specific serologic test for *M. pneumoniae*. It measures both IgM and IgG antibodies and in general seems to reflect both early and late humoral immunity (Fernald *et al.*, 1967b; Biberfeld, 1968). CF antibodies persist for weeks to months in children (Fernald *et al.*, 1975), and often for more than a year in adolescents and adults. The presence of IgM antibody may indicate a primary or recent reinfection (Biberfeld, 1971a), but individual variation makes this an unreliable means of evaluating a single titer (Umetsu *et al.*, 1975).

The indirect hemagglutination (IHA) test is performed with tanned erythrocytes coated with whole sonicated *M. pneumoniae* (Dowdle and Robinson, 1964; Lind, 1968). It measures IgM preferentially and rises sharply in early convalescence along with the cold agglutinins. It is technically difficult to control and has been used infrequently, since more sensitive tests have been developed.

Metabolic-inhibiting (MI) (Taylor-Robinson *et al.*, 1966) and growth-inhibiting (GI) (Fernald *et al.*, 1967a) antibodies are the most specific and biologically significant assays, because they depend on the inhibiting effect of antibody attached to the living cell membrane. Fresh serum factors, presumably complement, are also required. All the major classes of antibody are detected by this method (Fernald *et al.*, 1967b). The end point is judged by presence or absence of pH change due to glucose fermentation, as indicated by phenol red or other dyes.

A more sensitive modification of the GI test has been developed by focusing on the biological lesion produced in the mycoplasma membrane by antibody and complement (Brunner *et al.*, 1971). The complement-mediated lysis, or mycoplasmacidal test (MCT), is performed by incubating serial dilutions of serum with mycoplasmas and guinea pig complement and then assaying numbers of organisms lysed by quantitative culture of the reaction mixture (Gale and Kenny, 1970; Brunner *et al.*, 1972). The test is technically difficult, but is at least 10 times more sensitive than the standard CF and GI methods.

The most sensitive test for mycoplasma antibodies is the radioimmunoprecipitation (RIP) technique developed by Brunner and Chanock (1973). This method depends on coprecipitation of radiolabeled *M. pneumoniae*–antibody complexes with antiglobulin. Not only is it very sensitive, but also it allows detection of Ig class-specific antibodies, such as IgA in respiratory secretions (Brunner *et al.*, 1973b). Unfortunately, the biological significance of RIP antibody is unclear; like all precipitation tests it has no *in vivo* correlate. There is also evidence that levels of antibody detected by this assay may be stimulated by cross-reacting glycolipids in a variety of other microorganisms and natural sources (Plackett *et al.*, 1969; Gale and Kenny, 1970; Kenny and Newton, 1973).

The enzyme-linked immunosorbent assay (ELISA) method has been applied to measurement of antibody to mycoplasmas. Bruggman *et al.* (1977) were able to detect antibody in pigs experimentally infected with *M. suipneumoniae* several weeks before clinical manifestation of enzootic pneumonia. Horowitz and Cassell (1978) have applied the ELISA test to antibody to *M. pulmonis* in mice, and similar studies in *M. pneumoniae*-infected hamsters are in progress (D. A. Powell, personal communication).

In terms of clinical usage, only the cold hemagglutination and CF methods are feasible in most hospital laboratories. In the absence of a positive culture for *M. pneumoniae,* a fourfold rise in CF antibody may be taken as evidence of a recent infection. A single elevated CF titer with an accompanying cold hemagglutinin response also may be taken as evidence that the *M. pneumoniae* infection was recent (Jones and Stewart, 1974), provided that the patient is not a young child (Sussman *et al.*, 1966).

5.2. Assessment of Cell-Mediated Immunity

Assays for cell-mediated immunity to *M. pneumoniae* have been reviewed above. Skin test reactions to intradermally injected whole and lipid-depleted organisms appear to correlate with recent *M. pneumoniae* infection but hold little promise as acceptable clinical tools. *In vitro* lymphocyte stimulability also correlates with infection or immunization with *M. pneumoniae* (Fernald, 1972; Fernald and Glezen, 1973). In immunodeficient patients and in experimental studies this expensive and time-consuming assay may be indicated if a research laboratory is available to perform the test.

5.3. Mycoplasma Species Identification

A variety of immunological procedures has been utilized for identification and speciation of mycoplasma isolates. The most specific is the use of antiserum-saturated paper disks for identification of colonies grown on agar (Clyde, 1964). Complement fixation, immunodiffusion, and gel electrophoresis have also been employed to compare mycoplasmas.

A further immunodiagnostic procedure which has been tested experimentally by Del Giudice and Barile (1967) employs immunofluorescence for identification of mycoplasma colonies on agar culture plates. Exploitation of this technique could lead to more rapid and accurate identification of mycoplasmas from human material and perhaps eventual general availability of this service in well-equipped clinical laboratories. The same methodology has been applied to sputum samples, but problems of nonspecific fluorescence have not been overcome (Hers, 1962).

6. Immunoprophylaxis

6.1. Background of Vaccine Development Efforts

The history of research on *M. pneumoniae* is in essence a chronicle of efforts to develop a vaccine to control this common human respiratory infection. Because of these efforts, which began with the work of the Commission on Acute Respiratory Disease in the early 1940s, *M. pneumoniae* disease is one of the most thoroughly studied mycoplasma infections.

With the isolation and identification of the Eaton agent as a species of mycoplasma (Chanock *et al.,* 1962), efforts were immediately directed toward development of an attenuated vaccine strain to be given intranasally. It was soon determined that *in vitro* passage reduced not only virulence but also immunogenicity (Couch *et al.,* 1964; Smith *et al.,* 1967). Efforts to develop a killed vaccine were also disappointing; killed vaccines have yielded less than 70% reduction in pneumonia rates following experimental challenge or naturally acquired infection (Chanock *et al.,* 1967; Mogabgab, 1968, 1973; Wenzel *et al.,* 1976), although Mogabgab (1973) reported an 87% reduction in bronchitis due to *M. pneumoniae*. A further setback came with the observation of an adverse effect of killed vaccine in a group of volunteers (Smith *et al.,* 1967). Those men who failed to develop detectable antibody not only became infected when challenged but also experienced worse disease than antibody-negative, unvaccinated controls. This phenomenon has never been explained, although it has generated much speculation. Theories offered have been (1) that the lack of antibody response reflected lack of previous antigenic exposure, and, conversely, that vaccinees who developed serum antibodies and protective immuniy were responding anamnestically; (2) that the enhanced susceptibility to disease caused by *M. pneumoniae* infection related to stimulation of systemic (cell-mediated) immunity in the absence of local protective immunity in the lung; or (3) that, in view of the evidence that *M. pneu-*

moniae pneumonia is an expression of the host immune response (see previous section), the vaccine selectively sensitized volunteers on the basis of their varying states of local and systemic immunity. In fact, the reasons for the adverse reactions in this group of volunteers remain obscure (Craighead, 1975). No such problems have been observed in several large field trials, and the phenomenon has not been reproduced in the hamster model.

Efforts to produce safe and effective vaccines have involved methods to preserve the antigenicity of organisms during production of killed vaccines, thus yielding greater immunogenicity (Somerson *et al.,* 1973), as well as development of mutant temperature-restricted *M. pneumoniae* strains which grow only in the upper respiratory tract (Greenberg *et al.,* 1974). An alternative approach for a live vaccine, proposed by Lipman *et al.* (1969), is based on deletion of the cytadsorbing properties of a high-passage *M. pneumoniae* strain. This strain acts as a replicating, but biologically impotent, source of antigen in the hamster lung. A surface antigen related to the attachment property of *M. pneumoniae* is lacking in this strain (Hu *et al.,* 1975). Isolation and purification of this surface-active antigen could lead to preparation of a chemically defined specific vaccine.

6.2. Present Status of *M. pneumoniae* Vaccines

The only successful *M. pneumoniae* immunoprophylaxis to date has involved the use of whole organisms injected parenterally. Although it is clear from animal experimentation that parenteral immunization is less immunogenic than infection with live organisms (Fernald and Clyde, 1970), killed vaccines have reduced respiratory illness, including bronchitis, in some field trials by as much as 87% (Mogabgab, 1973). In a recent field trial Wenzel *et al.* (1976) noted a 68% reduction in *M. pneumoniae* pneumonia but no significant reduction in bronchitis and no effect on *M. pneumoniae* colonization rates. This is not an unexpected finding in view of the lack of local immune stimulation afforded by parenteral administration of a nonreplicating organism.

Because of the theoretical advantages of local immunization in the respiratory tract, much effort has gone into development of live

M. pneumoniae strains suitable for human use. Chanock and co-workers at the National Institute of Allergy and Infectious Diseases developed a series of temperature-restricted strains to test the feasibility of limiting infection with fully virulent organisms to the cooler environment of the upper respiratory tract (Brunner *et al.*, 1973a). Several candidate strains were developed and tested in the hamster model. In practice, protection was achieved only with those strains that produced pulmonary infection, again illustrating that immunogenicity can be equated with virulence. Strain H43, which did not infect hamsters, was tried in human volunteers; when it proved to be infectious, but apparently avirulent, a small challenge experiment was performed (Greenberg *et al.*, 1974). Infection of volunteers selected for antibody negativity by CF and MI tests resulted in colonization of the respiratory tract, generation of low-level serum and local antibody responses, but no detectable stimulation of circulating lymphocytes (Helms *et al.*, 1975). When immunized volunteers were challenged with a low-passage *M. pneumoniae* strain (PI 1428 in second passage), infection was reduced compared to that of unvaccinated controls. Serum antibodies and peripheral lymphocyte reactivity to *M. pneumoniae* was stimulated in controls but not in the vaccinees. Thus it appeared that the H43 *ts* mutant had potential as a live vaccine. Unfortunately, lack of clinical illness in challenged controls disallowed evaluation of protective efficacy. Present restrictions on human volunteer experimentation may prevent further controlled trials of this or other live vaccines.

At the time of this writing, no *M. pneumoniae* vaccines have been licensed for use. Because it appears to be an effective method of prophylaxis in young adults, the use of properly prepared, antigenically potent, killed vaccines, may be acceptable in selected populations at high risk such as military recruits. The potential risk of sensitization precludes the use of killed or live vaccines in children (Fernald *et al.*, 1975). An additional precaution to the use of live vaccines is raised by the report of Biberfeld and Sterner (1976a,b) that a state of anergy occurs following natural infection. Such nonspecific effects of mycoplasmas on the immune response will have to be considered in the design of future vaccine studies.

As it becomes increasingly difficult to contend with the multiple effects of whole organism vaccines, the possibility of immunizing with a specific defined antigen becomes more attractive. Continued research on identification and purification of a surface antigen, specifically involved in attachment of *M. pneumoniae* to respiratory epithelium, may lead to development of a more precise method of immunoprophylaxis.

7. Conclusions and Future Directions

Mycoplasmas, as extracellular infectious microorganisms, provide a distinct arena for study of the host immune response to surface infections. Because it is the only clearly defined human pathogen, *Mycoplasma pneumoniae* has been studied the most in this context. The immune response to this organism in the respiratory tract seems to occur in two functionally separate compartments. One, the generation of immune products directed at surface antigens of the living organisms, is probably involved in blocking attachment to host cells and promotion of phagocytosis. On reinfection it probably serves as the mediator of immune resistance.

The second component of the immune response to *M. pneumoniae* is the generation of a localized collection of immune and inflammatory cells, which is perceived clinically as disease. Certain autoimmune phenomena such as cold agglutinins and antitissue antibodies are also part of this response. This immunoinflammatory response of the host may have little to do with resistance to reinfection, although it obviously contributes to promoting clearance of organisms during the primary infection. Hypothetically, it should be possible to stimulate the protective phase of the host response to mycoplasmas without the potentially detrimental immunoinflammatory reaction. This could be accomplished by local immunization with purified antigens related to the attachment of organisms to host cells. Present and future research in this area may yield an acceptable method of immunoprophylaxis.

A major area of recent interest concerns the interactions of mycoplasmas with lymphocytes. It is becoming apparent that several species nonspecifically stimulate or suppress lymphocytes both *in vivo* and *in vitro*. Future studies of the pathogenesis of mycoplasma diseases must include careful evaluation of these nonspecific effects on the host immune response. Study of mycoplasma effects on cell membranes may also be of benefit to immunologists interested in control of lymphocyte function.

Although factual knowledge concerning the pathogenesis of *M. pneumoniae* disease in man is far from comprehensive, much information has been accummulated in the past 10 years. Based on this evidence we have proposed a hypothetical model to account for the various clinical expressions of *M. pneumoniae* infection from infancy to adulthood. Because of the evidence suggesting that asymptomatic infections in early childhood precede the appearance of clinically apparent pneumonia in the second decade of life, we question the wisdom of vaccine prophylaxis during childhood. However, in adolescents and adults, one can predict that recurrent disease is likely to occur. Field trials of killed vaccines have been demonstrated to be protective in the majority of recipients, presumably on the basis of boosting previously established immunity. Thus it seems reasonable, and not inconsistent with the precautions raised about childhood vaccination, to continue to support the use of killed *M. pneumoniae* vaccines for selected adult populations at high risk.

References

Arai, S., Hinuma, Y., Matsumoto, K., and Nakamura, T., 1971, Delayed hypersensitivity in hamsters infected with *Mycoplasma pneumoniae* as revealed by macrophage migration inhibition test, *Jpn. J. Microbiol.* **15**:509–514.

Bak, A. L., Black, F. T., Christiansen, C., and Freundt, E. A., 1969, Genome size of mycoplasmal DNA, *Nature (London)* **224**:1209–1210.

Bergquist, L. M., Lau, B. H. S., and Winter, C. E., 1974, Mycoplasma-associated immunosuppression: Effect on hemagglutinin response to common antigens in rabbits, *Infect. Immun.* **9**:410–415.

Biberfeld, G., 1968, Distribution of antibodies within 19s and 7s immunoglobulins following infection with *Mycoplasma pneumoniae*, *J. Immunol.* **100**:338–347.

Biberfeld, G., 1971a, Antibody responses in *Mycoplasma pneumoniae* infection in relation to serum immunoglobulins, especially IgM, *Acta. Pathol. Microbiol. Scand.* **79**:620–634.

Biberfeld, G., 1971b, Antibodies to brain and other tissues in cases of *Mycoplasma pneumoniae* infection, *Clin. Exp. Immunol.* **8**:319–333.

Biberfeld, G., 1973, Macrophage migration inhibition in response to experimental *Mycoplasma pneumoniae* infection in the hamster, *J. Immunol.* **110**:1146–1150.

Biberfeld, G., 1974, Cell-mediated immune responses following *Mycoplasma pneumoniae* infection in man. II. Leukocyte migration inhibition, *Clin. Exp. Immunol.* **17**:44–49.

Biberfeld, G., 1977, Activation of human lymphocyte subpopulations by *Mycoplasma pneumoniae*, *Scand. J. Immunol.* **6**:1145–1150.

Biberfeld, G., and Biberfeld, P., 1970, Ultrastructural features of *Mycoplasma pneumoniae*, *J. Bacteriol.* **102**:855–861.

Biberfeld, G., and Gronowicz, E., 1976, *Mycoplasma pneumoniae* is a polyclonal B-cell activator, *Nature (London)* **26**:238–239.

Biberfeld, G., and Norberg, R., 1974, Circulating immune complexes in *Mycoplasma pneumoniae* infection, *J. Immunol.* **112**:413–415.

Biberfeld, G., and Sterner, G., 1971, Antibodies in bronchial secretions following natural infection with *Mycoplasma pneumoniae*, *Acta. Pathol. Microbiol. Scand.* **79**:599–605.

Biberfeld, G., and Sterner, G., 1976a, Tuberculin anergy in patients with *Mycoplasma pneumoniae* infection, *Scand. J. Infect. Dis.* **8**:71–73.

Biberfeld, G., and Sterner, G., 1976b, Effect of *Mycoplasma pneumoniae* infection on cell-mediated immunity, *Infection* **4**:517–520.

Biberfeld, G., Biberfeld, P., and Sterner, G., 1974, Cell-mediated immune response following *Mycoplasma pneumoniae* infection in man. I. Lymphocyte stimulation, *Clin. Exp. Immunol.* **17**:29–41.

Bredt, W., 1974, Structure and motility, in: Les Mycoplasmes de L'homme, des Animaux, des Vegetaux et des Insects, *INSERM* **33**:47–52.

Bruggman, S., Keller, H., Bertschinger, H. V., and Engberg, B., 1977, Quantitative detection of antibodies to *Mycoplasma suipneumoniae* in pigs sera by an enzyme-linked immunosorbant assay, *Vet. Rec.* **110**:109–111.

Brunell, P. A., Dische, R. M., and Walker, M. B., 1969, *Mycoplasma*, amnionitis and respiratory distress syndrome, *J. Am. Med. Assoc.* **207**:2097–2099.

Brunner, H., and Chanock, R. M., 1973, A radioimmunoprecipitation test for detection of *Mycoplasma pneumoniae* antibody, *Proc. Soc. Exp. Biol. Med.* **143**:97–105.

Brunner, H., Razin, S., Kalica, A. R., and Chanock, R. M., 1971, Lysis and death of *Mycoplasma pneumoniae* by antibody and complement, *J. Immunol.* **106**:907–916.

Brunner, H., James, W. D., Horswood, R. L., and Chanock, R. M., 1972, Measurement of *Mycoplasma pneumoniae* mycoplasmacidal antibody in human serum, *J. Immunol.* **108**:1491–1498.

Brunner, H., Greenberg, H., James, W. D., Horswood, R. L., and Chanock, R. M., 1973a, Decreased virulence and protective effect of genetically stable temperature-sensitive mutants of *Mycoplasma pneumoniae, Ann. N.Y. Acad. Sci.* 225:436–452.

Brunner, H., Greenberg, H. B., James, W. D., Horswood, R. L., Couch, R. B., and Chanock, R. M., 1973b, Antibody to *Mycoplasma pneumoniae* in nasal secretions and sputa of experimentally infected human volunteers, *Infect. Immun.* 8:612–620.

Brunner, H., James, W. D., Horswood, R. L., and Chanock, R. M., 1973c, Experimental *Mycoplasma pneumoniae* infection of young guinea pigs, *J. Infect. Dis.* 127:315–318.

Brunner, H., Kalica, A. R., James, W. D., Horswood, R. L., and Chanock, R. M., 1973d, Ultrastructural lesions in *Mycoplasma pneumoniae* membranes produced by antibody and complement, *Infect. Immun.* 7:259–264.

Brunner, H., Dorner, I., Schiefer, H., Kraus, H., and Wellensiek, H. J., 1976, Lysis of *Acholeplasma laidlawii* by antibodies and complement, *Infect. Immun.* 13:1671–1677.

Chanock, R. M., Cook, M. K., Fox, H. H., Parrott, R. H., and Hubner, R. J., 1960, Serologic evidence of infection with Eaton agent in lower respiratory illness in childhood, *N. Engl. J. Med.* 262:648–654.

Chanock, R. M., Hayflick, L., and Barile, M. F., 1962, Growth on artifical medium of agent associated with atypical pneumonia and its identification as PPLO, *Proc. Natl. Acad. Sci. USA* 48:41–49.

Chanock, R. M., Smith, C. B., Friedewald, W. T., Gutekunst, R., Steinberg, P., Fuld, S., Jensen, K. E., Senterfit, L. B., and Prescott, B., 1967, *Mycoplasma pneumoniae* infection—Prospects for live and inactivated vaccines, in: *First International Conference on Vaccines Against Viral and Rickettsial Diseases of Man,* pp. 132–140, Pan American Health Organization, Sci. Publication No. 147, Washington, D.C.

Clyde, W. A., Jr., 1963, Hemolysis in identifying Eaton's pleuropneumonia-like organism, *Science* 139:55.

Clyde, W. A., Jr., 1964, Mycoplasma species identification based upon growth inhibition by specific antisera, *J. Immunol.* 92:958–965.

Clyde, W. A., Jr., 1971, Immunopathology of experimental *Mycoplasma pneumoniae* disease, *Infect. Immun.* 4:757–763.

Clyde, W. A., Jr., 1973, Models of *Mycoplasma pneumoniae* infection, *J. Infect. Dis.* 127:S69–72.

Clyde, W. A., Jr., 1975, Pathogenic mechanisms in mycoplasma diseases. in: *Microbiology—1975* (D. Schlessinger, ed.), pp. 143–146, American Society for Microbiology, Washington, D.C.

Cohen, G., and Somerson, N. L., 1967, *Mycoplasma pneumoniae*: Hydrogen peroxide secretion and its possible role in virulence. *Ann. N.Y. Acad. Sci.* 143:85–87.

Cole, B. C., Golightly-Rowland, L., and Ward, J. R., 1975a, Chronic proliferative arthritis of mice induced by *Mycoplasma arthritidis*: Demonstration of a cell mediated immune response to mycoplasma antigens *in vitro, Infect. Immun.* 11:1159–1161.

Cole, B. C., Golightly-Rowland, L., and Ward, J. R., 1975b, Arthritis of mice induced by *Mycoplasma pulmonis*: Humoral antibody and lymphocyte responses of CBA mice, *Infect. Immun.* 12:1083–1092.

Cole, B. C., Overall, J. C., Lombardi, P. S., and Glascow, L. A., 1976, Induction of interferon in bovine and human lymphocyte cultures by mycoplasmas, *Infect. Immun.* 14:88–94.

Cole, B. C., Aldridge, K. E., and Ward, J. R., 1977, Mycoplasma-dependent activation of normal lymphocytes: Mitogenic potential of mycoplasmas for mouse lymphocytes, *Infect. Immun.* 18:393–399.

Collier, A. M., 1972, Pathogenesis of *Mycoplasma pneumoniae* infection as studied in the human foetal trachea organ culture, in: *Pathogenic Mycoplasmas* (CBA Foundation Symposium), pp. 307–327, Associated Scientific Publishers, Amsterdam.

Collier, A. M., and Clyde, W. A., Jr., 1971, Relationships between *Mycoplasma pneumoniae* and human respiratory epithelium, *Infect. Immun.* 3:693–701.

Collier, A. M., and Clyde, W. A., Jr., 1974, Appearance of *Mycoplasma pneumoniae* in lungs of experimentally infected hamsters and sputum from patients with natural disease, *Am. Rev. Resp. Dis.* 110:765–773.

Collier, A. M., Clyde, W. A., Jr., and Denny, F. W., 1971, *Mycoplasma pneumoniae* in hamster tracheal organ culture: Immunofluorescent and electron microscopic studies, *Proc. Soc. Exp. Biol. Med.* 136:569–573.

Copperman, R., and Morton, H. E., 1966, Reversible inhibition of mitosis in lymphocyte cultures by non-viable mycoplasma, *Proc. Soc. Exp. Biol. Med.* 123:790–795.

Costea, N., Yakulis, V. J., and Heller, P., 1972, Inhibition of cold agglutinins (anti-I) by *M. pneumoniae* antigens, *Proc. Soc. Exp. Biol. Med.* 139:476–479.

Couch, R. B., 1973, *Mycoplasma pneumoniae*, in: *Viral and Mycoplasmal Infections of the Respiratory Tract* (V. Knight, ed.), pp. 217–235, Lea and Febiger, Philadelphia.

Couch, R. B., Cate, T. R., and Chanock, R. M., 1964, Infection with artificially propagated Eaton agent (*Mycoplasma pneumoniae*), *J. Am. Med. Assoc.* 187:442–447.

Craighead, J. E., 1975, Report of a workshop: Disease accentuation after immunization with inactivated microbial vaccines, *J. Infect. Dis.* 131:749–754.

Dajani, A. S., Clyde, W. A., Jr., and Denny, F. W., 1965, Experimental infection with *Mycoplasma pneumoniae* (Eaton's agent), *J. Exp. Med.* 121:1071–1084.

Del Giudice, R. A., Robillard, N. F., and Carski, T. R., 1967, Immunofluorescence identification of mycoplasma on agar by use of incident illumination, *J. Bacteriol.* 93:1205–1209.

Denny, F. W., Taylor-Robinson, D., and Allison, A. C., 1972, The role of thymus-dependent immunity in *Mycoplasma pulmonis* infections of mice, *J. Med. Microbiol.* 5:327–336.

Dowdle, W. R., and Robinson, R. Q., 1964, An indirect

hemagglutination test for diagnosis of *Mycoplasma pneumoniae* infections, *Proc. Soc. Exp. Biol. Med.* **116**:947–950.

Dunlop, E. M. C., Vaughn-Jackson, J. D., Darougar, S., and Jones, B. R., 1972, Chalamydial infection. Incidence in "non-specific" urethritis, *Br. J. Vener. Dis.* **48**:425–428.

Eaton, M. D., Meiklejohn, G., and Van Herick, W., 1944, Studies on the etiology of primary atypical pneumonia, *J. Exp. Med.* **79**:649–668.

Eckner, R. J., Han, T., and Kumar, V., 1974, Enhancement of murine leukemia by mycoplasmas; suppression of cell-mediated immunity but not humoral immunity, *Fed. Proc.* **33**:769 (abstr.).

Edward, D. G. 1974, Taxonomy of the class mollicutes, in: Les Mycoplasmes de L'homme, des Animaux, des Vegetaux et des Insectes, *INSERM* **33**:13–18.

Fabricant, J., 1968, Some pathological and epidemiological considerations of animal mycoplasmoses, *Yale J. Biol. Med.* **40**:449–453.

Fernald, G. W., 1969, Local immune mechanisms in respiratory infection due to *Mycoplasma pneumoniae*, in: *The Secretory Immunologic System* (D. H. Dayton *et al.*, eds.), pp. 215–227, U.S. Government Printing Office, Washington, D.C.

Fernald, G. W., 1972, *In vitro* response of human lymphocytes to *Mycoplasma pneumoniae, Infect. Immun.* **5**:552–558.

Fernald, G. W., and Clyde, W. A., Jr., 1970, Protective effect of vaccines in experimental *Mycoplasma pneumoniae* disease, *Infect. Immun.* **1**:559–565.

Fernald, G. W., and Clyde, W. A., Jr., 1974, Cell-mediated immunity in *M. pneumoniae* infections, in: Les Mycoplasmes de L'homme, des Animaux, des Vegetaux et des Insects, *INSERM* **33**:421–427.

Fernald, G. W., and Clyde, W. A., Jr., 1976, Pulmonary immune mechanisms in *Mycoplasma pneumoniae* disease, in: *Immunologic and Infectious Reactions in the Lung* (C. H. Kirkpatrick and H. Y. Reynolds, eds.), pp. 101–129, Marcel Dekker, New York.

Fernald, G. W., and Glezen, W. P., 1973, Humoral and cellular immune response to an inactivated *Mycoplasma pneumoniae* vaccine in children, *J. Infect. Dis.* **127**:498–504.

Fernald, G. W., Clyde, W. A., Jr., and Denny, F. W., 1967a, Factors influencing growth inhibition of *Mycoplasma pneumoniae* by immune sera, *Proc. Soc. Exp. Biol. Med.* **126**:161–166.

Fernald, G. W., Clyde, W. A., Jr., and Denny, F. W., 1967b, Nature of the immune response to *Mycoplasma pneumoniae, J. Immunol.* **98**:1028–1038.

Fernald, G. W., Clyde, W. A., Jr., and Bienenstock, J., 1972, Immunoglobulin-containing cells in lungs of hamsters infected with *Mycoplasma pneumoniae, J. Immunol.* **108**:1400–1408.

Fernald, G. W., Collier, A. M., and Clyde, W. A., Jr., 1975, Respiratory infections due to *Mycoplasma pneumoniae* in infants and children, *Pediatrics* **55**:327–335.

Foy, H. M., Nugent, C. G., Kenny, G. E., McMahan, R., and Grayston, J. T., 1971, Repeated *Mycoplasma pneumonia* after 4½ years, *J. Am. Med. Assoc.* **216**:671–672.

Foy, H. M., Ochs, H., Davis, S. D., Kenny, G. E., and Luce, R. R., 1973, *Mycoplasma pneumoniae* infections in patients with immunodeficiency syndromes: Report of four cases, *J. Infect. Dis.* **127**:388–393.

Freundt, E. A., 1974a, The Mycoplasmas, in: *Bergey's Manual of Determinative Bacteriology* (R. E. Buchanan and N. E. Gibbons, eds.), pp. 929–955, Williams and Wilkins, Baltimore.

Freundt, E. A., 1974b, Taxonomy and host relationships of mycoplasmas, in: Les Mycoplasmes de L'homme, des Animaux, des Vegetaux et des Insects, *INSERM* **33**:19–26.

Freundt, E. A., 1974c, Present status of the medical importance of mycoplasmas, *Pathol. Microbiol.* **40**:155–187.

Fubara, E. S., and Freter, R., 1973, Protection against enteric bacterial infection by secretory IgA antibodies, *J. Immunol.* **111**:395–403.

Gabridge, M. G., and Schneider, P. R., 1975, Cytotoxic effect of *Mycoplasma fermentans* on mouse thymocytes, *Infect. Immun.* **11**:460–465.

Gale, J. L., and Kenny, G. E., 1970, Complement dependent killing of *Mycoplasma pneumoniae* by antibody: Kinetics of the reaction, *J. Immunol.* **104**:1175–1183.

Ginsburg, H., and Nicolet, J., 1973, Extensive transformation of lymphocytes by a mycoplasma organism, *Nature (London), New Biol.* **246**:143–146.

Goldberg, S. S., Kraft, S. C., Peterson, R. D. A., and Rothberg, R. M., 1971, Relative absence of circulating antigen-reactive cells during oral immunization, *J. Immunol.* **107**:757–765.

Greenberg, H., Helms, C. M., Brunner, H., and Chanock, R. M., 1974, Asymptomatic infection of adult volunteers with a temperative sensitive mutant of *Mycoplasma pneumoniae, Proc. Natl. Acad. Sci. USA* **71**:4015–4019.

Griffin, J. P., and Klein, E. W., 1971, Role of sinusitis in primary atypical pneumonia, *Clin. Med.* **78**:23–27.

Helms, C., Grizzard, M., Fernald, G., Levine, M., Caplan, E., Greenberg, H., Woodward, W., and Chanock, R., 1975, Volunteer trials of a temperature-sensitive mutant of *Mycoplasma pneumoniae*, in: *Abstracts: Soc. Epidemiol. Res. Symp. Resp. Viruses*, Albany, N.Y., June 20.

Hers, J. F. Ph., 1962, Fluorescent antibody technique in respiratory viral diseases. in: Conference on Newer Respiratory Disease Viruses (C. G. Loosli, ed.), *Am. Rev. Resp. Dis.*, pp. 316–338.

Hollingdale, M. R., and Lemke, R. M., 1969, The antigens of *Mycoplasma hominis, J. Hyg.* **67**:585–602.

Horowitz, S. A., and Cassell, G. H., 1978, Application of the enzyme-linked immunosorbent assay (ELISA) for detection of antibodies to *Mycoplasma pulmonis, Infect. Immun.* **22**:161–170.

Hu, P. C., Collier, A. M., and Baseman, J. B., 1975, Alterations in metabolism of hamster trachea in organ culture following infection by virulent *Mycoplasma pneumoniae, Infect. Immun.* **11**:704–710.

Jansson, E., Makisara, P., Vaino, K., Vaino, U., Snellman, O., and Tuuri, S., 1971, An 8-year study on mycoplasma in rheumatoid arthritis, *Ann. Rheum. Dis.* **30**:506–508.

Jones, D. M., 1967, *Mycoplasma hominis* in abortion, *Br. Med. J.* **1**:338–340.

Jones, G. R., and Stewart, S. M., 1974, A prospective study of the persistence of *Mycoplasma pneumoniae* antibody levels, *Scott. Med. J.* **19**:129–133.

Jones, T. C., and Hirsch, J. G., 1971, The interaction *in vitro* of *Mycoplasma pulmonis* with mouse peritoneal macrophages and L-cells, *J. Exp. Med.* **133**:231–259.

Jurgenson, P. F., Olsen, G. N., Johnson, J. E., Swenson, E. W., Ayoub, E. M., Henny, C. S., and Waldman, R. H., 1973, Cell-mediated immunity in the lower respiratory tract to tuberculin, mumps and influenza virus, *J. Infect. Dis.* **128**:730–735.

Kahane, I., and Marchesi, V. T., 1973, Studies on the orientation of proteins in mycoplasma and erythrocyte membrances, *Ann. N.Y. Acad. Sci.* **225**:38–45.

Kaklamanis, E., and Pavlatos, M., 1972, The immunosuppressive effect of mycoplasma infection. I. Effect on the humoral and cellular response, *Immunology* **22**:695–702.

Kaltreider, H. B., 1976, Initiation of immune responses in the lower respiratory tract with red cell antigens, in: *Immunologic and Infectious Reactions in the Lung* (C. H. Kirkpatrick and H. Y. Reynolds, eds.), pp. 73–100, Marcel Dekker, New York.

Kaltreider, H. B., and Chan, M. K., 1976, The class-specific immunoglobulin composition of fluids obtained from various levels of the canine respiratory tract, *J. Immunol.* **116**:423–429.

Kaltreider, H. B., and Salmon, S. E., 1973, Immunology of the lower respiratory tract: Functional properties of bronchoalveolar lymphocytes obtained from the normal canine lung, *J. Clin. Invest.* **52**:2211–2217.

Kenny, G. E., and Grayston, J. T., 1965, Eaton pleuropneumonia-like organism (*Mycoplasma pneumoniae*) complement-fixing antigen, *J. Immunol.* **95**:19–25.

Kenny, G. E., and Newton, R. M., 1973, Close serological relationship between glycolipids of *Mycoplasma pneumoniae* and glycolipids of spinach, *Ann. N.Y. Acad. Sci.* **225**:54–61.

Kumagai, K., Iwabuchi, T., Hinuma, Y., Yuri, K., and Ishida, N., 1971, Incidence, species, and significance of *Mycoplasma* species in the mouth, *J. Infect. Dis.* **123**:16–21.

Leinikke, P., Pantzar, P., and Tykk, A. H., 1973, Antibody response in patients with acute pancreatitis to *Mycoplasma pneumoniae, Scand. J. Gastroenterol.* **8**:631–635.

Lemke, R. M., 1973, Serological reactions of mycoplasmas, *Ann. N.Y. Acad. Sci.* **225**:46–53.

Leventhal, B. G., Smith, C. B., Carbone, P. P., and Hersh, E. M., 1969, Lymphocyte transformation in response to *M. pneumoniae*, in: *Proceedings of the Third Annual Leukocyte Culture Conference* (W. O. Rieke, ed.), pp. 519–529, Appleton-Century-Crofts, New York.

Lind, K., 1968, An indirect haemagglutination test for serum antibodies against *Mycoplasma pneumoniae* using formalinized tanned sheep erythrocytes, *Acta. Pathol. Microbiol. Scand.* **73**:459–472.

Lipman, R. P., and Clyde, W. A., Jr., 1969, The interrelationship of virulence, cytadsorption, and peroxide formation in *Mycoplasma pneumoniae, Proc. Soc. Exp. Biol. Med.* **131**:1163–1167.

Lipman, R. P., Clyde, W. A., Jr., and Denny, F. W., 1969, Characteristics of virulent, attenuated and avirulent *Mycoplasma pneumoniae* strains, *J. Bacteriol.* **100**: 1037–1043.

Liu, C., Eaton, M. D., and Heyl, J. T., 1959, Studies on primary atypical pneumonia. II. Observations concerning the development and immunological characteristics of antibody in patients, *J. Exp. Med.* **109**:545–556.

Liu, C., Jayanetra, P., Voth, D. W., Muangmanee, L., and Cho, C. T., 1972, Potentiating effect of *Mycoplasma pneumoniae* infection on the development of pneumococcal septicemia in hamsters, *J. Infect. Dis.* **125**:603–612.

Lyell, A., Gordon, A. M., Dick, H. M., and Sommerville, R. G., 1967, Mycoplasmas and erythema multiforme, *Lancet* **2**:1116–1118.

Maisel, J. C., Babbitt, L. H., and John, T. J., 1967, Fatal *Mycoplasma pneumoniae* infection with isolation of organisms from lung, *J. Am. Med. Assoc.* **202**:287–290.

Manchee, R. J., and Taylor-Robinson, D., 1969, Studies on the nature of receptors involved in attachment of tissue culture cells to mycoplasmas, *Br. J. Exp. Pathol.* **50**:66–75.

Mårdh, P. A., and Ursing, B., 1973, Acute pancreatitis in *Mycoplasma pneumoniae* infections, *Br. Med. J.* **2**:240–241.

Mårdh, P. A., Skude, G., Akerman, M., and Ursing, B., 1974, *Mycoplasma pneumoniae* infection—A cause of acute pancreatitis and non-specific, reactive hepatitis in man and experimentally infected animals, *INSERM* **33**:403–409.

Martinez-Tello, F. J., Braun, D. G., and Blanc, W. A., 1968, Immunoglobulin production in bronchial mucosa and bronchial lymph nodes, particularly in cystic fibrosis of the pancreas, *J. Immunol.* **101**:989–1003.

McCormick, W. M., 1974, The role of genital mycoplasmas in human disease, in: *Les Mycoplasmes de L'homme, des Animaux, des Vegetaus et des Insectes, INSERM* **33**:381–387.

McCormick, W. M., Lee, Y., Lin, J., and Rankin, J. S., 1973, Genital mycoplasmas in postpartum fever, *J. Infect. Dis.* **127**:193–196.

Miller, T., and North, D., 1973, Studies of the local immune response to pyelonephritis in the rabbit, *J. Infect. Dis.* **128**:195–201.

Mizutani, H., 1975, The skin-reactive antigens of *Mycoplasma pneumoniae, Jpn. J. Microbiol.* **19**:157–162.

Mizutani, H., and Mizutani, H., 1975, The antigens participating in the macrophage migration inhibition to *Mycoplasma pneumoniae, Am. Rev. Resp. Dis.* **111:** 566–569.

Mizutani, H., Mizutani, H., Kitayama, T., Hayakawa, A., Nagayama, E., Kato, J., Nakamura, K., Tamura, H., and Izuchi, T., 1971, Delayed hypersensitivity in *Mycoplasma pneumoniae* infections, *Lancet* **1:**186–187.

Mogabgab, W. J., 1968, Protective effects of inactive *Mycoplasma pneumoniae* vaccine in military personnel 1964–1966, *Am. Rev. Resp. Dis.* **97:**359–365.

Mogabgab, W. J., 1973, Protective efficacy of killed *Mycoplasma pneumoniae* vaccine measured in large-scale studies in a military population, *Am. Rev. Resp. Dis.* **108:**899–908.

Naot, Y., Tully, J. G., and Ginsburg, H., 1977, Lymphocyte activation by various *Mycoplasma* strains and species, *Infect. Immun.* **18:**310–317.

Parkinson, C. F., and Carter, P. B., 1975, Phagocytosis of *Mycoplasma salivarium* by human polymorphonuclear leukocytes and monocytes, *Infect. Immun.* **11:**405–414.

Plackett, P., Marmion, B. P., Shaw, E. J., and Lemcke, R. M., 1969, Immunochemical analysis of *Mycoplasma pneumoniae*. 3. Separation and chemical identification of serologically active lipids, *Aust. J. Exp. Biol. Med. Sci.* **47:**171–195.

Powell, D. A., and Clyde, W. A., Jr., 1975, Opsonin-reversible resistance of *Mycoplasma pneumoniae* to *in vitro* phagocytosis by alveolar machrophages, *Infect. Immun.* **11:**540–550.

Purcell, R. H., and Chanock, R. M., 1967, Role of mycoplasmas in human respiratory disease, *Med. Clin. N. Am.* **51:**791–802.

Razin, S., Michmann, J., and Shymshoni, Z., 1964, The occurrence of mycoplasma in the oral cavity of dentulous and edentulous subjects, *J. Dent. Res.* **43:**402–405.

Razin, S., Prescott, B., James, W. D., Caldes, G., Valdesugo, J., and Chanock, R. M., 1971, Production and properties of antisera to membrane glycolipids of *Mycoplasma pneumoniae, Infect. Immun.* **3:**420–423.

Reed, S. E., 1972, Interaction between mycoplasmas and respiratory viruses studied in tracheal organ cultures, in: *Pathogenic Mycoplasmas* (Ciba Foundation Symposium), pp. 329–343, Associated Scientific Publishers, Amsterdam.

Richter, C. B., 1970, Electron microscopic pictures of *M. pulmonis* on ciliated epithelial cells, in: *Morphology of Experimental Respiratory Carcinogenesis* (P. Nettesheim, M. G. Hanna, Jr., and J. W. Deatherage, Jr., eds.), pp. 365–382, U.S.A.E.C. Symposium Series 21.

Rouse, B. T., and Warner, N. L., 1972, Depression of humoral antibody formation in the chicken by thymectomy and antilymphocyte serum, *Nature (London), New Biol.* **236:**79–80.

Sabin, A. B., 1941, The filtrable microorganisms of the pleuropneumonia group, *Bacteriol. Rev.* **5:**1–67.

Schiefer, H. G., Gerhardt, U., Brunner, H., and Krupe, M., 1974, Studies with lectins on the surface carbohy-

drate structures of mycoplasma membranes, *J. Bacteriol.* **120:**81–88.

Schiefer, H. G., Gerhardt, U., and Brunner, H., 1975, Immunological studies on the localization of phosphatidylglycerol in the membranes of *Mycoplasma hominis, Hoppe-Seylers Z. Physiol. Chem.* **356:**559–565.

Sethi, K. K., 1973, Diagnostic serology in human mycoplasmas, *Infection* **1:**236–240.

Shepard, M. C., 1970, Non-gonococcal urethritis associated with human strains of "T" mycoplasmas, *J. Am. Med. Assoc.* **211:**1335–1340.

Shulman, S. T., Bartlett, J., Clyde, W. A., Jr., and Ayoub, E. M., 1972, The unusual severity of mycoplasmal pneumonia in children with sickle-cell disease, *N. Engl. J. Med.* **287:**164–167.

Simberkoff, M. S., and Elsbach, P., 1971, The interaction *in vitro* between polymorphonuclear leukocytes and mycoplasma, *J. Exp. Med.* **134:**1417–1430.

Simberkoff, M., Thorbecke, S., and Thomas, L., 1969, Studies on PPLO infection. V. Inhibition of lymphocyte mitosis and antibody formation by mycoplasmal extracts, *J. Exp. Med.* **129:**1163–1181.

Smith, C. B., Friedewald, W. T., and Chanock, R. M., 1967, Inactivated *Mycoplasma pneumoniae* vaccine, *J. Am. Med. Assoc.* **199:**353–358.

Smith, P. F., Langworthy, T. A., and Mayberry, W. R., 1973, Lipids of mycoplasmas, *Ann. N.Y. Acad. Sci.* **225:**22–27.

Sobeslavsky, O., Syrucek, L., Bruckova, M., and Abrahamovic, M., 1965, The etiologic role of *Mycoplasma pneumoniae* in otitis media in children, *Pediatrics* **35:**652–657.

Sobeslavsky, O., Prescott, B., James, W. D., and Chanock, R. M., 1966, Isolation and characterization of fractions of *Mycoplasma pneumoniae, J. Bacteriol.* **91:** 2126–2138.

Sobeslavsky, O., Prescott, B., and Chanock, R. M., 1968, Adsorption of *Mycoplasma pneumoniae* to neuraminic acid receptors of various cells and possible role in virulence, *J. Bacteriol.* **96:**695–705.

Somerson, N. L., James, W. D., Walls, B. E., and Chanock, R. M., 1967, Growth of *Mycoplasma pneumoniae* on glass surface, *Ann. N.Y. Acad. Sci.* **143:**384–389.

Somerson, N. L., Senterfit, L. B., and Hamperian, V. V., 1973, Development of a *Mycoplasma pneumoniae* vaccine, *Ann. N.Y. Acad. Sci.* **225:**425–435.

Steinberg, P., White, R. J., Fuld, S. L., Gutekunst, R. R., Chanock, R. M., and Senterfit, L. B., 1969, Ecology of *Mycoplasma pneumoniae* infections in Marine recruits at Parris Island, S.C., *Am. J. Epidemiol.* **89:**62–73.

Sussman, S. J., Magoffin, R. L., Lennette, E. H., and Schieble, J., 1966, Cold agglutinins, Eaton agent, and respiratory infections of children, *Pediatrics* **38:**571–577.

Taylor, G., and Taylor-Robinson, D., 1975, The part played by cell-mediated immunity in mycoplasma respiratory infections, *Dev. Biol. Stand.* **28:**195–210.

Taylor, G., and Taylor-Robinson, D., 1976, Effects of active and passive immunization on *Mycoplasma pul-*

monis-induced pneumonia in mice, *Immunology* **30:**611–618.

Taylor, G., Taylor-Robinson, D., and Fernald, G. W., 1974, Reduction in the severity of *Mycoplasma pneumoniae*-induced pneumonia in hamsters by immunosuppressive treatment with antithymocyte sera, *J. Med. Microbiol.* **7:**343–347.

Taylor-Robinson, D., and Manchee, R. J., 1967a, Adherance of mycoplasmas to glass and plastic, *J. Bacteriol.* **94:**1781–1782.

Taylor-Robinson, D. and Manchee, R. J., 1967b, Spermadsorption and spermagglutination by mycoplasmas, *Nature (London)* **215:**484–487.

Taylor-Robinson, D., Purcell, R. H., Wong, D. C., and Chanock, R. M., 1966, A colour test for the measurement of antibody to certain mycoplasma species based upon the inhibition of acid production, *J. Hyg.* **64:**91–104.

Thomas, L., Davidson, M., and McCluskey, R. T., 1966, Studies of PPLO infection. I. The production of cerebral polyarteritis by *Mycoplasma gallisepticum* in turkeys; the neurotoxic property of the mycoplasma, *J. Exp. Med.* **123:**897–912.

Tully, J. G., and Smith, L. G., 1968, Postpartum septicemia with *Mycoplasma hominis, J. Am. Med. Assoc.* **204:**827–828.

Umetsu, M., Ogawa, S., Chiba, S., and Nakao, T., 1975, Immune responses in *Mycoplasma pneumoniae* infections, *Tohoku J. Exp. Med.* **116:**213–218.

Waldman, R. H., and Henny, C. S., 1971, Cell-mediated immunity and antibody response in the respiratory tract after local and systemic immunization, *J. Exp. Med.* **134:**482–494.

Wenzel, R. P., Craven, R. B., Davies, J. A., Hendley, J. O., Hamory, B. H. and Gwaltney, J. M., Jr., 1976, Field trial of an inactivated *Mycoplasma pneumoniae* vaccine. I. Vaccine efficacy, *J. Infect. Dis.* **134:**571–576.

Williams, R. C., and Gibbons, R. J., 1972, Inhibition of bacterial adherence by secretory immunoglobulin A: A mechanism of antigen disposal, *Science* **177:**697–699.

Zucker-Franklin, D., Davidson, M., and Thomas, L., 1966, The interaction of mycoplasmas with mammalian cells. I. HeLa cells, neutrophils, and eosinophils, *J. Exp. Med.* **124:**521–532.

18

Immunology of Chlamydial Infections

HAYES C. LAMONT and ROGER L. NICHOLS

1. A Perspective on Chlamydial Diseases

With its long recorded history, its high global prevalence, and its potential for causing partial or total blindness, trachoma ranks as one of the major afflictions of humanity (Bietti, 1974; Jones, 1975; Locatcher-Khorazo and Seegal, 1972; Nataf, 1952; Thygeson, 1971). The principal etiological agent of trachoma is an intracellular parasitic prokaryote, currently assigned to the genus *Chlamydia* (Becker, 1974, 1978; Moulder, 1964, 1966; Page, 1968; Storz, 1971; E. Weiss, 1971). The species designation of the trachoma organism is *C. trachomatis* (Page, 1968). Various serotypes of *C. trachomatis* also cause, besides trachoma-inclusion conjunctivitis (TRIC), some cases of nongonococcal urethritis and cervicitis (Dunlop, 1975; Fritsch *et al.*, 1910; Hobson and Holmes, 1977; Jones *et al.*, 1964; Lindner, 1910; Oriel *et al.*, 1978; Richmond and Sparling, 1976; Schachter *et al.*, 1976), some cases of infant pneumonia (Beem and Saxon, 1977; Frommell *et al.*, 1977; Schachter *et al.*, 1975), and lymphogranuloma venereum (LGV) (Abrams, 1968; Meyer, 1953; Rake and Jones, 1942; Willcox, 1975). Organisms assigned to the species *C. psittaci* are distinguished by their failure to store glycogen during growth

(Becker, 1978; Gordon and Quan, 1965; Jenkin and Fan, 1971): divers strains cause ornithosis (Bedson, 1958) and various diseases in nonhuman mammals, such as pneumonia, encephalitis, conjunctivitis, enteritis, abortion, and polyarthritis (Storz, 1971).

Unlike the rickettsiae, the chlamydiae are transmitted directly between vertebrate hosts, exhibit a characteristic change of form during their development within host cells, and lack the enzymatic capacity to generate adenosine triphosphate in phosphate transfer reactions. Their growth is inhibited by penicillin, D-cycloserine, tetracyclines, rifampicin, and other antibiotics (Becker, 1974, 1978; Litwin, 1959; Moulder, 1962, 1968; Storz, 1971; E. Weiss, 1971). Their intracellular multiplication, usually occurring first in mucosal epithelial cells and (in LGV and ornithosis) later in cells of the reticuloendothelial system, affords them intermittent protection from specific immunological responses (Mackaness, 1971) while possibly marking the host cells as targets for such responses (Metcalf and Helmsen, 1977; Metcalf and Kaufman, 1976; Prendergast and Henney, 1977; Snyderman and Pike, 1975). In theory, pathogenesis by chlamydiae may result from inhibition of host cell metabolism, lysis of host cells, release of host cell lysosomal enzymes, cytotoxicity of chlamydial products, hypersensitivity reactions to chlamydial antigens, autoimmunity to altered or unmasked host antigens, and/or lymphoid hyperplasia in refractory infections (Collier, 1967; Dawson, 1975; Dhermy *et al.*, 1967; Grayston,

HAYES C. LAMONT and ROGER L. NICHOLS
• Department of Microbiology, Harvard School of Public Health, Boston, Massachusetts 02115. *Present address of H. C. L.:* Department of Biology, Suffolk University, Boston, Massachusetts 02114.

1967; Grayston and Wang, 1975; Henley *et al.*, 1971; Manski and Whiteside, 1974; Metcalf and Helmsen, 1977; Metcalf and Kaufman, 1976; Mitsui *et al.*, 1962; Mondino *et al.*, 1977a; Nataf, 1952; Rahi and Garner, 1976; Silverstein, 1974; Silverstein and Prendergast, 1971; Smolin *et al.*, 1977; Storz, 1971; Taverne and Blyth, 1971; Woolridge *et al.*, 1967b). Acquired resistance of human hosts to chlamydial infections is usually weak and transient at best, so that infections tend to persist or to recur even while the hosts continue to produce serum and secretory antibodies (Bietti and Werner, 1967; Dunlop, 1975; Grayston and Wang, 1975; Meyer and Eddie, 1962; Schachter *et al.*, 1969; Willcox, 1975). Latent, inapparent chlamydial infections are common (Dunlop, 1975; Dunlop *et al.*, 1971; Kordová, 1978; Meyer, 1967; Oriel *et al.*, 1978; Storz, 1971).

Where trachoma is endemic, the prevalence of eye infections is usually high among infants, and older children typically suffer chronic infections or successive, aggravating episodes (Duke-Elder, 1965; Grayston, 1967; Grayston and Wang, 1975; Jones, 1975; Nichols *et al.*, 1967, 1971b; Woolridge *et al.*, 1967b). Mothers often infect their infants, sometimes by genital tract-to-eye transmission during childbirth (Duke-Elder, 1965; Pagès *et al.*, 1969; Shaaban *et al.*, 1972). Although all authorities agree that trachoma spreads mainly from eye to eye, and that it is mainly a disease of the poor, the actual mechanisms of transmission remain in doubt (Jones, 1975). Epidemiological data indicate that transmission occurs preferentially within families (Barenfanger, 1975; Grayston and Wang, 1975; Nichols *et al.*, 1971a,b), but Barenfanger (1975) found "no situation or practice within the family which would account for the familial aggregation of trachoma."

Recurrences of active, inflammatory trachoma, whether due to reinfection or to reactivation of a latent infection, tend eventually to entail conjunctival scarring, abrasion of the cornea, corneal neovascularization and scarring, and lasting visual impairment. Development of lymphoid follicles in the trachomatous conjunctiva evidences a vigorous local antibody response which may limit dissemination of infective particles; yet these conjunctival follicles, when they become foci of necrosis

and collagen deposition, are harbingers of blindness (Collier, 1967; Dhermy *et al.*, 1967; Duke-Elder, 1965; Nataf, 1952). It is possible, therefore, that immunological responses to the trachoma organism have both protective and pathogenic significance (Collier, 1967; Dawson, 1975; Grayston, 1967; Grayston and Wang, 1975; Silverstein, 1974; Silverstein and Prendergast, 1971; Woolridge *et al.*, 1967b).

Rather than being the certain consequence of a transient ocular infection with *C. trachomatis*, extensive scarring in trachoma thus appears to reflect an epidemiological pattern in which unknown factors associated with poverty favor intrafamilial eye-to-eye transmission and recurrent ocular infection. When public health measures and economic development combine to break the tight transmission cycle of endemic trachoma (Dawson *et al.*, 1976; Jones, 1975), the epidemiology of TRIC infections shifts toward a pattern of sexual transmission, persistent genital infections in sexually active adults, and transmission to the newborn from the cervix (Dawson, 1975; Grayston and Wang, 1975; Schachter *et al.*, 1976). In England and the United States, *C. trachomatis* has been isolated in cell culture from the urethras of about 40% of men with nongonococcal urethritis, and from an even greater proportion of cases of postgonococcal urethritis. The rate of isolation from women with cervicitis is about 30%, but the inflamed cervix often yields other potential pathogens along with chlamydiae. Many, if not most, cervical infections with *C. trachomatis* are asymptomatic, the isolation rate for normal, sexually active women being as high as 11% in some clinics in the United States (Schachter *et al.*, 1976). A genital TRIC infection may prime a person to develop damaging inflammation of the conjunctiva and cornea if the eye becomes infected secondarily (Grayston and Wang, 1975).

Although Reiter's syndrome, which preferentially affects young men possessing the HLA27 histocompatibility antigen, is sometimes accompanied by chlamydial infection of the urethra, there is no evidence proving that chlamydiae are the sole and primary infectious agents of this symptom complex (Dunlop, 1975; Schachter, 1976). LGV is a sexually transmitted chlamydial infection involving extension of the intracellular growth cycle beyond the genital tract epithelium to the regional lymphatics (Abrams, 1968; Willcox, 1975).

The full range of pathogenic and nonpathogenic chlamydial infections of the genital tract may well prove to be considerably greater than that revealed thus far (Dunlop, 1975; Hobson and Holmes, 1977; Oriel *et al.*, 1978; Richmond and Sparling, 1976; Schachter *et al.*, 1976). The apparent lack of acquired resistance to such infections gives special cause for concern.

2. Histopathology of Trachoma

At the present stage of research on chlamydial infections of humans, mechanisms of pathogenesis and the effects of immunological responses on pathogenesis are still largely unknown. Complementarity between parasite and host, latency, benign parasitism, lytic growth, toxicity, hyperplasia, protective immunity, hypersensitivity, necrosis, and scarring are finely interwoven in space–time, but most of the details of the weave appear blurred or disconnected. The histopathology of trachoma provides a space–time coordinate system in which other relevant data must be located (Collier, 1967; Dhermy *et al.*, 1967; Duke-Elder, 1965; Nataf, 1952; Taborisky, 1932).

The infected conjunctival epithelium in trachoma undergoes stratification, squamous metaplasia, and papillary hypertrophy. The superficial cells slough off readily, while mitotic activity increases in the basal layer. These changes, occurring in all persistent inflammations of the conjunctiva, can be attributed to nonspecific irritation (Duke-Elder, 1965; Theodore and Schlossman, 1958). Some epithelial cells contain chlamydial inclusions, and necrosis of epithelial cells is evident. Until recently, inclusions had not been seen in subepithelial cells (Collier, 1967; Mitsui and Suzuki, 1956); moreover, all attempts to infect the subepithelial tissue directly have failed (Thygeson, 1951; Thygeson and Richards, 1938). However, Gendre *et al.* (1975), studying thin sections of conjunctival biopsies with the electron microscope, found macrophages containing large numbers of *C. trachomatis* particles.

Immunological responses are conditioned in part by the distribution, persistence, and fate of antigens (Collier and Mogg, 1969; M. G. Hanna, Jr., *et al.*, 1969; Nossal and Ada, 1971); macrophages are apt to ingest particulate antigens and antigen–antibody complexes; and processing of chlamydial antigens by macrophages could be a step in toxigenesis (Davies *et al.*, 1976; Kordová *et al.*, 1973a; Taverne and Blyth, 1971) as well as in immunogenesis (Pearsall and Weiser, 1970; Stuart, 1970, 1975; Vernon-Roberts, 1972): therefore, tracing the fate of chlamydiae, of their antigens (Mields *et al.*, 1974), and of macrophages in subepithelial tissue is an essential task of future research. If trachoma organisms are as toxic to human conjunctival macrophages as they are to mouse peritoneal macrophages (Lawn *et al.*, 1973; Taverne and Blyth, 1971; Taverne *et al.*, 1974), such injury is likely to have effects on both pathology and immunology (Taverne and Blyth, 1971).

Infiltration of the trachomatous conjunctiva by granulocytes, lymphoid cells, and macrophages is superimposed on a normal abundance of subepithelial lymphocytes (Dhermy *et al.*, 1967). Lymphocytes and plasma cells predominate in the infiltrate, but the deep subepithelial tissue is also rich in mast cells and eosinophils. The presence of many polymorphonuclear neutrophil leukocytes (PMNs) beneath and within the epithelium, sometimes interpreted as evidence of secondary bacterial infection, is mainly a feature of the earliest stages of trachoma.

Aggregates of lymphocytes, reticular cells, and macrophages gradually develop into lymphoid follicles with germinal centers, thus presenting another histological correlate (in addition to plasma cell infiltration) of local antibody synthesis (Cottier *et al.*, 1967; Good *et al.*, 1969; M. G. Hanna, Jr., *et al.*, 1969; Jones, 1965, 1971; Nossal and Ada, 1971; Thorbecke and Lerman, 1976; Turk and Oort, 1967, 1969). Chronic irritation may be sufficient to account for this change, since eserine, atropine, and other chemical irritants applied repeatedly to the external eye can produce a follicular conjunctivitis resembling trachoma (Duke-Elder, 1965; Fromaget and Harriet, 1916; Theodore and Schlossman, 1958). The germinal centers are occupied mostly by mitotic figures, immunoblasts, reticular cells, and large macrophages (tingible body macrophages) containing phagocytized material in which nuclear debris is prominent. What happens in these germinal centers is crucial and poorly understood. One would like to know, for example, if any chlamydial components or products are concentrated in the germinal centers by antibody cytophilic for dendritic reticular cells (M. G. Hanna, Jr., and Szakal, 1968; M. G. Hanna, Jr., *et al.*, 1969; Nossal and Ada, 1971). Are some germinal centers responding to altered or unmasked host antigens (Chorzelski *et al.*, 1973; Henson *et al.*, 1974; Manski and Whiteside, 1974; Mondino *et al.*, 1977a; Rahi and Garner, 1976)? Are B memory cells proliferating and dying in the germinal centers (Grobler *et al.*, 1974; Humphrey, 1976; White, 1975)?

As the lymphoid follicles develop, the conjunctival lymphatic vessels dilate and become filled with small and large lymphocytes. Could some of these lymphocytes be B-memory cells that, having migrated from the adjacent follicles, are destined to seed distant lymphoid tissue?

In trachoma, as distinguished from other follicular conjunctivitides, necrosis of most of the cells present in germinal centers may succeed intense germinal center activity. A homogeneously staining eosinophilic material is seen in the spaces formerly occupied by living cells. The literature on germinal centers documents the death or injury of both immunoblasts and dendritic reticular cells as a normal feature of follicular responses (M. G. Hanna, Jr., and Szakal, 1968; Nossal and Ada, 1971; L. Weiss, 1972), the ultimate scavengers being tingible body macrophages (Fliedner, 1967; Odartchenko *et al.*, 1967; Vernon-Roberts, 1972). Thus central follicular necrosis appears to be the outcome not of a special pathogenetic mechanism but rather of continuing entrapment of antigen.

The sequel to central follicular necrosis in trachoma is subepithelial scarring, whereby the loose, lymphoidal connective tissue of the conjunctiva is replaced by inelastic masses of collagen fibers. Scarring of follicles is not an unusual feature of germinal center regression with necrosis (Ringertz and Adamson, 1950), and injured macrophages may release a factor that stimulates fibroblasts to lay down collagen (Davies *et al.*, 1976). If conjunctival scarring

becomes extensive, the eyelid turns inward so that the eyelashes abrade the cornea. This abrasion leads to ulceration, scarring, and opacification of the cornea. In addition, early infection and inflammation of the cornea itself result in exfoliation of corneal epithelium, ingrowth of granulation tissue with blood vessels (pannus), and development of lymphoid follicles near the limbus; persistent infiltration by lymphocytes and plasma cells follows an early PMN response (Duke-Elder, 1965).

If there is any major unifying pattern to be discerned in the histopathology of trachoma, it is the complementary relationship between a relatively inaccessible, possibly toxigenic, and thus persistent intracellular parasite on the one hand and, on the other hand, a sustained, local B-cell and antibody response to the persistent antigenic stimulation (Dhermy *et al.*, 1967; Silverstein, 1974; Silverstein and Prendergast, 1971). Although the links between the epithelial infection and the subepithelial lymphoid hyperplasia remain untraced, one can be fairly certain that there are decisive confrontations between chlamydiae and macrophages. In addition, one might adopt the working hypothesis that chlamydial antigen persists appreciably longer in subepithelial tissue than do live chlamydiae.

3. Interactions between Chlamydiae and Host Cells

3.1. Binding and Phagocytosis of Chlamydiae by Host Cells *in Vitro*

The first step in the establishment of the intracellular infection is attachment of the chlamydial elementary body to the surface of the host cell. Using ^{14}C-labeled elementary bodies, Becker *et al.* (1969) demonstrated that heparin inhibited attachment of TRIC elementary bodies to BSC_1 cells in monolayer culture. Since heparin is a strongly charged polyanion, they concluded that the attachment step involves electrostatic interaction. Kuo *et al.* (1973), using HeLa cells pretreated with polyelectrolytes, *N*-acetylneuraminic acid, or neuraminidase, obtained evidence suggesting that sialic acid residues on the cell surface may act as specific receptors for TRIC organisms, but not for LGV organisms. Heat-inactivated TRIC organisms in excess specifically blocked the TRIC receptors, while inactivated LGV organisms or inactivated influenza virus failed to do so. Kuo and Grayston (1976) found that the rate of attachment of TRIC and LGV organisms to HeLa 229 cells was temperature-dependent. Fluoride did not affect attachment but did inhibit intracellular growth of both TRIC and LGV organisms. Attachment appeared not to be critical in determining the differential susceptibility of HeLa 229 cells and fetal tonsil cells to infection with TRIC organisms.

Friis (1972) studied the entry of *C. psittaci* (meningopneumonitis strain) into mouse L cells (fibroblasts). The L cells phagocytosed not only intact chlamydiae but also chlamydiae inactivated by heat or neutralized by antiserum, as demonstrated by electron microscopy. Following ingestion, intact chlamydiae remained segregated from lysosomes in a phagocytic vacuole throughout their developmental cycle, whereas heat-inactivated organisms or those neutralized by homologous antiserum appeared in phagolysosomes within 12 hr after attachment. By infecting the L cells in the presence of chloramphenicol, Friis showed that the intracellular chlamydiae were protected from lysosomal attack even when unable to synthesize new protein. Failure of host cell lysosomes to fuse with phagosomes containing *Chlamydia* cells has also been demonstrated by other investigators (Kordová and Wilt, 1972; Kordová *et al.*, 1971, 1972a,b, 1973a,b, 1975; Lawn *et al.*, 1973; Taverne *et al.*, 1974; Todd and Storz, 1975; Wyrick and Brownridge, 1978). We shall discuss below a proposed mechanism (Moulder *et al.*, 1976) for the failure of lysosomal fusion in "successful" chlamydial infections.

Byrne (1976) and Byrne and Moulder (1978) showed that HeLa 229 cells and L cells phagocytosed *C. trachomatis* (LGV strain) and *C. psittaci* (6BC psittacosis strain) 10–100 times more efficiently than they phagocytosed *Escherichia coli* or polystyrene latex spheres 0.5–1.0 μm in diameter. Whereas ultraviolet irradiation of the chlamydiae sufficient to prevent multiplication did not reduce the efficiency with which they were phagocytosed, heating the chlamydiae for 3 min at 60°C or exposing them to homologous rabbit antiserum inhibited phagocytosis (in contrast with the behavior of Friis's meningopneumonitis strain/L-cell sys-

tem). Phagocytosis was not affected by exposure of the chlamydiae to proteases or detergent but was inhibited when host cells had been exposed to proteases. Preincubation of host cells with cycloheximide also inhibited phagocytosis. Byrne and Moulder (1978) conclude that each chlamydial cell specifies its own attachment and ingestion by virtue of possessing surface ligands with high affinity for normal, ubiquitous configurations on the surface of host cells. They suggest that such surface ligands, permitting parasite-specified phagocytosis by nonprofessional phagocytes, represent evolutionary adaptations to intracellular existence.

Lawn *et al.* (1973) found striking differences between mouse peritoneal macrophages and BHK21 (baby hamster kidney) cells in their interactions with *C. trachomatis* cells. Macrophages phagocytosed unselectively, ingesting latex particles as well as chlamydial elementary bodies and reticulate bodies. Lysosomes fused with phagosomes containing ingested chlamydiae, and the parasites were digested. The macrophages exhibited cytopathic effects (Taverne and Blyth, 1971). BHK21 cells, in contrast, phagocytosed the elementary bodies selectively, totally excluding latex particles: this selectivity is consistent with the concept of parasite-specified phagocytosis by nonprofessional phagocytes (Byrne and Moulder, 1978). Ingested elementary bodies remained sequestered from lysosomes and underwent typical developmental changes.

3.2. Cytopathic and Other Modes of Infection *in Vitro*

The pathogenicity of chlamydiae is still not well understood. Some productive chlamydial infections are apparently nonlytic, that is, the chlamydiae establish a mode of growth and of egress which leaves their host cells alive (Kordová *et al.*, 1972a,b). Fast, highly lytic infections may become slow (latent) and benign (Meyer and Eddie, 1951, 1962; Morgan, 1956; Moulder, 1964). Officer and Brown (1961) maintained a chronic infection with egg-grown *C. psittaci* 6BC in a culture of Chang's human liver cells. During a period of 1 year, they observed selection, first of a more virulent chlamydial variant and then of a more resistant host cell variant. When an infected cell divided mitotically, one of the two daughter cells sometimes emerged from the division uninfected. Some cells containing well-developed inclusion bodies appeared to release or to destroy the parasites without undergoing lysis.

Kordová and co-workers have produced cytopathic and noncytopathic infections in cell culture with different strains of *C. psittaci* 6BC. When mouse L cells or peritoneal macrophages were infected with organisms that had been passaged in L cells, cytopathic effects occurred following disintegration of host cell lysosomes and intracellular redistribution of lysosomal acid phosphatase (Kordová and Wilt, 1972; Kordová *et al.* 1971, 1973a). The cytopathic effects included agglutination, rounding up of cells, detachment from cover slips, uptake of trypan blue, cytoplasmic granulation and vacuolation, nuclear pyknosis, and lysis. Similar injury was observed after exposure of macrophages to heat-inactivated, chlamydia-free material from infected L cells. Pretreatment of the infectious organisms with homologous antiserum neutralized their cytopathic effect (Kordová and Wilt, 1972).

Taverne *et al.* (1974) obtained similar results when they infected mouse peritoneal macrophages with *C. trachomatis*. In their system, ingestion of heat-killed trachoma organisms did not induce redistribution of acid phosphatase or cytopathic effects. Todd and Storz (1975), in an ultrastructural and enzymological study of *C. psittaci* (polyarthritis strain), showed that maturation of chlamydiae in bovine fetal spleen cells was accompanied by intracellular dispersal of lysosomal acid phosphatase, disintegration of host cell constituents, and lysis. They and others (Kordová *et al.*, 1973a; Taverne *et al.*, 1974) have suggested that at least some of the pathology of chlamydial infections may be due to host cell autodigestion by released lysosomal enzymes.

Since the lysosomes of any dead or dying animal cell tend to disintegrate, the hypothesis of lysosome-mediated host cell injury is hard to verify. Moulder *et al.* (1976) investigated the immediate toxicity for L cells of high multiplicities of *C. psittaci* 6BC that had been passaged in L cells. These workers demonstrated that the concentrations of free and of bound intracellular acid phosphatase did not change until uptake of trypan blue signaled the onset of death in the infected host cell population.

In the presence of chloramphenicol, which prevented multiplication of the parasites, cell death was delayed, but the delay decreased as the multiplicity of infection increased. Using inhibition of L-cell attachment and spreading on plastic as an assay for immediate toxicity following infection, Moulder's group found that such inhibition occurred without any prior or concomitant changes in the rates of oxygen consumption, glucose utilization, or lactate production. The concentration of cAMP (cyclic adenylate) also remained constant after infection, and analogues of cAMP failed to affect the expression of immediate toxicity.

Continuing studies by Moulder and others (Byrne, 1978; Chang and Moulder, 1978; Horoschak and Moulder, 1978; Kellogg *et al.*, 1977), employing various multiplicities of infectious or ultraviolet-killed *C. psittaci* 6BC, further characterized toxic injury of L cells: injury was manifested by failure to exclude trypan blue, by leakage of lactic dehydrogenase and of potassium, magnesium, and inorganic phosphate ions, by inhibition of protein and DNA synthesis and of cell division, and eventually by cell disintegration. Infectious inocula and high multiplicities of infection caused greater damage, and acted more rapidly, than did ultraviolet-killed inocula and low multiplicities. Heat-killed chlamydiae were not measurably toxic, and infected L cells did not release any soluble toxic factor. Infectious, but not ultraviolet-killed, chlamydiae stimulated host cell glycolysis, and this stimulatory effect was blocked by cycloheximide.

Moulder *et al.* (1976) have proposed that the primary early lesion induced by *C. psittaci* or by *C. trachomatis* in the host cell lines studied is an alteration of the host cell plasma membrane. Each act of ingestion would independently produce a membrane lesion, and the discrete lesions would affect host cell functions additively. Membrane lesions could be responsible not only for a variety of permeability changes but also for parasite-specified phagocytosis and failure of lysosomal fusion. The cascade of secondary injurious effects would lead to cell death, which, *in vivo*, might lead in turn to quick death of massively inoculated mice (Manire and Meyer, 1950a; Rake and Jones, 1944). However, in natural infections at low multiplicity, an infected cell would initially suffer very few membrane lesions and would thus support multiplication of the parasites before dying.

If the capacity of chlamydial elementary bodies to modify the host cell plasma membrane is nicely commensurate with the parasite's need to multiply, then the persistent, localized infections that typify the natural lifestyle of some strains of *Chlamydia* may well reflect a perfect, steady-state balance among parasite multiplication, induction of host cell membrane lesions, host cell death, multiplication of neighboring uninfected cells, and host defense mechanisms. One possible unbalancing host response that does not fit into the category of immunological mechanisms is a change of epithelial cell type which would present the parasite with a relatively unreceptive host cell plasma membrane. We suggest that the epidermoid metaplasia seen in some cases of trachoma (Duke-Elder, 1965) might have, fortuitously, just this effect. In addition, the slowing metabolism of the most superficial epidermoid cells might support chlamydial multiplication only at a diminished rate. Immunological mechanisms could then finish off the infection, but a less dramatic possibility is persistent slow replication, blurring into latency (see below).

Kordová *et al.* (1972a,b) produced noncytopathic infections of L cells and of mouse peritoneal macrophages with *C. psittaci* 6BC that had been passaged in chicken eggs rather than in L cells. Lysosomes retained their integrity at all stages of chlamydial development. Infected L cells grew and divided faster than uninfected control cells. Infected macrophages displayed a greater capacity than uninfected ones to spread and to transform into giant cells. Cells of either type, stained with May-Grünwald-Giemsa, exhibited pseudopodiumlike cytoplasmic extrusions which contained chlamydial particles. The authors concluded that the host cell, by pinching off bits of its own cytoplasm, released chlamydiae without undergoing lysis. Unfortunately, they did not report on their observations of living infected cells by phase contrast microscopy, so that the significance of the cytoplasmic extrusions of fixed cells remains in doubt. Certainly the possible maintenance of noncytopathic chlamydial infections by continuous release of cytoplasm (cf. Doughri *et al.*, 1972) or by exocytosis is of utmost importance in the context of immunology. Also worth considering is the possibility that, *in vivo*, the host cell modifications described would eventually cause tissue pathology.

L-cell-grown *C. psittaci* 6BC, when inoculated intraperitoneally into mice, not only failed to replicate but also induced cytopathic effects in macrophages (Kordová *et al.*, 1975). The egg-attenuated strain, in contrast, grew within peritoneal macrophages *in vivo* without appearing to cause damage (Kordová *et al.*,1973b). Both strains induced cytolysis of PMNs.

In another study of encounters between chlamydiae and professional phagocytes (Wyrick and Brownridge, 1978; Wyrick *et al.*, 1978), L-cell-grown *C. psittaci* (meningopneumonitis strain), offered at a low multiplicity of infection (1 : 1) to mouse peritoneal macrophages *in vitro*, was rapidly phagocytized, and proceeded to undergo a typical chlamydial growth cycle with eventual production of infectious elementary bodies. In contrast, at a high multiplicity of infection (100 : 1), although phagocytosis was again rapid, immediate damage to the macrophages greatly reduced survival of the ingested elementary bodies. Pretreatment of elementary bodies with heat or with homologous antibody abolished or reduced immediate toxicity to macrophages, and restored "normal" fusion of lysosomes with the phagosomes in which the treated elementary bodies were enclosed.

No matter how many different kinds of microbes may claim the satisfaction of reproducing in macrophages (Stuart, 1970), the picture will probably never cease to amaze. LGV and *C. psittaci* infections of humans may involve chlamydial growth in macrophages, whereas natural infections with TRIC organisms seem to be confined to epithelial cells. However, macrophages laden with chlamydial particles have been seen with the electron microscope in subepithelial tissue of the trachomatous conjunctiva (Gendre *et al.*, 1975).

Strictly speaking, a latent infection differs from the productive, noncytopathic type of infection described above in that the latent infectious agent is present in the host but does not multiply rapidly enough to provide free infectious particles for laboratory culture or to cause detectable pathological tissue changes. In nature, reactivation of a latent infection is hard to distinguish from reinfection. *In vitro*, however, latency of *C. psittaci* infections has been amply demonstrated (Moulder, 1964). Experimental conditions can be imposed such that the chlamydiae enter host cells and persist intact without multiplying. Penicillin, D-cyclo-serine, sulfadiazine, aminopterin, and starva-tion have been used for this purpose, the du-ration of latency being as long as 28 days. When the growth-inhibiting condition is re-versed, normal intracellular development of the chlamydiae resumes. Hatch (1975) showed that a latent *C. psittaci* 6BC infection in starved, nongrowing L cells could be activated by addition of either isoleucine or cyclohexi-mide. He concluded that the parasite and the L-cell host compete for the isoleucine in the soluble pool of the host cell. In natural, un-treated chlamydial infections, nutritional fac-tors could well be most significant in control-ling latency and activation. As we proposed above, a change of host cell type could alter the nutritional status of the parasite. One might expect antibiotic treatment to sway the parasite–host balance toward either latency or cure.

It is clear that predominantly *in vitro* studies have yielded, and will continue to yield, es-sential information about diverse modes of chlamydial infection (Kordová, 1978). Hardly begun, however, is the task of showing exactly where and when any particular mode of infec-tion comes into play during chlamydial infec-tions of humans.

3.3. Chlamydial Toxicity *in Vivo*

In mice, intravenous inoculation of ex-tremely high doses of certain virulent chla-mydial strains causes toxic death within 2–20 hr (Bietti and Werner, 1967; Manire and Meyer, 1950a; Rake and Jones, 1944). Pro-cedures which destroy the infectivity of the elementary bodies also abolish their toxicity. In the case of trachoma organisms, prelimi-nary intraabdominal immunization with for-maldehyde-, phenol-, or ether-inactivated chlamydiae renders the mice resistant to in-travenous challenge (Bell and Theobald, 1962). When Murray *et al.* (1958) demonstrated the toxic death phenomenon for a trachoma agent,

they noted that the dead mice showed hem-orrhagic exudation into the lumen of the upper small intestine and, frequently, moderate congestion of the lungs.

It is not clear how experimental toxic death is related to pathogenesis in natural chlamydial infections. Taverne *et al.* (1964) compared tox-icities of strains of TRIC agents differing in virulence for the chicken embryo. Finding that particle-to-toxin ratios were similar for all strains tested, they concluded that differences in the amount of toxin per elementary body probably could not account for the differing virulences of the strains.

Mitsui *et al.* (1962) recovered a noninfec-tive, toxic filtrate from homogenates of yolk sac infected with trachoma organisms. Instil-lation of this filtrate 36 times per day into the right eye of each of two human volunteers caused subacute follicular conjunctivitis from which no chlamydiae could be isolated. The volunteers' left eyes, instilled with a filtrate of normal yolk sac, showed no pathology. The authors concluded that the chlamydial cells or the host epithelial cells probably produced a free toxic substance which caused trachoma-tous inflammation of the subepithelial tissue. It remains to be discovered which human cells are the target cells for direct cytotoxic action in natural chlamydial infections and which are damaged by substances released from the pri-mary target cells. Also, a careful semantic dis-tinction among nonspecific irritants (Duke-Elder, 1965; Theodore and Schlossman, 1958), toxins, and nontoxic antigens is essential in discussions of pathogenetic mechanisms.

4. Chlamydial Antigens

4.1. Group-Specific Antigens

Chlamydial group- or family-specific anti-gens, usually detected by complement fixation (CF) in clinical practice, are heat-stable and common to all members of the genus *Chla-mydia* (Bedson, 1932, 1933, 1936; Bedson *et al.*, 1949). Chemicals used to extract group-specific antigens from boiled chlamydial sus-pensions have included water, acid, alkali, ether, deoxycholate, sodium dodecylsulfate, phenol, and urea (Bietti and Werner, 1967;

Storz, 1971). Benedict and O'Brien (1956) used sodium dodecylsulfate to extract a water-soluble group antigen from purified chlamydial elementary bodies. Following partial purification by repeated acid precipitation, treatment with 5% phenol yielded two antigenically active fractions. The phenol-insoluble group antigen, a lipopolysaccharide, contained lecithin and was inactivated by oxidation with periodate. The phenol-soluble group antigen, mainly protein, was insensitive to periodate.

Jenkin et al. (1961) found periodate-sensitive and periodate-resistant group antigens in deoxycholate extracts of chlamydiae. Group antigens were not present in cell walls of the meningopneumonitis and feline pneumonitis strains of C. psittaci. Using Jenkin's method to prepare cell walls of several chlamydial strains as immunogens, Schachter (1968) demonstrated significant activity against group antigens in the sera of guinea pigs immunized with these cell walls. Periodate abolished most of the reactivity of the test antigens. It is essential to note that Jenkin's group used intact elementary bodies as immunogens and cell walls as test antigens, while Schachter used cell walls as immunogens and intact elementary bodies as test antigens. Despite such differences in technique, the data indicate that cell walls do not contain the bulk of the chlamydial group antigens.

Dhir et al. (1971a) recovered a water-soluble polysaccharide antigen by alkali saponification of CF-reactive, lipopolysaccharide group antigen preparations from three trachoma strains. Antibody that fixed complement in combination with the crude antigen failed to fix complement when combined with the polysaccharide antigen. The polysaccharide gave a reaction of identity with several trachoma strains on immunodiffusion plates. Dhir et al. (1972) purified this antigen by DEAE-cellulose chromatography. Gel filtration indicated a molecular weight between 200,000 and 2,000,000. Antigenic activity was destroyed both by 0.005 M periodate and by mild acid hydrolysis. Acid hydrolysis released an acidic component which behaved chemically and chromatographically like 2-keto-3-deoxyoctanoic acid but which probably differs sterically from the 2-keto-3-deoxyoctanoic acid of Salmonella lipopolysaccharides.

4.2. Species-Specific and Type-Specific Antigens

The genus Chlamydia currently includes two species, C. trachomatis and C. psittaci, also designated subgroup A and subgroup B (not to be confused with serotypes A and B), respectively. Cells of C. trachomatis form compact, glycogen-containing inclusions in the cytoplasm of host cells and are sensitive to sulfadiazine, in contrast to cells of C. psittaci strains other than the sulfadiazine-sensitive psittacosis 6BC strain (Becker, 1974, 1978; Gordon and Quan, 1965; Jenkin and Fan, 1971; Lin and Moulder, 1966; Storz, 1971). A number of serological tests can distinguish not only between the species but also between types within each species. Bedson et al. (1949) identified CF antibodies against species-specific antigens in sera from human cases of LGV and ornithosis. These antibodies remained after antibodies against group antigens had been adsorbed out with steamed chlamydial cells. Manire and Meyer (1950b) distinguished six chlamydial serotypes by a toxin neutralization test in which incubation of infectious organisms with antibody prevented toxic death of mice. Neutralization of infectivity has also been used to demonstrate type-specific antigens (Banks et al., 1970). The CF reaction resolved C. psittaci isolates from cattle, sheep, and cats into seven serotypes (Fraser and Berman, 1965), and the mouse toxicity prevention test differentiated six serotypes from human ocular and genital infections alone (Alexander et al., 1967).

At present, the most specific, most sensitive, and most convenient method for typing isolates or sera from chlamydial infections is indirect immunofluorescence (L. Hanna et al., 1972; McComb and Nichols, 1969; Nichols and McComb, 1962; Nichols et al., 1971a; Wang, 1971; Wang and Grayston, 1970). Fifteen antigenic types reactive in the indirect fluorescent antibody (FA) test have been distinguished thus far within the TRIC-LGV spectrum of C. trachomatis strains. These serotypes are lettered A, B, Ba, C through K, L_1, L_2, and L_3. The three L types are associated with LGV. Patterns of cross-reactivity among the 15 serotypes are indicated in Figure 1. The types fall into distinct epidemiological patterns

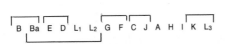

Figure 1. Patterns of cross-reactivity among TRIC-LGV serotypes. Reproduced from Grayston and Wang (1975) by courtesy of the authors, *The Journal of Infectious Diseases*, and The University of Chicago Press. Copyright © 1975 by the University of Chicago. All rights reserved.

as shown in Table 1 for isolates from the eyes and genital tracts of 453 persons. Types A, B, and C, for example, occur predominantly in the eye in populations with endemic trachoma. Types D, E, F, and G are the most frequent genital isolates in both trachoma-endemic and nonendemic areas (Grayston and Wang, 1975; Wang, 1971; Wang and Grayston, 1971).

A clear, consistent picture of the chemistry of type-specific chlamydial antigens has not yet emerged. Even their heat-lability cannot be considered a defining feature, since the type-specific cell wall antigens described by Jenkin *et al.* (1961) were not destroyed by heating at 100°C. Type-specific antigens are consistently resistant to oxidation by periodate (Jenkin *et al.*, 1961; Ross and Gogolak, 1957; Sacks *et al.*, 1978a; Sigel and Pollikoff, 1953), indicating that their determinant groups lack polyhydroxy residues (sugars and sugar derivatives). Dhir *et al.* (1971b) reported that various single lipid solvents, detergents, and proteolytic enzymes failed to affect type-specific antigens. Acid and alkaline hydrolysis both destroyed antigenic activity in the FA test, as did chloroform–methanol–water partitioning. After treatment of antigenic material at pH 12.5, the alkali-soluble fraction adsorbed FA-reactive antibody, blocked mouse toxicity protection, and was active in CF tests both before and after exposure to periodate. The lipid extract from chloroform–methanol–water partitioning was similarly active except in adsorption. Dhir *et al.* (1971b) suggest that "one specific antigen may be a lipoid hapten which is strongly bound to a protein."

Caldwell *et al.* (1975a,b) used two-dimensional immunoelectrophoresis to resolve water-soluble, species-specific chlamydial antigens that had been extracted with the nonionic detergent Triton X-100 from organisms grown in cell culture. A LGV strain of *C. trachomatis* and a meningopneumonitis strain of *C. psittaci* yielded, respectively, 19 and 16 distinct components, of which only one pair showed reciprocal cross-reactivity; in contrast, the antigens of a trachoma strain were very similar to the LGV antigens. One of the LGV antigens was excised (as antigen–antibody complexes) from the agarose gel of electrophorograms and was used to immunize rabbits. The resulting antiserum reacted with TRIC-LGV strains but not with the mouse pneumonitis strain of *C. trachomatis* or the meningopneumonitis strain of *C. psittaci*. Precipitins with specificity for the LGV antigen were identified in 15 of 18 sera from patients having diagnosed LGV or TRIC infections.

The LGV antigen was purified by immunoadsorption with rabbit antiserum γ-globulins that had been coupled to the *N*-hydroxysuccinimide ester derivative of agarose. The purified antigen was a heat-labile protein, resistant to periodate oxidation, with an apparent molecular weight of 155,000 (Caldwell and Kuo, 1977a). Antibody reacting with the purified antigen in counterimmunoelectrophoresis was found in 43 of 45 sera from patients with LGV, whereas no positive reactions were given by sera from 50 patients with nongonococcal urethritis, 38 of whom had antibody reacting with whole fixed TRIC organisms in the indirect FA test (Caldwell and Kuo, 1977b).

TABLE 1.   Results of Serotyping of TRIC-LGV Isolates from the Eyes and Genital Tracts of 453 Persons from around the World[a]

Isolates	A	B	Ba	CJ	ED	GF	H	I	K	L₁	L₂	L₃
Ocular strains												
Trachoma endemic	10	25	12	79	4	1						
Trachoma nonendemic		1	3	3	26	11	1	4	1			
Genital strains		11		9	113	76	16	12	17	3	12	3

[a] Reproduced from Grayston and Wang (1975) by courtesy of the authors, *The Journal of Infectious Diseases*, and The University of Chicago Press. Copyright © 1975 by the University of Chicago. All rights reserved.

Caldwell and Kuo suggested that counterimmunoelectrophoresis with their purified *C. trachomatis* antigen would be a useful serologic test for diagnosis of LGV.

Partial purification of water-soluble, type-specific antigens from human ocular strains of *C. trachomatis* has been achieved by two different methods. In the first procedure, Sacks *et al.* (1978a) labeled surface components of yolk-sac-grown, renografin-purified type B organisms with radioiodine (^{125}I) and then extracted the organisms with Triton X-100. The heterogeneous antigen solution was resolved by gel filtration through Sepharose 6B. Radioimmunoassay was used to test all filtration fractions for binding with rabbit antisera raised against immunogens extracted from homologous- and heterologous-type organisms that had been propagated in BHK21 cells. A fraction exhibiting only homologous binding served subsequently as tracer for the isolation of larger quantities of type-B-specific antigen. Under conditions of antibody excess in the radioimmunoassay, homologous rabbit antiserum bound 3–4 times as much purified antigen as did heterologous and control antisera. The reactivity of the antigen was destroyed by proteolytic enzymes and by heating at 56°C for 30 min but was not affected by periodate. Molecular filtration gave an apparent molecular weight of 28,000.

In the second isolation procedure, Sacks and MacDonald (1979) extracted ^{125}I-labeled, type A trachoma organisms with Nonidet P-40 and sonicated them. The extracted antigens were precipitated with homologous rabbit antiserum and goat antirabbit Fc. The precipitates, after having been washed, were dissolved in buffered 4% sodium dodecylsulfate at 100°C. The resulting solutions of test antigen were analyzed by electrophoresis in polyacrylamide gels containing 0.1% sodium dodecylsulfate. A type-A-specific electrophoretic peak appeared which was specifically eliminated by immunoadsorbent chromatography of the test antigen with purified immunoglobulin G (IgG) fractions from homologous rabbit antisera. Comparison of the type-specific peak with those of protein standards indicated an approximate molecular weight of 27,000.

In the Triton X-100/Sepharose 6B procedure (Sacks *et al.,* 1978a), less than 4% of the total radioactivity of the major elution peak was specifically bound by homologous antibody in excess. In the alternate procedure (Sacks and MacDonald, 1979), the type-specific electrophoretic peak represented less than 1% of the total radioactivity precipitated with homologous rabbit antiserum and antirabbit Fc in the early immunoprecipitation step. Modifications of technique will probably improve the purity and yield of type-specific antigens. The possibility of type-specific chlamydial antigens becoming available for clinical laboratory procedures and for vaccination trials, as well as for basic research, is very exciting.

In a few preliminary studies, researchers have sought to characterize those chlamydial antigens that elicit cell-mediated immunologic responses. Kuo *et al.* (1971b,c) sensitized guinea pigs with inactivated TRIC, LGV, or meningopneumonitis organisms and then assayed variously treated antigen preparations by skin testing and by *in vitro* lymphocyte transformation. The effects of the pretest treatments of antigen indicated that the active moiety was a species-specific, heat-stable protein, extractable with weak acid. Sayed *et al.* (1972) sensitized guinea pigs and mice with live LGV organisms and then tested for cell-mediated immunity with a commercial Frei test antigen. The test antigen was fractionated by electrofocusing (following sonication) in order to isolate and identify antigenic components. Of 42 fractions, 17 were inhibitory in the mouse macrophage spreading inhibition test: the four most active fractions, which caused inhibition ranging from 57% to 69%, had relatively small amounts of nitrogen, relatively high ratios of nonreducing sugars to nitrogen, and extreme values of isoelectric points. Subsequent work (Sayed *et al.,* 1976) showed that the protein and carbohydrate content of the most active electrofocused fractions in the macrophage spreading inhibition test were different for TRIC and LGV organisms.

5. Cellular and Humoral Immunological Responses to Chlamydiae

Obviously one cannot treat the spectrum of host responses to infection as a topic independent of antigenic diversity. Our purpose in making this artificial separation is to shift emphasis now to resistance and pathogenesis in chlamydial infections. In surveying the known modes of immunological response to chlamydiae, we hope to bring out the various possible means by which such responses might hinder or promote the disease process.

5.1. Evidence of Cell-Mediated Immunity

Most persons having active or healed trachoma displayed delayed-type hypersensitivity when challenged intradermally with trachoma antigens (Bietti and Werner, 1967; Ghione et al., 1974; Grayston et al., 1960). Some responded similarly to ornithosis antigens. The group specificity of the skin test precluded its use for diagnosis of trachoma. Sensitivity to trachoma antigens could be passively transferred with suspensions of leukocytes from trachoma patients (D'Ermo et al., 1964). Soldati et al. (1971) demonstrated significant blast transformation, on challenge with trachoma agent, in cultures of lymphocytes from nontrachomatous persons who had received killed trachoma vaccine intramuscularly 45–90 days previously.

Repeated intraperitoneal inoculations of mice with trachoma organisms activated the peritoneal macrophages so that in vivo replication of chlamydiae in these macrophages, observed (although in decline) after each of the first three inoculations, did not occur after subsequent inoculations (Soldati et al., 1971). It was not proven in this experiment that the increasing capacity of macrophages to kill ingested chlamydiae reflected cell-mediated immunity (CMI) rather than promotion of lysosomal fusion by antibody (Friis, 1972; Wyrick and Brownridge, 1978; Wyrick et al., 1978). Trachoma and psittacosis antigens induced group-specific, delayed-type hypersensitivity in guinea pigs (Kassira, 1971; Kuo and Grayston, 1974; Kuo et al., 1971b,c). Ronald Watson et al. (1973b) showed that guinea pigs also develop delayed-type hypersensitivity to the agent of guinea pig inclusion conjunctivitis (Murray, 1964). Use of a single injection of cyclophosphamide to deplete the B-lymphocyte population of guinea pigs indicated that T lymphocytes may mediate early development of specific resistance to guinea pig inclusion conjunctivitis (Modabber et al., 1976). The cyclophosphamide treatment left the T-cell areas of the spleen and lymph nodes well populated, and

the delayed skin reaction unchanged, but it depleted the B-cell areas and delayed the appearance of serum antibodies and of lacrimal secretory IgA antibody. Although disappearance of chlamydial inclusions from conjunctival epithelial cells was also delayed, showing that complete recovery probably required antibody, an early phase of partial recovery was consistent with a role for effector T cells.

Sacks et al. (1978b) demonstrated CMI to trachoma antigens in owl monkeys. Water-soluble antigen was obtained by extracting homogenates of infected BHK21 cells with Triton X-100 at pH 10. Following experimental infection of the monkeys' eyes with trachoma organisms, the antigen was used in a leukocyte migration inhibition test and in a skin test for delayed-type hypersensitivity. The onset of inhibition of leucocyte migration, occurring by the ninth day after inoculation, accompanied clearance of inclusions from the monkeys' conjunctival cells, whereas titers of plasma and eye secretion antibodies did not rise until a few days later. Two months after the primary infection, all test animals were resistant to reinfection and showed persistence of both CMI and humoral immunity. Sacks et al. (1978b) conclude that CMI was probably the principal mechanism effecting recovery from primary infection in these experiments, but they also consider the possibility that binding of local antibodies to trachoma organisms precluded early detection of such antibodies.

In the Frei test for LGV, killed LGV antigen is injected intradermally and elicits a group-specific, delayed-type hypersensitivity reaction (Bedson et al., 1949; Frei, 1925; Hilleman et al., 1958). Many patients who have had a chlamydial infection other than LGV show positive Frei tests. False-negative Frei tests are also frequent (Willcox, 1975). Thus, for diagnosis of LGV, the Frei test is less reliable than the CF or indirect FA tests (Grayston and Wang, 1975; Schachter et al., 1969, 1976; Wang and Grayston, 1971, 1974; Wang et al., 1973; Willcox, 1975).

Because plasma cells persistently infiltrate the trachomatous conjunctiva and cornea along with lymphocytes and macrophages, and because, in the typical sequence of pathological changes, lymphoid follicles also appear, one can readily infer from the histopathological picture of trachoma that local B-cell proliferation and local antibody synthesis are major features of the disease. It is much more difficult to assess the relative contribution of CMI to the histopathology (Dvorak *et al.*, 1974; Friedlander and Dvorak, 1977; Friedlander *et al.*, 1978). Assuming that effector T lymphocytes are present, how might they be involved in protecting or injuring the host? Infected epithelial cells could be targets of lymphotoxin. Inhibition of macrophage migration and induction of macrophage proliferation by lymphokines would keep macrophages available locally as potential cellular hosts, or victims, or killers of the intracellular parasites. Activation of macrophages would promote killing of chlamydiae within phagolysosomes (David, 1976; Hadden *et al.*, 1978; Mackaness, 1971; Prendergast and Henney, 1977; Sayed *et al.*, 1972; Soldati *et al.*, 1971; Snyderman and Pike, 1975; Stuart, 1970, 1975). Some antigenic material, resisting digestion by lysosomal enzymes, might persist and might continue to stimulate the immune system even after all live chlamydiae had been eliminated (Ginsburg *et al.*, 1976). Thus far, there is no evidence that any of these expressions and consequences of CMI actually occur in natural trachoma or in other chlamydial infections of humans.

5.2. Interferon

Several laboratories have reported on the induction and effects of interferon in cells infected by chlamydiae (L. Hanna *et al.*, 1966, 1967; Jenkin and Lu, 1967; Kazar *et al.*, 1971; Merigan and Hanna, 1966; Mordhorst *et al.*, 1967; Oh *et al.*, 1971; Sueltenfuess and Pollard, 1963). Lavelle Hanna *et al.* (1966) infected mouse L cells with Newcastle disease virus in order to induce formation of interferon. This interferon, but not interferon induced in human neonate fibroblasts, inhibited growth of an inclusion conjunctivitis strain of *C. trachomatis* in L cells. Conversely, mouse L cells or mice infected with *C. trachomatis* produced an interferon that inhibited growth of bovine vesicular stomatitis virus in L cells (Merigan and Hanna, 1966). The interferon induced by *C. trachomatis* had a molecular weight of about 50,000, thus contrasting with virus-induced interferons which have molecular weights of 36,000 or less. Kazar *et al.*

(1971) showed that mouse interferon inhibited replication of *C. trachomatis* in L cells without affecting prior phagocytosis of the chlamydial elementary bodies by the L cells.

High levels of artificially induced interferon in the serum and aqueous humor of rabbits failed to inhibit growth of trachoma agent in their ocular tissues following inoculation of the anterior chamber (Oh *et al.*, 1971). Although the infection in this case was in an unnatural location in an unnatural host, one cannot take lightly an apparent failure of interferon to protect *in vivo*. We know of no persuasive evidence indicating that interferon production plays a significant role in resistance to natural chlamydial infections.

5.3. Complement-Fixing Antibodies

Fixation and activation of complement by antigen–antibody complexes may promote opsonization, immune adherence, PMN chemotaxis, bacteriolysis, and other processes (Müller-Eberhard, 1975; Volanakis, 1975). When, for example, complement fixation is a prerequisite for neutralization of infectivity, the neutralizing antibodies are properly included in the general category of CF antibodies. In the commonest test for CF antibodies, these antibodies inhibit complement-mediated hemolysis. Used routinely to detect antibodies against chlamydial group antigens, the CF test has also been applied (although less routinely) to serotyping.

Serum CF antibodies are not reliable correlates of disease in trachoma patients (Woolridge and Grayston, 1962). Bietti and Werner (1967) reviewed evidence indicating that from 40% to 75% of trachoma patients lack serum CF antibodies against chlamydial group antigen. The percentage of positive sera increases with the age of the patients. Bietti and Werner suggest that chlamydiae other than TRIC agents stimulate production of CF antibodies which subsequently modify the clinical course of the ocular disease. Apparently the group antigens of TRIC organisms are only weakly immunogenic for CF antibodies but may cause the titer of such antibodies, if they are already present, to increase. Modifications of procedures used to kill, disintegrate, and purify chlamydial elementary bodies have yielded antigen preparations that show, in addition to group specificity, varying degrees of species or type specificity with respect to CF antibodies (Bedson et al., 1949; Fraser and Berman, 1965; Jenkin et al., 1961; Ross and Gogolak, 1957; Schachter, 1968). Serological methods can be varied. Lycke and Peterson (1976) developed a hemolysis-in-gel test in which the targets for CF antibodies were tannic-acid-treated sheep erythrocytes coated with C. trachomatis antigen from infected McCoy cells.

Most LGV patients with active disease develop serum CF antibodies against chlamydial group antigens (Abrams, 1968; Meyer and Eddie, 1962; Grayston and Wang, 1975; Schachter et al., 1969). Although titers tend to fall or to vanish when antibiotic treatment results in clinical cure, many persons who have significant antibody titers present neither physical evidence nor a history of disease. Children and young adolescents rarely have antibodies; hence it is possible that sexual transmission of the LGV agent can lead to persistent, asymptomatic, immunogenic infections (Grant et al., 1962). It is also possible that some of the seropositive individuals have had asymptomatic, immunogenic genital tract infections with TRIC agents (Willcox, 1975).

Using a group-specific antigen from a strain of C. psittaci causing abortion in sheep, Schmatz et al. (1977) detected antichlamydial CF antibodies in serum samples from 10% of 1075 randomly chosen blood donors and 26% of 524 randomly chosen "sick" patients. In general, the seropositive patients had significantly higher titers than did the seropositive blood donors. Schmatz and co-workers suggest that more attention be paid to a possible etiological role of chlamydiae in pathological conditions of unknown origin. Their results are also consistent with transient chlamydial superinfection of persons whose resistance has been lowered by some unrelated pathologic process.

Determination of CF antibody titers has been applied almost exclusively to diagnosis and epidemiology of chlamydial infections. There is, however, absolutely no direct evidence that complement-mediated immunological reactions play even a minor role in resistance to or in pathogenesis of natural chlamydial infections. Assays for complement-mediated neutralization of infectivity have provided indirect evidence for a protective role. Howard (1975) assayed neutralization of C. trachomatis by the decrease in inclusion-forming units in cultured BHK21 cells. Rabbit antisera, human antisera, and human eye secretions displayed specific neutralizing activity that depended on the presence of a heat-labile component (presumably complement) of normal guinea pig serum. On the other hand, resistance of guinea pigs to guinea pig inclusion conjunctivitis failed to correlate with the presence of serum CF antibodies, even though serum antibodies were active in complement-mediated neutralization when incubated with infectious organisms prior to inoculation of the conjunctiva (Murray et al., 1973). Thus one may be comforted by the evidence that chlamydiae can induce their natural hosts to make neutralizing CF antibodies and discomforted by the evidence that, in infections occurring naturally, the chlamydiae probably escape the influence of such antibodies.

Regardless of whether or not complement-mediated neutralization of pathogenic chlamydiae occurs in vivo under natural conditions, one must also consider the possibility of complement-mediated immunopathogenesis. In trachoma, for example, inflammatory cells and new blood vessels from the limbus invade the substantia propria of the cornea (Nataf, 1952). When trachoma organisms are inoculated into the anterior chamber of the rabbit eye (Oh and Tarizzo, 1969), intravenous injection of a synthetic polyriboinosinic acid–polyribocytidylic acid complex (an interferon inducer) suppresses opacification and neovascularization of the cornea without suppressing growth of chlamydiae in the ocular tissues (Oh et al., 1971). Collier (1967) has remarked that pannus formation in trachoma resembles immunological vasculitis (Arthus-type reaction, e.g., Parish, 1972) induced experimentally by injection of soluble antigens into the corneas of previously immunized rabbits (Germuth et al., 1962; Klintworth, 1977; Rahi and Garner, 1976). PMN chemotaxis could be caused either by operation of the major complement pathway or by properdin activation leading to stimulation of the alternate pathway of complement (Mondino et al., 1977b). Although rat PMNs may release angiogenic factors (Fromer and Klintworth, 1976), normal vascularization of healing wounds in guinea pigs does not require PMNs (Simpson and Ross, 1972). According to Duke-Elder (1965), neovascularization of the trachomatous cornea is most closely preceded not by PMN infiltration, but by infiltration of lymphocytes and plasma cells, as if the corneal subepithelial tissue, like that of the conjunctiva (Jones, 1965), were being made into accessory lymphoid tissue. Clearly, the uncertain role of immunological vasculitis challenges those engaged in research on chlamydial diseases to test specific immunopathological models.

Most laboratories titrate group-specific antichlamydial antibodies by one or another method involving CF. The search continues, however, for convenient group-specific assays that do not require CF. Lewis *et al.* (1977) developed an enzyme-linked immunosorbent assay (ELISA) in which conjugated horseradish peroxidase catalyzed a color change. Antigen was dried and fixed in the wells of microtiter plates; it was then exposed to dilutions of human antisera. The indicator layer was sheep antihuman IgG conjugated with horseradish peroxidase. Peroxidase activity changed the color of a solution containing hydrogen peroxide and 5-amino-2-hydroxybenzoic acid. The ELISA was more rapid and more sensitive than the CF test; other advantages included stability of the dried antigen for over 1 year at $-65°C$, and the possibility of automatic spectrophotometry (Clem and Yolken, 1978).

5.4. Antibodies (Possibly Non-CF) Neutralizing Chlamydial Infectivity or Toxicity

Various host cell systems have been used to assay neutralization of chlamydial infectivity. Reeve and Graham (1962) counted inclusions in HeLa cell cultures in order to titrate the neutralizing activity of rabbit antisera against TRIC agents. Banks *et al.* (1970), using hyperimmune chicken antisera against chlamydiae isolated from avian species, counted plaques in monolayers of mouse L cells. Nichols *et al.* (1973) counted inclusions in conjunctival smears from owl monkeys whose conjunctivae had been inoculated with a type A trachoma agent. Partial neutralization of this organism was achieved by incubation with

pooled eye secretions from Saudi Arabian children having active or inactive trachoma. Using the same host system, Barenfanger and MacDonald (1974b) demonstrated neutralization of trachoma organisms by pooled eye secretions and pooled plasma from Saudi Arabian children with active trachoma. When the eye secretion pool was fractionated by precipitation with 50% saturated ammonium sulfate, neutralizing activity was recovered only in the precipitating (Ig) fraction, and the neutralization was type-specific. Monkeys inoculated with fully infective trachoma agent developed much higher titers of FA-reactive antibodies in their eye secretions and sera than did those inoculated with neutralized trachoma agent. Perhaps the most striking feature of this experiment was that the children who served as sources of neutralizing antibody had active trachoma, i.e., the antibody did not protect them from persistent infection. It should be noted that the children's eye secretions and plasmas were not heated in either of these studies of owl monkeys, leaving open the possibility of complement activation.

As mentioned earlier in this chapter, the mouse toxicity prevention test was a major predecessor of the FA test for identification of chlamydial serotypes. Wang (1971), studying mice that had been immunized intravenously with TRIC antigens, found complete agreement between resistance to toxic death and FA reactivity of the mouse antisera in terms of type specificity, dose response, time response, and correlation of protection with type-specific antibody titers. He concluded that humoral antibody was responsible for type-specific acquired resistance to toxic death in mice.

By what means might neutralization have been effected in the experiments that we have summarized? Complement-mediated lysis of chlamydiae, although never (to our knowledge) reported in the literature, is a possibility more attractive for antibodies to group-specific lipopolysaccharides than for antibodies to type-specific proteins. It seems likely that antibodies inhibit attachment of elementary bodies to host cells that are not professional phagocytes (Gibbons, 1974; Byrne and Moulder, 1978). On the other hand, when professional phagocytes are clearly available, as they are in the mouse toxicity prevention test, opsonization may enhance their natural and unselective tendency to ingest chlamydiae (Lawn *et al.*, 1973; Pearsall and Weiser, 1970; Scribner and Fahrney, 1976; Stuart, 1970; Vernon-Roberts, 1972; Wyrick *et al.*, 1978). If antibody-coated chlamydiae are ingested into phagosomes, the antibody prevents the parasites from inhibiting lysosomal fusion; consequently, the phagosomes fuse with lysosomes, and the parasites are digested (Friis, 1972; Wyrick and Brownridge, 1978; Wyrick *et al.*, 1978). Other possible mechanisms, such as antibody-dependent toxic lysis by nonsensitized lymphocytes (Wunderlich *et al.*, 1971), seem to be beyond the scope of this discussion.

5.5. Agglutinating Antibodies

Having purified intact elementary bodies of psittacosis agent from infected mouse spleen, Bedson (1932) demonstrated their agglutination by a guinea pig antipsittacosis serum. Although none of his sera had an agglutinating titer greater than 1 : 8, Lazarus and Meyer (1939) refined his technique and obtained titers as high as 1 : 320. Subsequently, others reported success in demonstrating antichlamydial serum agglutinins (Storz, 1971). Only group-specific reactivity was observed. Bernkopf *et al.* (1960) purified trachoma agent from infected yolk sac by extraction of contaminating material with a fluorocarbon. They used dark-field microscopy to assess agglutination of the purified, noninfectious elementary bodies by sera of immunized rabbits and of trachoma patients. Of 48 active trachoma cases, 88% were seropositive by the agglutination test, while only 54% were seropositive in CF tests with trachoma antigen.

Gerloff and Watson (1967) developed a "radioisotope precipitation" (RIP) test for chlamydial group-specific antibody. Their radioactive antigen was purified meningopneumonitis agent labeled with ^{32}P during growth in mouse fibroblasts. As in the RIP test for poliomyelitis antibody, rabbit antiglobulin was used to clump the suspended, antibody-coated elementary bodies. (Since the antigen is particulate, the reaction is an agglutination rather than a precipitation.) Gerloff and Watson applied the test to sera from patients with clinical chlamydial infection, from persons occupa-

tionally exposed to animals with chlamydial infections, from children who had presumably experienced minimal exposure, and from persons with histories of chronic carditis. When CF tests were also performed on sera from members of these groups, the RIP test was 2–32 times more sensitive than the CF test, and the two tests appeared to detect different antibodies. More recent studies on the epidemiology of TRIC and LGV infections have confirmed that the RIP test, though laborious, is a very sensitive assay for group-specific antibodies (Dwyer *et al.*, 1972; Jones, 1974; Reeve *et al.*, 1974).

5.6. Antibodies Effecting or Inhibiting Hemagglutination

Chlamydial antigens have been used to sensitize untreated (Dhir *et al.*, 1971a) or tannic-acid-treated erythrocytes for passive hemagglutination. Studies of sera from human patients with histories of chlamydial infection revealed that the passive hemagglutination test and the CF test detected different antibodies (Benedict and O'Brien, 1958). The passive hemagglutination test distinguished between a trachoma strain and an inclusion conjunctivitis strain of *C. trachomatis* (Turner and Gordon, 1964). Treatment of sheep erythrocytes with 1% glutaraldehyde before sensitization markedly increased their stability during storage at 4°C or −50°C (Lewis *et al.*, 1972, 1975). If, in the future, type-specific chlamydial antigens can be routinely isolated (Sacks and MacDonald, 1979; Sacks *et al.*, 1978a), and then used to sensitize erythrocytes or other particles, passive agglutination may lend itself to rapid typing of antichlamydial antisera.

Lipid-containing hemagglutinating antigens, related to the group antigens, can be separated from chlamydial elementary bodies by disruption and centrifugation. Sera from immune animals inhibit the antigen-mediated hemagglutination (Gogolak and Ross, 1955; Henneberg *et al.*, 1966; Hilleman *et al.*, 1951; Jenkin *et al.*, 1970; Sayed and Wilt, 1971; Tamura and Manire, 1974; Zakay-Rones *et al.*, 1968).

5.7. Precipitating Antibodies

The Ouchterlony double immunodiffusion technique has demonstrated the diversity of water-soluble, precipitable chlamydial antigens. Methods for extracting test antigens have included treatment of chlamydiae with Genetron or deoxycholate, as well as sonication. Both group- and type-specific antigens have been identified (Barron and Collins, 1967; Barron *et al.,* 1972; Collins and Barron, 1970; Katzenelson and Bernkopf, 1967; Kuo *et al.,* 1971a; Parikh and Shechmeister, 1964).

The conjunctival response in trachoma and inclusion conjunctivitis includes growth of lymphoid follicles with germinal centers and infiltration by plasma cells in large numbers (Badir *et al.,* 1953; Collier, 1967; Dhermy *et al.,* 1967; Duke-Elder, 1965; Maslova-Khoroshilova *et al.,* 1974; Nataf, 1952). A variety of other infectious agents and of chemical irritants also induce this response (Duke-Elder, 1965; Jones, 1971; Rahi and Garner, 1976; Theodore and Schlossman, 1958). The histopathological picture is consistent with local antibody production in an accessory lymphoid organ (Jones, 1965, 1971).

Seeking evidence of local antibody production in nonchlamydial conjunctivitides, Jones (1971) ground up biopsy specimens of follicle-bearing conjunctivae from patients with conjunctivitis due to molluscum contagiosum, adenovirus, or cat scratch disease. Double immunodiffusion tests showed that, in each of nine cases, the conjunctival biopsy contained precipitating antibody directed against the specific causal agent. The conjunctival antibody titer was higher than the serum antibody titer in seven of these nine positive cases. Clinically normal conjunctivae contained no detectable precipitating antibody. Jones suggests that lymphoid cells in the inflamed conjunctivae synthesize antibody locally and that this antibody may be protective, or immunopathogenic, or both. Although his studies offer no evidence of local synthesis of precipitating antibodies in chlamydial disease, antibody reacting specifically with trachoma organisms in indirect FA tests does appear in eye secretions of trachoma patients, and will be discussed presently.

5.8. Antibodies Reacting in Immunofluorescence Tests

At present, immunofluorescence is the serological technique that offers the most ac-

ceptable combination of sensitivity, specificity, and convenience. It has been applied mainly to detection of chlamydial antigen in infected tissue, to serotyping of isolates from infected tissue, and to titration of type-specific antibodies in sera and secretions. Each of these applications is surveyed below.

5.8.1. Detection of Chlamydial Antigen in Infected Tissue

Buckley *et al.* (1955) used Coons's indirect FA method (Coons and Kaplan, 1950; Coons *et al.,* 1950) to identify developmental forms of the psittacosis agent in cultured embryonic mouse liver cells. Fluorescein isocyanate was conjugated to horse antihuman γ-globulin, while human antipsittacosis serum provided the specific link between antigen and fluorescent antibody. Although Giemsa staining failed to reveal unequivocal chlamydial inclusions up to 3 hr following inoculation, the FA technique indicated that psittacosis antigen was present in typical developmental forms in the cytoplasm of infected cells throughout the chlamydial growth cycle.

Nichols and McComb (1962) used the direct FA technique to demonstrate trachoma, LGV, and psittacosis antigens in yolk sac preparations and in cultured cells. They also examined conjunctival smears from children living in an area where trachoma is endemic. Their basic FA test showed only group specificity but could distinguish between certain strains provided that antisera were initially cross-adsorbed. The advantages of the FA method for detecting antigen in infected cells were best illustrated when conjunctival inocula from 62 children were carried through three or more yolk sac passages: the mean number of passages required to confirm growth of trachoma agent was 3.7 using the Macchiavello stain and only 2.0 using FA. Subsequent work by Nichols's group showed that the FA stain with conjugated LGV antiserum was more easily read and more reliable than the Giemsa stain in identification of trachoma agent in conjunctival scrapings (Nichols *et al.,* 1963, 1967). Surman *et al.* (1967), studying trachoma among Aboriginal school children in South Australia, obtained a less sensitive FA stain with conjugated psittacosis antiserum.

Ashley *et al.* (1975) used group-specific rabbit antibody against *C. trachomatis,* followed by ferritin-conjugated goat antirabbit globulin, to identify elementary bodies in clinical swab specimens and McCoy cells with the electron microscope. Applied to the swab specimens, their indirect immunoferritin technique was comparable in sensitivity to isolation methods.

5.8.2. Serotyping of Isolates from Infected Tissue

Immunofluorescent typing of chlamydial isolates has been refined to the extent that it is now a valuable epidemiological tool. Using adsorbed human antisera in an indirect test, Nichols and McComb (1964) identified two main TRIC serotypes. Katzenelson and Bernkopf (1965), in a direct FA test, also distinguished two serotypes. Bell and McComb (1967), using guinea pig early antiserum (7–10 days after intracardial inoculation), identified three TRIC serotypes. More or less concurrently, use of the mouse toxicity prevention test had permitted identification of seven cross-protecting TRIC serotypes, four from ocular trachoma and three from genital TRIC infections (Alexander et al., 1967; Wang and Grayston, 1963).

In 1970, Wang and Grayston succeeded in distinguishing six TRIC serotypes and two LGV serotypes by an indirect FA technique. They used dip pen points to place spots of different antigens from infected yolk sacs in a space small enough to be covered by a single drop of mouse antiserum. Their procedure included thorough cross-testing of unknown isolates and prototype antigens, as well as comparison with the results of the mouse toxicity prevention test (Wang, 1971; Wang and Grayston, 1970, 1971). By 1974, they and their associates had differentiated 15 serotypes of TRIC-LGV organisms (Grayston and Wang, 1975; Kuo et al., 1974; see above discussion of chlamydial type-specific antigens). They developed, in addition, a simpler and less precise method in which unknown chlamydial isolates, grown in HeLa 229 cells, were used as immunogens in mice. Mouse antisera obtained 4 days after inoculation (containing IgM antibodies) were tested against prototype TRIC-LGV antigens by the indirect FA technique. The pattern of reactivity of an early mouse antiserum thus identified the immunizing chlamydial serotype (Wang et al., 1973).

Some laboratories have used McCoy (mouse heteroploid, Gordon et al., 1972) cells or BHK cells for primary isolation and FA typing of clinical specimens of C. trachomatis (Blyth and Taverne, 1974; Darougar et al., 1971; Gordon et al., 1971, 1972; McComb and Puzniak, 1974). Variations and improvements in cell culture techniques continue to appear (Johnson and Hobson, 1976; Ripa and Mårdh, 1977; Rota and Nichols, 1973; Sompolinsky and Richmond, 1974; Thomas et al., 1977; Wentworth and Alexander, 1974).

Using adsorbed donkey antisera in an indirect FA test, Nichols et al. (1971a) typed 338 trachoma strains isolated from Saudi Arabian children. Every isolation yielded a single serotype: 37% were type A, 38% were type B, and 25% were type C. Individual localities, between which there was considerable social interchange, exhibited widely divergent frequency distributions of serotypes. The serotype remained unchanged in 90% of 170 paired successive isolations from 72 individual children. Of 40 children in 27 families, 78% shared their serotype with their sibling or siblings. Individual families tended to carry single serotypes for years. From these epidemiological findings, Nichols and his co-workers concluded that, in the population studied, trachoma spread mainly within families and tended to persist as a chronic infection.

5.8.3. Titration of Antibodies in Sera and Secretions

Immunofluorescence can be used to titrate antibodies in clinical specimens of serum or of body secretions. Nichols and McComb (1962) compared CF and direct FA titers in serial sera from two human volunteers infected with trachoma. Titers obtained by the two methods rarely differed by a factor greater than 4. Similarly, Isa et al. (1968, 1969) compared CF and indirect FA titers of serial sera from volunteers infected with inclusion conjunctivitis. Although CF antibodies were sometimes detected one to two weeks earlier than antibodies reactive in the FA test, both tests revealed peak titers about 4 weeks after inoculation. The CF and FA-reactive antibodies were mostly of the IgG class, and none were IgM. Cross-adsorption of antisera indicated that the two methods defined two distinct populations of antibodies which reacted with different antigenic determinant groups.

Jawetz *et al.* (1971) found no serum IgM antibodies in human ocular TRIC infections, even when sera were obtained as early as 4 days after clinical signs appeared.

Since the adoption of indirect FA methods for routine typing of antibodies to chlamydial antigens (L. Hanna *et al.*, 1972; McComb and Nichols, 1969; Wang, 1971; Wang and Grayston, 1970), a few modifications for rapid screening have been reported (Richmond and Caul, 1975; Thomas *et al.*, 1976; Treharne *et al.*, 1977; Wang *et al.*, 1975). In general, FA titration studies of human type-specific antibodies to TRIC or LGV agents have focused on the following questions: How is antibody titer related temporally to the presence of clinical disease? How is antibody specificity related to the serotype of the infecting organism? What roles do antibodies play in immunological defense or in immunopathogenesis? In which immunoglobulin classes are antibodies found? What are the relationships between serum antibodies and eye secretion antibodies? What is the geographical distribution of antibody patterns?

Grayston and Wang (1975) studied a group of families for 3½ years in an area of Taiwan where trachoma was endemic and severe.

Table 2 presents their summarized data from a family of nine that was typical of families in which new disease failed to develop. In 1971, every member of the family had serum antibody against type C and no other type, although types B and C were both present in the population studied. All individuals, except the mother, also had antibody to type C in their tears. Isolation attempts yielded trachoma organisms from the conjunctiva of only one child. By 1974, none of the children displayed active trachoma, and most showed falls in the antibody titers of both serum and tears. Table 3 presents data on a girl from a different family who was 1 year old at initial examination. At a time when the patient had papillae indicating acute inflammation, before conjunctival swabs yielded an isolate, antibody to type B appeared in her tears. Three months later, when the first and only positive isolation (type B) was made, antibody was present in both serum and tears. Antibody was still present in 1973, in the absence of clinical disease and of culturable trachoma organisms. By 1974, no antibody could be detected in the tears.

These data show that clinically active trachoma can be present when no chlamydiae can be cultured from the conjunctiva. Active tra-

TABLE 2. Results of Clinical and Laboratory Examinations for Trachoma (over a 3-Year Period) of Members of a Family Living in One Household in Rural Southwestern Taiwan[a]

| Age (sex) | Diagnosis[b] | | Microimmunofluorescent antibody | | | | | Isolation[e] | |
	1971	1974	Type	Serum[c] 1971	Serum[c] 1974	Tears[d] 1971	Tears[d] 1974	1971	1974
39 (F)	IV	III	C	16	—	0	0	—	—
37 (M)	IV	IV	C	128	—	2+	160	—	—
16 (F)	III	—	C	512	—	2+	—	0	—
14 (F)	III	IV	C	32	8	3+	10	0	—
12 (M)	IV	IV	C	32	16	40	40	0	0
10 (F)	II, + +	IV	C	128	32	160	10	0	0
9 (F)	II, + +	NP	C	512	128	160	10	+	0
6 (F)	II, + +	NP	C	16	0	160	40	0	0
4 (M)	NP	NP	C	256	0	160	0	0	0

[a] Reproduced from Grayston and Wang (1975) by courtesy of the authors, *The Journal of Infectious Diseases*, and The University of Chicago Press. Copyright © 1975 by the University of Chicago. All rights reserved.

[b] Clinical diagnosis is classified by the World Health Organization classification: I, trachoma at onset; II, active trachoma; III, active and scarring trachoma; IV, inactive trachoma with residual scars and/or pannus. NP, "Nothing particular," or no clinical findings of trachoma. + + Stands for papillae and indicates acute, relatively severe infections.

[c] Reciprocal of serum dilution: 0 = <8.

[d] Titers are expressed as the reciprocal of the tear specimen dilution (0 = >10) or +, 2 +, 3 + (intensity of fluorescence at original 1 : 10 dilution).

[e] Isolation was from conjunctival swabs, and organisms were isolated in egg yolk sac or tissue culture: 0, culture negative; +, isolate obtained not typed.

TABLE 3.   Results of a Series of Examinations of a 1-Year-Old Taiwanese Girl Who Developed Stage I Trachoma[a,b]

		Micro-immunofluorescent antibody			
Date	Diagnosis	Type	Serum	Eye	Isolation
11/70	NP	—	0	0	—
2/71	NP	—	0	0	0
6/71	NP, + +	B	—	120	0
9/71	NP, + +	B	128	160	B
1/72	I, + +	B	—	3+	—
6/72	I	B	—	40	—
1/73	NP	B	64	80	0
1/74	NP	B	32	0	0
7/74	NP	—	—	0	—

[a] Reproduced from Grayston and Wang (1975) by courtesy of the authors, *The Journal of Infectious Diseases*, and The University of Chicago Press. Copyright © 1975 by the University of Chicago. All rights reserved.
[b] Note: See footnotes to Table II for explanation of notations.

choma correlates better with presence of antibody, especially eye secretion antibody, than with positive isolation of *C. trachomatis*. In some endemic areas, however, there is a high percentage of antibody secretors among asymptomatic children (Zakay-Rones *et al.*, 1972). As Grayston and Wang (1975) suggest, the observed correlations are consistent with (but do not prove) a role of the immunological response in the pathogenesis of trachoma. According to their view, the immunological response to infection of conjunctival and corneal epithelium by a TRIC organism causes more tissue damage than does any direct effect (such as lytic growth or cytotoxicity) of the parasite. Earlier studies of matched specimens of serum and tears from trachoma patients, by Lavelle Hanna *et al.* (1973a,b), support this view while casting doubt on the role of eye secretion antibodies in resistance to chlamydial infection of the outer eye. It is possible but unproven that, while secretion antibodies hinder the initial attachment of chlamydial elementary bodies to superficial epithelial cells, the epithelium, once invaded, keeps both intracellular and extracellular chlamydiae out of contact with antibody. Indeed, one cannot assume that immunoglobulins have easy access to the scanty extracellular space of a metaplastic, epidermoid epithelium.

The role of serum antibody in oculogenital chlamydial infections is obscure. In owl monkeys, titers of both serum antibodies and eye secretion antibodies correlated well with ocular resistance to challenge six months after a primary ocular infection with trachoma agent (Fraser *et al.*, 1975). However, when serum containing FA-reactive antitrachoma antibody was passively transferred from immune owl monkeys to nonimmune monkeys, the recipient animals were not protected against infectious challenge with homologous trachoma agent, and they yielded no detectable eye secretion antibody until the intensity of infection was waning (Orenstein *et al.*, 1973). In the guinea pig inclusion conjunctivitis model, passively transferred serum antibody similarly failed to modify the ocular disease and appeared not to be the source of eye secretion antibody (R. R. Watson *et al.*, 1973a). Howard *et al.* (1976), studying immunity to reinfection with guinea pig inclusion conjunctivitis agent in the urethra and eyes of male guinea pigs, found that an eye infection induced solid immunity in both the eye and the urethra, whereas a urethral infection induced protective immunity only in the urethra. Infection at either site elicited production of serum antibody. In the guinea pig model, therefore, serum antibody clearly fails to protect, and dissemination of antigen, lymphoid cells, or other factors responsible for local immunity occurs more readily from the conjunctiva than from the wall of the urethra.

Indirect FA tests have shown that human eye secretion antibodies against trachoma organisms usually represent at least three Ig classes, namely, IgG, IgM, and IgA (Barenfanger and MacDonald, 1974a; Collier *et al.*, 1972; Hathaway and Peters, 1971; Jawetz *et al.*, 1971; Peters *et al.*, 1971), and possibly also a fourth, IgE (Hathaway and Peters, 1971). Although, in early studies, IgG antibody was found more consistently and at higher titers than were antibodies of the other classes (Hathaway and Peters, 1971; Collier *et al.*, 1972), use of highly specific goat antihuman Igs from adsorbed antisera revealed the predominance of secretory IgA antibody in eye secretions of Saudi Arabian infants with trachoma (Barenfanger and MacDonald, 1974a). This finding is consistent with local synthesis of antibody (Bluestone *et al.*, 1975; Franklin *et al.*, 1973; Jones, 1971; Shimada and Silverstein, 1975). After administering purified inactive trachoma elementary bodies topically to the conjunctival sac of guinea pigs, Zakay-Rones *et al.* (1972) showed by FA methods that antibody-containing cells were present in frozen sections of conjunctiva. In studies of guinea pig inclusion conjunctivitis, presence of secretory IgA antibody in eye secretions correlated with ocular resistance to reinfection (Murray *et al.*, 1973; Modabber *et al.*, 1976).

Despite these hints of import, the actual role of eye secretion antibodies in human eye infections with *C. trachomatis* remains to be elucidated: blocking attachment of elementary bodies to superficial epithelial cells is the least devious role (Byrne and Moulder, 1978; Dawson, 1976; Gibbons, 1974, 1977; Tramont, 1977; Williams and Gibbons, 1972). Since abnormally large numbers of mast cells are found in the connective tissue of the trachomatous conjunctiva (Dhermy *et al.*, 1967), the presence of IgE antibody in eye secretions, if confirmed, offers the possibility that subepithelial anaphylactic reactions (Ishizaka and Ishizaka, 1971) contribute to the pathology of trachoma.

From these studies of eye secretion antibody Ig classes, from the positive correlation between eye secretion antibody titer and severity of inflammation (Grayston and Wang, 1975; L. Hanna *et al.*, 1973a,b), and from the histopathology (Collier, 1967; Dhermy *et al.*, 1967; Duke-Elder, 1965) emerges a picture of exuberant local synthesis of antibodies during the most florid stage of trachoma (Jones, 1971; Silverstein, 1974; Silverstein and Prendergast, 1971). It is interesting that concentrations of IgG and IgA (*not* antibody titers or protein concentration), measured by radial immunodiffusion, are typically lower in tears of trachoma patients than in tears of normal controls (McClellan *et al.*, 1974; Sen *et al.*, 1977), as if epithelial secretion of secretory IgA were impaired. IgA-producing lymphoid cells greatly outnumber IgG- and IgM-producing cells in the connective tissue of normal human lacrimal glands (Franklin *et al.*, 1973). In rabbits immunized by injection of soluble proteins into the vitreous humor, IgA-producing cells predominate in the lacrimal glands, whereas they are modestly outnumbered by IgG-producing cells in the perilimbal conjunctiva (Shimada and Silverstein, 1975). IgA-producing cells

predominate in normal and inflamed human conjunctivae, and the population densities (cells per unit area of a section) of all Ig-producing cells tend to increase at least three- to fivefold during inflammation (Bloch-Michel *et al.*, 1977). When the appropriate studies are carried out, trachomatous conjunctivae with heavy plasma cell infiltration and active lymphoid follicles will probably be found to have very high subepithelial concentrations of monomeric and dimeric nonsecretory IgA (Heremans, 1974; Lamm, 1976; Parkhouse and Della Corte, 1974), much of which diffuses into lymph and blood instead of undergoing secretion by goblet cells. Part of this vigorous response may be directed nonspecifically to synthesis of antibodies against antigens other than chlamydial antigens (Shimada and Silverstein, 1975; J. Watson *et al.*, 1977).

Human antisera formed against TRIC-LGV agents exhibit various degrees of specificity in indirect FA tests. Dwyer *et al.* (1972) found that antisera induced by TRIC type A, B, or C were more specific than those formed against type D, E, F, or G. Anti-LGV sera were the most broadly reactive. A subsequent study by Briones *et al.* (1974) indicated that antisera against type A, C, or F were most specific. Following ocular infection of volunteers with type D or F, the prominence of cross-reactive antibodies increased with time. When volunteers were infected with different types sequentially, antibody to the first infecting type was recalled to a higher level by the second, heterotypic infection. In Tunisia, where most cases of trachoma are caused by type A organisms, the tears and sera of a small proportion of cases (less than 10%) possess antibodies to type B as well as to type A. Sequential acquisition of antibodies differing in type specificity has been demonstrated in a few of these cases (L. Hanna *et al.*, 1976).

Table 4 illustrates the distribution of FA-reactive serum antibodies in two population groups on Taiwan (Grayston and Wang, 1975). Among U.S. airmen and Taiwanese prostitutes, the predominance of antibodies to TRIC types D and E is typical of sexually transmitted chlamydial infection. About a quarter of the prostitutes had antibodies to type B or C, indicating that these women were previously exposed to endemic trachoma.

The importance of chlamydiae as frequent

TABLE 4. FA-Reactive Antibodies to TRIC-LGV Antigens in Sera of Two Population Groups on Taiwan[a]

Group (median age)	Number tested (% with antibody)	Percentage with one type	Percentage with indicated immunotype[b]						
			C(J)	B	EDL₁L₂	F(G)	H	I	L₃(K)
Prostitutes (24 years)	224 (78)	52	22	26	81	19	4	6	0
U.S. airmen (22 years)	378 (27)	97	7	0	73	6	0	10	8

[a] Reproduced from Grayston and Wang (1975) by courtesy of the authors, *The Journal of Infectious Diseases*, and The University of Chicago Press. Copyright © 1975 by the University of Chicago. All rights reserved.
[b] Types J, G, and K were not used as antigen in these tests.

etiological agents of nongonococcal urethritis has been demonstrated not only by isolation of infective organisms (Schachter *et al.,* 1976) but also by indirect FA serology. For example, in a Washington, D.C., venereal disease clinic population, 25% of tested patients yielded TRIC or LGV chlamydiae from their urogenital tracts, but 80% had FA-reactive serum antibodies. Twenty percent of the population had antichlamydial IgM antibodies (Philip *et al.,* 1974). In another study, Reeve *et al.* (1974) performed FA tests on 103 London men with nongonococcal urethritis. Of 74 men who yielded a chlamydial isolate, 86% had FA-reactive IgG antibodies and 28% had IgM antibodies (Table 5), as compared with figures of 24% and 3%, respectively, for the 29 men from whom no chlamydiae were isolated. Oriel *et al.* (1975) demonstrated positive FA titers in sera from 15 London men all of whom developed postgonococcal urethritis after chlamy-

diae had been isolated during treatment of the gonorrhea with gentamicin.

6. Immunological Prevention of Chlamydial Infections

6.1. Field Trials of Vaccines

Field trials of trachoma vaccines have been carried out in Taiwan, the Punjab, Saudi Arabia, Ethiopia, the Gambia, and the Soviet Union (reviewed by Becker, 1974; Bietti and Werner, 1967; Collier, 1966; Dawson and Schachter, 1974; Ghione *et al.,* 1974; Storz, 1971). In most such trials, killed vaccines were given intramuscularly or subcutaneously. A reduction in incidence of clinical trachoma or (when a vaccinated person later acquired trachoma) in conjunctival inclusion counts up to 2½ years following vaccination was observed in some trials (Table 6, from Dhir *et al.,* 1967),

TABLE 5. Chlamydial Antibodies in Nonspecific Urethritis[a]

Clinical category	Chlamydia isolated	Number tested	Serological tests[b]							
			RIP			IF				
						IgG			IgM	
			Positive			Positive			Positive	
			Number[c]	Percent	GMT[d]	Number[c]	Percent	GMT[d]	Number[c]	Percent
A. Nonspecific urethritis (NSU)	Yes	74	70	94	156	64	86	26	21	28
B. NSU	No	29	16	55	70	7	24	16	1	3
C. No urethritis	Not done	37	20	54	55	14	38	10	0	0

[a] Reproduced from Reeve *et al.* (1974) by courtesy of the authors and the Editor of the *British Journal of Venereal Diseases*.
[b] RIP, Radioisotope precipitation test; IF, microimmunofluorescence test.
[c] Figures represent numbers of patients having serum titers of 1:32 or more (RIP test) and 1:8 or more (IF test).
[d] Geometric mean titer (reciprocal).

	Gradient	Genetron	Placebo
Converts to trachoma (cumulative total)	9	17	32
Examined at 1 year (including cumulative converters)	90	92	87
Cumulative conversion rate (%)	10.0	18.5	36.8
Effectiveness (%)	73	50	

[a] Reproduced from Dhir *et al.* (1967) by courtesy of the authors and the Editor of the *American Journal of Ophthalmology*.
[b] Explanation: The vaccines were purified with either Genetron or a sucrose–KCl density gradient and were inactivated with formalin. Initial injections were given to children having no clinical evidence of trachoma. These children received booster injections approximately 3 months after their initial vaccinations.

but protection waned thereafter. In a few vaccinated groups, trachoma was more frequent or more severe than among controls who received no vaccine (Grayston and Wang, 1975; Sowa *et al.*, 1969; Woolridge *et al.*, 1967a); thus it appeared that certain trachoma vaccines or vaccination procedures could induce hypersensitivity. Similar instances of apparent hypersensitivity were observed following infectious challenge of vaccinated or otherwise presensitized Taiwan monkeys (Alexander and Chiang, 1967; Grayston, 1967; Grayston *et al.*, 1971; Wang *et al.*, 1967). It should be noted that "hypersensitivity" of these human and simian antigen recipients was evidenced by unexpected or accelerated development of ocular inflammation on subsequent infection with live organisms. As we hope to have made clear in this chapter, the follicles and pannus of trachoma need not be expressions of any classical hypersensitivity mechanisms. They may represent merely the gathering and proliferation of lymphoid cells in areas where cytophilic antitrachoma antibodies, bound at the surfaces of reticular cells, have captured antigen (M. G. Hanna, Jr., and Szakal, 1968; M. G. Hanna, Jr., *et al.*, 1969; Humphrey, 1976; Nossal and Ada, 1971; White, 1975). Persistence of infection or of nonviable antigen could prolong the cycle of antigen capture, B-cell proliferation, and antibody synthesis (Silverstein, 1974; Silverstein and Prendergast, 1971).

The possibility of administering live or killed trachoma vaccines orally, in an effort to stimulate precursors of IgA-producing cells in gut-associated lymphoid tissue (Cooper *et al.*, 1974; Michalek *et al.*, 1976; Rothberg *et al.*, 1974), has not been explored. In the guinea pig model, a live oral vaccine induced partial protective immunity of the eyes and the vagina against the agent of guinea pig inclusion conjunctivitis (Nichols *et al.*, 1978).

6.2. Speculations on the Future of Vaccines

The incidence and severity of trachoma tend to decline as standards of living and motivation to avoid disease increase (Dawson *et al.*, 1976; Grayston and Wang, 1975; Jones, 1975). Antibiotic therapy can reduce the incidence of blinding sequelae by diminishing the severity of the disease and by shortening its duration. Because no trachoma vaccine has afforded protection to human recipients for more than 3 years, and because such protection has been far from complete, mass vaccination must be carefully weighed against other approaches (Dawson and Schachter, 1974; Jones, 1975). Collier (1972) has estimated that, depending on production methods, the cost of trachoma vaccine could be as little as $0.71 per dose or as much as $27.23 per dose, whereas tetracycline costs $0.20 or less per cycle of treatment. Clearly, then, development of a universally acceptable vaccine will require intensification of research on purified trachoma antigens, on stimulation of local immunity, and on mechanisms of acquired resistance and of pathogenesis in chlamydial infections.

7. Conclusion

Of the estimated 400 million people who have trachoma, 6 million are totally blind. Symptomatic and asymptomatic chlamydial infections of the genital tract are common. The phenomenal success of chlamydiae as intracellular parasites of humans is associated with their capacity to persist in their hosts, and probably to reinfect, despite the presence of serum antibodies, of antibodies in secretions, and of cell-mediated immunologic reactivity.

The pathogenesis of blinding trachoma appears to involve a massive B-lymphocyte and plasma cell response in the conjunctiva and cornea. By comparison, the still unknown contribution of effector T lymphocytes to the pathology is likely to be small. The pathways of chlamydial antigens, the role of macrophages, and the specificity of local immunological responses in human infections are among the essential concerns of future research. Continuing improvements in purification of chlamydial antigens will undoubtedly avail laboratory diagnosis and basic research, but the ambiguous immunological picture of trachoma does not inspire confident prophecies of a universally acceptable vaccine.

NOTE ADDED IN PROOF. The following superb monograph, which came into our hands after we had submitted our final draft of this chapter, will be indispensable to any student of the chlamydiae: Schachter, J., and Dawson, C. R., 1978, *Human Chlamydial Infections,* PSG Publishing Co., Littleton, Massachusetts.

References

Abrams, A. J., 1968, Lymphogranuloma venereum, *J. Am. Med. Assoc.* **205:**199–202.

Alexander, E. R., and Chiang, W. T., 1967, Infection of pregnant monkeys and their offspring with TRIC agents, *Am. J. Ophthalmol.* **63:**1145–1153.

Alexander, E. R., Wang, S. P., and Grayston, J. T., 1967, Further classification of TRIC agents from ocular trachoma and other sources by the mouse toxicity prevention test, *Am. J. Ophthalmol.* **63:**1469–1478.

Ashley, C. R., Richmond, S. J., and Caul, E. O., 1975, Identification of the elementary bodies of *Chlamydia trachomatis* in the electron microscope by an indirect immunoferritin technique, *J. Clin. Microbiol.* **2:**327–331.

Badir, G., Wilson, R. P., and Lyons, F. M., 1953, The histopathology of trachoma, *Bull. Egypt. Ophthalmol. Soc.* **46:**97–129.

Banks, J., Eddie, B., Sung, M., Sugg, N., Schachter, J., and Meyer, K. F., 1970, Plaque reduction technique for demonstrating neutralizing antibodies for *Chlamydia, Infect. Immun.* **2:**443–447.

Barenfanger, J., 1975, Studies on the role of the family unit in the transmission of trachoma, *Am. J. Trop. Med. Hyg.* **24:**509–515.

Barenfanger, J., and MacDonald, A. B., 1974a, Determination of immunoglobulin classes of anti-trachoma antibodies in various epidemiological groups of trachoma patients, Part 3 of Studies on the humoral antibody response to trachoma in humans, by J. Barenfanger, S.D. thesis, Harvard School of Public Health, Boston.

Barenfanger, J., and MacDonald, A. B., 1974b, The role of immunoglobulin in the neutralization of trachoma infectivity, *J. Immunol.* **113:**1607–1617.

Barron, A. L., and Collins, A. R., 1967, Studies on trachoma agent by double diffusion gel precipitation, *Am. J. Ophthalmol.* **63:**1487–1491.

Barron, A. L., Caste, P. G., Paul, B., and Page, L. A., 1972, Detection of chlamydial antibodies in animal sera by double diffusion in gel, *Appl. Microbiol.* **23:**770–774.

Becker, Y., 1974, The agent of trachoma, in: *Monographs in Virology,* Vol. 7, Karger, Basel.

Becker, Y., 1978, The chlamydia: Molecular biology of procaryotic obligate parasites of eucaryocytes, *Microbiol. Rev.* **42:**274–306.

Becker, Y., Hochberg, E., and Zakay-Rones, Z., 1969, Interaction of trachoma elementary bodies with host cells, *Isr. J. Med. Sci.* **5:**121–124.

Bedson, S. P., 1932, The nature of the elementary bodies in psittacosis, *Br. J. Exp. Pathol.* **13:**65–72.

Bedson, S. P., 1933, Immunological studies with the virus of psittacosis, *Br. J. Exp. Pathol.* **14:**162–170.

Bedson, S. P., 1936, Observations bearing on the antigenic composition of psittacosis virus, *Br. J. Exp. Pathol.* **17:**109–121.

Bedson, S. P., 1958, The Harben Lectures, 1958: The psittacosis-lymphogranuloma group of infective agents. Lecture I. The history and the characters of these agents, *J. R. Inst. Public Health Hyg.* **22:**67–78.

Bedson, S. P., Barwell, C. F., King, E. J., and Bishop, L. W. J., 1949, Laboratory diagnosis of lymphogranuloma venereum, *J. Clin. Pathol.* **2:**241–249.

Beem, M. O., and Saxon, E. M., 1977, Respiratory tract colonization and a distinctive pneumonia syndrome in infants infected with *Chlamydia trachomatis, N. Engl. J. Med.* **296:**306–310.

Bell, S. D., Jr., and McComb, D. E., 1967, Differentiation of trachoma Bedsoniae *in vitro, Proc. Soc. Exp. Biol. Med.* **124:**34–39.

Bell, S. D., Jr., and Theobald, B., 1962, Differentiation of trachoma strains on the basis of immunization against toxic death of mice, *Ann. N.Y. Acad. Sci.* **98:**337–345.

Benedict, A. A., and O'Brien, E., 1956, Antigenic studies on the psittacosis L. G. V. group of viruses. II. Characterization of complement fixing antigens extracted with sodium lauryl sulfate, *J. Immunol.* **76:**293–300.

Benedict, A. A., and O'Brien, E., 1958, A passive hemagglutination reaction for psittacosis, *J. Immunol.* **80:**94–99.

Bernkopf, H., Nishmi, M., Maythar, B., and Feitelberg, I., 1960, Dark-field agglutination of fluorocarbon-treated trachoma virus by serums of trachoma patients and immunized rabbits, *J. Infect. Dis.* **106:**83–86.

Bietti, G.-B., 1974, Trachoma as a cause of visual impairment and blindness, *Rev. Int. Trach.* **51**(3):59–76.

Bietti, G., and Werner, G. H., 1967, *Trachoma: Prevention and Treatment,* Thomas, Springfield, Ill.

Bietti, G. B., Freyche, M. J., and Vozza, R., 1962, La diffusion actuelle du trachome dans le monde, *Rev. Int. Trach.* **39:**113–310.

Bloch-Michel, E., Audoin-Berault, J., Diebold, J., Herman, D., Dry, J., and Campinchi, R., 1977, Étude en immunofluorescence des plasmocytes de la conjonctive allergique en particulier des cellules formatrices des immunoglobulines E (IgE), *Arch. Ophtalmol. (Paris)* **37:**89–100.

Bluestone, R., Easty, D. L., Goldberg, L. S., Jones, B. R., and Pettit, T. H., 1975, Lacrimal immunoglobulins and complement quantified by counter-immunoelectrophoresis, *Br. J. Ophthalmol.* **59:**279–281.

Blyth, W. A., and Taverne, J., 1974, Cultivation of TRIC agents: A comparison between the use of BHK-21 and irradiated McCoy cells, *J. Hyg.* **72:**121–128.

Briones, O. C., Hanna, L., Jawetz, E., Dawson, C. R., and Ostler, H. B., 1974, Type-specific antibodies in human *Chlamydia trachomatis* infections of the eye, *J. Immunol.* **113:**1262–1270.

Buckley, S. M., Whitney, E., and Rapp, F., 1955, Identification by fluorescent antibody of developmental forms of psittacosis virus in tissue culture, *Proc. Soc. Exp. Biol. Med.* **90:**226–230.

Byrne, G. I., 1976, Requirements for ingestion of *Chlamydia psittaci* by mouse fibroblasts (L cells), *Infect. Immun.* **14:**645–651.

Byrne, G. I., 1978, Kinetics of phagocytosis of *Chlamydia psittaci* by mouse fibroblasts (L cells): Separation of the attachment and ingestion stages, *Infect. Immun.* **19:**607–612.

Byrne, G. I., and Moulder, J. W., 1978, Parasite-specified phagocytosis of *Chlamydia psittaci* and *Chlamydia trachomatis* by L and HeLa cells, *Infect. Immun.* **19:**598–606.

Caldwell, H. D., and Kuo, C.-C., 1977a, Purification of a *Chlamydia trachomatis*-specific antigen by immunoadsorption with monospecific antibody, *J. Immunol.* **118:**437–441.

Caldwell, H. D., and Kuo, C.-C., 1977b, Serologic diagnosis of lymphogranuloma venereum by counterimmunoelectrophoresis with a *Chlamydia trachomatis* protein antigen, *J. Immunol.* **118:**442–445.

Caldwell, H. D., Kuo, C. C., and Kenny, G. E., 1975a, Antigenic analysis of chlamydiae by two-dimensional immunoelectrophoresis. I. Antigenic heterogeneity between *C. trachomatis* and *C. psittaci, J. Immunol.* **115:**963–968.

Caldwell, H. D., Kuo, C. C., and Kenny, G. E., 1975b, Antigenic analysis of chlamydiae by two-dimensional immunoelectrophoresis. II. A trachoma-LGV-specific antigen, *J. Immunol.* **115:**969–975.

Chang, G. T., and Moulder, J. W., 1978, Loss of inorganic ions from host cells infected with *Chlamydia psittaci, Infect. Immun.* **19:**827–832.

Chorzelski, T. P., Jablońska, S., and Beutner, E. H., 1973, Clinical significance of pemphigus antibodies, in: *Immunopathology of the Skin: Labeled Antibody Studies* (E. H. Beutner, T. D. Chorzelski, S. F. Bean, and R. E. Jordan, eds.), pp. 25–43, Dowden, Hutchinson and Ross, Inc., Stroudsburg, Pa.

Clem, T. R., and Yolken, R. H., 1978, Practical color-imeter for direct measurement of microplates in enzyme immunoassay systems, *J. Clin. Microbiol.* **7:**55–58.

Collier, L. H., 1966, The present status of trachoma vaccination studies, *Bull. WHO* **34:**233–241.

Collier, L. H., 1967, The immunopathology of trachoma: Some facts and fancies, *Arch. Gesamte Virusforsch.* **22:**280–293.

Collier, L. H., 1972, Some aspects of trachoma control and provisional estimates of the cost of vaccine production, *Isr. J. Med. Sci.* **8:**1114–1123.

Collier, L. H., and Mogg, A. E., 1969, Dissemination and immunogenicity of live TRIC agent in baboons after parenteral injection. II. Experiments with a "slow-killing" strain, *J. Hyg.* **67:**449–455.

Collier, L. H., Sowa, J., and Sowa, S., 1972, The serum and conjunctival antibody response to trachoma in Gambian children, *J. Hyg.* **70:**727–740.

Collins, A. R., and Barron, A. L., 1970, Demonstration of group- and species-specific antigens of chlamydial agents by gel diffusion, *J. Infect. Dis.* **121:**1–8.

Coons, A. H., and Kaplan, M. H., 1950, Localization of antigen in tissue cells. II. Improvements in a method for the detection of antigen by means of fluorescent antibody, *J. Exp. Med.* **91:**1–13.

Coons, A. H., Snyder, J. C., Cheever, F. S., and Murray, E. S., 1950, Localization of antigen in tissue cells. IV. Antigens of rickettsiae and mumps virus, *J. Exp. Med.* **91:**31–38.

Cooper, M. D., Kincade, P. W., Bockman, D. E., and Lawton, A. R., 1974, Origin, distribution and differentiation of IgA-producing cells, in: *The Immunoglobulin A System* (J. Mestecky and A. R. Lawton, eds.), pp. 13–22, *Advances in Experimental Medicine and Biology,* Vol. 45, Plenum Press, New York.

Cottier, H., Keiser, G., Odartchenko, N., Hess, M., and Stoner, R. D., 1967, *De novo* formation and rapid growth of germinal centers during secondary antibody responses to tetanus toxoid in mice, in: *Germinal Centers in Immune Responses* (H. Cottier, N. Odartchenko, R. Schindler, and C. C. Congdon, eds.), pp. 270–276, Springer-Verlag, Berlin.

Darougar, S., Kinnison, J. R., and Jones, B. R., 1971, Simplified irradiated McCoy cell culture for isolation of *Chlamydia,* in: *Trachoma and Related Disorders* (R. L. Nichols, ed.), pp. 63–70, *International Congress Series No. 223,* Excerpta Medica, Amsterdam.

David, J. R., 1976, Macrophage activation by lymphocyte mediators, in: *Infection and Immunology in the Rheumatic Diseases* (D. C. Dumonde, ed.), pp. 25–29, Blackwell Scientific Publications, Oxford.

Davies, P., Allison, A. C., Dym, M., and Cardella, C., 1976, The selective release of lysosomal enzymes from mononuclear phagocytes by immune complexes and other materials causing chronic inflammation, in: *Infection and Immunology in the Rheumatic Diseases* (D. C. Dumonde, ed.), pp. 365–373, Blackwell Scientific Publications, Oxford.

Dawson, C. R., 1975, Lids, conjunctiva, and lacrimal apparatus: Eye infections with *Chlamydia, Arch. Ophthalmol. (Chicago)* **93**:854–862.

Dawson, C. R., 1976, How does the external eye resist infection? *Invest. Ophthalmol.* **15**:971–974.

Dawson, C. R., and Schachter, J., 1974, Trachoma—Antibiotics or vaccine, *Invest. Ophthalmol.* **13**:85–86.

Dawson, C. R., Daghfous, T., Messadi, M., Hoshiwara, I., and Schachter, J., 1976, Severe endemic trachoma in Tunisia, *Br. J. Ophthalmol.* **60**:245–252.

D'Ermo, F., Lanzieri, M., and Contini, A., 1964, Recherches immunologiques sur le virus du trachome, *Rev. Int. Trach.* **41**:262–281.

Dhermy, P., Coscas, G., Nataf, R., and Levaditi, J. C., 1967, Histopathologie des follicules au cours du trachome et des conjonctivites folliculaires, *Rev. Int. Trach.* **44**:295–397.

Dhir, S. P., Agarwal, L. P., Detels, R., Wang, S.-P., and Grayston, J. T., 1967, Field trial of two bivalent trachoma vaccines in children of Punjab Indian villages, *Am. J. Ophthalmol.* **63**:1639–1644.

Dhir, S. P., Kenny, G. E., and Grayston, J. T., 1971a, Characterization of the group antigen of *Chlamydia trachomatis, Infect. Immun.* **4**:725–730.

Dhir, S. P., Wang, S.-P., and Grayston, J. T., 1971b, Type-specific antigens of trachoma organisms, in: *Trachoma and Related Disorders* (R. L. Nichols, ed.), pp. 133–141, *International Congress Series* No. 223, Excerpta Medica, Amsterdam.

Dhir, S. P., Hakomori, S., Kenny, G. E., and Grayston, J. T., 1972, Immunochemical studies on chlamydial group antigen (presence of a 2-keto-3-deoxycarbohydrate as immunodominant group), *J. Immunol.* **109**:116–122.

Doughri, A. M., Storz, J., and Altera, K. P., 1972, Mode of entry and release of chlamydiae in infections of intestinal epithelial cells, *J. Infect. Dis.* **126**:652–657.

Duke-Elder, S., 1965, *System of Ophthalmology* (S. Duke-Elder, ed.), Vol. 8, *Diseases of the Outer Eye*, Part 1, Henry Kimpton, London.

Dunlop, E. M. C., 1975, Non-specific genital infection: Laboratory aspects, in: *Recent Advances in Sexually Transmitted Diseases*, No. 1 (R. S. Morton and J. R. W. Harris, eds.), pp. 267–295, Churchill Livingstone, Edinburgh.

Dunlop, E. M. C., Hare, M. J., Darougar, S., and Jones, B. R., 1971, Chlamydial isolates from the rectum in association with chlamydial infection of the eye or genital tract. II. Clinical aspects, in: *Trachoma and Related Disorders* (R. L. Nichols, ed.), pp. 507–512, *International Congress Series* No. 223, Excerpta Medica, Amsterdam.

Dvorak, H. F., Mihm, M. C., Jr., Dvorak, A. M., Johnson, R., Manseau, E. J., Morgan, E., and Colvin, R. B., 1974, Morphology of delayed type hypersensitivity reactions in man. I. Quantitative description of the inflammatory response, *Lab. Invest.* **31**:111–130.

Dwyer, R. St. C., Treharne, J. D., Jones, B. R., and Herring, J., 1972, Chlamydial infection: Results of micro-immunofluorescence tests for the detection of type-specific antibody in certain chlamydial infections, *Br. J. Vener. Dis.* **48**:452–459.

Fliedner, T. M., 1967, On the origin of tingible bodies in germinal centers, in: *Germinal Centers in Immune Responses* (H. Cottier, N. Odartchenko, R. Schindler, and C. C. Congdon, eds.), pp. 218–222, Springer-Verlag, Berlin.

Franklin, R. M., Kenyon, K. R., and Tomasi, T. B., 1973, Immunohistologic studies of human lacrimal gland: Localization of immunoglobulins, secretory component and lactoferrin, *J. Immunol.* **110**:984–992.

Fraser, C. E. O., and Berman, D. T., 1965, Type-specific antigens in the psittacosis-lymphogranuloma venereum group of organisms, *J. Bacteriol.* **89**:943–948.

Fraser, C. E. O., McComb, D. E., Murray, E. S., and MacDonald, A. B., 1975, Immunity to chlamydial infections of the eye. IV. Immunity in owl monkeys to reinfection with trachoma, *Arch. Ophthalmol. (Chicago)* **93**:518–521.

Frei, W., 1925, Eine neue Hautreaktion bei "Lymphogranuloma inguinale," *Klin. Wochenschr.* **4**:2148–2149.

Friedlander, M. H., and Dvorak, H. F., 1977, Morphology of delayed-type hypersensitivity reactions in the guinea pig cornea, *J. Immunol.* **118**:1558–1563.

Friedlander, M. H., Howes, E. L., Jr., Hall, J. M., Krasnobrod, H., and Wormstead, M. A., 1978, Histopathology of delayed hypersensitivity reactions in the guinea pig uveal tract, *Invest. Ophthalmol. Vis. Sci.* **17**:327–335.

Friis, R. R., 1972, Interaction of L cells and *Chlamydia psittaci*: Entry of the parasite and host responses to its development, *J. Bacteriol.* **110**:706–721.

Fritsch, H., Hofstätter, A., and Lindner, K., 1910, Experimentelle Studien zur Trachomfrage, *Arch. Ophthalmol. (Leipzig)* **76**:547–558.

Fromaget, C., and Harriet, 1916, Conjonctivites et pseudotrachomes provoqués par l'émétine, *Ann. Ocul.* **153**:388–395.

Fromer, C. H., and Klintworth, G. K., 1976, An evaluation of the role of leukocytes in the pathogenesis of experimentally induced corneal vascularization. III. Studies related to the vasoproliferative capability of polymorphonuclear leukocytes and lymphocytes, *Am. J. Pathol.* **82**:157–170.

Frommell, G. T., Bruhn, F. W., and Schwartzman, J. D., 1977, Isolation of *Chlamydia trachomatis* from infant lung tissue, *N. Engl. J. Med.* **296**:1150–1152.

Gendre, Ph., Vérin, Ph., and Vildy, A., 1975, Étude du trachome en microscopie électronique, *Arch. Ophtalmol. (Paris)* **35**:981–1004.

Gerloff, R. K., and Watson, R. O., 1967, The radioisotope precipitation test for psittacosis group antibody, *Am. J. Ophthalmol.* **63**:1492–1498.

Germuth, F. G., Maumenee, A. E., Senterfit, L. B., and Pollack, A. D., 1962, Immunohistologic studies on antigen–antibody reactions in the avascular cornea. I. Reactions in rabbits actively sensitized to foreign protein, *J. Exp. Med.* **115**:919–928.

Ghione, M., Werner, G.-H., and Cerulli, L., 1974, Problèmes immunologiques du trachome, *Rev. Int. Trach.* **51**(1):3–49.

Gibbons, R. J., 1974, Bacterial adherence to mucosal surfaces and its inhibition by secretory antibodies, in: *The Immunoglobulin A System* (J. Mestecky and A. R. Lawton, eds.), pp. 315–325, *Advances in Experimental Medicine and Biology,* Vol. 45, Plenum Press, New York.

Gibbons, R. J., 1977, Adherence of bacteria to host tissue, in: *Microbiology—1977* (D. Schlessinger, ed.), pp. 395–406, American Society for Microbiology, Washington, D.C.

Ginsburg, I., Neeman, N., Gallily, R., and Lahav, M., 1976, Degradation and survival of bacteria in sites of allergic inflammation, in: *Infection and Immunology in the Rheumatic Diseases* (D. C. Dumonde, ed.), pp. 43–59, Blackwell Scientific Publications, Oxford.

Gogolak, F. M., and Ross, M. R., 1955, The properties and chemical nature of the psittacosis virus hemagglutinin, *Virology* **1**:474–496.

Good, R. A., Cain, W. A., Perey, D. Y., Dent, P. B., Meuwissen, H. J., Rodey, G. E., and Cooper, M. D., 1969, Studies on the nature of germinal centers, in: *Lymphatic Tissue and Germinal Centers in Immune Response* (L. Fiore-Donati and M. G. Hanna, Jr., eds.), pp. 33–47, *Advances in Experimental Medicine and Biology,* Vol. 5, Plenum Press, New York.

Gordon, F. B., and Quan, A. L., 1965, Occurrence of glycogen in inclusions of the psittacosis–lymphogranuloma venereum–trachoma agents, *J. Infect. Dis.* **115**:186–196.

Gordon, F. B., Nichols, R. L., and Quan, A. L., 1971, Immunotyping of *Chlamydia trachomatis* with fluorescent antibody: Retention of immunospecificity in cell culture passage, and typing with infected cell monolayers, in: *Trachoma and Related Disorders* (R. L. Nichols, ed.), pp. 358–362, *International Congress Series* No. 223, Excerpta Medica, Amsterdam.

Gordon, F. B., Dressler, H. R., Quan, A. L., McQuilkin, W. T., and Thomas, J. I., 1972, Effect of ionizing irradiation on susceptibility of McCoy cell cultures to *Chlamydia trachomatis, Appl. Microbiol.* **23**:123–129.

Grant, L. S., Burgoon, C. F., Sutherland, E. S., and Sigel, M. M., 1962, Background information, in: *Lymphogranuloma Venereum: Epidemiological, Clinical, Surgical and Therapeutic Aspects Based on a Study in the Caribbean* (M. M. Sigel, ed.), pp. 1–12, University of Miami Press, Coral Gables, Fla.

Grayston, J. T., 1967, Immunization against trachoma, in: *First International Conference on Vaccines against Viral and Rickettsial Diseases of Man,* pp. 546–559, World Health Organization.

Grayston, J. T., and Wang. S. P., 1975, New knowledge of chlamydiae and the diseases they cause, *J. Infect. Dis.* **132**:87–105.

Grayston, J. T., Wang, S. P., Woolridge, R. L., Yang, Y. F., and Johnston, P. B., 1960, Trachoma—Studies of etiology, laboratory diagnosis and prevention, *J. Am. Med. Assoc.* **172**:1577–1586.

Grayston, J. T., Kim, K. S. W., Alexander, E. R., and Wang, S. P., 1971, Protective studies in monkeys with trivalent and monovalent trachoma vaccines, in: *Trachoma and Related Disorders* (R. L. Nichols, ed.), pp. 377–385, *International Congress Series* No. 223, Excerpta Medica, Amsterdam.

Grobler, P., Buerki, H., Cottier, H., Hess, M. W., and Stoner, R. D., 1974, Cellular bases for relative radioresistance of the antibody-forming system at advanced stages of the secondary response to tetanus toxoid in mice, *J. Immunol.* **112**:2154–2165.

Hadden, J. W., Sadlik, J. R., and Hadden, E. M., 1978, The induction of macrophage proliferation *in vitro* by a lymphocyte-produced factor, *J. Immunol.* **121**:231–238.

Hanna, L., Merigan, T. C., and Jawetz, E., 1966, Inhibition of TRIC agents by virus-induced interferon, *Proc. Soc. Exp. Biol. Med.* **122**:417–421.

Hanna, L., Merigan, T. C., and Jawetz, E., 1967, Effect of interferon on TRIC agents and induction of interferon by TRIC agents, *Am. J. Ophthalmol.* **63**:1115–1119.

Hanna, L., Jawetz, E., Nabli, B., Hoshiwara, I., Ostler, B., and Dawson, C., 1972, Titration and typing of serum antibodies in TRIC infections by immunofluorescence, *J. Immunol.* **108**:102–107.

Hanna, L., Jawetz, E., Briones, O. C., Keshishyan, H., Hoshiwara, I., Ostler, H. B., and Dawson, C. R., 1973a, Antibodies to TRIC agents in tears and serum of naturally infected humans, *J. Infect. Dis.* **127**:95–98.

Hanna, L., Jawetz, E., Briones, O., Ostler, H. B., Keshishyan, H., and Dawson, C. R., 1973b, Antibodies to TRIC agents in matched human tears and sera, *J. Immunol.* **110**:1464–1469.

Hanna, L., Jawetz, E., and Dawson, C. R., 1976, Antibodies to two immunotypes of *Chlamydia trachomatis* in individuals with trachoma, *Infect. Immun.* **14**:429–432.

Hanna, M. G., Jr., and Szakal, A. K., 1968, Localization of ^{125}I-labeled antigen in germinal centers of mouse spleen: Histologic and ultrastructural autoradiographic studies of the secondary immune reaction, *J. Immunol.* **101**:949–962.

Hanna, M. G., Jr., Szakal, A. K., and Walburg, H. E., Jr., 1969, The relation of antigen and virus localization to the development and growth of lymphoid germinal centers, in: *Lymphatic Tissue and Germinal Centers in Immune Response* (L. Fiore-Donati and M. G. Hanna, Jr., eds.), pp. 149–165, *Advances in Experimental Medicine and Biology,* Vol. 5, Plenum Press, New York.

Hatch, T. P., 1975, Competition between *Chlamydia psittaci* and L cells for host isoleucine pools: A limiting factor in chlamydial multiplication, *Infect. Immun.* **12**:211–220.

Hathaway, A., and Peters, J. H., 1971, Characterization of antibodies to trachoma in human eye secretions, in: *Trachoma and Related Disorders* (R. L. Nichols, ed.), pp. 260–268, *International Congress Series* No. 223, Excerpta Medica, Amsterdam.

Henley, W. L., Shore, B., and Leopold, I. H., 1971, Inhibition of leucocyte migration by corneal antigen in chronic viral keratitis, *Nature (London), New Biol.* **233**:115.

Henneberg, G., Jordanski, H., Kauffman, H., and Antoniadis, G., 1966, Experimente mit Miyagawanellen Haemagglutinin und Haemagglutinationshemmteste, *Zentralbl. Bakteriol. I. Abt. (Orig.)* **200**:325–347.

Henson, D., Helmsen, R., Becker, K. E., Strano, A. J., Sullivan, M., and Harris, D., 1974, Ultrastructural localization of herpes simplex virus antigens on rabbit corneal cells using sheep antihuman IgG antihorse ferritin hybrid antibodies, *Invest. Ophthalmol.* **13**:819–827.

Heremans, J. F., 1974, The IgA system in connection with local and systemic immunity, in: *The Immunoglobulin A System* (J. Mestecky and A. R. Lawton, eds.), pp. 3–11, *Advances in Experimental Medicine and Biology,* Vol. 45, Plenum Press, New York.

Hilleman, M. R., Haig, D. A., and Helmold, R. J., 1951, The indirect complement fixation, hemagglutination and conglutinating complement absorption tests for viruses of the psittacosis-lymphogranuloma venereum group, *J. Immunol.* **66**:115–130.

Hilleman, M. R., Greaves, A. B., and Werner, J. H., 1958, Group-specificity of psittacosis-lymphogranuloma venereum group skin test antigens in lymphogranuloma venereum patients, *J. Lab. Clin. Med.* **52**:53–57.

Hobson, D., and Holmes, K. K. (eds.), 1977, *Nongonococcal Urethritis and Related Infections,* American Society for Microbiology, Washington, D.C.

Horoschak, K. D., and Moulder, J. W., 1978, Division of single host cells after infection with chlamydiae, *Infect. Immun.* **19**:281–286.

Howard, L. V., 1975, Neutralization of *Chlamydia trachomatis* in cell culture, *Infect. Immun.* **11**:698–703.

Howard, L. V., O'Leary, M. P., and Nichols, R. L., 1976, Animal model studies of genital chlamydial infections: Immunity to reinfection with guinea-pig inclusion conjunctivitis agent in the urethra and eye of male guinea-pigs, *Br. J. Vener. Dis.* **52**:261–265.

Humphrey, J. H., 1976, The still unsolved germinal centre mystery, in: *Immune Reactivity of Lymphocytes: Development, Expression, and Control* (M. Feldman and A. Globerson, eds.), pp. 711–723, *Advances in Experimental Medicine and Biology,* Vol. 66, Plenum Press, New York.

Isa, A. H., Hanna, L., Linscott, W. D., and Jawetz, E., 1968, Experimental inclusion conjunctivitis in man. IV. The nature of the antibody response, *J. Immunol.* **101**:1154–1158.

Isa, A. H., Hanna, L., and Jawetz, E., 1969, Diversity of human antibody to TRIC agents (Chlamydiae) detected by different serological procedures, *Proc. Soc. Exp. Biol. Med.* **130**:1087–1092.

Ishizaka, K., and Ishizaka, T., 1971, Immunoglobulin E and homocytotropic properties, in: *Progress in Immunology: First International Congress of Immunology* (B. Amos, ed.), pp. 859–874, Academic Press, New York.

Jawetz, E., 1964, Agents of trachoma and inclusion conjunctivitis, *Annu. Rev. Microbiol.* **18**:301–334.

Jawetz, E., Dawson, C. R., Schachter, J., Juchau, V., Nabli, B., and Hanna, L., 1971, Immunoglobulin nature of antibodies in chlamydial infections, in: *Trachoma and Related Disorders* (R. L. Nichols, ed.), pp. 233–242, *International Congress Series* No. 223, Excerpta Medica, Amsterdam.

Jenkin, H. M., and Fan, V. S. C., 1971, Contrast of glycogenesis of *Chlamydia trachomatis* and *Chlamydia psittaci* strains in HeLa cells, in: *Trachoma and Related Disorders* (R. L. Nichols, ed.), pp. 52–59, *International Congress Series* No. 223, Excerpta Medica, Amsterdam.

Jenkin, H. M., and Lu, Y. K., 1967, Induction of interferon by the Bour strain of trachoma in HeLa 229 cells, *Am. J. Ophthalmol.* **63**:1110–1115.

Jenkin, H. M., Ross, M. R., and Moulder, J. W., 1961, Species-specific antigens from the cell walls of the agents of meningopneumonitis and feline pneumonitis, *J. Immunol.* **86**:123–127.

Jenkin, H. M., Makino, S., Townsend, D., Riera, M. C., and Barron, A. L., 1970, Lipid composition of the hemagglutinating active fraction obtained from chick embryos infected with *Chlamydia psittaci* 6BC, *Infect. Immun.* **2**:316–319.

Johnson, F. W. A., and Hobson, D., 1976, Factors affecting the sensitivity of replicating McCoy cells in the isolation and growth of chlamydia A (TRIC agents), *J. Hyg.* **76**:441–451.

Jones, B. R., 1965, cited by S. Duke-Elder, *System of Ophthalmology* (S. Duke-Elder, ed.), Vol. 8, *Diseases of the Outer Eye,* Part 1, pp. 4–5, Henry Kimpton, London.

Jones, B. R., 1971, Immunological specificity of follicles in conjunctivitis due to molluscum contagiosum, adenovirus and cat scratch disease, in: *Trachoma and Related Disorders* (R. L. Nichols, ed.), pp. 243–253, *International Congress Series* No. 223, Excerpta Medica, Amsterdam.

Jones, B. R., 1974, Laboratory tests for chlamydial infection: Their role in epidemiological studies of trachoma and its control, *Br. J. Ophthalmol.* **58**:438–454.

Jones, B. R., 1975, The prevention of blindness from trachoma, *Tr. Ophthalmol. Soc. U.K.* **95**:16–33.

Jones, B. R., Al-Hussaini, M. K., and Dunlop, E. M. C., 1964, Genital infection in association with TRIC virus infection of the eye. I. Isolation of virus from urethra, cervix, and eye. Preliminary report, *Br. J. Vener. Dis.* **40**:19–24.

Kassira, E. N., 1971, Delayed-type hypersensitivity for differentiation of chlamydial agents, in: *Trachoma and Related Disorders* (R. L. Nichols, ed.), pp. 177–184, *International Congress Series* No. 223, Excerpta Medica, Amsterdam.

Katzenelson, E., and Bernkopf, H., 1965, Serologic differentiation of trachoma strains and other agents of the psittacosis-lymphogranuloma venereum-trachoma group with the aid of the direct fluorescent antibody method, *J. Immunol.* **94**:467–474.

Katzenelson, E., and Bernkopf, H., 1967, Studies of PLT agents with the aid of the agar immune diffusion technique, *Am. J. Ophthalmol.* **63**:1483–1487.

Kazar, J., Gillmore, J. D., and Gordon, F. B., 1971, The effect of interferon and interferon inducers on infections with a nonviral intracellular microorganism, *Chlamydia trachomatis, Infect. Immun.* **3**:825–832.

Kellogg, K. R., Horoschak, K. D., and Moulder, J. W., 1977, Toxicity of low and moderate multiplicities of *Chlamydia psittaci* for mouse fibroblasts (L cells), *Infect. Immun.* **18**:531–541.

Klintworth, G. K., 1977, The contribution of morphology to our understanding of the pathogenesis of experimentally produced corneal vascularization, *Invest. Ophthalmol. Vis. Sci.* **16**:281–285.

Kordová, N., 1978, Chlamydiae, rickettsiae, and their cell wall defective variants, *Can. J. Microbiol.* **24**:339–352.

Kordová, N., and Wilt, J. C., 1972, Lysosomes and the "toxicity" of Rickettsiales. I. Cytochemical studies of macrophages inoculated *in vitro* with *C. psittaci* 6BC, *Can. J. Microbiol.* **18**:457–464.

Kordová, N., Wilt, J. C., and Sadiq, M., 1971, Lysosomes in L cells infected with *Chlamydia psittaci* 6BC strain, *Can. J. Microbiol.* **17**:955–959.

Kordová, N., Poffenroth, L., and Wilt, J. C., 1972a, Lysosomes and the "toxicity" of Rickettsiales. II. Noncytocidal interactions of egg-grown *C. psittaci* 6BC and *in vitro* macrophages, *Can. J. Microbiol.* **18**:869–873.

Kordová, N., Poffenroth, L., and Wilt, J. C., 1972b, Lysosomes and the "toxicity" of Rickettsiales. III. Response of L cells infected with egg-attenuated *C. psittaci* 6BC strain, *Can. J. Microbiol.* **18**:1343–1348.

Kordová, N., Hoogstraten, J., and Wilt, J. C., 1973a, Lysosomes and the "toxicity" of Rickettsiales. IV. Ultrastructural studies of macrophages infected with a cytopathic L cell-grown *C. psittaci* 6BC strain, *Can. J. Microbiol.* **19**:315–320.

Kordová, N., Wilt, J. C., and Poffenroth, L., 1973b, Lysosomes and the "toxicity" of Rickettsiales. V. *In vivo* relationship of peritoneal phagocytes and egg-attenuated *C. psittaci* 6BC, *Can. J. Microbiol.* **19**:1417–1423.

Kordová, N., Wilt, J. C., and Martin, C., 1975, Lysosomes and the "toxicity" of Rickettsias. VI. *In vivo* response of mouse peritoneal phagocytes to L-cell-grown *Chlamydia psittaci* 6BC strain, *Can. J. Microbiol.* **21**:323–331.

Kuo, C.-C., and Grayston, J. T., 1974, Studies on delayed hypersensitivity with trachoma organisms. III. Lymphokines, *J. Immunol.* **112**:540–545.

Kuo, C.-C., and Grayston, J. T., 1976, Interaction of *Chlamydia trachomatis* organisms and HeLa 229 cells, *Infect. Immun.* **13**:1103–1109.

Kuo, C.-C., Kenny, G. E., and Wang, S.-P., 1971a, Trachoma and psittacosis antigens in agar gel double immunodiffusion, in: *Trachoma and Related Disorders* (R. L. Nichols, ed.), pp. 113–123, *International Congress Series* No. 223, Excerpta Medica, Amsterdam.

Kuo, C.-C., Wang, S.-P., and Grayston, J. T., 1971b, Studies on delayed hypersensitivity with trachoma organisms. I. Induction of delayed hypersensitivity in guinea pigs and characterization of trachoma allergens, in: *Trachoma and Related Disorders* (R. L. Nichols, ed.), pp. 158–167, *International Congress Series* No. 223, Excerpta Medica, Amsterdam.

Kuo, C.-C., Wang, S.-P., and Grayston, J. T., 1971c, Studies on delayed hypersensitivity with trachoma organisms. II. Demonstration of lymphocyte transformation *in vitro* by a microtechnique of peripheral blood lymphocyte culture, in: *Trachoma and Related Disorders* (R. L. Nichols, ed.), pp. 168–176, *International Congress Series* No. 223, Excerpta Medica, Amsterdam.

Kuo, C.-C., Wang, S.-P., and Grayston, J. T., 1973, Effect of polycations, polyanions, and neuraminidase on the infectivity of trachoma-inclusion conjunctivitis and lymphogranuloma venereum organisms in HeLa cells: Sialic acid residues as possible receptors for trachoma-inclusion conjunctivitis, *Infect. Immun.* **8**:74–79.

Kuo, C.-C., Wang, S.-P., Grayston, J. T., and Alexander, E. R., 1974, TRIC type K, a new immunologic type of *Chlamydia trachomatis, J. Immunol.* **113**:591–596.

Lamm, M. E., 1976, Cellular aspects of immunoglobulin A, *Adv. Immunol.* **22**:223–290.

Lawn, A. M., Blyth, W. A., and Taverne, J., 1973, Interactions of TRIC agents with macrophages and BHK-21 cells observed by electron microscopy, *J. Hyg.* **71**:515–528.

Lazarus, A. S., and Meyer, K. F., 1939, The virus of psittacosis. III. Serological investigations, *J. Bacteriol.* **38**:171–198.

Lewis, V. J., Thacker, W. L., and Engelman, H. M., 1972, Indirect hemagglutination test for chlamydial antibodies, *Appl. Microbiol.* **24**:22–25.

Lewis, V. J., Engelman, H. M., and Thacker, W. L., 1975, Preparation of stable sensitized erythrocytes for detection of chlamydial antibodies, *J. Clin. Microbiol.* **1**:110–111.

Lewis, V. J., Thacker, W. L., and Mitchell, S. H., 1977, Enzyme-linked immunosorbent assay for chlamydial antibodies, *J. Clin. Microbiol.* **6**:507–510.

Lin, H. S., and Moulder, J. W., 1966, Patterns of response to sulfadiazine, D-cycloserine and D-alanine in members of the psittacosis group, *J. Infect. Dis.* **116**:372–376.

Lindner, K., 1910, Zur Aetiologie der gonokokkenfreien Urethritis, *Wien. Klin. Wochenschr.* **23**:283–284.

Litwin, J., 1959, The growth cycle of the psittacosis group of microorganisms, *J. Infect. Dis.* **105**:129–160.

Locatcher-Khorazo, D., and Seegal, B. C., 1972, *Microbiology of the Eye*, C. V. Mosby Co., St. Louis, Mo.

Lycke, E., and Peterson, M., 1976, Hemolysis-in-gel test for demonstration of *Chlamydia* antibodies, *J. Clin. Microbiol.* **4:**450–452.

Mackaness, G. B., 1971, Resistance to intracellular infection, *J. Infect. Dis.* **123:**439–445.

Manire, G. P., and Meyer, K. F., 1950a, The toxins of the psittacosis-lymphogranuloma group of agents. I. The toxicity of various members of the PLV group, *J. Infect. Dis.* **86:**226–232.

Manire, G. P., and Meyer, K. F., 1950b, The toxins of the psittacosis-lymphogranuloma group of agents. III. Differentiation of strains by the toxin neutralization test, *J. Infect. Dis.* **86:**241–250.

Manski, W., and Whiteside, T. L., 1974, Cell-surface receptors of normal, regenerating, and cultured corneal epithelial and endothelial cells, *Invest. Ophthalmol.* **13:**935–944.

Maslova-Khoroshilova, I. P., Muravieva, T. V., and Zatsepina, N. D., 1974, Morphological substrate of immune reactions in the conjunctiva in paratrachoma and trachoma, *Rev. Int. Trach.* **51**(3):7–28.

McClellan, B. H., Bettman, J. W., Jr., and Allansmith, M. R., 1974, Tear and serum immunoglobulin levels in Navajo children with trachoma, *Am. J. Ophthalmol.* **78:**106–109.

McComb, D. E., and Nichols, R. L., 1969, Antibodies to trachoma in eye secretions of Saudi Arab children, *Am. J. Epidemiol.* **90:**278–284.

McComb, D. E., and Puzniak, C. I., 1974, Micro cell culture method for isolation of *Chlamydia trachomatis, Appl. Microbiol.* **28:**727–729.

Merigan, T. C., and Hanna, L., 1966, Characteristics of interferon induced *in vitro* and *in vivo* by a TRIC agent, *Proc. Soc. Exp. Biol. Med.* **122:**421–424.

Metcalf, J. F., and Helmsen, R., 1977, Immunoelectron microscopic localization of herpes simplex virus antigens in rabbit cornea with antihuman IgG-antiferritin hybrid antibodies, *Invest. Ophthalmol. Vis. Sci.* **16:**779–786.

Metcalf, J. F., and Kaufman, H. E., 1976, Herpetic stromal keratitis: Evidence for cell-mediated immunopathogenesis, *Am. J. Ophthalmol.* **82:**827–834.

Meyer, K. F., 1953, Psittacosis group, *Ann. N.Y. Acad. Sci.* **56:**545–556.

Meyer, K. F., 1967, The host spectrum of psittacosis-lymphogranuloma venereum (PL) agents, *Am. J. Ophthalmol.* **63:**1225–1246.

Meyer, K. F., and Eddie, B., 1951, Human carrier of the psittacosis virus, *J. Infect. Dis.* **88:**109–125.

Meyer, K. F., and Eddie, B., 1962, Immunity against some bedsonia in man resulting from infection and in animals from infection or vaccination, *Ann. N.Y. Acad. Sci.* **98:**288–313.

Michalek, S. M., McGhee, J. R., Mestecky, J., Arnold, R. R., and Bozzo, L., 1976, Ingestion of *Streptococcus mutans* induces secretory immunoglobulin A and caries immunity, *Science* **192:**1238–1240.

Mields, W., Hentschke, J., Becker, W., and Teufel, P., 1974, Die Immunperoxidase-Methode zum Nachweis von Virus- und Chlamydien-Antigenen. II. Mitteilung: Darstellung des Entwicklungszyklus von *Chlamydia psittaci* in Peritonealmakrophagen infizierter Mäuse, *Zentralbl. Vet. Med. B* **21:**48–58.

Mitsui, Y., and Suzuki, A., 1956, Electron microscopy of trachoma virus in section, *Arch. Ophthalmol. (Chicago)* **56:**429–448.

Mitsui, Y., Higai, H., and Kitamuro, T., 1962, Free toxic substance of trachoma virus, *Arch. Ophthalmol. (Chicago)* **68:**651–653.

Modabber, F., Bear, S. E., and Cerny, J., 1976, The effect of cyclophosphamide on the recovery from a local chlamydial infection: Guinea-pig inclusion conjunctivitis (GPIC), *Immunology* **30:**929–933.

Mondino, B. J., Brown, S. I., Rabin, B. S., and Lemp, M. A., 1977a, Autoimmune phenomena of conjunctiva and cornea: A case report, *Arch. Ophthalmol. (Chicago)* **95:**468–473.

Mondino, B. J., Rabin, B. S., Kessler, E., Gallo, J., and Brown, S. I., 1977b, Corneal rings with gram-negative bacteria, *Arch. Ophthalmol. (Chicago)* **95:**2222–2225.

Mordhorst, C. H., Reinicke, V., and Schonne, E., 1967, *In ovo* inhibition by concentrated chick interferon of the growth of TRIC agents, *Am. J. Ophthalmol.* **63:**1107–1109.

Morgan, H. R., 1956, Latent viral infection of cells in tissue culture. I. Studies on latent infection of chick embryo tissues with psittacosis virus, *J. Exp. Med.* **103:**37–47.

Moulder, J. W., 1962, *The Biochemistry of Intracellular Parasitism,* University of Chicago Press, Chicago.

Moulder, J. W., 1964, *The Psittacosis Group as Bacteria,* Wiley, New York.

Moulder, J. W., 1966, The relation of the psittacosis group (chlamydiae) to bacteria and viruses, *Annu. Rev. Microbiol.* **20:**107–130.

Moulder, J. W., 1968, The life and death of the psittacosis virus, *Hosp. Pract.* **3:**35–45.

Moulder, J. W., 1974, Intracellular parasitism: Life in an extreme environment, *J. Infect. Dis.* **130:**300–306.

Moulder, J. W., Hatch, T. P., Byrne, G. I., and Kellogg, K. R., 1976, Immediate toxicity of high multiplicities of *Chlamydia psittaci* for mouse fibroblasts (L cells), *Infect. Immun.* **14:**277–289.

Müller-Eberhard, H. J., 1975, Complement, *Annu. Rev. Biochem.* **44:**697–724.

Murray, E. S., 1964, Guinea pig inclusion conjunctivitis virus. I. Isolation and identification as a member of the psittacosis-lymphogranuloma-trachoma group, *J. Infect. Dis.* **114:**1–12.

Murray, E. S., Snyder, J. C., and Bell, S. D., Jr., 1958, A note on the toxicity for white mice and gerbilles of a strain of elementary bodies isolated from a patient with trachoma in eastern Saudi Arabia, *Proc. 6th Int. Congr. Trop. Med. Malar. (Lisbon)* **5:**530–535.

Murray, E. S., Charbonnet, L. T., and MacDonald, A. B., 1973, Immunity to chlamydial infections of the eye.

I. The role of circulatory and secretory antibodies in resistance to reinfection with guinea pig inclusion conjunctivitis, *J. Immunol.* **110:**1518–1525.

Nataf, R., 1952, *Le Trachome,* Masson et Cie., Paris.

Nichols, R. L., and McComb, D. E., 1962, Immunofluorescent studies with trachoma and related antigens, *J. Immunol.* **89:**545–554.

Nichols, R. L., and McComb, D. E., 1964, Serologic strain differentiation in trachoma, *J. Exp. Med.* **120:**639–654.

Nichols, R. L., McComb, D. E., Haddad, N., and Murray, E. S., 1963, Studies on trachoma. II. Comparison of fluorescent antibody, Giemsa, and egg isolation methods for detection of trachoma virus in human conjunctival scrapings, *Am. J. Trop. Med. Hyg.* **12:**223–229.

Nichols, R. L., Bobb, A. A., Haddad, N. A., and McComb, D. E., 1967, Immunofluorescent studies of the microbiologic epidemiology of trachoma in Saudi Arabia, *Am. J. Ophthalmol.* **63:**1372–1408.

Nichols, R. L., von Fritzinger, K., and McComb, D. E., 1971a, Epidemiological data derived from immunotyping of 338 trachoma strains isolated from children in Saudi Arabia, in: *Trachoma and Related Disorders* (R. L. Nichols, ed.), pp. 337–357, *International Congress Series* No. 223, Excerpta Medica, Amsterdam.

Nichols, R. L., Murray, E. S., Scott, P. P., and McComb, D. E., 1971b, Trachoma isolation studies in Saudi Arabia from 1957 through 1969, in: *Trachoma and Related Disorders* (R. L. Nichols, ed.), pp. 517–528, *International Congress Series* No. 223, Excerpta Medica, Amsterdam.

Nichols, R. L., Oertley, R. E., Fraser, C. E. O., MacDonald, A. B., and McComb, D. E., 1973, Immunity to chlamydial infections of the eye. VI. Homologous neutralization of trachoma infectivity for the owl monkey conjunctivae by eye secretions from humans with trachoma, *J. Infect. Dis.* **127:**429–432.

Nichols, R. L., Murray, E. S., and Nisson, P. E., 1978, Use of enteric vaccines in protection against chlamydial infections of the genital tract and the eye of guinea pigs, *J. Infect. Dis.* **138:**742–746.

Nossal, G. J. V., and Ada, G. L., 1971, *Antigens, Lymphoid Cells, and the Immune Response,* Academic Press, New York.

Odartchenko, N., Lewerenz, M., Sordat, B., Roos, B., and Cottier, H., 1967, Kinetics of cellular death in germinal centers of mouse spleen, in: *Germinal Centers in Immune Responses* (H. Cottier, N. Odartchenko, R. Schindler, and C. C. Congdon, eds.), pp. 212–217, Springer-Verlag, Berlin.

Officer, J. E., and Brown, A., 1961, Serial changes in virus and cells in cultures chronically infected with psittacosis virus, *Virology* **14:**88–99.

Oh, J. O., and Tarizzo, M. L., 1969, Ocular lesions induced by the trachoma agent in rabbits, *J. Bacteriol.* **97:**1042–1047.

Oh, J. O., Ostler, H. B., and Schachter, J., 1971, Effects of interferon inducers on ocular lesions produced by trachoma agent in rabbits, in: *Trachoma and Related*

Disorders (R. L. Nichols, ed.), pp. 533–539, *International Congress Series* No. 223, Excerpta Medica, Amsterdam.

Orenstein, N. S., Mull, J. D., and Thompson, S. E., III, 1973, Immunity to chlamydial infections of the eye. V. Passive transfer of antitrachoma antibodies to owl monkeys, *Infect. Immun.* **7:**600–603.

Oriel, J. D., Reeve, P., Thomas, B. J., and Nicol, C. S., 1975, Infection with *Chlamydia* group A in men with urethritis due to *Neisseria gonorrhoeae, J. Infect. Dis.* **131:**376–382.

Oriel, J. D., Johnson, A. L., Barlow, D., Thomas, B. J., Nayyar, K., and Reeve, P., 1978, Infection of the uterine cervix with *Chlamydia trachomatis, J. Infect. Dis.* **137:**443–451.

Page, L. A., 1968, Proposal for the recognition of two species in the genus *Chlamydia* Jones, Rake, and Stearns, 1945, *Int. J. Syst. Bacteriol.* **18:**51–66.

Pagès, R., Paque, A., and Dernoncourt, Y., 1969, Presence of inclusion bodies morphologically identical with those of trachoma in the mucous membrane of the uterine cervix of 50% of female sufferers from trachoma examined, *Rev. Int. Trach.* **46**(2):175–181.

Parikh, G., and Shechmeister, I. L., 1964, Interaction of meningopneumonitis virus with white blood cells. II. Antigenic subunits of meningopneumonitis virus, *Virology* **22:**177–185.

Parish, W. E., 1972, Host damage resulting from hypersensitivity to bacteria, in: *Microbial Pathogenicity in Man and Animals* (H. Smith and J. H. Pearce, eds.), pp. 157–192, *Symposia of the Society for General Microbiology,* Vol. 22, Cambridge University Press, Cambridge.

Parkhouse, R. M. E., and Della Corte, E., 1974, Assembly and secretion of immunoglobulin A, in: *The Immunoglobulin A System* (J. Mestecky and A. R. Lawton, eds.), pp. 139–149, *Advances in Experimental Medicine and Biology,* Vol. 45, Plenum Press, New York.

Pearsall, N. N., and Weiser, R. S., 1970, *The Macrophage,* Lea and Febiger, Philadelphia, Pa.

Peters, J. H., Murray, E. S., Fraser, C. E. O., McComb, D. E., Nichols, R. L., Hathaway, A., Baldwin, E., Radcliffe, F., Charbonnet, L., and von Fritzinger, K., 1971, Development of local and systemic immunity in trachoma of man and animals, in: *Secretory Immunologic System* (D. H. Dayton, Jr., P. A. Small, Jr., R. M. Chanock, H. E. Kaufman, and T. B. Tomasi, Jr., eds.), pp. 341–358, U.S. Department of Health, Education, and Welfare, Washington, D.C.

Philip, R. N., Casper, E. A., Gordon, F. B., and Quan, A. L., 1974, Fluorescent antibody responses to chlamydial infection in patients with lymphogranuloma venereum and urethritis, *J. Immunol.* **112:**2126–2134.

Prendergast, R. A., and Henney, C. S., 1977, Cellular immune reactions, in: *The Lymphocyte: Structure and Function,* Part 1 (J. J. Marchalonis, ed.), pp. 257–277, Dekker, New York.

Rahi, A. H. S., and Garner, A., 1976, *Immunopathology of the Eye,* Blackwell Scientific Publications, Oxford.

Rake, G., and Jones, H. P., 1942, Studies on lymphogranuloma venereum. I. Development of the agent in the yolk sac of the chicken embryo, *J. Exp. Med.* **75:**323–338.

Rake, G., and Jones, H. P., 1944, Studies on lymphogranuloma venereum. II. The association of specific toxins with agents of the lymphogranuloma-psittacosis group, *J. Exp. Med.* **79:**463–486.

Reeve, P., and Graham, D. M., 1962, A neutralization test for trachoma and inclusion blennorrhoea viruses grown in HeLa cell cultures, *J. Gen. Microbiol.* **27:**177–180.

Reeve, P., Gerloff, R. K., Casper, E., Philip, R. N., Oriel, J. D., and Powis, P. A., 1974, Serological studies on the role of *Chlamydia* in the aetiology of non-specific urethritis, *Br. J. Vener. Dis.* **50:**136–139,

Richmond, S. J., and Caul, E. O., 1975, Fluorescent antibody studies in chlamydial infections, *J. Clin. Microbiol.* **1:**345–352.

Richmond, S. J., and Sparling, P. F., 1976, Genital chlamydial infections, *Am. J. Epidemiol.* **103:**428–435.

Ringertz, N., and Adamson, C. A., 1950, The lymph-node response to various antigens: An experimental-morphological study, *Acta Microbiol. Scand. Suppl.* **86:**1–69.

Ripa, K. T., and Mårdh, P.-A., 1977, Cultivation of *Chlamydia trachomatis* in cycloheximide-treated McCoy cells, *J. Clin. Microbiol.* **6:**328–331.

Ross, M. R., and Gogolak, F. M., 1957, The antigenic structure of psittacosis and feline pneumonitis viruses. I. Isolation of complement-fixing antigens with group and species specificity, *Virology* **3:**343–364.

Rota, R. R., and Nichols, R. L., 1973, *Chlamydia trachomatis* in cell culture. I. Comparison of efficiencies of infection in several chemically defined media, at various pH and temperature values, and after exposure to diethylaminoethyl-dextran, *Appl. Microbiol.* **26:**560–565.

Rothberg, R. M., Kraft, S. C., and Michalek, S. M., 1974, The establishment of systemic immunity following antigenic stimulation of the lymphoid tissue of the gastrointestinal mucosa, in: *The Immunoglobulin A System* (J. Mestecky and A. R. Lawton, eds.), pp. 473–478, *Advances in Experimental Medicine and Biology,* Vol. 45, Plenum Press, New York.

Sacks, D. L., and MacDonald, A. B., 1979, Isolation of a type-specific antigen from *Chlamydia trachomatis* by sodium dodecyl sulfate-polyacrylamide gel electrophoresis, *J. Immunol.* **122:**136–139.

Sacks, D. L., Rota, T. R., and MacDonald, A. B., 1978a, Isolation and partial characterization of a type-specific antigen from *Chlamydia trachomatis, J. Immunol.* **121:**204–208.

Sacks, D. L., Todd, W. J., and MacDonald, A. B., 1978b, Cell-mediated immune responses in owl monkeys (*Aotus trivergatus*) to soluble antigens of *Chlamydia trachomatis, Clin. Exp. Immunol.* **33:**57–64.

Sayed, H., and Wilt, J. C., 1971, Purification and properties of a chlamydial hemagglutinogen, *Can. J. Microbiol.* **17:**1509–1515.

Sayed, H. I., Nicks, R., and Wilt, J. C., 1972, Cellular-mediated immunity to the lymphogranuloma venereum agent, *Can. J. Microbiol.* **18:**385–390.

Sayed, H., Fung, K., and Wilt, J. C., 1976, Differences in physicochemical and antigenic properties of chlamydial strains, *Can. J. Microbiol.* **22:**937–941.

Schachter, J., 1968, Serologic response to Bedsonia cell walls, *Rev. Int. Trach.* **45:**311–318.

Schachter, J., 1976, Can chlamydial infections cause rheumatic disease? in: *Infection and Immunology in the Rheumatic Diseases* (D. C. Dumonde, ed.), pp. 151–157, Blackwell Scientific Publications, Oxford.

Schachter, J., Smith, D. E., Dawson, C. R., Anderson, W. R., Deller, J. J., Jr., Hoke, A. W., Smartt, W. H., and Meyer, K. F., 1969, Lymphogranuloma venereum. I. Comparison of the Frei test, complement fixation test, and isolation of the agent, *J. Infect. Dis.* **120:**372–375.

Schachter, J., Lum, L., Gooding, C. A., and Ostler, B., 1975, Pneumonitis following inclusion blennorrhea, *J. Pediatr.* **87:**779–780.

Schachter, J., Causse, G., and Tarizzo, M. L., 1976, Chlamydiae as agents of sexually transmitted diseases, *Bull. WHO* **54:**245–254.

Schmatz, H.-D., Brunner, H., Schmatz, S., and Sailer, J., 1977, Seroepidemiologische Untersuchungen zum Vorkommen von Chlamydien-Antikörpern beim Menschen, *Infection* **5:**6–8.

Scribner, D. J., and Fahrney, D., 1976, Neutrophil receptors for IgG and complement: Their roles in the attachment and ingestion phases of phagocytosis, *J. Immunol.* **116:**892–897.

Sen, D. K., Sarin, G. S., and Saha, K., 1977, Immunoglobulins in tears in trachoma patients, *Br. J. Ophthalmol.* **61:**218–220.

Shaaban, M. M., Shokeir, A. A., Wasfy, I. A., and Al-Hussaini, M. K., 1972, Female genital infection with TRIC agents in a trachomatous population, *J. Obstet. Gynaecol. Br. Commonw.* **79:**360–362.

Shimada, K., and Silverstein, A. M., 1975, Local antibody formation within the eye: A study of immunoglobulin class and antibody specificity, *Invest. Ophthalmol.* **14:**573–583.

Sigel, M. M., and Pollikoff, R., 1953, Reduction of group reactivity of complement-fixing antigen of meningopneumonitis virus by potassium periodate, *Proc. Soc. Exp. Biol. Med.* **84:**517–520.

Silverstein, A. M., 1974, The immunologic modulation of infectious disease pathogenesis, *Invest. Ophthalmol.* **13:**560–574.

Silverstein, A. M., and Prendergast, R. A., 1971, Lymphofollicular hyperplastic responses in ectopic locations: Trachoma as a paradigm, in: *Morphological and Functional Aspects of Immunity* (K. Lindahl-Kiessling, G. Alm, and M. G. Hanna, Jr., eds.), pp. 583–594, *Advances in Experimental Medicine and Biology,* Vol. 12, Plenum Press, New York.

Simpson, D. M., and Ross, R., 1972, The neutrophilic leukocyte in wound repair: A study with antineutrophil serum, *J. Clin. Invest.* **51:**2009–2023.

Smolin, G., Hall, J. M., Okumoto, M., and Ohno, S., 1977, High doses of subconjunctival corticosteroid and antibody-forming cells in the eye and draining lymph nodes, *Arch. Ophthalmol. (Chicago)* **95:**1631–1633.

Snyderman, R., and Pike, M. C., 1975, The role of lymphokines in delayed hypersensitivity reactions, in: *Immunopharmacology* (M. E. Rosenthale and H. C. Mansmann, Jr., eds.), pp. 31–45, *Monographs of the Physiological Society of Philadelphia,* Vol. 1, Spectrum Publications, Holliswood, N.Y..

Soldati, M., Verini, M. A., Isetta, A. M., and Ghione, M., 1971, Immunization researches in the field of trachoma: Some laboratory and clinical contributions, in: *Trachoma and Related Disorders* (R. L. Nichols, ed.), pp. 407–417, *International Congress Series* No. 223, Excerpta Medica, Amsterdam.

Sompolinsky, D., and Richmond, S., 1974, Growth of *Chlamydia trachomatis* in McCoy cells treated with cytochalasin B, *Appl. Microbiol.* **28:**912–914.

Sowa, S., Sowa, J., Collier, L. H., and Blyth, W. A., 1969, Trachoma vaccine field trials in the Gambia, *J. Hyg.* **67:**699–717.

Storz, J., 1971, *Chlamydia and Chlamydia-Induced Diseases,* Thomas, Springfield, Ill.

Stuart, A. E., 1970, *The Reticulo-endothelial System,* E. and S. Livingstone, Edinburgh.

Stuart, A. E., 1975, The reticulo-endothelial system, in: *Clinical Aspects of Immunology,* 3rd ed. (P. G. H. Gell, R. R. A. Coombs, and P. J. Lachmann, eds.), pp. 365–409, Blackwell Scientific Publications, Oxford.

Sueltenfuess, E. A., and Pollard, M., 1963, Cytochemical assay of interferon produced by duck hepatitis virus, *Science* **139:**595–596.

Surman, P. G., Hardy, D., and Howarth, W. H., 1967, The immunofluorescent staining technique applied to trachomatous eye smears in aboriginal school children in South Australia, *Am. J. Ophthalmol.* **63:**1361–1372.

Taborisky, J., 1932, Über die mikroskopische Diagnose des Trachoms, *Folia Ophthalmol. Orient.* **1:**34–52.

Tamura, A., and Manire, G. P., 1974, Hemagglutinin in cell walls of *Chlamydia psittaci, J. Bacteriol.* **118:**144–148.

Taverne, J., and Blyth, W. A., 1971, Interactions between trachoma organisms and macrophages, in: *Trachoma and Related Disorders* (R. L. Nichols, ed.), pp. 88–107, *International Congress Series* No. 223, Excerpta Medica, Amsterdam.

Taverne, J., Blyth, W. A., and Reeve, P., 1964, Toxicity of the agents of trachoma and inclusion conjunctivitis, *J. Gen. Microbiol.* **37:**271–275.

Taverne, J., Blyth, W. A., and Ballard, R. C., 1974, Interactions of TRIC agents with macrophages: Effects on lysosomal enzymes of the cell, *J. Hyg.* **72:**297–309.

Theodore, F. H., and Schlossman, A., 1958, *Ocular Allergy,* Williams and Wilkins, Baltimore.

Thomas, B. J., Reeve, P., and Oriel, J. D., 1976, Simplified serological test for antibodies to *Chlamydia trachomatis, J. Clin. Microbiol.* **4:**6–10.

Thomas, B. J., Evans, R. T., Hutchinson, G. R., and Taylor-Robinson, D., 1977, Early detection of chlamydial inclusions combining the use of cycloheximide-treated McCoy cells and immunofluorescence staining, *J. Clin. Microbiol.* **6:**285–292.

Thorbecke, G., and Lerman, S. P., 1976, Germinal centers and their role in immune responses, in: *The Reticuloendothelial System in Health and Disease: Functions and Characteristics* (S. M. Reichard, M. R. Escobar, and H. Friedman, eds.), pp. 83–100, *Advances in Experimental Medicine and Biology,* Vol. 73A, Plenum Press, New York.

Thygeson, P., 1951, The trachoma-psittacosis-lymphogranuloma venereum group of viruses: The Chlamydozoaceae, *Am. J. Ophthalmol.* **34**(5):7–34 (Part II).

Thygeson, P., 1971, Historical review of oculogenital disease, *Am. J. Ophthalmol.* **71:**975–985.

Thygeson, P., and Richards, P., 1938, Nature of the filtrable agent of trachoma, *Arch. Ophthalmol. (Chicago)* **20:**569–584.

Todd, W. J., and Storz, J., 1975, Ultrastructural cytochemical evidence for the activation of lysosomes in the cytocidal effect of *Chlamydia psittaci, Infect. Immun.* **12:**638–646.

Tramont, E. C., 1977, Inhibition of adherence of *Neisseria gonorrhoeae* by human genital secretions, *J. Clin. Invest.* **59:**117–124.

Treharne, J. D., Darougar, S., and Jones, B. R., 1977, Modification of the microimmunofluorescence test to provide a routine serodiagnostic test for chlamydial infection, *J. Clin. Pathol.* **30:**510–517.

Turk, J. L., and Oort, J., 1967, Germinal center activity in relation to delayed hypersensitivity, in: *Germinal Centers in Immune Responses* (H. Cottier, N. Odartchenko, R. Schindler, and C. C. Congdon, eds.), pp. 311–316, Springer-Verlag, Berlin.

Turk, J. L., and Oort, J., 1969, Further studies on the relation between germinal centers and cell-mediated injury, in: *Lymphatic Tissue and Germinal Centers in Immune Response* (L. Fiore-Donati and M. G. Hanna, Jr., eds.), pp. 317–326, *Advances in Experimental Medicine and Biology,* Vol. 5, Plenum Press, New York.

Turner, W., and Gordon, F. B., 1964, Indirect hemagglutination with the trachoma agent and related microorganisms, *J. Bacteriol.* **87:**1251–1252.

Vernon-Roberts, B., 1972, The macrophage, Cambridge Univ. Press.

Volanakis, J. E., 1975, The human complement system, *J. Oral Pathol.* **4:**195–221.

Wang, S.-P., 1971, A microimmunofluorescence method. Study of antibody response to TRIC organisms in mice, in: *Trachoma and Related Disorders* (R. L. Nichols, ed.), pp. 273–288, *International Congress Series* No. 223, Excerpta Medica, Amsterdam.

Wang, S.-P., and Grayston, J. T., 1963, Classification of

trachoma virus strains by protection of mice from toxic death, *J. Immunol.* **90:**849–856.

Wang, S.-P., and Grayston, J. T., 1970, Immunologic relationship between genital TRIC, lymphogranuloma venereum, and related organisms in a new microtiter indirect immunofluorescence test, *Am. J. Ophthalmol.* **70:**367–374.

Wang, S.-P., and Grayston, J. T., 1971, Classification of TRIC and related strains with microimmunofluorescence, in: *Trachoma and Related Disorders* (R. L. Nichols, ed.), pp. 305–321, *International Congress Series* No. 223, Excerpta Medica, Amsterdam.

Wang, S.-P., and Grayston, J. T., 1974, Human serology in *Chlamydia trachomatis* infection with microimmunofluorescence, *J. Infect. Dis.* **130:**388–397.

Wang, S.-P., Grayston, J. T., and Alexander, E. R., 1967, Trachoma vaccine studies in monkeys, *Am. J. Ophthalmol.* **63:**1615–1630.

Wang, S.-P., Kuo, C.-C., and Grayston, J. T., 1973, A simplified method for immunological typing of trachoma-inclusion conjunctivitis-lymphogranuloma venereum organisms, *Infect. Immun.* **7:**356–360.

Wang, S.-P., Grayston, J. T., Alexander, E. R., and Holmes, K. K., 1975, Simplified microimmunofluorescence test with trachoma-lymphogranuloma venereum (*Chlamydia trachomatis*) antigens for use as a screening test for antibody, *J. Clin. Microbiol.* **1:**250–255.

Watson, J., Kelly, K., and Largen, M., 1977, Genetic and cellular aspects of host response to endotoxin, in: *Microbiology—1977* (D. Schlessinger, ed.), pp. 298–303, American Society for Microbiology, Washington, D.C.

Watson, R. R., Mull, J. D., MacDonald, A. B., Thompson, S. E., III, and Bear, S. E., 1973a, Immunity to chlamydial infections of the eye. II. Studies of passively transferred serum antibody in resistance to infection with guinea pig inclusion conjunctivitis, *Infect. Immun.* **7:**597–599.

Watson, R. R., MacDonald, A. B., Murray, E. S., and Modabber, F. Z., 1973b, Immunity to chlamydial infections of the eye. III. Presence and duration of delayed hypersensitivity to guinea pig inclusion conjunctivitis, *J. Immunol.* **111:**618–623.

Weiss, E., 1971, Evolution of *Chlamydia*, in: *Trachoma and Related Disorders* (R. L. Nichols, ed.), pp. 3–12, *International Congress Series* No. 223, Excerpta Medica, Amsterdam.

Weiss, L., 1972, *The Cells and Tissues of the Immune System: Structure, Functions, Interactions*, Prentice-Hall, Englewood Cliffs, N.J.

Wentworth, B. B., and Alexander, E. R., 1974, Isolation of *Chlamydia trachomatis* by use of 5-iodo-2-deoxyuridine-treated cells, *Appl. Microbiol.* **27:**912–916.

White, R. G., 1975, Immunological functions of lymphoreticular tissues, in: *Clinical Aspects of Immunology,* 3rd ed. (P. G. H. Gell, R. R. A. Coombs, and P. J. Lachmann, eds.), pp. 411–445, Blackwell Scientific Publications, Oxford.

Willcox, R. R., 1975, Lymphogranuloma venereum, in: *Recent Advances in Sexually Transmitted Diseases,* No. 1 (R. S. Morton and J. R. W. Harris, eds.), pp. 188–193, Churchill Livingstone, Edinburgh.

Williams, R. C., and Gibbons, R. J., 1972, Inhibition of bacterial adherence by secretory immunoglobulin A: A mechanism of antigen disposal, *Science* **177:**697–699.

Wilt, P. C., Kordová, N., and Wilt, J. C., 1972, Preliminary characterization of a chlamydial agent isolated from embryonated snow goose eggs in northern Canada, *Can. J. Microbiol.* **18:**1327–1332.

Woolridge, R. L., and Grayston, J. T., 1962, Further studies with a complement fixation test for trachoma, *Ann. N.Y. Acad. Sci.* **98:**314–324.

Woolridge, R. L., Grayston, J. T., Chang, I. H., Cheng, K. H., Yang, C. Y., and Neave, C., 1967a, Field trial of a monovalent and of a bivalent mineral oil adjuvant trachoma vaccine in Taiwan school children, *Am. J. Ophthalmol.* **63:**1645–1653.

Woolridge, R. L., Grayston, J. T., Perrin, E. B., Yang, C. Y., Cheng, K. H., and Chang, I. H., 1967b, Natural history of trachoma in Taiwan school children, *Am. J. Ophthalmol.* **63:**1313–1320.

Wunderlich, J. R., Rosenberg, E. B., and Connolly, J. M., 1971, Human lymphocyte-dependent cytotoxic antibody and mechanisms of target cell destruction *in vitro*, in: *Progress in Immunology: First International Congress of Immunology* (B. Amos, ed.), pp. 473–482, Academic Press, New York.

Wyrick, P. B., and Brownridge, E. A., 1978, Growth of *Chlamydia psittaci* in macrophages, *Infect. Immun.* **19:**1054–1060.

Wyrick, P. B., Brownridge, E. A., and Ivins, B. E., 1978, Interaction of *Chlamydia psittaci* with mouse peritoneal macrophages, *Infect. Immun.* **19:**1061–1067.

Zakay-Rones, Z., Katzenelson, E., and Levy, R., 1968, Hemagglutinin of trachoma agent, *Isr. J. Med. Sci.* **4:**305–306.

Zakay-Rones, Z., Levy, R., and Maythar, B., 1972, Local antibodies to trachoma agent, *Isr. J. Med. Sci.* **8:**1130–1133.

19

Mechanisms of Resistance in the Systemic Mycoses

DEXTER H. HOWARD

1. Introduction

1.1. Natural and Acquired Resistance

Infection by zoopathogenic fungi frequently results only in inapparent, subclinical, or completely benign disease (Rippon, 1974). Malignant consequences from such infections are quite rare (Salvin, 1972). Thus animals must have very efficient ways of dealing with potentially invasive and destructive fungi. This efficiency is further exemplified by the fact that immunologically compromised hosts are dreadfully susceptible to a large number of species of fungi which have no obvious effect on normal individuals (Chick *et al.*, 1975). It is, then, not surprising that the literature is replete with descriptions of the ways that physiologically normal animals resist the penetration or preclude the multiplication of fungi in vital tissues (Austwick, 1972; Salvin, 1972).

Reinfections after recovery from some mycotic infections are considered to be extremely rare (Wilson, 1957), and enhanced resistance can be established in experimental animals by a wide variety of means (Beaman *et al.*, 1979; Dobias, 1964; Feit and Tewari, 1974; Kong and Levine, 1967; Levine *et al.*, 1970; Louria, 1960; Louria *et al.*, 1963b; Salvin, 1972). Thus a great body of available evidence documents the fact that both natural and acquired resistance are prominent features of the response of hosts to zoopathogenic fungi.

For the most part, work on experimental mycoses has amply documented the efficiency of animals in dealing with fungi. Although immune serum has been shown to convey protection in some studies (Gadebusch, 1958; Mourad and Friedman, 1968; Pearsall and Lagunoff, 1974), the effects appear to be mediated indirectly through augmentation of other mechanisms, and antibodies are not believed to play a key role in the mechanism of acquired resistance in most mycoses (Salvin, 1960). Indeed, cellular events seem to be of central importance in both natural and acquired resistance. Early work by Salvin (1954) established that the liver, spleen, and kidneys were prominent organs instrumental in clearing *Histoplasma capsulatum* from the tissues of experimental animals after sublethal infection. Inoculation of animals by any one of several routes was followed by obvious proliferation of cells of the reticuloendothelial system. Kuppfer's cells of the liver became heavily parasitized, and macrophages in other organs were engorged with yeast cells. The numbers of fungi were reduced over the course of several weeks, but viable organisms often persisted for long periods in host tissue (Louria *et al.*, 1959; Salvin, 1972). Subsequent work has shown that procedures which alter the proper functioning of cells of the reticuloendothelial system have disastrous consequences in experimental murine histoplasmosis (Berry, 1969).

DEXTER H. HOWARD • Department of Microbiology and Immunology, School of Medicine, University of California, Los Angeles, California 90024.

The work with *H. capsulatum* briefly described in the preceding paragraph has been extended to other systemic mycoses (e.g., Baine *et al.*, 1974; Louria, 1960; Louria *et al.*, 1963a,b; Sawyer *et al.*, 1976). It would be beyond the intended scope of this chapter to examine the pertinent literature with each of the fungi capable of causing systemic involvement. Furthermore, reviews of that literature are available (e.g., see Baker, 1971; Salvin, 1963, 1972). All lines of evidence have confirmed abundantly that natural and acquired resistance in the systemic mycoses are predominantly cell-mediated events. Accordingly, I propose to review the current state of our knowledge regarding the interaction of zoopathogenic fungi and phagocytic cells, to describe some cellular mechanisms mediating antifungal effects, and to give an account of the central importance of lymphocytes in mechanisms of acquired resistance.

1.2. Historical Antecedents

Metchnikoff studied a yeast infection of the freshwater crustacean *Daphnia magna* and observed that the blastospores and the needle-shaped ascospores of the fungus [now called *Metchnikowia biscuspidata* but named by him *Monospora bicuspidata* (Lodder, 1970)] were phagocytosed by leukocytes in the body cavity of the daphnia, after which the spores underwent degenerative changes (Metchnikoff, 1893). Morphological alterations were thus used to document the death of *M. bicuspidata* within the leukocytes of *D. magna*, and similar changes have been employed subsequently by investigators interested in the interaction of other fungi with phagocytes.

1.3. Background Information

Observations on the histopathology of the mycoses have provided evidence for the destruction of fungi within phagocytes through the morphological and tinctorial alterations noted (Baker, 1971; Gadebusch, 1972; Tashdjian *et al.*, 1971). No effort has been made to review all instances of these sorts of alterations recorded by numerous investigators since such observations would not distinguish the relative contributions of the many factors which compose the inflammatory response

(Dubos, 1954). This type of information is presented in a comprehensive consideration of the histopathology of the mycoses edited by R. D. Baker (1971).

Fungi have not so often been the subjects of experimental studies on the interaction of microbes and phagocytes as have been bacteria (Laskin and Lechevalier, 1972; Mackaness and Blanden, 1967; Pearsall and Weiser, 1970; Solotorovsky and Soderberg, 1972). This situation has changed somewhat in the last few years (Diamond *et al.*, 1972; Gadebusch, 1972; Howard, 1973a,b, 1975; Laskin and Lechevalier, 1972; Lehrer, 1970; Lehrer and Cline, 1969; Lehrer and Jan, 1970), and the current interest in fungi stems, at least in part, from a recognition of their importance as opportunistic pathogens.

Two types of phagocytes are predominantly involved in cellular defense mechanisms: polymorphonuclear leukocytes and mononuclear phagocytes. Polymorphonuclear neutrophils (PMNs) arise from stem cells in the bone marrow by a series of maturational steps and when released into the circulation are actively phagocytic, remarkably microbicidal, and nonreplicating (Bainton *et al.*, 1971). PMNs do not survive long in cell culture, but conditions have been devised so that the fate of microbes within them can be studied *in vitro* (Klebanoff, 1970; Klebanoff and Clark, 1978).

Mononuclear phagocytes (MNs) derive from actively dividing promonocytes in the bone marrow and are released into the bloodstream (Cohen and Cline, 1971; Nichols *et al.*, 1971; Van Furth and Cohn, 1968). These circulating MNs (CMNs) may differentiate into macrophages found in many areas of the body (Cohn, 1975). Those macrophages located in the lungs (AMNs) or the peritoneal cavity (PECs) have been chosen frequently for study of particle fate because of their accessibility. In contrast to PMNs, MNs survive for considerable periods in cell culture. Furthermore, MNs mature in response to environmental stimuli of various kinds (Cohn, 1975). Assessment of the fate of a microbe within MNs is thus determined, at least in part, by what type of MN phagocyte is studied, e.g., a circulating monocyte, a tissue histiocyte, a peritoneal macrophage, or a mononuclear cell exposed to lymphocytes from immunized animals (Artz and Bullock, 1979a,b; Howard *et al.*, 1971).

Lymphocytes clearly are mediator cells of acquired resistance. Information on the biology of this type of cell is vast, and techniques for cell manipulation have been discussed in detail (Bloom and David, 1976).

2. Polymorphonuclear Leukocytes

2.1. Fate of Fungi within PMNs

Fungi whose fate in neutrophils has been studied are shown in Table 1. The lethal effect of PMN phagocytes has been displayed for a broad range of fungi. The single obvious exception to the rather uniform antifungal activity of PMNs was the insusceptibility of conidiospores of *Aspergillus fumigatus,* which remained viable after 3 hr within human PMNs. The failure of PMNs to deal with *A. fumigatus* was related to the fact that the spo-

res were insensitive to a myeloperoxidase (MPO)–H_2O_2 system mediated *in vitro* by chloride ions but were sensitive to such a system when it was supplied with iodide ions (Lehrer and Jan, 1970). However, the insusceptibility of conidiospores to the nonoxidative antifungal systems also present in intact PMNs (Lehrer, 1972) suggests that dormant conidiospores are not so sensitive to killing by PMNs as are metabolically more active blastospores. Unpublished data from my laboratory show that conidiospores of *H. capsulatum* are somewhat more resistant to H_2O_2 than are the blastospores of the fungus. Moreover, as the conidiospores germinate, their sensitivity to peroxide increases to a level comparable to that of blastospores. The same disparity in sensitivity between dormant and germinating conidiospores was even more obvious in a *Penicillium* sp. subsequently studied in my laboratory (unpublished observation).

TABLE 1. Antifungal Activity of PMN Leukocytes[a]

Fungus	Antifungal activity[b]	Animal sources	References
Aspergillus fumigatus (conidia)	−	Human	Lehrer and Jan (1970)
Blastomyces dermatitidis	+	Human	Sixbey *et al.* (1979)
Candida albicans	+	Human	Albrecht (1968), Belcher *et al.* (1973), Brune *et al.* (1973), Lehrer (1972), Lehrer and Cline (1969), Louria and Brayton (1964), Schmid and Brune (1974), Leijh *et al.* (1977), Schuit (1979)
	+	Guinea pig	Howard (1973a), Arai *et al.* (1977)
	+	Chicken	Brune *et al.* (1973)
	+	Pig	Brune *et al.* (1973)
	+	Rabbit	Venkataraman *et al.* (1973)
C. krusei	+	Human	Lehrer (1972)
C. parapsilosis	+	Human	Lehrer (1972)
C. pseudotropicalis	+	Human	Lehrer (1972)
C. tropicalis	+	Human	Lehrer (1971, 1972), Louria and Brayton (1964), Schuit (1979)
Coccidioides immitis (endospores)	?	Dog	Wegner *et al.* (1972)
Cryptococcus neoformans	+	Rabbit	Gadebusch (1972)
	+	Human	Diamond *et al.* (1972), Tacker *et al.* (1972)
Histoplasma capsulatum	+	Human	Holland (1971)
	+	Guinea pig	Howard (1973a)
	+	Mouse	Unpublished observation
Paracoccidioides brasiliensis	+	Human	Resprepo-M and Velez (1975), Golman Yahr *et al.* (1979)
Saccharomyces cerevisiae	+	Human	Schuit (1979)
Torulopsis glabrata	+	Human	Lehrer (1972), Thong *et al.* (1979)

[a] This table is a modification of one presented at the Third International Conference on the Mycoses, São Paulo, Brazil, August 27–29, 1974 (Howard, 1975).
[b] +, Fungus killed (scored as positive regardless of percent killed); −, fungus not killed; ?, spores ingested but fate was not studied.

2.2. Antifungal Mechanisms within PMNs

A number of antimicrobial systems operative within PMNs have been described (Babior, 1978; Bellanti and Dayton, 1975; DeChatelet, 1975; Klebanoff, 1971, 1975; Klebanoff and Clark, 1978; Spitznagel, 1977). It is convenient to divide such mechanisms into two sorts: nonoxidative and oxidative (Table 2). Among nonoxidative systems are the following: acid pH (Dubos, 1954); hydrolytic enzymes, including lysozyme, acid phosphatase, and β-glucuronidase (Dubos, 1954; Klebanoff, 1975; Van Furth and Cohn, 1968); and cationic proteins (Gadebusch and Johnson, 1966; Olsson and Venge, 1974) other than the aforementioned enzymes but including phagocytin (Hirsch, 1956), histones (Hirsch, 1958), and lactoferrin (Kirkpatrick *et al.,* 1971b). Oxidative mechanisms include the following: H_2O_2 (Lehrer, 1969); myeloperoxidase and other peroxidases (Babior, 1978; Brune *et al.,* 1973; DeChatelet, 1975; Klebanoff, 1970, 1975; Klebanoff and Hamon, 1972; Klebanoff, and Clark, 1978; McRipley and Sbarra, 1967); ascorbic acid (Drath and Karnovsky, 1974, 1975); and superoxide anion, hydroxyl radicals, and singlet oxygen (Allen *et al.,* 1974; Babior, 1978; DeChatelet, 1975; DeChatelet *et al.,* 1975; Johnston *et al.,* 1975; Klebanoff, 1974, 1975; Klebanoff and Clark, 1978; Mandell, 1975; Rosen and Klebanoff, 1979).

2.2.1. Oxidative Antifungal Systems

Fungi are sensitive to H_2O_2, and their sensitivity is increased by the presence of halide ions (Howard, 1973a; Lehrer, 1969). One previously unpublished example of this sort of activity is shown in Table 3, where the sensitivity of *Torulopsis glabrata* to H_2O_2 and iodide is recorded. Hydrogen peroxide at 2.5×10^{-4} M in the presence of 2.5×10^{-4} M KI killed a large proportion of the yeast cells. These reagents by themselves are harmless at the concentration tested (Table 3).

Spores differ in their sensitivity to peroxide and halide. A comparative study of the sensitivity of the blastospores of the yeast *T. glabrata,* the blastospores of the dimorphic fungus *H. capsulatum,* and the conidiospores of *Chrysosporium* sp. has been published (Howard, 1977). The most sensitive of these types of spores were the blastospores of *H. capsulatum,* followed by the blastospores of *T. glabrata,* and then the conidiospores of *Chrysosporium* sp. However, the differences are not any larger than similar quantitative differences that have been reported among some species of *Candida* (Lehrer, 1971, 1972). Perhaps more instructive in this regard were the unpublished observations alluded to in a preceding paragraph. In these studies it was noted that dormant conidiospores of *H. capsulatum* and of a *Penicillium* sp. were less sensitive to peroxide and halide than were germlings of those fungi.

The most extensively examined of the antifungal properties of PMNs is the MPO-mediated system (Howard, 1973a; Lehrer, 1969). An example of the activity of this system has been published (Howard, 1977). Yeast cells of *C. albicans* and *H. capsulatum* are killed in a reaction mixture composed of granule lysates from mouse PMNs, H_2O_2, and chloride or iodide ions. The mechanisms by which the MPO-mediated system kills are not completely known, but several possibilities have been explored. When iodide is the halide, iodination of microorganisms occurs, and such halogenization of the microbial proteins may explain in part the microbicidal effects (Babior, 1978; Klebanoff, 1970; Klebanoff and Hamon, 1972;

TABLE 2. Antifungal Systems of Polymorphonuclear Leukocytes[a]

Oxidative	Nonoxidative
H_2O_2	Acid
Myeloperoxidase + H_2O_2 + halide	Hydrolytic enzymes, e.g., lysozyme
Ascorbic acid + peroxidase + copper	Cationic proteins, e.g., phagocytin
Superoxide anion	Lactoferrin
Hydroxyl radicals	
Singlet oxygen	

[a] The systems are not mutually exclusive. For example, some hydrolytic enzymes (lysozyme) and myeloperoxidase also migrate as cationic proteins.

TABLE 3. Augmentation by KI of the Fungicidal Effect of H_2O_2 on *Torulopsis glabrata*

	Percent dead yeast cells at indicated molar concentrations of reactants[a]				
	H_2O_2 (M)				
KI (M)	None	2.5×10^{-2}	2.5×10^{-3}	2.5×10^{-4}	2.5×10^{-5}
None	—	0	0	0	0
2.5×10^{-3}	0	100	97	97	91
2.5×10^{-4}	0	100	89	78	4
2.5×10^{-5}	0	14	0	0	0

[a] Diluent was 10^{-2} M phosphate buffer. Cells were harvested from overnight growth on glucose peptone agar slants and used at a concentration of 5×10^6 yeasts/ml. Five-tenths milliliter of cells was added to 0.5 ml of each reactant (final concentration shown), and total volume was raised to 2.0 ml with phosphate buffer. Tests were read after 3 hr incubation at 37°C. Death assessed by eosin-y dye exclusion (Howard, 1973a).

Olsson *et al.*, 1975). However, this apparently is not the mechanism of PMN candidacidal activity (Lehrer, 1972). When chloride is the halide, hypochlorous acid is evolved (De-Chatelet, 1975; Harrison and Schultz, 1976; Klebanoff, 1975; Klebanoff and Hamon, 1972; Sbarra *et al.*, 1972), and one of the effects of hypochlorous acid is the generation of toxic aldehydes from cell wall components of the microbe (Klebanoff, 1975). Further work has yielded data which show that peptides are oxidatively cleaved, and this also could play a role in the microbicidal activity of leukocytes (Selvaraj *et al.*, 1974). A recent suggestion is that the MPO system generates singlet oxygen which kills microbes (see last paragraph of this section).

Drath and Karnovsky (1974) have reminded us of another peroxide-mediated bactericidal system in PMNs involving ascorbic acid and copper. Several years ago Ericsson and Lundbeck (1955) showed that this system kills *Candida albicans* and *Torulopsis* sp. However, the ascorbic acid system is not so potent as the one involving MPO–H_2O_2–halide (Drath and Karnovsky, 1974).

Recently attention has focused on the interaction of superoxide anions, hydroxyl radicals, and singlet oxygen in the microbicidal effects of PMNs (Allen *et al.*, 1974; Babior, 1978; DeChatelet *et al.*, 1975; Drath and Karnovsky, 1975; Fridovich, 1972, 1974; Johnston *et al.*, 1975; Klebanoff, 1975; Rosen and Klebanoff, 1979). These powerful substances would kill fungi (Shimizu *et al.*, 1979), but whether they act directly or indirectly by generating

additional H_2O_2 to interact with the MPO system has not been established (Klebanoff, 1975; Rosen and Klebanoff, 1979). A number of authors have provided excellent reviews of the subject of oxidative antimicrobial mechanisms in PMNs (Babior, 1978; Klebanoff, 1975; Klebanoff and Clark, 1978; Spitznagel, 1977; Rosen and Klebanoff, 1979). Each discusses the oxidative systems in considerable detail, and their excellent coverage should be consulted for more information. Whatever the precise mode of action, it is clear that defects in one or another of the oxidative antimicrobial systems of PMNs can be correlated with a patient's inability to deal efficiently with pathogens (Babior, 1978; Klebanoff, 1971; Lehrer, 1970).

2.2.2. Nonoxidative Antifungal Systems from PMNs

The sensitivity of fungi to each of the non-oxidative factors listed in Table 2 is not equally well known. In general, zoopathogenic fungi are not particularly sensitive to the pH levels reported to exist in phagocytic vacuoles, and their response to phagocytin has not been evaluated. It has long been known that lysine-rich histones kill *Cryptococcus neoformans* (Gadebusch and Johnson, 1966). Lysozyme is reported to be fungicidal to several *Candida* species (Kamaya, 1970), to *Cr. neoformans* (Gadebusch and Johnson, 1966), and to *Coccidioides immitis* (Collins and Pappagianis, 1973). The mechanism of the action of lysozyme against fungi has not been determined, and there is one contradictory report on the sensitivity to it of *C. albicans* (Kozinn *et al.,* 1964). The specific substrate of lysozyme is not present in fungal cell walls.

The existence of antifungal mechanisms independent of the direct effects of oxidative systems is proven by four observations: (1) NaN$_3$ treatment, which inactivates oxidative systems such as MPO, does not remove the anticryptococcal effects of leukocytes (Diamond *et al.,* 1972; Lehrer, 1975); (2) MPO-deficient cells are still antifungal (Brune *et al.,* 1973; Lehrer, 1970, 1972); (3) certain fungi somewhat resistant to H$_2$O$_2$ are nevertheless killed by leukocytes (Lehrer, 1972); (4) leukocytes contain cationic proteins other than MPO which are actively fungicidal (Gadebusch and Johnson, 1966; Howard, 1975; Zeya and Spitznagel, 1966). With regard to the last point, human PMNs contain cationic proteins other than MPO which kill *H. capsulatum* (Howard, 1975). One such protein occurs at the place on polyacrylamide gels that one would expect to find lysozyme, and it can be shown that *H. capsulatum* is sensitive to this enzyme even though it is not lysed by it (unpublished observations).

Several investigators have used *C. albicans* and *C. parapsilosis* in studies on the antimicrobial effects of cationic proteins from human (Lehrer *et al.,* 1975; Olsson and Venge, 1974), guinea pig (Lehrer *et al.,* 1975; Zeya and Spitznagel, 1966), and rabbit (Lehrer *et al.,* 1975) leukocytes. Cationic proteins which kill *H. capsulatum* occur at approximately the same position on polyacrylamide gels as do the candidacidal protein (Howard, 1975), and similar components of mammalian granulocytes active against *Cr. neoformans* have been described (Lehrer and Ladra, 1977). Among the antifungal components of the human neutrophil is a protein, more cathodal than lysozyme, with chymotrypsinlike activity (Drazin and Lehrer, 1977; Lehrer *et al.,* 1975; Lehrer and Ladra, 1977; Rindler and Braunsteiner, 1973). The chymotrypsinlike cationic protein (CLCP) from human neutrophils binds specifically to the surface of *C. parapsilosis* and can be adsorbed preferentially by yeast cells that are mixed with whole extracts of neutrophil granules (Drazin and Lehrer, 1977). The enzyme activity of CLCP was unrelated to its candidacidal activity, and the mechanism by which it kills fungi remains to be determined (Drazin

and Lehrer, 1977). The highly cationic proteins of rabbit and guinea pig granules did not show chymotrypsinlike activity, but some of them did kill *C. parapsilosis* (Lehrer *et al.,* 1975).

Another cationic protein, the iron-binding lactoferrin (Leffell and Spitznagel, 1972), inhibits the growth of *C. albicans* (Kirkpatrick *et al.,* 1971b). Since serum transferrin inhibits the growth of many species of fungi in culture media (Baum and Artis, 1961; Esterly *et al.,* 1967; Gale and Welch, 1961; Howard, 1961; King *et al.,* 1975; Summers and Hasenclever, 1964), it is likely that these fungi would also be susceptible to the action of lactoferrin in PMNs (see Section 2.4 for a more complete discussion).

2.3. Extracellular Activity of Antifungal Systems Derived from PMNs

The data shown in Table 4 document the fact that many different fungi and spore types are sensitive to the fungicidal effects of peroxidases derived from PMNs and tested *in vitro.* One might reasonably speculate that fungal structures too large for PMN engulfment, e.g., spherules of *C. immitis,* or the hyphal elements of *Aspergillus* or *Rhizopus* nevertheless would be susceptible to killing by fungicidal systems present within PMNs and released into the internal milieu of the responding host. Such speculation is encouraged by the observation that PMNs cluster about large cells of *Cr. neoformans* (Kalina *et al.,* 1971), the filamentous forms of *C. albicans,* and the hyphae of *Aspergillus* and *Rhizopus* (Diamond *et al.,* 1978a,b). Granulocytes release both H$_2$O$_2$ (Root *et al.,* 1975) and cationic proteins (Venge and Olsson, 1975), and the damage to the hyphal forms of *C. albicans* is believed to be related to such release (Diamond *et al.,* 1978a).

2.4. Role of Serum Factors in Intracellular Fate

Fresh serum is essential for proper phagocytosis of fungi by PMNs (Howard, 1973a; Lehrer and Cline, 1969; Leijh *et al.,* 1977), but reports of direct damage to fungi by antifungal antibodies are uncommon (e.g., see Grappel and Calderone, 1976; Neill *et al.,* 1949).

Diamond *et al.* (1975) have exhaustively ex-

TABLE 4. Antifungal Activity of Peroxidases

Fungus	Type of spore	Peroxidase[a,b]		References
		Human	Animal	
Aspergillus niger	Conidiospore	+	NR	Lehrer (1969)
A. fumigatus	Conidiospore	+	NR	Lehrer (1969)
Candida albicans	Blastospore	+	+	Howard (1973a), Lehrer (1969)
C. krusei	Blastospore	+	NR	Lehrer (1969)
C. parapsilosis	Blastospore	+	NR	Lehrer (1969)
C. stellatoidea	Blastospore	+	NR	Lehrer (1969)
C. pseudotropicalis	Blastospore	+	NR	Lehrer (1969)
C. tropicalis	Blastospore	+	NR	Klebanoff (1970), Lehrer (1969)
Cryptococcus neoformans	Blastospore	+	NR	Diamond *et al.* (1972), Tacker *et al.* (1972)
Geotrichum candidium	Arthrospore	+	NR	Lehrer (1969)
Histoplasma capsulatum	Blastospore	+	+	Howard (1973a), Lehrer (1969)
Rhodotorula sp.	Blastospore	+	NR	Lehrer (1969)
Saccharomyces cerevisiae	Blastospore	+	NR	Lehrer (1969)

[a] +, Fungus killed; −, fungus not killed; NR, no report discovered.
[b] Peroxidase = myeloperoxidase derived from PMN granules and tested *in vitro* with H_2O_2 and iodide.

amined the role of complement in host defenses against *Cr. neoformans*. They discovered that 40–70% of the late components, i.e., C′3–9, of complement were adsorbed from guinea pig and human sera by *Cr. neoformans* or by the polysaccharide from its capsule. The late components were required for phagocytosis, and serum with low levels of these components did not allow *Cr. neoformans* to be phagocytosed. Spinal fluid, which does not contain complement, does not opsonize *Cr. neoformans*. The early components of complement, C′1,4,2, were required for optimum kinetics of phagocytosis. These workers went on to show that certain additive nonspecific factors such as properdin influenced phagocytosis and intracellular fate of *Cr. neoformans*. However, early work by Gadebusch (1961) did not supply convincing evidence that properdin played a significant role in modifying experimental cryptococcosis. Nevertheless, it is clear that serum factors control the kinetics of entry of fungi into PMNs and may also influence the intracellular killing in some instances. Moreover, polysaccharides derived from *C. immitis* depress the properdin system and inactivate complement of mice (McNall *et al.*, 1960). The resistance of mice injected

with this polysaccharide is reduced for a period of 2–4 days after injection.

The immune state of the host has not frequently been shown to influence the fate of fungi with PMNs. However, there is one recent report in which the greatest killing of *C. albicans* was observed in neutrophils and serum from immunized animals (Venkataraman *et al.*, 1973). The increased effect was not obviously related to humoral factors alone. Morelli and Rosenberg (1971) have established that phagocytosis by blood leukocytes was enhanced by specific antibody and a complete hemolytic complement system. However, the extent of killing within mouse peritoneal exudate cells was not influenced by antibody, complement, or the complement status of the animals supplying the cells.

Animal serum incorporated into culture media inhibits the growth of many species of fungi (Baum and Artis, 1961; Gale and Welch, 1961; Howard, 1961; Howard and Otto, 1967; Igel and Bolande, 1966; King *et al.*, 1975; Newcomer *et al.*, 1968; Otto and Howard, 1976; Reiss and Szilagyi, 1967; Roth *et al.*, 1959; Roth and Goldstein, 1961; Shiraishi and Arai, 1979; Summers and Hasenclever, 1964; Weinberg, 1974). Such growth suppression is caused most often by serum transferrin, which binds iron and makes it unavailable for the nutrition of the microorganism (Caroline *et al.*, 1964; Davis and Denning, 1972; Elin and Wolff, 1973; Esterly *et al.*, 1967; Hendry and Bakerspigel, 1969; King *et al.*, 1975; Landau *et al.*, 1964; Shiraishi and Arai, 1979; Summers and Hasenclever, 1964). Although factors other than transferrin may account for certain aspects of serum-induced fungistasis in some organisms (Esterly *et al.*, 1967; Reiss *et al.*, 1975), it is clear that addition of iron to serum-containing media commonly reverses the fungistatic activity of those media (Davis and Denning, 1972; Elin and Wolff, 1973; King *et al.*, 1975; Summers and Hasenclever, 1964). These observations indicate that serum transferrin and the lactoferrin of PMNs may be important in limiting the replication of fungi *in vivo* (Kirkpatrick *et al.*, 1971b).

3. Mononuclear Phagocytes

3.1. Fate of Fungi within Normal MNs

Three types of cells figure prominently in studies on the interaction of microorganisms and MN phagocytes: circulating monocytes (CMNs), alveolar macrophages (AMNs), and peritoneal macrophages (PECs). Data on the fate of fungi within such cells are summarized in Table 5. Generally fungi are readily phagocytosed by PEC in cell culture. Nevertheless, engulfment may be sponsored by both heat-labile and heat-stable factors (Kozel and Mastroianni, 1976; Morrison and Cutler, 1977; Swanson and Kozel, 1978).

3.1.1. CMNs

Human CMNs kill *Cr. neoformans* (Diamond *et al.*, 1972), but when the monocytes are maintained in cell culture and become macrophages they lose their cryptococcocidal capacity (Diamond and Bennett, 1973; Gentry and Remington, 1971). *H. capsulatum* and *C. albicans* are killed by human CMNs (Holland, 1971; Lehrer, 1975; Leijh *et al.*, 1977), but both of these fungi survive and multiply within mouse PECs (Howard, 1965; Stanley and Hurley, 1969; Taschdjian *et al.*, 1971). The same difference in intracellular fate has been recorded for *Saccharomyces cerevisiae* and *C.*

tropicalis within CMNs and PECs (Howard, 1959; Schuit, 1979; Stanley and Hurley, 1969). Some fungi, however, are readily killed by both CMNs and PECs (Lehrer, 1975; Stanley and Hurley, 1969) (Table 5).

3.1.2. AMNs

Kong and Levine (1967) report that *C. immitis* arthrospores and spherules were found in lung macrophages, but the actual intracellular death or digestion of the fungus was not determined. Masshof and Adams (1957) found *C. albicans* in AMNs and giant cells of rabbits after intrabronchial instillation. The yeast appeared to disintegrate within the macrophages but survived and multiplied in the giant cells. Peterson and Calderone (1977) reported that growth of *C. albicans* was inhibited by rabbit AMNs. Tacker and Bulmer reported that *Cr. neoformans* was not killed by guinea pig AMNs (Bulmer and Tacker, 1975; Tacker and Bulmer, 1972); however, Epstein *et al.* (1967) showed that spores of *A. flavus* were killed within mouse AMNs. Sanchez and Carbonell (1975) reported that AMNs did not kill *H. capsulatum*. Thus differences in intracellular behavior within AMNs have been discovered among various species of fungi (Table 5).

3.1.3. PECs

Cultured PECs seemingly have a lesser capacity to deal with fungi than do other types of mononuclear cells. *Blastomyces dermatitidis* (Howard and Herndon, 1960), *C. albicans* (Stanley and Hurley, 1969), *C. tropicalis* (Stanley and Hurley, 1969), *Cr. neoformans* (Gentry and Remington, 1971; Mitchell and Friedman, 1972), *H. capsulatum* (Howard, 1959, 1964, 1965), and *Saccharomyces cerevisiae* (Howard, 1959) have been reported to survive and multiply within PECs maintained in cell culture. In contrast, *C. guilliermondii* (Donaldson *et al.*, 1956; Stanley and Hurley, 1969) and some isolates of *C. pseudotropicalis* (unpublished observations) apparently are killed while *C. krusei*, *C. parapsilosis*, some other isolates of *C. pseudotropicalis*, and *T. glabrata* have a limited ability to grow within cultured macrophages (Howard and Otto, 1967; Stanley and Hurley, 1969). A recent report suggests that intracellular death of *C. albicans* within cultured monocytes has to be measured in the first 60 min after phagocytosis, since

TABLE 5. Fate of Fungi in Mononuclear Phagocytes[a]

Species of fungus	Type of MN phagocyte[b]			References
	CMN	AMN	PEC	
Absidia ramosa	+	+	NR	Smith (1976)[c]
Aspergillus flavus	NR	+	NR	Epstein *et al.* (1967)
A. fumigatus	NR	NR	+	White (1977)
Blastomyces dermatitidis	NR	NR	−	Howard and Herndon (1960)
Candida albicans	+	+	−	Arai *et al.* (1977), Lehrer (1975), Leijh *et al.* (1977), Stanley and Hurley (1969), Peterson and Calderone (1977), Patterson-Delafield and Lehrer (1979), Schuit (1979), Taschdjian *et al.* (1971)
C. guilliermondii	NR	NR	+	Stanley and Hurley (1969), Donaldson *et al.* (1956)
C. pseudotropicalis	+	NR	+	Lehrer (1975), Stanley and Hurley (1969)
C. parapsilosis	+	NR	±	Lehrer (1975), Stanley and Hurley (1969)
C. krusei	NR	NR	±	Stanley and Hurley (1969)
C. tropicalis	+	NR	−	Schuit (1979), Stanley and Hurley (1969)
Cryptococcus neoformans	+	−	−	Bulmer and Tacker (1975), Diamond and Bennett (1973), Diamond *et al.* (1972, 1975), Gentry and Remington (1971), Mitchell and Friedman (1972), Tacker and Bulmer (1972)
Coccidioides immitis	NR	?	NR	Kong and Levine (1967)
Histoplasma capsulatum	+	−	−	Dumont and Robert (1970), Holland (1971), Howard (1959, 1964, 1965), Sanchez and Carbonell (1975)
Saccharomyces cerevisiae	+	NR	±	Howard (1959), Schuit (1979)
Torulopsis glabrata	NR	NR	±	Howard and Otto (1967)

[a] Results summarized from the literature.
[b] NR, No report discovered; +, killed; −, not killed (intracellular growth observed); ±, limited intracellular growth; ?, observed but fate not determined.
[c] Results suggestive but no direct observations.

thereafter growth of the remaining viable yeasts makes further assessment of the killing process impossible (Van Zwet *et al.*, 1975). Moreover, PECs lose their antifungal capacities in cell culture (Howard *et al.*, 1971). Inasmuch as these facts were not always appreciated in the studies recorded in Table 5, some of the conclusions may have to be reassessed.

3.2. Acquired Immunity in the Mycoses

It is generally agreed that lymphocytes are crucial in various aspects of acquired immunity (Bloom and David, 1976). Cutaneous reac-

tivity of the delayed type consistently accompanies most of the systemic mycoses (Rifkind *et al.*, 1976; Rippon, 1974) and can be consistently displayed in experimental infections (Domer and Moser, 1978; Giger *et al.*, 1978; Poulain *et al.*, 1978; Spencer and Cozad, 1973). In coccidioidomycosis such reactivity is transferable to normal individuals by means of a dialyzable extract of lymphocytes obtained from donors with positive skin tests (Rapaport *et al.*, 1960). In candidiasis, coccidioidomycosis, cryptococcosis, histoplasmosis, and sporotrichosis lymphocytes from skin-test-positive individuals respond *in vitro* to specific antigen (Alford and Goodwin, 1973; Belcher *et al.*, 1975; Cox *et al.*, 1976, 1977; Cox and Vias, 1977; Fromtling *et al.*, 1979; Graybill and Alford, 1974; Hall *et al.*, 1978; Kirkpatrick *et al.*, 1971a; Landau and Newcomer, 1967; Musatti *et al.*, 1976; Opelz and Scheer, 1975; Rocklin *et al.*, 1970; Rogers and Balish, 1978; Zweiman *et al.*, 1969). Macrophages are responsive to factors released from sensitized lymphocytes by fungal antigens (Deighton *et al.*, 1977, Kashkin *et al.*, 1977; Pague *et al.*, 1969; Thor and Dray, 1968).

Macrophages from immunized animals restrict the growth of *H. capsulatum* (Hill and marcus, 1960; Miya and Marcus, 1961; Wu and Marcus, 1960; Miya and Marcus, 1961; Wu and Marcus, 1964) and *Cr. neoformans* (Diamond, 1977; Gentry and Remington, 1971). The lymphocyte is the mediator cell and the macrophage the effector cell of this phenomenon (Abrahams, 1965; Abrahams *et al.*, 1971; Howard *et al.*, 1971). Partially purified lymphocytes activate macrophages to suppress the intracellular growth of *H. capsulatum* (Howard *et al.*, 1971). How this suppression is brought about is not known, but it is accompanied by depression of protein synthesis of the fungus (Howard, 1973b). Lymphocytes from immunized animals can transfer immunity to inexperienced recipients (Beaman *et al.*, 1977, 1979; Tewari *et al.*, 1977), and work on experimental infections in nude mice clearly implicates the decisive importances of cell-mediated effects (Cutler, 1976; Graybill and Drutz, 1978; Williams *et al.*, 1978).

It seems likely that soluble factors derived from sensitized lymphocytes by immunological or pharmacological methods (Cahall and Youmans, 1975; Fowles *et al.*, 1973; Pantalone and Page, 1975; Patterson and Youmans, 1970; Youmans, 1971) will be found to arm macrophages to an antihistoplasma capacity. Nevertheless, in spite of intensive efforts, solid data on this point are still lacking (Howard and Otto, 1977). It is interesting to note that a similar difficulty in obtaining lymphokines which arm macrophages from mouse cells has been experienced with the *Toxoplasma gondii* system (Jones *et al.* 1975). The difficulty was overcome when human material was employed and the growth of *T. gondii* was inhibited in normal human monocytes treated with a product released after exposure of T lymphocytes from immune subjects to toxoplasma antigen (Borges and Johnson, 1975).

3.3. Antibody-Dependent Cell-Mediated Antifungal Effects

It has been observed repeatedly that antibodies against fungi either derived from patients or raised in experimental animals do not markedly affect the viability of fungi *in vitro* or seemingly facilitate acquired immunity (Diamond 1974; Grappel and Calderone, 1976; Salvin, 1960). However, Gadebusch (1972) showed that *Cr. neoformans* was killed by histiocytes and antibody in a fashion which suggested death before phagocytosis. This early observation has received confirmation and extension by Diamond's report (1974) in which he established that human CMNs in the presence of specific antibody killed *Cr. neoformans*. The anticryptococcal effect was extracellular because the experiments were performed in the presence of cytochalasin B, which effectively inhibited phagocytosis of the cryptococci but did not block antibody-dependent cell-mediated cytotoxicity. Preliminary studies indicated that human antibody could act in the system. The IgG fraction from a high-titer human system was separated and was very efficient in the presence of mononuclear cells in killing *Cr. neoformans*. Several types of blood leukocytes, except T cells, are capable of this type of antibody-dependent antifungal activity (Diamond and Allison, 1976). Such extracellular events are particularly interesting in that they present possible mechanisms for killing fungal forms generally considered too large for phagocytosis, e.g., the spherules of *C. immitis*, the pseudohyphae and hyphae of *C. albicans*, and hyphal elements of *Aspergillus* sp. or *Rhizopus* sp.

3.4. Antifungal Effects of Irritant-Induced PECs

Inflammatory substances are frequently injected intraperitoneally into animals in order to evoke macrophages. The cells harvested have heightened microbicidal properties (Pearsall and Weiser, 1970; Reikvam *et al.*, 1975; Reikvam and Hoiby, 1975). Substances used as irritants have included oil (Elberg *et al.*, 1960), glycogen (Elberg *et al.*, 1960), casein (Elberg *et al.*, 1960), bacterial endotoxin (Mackaness and Blanden, 1967), polyanions (Remington and Merigan, 1970), and immunoadjuvants (Mackaness and Blanden, 1967; Sorrell *et al.*, 1978). Generally PECs have to be irritant-induced in animals other than mice because mice are the only widely used animal with a large resident population of PECs (David, 1975). Thus in most instances in studies made with PECs from species of donor animals other than mice the PECs are to some degree "activated" and accordingly will have heightened antimicrobial abilities. Moreover, the type of incitant will affect the lysosomal enzymes expressed (Mørland and Mørland, 1978).

Bacterial endotoxin is cytotoxic to mouse PECs (Shands *et al.*, 1974), but intravenous adminstration does stimulate animals without killing peritoneal macrophages. However, macrophages from mice injected i.v. with 200 μg LPS from *Salmonella typhosa* 18 hr before harvest did not inhibit intracellular growth of *H. capsulatum* (Howard, 1975). Likewise, injection of glycogen i.p. into mice evokes a large number of macrophages, but intracellular growth of *H. capsulatum* is not modified in such cells (Howard *et al.*, 1971).

Synthetic polyanions, especially poly(I) · poly(C), protect mice against intracellular bacterial infections (Remington and Merigan, 1970; Weinstein *et al.*, 1970). Furthermore, Gober *et al.*, (1972) reported suppression of intracellular growth of *Shigella flexneri* in cell cultures treated with this substance. However, Thalinger and Mandell (1972) did not observe enhanced killing of *Escherichia coli* by mouse PECs exposed to poly(I) · poly(C). The polyanion did not affect intracellular growth of *H. capsulatum* within mouse PEC harvested from animals injected with it or within such cells maintained in cultures containing it (Howard, 1975). This result is in keeping with that of Worthington and Hasenclever (1972), who reported that poly(I) · poly(C) increased the severity of certain experimental fungal infections and had no obvious effect on others.

In contrast to these negative results, sodium caseinate (Difco) induces a population of macrophages with antihistoplasma effects (Howard, 1975). The results are reminiscent of a similar finding by Elberg *et al.* (1960), who reported that such cells were more resistant to the destructive intracellular growth of *Mycobacterium tuberculosis*. Further studies have revealed that the effect is substantially removed by washing and that partially purified lymphocytes from caseinate-induced exudates will activate macrophages from nonstimulated animals (unpublished data). Lymphocytes which mediate immunity to infection with *Listeria monocytogenes* in mice have been reported to occur in casein-induced peritoneal exudates by others (North and Spitalny, 1974).

3.5. Antifungal Mechanisms in MNs

3.5.1. Cells from Normal Animals

Activated mouse PECs can be triggered to release H_2O_2 (Nathan and Root, 1977), and the well-described MPO of PMN cells is also found in MN cells (Cotran and Litt, 1970; Daems and Brederoo, 1971; Lepper and Hart, 1976). The presence of MPO as revealed by histochemical techniques depends on the stage of differentiation of the cells and on the animal species. However, biochemical determinations have often been at variance with histochemical ones. For example, rabbit AMNs and PECs, previously reported to have no peroxidase, have been shown to contain the enzyme when tests were performed biochemically (Paul *et al.*, 1973; Romeo *et al.*, 1973). However, contradictory results continue to be reported with some mononuclear cells (e.g., Biggar and Sturgess, 1976). Nevertheless, the MPO system reported in human CMNs kills *C. albicans* and *C. parapsilosis* (Lehrer, 1975). Other microbicidal materials such as the antimycobacterial substances which have been extracted from macrophages (Kochan and Golden, 1974) have not been studied in relation to fungi, but cationic proteins from human CMNs have candidacidal effects (Lehrer, 1975). Lysosomal extracts from rabbit alveolar macrophages inhibit amino acid uptake by *C. albicans* (Peterson and Calderone, 1977, 1978).

3.5.2. Cells from Immunized Animals

Efforts to extract inhibitory substances from immunologically activated macrophages have not been consistently successful (Laskin and Lechevalier, 1972). A recent report, however, shows that such a substance capable of killing *L. monocytogenes* is released by monolayers of PECs from BCG-immunized guinea pigs following incubation with PPD in cell culture (Bast *et al.*, 1974). Such lymphokines have been reported to kill yeast cells (Pearsall *et al.*, 1973).

3.5.3. Growth of Facultative Intracellular Parasites within Cultured PECs

Engulfment of particles by cultured PECs is generally followed by the fusion of lysosomes with the phagosomes to effect the delivery of lysosomal enzymes into the phagolysosome. But with some bacteria, e.g., *Mycobacterium tuberculosis* (Armstrong and Hart, 1971; Hart *et al.*, 1972), and with the protozoan *Toxoplasma gondii* (Jones *et al.*, 1972) lysosomal fusion does not take place. This failure of fusion has been suggested as one mechanism whereby intracellular parasites avoid exposure to the antimicrobial effects of lysosomal contents. The sulfatides extracted from *M. tuberculosis* inhibited phagolysosome fusion in cultured PEC which had engulfed *S. cerevisiae* (Goren *et al.*, 1976). In contrast, however, some intracellular pathogens, e.g., *Listeria monocytogenes* (Pesonti, 1978) and *M. lepraemurium* (Draper *et al.*, 1979), promote lysosomal fusion and nevertheless survive within cultured PECs. Moreover, lysosomal fusion will take place with phagosomes containing tubercle bacilli coated with specific immune serum, and the bacilli survive and mutiply even though presumably in the presence of antimicrobial substances. Likewise, yeast cells of *H. capsulatum* coated with high-titer immune serum replicate at an undiminished rate in guinea pig PECs (Howard, 1965). Thus the successful multiplication of facultative intracellular parasites in PECs cultured *in vitro* cannot always be explained by failure of delivery of microbicidal substances into the phagosomes. Clearly, certain pathogens survive within cells possessed of potent antimicrobial substances and seemingly replicate while in contact with such substances.

4. Conclusion

Cellular events are of crucial importance in both natural and acquired resistance to zoopathogenic fungi. The fate of fungi within phagocytes has been reviewed. PMN leukocytes and MN phagocytes are involved predominantly in this type of host–fungus interaction. PMN leukocytes kill blastospores of fungi, but the sensitivity of other types of spores is not so well established. Microbicidal substances within PMNs have been described and, in many instances, the sensitivity of fungi to them has been recorded.

Three types of MN phagocytes have been studied: circulating monocytes (CMNs), alveolar macrophages (AMNs), and peritoneal exudate cells (PECs). The fate of fungi within these cells is different. CMNs kill *C. albicans*, *C. tropicalis*, *C. pseudotropicalis*, *C. parapsilosis*, *Cr. neoformans*, *H. capsulatum*, and *Saccharomyces cerevisiae*; the fate of other fungi in this cell has not been recorded. Some fungi are killed in AMNs, while others survive. The fate of organisms within PECs depends on the species of fungus, the immune state of the animal from which the cells were obtained, and whether or not an irritant was used to evoke them. The mechanisms of fungicidal activity of MN phagocytes are not so well documented as are those of PMNs.

ACKNOWLEDGMENTS

The work from my laboratory was supported by U.S. Public Health Service Grants AI-07461 and AI-15120, and was done with the collaborative efforts of Mlles. E. Nagatani, V. Otto, J. Pang, and S. Munnerlyn, and Mr. M. Zapf. I am grateful to my secretary, Ms. J. Fung, and to my wife, Lois, for the numerous typings and readings that a work of this sort requires.

Some of the material covered in this chapter was first prepared and presented in a paper entitled "The interaction of zoopathogenic fungi and mammalian phagocytes" at the seminar "Mechanisms of Host Resistance to Fungi," Annual Meeting, American Society for Microbiology, Chicago, Illinois, May 12–17, 1974.

A major portion of the chapter was prepared while I was on sabbatical leave in the laboratory of Dr. Phyllis Stockdale at the Commonwealth Mycological Institute, Kew, Surrey, England (1974–1975). Portions of it have been presented to the British Mycopathological Society, Glasgow, Scotland (March 25, 1975); to the Service de Mycologie, Institut Pasteur, Paris, France (April 7, 1975); at the Sixth Congress of the International Society for Human and Animal Mycology, Tokyo, Japan (July 4, 1975); and at the First Asilomar Conference of the Northern California Branch of the American Society for Microbiology entitled "Pathogenic Mechanisms in Microbial Disease," Asilomar, California (November 7–9, 1975). I herewith express my appreciation to each of these groups for inviting me to speak.

I apologize to any investigators whose contributions to an understanding of the intracellular fate of fungi have been overlooked in this chapter.

References

Abrahams, I., 1965, Further studies on acquired resistance in murine cryptococcosis: Enhancing effect of *Bordetella pertussis, J. Immunol.* **96**:525–529.

Abrahams, I., Stoffer, H. R., and Payette, K. M., 1971, Cellular immunity in experimental cryptococcosis: Contribution of macrophages and lymphocytes, in: *Comptes Rendus International Society Human and Animal Mycology*, pp. 258–259, Pasteur Institute, Paris (abstract).

Albrect, L. R., 1968, Innate resistance to *Candida albicans*, Ph.D. thesis, University of North Carolina, Chapel Hill.

Alford, R. H., and Goodwin, R. A., 1973, Variation in lymphocyte reactivity to histoplasmin during the course of chronic pulmonary histoplasmosis, *Am. Rev. Resp. Dis.* **108**:85–92.

Allen, R. C., Yevich, S. J., Orth, R. W., and Stelle, R. H., 1974, The superoxide anion and singlet molecular oxygen: Their role in the microbicidal activity of PMN, *Biochem. Biophys. Res. Commun.* **60**:909–915.

Arai, T., Mikami, Y., and Yokoyama, K., 1977, Phagocytosis of *Candida albicans* by rabbit alveolar macrophages and guinea pig neutrophils, *Sabouraudia* **15**:171–177.

Armstrong, J. A., and Hart, D'Arcy P., 1971, Response of cultured macrophages to *Mycobacterium tuberculosis*, with observations on fusion of lysosomes with phagosomes, *J. Exp. Med.* **134**:713–740.

Armstrong, J. A., and Hart, D'Arcy P., 1975, Phagosome–lysosome interactions in cultured macrophages infected with virulent tubercle bacilli, *J. Exp. Med.* **142**:1–16.

Artz, R. P., and Bullock, W. E., 1979a, Immunoregulatory responses in experimental disseminated histoplasmosis: Lymphoid organ histopathology and serological studies, *Infect. Immun.* **23**:884–892.

Artz, R. P., and Bullock, W. E., 1979b, Immunoregulatory responses in experimental disseminated histoplasmosis: Depression of T-cell-dependent and T-effector responses by activation of splenic suppressor cells, *Infect. Immun.* **23**:893–902.

Austwick, P. K. C., 1972, The pathogenicity of fungi, in: *Microbial Pathogenicity in Man and Animals* (H. Smith and J. H. Pearce, eds.), pp. 251–268, Cambridge University Press, Cambridge.

Babior, B. M., 1978, Oxygen-dependent microbial killing by phagocytes, *N. Engl. J. Med.* **298**:659–668, 721–725.

Baine, W. B., Koenig, M. G., and Goodman, J. S., 1974, Clearance of *Candida albicans* from the bloodstream of rabbits, *Infect. Immun.* **10**:1420–1425.

Bainton, D. F., Ullyot, J. L., and Farquhar, M. G., 1971, The development of neutrophilic polymorphonuclear leukocytes in human bone marrow, *J. Exp. Med.* **134**:907–934.

Baker, R. D. (ed.), 1971, *Human Infection with Fungi, Actinomycetes and Algae*, Springer-Verlag, New York, 1191 pp.

Bast, R. C., Cleveland, R. P., Littman, B. H., Zbar, B., and Rapp, H. J., 1974, Acquired cellular immunity: Extracellular killing of *Listeria monocytogenes* by a product of immunologically activated macrophages, *Cell. Immunol.* **10**:248–259.

Baum, G. L., and Artis, D., 1961, Growth inhibition of *Cryptococcus neoformans* by cell free serum, *Am. J. Med. Sci.* **241**:613–616.

Beaman, L., Pappagianis, D., and Benjamini, E., 1977, The significance of T cells in resistance to experimental murine coccidioidomycosis, *Infect. Immun.* **17**:580–585.

Beaman, L., Pappagianis, D., and Benjamini, E., 1979, Mechanism of resistance to infection with *Coccidioides immitis* in mice, *Infect. Immun.* **23**:681–685.

Belcher, R. W., Carney, J. F., and Monahan, F. G., 1973, An electron microscopic study of phagocytosis of *Candida albicans* by polymorphonuclear leukocytes, *Lab. Invest.* **29**:620–627.

Belcher, R. W., Palazij, R., and Wolinsky, E., 1975, Immunologic studies in patients with sarcoidosis and cryptococcosis, *Arch. Dermatol.* **111**:711–716.

Bellanti, J. A., and Dayton, D. H. (eds.), 1975, *The Phagocytic Cell in Host Resistance*, Raven, New York, 348 pp.

Berry, C. L., 1969, The production of disseminated histoplasmosis in the mouse: The effects of changes in reticulo-endothelial function, *J. Pathol.* **97**:441–457.

Biggar, W. D., and Sturgess, J. M., 1976, Peroxidase activity of alveolar macrophages, *Lab. Invest.* **34**:31–42.

Bloom, B. R., and David, J. (eds), 1976, *In Vitro Methods in Cell-Mediated and Tumor Immunity*, Academic Press, New York, 748 pp.

Borges, J. S., and Johnson, W. D., Jr., 1975, Inhibition of multiplication of *Toxoplasma gondii* by human monocytes exposed to T-lymphocyte products, *J. Exp. Med.* **141**:483–496.

Brune, K., Schmid, L., Glatt, M., and Minder, B., 1973,

Correlation between antimicrobial activity and peroxidase content of leukocytes, *Nature (London)* **245:** 209–210.

Bulmer, G. S., and Tacker, J. R., 1975, Phagocytosis of *Cryptococcus neoformans* by alveolar macrophages, *Infect. Immun.* **11:**73–79.

Cahall, D. L., and Youmans, G. P., 1975, Conditions for production, and some characteristics, of mycobacterial growth inhibitory factor produced by spleen cells from mice immunized with viable cells of the attenuated H37Ra strain of *Mycobacterium tuberculosis, Infect. Immun.* **12:**833–840.

Caroline, L., Taschdjian, C. L., Kozinn, P. J., and Schade, A. L., 1964, Reversal of serum fungistasis by addition of iron, *J. Invest. Dermatol.* **42:**415–419.

Chick, E. W., Balows, A., and Furcolow, M. L. (eds.), 1975, *Opportunistic Fungal Infections,* Thomas, Springfield, 359 pp.

Clark, R. A., and Klebanoff, S. J., 1975, Neutrophil-mediated tumor-cell cytotoxicity: Role of the peroxidase system, *J. Exp. Med.* **141:**1442–1447.

Cohen, A. B., and Cline, M. J., 1971, The human alveolar macrophage: Isolation, cultivation *in vitro,* and studies of morphologic and function characteristics, *J. Clin. Invest.* **50:**1390–1398.

Cohn, Z. A., 1975, Macrophage physiology, *Fed. Proc.* **34:**1725–1729.

Collins, M., and Pappagianis, D., 1973, Effects of lysozyme and chitinase on the spherules of *Coccidioides immitis in vitro, Infect. Immun.* **7:**817–822.

Cotran, R. S., and Litt, M., 1970, Ultrastructural localization of horseradish peroxidase and endogenous peroxidase activity in guinea pig peritoneal macrophages, *J. Immunol.* **105:**1536–1546.

Cox, R. A., and Vias, J. R., 1977, Spectrum of *in vivo* and *in vitro* cell-mediated responses in coccidioidomycosis, *Cell. Immunol.* **31:**130–141.

Cox, R. A., Vivas, J., Grass, A., Lecara, G., Miller, E., and Brummer, E., 1976, *In vivo* and *in vitro* cell-mediated responses in coccidioidomycosis. I. Immunologic responses of persons with primary asymptomatic infections, *Am. Rev. Resp. Dis.* **114:**937–943.

Cox, R. A., Brummer, E., and Lecara, G., 1977, *In vitro* lymphocyte responses of coccidioidin skin test-positive and -negative persons to coccidioidin, spherulin, and a *Coccidioides* cell wall antigen, *Infect. Immun.* **15:** 751–755.

Cutler, J. E., 1976, Acute systemic candidiasis in normal and congenitally thymic-deficient (nude) mice, *J. Reticuloendothel. Soc.* **19:**121–124.

Daems, W. T., and Brederoo, P., 1971, The fine structure and peroxidase activity of resident and exudate peritoneal macrophages in the guinea pig, in: *The Reticuloendothelial System and Immune Phenomena* (N. R. DiLuzio and K. Flemming, eds.), pp. 19–31, Plenum Press, New York.

David, J. R., 1975, Macrophages activation by lymphocyte mediators, *Fed. Proc.* **34:**1730–1736.

Davis, R. R., and Denning, T. J. V., 1972, Growth and form in *Candida albicans, Sabouraudia* **10:**180–188.

DeChatelet, L. R., 1975, Oxidative bactericidal mechanisms in polymorphonuclear leukocytes, *J. Infect. Dis.* **131:**295–303.

DeChatelet, L. R., Mullikin, D., and McCall, C. E., 1975, The generation of superoxide anion by various types of phagocytes, *J. Infect. Dis.* **131:**443–446.

Deighton, F., Cox, R. A., Hall, N. K., and Larsh, H. W., 1977, *In vivo* and *in vitro* cell-mediated immune response to a cell wall antigen of *Blastomyces dermatitidis, Infect. Immun.* **15:**429–435.

Diamond, R. D., 1974, Antibody-dependent killing of *Cryptococcus neoformans* by human peripheral blood mononuclear cells, *Nature (London)* **247:**148–150.

Diamond, R. D., 1977, Effects of stimulation and suppression of cell-mediated immunity on experimental cryptococcosis, *Infect. Immun.* **17:**187–194.

Diamond, R. D., and Allison, A. C., 1976, Nature of the effector cells responsible for antibody-dependent cell-mediated killing of *Cryptococcus neoformans, Infect. Immun.* **14:**716–720.

Diamond, R. D., and Bennett, J. E., 1973, Growth of *Cryptococcus neoformans* within human macrophages *in vitro, Infect. Immun.* **7:**231–236.

Diamond, R. D., Root, R. K., and Bennett, J. E., 1972, Factors influencing killing of *Cryptococcus neoformans* by human leukocytes *in vitro, J. Infect. Dis.* **125:**367–376.

Diamond, R. D., May, J. E., Kane, M., Frank, M. M., and Bennett, J. E., 1975, The role of the late complement components and the alternate complement pathway in experimental cryptococcosis, *Proc. Soc. Exp. Biol. Med.* **144:**312–315.

Diamond, R. D., Krzesicki, R., and Jao, W., 1978a, Damage to pseudohyphal forms of *Candida albicans* by neutrophils in absence of serum *in vitro, J. Clin. Invest.* **61:**349–359.

Diamond, R. D., Krzesicki, R., Epstein, B., and Jao, W., 1978b, Damage to hyphal forms of fungi by human leukocytes *in vitro, Am. J. Pathol.* **91:**313–324.

Dobias, B., 1964, Specific and nonspecific immunity in *Candida* infections, *Acta Med. Scand. Suppl.* **421,** 77 pp.

Domer, J. E., and Moser, S. A., 1978, Experimental murine candidiasis: Cell-mediated immunity after cutaneous challenge, *Infect. Immun.* **20:**88–98.

Donaldson, D. M., Marcus, S., Gyi, K. K., and Perkins, E. H., 1956, The influence of immunization and total body X-irradiation on intracellular digestion by peritoneal phagocytes, *J. Immunol.* **76:**192–199.

Draper, P., Hart, D'Arcy P., and Young, M. R., 1979, Effects of anionic inhibitors of phagosome–lysosome fusion in cultured macrophages when the ingested organism is *Mycobacterium lepraemurium, Infect. Immun.* **24:**558–561.

Drath, D. B., and Karnovsky, M. L., 1974, Bactericidal activity of metal-mediated peroxide ascorbate systems, *Infect. Immun.* **10:**1077–1083.

Drath, D. B., and Karnovsky, M. L., 1975, Superoxide production by phagocytic leukocytes, *J. Exp. Med.* **141**:257–263.

Drazin, R. E., and Lehrer, R. I., 1977, Fungicidal properties of a chymotrypsin-like cationic protein from human neutrophiles: Adsorption to *Candida parapsilosis, Infect. Immun.* **17**:382–388.

Dubos, R. J., 1954, *Biochemical Determinants of Microbial Diseases,* Harvard University Press, Cambridge, Mass., 152 pp.

Dumont, A., and Robert, A., 1970, Electron microscopic study of phagocytosis of *Histoplasma capsulatum* by hamster peritoneal macrophages, *Lab. Invest.* **23**: 278–286.

Elberg, S. S., Mascarenhas, P., and Fong, J., 1960, Response of peritoneal exudate cells to *Brucella melitensis*: Influence of nature of inflammatory irritant, *Proc. Soc. Exp. Biol. Med.* **104**:295–297.

Elin, R. J., and Wolff, S. M., 1973, Effect of pH and iron concentration on growth of *Candida albicans* in human serum, *J. Infect. Dis.* **127**:705–708.

Epstein, S. M., Verney, E., Miale, T. D., and Sidransky, H., 1967, Studies on the pathogenesis of experimental pulmonary aspergillosis, *Am. J. Pathol.* **51**:769–788.

Ericsson, Y., and Lundbeck, H., 1955, Antimicrobial effect *in vitro* of ascorbic acid oxidation, I. Effect on bacteria, fungi and viruses in pure culture, *Acta Pathol. Microbiol. Scand.* **37**:493–506.

Esterly, N. B., Brammer, S. B., and Crounse, R. G., 1967, The relationship of transferrin and iron to serum inhibition of *Candida albicans, J. Invest. Dermatol.* **49**:437–442.

Feit, C., and Tewari, R. P., 1974, Immunogenicity of ribosomal preparations from yeast cells of *Histoplasma capsulatum, Infect. Immun.* **10**:1091–1097.

Fowles, R. E., Jajardo, I. M., Leibowitch, J. L., and David, J. R., 1973, The enhancement of macrophage bacteriostasis by products of activated lymphocytes, *J. Exp. Med.* **138**:952–964.

Fridovich, I., 1972, Superoxide radical and superoxide dismutase, *Acc. Chem. Res.* **5**:321–326.

Fridovich, I., 1974, Superoxide radical on the bactericidal action of phagocytes, *N. Engl. J. Med.* **290**:624–625.

Fromtling, R. A., Blackstock, R., Hall, N. K., and Bulmer, G. S., 1979, Kinetics of lymphocyte transformation in mice immunized with viable avirulent forms of *Cryptococcus neoformans, Infect. Immun.* **24**:449–453.

Gadebusch, H. H., 1958, Passive protection against *Cryptococcus neoformans, Proc. Soc. Exp. Biol. N.Y.* **98**:611–614.

Gadebusch, H. H., 1961, Natural host resistance to infection with *Cryptococcus neoformans,* I. The effect of the properdin system on the experimental disease, *J. Infect. Dis.* **109**:147–153.

Gadebusch, H. H., 1972, Mechanisms of native and acquired resistance to infection with *Cryptococcus neoformans,* in: *Macrophages and Cellular Immunity* (A.

I. Laskin and H. Lechevalier, eds.), pp. 3–12, CRC Press, Cleveland.

Gadebusch, H. H., and Johnson, A. G., 1966, Natural host resistance to infection with *Cryptococcus neoformans,* IV. The effect of some cationic proteins on the experimental disease, *J. Infect. Dis.* **116**:551–565.

Gale, G. R., and Welch, A. M., 1961, Studies on opportunistic fungi. I. Inhibition of *Rhizopus oryzae* by human serum, *Am. J. Med. Sci.* **241**:604–612.

Gentry, L. O., and Remington, J. S., 1971, Resistance against *Cryptococcus* conferred by intracellular bacteria and protozoa, *J. Infect. Dis.* **123**:22–31.

Giger, D. K., Domer, J. E., Moser, S. A., and McQuitty, J. T., Jr., 1978, Experimental murine candidiasis: Pathological and immune responses in T lymphocyte-depleted mice, *Infect. Immun.* **21**:729–737.

Gober, L. L., Friedman-Kien, A. E., Havell, E. A., and Vilcek, J., 1972, Suppression of the intracellular growth of *Shigella flexneri* in polycytidylic acid, *Infect. Immun.* **5**:370–376.

Goihman-Yahr, M., Essenfeld-Yahr, E., Albornoz, M. C., Yarzabal, L., Gomez, H. M. de, San Martin, B., Ocanto, A., and Convit, J., 1979, A new method to estimate digestion of *Paracoccidioides brasiliensis* by phagocytic cells *in vitro, J. Clin. Microbiol.* **10**:365–370.

Goren, M. B., Hart, D'Arcy P., Young, M. R., and Armstrong, J. A., 1976, Prevention of phagosome–lysosome fusion in cultured macrophages by sulfatides of *Mycobacterium tuberculosis, Proc. Natl. Acad. Sci. USA* **73**:2510–2514.

Grappel, S. F., and Calderone, R. A., 1976, Effect of antibodies on the respiration and morphology of *Candida albicans, Sabouraudia* **14**:51–60.

Graybill, J. R., and Alford, R. H., 1974, Cell-mediated immunity in cryptococcosis, *Cell. Immunol.* **14**:12–21.

Graybill, J. R., and Drutz, D. J., 1978, Host defense in cryptococcosis. II. Cryptococcosis in the nude mouse, *Cell. Immunol.* **40**:263–274.

Hall, N. K., Deighton, F., and Larsh, H. E., 1978, Use of an alkali-soluble water-soluble extract of *Blastomyces dermatitidis* yeast-phase cell walls and isoelectrically focused components in peripheral lymphocyte transformations, *Infect. Immun.* **19**:411–415.

Harrison, J. E., and Schutz, J., 1976, Studies on the chlorinating activity of myeloperoxidase, *J. Biol. Chem.* **251**:1371–1374.

Hart, D'Arcy P., Armstrong, J. A., Brown, C. A., and Draper, P., 1972, Ultrastructural study of the behavior of macrophages toward parasitic mycobacteria, *Infect. Immun.* **5**:803–807.

Hendry, A. T., and Bakerspigel, A., 1969, Factors affecting serum inhibited growth of *Candida albicans* and *Cryptococcus neoformans, Sabouraudia* **7**:219–229.

Hill, G. A., and Marcus, S., 1960, Study of cellular mechanisms in resistance to systemic *Histoplasma capsulatum* infection, *J. Immunol.* **85**:6–13.

Hirsch, J. G., 1956, Phagocytin: A bactericidal substance

from polymorphonuclear leukocytes, *J. Exp. Med.* **113**:589–611.

Hirsch, J. G., 1958, Bactericidal action of histone, *J. Exp. Med.* **108**:925–944.

Holland, P., 1971, Circulating human phagocytes and *Histoplasma capsulatum*, in: *Histoplasmosis: Proceedings of the 2nd National Conference* (L. Ajello, E. W. Chick, and M. L. Furcolow, eds.), pp. 380–383, Thomas, Springfield.

Howard, D. H., 1959, Observations on tissue cultures of mouse peritoneal exudates inoculated with *Histoplasma capsulatum*, *J. Bacteriol.* **78**:69–78.

Howard, D. H., 1961, Some factors which affect the initiation of growth of *Cryptococcus neoformans*, *J. Bacteriol.* **82**:430–435.

Howard, D. H., 1964, Intracellular behavior of *Histoplasma capsulatum*, *J. Bacteriol.* **87**:33–38.

Howard, D. H., 1965, Intracellular growth of *Histoplasma capsulatum*, *J. Bacteriol.* **87**:518–523.

Howard, D. H., 1973a, Fate of *Histoplasma capsulatum* in guinea pig polymorphonuclear leukocytes, *Infect. Immun.* **8**:412–419.

Howard, D. H., 1973b, Further studies on the inhibition of *Histoplasma capsulatum* within macrophages from immunized animals, *Infect. Immun.* **8**:577–581.

Howard, D. H., 1975, The role of phagocytic mechanisms in defense against *Histoplasma capsulatum*, in: *Proceedings of the Third International Symposium on Mycoses*, 27–29 August 1974, São Paulo, Brazil, Scientific Publication No. 304, pp. 50–59, Pan American Health Organization, Washington, D.C.

Howard, D. H., 1977, Fungicidal systems derived from phagocytic cells, in: *Recent Advances in Medical and Veterinary Mycology*, pp. 197–202, University of Tokyo Press, Tokyo.

Howard, D. H., and Herndon, R. L., 1960, Tissue cultures of mouse peritoneal exudates inoculated with *Blastomyces dermatitidis*, *J. Bacteriol.* **80**:522–527.

Howard, D. H., and Otto, V., 1967, The intracellular behavior of *Torulopsis glabrata*, *Sabouraudia* **5**:235–239.

Howard, D. H., and Otto, V., 1977, Experiments on lymphocyte-mediated cellular immunity in murine histoplasmosis, *Infect. Immun.* **16**:226–231.

Howard, D. H., Otto, V., and Gupta, R. K., 1971, Lymphocyte-mediated cellular immunity in histoplasmosis, *Infect. Immun.* **4**:605–610.

Igel, H. J., and Bolande, R. P., 1966, Humoral defense mechanisms in cryptococcosis: Substances in normal human serum, saliva, and cerebrospinal fluid affecting the growth of *Cryptococcus neoformans*, *J. Infect. Dis.* **116**:75–83.

Johnston, R. B., Jr., Keele, B. B., Jr., Misra, H. P., Lehmeyer, J. E., Webb, L. S., Baehner, R. L., and Rajagopalian, K. V., 1975, The role of superoxide anion generation in phagocytic bactericidal activity, *J. Clin. Invest.* **55**:1357–1372.

Jones, T. C., and Hirsch, J. G., 1972, The interaction between *Toxoplasma gondii* and mammalian cells, *J. Exp. Med.* **136**:1173–1194.

Jones, T. C., Yeh, S., and Hirsch, J. G., 1972, The interaction between *Toxoplasma gondii* and mammalian cells. I. Mechanism of entry and intracellular fate of the parasite, *J. Exp. Med.* **136**:1157–1172.

Jones, T. C., Len, L., and Hirsch, J., 1975, Assessment *in vitro* of immunity against *Toxoplasma gondii*, *J. Exp. Med.* **141**:466–482.

Kalina, M., Kletter, Y., Shahar, A., and Aronson, M., 1971, Acid phosphatase release from intact phagocytic cells surrounding a large-size parasite, *Proc. Soc. Exp. Biol. Med.* **136**:407–410.

Kamaya, T., 1970, Lytic action of lysozyme on *Candida albicans*, *Mycopathol. Mycol. Appl.* **42**:197–207.

Kashkin, K. P., Kikholetov, S. M., and Lipnitsky, A. V., 1977, Studies on mediators of cellular immunity in experimental coccidioidomycosis, *Sabouraudia* **15**:59–68.

King, R. D., Khan, H. A., Faye, J. C., Greenberg, J. H., and Jones, H. E., 1975, Transferrin, iron and dermatophytes. I. Serum dermatophyte inhibitory component definitively identified as unsaturated transferrin, *J. Lab. Clin. Med.* **86**:204–212.

Kirkpatrick, C. H., Chandler, J. W., Jr., Smith, T. K., and Newberry, W. M., Jr., 1971a, Cellular immunologic studies in histoplasmosis, in: *Histoplasmosis* (L. Ajello, E. W. Chick, and M. L. Furcolow, eds.), pp. 371–379, Thomas, Springfield.

Kirkpatrick, C. H., Green, I., and Rich, R. R., 1971b, Inhibition of growth of *Candida albicans* by iron-unsaturated lactoferrin: Relation to host-defense mechanisms in chronic mucocutaneous candidiasis, *J. Infect. Dis.* **124**:539–544.

Klebanoff, S. J., 1970, Myeloperoxidase: Contribution to microbicidal activity of intact leukocytes, *Science* **169**:1095–1097.

Klebanoff, S. J., 1971, Intraleukocytic microbicidal defects, *Annu. Rev. Med.* **22**:39–62.

Klebanoff, S. J., 1974, Role of superoxide anion in the myeloperoxidase-mediated antimicrobial system, *J. Biol. Chem.* **249**:3724–3728.

Klebanoff, S. J., 1975, Antimicrobial mechanisms in neutrophilic polymorphonuclear leukocytes, *Semin. Hematol.* **12**:117–142.

Klebanoff, S. J., and Clark, R. O., 1978, *The Neutrophil: Function and Clinical Disorders*, North-Holland, Amsterdam, 810 pp.

Klebanoff, S. J., and Hamon, C. B., 1972, Role of myeloperoxidase-mediated antimicrobial systems in intact leukocytes, *J. Reticuloendothel. Soc.* **12**:170–196.

Kochan, I., and Golden, C. A., 1974, Immunological nature of antimycobacterial phenomenon in macrophages, *Infect. Immun.* **9**:249–254.

Kong, Y. M., and Levine, H. B., 1967, Experimentally induced immunity in the mycoses, *Bacteriol. Rev.* **31**:35–53.

Kozel, T. R., and Mastroianni, R. P., 1976, Inhibition of

phagocytosis by cryptococcal polysaccharide: Dissociation of the attachment and ingestion phases of phagocytosis, *Infect. Immun.* **14**:62–67.

Kozinn, P. J., Caroline, L., and Taschdjian, C. L., 1964, Conjunctiva contains factor inhibiting growth of *Candida albicans*, *Science* **146**:1479–1480.

Landau, J. W., and Newcomer, V. D., 1967, Cytolytic plasma factor in experimental coccidioidomycosis, *J. Bacteriol.* **94**:918–923.

Landau, J. W., Dabrowa, N., Newcomer, V. D., and Rowe, J., 1964, The relationship of serum transferrin and iron to the rapid formation of germ tubes by *Candida albicans*, *J. Invest. Dermatol.* **43**:473–482.

Laskin, A. I., and Lechevalier, H. (eds.), 1972, *Macrophages and Cellular Immunity*, CRC Press, Cleveland.

Leffell, M. S., and Spitznagel, J. K., 1972, Association of lactoferrin with lysozyme in granules of human polymorphonuclear leukocytes, *Infect. Immun.* **6**:761–765.

Lehrer, R. I., 1969, Antifungal effects of peroxidase systems, *J. Bacteriol.* **99**:361–365.

Lehrer, R. I., 1970, Measurement of candidacidal activity of specific leukocyte types in mixed cell populations. I. Normal myeloperoxidase-deficient, and chronic granulomatous disease neutrophils, *Infect. Immun.* **2**:42–47.

Lehrer, R. I., 1971, Inhibition by sulfanamides of the candidacidal activity of human neutrophils, *J. Clin. Invest.* **59**:2498–2505.

Lehrer, R. I., 1972, Functional aspects of a second mechanism of candidacidal activity of human neutrophils, *J. Clin. Invest.* **51**:2566–2572.

Lehrer, R. I., 1975, The fungicidal mechanisms of human monocytes. I. Evidence for myeloperoxidase-linked and myeloperoxidase-independent candidacidal mechanisms, *J. Clin. Invest.* **55**:330–346.

Lehrer, R. I., and Cline, M. J., 1969, Interaction of *Candida albicans* with human leukocytes and serum, *J. Bacteriol.* **98**:996–1004.

Lehrer, R. I., and Jan, R. G., 1970, Interaction of *Aspergillus fumigatus* spores with human leukocytes and serum, *Infect. Immun.* **1**:345–350.

Lehrer, R. I., and Ladra, K. M., 1977, Fungicidal components of mammalian granulocytes active against *Cryptococcus neoformans*, *J. Infect. Dis.* **136**:96–99.

Lehrer, R. I., Ladra, K. M., and Hake, R. B., 1975, Nonoxidative fungicidal mechanisms of mammalian granulocytes: Demonstration of components with candidacidal activity in human, rabbit, and guinea pig leukocytes, *Infect. Immun.* **11**:1226–1234.

Leijh, P. C. J., Barselear, M. T. van den, and van Furth, R., 1977, Kinetics and phagocytosis and intracellular killing of *Candida albicans* by human granulocytes and monocytes, *Infect. Immun.* **17**:313–318.

Lepper, A. W. D., and Hart, P. D'Arcy, 1976, Peroxidase staining in elicited and nonelicited mononuclear cells from BCG-sensitized and nonsensitized mice, *Infect. Immun.* **14**:522–526.

Levine, H. B., Pappagianis, D., and Cobb, J. M., 1970,

Development of vaccines from coccidioidomycosis, *Mycopathol. Mycol. Appl.* **41**:177–185.

Lodder, J. (ed.), 1970, *The Yeasts: A Taxonomic Study*, North-Holland, Amsterdam, 1385 pp.

Louria, D. B., 1960, Specific and non-specific immunity in experimental cryptococcosis in mice, *J. Exp. Med.* **111**:643–665.

Louria, D. B., and Brayton, R. G., 1964, Behavior of *Candida* cells within leukocytes, *Proc. Soc. Exp. Biol. Med.* **115**:93–98.

Louria, D. B., Feder, N., Mitchell, W., and Emmons, C. W., 1959, Influence of fungus strain and lapse of time in experimental histoplasmosis and of volume of inoculum in cryptococcosis upon recovery of the fungi, *J. Lab. Clin. Med.* **53**:311–317.

Louria, D. B., Brayton, R. G., and Finkel, G., 1963a, Studies on the pathogenesis of experimental *Candida albicans* infection in mice, *Sabouraudia* **2**:271–283.

Louria, D. B., Kaminski, T., and Finkel, G., 1963b, Further studies on immunity in experimental cryptococcosis, *J. Exp. Med.* **117**:509–520.

Mackaness, G. B., and Blanden, R. V., 1967, Cellular immunity, *Prog. Allergy* **11**:89–140.

Mandell, G. L., 1975, Catalase, superoxide dismutase, and virulence of *Staphylococcus aureus*, *J. Clin. Invest.* **55**:561–566.

Masshof, W., and Adams, W., 1957, Histomorphologie der experimentallen *Candida*-Infektion, *Arch. Klin. Exp. Dermatol.* **204**:416–446.

McNall, E. G., Sorensen, L. J., Newcomer, V. D., and Sternberg, T. H., 1960, The role of specific antibodies and properdine in coccidioidomycosis, *J. Invest. Dermatol.* **34**:213–217.

McRipley, R. J., and Sbarra, A. J., 1967, Role of the phagocyte in host–parasite interactions. XII. Hydrogen peroxide–myeloperoxidase bactericidal system in the phagocyte, *J. Bacteriol.* **94**:1425–1430.

Metchnikoff, E., 1893, *Lectures on the Comparative Pathology of Inflammation*, pp. 82–87 (trans. from French by F. A. Starling and E. H. Starling), Kegan Paul, Trench, Trübner & Co., London, Reprint: Dover Publications, New York, 1968.

Mitchell, T. G., and Friedman, L., 1972, *In vitro* phagocytosis and intracellular fate of variously encapsulated strains of *Cryptococcus neoformans*, *Infect. Immun.* **5**:491–498.

Miya, F., and Marcus, S., 1961, Effect of humoral factors on *in vitro* phagocytic and cytopeptic activities of normal and "immune" phagocytes, *J. Immunol.* **85**:652–668.

Morelli, R., and Rosenberg, L. T., 1971, The role of complement in the phagocytosis of *Candida albicans* by mouse peripheral blood leukocytes, *J. Immunol.* **107**:476–480.

Mørland, B., and Mørland, J., 1978, Selective induction of lysosomal enzyme activities in mouse peritoneal macrophages, *J. Reticuloendothel. Soc.* **23**:469–477.

Morrison, R. P., and Cutler, J. E., 1977, Serum factors

required by macrophages for phagocytosis of *Candida albicans, Abstracts of the Annual Meeting of the American Society for Microbiology,* New Orleans, p. 124.

Mourad, S., and Friedman, L., 1968, Passive immunization of mice against *Candida albicans, Sabouraudia* 6:103–105.

Musatti, C. C., Rezkallah, M. T., Mendes, E., and Mendes, N. F., 1976, *In vivo* and *in vitro* evaluation of cell-mediated immunity in patients with paracoccidioidomycosis, *Cell. Immunol.* 24:365–378.

Nathan, C. F., and Root, R. K., 1977, Hydrogen peroxide release from mouse peritoneal macrophages. *J. Exp. Med.* 146:1648–1662.

Neill, J. M., Castillo, C. G., Smith, R. H., Kapros, C. E., 1949, Capsular reactions and soluble antigens of *Torula histolytica* and *Sporotrichum schenckii, J. Exp. Med.* 89:93–106.

Newcomer, V. D., Landau, J. W., Dabrowa, N., and Fenster, M. L., 1968, Effects of human body fluids on *Candida albicans,* in: *Proceedings of the XIIIth International Congress of Dermatology, Munich, 1967,* pp. 813–817, Springer-Verlag, Berlin.

Nichols, B. A., Bainton, D. F., and Farquhar, M. G., 1971, Differentiation of monocytes, *J. Cell Biol.* 50: 498–515.

North, R. J., and Spitalny, G., 1974, Inflammatory lymphocyte in cell-mediated antibacterial immunity: Factors governing the accumulation of mediator T cells in peritoneal exudates, *Infect. Immun.* 10:489–498.

Olsson, I., and Venge, P., 1974, Cationic proteins of human granulocytes. II. Separation of the cationic proteins of the granules of leukemic myeloid cells, *Blood* 44:235–246.

Olsson, I., Olofsson, T., and Odeberg, H., 1975, Myeloperoxidase-mediated iodination in granulocytes, *Scand. J. Haematol.* 9:483–491.

Opelz, G., and Scheer, M. I., 1975, Cutaneous sensitivity and *in vitro* responsiveness of lymphocytes in patients with disseminated coccidioidomycosis, *J. Infect. Dis.* 132:250–255.

Otto, V., and Howard, D. H., 1976, Further studies on the intracellular behavior of *Torulopsis glabrata, Infect. Immun.* 14:433–438.

Pague, R. E., Kniskern, P. J., Dray, S., and Buram, P., 1969, *In vitro* studies with "transfer factor": Transfer of the cell-migration inhibition correlate of delayed hypersensitivity in humans with cell lysates from humans sensitized to histoplasmin, coccidioidin, or PPD, *J. Immunol.* 103:1014–1021.

Pantalone, R. M., and Page, R. C., 1975, Lymphokine-induced production and release of lysosomal enzymes by macrophages, *Proc. Natl. Acad. Sci. USA* 72: 2091–2094.

Patterson, R. J., and Youmans, G. P., 1970, Demonstration in tissue culture of lymphocyte-mediated immunity to tuberculosis, *Infect. Immun.* 1:600–603.

Patterson-Delafield, J., and Lehrer, R. I., 1979, Cationic proteins: Potential microbicidal mechanism for rabbit

alveolar macrophages, *Abstracts of the Annual Meeting of the American Society for Microbiology,* Los Angeles, p. 26.

Paul, B. B., Strauss, R. R., Jacobs, A. A., and Sbarra, A. J., 1970, Function of H_2O_2, myeloperoxidase and hexose monophosphate shunt in phagocytizing cells from different species, *Infect. Immun.* 1:338–344.

Paul, B. B., Strauss, R. R., Selvaraj, R. J., and Sbarra, A. J., 1973, Peroxidase mediated antimicrobial activities of alveolar macrophage granules, *Science* 181:849–850.

Pearsall, N. N., and Lagunoff, D., 1974, Immunological responses to *Candida albicans.* I. Mouse-thigh lesion as a model for experimental condidiasis, *Infect. Immun.* 9:999–1002.

Pearsall, N. N., and Weiser, R. S., 1970, *The Macrophage,* Lea and Febiger, Philadelphia, 204 pp.

Pearsall, N. N., Sundseno, J. S., and Weiser, R. S., 1973, Lymphokine toxicity for yeast cells, *J. Immunol.* 110:1444–1446.

Pesonti, E. L., 1978, Suramin effects on macrophage phagolysosome formation and antimicrobial activity, *Infect. Immun.* 20:503–511.

Peterson, E. M., and Calderone, R. A., 1977, Growth inhibition of *Candida albicans* by rabbit alveolar macrophages, *Infect. Immun.* 15:910–915.

Peterson, E. M., and Calderone, R. A., 1978, Inhibition of specific amino acid uptake in *Candida albicans* by lysosomal extracts from rabbit alveolar macrophages, *Infect. Immun.* 21:506–513.

Poulain, D., Vernes, A., and Biguet, J., 1978, Experimental study of cell-mediated immunity in dermatophytosis, *Mycopathologia* 63:81–88.

Rapaport, F. T., Lawrence, H. S., Millar, J. W., Pappagianis, D., and Smith, C. E., 1960, Transfer of delayed hypersensitivity to coccidioidin in man, *J. Immunol.* 84:358–367.

Reikvam, A., and Hoiby, E. A., 1975, Phagocytosis and microbicidal capacity of mouse macrophages nonspecifically activated *in vitro, Acta Pathol. Microbiol. Scand.* 83:121–128.

Reikvam, A., Grammeltvedt, R., and Hoiby, E. A., 1975, Activated mouse macrophages: Morphology, lysosomal biochemistry, and microbicidal properties of *in vivo* and *in vitro* activated cells, *Acta. Pathol. Microbiol. Scand.* 83:129–138.

Reiss, F., and Szilagyi, G., 1967, The effect of mammalian and avian sera on the growth of *Cryptococcus neoformans, J. Invest. Dermatol.* 48:264–265.

Reiss, F., Szilagyi, G., and Mayer, F., 1975, Immunological studies of the anticryptococcal factor of normal human serum, *Mycopathologia* 55:175–178.

Remington, J. S., and Merigan, T. C., 1970, Synthetic polyanions protect mice against intracellular bacterial infection, *Nature (London)* 226:361–363.

Resprepo-M., A., and Velez, A. H., 1975, Effectos de la fagocitosis *in vitro* sobre el *Paracoccidioides brasiliensis, Sabouraudia* 13:10–21.

Rifkind, D., Frey, J. A., Davis, J. R., Peterson, E. A.,

and Dinowitz, M., 1976, Delayed hypersensitivity to fungal antigens in mice. I. Use of the intradermal skin and footpad swelling test as assays of active and passive sensitization, *J. Infect. Dis.* **133**:50–56.

Rindler, R., and Braunsteiner, H., 1973, Soluble proteins from human leukocyte granules. I. Esterase activity of cationic proteins, *Blut* **27**:26–32.

Rippon, J. W., 1974, *Medical Mycology*, Saunders, Philadelphia, 587 pp.

Rocklin, R. E., Chilgren, R. A., Hong, R., and David, J. R., 1970, Transfer of cellular hypersensitivity in chronic mucocutaneous candidiasis monitored *in vivo* and *in vitro*, Cell. *Immunol.* **1**:290–299.

Rogers, T. J., and Balish, E., 1978, Effect of systemic candidasis on blastogenesis of lymphocytes from germfree and conventional rats, *Infect. Immun.* **20**:142–150.

Romeo, D., Cramer, R., Marzi, T., Spranzo, M. R., Zabucchi, G., and Rossi, F., 1973, Peroxidase activity of alveolar and peritoneal macrophages, *J. Reticuloendothel. Soc.* **13**:399–409.

Root, R. K., Metcalf, J., Oshino, N., and Chance, B., 1975, H_2O_2 release from human granulocytes during phagocytosis. I. Documentation, quantitation, and some regulating factors, *J. Clin. Invest.* **55**:945–955.

Rosen, H., and Klebanoff, S. J., 1979, Bactericidal activity of a superoxide anion-generating systems, *J. Exp. Med.* **149**:27–39.

Roth, F. J., Jr., and Goldstein, M. I., 1961, Inhibition of growth of pathogenic yeasts by human serum, *J. Invest. Dermatol.* **36**:383–387.

Roth, F. J., Jr., Boyd, C. C., Sagami, S., and Blank, H., 1959, An evaluation of the fungistatic activity of serum, *J. Invest. Dermatol.* **32**:549–555.

Salvin, S. B., 1954, Cultural and serologic studies on nonfatal histoplasmosis in mice, hamsters, and guinea pigs, *J. Infect. Dis.* **94**:22–29.

Salvin, S. B., 1960, Resistance of animals and man to histoplasmosis, in: *Histoplasmosis* (H. C. Sweany, ed.), pp. 99–112, Thomas, Springfield.

Salvin, S. B., 1963, Immunological aspects of the mycoses, *Progr. Allergy* **7**:213–328.

Salvin, S. B., 1972, Immunity in the systemic mycoses, in: *Immunogenicity* (F. Borek, ed.), pp. 225–259, North Holland Publishing Co., Amsterdam.

Sanchez, S., and Carbonell, L. M., 1975, Immunological studies on *Histoplasma capsulatum*, *Infect. Immun.* **11**:387–394.

Sawyer, R. T., Moon, R. J., and Beneke, E. S., 1976, Hepatic clearance of *Candida albicans* in rats, *Infect. Immun.* **14**:1348–1355.

Sbarra, A. J., Paul, B. B., Jacobs, A. A., Strauss, R. R., and Mitchell, G. W., Jr., 1972, Role of the phagocyte in host-parasite interactions. XXXVIII. Metabolic activities of the phagocyte as related to antimicrobial action, *J. Reticuloendothel. Soc.* **12**:109–126.

Schmid, L., and Brune, K., 1974, Assessment of phagocytic and antimicrobial activity of human granulocytes, *Infect. Immun.* **10**:1120–1126.

Schuit, K. E., 1979, Phagocytosis and intracellular killing of pathogenic yeasts by human monocytes and neutrophils, *Infect. Immun.* **24**:932–938.

Selvaraj, R. J., Paul, B. B., Strauss, R. R., Jacobs, A. A., and Sbarra, A. J., 1974, Oxidative peptide cleavage and decarboxylation by the MPO-H_2O_2 · Cl antimicrobial system, *Infect. Immun.* **9**:255–260.

Shands, J. W., Peavy, D. L., Gormus, B. J., and McGraw, J., 1974, *In vitro* and *in vivo* effects of endotoxin on mouse peritoneal cells, *Infect. Immun.* **9**:106–112.

Shimizu, M., Egashira, T., and Takahama, V., 1979, Inactivation of *Neurospora crassa* conidia by singlet molecular oxygen generated by a photosensitized reaction, *J. Bacteriol.* **138**:293–296.

Shiraishi, A., and Arai, T., 1979, Antifungal activity of transferrin, *Sabouraudia* **17**:79–83.

Sixbey, J. W., Fields, B. T., Sun, C. N., Clark, R. A., and Nolan, C. M., 1979, Interactions between human granulocytes and *Blastomyces dermatitidis*, *Infect. Immun.* **23**:41–44.

Smith, J. M. B., 1976, *In vivo* development of spores of *Absidia ramosa*, *Sabouraudia* **14**:11–15.

Solotorovsky, M., and Soderberg, L. S. F., 1972, Host–parasite interactions with macrophages in culture, in: *Macrophages and Cellular Immunity* (A. I. Laskin and H. Lechevalier, eds.), pp. 77–123, CRC Press, Cleveland.

Sorrell, T. C., Lehrer, R. I., and Cline, M. J., 1978, Mechanism of nonspecific macrophage-mediated cytotoxicity: Evidence for lack of dependence upon oxygen, *J. Immunol.* **120**:347–352.

Spencer, H. D., and Cozad, G. C., 1973, Role of delayed hypersensitivity in blastomycosis in mice, *Infect. Immun.* **7**:329–334.

Spitznagel, J. K., 1977, Bactericidal mechanisms of the granulocyte, in: *The Granulocyte: Function and Clinical Utilization*, pp. 103–131, Alan R Liss, New York.

Stanley, V. C., and Hurley, R., 1969, The growth of *Candida albicans* in mouse peritoneal macrophages, *J. Pathol.* **97**:357–366.

Steele, R. W., Cannady, P. B., Jr., Moore, W. L., Jr., and Gentry, L. O., 1976, Skin test and blastogenic responses to *Sporotrichum schenkii*, *J. Clin. Invest.* **57**:156–160.

Summers, D. F., and Hasenclever, H. F., 1964, *In vitro* inhibition of yeast growth by mouse ascites fluid and serum, *J. Bacteriol.* **87**:1–7.

Swanson, F. J., and Kozel, T. R., 1978, Phagocytosis of *Cryptococcus neoformans* by normal and thioglycolate-activated macrophages, *Infect. Immun.* **21**:714–720.

Tacker, J. R., and Bulmer, G. S., 1972, Pathogenesis of cryptococcosis: Initial events involving the lungs, in: *Abstracts of the Annual Meeting of the American Society for Microbiology*, p. 133.

Tacker, J. R., Farhi, F., and Bulmer, G. S., 1972, Intracellular fate of *Cryptococcus neoformans*, *Infect. Immun.* **6**:162–167.

Taschdjian, C. L., Toni, E. F., Hsu, K. C., Seelig, M. S.,

Cuesta, M. B., and Kozinn, P. J., 1971, Immunofluorescent studies on *Candida* in human reticuloendothelial phagocytes, *Am. J. Clin. Pathol.* **56:**50–58.

Tewari, R. P., Sharma, D., Solotorovsky, M., Lafemina, R., and Balint, J., 1977, Adoptive transfer of immunity from mice immunized with ribosomes or live yeast cells of *Histoplasma capsulatum, Infect. Immun.* **15:**789–795.

Thalinger, K. K., and Mandell, G. L., 1972, Failure of poly(I-C) to enhance killing of *Escherichia coli* by mouse peritoneal macrophages, *J. Reticuloendothel. Soc.* **12:**343–346.

Thong, Y. H., Ness, D., and Ferrante, A., 1979, Effect of bilirubin on the fungicidal capacity of human neutrophils, *Sabouraudia* **17:**125–129.

Thor, D. E., and Dray, S., 1968, A correlate of human delayed hypersensitivity: Specific inhibition of capillary tube migration of sensitized human lymph node cells by tuberculin and histoplasmin, *J. Immunol.* **101:**51–61.

Van Furth, R., and Cohn, Z. A., 1968, The origin and kinetics of mononuclear phagocytes, *J. Exp. Med.* **128:**415–435.

Van Furth, R., Hirsch, J. G., and Fedorko, M. E., 1970, Morphology and peroxidase cytochemistry of mouse promonocytes, monocytes, and macrophages, *J. Exp. Med.* **132:**794–812.

Van Zwet, T. L., Thompson, J., and Van Furth, R., 1975, Effects of glucocorticosteroids on the phagocytosis and intracellular killing by peritoneal macrophages, *Infect. Immun.* **12:**699–705.

Venge, P., and Olsson, I., 1975, Cationic proteins of human granulocytes. VI. Effects on the complement system and mediation of chemotactic activity, *J. Immunol.* **115:**1505–1508.

Venkataraman, M., Mohapatra, L. N., and Bhoyan, U. N., 1973, Phagocytosis of *Candida albicans* by rabbit neutrophils, *Sabouraudia* **9:**183–191.

Wegner, D. W., Reed, R. E., Trantman, R. J., Beavers, C. D., 1972, Some evidence for the development of a phagocytic response by polymorphonuclear leukocytes recovered from the venous blood of dogs inoculated with *Coccidioides immitis* or vaccinated with an irradiated spherule vaccine, *Am. Rev. Resp. Dis.* **105:**845–849.

Weinberg, E. D., 1974, Iron and susceptibility to infectious diseases, *Science* **184:**952–956.

Weinstein, M. M., Waitz, J. A., and Came, P. E., 1970, Induction of resistance to bacterial infections of mice with poly I · poly C, *Nature (London)* **226:**170.

White, L. O., 1977, Germination of *Aspergillus fumigatus* conidia in the lungs of normal and cortisone-treated mice, *Sabouraudia* **15:**37–41 [author describes work on germination of spores within murine peritoneal macrophages in the Discussion section of this paper].

Williams, D. M., Graybill, J. R., and Drutz, D. R., 1978, *Histoplasma capsulatum* infection in nude mice, *Infect. Immun.* **21:**973–977.

Wilson, J. W., 1957, *Clinical and Immunologic Aspects of Fungous Diseases,* Thomas, Springfield, 280.

Worthington, M., and Hasenclever, H. F., 1972, Effect of an interferon stimulator, polyinosinic: polycytidylic acid, on experimental fungus infection, *Infect. Immun.* **5:**199–202.

Wu, W. G., and Marcus, S., 1964, Humoral factors and cellular resistance. II. The role of complement and properdin in phagocytosis and cytopepsis by normal and "immune" macrophages, *J. Immunol.* **92:**397–403.

Youmans, G. P., 1971, The role of lymphocytes and other factors in antimicrobial cellular immunity, *J. Reticuloendothel. Soc.* **10:**100–119.

Zeya, H. I., and Spitznagel, J. K., 1966, Cationic proteins of polymorphonuclear leukocyte lysosomes. II. Composition, properties, and mechanism of antibacterial action, *J. Bacteriol.* **91:**755–762.

Zweiman, B., Pappagianis, D., Maisbach, H., and Hildreth, E. A., 1969, Coccidioidin delayed hypersensitivity: Skin test and *in vitro* lymphocyte reactivities, *J. Immunol.* **102:**1284–1289.

20

Immunology of Surface Fungi
Dermatophytes

SARAH F. GRAPPEL

1. Introduction

The majority of cutaneous fungus infections in man are caused by a group of filamentous fungi known as dermatophytes. These fungi, species belonging to the genera *Epidermophyton, Microsporum,* and *Trichophyton,* usually infect only the nonliving superficial keratinized layers of skin, hair, and nails. Although they have occasionally been isolated from the bloodstream, they rarely have been reported to cause systemic disease.

Other species of fungi which may cause infections limited to the keratinized layers of the epidermis and its appendages (dermatomycoses) include *Pityrosporum orbiculare,* tinea versicolor, and *Cladosporium werneckii,* tinea nigra. These fungi do not usually induce significant tissue responses in the host, and very little is known about immunity in these infections. *Candida* is discussed in Chapter 22.

Detailed descriptions of all these species, including the dermatophytes and the infections which they produce, can be found in textbooks on medical mycology, including those by Rippon (1974), Conant *et al.* (1971), Emmons *et al.* (1970), and Hildick-Smith *et al.* (1964).

The only significant information available on immune mechanisms in the restricted sur-face infections caused by filamentous fungi comes from investigations on dermatophytosis. This chapter will therefore be limited to the dermatophytes.

Reviews which have covered immunological aspects of dermatophytes and dermatophytosis include those by Bloch (1928), Götz (1962), Sulzberger, (1940), Huppert (1962), Lepper (1969), and Grappel *et al.* (1974). Grappel *et al.* (1974) reviewed both the early and recent literature which illustrates the variety of immune phenomena that occur in dermatophytosis. The chemical and antigenic composition of the dermatophyte group was discussed in detail.

This chapter will deal primarily with our present understanding of the disease process in dermatophytosis. Selected references which contribute to our knowledge of the factors involved in the pathogenicity of the dermatophyte and the host's defense mechanisms will be included.

2. Evolutionary Aspects

2.1. Dermatophytes

Beginning with Sabouraud's (1910) classic description of the dermatophyte group, several reviews have been written on these fungi and their apparent evolutionary progression from soil saprophytes to true parasites of man. The older reviews include those by Tate

SARAH F. GRAPPEL • Skin and Cancer Hospital, Temple University Health Sciences Center, Philadelphia, Pennsylvania 19140. *Present address:* Smith Kline & French Laboratories, Philadelphia, Pennsylvania 19101.

(1929a,b) and Gregory (1935) and more recently Vanbreuseghem (1961), Grin and Ozegovic (1963), Hildick-Smith *et al.* (1964), Balabanoff (1965), Ajello (1974), and Rippon (1974).

The relationship of the asexual dermatophytes, members of the fungi imperfecti or deuteromycetes, to the soil-inhabiting keratinophilic ascomycetes, the gymnoascaceae, was established by the works of Stockdale (1961) and Dawson and Gentles (1961). These investigators demonstrated the existence of perfect or sexual ascogenous forms of several of the geophilic species. The dermatophytes are now represented in the gymnoascaceae by two genera, *Anthroderma* and *Nannizzia*.

Further evidence of their relationship to the soil ascomycetes is their production of penicillinlike antibiotics (Peck and Hewitt, 1945; Uri *et al.*, 1963) and their production of aflatoxinlike compounds (Kaliciński *et al.*, 1975).

Dermatophyte species may be grouped according to their source as geophilic (soil), zoophilic (animal), or anthropophilic (man). The geophilic species are most closely related to the soil ascomycetes. They exist as saprophytes in the soil and can be induced to form the perfect stage most readily. Only a few of the geophilic dermatophytes have been shown to be pathogenic for man or animals. They are contracted directly from the soil and cause mainly transient infections.

The zoophilic species are only occasionally found in soil, usually only in association with keratinaceous animal debris. Perfect stages have been reported for only a few of the zoophilic species. Man is usually infected by zoophilic dermatophytes by direct contact with the infected animal host. Infections due to these species are usually highly inflammatory and circumscribed and may heal spontaneously.

The adaptation of the dermatophytes to their host is demonstrated to the highest degree among the anthropophilic species. These dermatophytes are not found in nature but live only on man and are transmitted from man to man. Perfect stages have not been induced in any of the anthropophilic dermatophytes. These species rarely cause infection in animals.

Grin and Ozegovic (1963) showed that none of the anthropophilic species studied and only *Trichophyton mentagrophytes,* of the zoo-

philic species investigated could survive in the presence of the microflora of the soil. However, the geophilic species *Microsporum gypseum* was not inhibited by the soil microflora. Their study made it apparent that the parasitic dermatophytes do not survive well in nature and are highly dependent on their hosts.

Dermatophytes are aerobic organisms. They are sensitive to both extreme CO_2 and O_2 tension. They are not fastidious in their nutritional requirements for growth on artificial media. They do not require keratinaceous substrates and grow at a broad range of both pH, their optima being somewhat below 7.0, and temperature, their optima being between 25°C and 35°C (Stockdale, 1953).

Although *in vivo* they require a moist environment, their growth is usually restricted to keratinaceous structures, where they may enjoy an advantage over the resident microflora due to their production of keratinolytic enzymes, their preference for lower temperatures, and their production of alkalinity.

2.2. Hosts

Dermatophyte infections have been reported only in the warm-blooded classes of the higher vertebrates, the Mammalia and Aves. Both of these classes produce both hard and soft keratins. Keratin production is the major role of the epidermis in these species, specialized appendages such as hair or feathers being important in the regulation of body temperature as well as protection.

The evolution of keratins has been reviewed by Fraser *et al.* (1972). The fact that dermatophyte infections are not reported in lower vertebrates may be due in part to the relative absence of keratin, in particular hard keratin. In addition, their lower body temperature may play a role in the failure of these fungi to establish a harmonious host–parasite relationship. For example, although the Repitlia have scale keratin resembling that of the feather keratin of birds, dermatophyte infections are not reported in this class. In establishing a harmonious relationship with their host, the inhibition of dermatophytes at temperatures of 37°C and above may be important (Lorincz and Sun, 1963). In warm-blooded hosts, they fail to cause systemic infection and do not kill their host. They survive in areas lacking blood vessels where they are protected from host defenses.

All of the susceptible higher vertebrates have fully developed immune systems. However, those parasitic dermatophytes which live in the horny layers of skin may develop a chronic infection devoid of a significant cellular immune response.

3. Biochemical and Immunochemical Aspects of Dermatophytes

3.1. Factors Contributing to Pathogenesis and Invasiveness

The dermatophytes are universally accepted as primary pathogens of previously healthy skin, nails, and hair (English, 1976). The ability of these fungi to establish themselves in the fully keratinized, nonviable portions of epidermis or its appendages is believed to be mainly due to proteolytic enzymes which allow them to penetrate and grow in keratinized tissue. However, although many workers have shown that dermatophytes can digest keratin *in vitro* (Chattaway *et al.,* 1963; Schönborn, 1967; Yu *et al.,* 1968, 1969a, 1971; Weary and Canby, 1969; Page and Stock, 1974), the role of keratinolysis in their penetration of skin, hair, and nails *in vivo* is still not clear-cut.

Raubitschek (1961) suggested that, in the host, dermatophytes digest intercellular cement and not keratin. He proposed that the subsequent mechanical breaking apart of keratinized cells results in the clinical signs of scaling and breakage of hairs seen in ringworm. However, studies with the scanning electron microscope (Tosti *et al.,* 1970) have provided evidence that dermatophytes may initially work their way into hair by dissolving nonkeratinous material, thus disassembling the hair framework. In advanced stages of invasion, keratin fibrils disintegrate and may even disappear, leaving ghost hairs. These investigators concluded that such complete destruction of keratin cannot be purely mechanical but must be due to the organism's keratinolytic activity. In addition, light microscopic studies of tinea unguium show tunnels in the nail which could only result from digestion of keratin (Sowinski, 1971).

Using fluorescent antibody tests, Collins *et*

al. (1973) demonstrated the production of a keratinase from *T. mentagrophytes* var. *granulosum* in lesions produced in guinea pigs. Incorporation of griseofulvin into keratinaceous substrates interfers with the hydrolytic activity of this enzyme (Yu and Blank, 1973).

The species of dermatophytes differ in their parasitic patterns. This is especially apparent in the different patterns of hair invasion, although invasion of smooth skin and nail may also differ. The differences in their invasion, as well as in their host specificities, have been attributed to the specificity of the proteolytic enzymes or keratinases produced (Yu *et al.,* 1972b).

Although the growth of the fungus is confined to the stratum corneum in dermatophytic infections of the skin, the pathological changes produced occur chiefly in the deeper layers of the epidermis and dermis. Graham (1972) described the histopathological changes which occur in dermatophytosis in detail.

Enzymes as well as antigens, mainly soluble glycopeptides, released by the dermatophyte may be responsible for the marked inflammation which may occur in the disease process. Zoophilic dermatophytes are the main cause of highly inflammatory infections in man, often causing kerion celsi. Such inflammatory reactions are usually associated with eventual regression of the infection. The anthropophilic species cause kerion celsi less often. In general, a less inflammatory, more chronic-type infection occurs which may become more widespread.

Minocha *et al.* (1972) correlated the proteolytic activity of dermatophytes with the clinical characteristics of the lesions produced. A direct relationship was found between the proteolytic activity of zoophilic strains of *T. mentagrophytes* and inflammation. Proteolytic activity was lower in the extracts of the anthropophilic *T. rubrum* strains and lowest in extracts of isolates from patients with extensive noninflammatory cutaneous lesions. Rippon (1967, 1975) found a similar correlation with the elastase activity of cultures isolated. Anthropophilic strains were usually elastase negative.

Antigenic components of these fungi may also induce secondary allergic eruptions, known as dermatophytids, which also contribute to the pathological changes associated with dermatophytosis. Evidence available indicates that the antigens responsible for these reactions are probably polysaccharide or glycopeptide in nature (Bloch, 1928; Henrici, 1939).

The pathogenicity of the anthropophilic species in man is increased by their ability to induce a specific anergy, i.e., suppress the cell-mediated immune response of the host. The evidence for suppression of the immune response by several other microorganisms has recently been reviewed by Schwab (1975).

3.2. Factors Contributing to Induction of Inflammation

The first studies on cutaneous hypersensitivity in dermatophytosis were carried out by Plato in 1902 (Neisser, 1902). The antigen that he prepared was a crude extract of mycelia of *Trichophyton* species which he called "trichophytin." Bloch and Massini (1909) were the first to show that the inflammatory response and clearing of the infection by dermatophytes corresponded to the development of delayed-type cutaneous hypersensitivity to "trichophytin" both in experimental animals and in man.

Bloch *et al.* (1925) first identified the active component of "trichophytin" as a nitrogen-containing polysaccharide. Although numerous investigators later attempted to isolate such antigens, most of their preparations were crude fractions which elicited "trichophytin" reactions in sensitized animals. These preparations included nitrogen-containing crude polysaccharides (Barker and Trotter, 1960), proteins (Meyer *et al.*, 1952), lipids (Sampei, 1950), and ribonucleic acids (Y. Ito, 1965a,b).

The antigenic components which have been purified and studied have been glycopeptides (= peptidopolysaccharides), polysaccharides, and keratinases. The first highly purified glycopeptides studied were isolated from *T. mentagrophytes* by Barker *et al.* (1962, 1963, 1967). These were galactomannan peptides prepared from ethylene glycol extracts of mycelia by fractional precipitation with cetyltrimethyl-ammonium bromide and subsequent chromatographic separation on DEAE-Sephadex A-50. Similar glycopeptides were later isolated from *T. rubrum* and *M. canis* by these investigators (Basarab *et al.*, 1968).

These glycopeptides elicited both immedi-

ate and delayed-type cutaneous hypersensitivity reactions in guinea pigs sensitized both by infection and by immunization with crude ethylene glycol extracts. Degradation of the carbohydrate portion of the glycopeptides diminished the immediate-type reaction, while degradation of the peptide portion by proteolytic enzymes diminished the delayed reaction (Barker *et al.*, 1962, 1967; Basarab *et al.*, 1968). Based on cutaneous hypersensitivity reactions in guinea pigs sensitized by immunization, these investigators concluded that the glycopeptides were not species specific. Other microbial polysaccharides, with structural features similar to those of the glycopeptides, elicited immediate-type reactions in such sensitized guinea pigs.

The purified galactomannan peptides from *T. mentagrophytes* also elicited delayed cutaneous hypersensitivity reactions in patients with dermatophytosis (Wood and Cruickshank, 1962; Jones *et al.*, 1973a) and in volunteers experimentally infected with *T. mentagrophytes* (Jones *et al.*, 1974a). Ottaviano *et al.* (1974) showed that similar glycopeptides could be isolated from *T. mentagrophytes* grown on a synthetic medium. Their preparations elicited less nonspecific reactions both in sensitized guinea pigs and in human volunteers.

The inflammatory response and the clearing of the infection were related to the presence of delayed-type cutaneous hypersensitivity to the galactomannan peptide. Individuals in whom only immediate-type reactions or both immediate and delayed-type cutaneous reactions were elicited by the glycopeptide had more chronic infections (Wood and Cruickshank, 1962; Jones *et al.*, 1973a, 1974a,b,c).

Glycopeptides which were later purified by other procedures were also galactomannan peptides and also had "trichophytin" activity (Nozawa *et al.*, 1970, 1971; Arnold *et al.*, 1976).

Nozawa *et al.* (1970, 1971) separated their polysaccharide–peptide complexes from phenol–water extracts of defatted *T. mentagrophytes* mycelia by gel filtration and DEAE-cellulose chromatography. Their galactomannan peptides elicited both immediate and delayed-type cutaneous hypersensitivity reactions in patients with trichophytosis. Proteolytic digestion of the polysaccharide–peptide complexes decreased the delayed hypersensitivity reaction but did not affect the immediate hypersensitivity reaction elicited in the patients or the precipitation reaction with rabbit hyperimmune serum.

The peptidopolysaccharides prepared by Arnold *et al.* (1976) from trichloracetic acid extracts of *T. mentagrophytes* var. *granulosum* mycelia were easily separated by gel filtration and DEAE-cellulose chromatography. These galactomannan peptides elicited delayed-type hypersensitivity reactions both in patients with dermatophytosis and in guinea pigs experimentally infected with *T. mentagrophytes* var. *granulosum*. No circulating antibodies to these glycopeptides were detected in sera from the patients or the infected guinea pigs (Grappel *et al.*, unpublished).

Nitrogen-free neutral polysaccharides were first isolated by Bishop *et al.* (1962, 1965, 1966a,b) from five species of dermatophytes, *T. granulosum, T. interdigitale, M. quinckeanum, T. rubrum,* and *T. schoenleinii*. Three polysaccharides, two galactomannans, and a glucan were obtained from each species. Similar polysaccharides were later isolated from four additional species, *M. praecox, T. ferrugineum, T. sabouraudi,* and *T. tonsurans* (Grappel *et al.*, 1969).

The polysaccharides were shown to be antigenic and were compared serologically with antisera to the nine species of dermatophytes (Grappel *et al.*, 1967, 1968a,b, 1970). These N-free neutral polysaccharides did not elicit any cutaneous hypersensitivity reactions in guinea pigs sensitized by infection (Saferstein *et al.* 1968).

Patients were not tested for dermal reactivity; however, low titers of circulating antibodies to these polysaccharides, probably IgM, were detected in sera from patients with dermatophytosis by a sensitive charcoal agglutination test (Grappel *et al.*, 1971c, 1972).

A nitrogen-free pyruvated glucan, later purified from ethylene glycol extracts of *M. quinckeanum* by Fielder *et al.* (1972), did not elicit the delayed-type cutaneous hypersensitivity reaction associated with inflammation and clearing of the infection but did elicit immediate-type cutaneous hypersensitivity reactions in guinea pigs sensitized by infection with *M. Quinckeanum*. Glucans have also been purified from ethylene glycol extracts of

four species of dermatophytes, *T. mentagrophytes, T. rubrum, M. canis,* and *T. schoenleinii,* by How *et al.* (1972, 1973). Their glucan from *T. rubrum* contained 0.1% nitrogen and differed in structure from the glucans of the other three species as well as the glucans isolated by other investigators. Immunization with the *T. rubrum* glucan induced immediate but not delayed-type hypersensitivity in guinea pigs. No studies were carried out on the dermal reactivity of infected guinea pigs or patients.

Induction of humoral antibodies, especially IgE, in man by polysaccharides of the dermatophyte may be one way in which the fungus counteracts the cellular immune responses of the host. Circulating antibodies are usually found in patients with chronic dermatophytosis. Experimental infection in man with both *T. rubrum* and *T. mentagrophytes* showed that delayed-type cutaneous reactivity disappeared following the appearance of the immediate-type cutaneous reaction due to IgE (K. Ito, 1963; Jones *et al.*, 1974b). Increased levels of IgE have been associated with the inhibition of leukocyte chemotaxis and chronicity in cutaneous infections due to other microorganisms (Hill and Quie, 1975). In addition, stimulation of B cells by the polysaccharides may maintain a suppressor B-cell population which suppresses potentially reactive T-cell clones. This mechanism of suppression was suggested by Turk (1976) in explaining the anergy which develops in patients with lepromatous leprosy. Walters *et al.* (1976) found evidence of serum blocking factors, probably antigen–antibody complexes, which interfered with effector lymphocytes in patients with chronic infections.

In addition to the purified glycopeptides, proteolytic enzymes involved in invasiveness of the dermatophytes have been shown to contribute to the induction of inflammation and clearing mechanisms of the host.

Elastase activity has been reported in species which produce the more imflammatory infections both in experimental animals (Rippon and Varadi, 1968) and in man (Rippon, 1967; H. Blank *et al.*, 1969). The more severe the inflammatory response, the less persistent was the infection in guinea pigs (Rippon and Garber, 1969). These investigators speculated on the role of antibodies to the enzymes in the clearing of the infection. Although elastase activity was demonstrated in infected tissues, the elastases were not isolated nor were immune responses demonstrated.

Keratinolytic enzymes (keratinases I and II) isolated from *T. mentagrophytes* var. *granulosum* by Yu *et al.* (1968, 1969b, 1971) also had elastase activity and were shown to be immunogenic. Keratinase I was an extracellular protein with a molecular weight of 48,000, and keratinase II was a mycelial glycoprotein with a molecular weight of 440,000. Both of these enzymes were shown to elicit delayed-type cutaneous hypersensitivity reactions in guinea pigs sensitized by infection with *T. mentagrophytes* var. *granulosum,* as well as in patients with dermatophytosis (Grappel and Blank, 1972; Grappel *et al.*, unpublished). The cell-mediated nature of the cutaneous reactions to the keratinases was confirmed *in vitro,* using macrophage migration inhibition tests (Eleuterio *et al.*, 1973).

Complement-fixing antibodies to keratinase II, detectable in sera of approximately 50% of infected guinea pigs, did not usually persist in the circulation (Grappel, 1976). However, local antibody reactions to keratinase II were demonstrated in biopsy sections of guinea pig skin previously infected with *T. mentagrophytes* (Collins *et al.*, 1973). Such antibodies may play a role in the local immunity associated with recovery from infection. Austwick (1972) speculated that such antibodies diffusing into the hair could be responsible for the degenerative changes observed in the intrapilary hyphae in healing ringworm infections. Zaslow and Derbes (1969) also detected γ-globulins in sections of deep inflammatory tinea capitis lesions, kerion celsi.

Antibodies prepared by immunization of rabbits with active keratinases cause a retardation in growth and an alteration in the structure of *T. mentagrophytes* var. *granulosum* in culture (Grappel *et al.*, 1971a). This species has been widely used for studies on "protective antigens" because of the relative resistance which follows infection in man.

3.3. Antigens Which Stimulate Immunity

The cell-mediated hypersensitivity which develops during infection, and is associated with inflammation and clearing of the infec-

tion, persists and is associated with a relative resistance to reinfection. The same antigens which induce inflammation therefore may also stimulate a generalized cell-mediated immunity to reinfection, as well as a local immunity, possibly mediated by antibody. Jones *et al.* (1974a,b,c) could predict susceptibility to infection in human volunteers by their dermal reactivity to a galactomannan peptide.

The ability of both immunogenic enzymes and glycopeptides to induce cell-mediated hypersensitivity in guinea pigs (Grappel and Blank, 1972; Basarab *et al.*, 1968), and to elicit such reactions both in guinea pigs sensitized by infection (Cruickshank *et al.*, 1960; Grappel and Blank, 1972; Grappel, unpublished) and in patients with dermatophytosis (Grappel, unpublished; Jones *et al.*, 1973a), suggested that both of these types of antigens may be capable of inducing a generalized immunity to infection.

Experiments in guinea pigs have shown that prior immunization with active keratinases does not consistently alter the course of an infection with *T. mentagrophytes* var. *granulosum* at sites distant from the site of immunization (Grappel, unpublished). However, prior immunization of guinea pigs with peptidopolysaccharides prepared by Arnold *et al.* (1976) did decrease both the extent and duration of *T. mentagrophytes* var. *granulosum* infections at sites distant from the site of immunization (Grappel, unpublished).

3.4. Genetic Features Associated with Virulence

Heterothallism (sexual reproduction by two different thalli) in the dermatophytes was first proven by Stockdale in 1961. Weitzman (1964) showed that the mating system was based upon one locus with a single pair of alleles, designated as $A(+)$ and $a(-)$. The same basic system has been shown to occur among all of the dermatophytes studied and has allowed investigations of the genetic basis of virulence and its relationship to factors such as protease activity (Kwon-Chung, 1974).

The genetic relationship between enzymes which help establish the dermatophyte in the host tissue and mating-type alleles was first studied by Rippon (1967) in *N. fulva,* the perfect form of *M. fulvum.* His results indicated that mating type and elastase activity were determined by two alleles and that the loci for these were closely linked. Weitzman *et al.* (1971) could find no such correlation between elastase activity and mating type in *N. fulva.*

Later studies by Rippon and Garber (1969) showed that elastase production might also be related to mating type in *A. benhamiae,* the perfect form of *T. mentagrophytes.* The type of lesion (severe inflammatory or noninflammatory) produced in the guinea pig was related to the production of the enzyme, the activity of which was actually demonstrated in the infected tissue. The severe inflammatory lesion was produced by the *a*(−) strain, which was elastase positive, while the less inflammatory, more chronic infections were produced by the *A*(+), elastase-negative strain. A survey of cultures of *T. mentagrophytes* var. *granulosum* obtained from infected U.S. soldiers in Southeast Asia confirmed his earlier observation (Rippon, 1975). All of the cultures from severe inflammatory lesions were of the minus mating type (*a*) and produced elastase. None of the anthropophilic *T. rubrum* or E. floccosum strains isolated had elastase activity. They were all (−) strains based on mating reactions with *A. simii.*

Hejtmánek and Lenhart (1970) correlated virulence in the dermatophytes with morphology and growth rate. They found the mutation in two loci consistently led to loss of virulence. The loss of virulence was always associated with a decrease in growth rate.

3.5. Interaction of Dermatophytes with Normal Flora

There is no evidence to suggest that dermatophytes make the skin an unfavorable site for multiplication of any of its normal bacterial flora (Noble and Somerville, 1974). However, quantitative changes, including increased colonization by staphylococci and decreases in micrococci, have been reported (Bibel, and Lebrun, 1975). *Staphylococcus aureus* has also been reported in ringworm lesions, and this pathogen has been implicated in the instigation of symptoms (Marples and Bailey, 1957).

Many dermatophytes produce penicillinlike antibiotics which may provide a selective pressure for the normal cutaneous bacterial flora.

Several investigators have reported increased resistance to penicillin in the bacterial flora of infected subjects or experimental animals. Bibel and LeBrun (1975) found that penicillin-resistant microorganisms increased during the course of experimental infections with *T. mentagrophytes* but diminished when the infection cleared. These investigators suggested that ringworm lesions may be an important reservoir for penicillin-resistant strains of pathogenic or opportunistic *Staphylococcus* and *Micrococcus* species.

The resident *Pityrosporum* species, as well as the skin bacteria, influence the lipid content of the surface film, especially on the scalp (Noble and Somerville, 1974). Weary (1968) reported the elaboration of a substance by *P. ovale* which inhibited all of the dermatophyte species tested *in vitro.* It was characterized as chloroform soluble and nondialyzable. No attempts were made to determine its significance in dermatophytosis.

4. Dermatophyte–Host Interactions

4.1. Natural Infections

The dermatophytes have been described by some investigators as scarcely more than saprophytes, living and growing in dead tissue. However, neither the restricted morphology of their parasitic state *in vivo* nor their parasitic patterns of invasion of keratinaceous tissue *in vivo* is reproduced by the dermatophytes *in vitro.*

Although the infection begins in the horny layer of the skin in most types of dermatophytosis, the ultimate disease picture depends on the host and the anatomical site of infection, as well as on the species of dermatophyte.

Man is the primary and almost the exclusive host of the anthropophilic species of dermatophytes. Different species may be associated with different geographic locations, as well as different anatomical sites on the body. These infections may become epidemic both by direct contact of individuals and by contact with contaminated fomites. The lesions tend to be very superficial, with minimal inflammation, and the fungus is usually easily demonstrated. Delayed cutaneous hypersensitivity reactions to "trichophytin" are often negative, and there is little or no tendency for the lesion to heal spontaneously. The exception is prepubertal tinea capitis, which usually clears at puberty. With the possible exception of tinea capitis, most of these infections do not respond well to therapy.

Infections of the smooth skin are most often caused by *T. rubrum, T. mentagrophytes* var. *interdigitale* (= downy variety) and *E. floccosum,* the most common form of infection being tinea pedis (F. Blank *et al.,* 1974).

In the United States *T. rubrum* has become the most common agent of dermatophytosis in adults, including chronic tinea pedis, tinea corporis, tinea cruris, and tinea unguium (F. Blank and Mann, 1975). Infections with invasion of hair follicles are most common on the scalp and are usually caused by other species. Prepubertal tinea capitis is usually caused by *M. audouinii* or *T. tonsurans* var. *sulfureum* in this country. Abroad, *T. violaceum* is a common cause of tinea capitis and *T. schoenleinii* is the cause of chronic favis of both the scalp and smooth skin. Different patterns of hair invasion are seen with each of these species (Graham, 1972).

Infections of animals with the anthropophilic species have been only rarely reported. In general, these have been due to contact with infected humans. Chakraborty *et al.* (1954), Kushida and Watanabe (1975), and Kaplan and Georg (1957) reported on dogs infected with *T. rubrum* and *M. audouinii.* The lesions produced in animals by these species are usually deep and inflammatory and tend to heal spontaneously.

Man is also a frequent host for zoophilic species of dermatophytes (F. Blank, 1955). However, the zoophilic species are associated with specific animal species as their primary host (Dawson, 1968). In their primary hosts (e.g., *M. canis* in the cat, *T. mentagrophytes* var. *granulosum* in mice and rats), the characteristics of the diseases due to the zoophilic species are comparble to those of the diseases due to anthropophilic species in man. The infections are highly contagious among the animal species. The lesions tend to be very superficial, with little inflammation, and the fungus is easily demonstrated in the lesions. Delayed-type cutaneous reactions to "trichophytin" may be absent, and there is little tend-

ency for spontaneous healing. Such infections are relatively resistant to therapy.

Infections due to zoophilic species of dermatophytes have been described in many animal species including farm animals (cattle, horses, pigs, sheep, goats, fowl), domestic animals (dogs, cats), fur-bearing animals (chincillas, foxes, hares, mink, muskrats, nutria, squirrels), laboratory animals (mice, rats, guinea pigs, rabbits), and wild animals (hedgehogs, porcupines, primates, voles) (Dawson, 1968).

Infection of man with zoophilic species occurs frequently, but these infections have a strong tendency to clear spontaneously and are not usually highly contagious. The lesions tend to be highly inflammatory, even to the extent of tissue destruction. Microorganisms may be scarce in the lesions and difficult to demonstrate by direct examination in the later stages of infection. A strong delayed-type cutaneous hypersensitivity reaction to "trichophytin" usually develops, and these infections usually respond well to therapy.

The large-scale epidemics of severe, often debilitating inflammatory dermatophytosis, which occurred in the U.S. troops in Southeast Asia, were due to the zoophilic species, *T. mentagrophytes* var. *granulosum* (H. Blank *et al.,* 1969; Allen and Taplin, 1973).

In all forms of dermatophytosis in an immunocompetent host, only the keratinaceous nonliving tissue is usually colonized or invaded. However, although these dermatophytes do not normally invade living tissue *in vivo,* they may grow in close proximity to living cells. Growth in this situation is believed to account for their reduced morphology, i.e., the suppression of conidia formation characteristic of their *in vitro* growth. Some species are believed to be better adapted to parasitism than others. Such species are believed to have an improved ability to survive in close proximity to living cells. In toenails *T. interdigitale* (= *T. mentagrophytes* var. *interdigitale*) can colonize the hard surface keratin, causing leukonychia trichophytica, a strictly surface growth which results in white patches on the nail. In contrast, *T. rubrum* always grows in the inner layers of the nail areas where there is mainly soft keratin, in close proximity to living cells. *T. interdigitale* rarely spreads to other parts of the body, whereas *T. rubrum* spreads readily to all parts of the body (English, 1976).

Although the dermatophytes do not usually grow in living tissue, numerous isolations of these fungi from the blood and lymph nodes of patients with various forms of dermatophytosis have been recorded in the earlier literature. Gregory (1935) reviewed several of these cases which included patients with tinea capitis, favus, and tinea pedis due to several dermatophyte species. Sulzberger (1928) showed that following cutaneous inoculation of guinea pigs with *A. quinckeanum* (= *M.* or *T. quinckeanum*), the fungus could be cultured from blood for 2 days. Fungi were again released into the bloodstream at the height of the inflammatory process (12 days), which marked the beginning of healing of the lesion.

Reports of invasion of living tissue by the dermatophytes are rare and are often accompanied by some underlying disease. The most common form of deeper invasion below the stratum corneum is the invasion of the dermis as a result of the rupture of hair follicles in lesions known as Majocchi's granuloma. These infections are usually caused by *T. rubrum* and often occur on the lower legs. Wilson *et al.* (1954), who described such subcutaneous granulomatous infections of the leg, observed "bizarre" forms of the dermatophyte in lesions. Blank and Smith (1960) also found abnormal forms of the dermatophyte in a patient with such widespread granulomatous lesions due to *T. rubrum*. Elevated serum γ-globulins and decreased cell-mediated reactions have been reported in such cases. Precipitins are often found in sera of patients with infections due to *T. rubrum* (Grappel *et al.,* 1974). Such antibodies cause structural changes in dermatophytes *in vitro* (Grappel *et al.,* 1971a).

More extreme cases of invasiveness have also been recorded in the literature. A series of reports by Aravysky (1959, 1961, 1964) described patients with lesions in bone, with central nervous system involvement and with lesions in the brain. The dermatophyte was demonstrated in granulomatous foci. In each of these cases anthropophilic species were isolated. Unfortunately, no information on fungistatic serum factors, immunological competence, or possible underlying diseases was reported.

Sternberg *et al.* (1952) produced deep infections in three strains of mice by intraperitoneal injection of *T. rubrum*. A pathological process culminating in chronic granulomatous lesions in the omentum, liver, spleen, and muscles was observed. *T. rubrum* could be demonstrated in the granulomatous lesions and reisolated 25 days after inoculation. Its adaptation to the deep tissue environment was accompanied by some structural changes to unicellular forms. None of the mice had delayed-type dermal reactivity to "trichophytin."

4.2. Experimental Infections

Several laboratory and domestic animals have been used to study dermatophyte pathogenicity. However, because of its superficial nature, dermatophytosis has also been studied by experimental infections in man.

4.2.1. Animals

Bloch and co-workers used most of the common laboratory animals and a variety of dermatophyte species for studies on the pathology, hypersensitivity, and immunity associated with dermatophytosis (Bloch, 1928). However, *T. gypseum* (= *T. mentagrophytes* var. *granulosum*) and *A. quinckeanum* (= *M.* or *T. quinckeanum*) were used for most of the experimental infections in animals, the animal of choice being the guinea pig.

The course of infection in guinea pigs inoculated cutaneously with *T. gypseum* closely resembled dermatophytosis in man infected with this species. The course could be divided into four distinct phases: (1) incubation, 4–6 days; (2) spreading, 7–10 days; (3) climax, 12–15 days; and (4) clearing, from the 16th to about the 35th day, when the skin appears normal.

DeLamater and Benham (1938a) described the course of infection in guinea pigs, rabbits, and cats with several strains of dermatophytes. The course of infection varied somewhat with different species of dermatophytes. In general, the anthropophilic species tested were relatively nonpathogenic for animals. Silva *et al.* (1955) were able to produce lesions in guinea pigs with some strains of *T. rubrum*; the infections were short lived.

Most of the earlier procedures for production of experimental dermatophytosis in laboratory animals employed large inocula which were not quantitated prior to inoculation. Methods for producing infections in guinea pigs have recently been improved and standardized. Tagami *et al.* (1973) used a quantitated inoculum of *T. mentagrophytes* microconidia. Greenberg *et al.* (1976) further improved the method of infection in that the epidermis of the infection site was neither traumatized nor epilated.

If routes of inoculation other than the cutaneous were used, either no infections or only cutaneous lesions were produced in experimental animals. Saeves (1915) was the first to produce disseminated lesions on the skin by intracardiac inoculation of guinea pigs. The lesions resembled those produced by cutaneous inoculation. Later, Sulzberger (1929) showed that only skin lesions were produced, and only at traumatized areas, following intracardiac injection of guinea pigs with *A. quinckeanum* (= *M.* or *T. quinckeanum*). Although no foci of fungi or lesions were visible in any internal organs, the dermatophyte could be cultured from some internal organs up to 12 days following inoculation.

More recently, Lepper (1974) injected cows intradermally with viable units of *T. verrucosum*. Invasion of the keratinized portions of the skin did not occur. Instead, a marked cellular response resulted in the destruction of the fungal elements.

4.2.2. Man

In a review of the literature on experimental dermatophyte infections in man, Knight (1972) described the species which have been used to produce such infections, the types of inocula used, and the physical state of the skin necessary for the infection to take. Such infections have been produced on the skin of human subjects for many years, starting with the work of Bloch and Massini (1909).

T. mentagrophytes var. *granulosum* has been used most extensively for human infections. Infections with this zoophilic species are easy to obtain and reproducible, and they usually heal spontaneously within 60 days. Anthropophilic species, such as *T. rubrum,* have also been used by several investigators. However, infections by these species are more difficult to produce consistently and, when they are produced, the lesion may be chronic, lasting many months.

The site of infection is also important. Some areas, such as the groin and the feet are more difficult to clear, i.e., infections are more severe and of longer duration. In addition, some species do not seem to infect certain areas of the body. For example, Kligman (1952) could not infect the scalp of adults with *T. mentagrophytes.*

It was realized initially that simple application of the fungus to normal skin was not sufficient to produce infection. Superficial abrasion was noted to increase the chances of infection by keeping spores within the stratum corneum, where the humidity is higher. However, occlusion of the infection site to prevent water evaporation made abrasion of the surface unnecessary.

In most of the earlier studies, massive doses of spores or fungal elements were used in efforts to produce infections. The outbreak of *T. mentagrophytes* var. *granulosum* epidemics in U.S. troops in Southeast Asia aroused new interest in studies on the disease process in man. As a result, new procedures for standardization of inocula and improved methods of infection of volunteers with *T. mentagrophytes* var. *granulosum* were devised by Reinhardt *et al.* (1974). Using their improved methods, i.e., quantitated spore suspensions and occlusive bandages, these investigators were able to produce consistent infections on the forearms of volunteers using as few as six microaleurospores (Jones *et al.,* 1974a).

In general, experimental infections, both in man and in animals, tend to run a shorter course than naturally acquired infections with the same dermatophyte species. This may be due to the various inocula used, as well as to the different sites of infection. Greenberg *et al.* (1976) showed that infections initiated with larger numbers of spores resolved more quickly.

4.3. Infection in Susceptible Hosts

The increased severity of infection in immunosuppressed hosts suggests that immunological factors are involved in the control of dermatophytosis. More specifically, chronic dermatophytosis, or an increased susceptibility to infection, has usually been associated with a disturbance in cell-mediated immunity or T-cell reactivity, as manifested by the absence of delayed-type cutaneous hypersensitivity to "trichophytin." An enhancement of B-cell reactivity as manifested by type I immediate cutaneous hypersensitivity and circulating antibodies may also occur in patients with chronic infections.

The results of tests for dermal reactivity to a variety of antigens have indicated that cellular anergy in patients with chronic dermatophytosis is most often specific for the infecting organism (Hanifin *et al.*, 1974; Sorensen and Jones, 1976; Walters *et al.*, 1974). However, Sorensen and Jones (1976) showed that, in some patients, cell-mediated hypersensitivity reactions to other antigens may also be somewhat decreased. Two of 38 (5%) patients were anergic to all skin test antigens. In the majority of their patients the delayed-type cutaneous reaction was diminished and was usually preceded by an immediate-type reaction to "trichophytin."

Walters *et al.* (1974) demonstrated blocking factors in the sera of patients chronically infected. Such blocking factors did not affect lymphocyte reactivity to tuberculin (PPD). All of the patients, whether they had chronic or acute dermatophytosis, possessed cell-mediated hypersensitivity which could be measured *in vitro*. These investigators concluded that the continued release of antigens in chronic infection allows the formation of antigen–antibody complexes in serum which may interfere with the manifestation of cell-mediated immunity *in vivo*. Sera from patients with acute dermatophytosis were not tested for "unblocking factors."

An association of chronic dermatophytosis with elevated serum levels of IgE, as well as with other classes of circulating antibodies to dermatophytes, including IgM with affinity for epithelial tissue, has been noted by several investigators (Grappel *et al.*, 1972; Peck *et al.*, 1972; Hopfer *et al.*, 1975; Lobitz *et al.*, 1972). Lobitz *et al.* (1972) reported a chronic widespread *T. rubrum* infection in a patient with depressed cell-mediated immunity and with a lifelong history of atopic dermatitis. Increased susceptibility of individuals with hyperimmunoglobulinemia E, even those with normal *in vitro* T-lymphocyte responses, has been reported in cutaneous infections due to other microorganisms (Hill and Quie 1975; Buckley *et al.*, 1972). Hill and Quie (1975) suggested that IgE can inhibit neutrophil function by causing the release of histamine, which in turn is capable of inhibiting neutrophil chemotaxis. Dysproteinemia, consisting of elevated γ-globulin and decreased albumin levels, has also been reported in sera of patients with chronic *T. rubrum* infections and cutaneous anergy to "trichophytin" (Desai *et al.*, 1962).

Patients with chronic dermatophytosis do not usually develop severe infections with viruses, bacteria, or other fungi. Their defective cell-mediated immune response therefore does not appear to reflect a primary immunodeficiency (Fudenberg *et al.*, 1971; Bean and South, 1973). However, depressed T-cell reactivity to phytohemagglutinnin has also been reported in patients with chronic *T. rubrum* (Abraham *et al.*, 1975).

Suppressor T cells have been detected in patients who developed disseminated or widespread cutaneous infection due to several other fungi (Stobo *et al.*, 1976). T-cell reactivity, but not B-cell reactivity, was suppressed. Although the suppressor T-cells could have been generated in response to specific fungal antigens, these investigators suggested that soluble factors released might mediate suppression regardless of antigen specificity. The presence of suppressor T or B cells in dermatophytosis has not been investigated. A high antigen load might also maintain a population of suppressor B cells which could suppress responsive T-cell clones (Turk, 1976).

This theory would explain the absence of lymphocyte transformation *in vitro* in chronically infected patients. Suppressor cells would also explain the apparent specific anergy which may appear early in the course of infection, as well as the generalized depression of T-cell reactivity which is found in chronic, widespread infection.

Marmor and Barnett (1968) reported a case of widespread *E. flocossum* with extensive granuloma formation of the face and scalp in a 21-year-old woman. She demonstrated cutaneous anergy to common skin tests, as well as diminished skin homograft rejection. In addition, she could not be sensitized actively or passively by the transfer of lymphocytes. Although she had chronic superficial fungus infections, she showed no signs of systemic disease. All noncutaneous immunological parameters were normal. The tolerance to dermatophyte antigens was accompanied by tolerance to nonfungal antigens, possibly due to suppressors cells which depress T-cell reactivity. Chronic widespread *E. flocossum* infection, which was resistant to treatment, has also been reported in a patient who later developed a lymphoma (Levene, 1973).

5. Defense Mechanisms

Because of the prevalence of the dermatophytes, essentially all people are exposed to these fungi during their lives. Despite the fact that a large percentage of individuals develop clinical symptoms of disease, only a minority develop widespread or chronic infection.

5.1. Natural Factors

In man the principal problems of epidemiology and contagion have been concerned with the infections due to anthropophilic species.

The very high incidence of multiple infection among certain genetically related groups suggests that hereditary factors may be involved in the susceptibility of individuals to *T. rubrum* infections (Many *et al.*, 1960). *T. rubrum* and/or *E. floccosum* infections also occur in patients susceptible to cutaneous infections with other fungi, including *C. albicans* and *M. furfur* (Partridge, 1955). Hanifin *et al.* (1974) speculated that the "symbiosis" between the human host and *T. rubrum* could be due to host-determined genetic defects in recognition of dermatophyte antigens. Evidence for such defects has been found in lepromatous leprosy (Godal *et al.*, 1971). However, little is known about the genetic basis of resistance in human dermatophytosis, except for the familial predisposition to atopy. As already discussed, atopic individuals have a greater tendency to develop chronic, widespread infections (Jones *et al.*, 1973a, 1974b).

An association between the human leukocyte antigen types, specific IgE antibody responses, and some dermatological diseases has been reported (McDevitt, 1976). No attempts have been made to relate particular HLA types to susceptibility to chronic der-

matophytosis. However, studies in mice have led some investigators to conclude that the genotype of the host is of decisive importance for the development of dermatophytosis (Schmitt *et al.*, 1962; Hejtamanek and Lenhart, 1971). The necessity for active keratinization in order for dermatophytes to infect animals with skin cycles, such as occurs in mice, makes interpretation of these investigations difficult (Kligman, 1956).

Differences in the incidence of human infections with anthropophilic species have been noted according to age, ethnic origin, and sex (Blank, *et al.*, 1974; Blank and Mann, 1975). Rothman *et al.* (1947) explained the spontaneous cure of tinea capitis at puberty as being due to an increase in the fungistatic fatty acids in sebum of adults, an explanation not generally accepted. Kligman and Ginsberg (1950) observed no increase in the fungistatic activity of fatty acids in adult sebum, and Kligman (1952) also found that he could produce experimental tinea capitis in adults as well as in children.

In guinea pigs and cattle, both DeLamater (1942) and Lepper (1974) showed that age did not affect susceptibility to infection; however, young animals developed more prolonged or progressive infections, which were related to the development of a lower level of cell-mediated cutaneous hypersensitivity.

A lower rate of desquamation of skin may also increase susceptibility and lead to more chronic widespread infection in man (Rothman and Lorincz, 1963). Noble and Somerville (1974) reported that superficial fungus infections are less common in patients with psoriasis, presumably because of the increased turnover of skin cells.

In addition, environmental factors influence the incidence of dermatophytosis (Barlow *et al.*, 1961). As already mentioned, the establishment of dermatophytes in the stratum corneum is facilitated by high moisture as well as trauma. The incidence of tinea pedis (athletes foot) usually increases during the summer.

Chronic widespread infections have been shown to occur in hosts whose general resistance has been reduced. Underlying disease such as Cushing's syndrome, or adrenal hypercorticism (Canizares *et al.*, 1959; Nelson and McNiece, 1959; Pillsbury and Jacobson, 1955), malignant lymphoma (Levene, 1973;

Lewis *et al.*, 1953), rheumatoid arthritis (Blank and Smith, 1960), or diabetes (Mandel, 1960), as well as treatment with immunosuppressive agents (Canizares *et al.*, 1959; Lavalle, 1975; Burgoon *et al.*, 1974; Marks and Dawber, 1972; Goss *et al.*, 1963), has been associated with widespread intractable infections. Graham (1972) suggested that *T. rubrum* should also be considered as an opportunistic organism which takes advantage of a wide spectrum of systemic illnesses, in some instances masking the underlying disease that has altered the host–parasite relationship.

Both Lavalle (1975) and Marks and Dawber (1972) reported that even topical treatment with corticosteroids enhanced the growth of dermatophytes. In addition, such treatment may lead to lesions in the dermis (Lavalle, 1975). Burgoon *et al.* (1974) were the first to report a case of mycetoma due to a dermatophyte, *T. rubrum*. Their patient had received longterm systemic treatment with steroids. Goss *et al.* (1963) showed that widespread dermatophyte infections could also be produced in guinea pigs given very high levels of steroids.

The restriction of dermatophyte growth to the keratinized tissue is believed by some investigators to be due mainly to a fungistatic substance normally present in sera of man and animals (Hildick-Smith, 1964). This substance, referred to as "serum factor," has been offered as the principal mechanism preventing fungal elements which enter the bloodstream from multiplying there or in any of the internal organs. Both the existence and significance of this factor are highly controversial in light of the many conflicting reports.

The antidermatophytic activity of normal serum has been demonstrated both *in vitro* and *in vivo* by several investigators (Peck *et al.*, 1940; Lorincz *et al.*, 1958; Roth *et al.*, 1959; Barlow *et al.*, 1961; Goodman *et al.*, 1961; Carlisle *et al.*, 1974; King *et al.*, 1975). In addition, these investigators have shown that the "serum factor" is present at birth, does not change appreciably with age, and is present in sera of individuals regardless of whether they have any history of dermatophytosis, including those with relative acquired immunity and those with chronic infection (Roth *et al.*, 1959; Desai and Harvey, 1967; Carlisle *et al.*, 1974).

Although dermatophytes do not usually grow in the internal organs of the body, they can easily be cultured on these organs *in vitro* (W. Jadassohn, 1928). Blank *et al.* (1959) infected human skin in tissue culture in order to simulate infection. Hyphae readily invaded all layers of the skin when no serum was present, but growth of the dermatophyte was restricted to the keratinized layers when fresh serum was added to the culture medium.

Lorincz *et al.* (1958) and Goodman *et al.* (1961) showed that the growth of *T. mentagrophytes* and *M. gypseum* was inhibited in dialysis bags implanted in the peritoneal cavities of mice or dogs. The growth of these species resumed when cultured on media *in vitro*. Goodman *et al.* (1961) could not demonstrate inhibition of these species by hemodialysates *in vitro*. They suggested that *in vivo* the difference in temperature or the presence of a dialyzable substance released by cellular reactions may actually have been responsble for the fungistatic effect.

Rippon and Scherr (1959) did not observe inhibition of growth but found structural alterations in the anthropophilic species *M. audouinii* and *T. rubrum* when these species were grown in dialysis bags planted in the peritoneal cavities of rabbits. A change in morphology to a yeastlike growth, especially with *T. rubrum,* was accompanied by an increase in pathogenicity, resembling the yeast phase of some dimorphic fungi. They believed that the dialysis bag protected these species from the host's defenses.

Sternberg *et al.* (1952) produced deep tissue granulomatous infections with *T. rubrum* in mice which did not have cell-mediated immune responses to "trichophytin."

The "serum factor" has been characterized as an unstable, dialyzable, heat-labile component of fresh serum and tissue fluids (Lorincz *et al.*, 1958; H. Blank *et al.*, 1959; Goodman *et al.*, 1961). In addition, H. Blank *et al.* (1959) showed that neither γ-globulin, albumin, nor Cohn fraction II, III, or IV had any inhibitory activity in their tissue culture system.

Although some rare instances of deeper invasion by the dermatophytes in man have been reported in the literature, information on serum factors in most of those patients is not available. Blank and Smith (1960) measured the antidermatophytic activity of serum from their patient with widespread granulomatous dermal nodules and subcutaneous abscesses due to *T. rubrum*. They reported an abnormally low titer of "serum factor" in that patient.

King *et al.* (1975) showed that normal serum transferrin, which is unsaturated, inhibits the growth of dermatophytes. Removal of transferrin from serum resulted in the loss of antidermatophyte activity in their studies. Other investigators have implicated iron-binding transferrin in the inhibition of *Candida albicans* by normal serum (Caroline *et al.*, 1964; Esterly *et al.*, 1967). However, this nondialyzable, heat-stable (56°C) protein may be different from the "serum factor" described in earlier investigations.

Normal sera from man and animals, including guinea pigs and rabbits, inhibit the proteolytic enzymes (keratinases) isolated from *T. mentagrophytes* var. *granulosum*. The natural inhibitor has been isolated from human serum and identified as α_2 (Yu *et al.*, 1972a). It is present in sera of both man and experimental animals regardless of their history of dermatophytosis (Grappel and Blank, 1972; Grappel, 1976, and unpublished). A natural inhibitor of the proteolytic enzymes of the dermatophytes may play a role in inhibiting their growth in serum and thus restricting their growth to the nonliving keratinous tissue. Unfortunately, sera from patients with deep tissue invasion were not examined for the presence of a natural inhibitor of the enzymes, nor were any studies on inhibition of dermatophyte growth by α_2-macroglobulin carried out.

Body temperature may also be an important factor in the restriction of the growth of dermatophytes. Lorincz and Sun (1963) showed that the growth of several strains was inhibited at temperatures of 37°C, while temperatures of 39°C were lethal for most strains. In addition, infections could not be established on the tails of rats if the tails were kept at 41°C.

5.2. Acquired Immunity

Cutaneous infection with a dermatophyte may result in a relative acquired resistance to reinfection. In man resistance may vary depending on several factors, including the strain of dermatophyte, zoophilic vs. anthropophilic, and the anatomical site of infection, smooth skin, hair, or nails. As previously mentioned, human infections with zoophilic species usually result in highly inflammatory lesions. These usually heal spontaneously and are followed by a state of relative acquired immunity to reinfection. The infections caused by anthropophilic species are usually more chronic and less circumscribed, and they generally result in less resistance to reinfection.

The original experimental infections produced by Bloch, both in animals and in man, revealed that cutaneous inoculation with zoophilic species resulted in a generalized relative resistance to reinfection, which was not species specific (Bloch, 1908; Bloch and Massini, 1909). The infections in man, even with zoophilic species, were less circumscribed and more chronic than those produced in guinea pigs. However, they usually healed spontaneously within 3 months. Reinfection resulted in a highly accelerated, less severe course of disease in which no fungi were isolated.

Other investigators could demonstrate a strong local immunity, only at the previously infected site following experimental infections of the smooth skin with zoophilic species (Sutter, 1917; Greenbaum, 1924; Epstein and Grünmandel, 1930).

The most recent studies on acquired resistance in man following experimental infection of smooth skin with a zoophilic species (*T. mentagrophytes* infections on the forearm) revealed only a generalized relative immunity to reinfection (Jones *et al.*, 1974). Immunity was manifested in the second infection by the requirement of a larger inoculum to initiate infection and an accelerated course in which there were less severe inflammation and a decrease in peripheral spreading.

Several investigators have pointed out that such resistance does not always follow the more chronic infections in man, which are usually caused by anthropophilic species (Barlow and Chattaway, 1958; Rivalier, 1960). Desai *et al.* (1963) could not demonstrate acquired immunity to experimental infections of the smooth skin by *T. rubrum*. Silva *et al.* (1955) infected patients who already had lesions due to *T. rubrum* at sites not previously infected. The first experimental infections lasted 2–4 months. Reinfection of the patients, either at the sites of previous experimental infections or at distant sites, resulted in lesions indistinguishable from the first infections but which persisted almost twice as long. In each case, the fungus was cultured from the lesions, and there was no effect on the original "natural" infections which were still present.

Barlow and Chattaway (1958) pointed out that species which grow only in the horny layer of the skin, usually the sole of the foot, do not give rise to the local immunity that may follow infection by species which invade hair follicles causing acute inflammatory reactions.

Resistance to reinfection has been demonstrated in "natural" tinea capitis infections in children (Tschernogubow and Muskatblüt, 1929; Friedman and Derbes, 1960), as well as in experimental tinea capitis (Kligman, 1952).

Studies on acquired immunity in several species of animals have also been carried out since Bloch's (1908) original investigations. In contrast to Bloch's findings, most of the results of subsequent investigations on immunity in guinea pigs have indicated that immunity is complete or greatest only at the site of previous infection, while generalized immunity is of a lower grade (Sutter, 1917; Greenbaum, 1924; Kogoj, 1926; DeLamater and Benham, 1938b; Bonk *et al.,* 1962).

Kielstein (1968) and Lepper (1972) reported the development of a generalized resistance to reinfection in cattle following a primary experimental infection. Resistance persisted 1 year or more. Kligman (1956) found no evidence of acquired resistance or cutaneous sensitization in mice or rats.

5.2.1. Cellular Immunity

The appearance of the delayed-type cutaneous hypersensitivity to "trichophytin," a marker of cell-mediated immunity, is closely associated with recovery and the accelerated host response to reinfection both in man and animals.

The suppurative type of inflammatory response, of which kerion celsi is the extreme example, is usually correlated with spontaneous resolution of ringworm lesions and acquired resistance and is accompanied by delayed-type cutaneous hypersensitivity. The granulomatous type of inflammatory response, such as is often seen with *T. rubrum, T. schoenleinii,* and other species causing chronic widespread infections in man, is not associated with recovery or acquired resist-

ance and is often found in individuals who are without delayed-type cutaneous reactivity to "trichophytin." Bloch and Massini (1909) showed that experimental infection of both man and guinea pigs with zoophilic species induced delayed-type cutaneous reactivity to "trichophytin," which became apparent 7–10 days following cutaneous inoculation, corresponding to the height of infection. Other investigators showed that the level of cutaneous reactivity reached its maximum after the infection cleared. The hypersensitivity persisted up to 3 years and was not species specific (Sutter, 1917; DeLamater and Benham, 1938b; DeLamater, 1941).

In man, as well as in guinea pigs, repeated inoculation led to a state of relative anergy to "trichophytin" at the sites of previous infections. The inflammatory response to dermatophytes inoculated at such sites was markedly decreased (Sutter, 1917; DeLamater and Benham, 1938b).

The development of cutaneous hypersensitivity has also been reported in man following experimental infection with *T. rubrum* (K. Ito, 1963). The delayed-type cutaneous reactivity developed 14 days after inoculation but disappeared following the development of immediate-type reactivity 35 days after inoculation. Jones *et al.* (1974a) showed a similar development of delayed cutaneous hypersensitivity following inoculation of volunteers with quantitated inocula of *T. mentagrophytes* var. *granulosum*. Most subjects who were "immunological virgins" converted from negative to positive delayed hypersensitivity skin tests between 10 and 17 days, at which time the infected sites became intensely inflamed and pruritic and peripheral spreading of the infection ceased. Lesions reached a greater diameter in subjects who took longer to convert. The cell-mediated reaction in the dermis consisted of infiltrates of macrophages and lymphocytes.

Delayed-type cutaneous hypersensitivity also developed in atopic individuals who were experimentally infected with this species (Jones *et al.,* 1974b). However, one atopic individual out of the three infected also developed immediate-type hypersensitivity 32 days following infection, which was followed by a decrease in the inflammation of the lesions and a decrease in cell-mediated hypersensitivity.

The two subjects who developed only cell-mediated hypersensitivity cleared in the normal time. However, the infection in the subject who developed immediate-type reactivity became chronic and spread to the subject's feet. The ability of a previous immediate-type reaction, produced by passive sensitization to "trichophytin," to block the cell-mediated cutaneous reaction was also demonstrated in this study.

Jones *et al.* (1974a) speculated on the role of the cellular immune response in the clearing of infection. They found no evidence that the macrophages or lymphocytes in the dermis had any direct effect on the dermatophyte. Instead, they believed that the production of factors which mediate inflammation by macrophages and lymphocytes in the dermis results in damage to host tissue and impairment of the dermal–epidermal barrier. Impairment of the barrier would allow serum containing the fungistatic "serum factor" to percolate into the stratum corneum. The "static" dermatophyte could then be shed in the outward growth of the epidermis, which would also be increased by inflammation.

This theory would explain the halt in spreading of the infection at the time of the development of cell-mediated hypersensitivity, as well as the variable persistence of the organism in tissue.

Lepper (1972) also observed that the development of delayed-type hypersensitivity 14 days after inoculation with *T. verrucosum* was associated with the elimination of infection in cattle. Lepper (1974) also studied the cellular components of the inflammatory response to a primary cutaneous infection both in cattle and in guinea pigs, as well as to an intradermal injection of live mycelia in cattle. In the primary cutaneous infection a well-defined pattern of hypersensitivity responses to antigenic components of the dermatophytes was observed both in cattle and guinea pigs. The inflammatory response to cutaneous infection with *T. verrucosum* was more intense in the guinea pigs. Fully activated macrophages containing phosphatase-rich lysosomes were more numerous in infiltrates during the climax of the the inflammatory response in the guinea pig than in cattle cutaneously infected. Nonfollicular microabscess formation and breakdown occurred which probably resulted in large amounts of particulate antigen in the dermis. Intradermal inoculation of cattle with *T. verrucosum* resulted in a polymorphonuclear reaction similar to a foreign body reaction which caused necrosis and rupture of the epidermis and was accompanied by the death of the dermatophyte in the dermis.

Patients with chronic *T. rubrum* infections frequently have a negative delayed-type or a retarded delayed-type reaction to "trichophytin" (Lewis and Hopper, 1948; Hanifin *et al.*, 1974; Abraham *et al.*, 1975). The retarded delayed-type reaction has been found in patients with dermatophytid eruptions (Cruickshank, 1966; Wood and Cruickshank, 1962).

Jones *et al.* (1973a) found that, regardless of the infecting species, only 7% of patients with only delayed-type hypersensitivity had recurrent dermatophyte infections, while 75% of those with only immediate-type of both delayed- and immediate-type reactivity had recurrent dermatophyte infections.

Several investigators have used *in vitro* correlates of cell-mediated immunity in order to learn more about resistance to dermatophyte infections. Hanifin *et al.* (1974) demonstrated lymphocyte transformation with peripheral blood lymphocytes from patients infected with *T. mentagrophytes* who had delayed-type cutaneous hypersensitivity. Lymphocytes from patients with *T. rubrum* infections who had only immediate-type cutaneous reactivity were not transformed, regardless of whether the cells were incubated with *T. rubrum* or *T. mentagrophytes* antigens. The cellular anergy of their paients with *T. rubrum* appeared to be specific for "trichophytin," and no evidence of serum factors which could block lymphocyte transformation was found.

Other investigators (Svejgaard *et al.*, 1976) found no difference in *in vitro* lymphocyte transformation responses to dermatophyte antigens with cells from patients with acute or chronic *T. rubrum* infections. However, they did find a general depression of lymphocyte responses to mitogens and nondermatophyte antigens in a few patients with chronic infections due to *T. mentagrophytes*. Abraham *et al.* (1975) also found evidence of a general depression of T-lymphocyte reactivity in patients with *T. rubrum* who had no delayed-type cutaneous reactions to "trichophytin."

Using an *in vitro* leukocyte adherence inhibition test, devised originally for the detection of cell-mediated immunity to tumors, Walters *et al.* (1974) found that patients suffering from both acute and chronic dermatophyte infections had specific cell-mediated immunity against their infecting organism. However, sera from chronically infected patients specifically blocked the activity of their own leukocytes or those of other patients with the same infecting species. Their results are in conflict with those obtained by the *in vitro* tests used by Hanifin *et al.* (1974). However, these findings offer some explanation for the state of apparent specific cellular anergy and the chronicity of dermatophytosis in patients without central immunologic deficiencies.

Each of the *in vitro* studies described was performed with different types of antigen preparations. These differences, as well as the different test procedures used, probably contribute to some of the contradictory results.

5.2.2. Humoral Immunity

Immediate-type cutaneous hypersensitivity reactions to "trichophytin" and circulating antibodies have been found to be exceptionally prevalent in patients with chronic *T. rubrum* infections (Desai *et al.*, 1966; Sulzberger, 1940; Lewis *et al.*, 1958; Wood and Cruickshank, 1962; Grappel *et al.*, 1972; Hanifin *et al.*, 1974).

Desai *et al.* (1966) found immediate-type cutaneous hypersensitivity to "trichophytin" in 85% of patients infected with *T. rubrum*. Immediate-type reactions have been reported to occur more frequently in inviduals with recurrent infections, 40% of whom were shown to be atopic (Jones *et al.*, 1973a, 1974b,c), in atopic individuals (Marcussen, 1937;, Jones *et al.*, 1973a, 1974b,c), in individuals with recurrent erysipelaslike eruptions (Sulzberger *et al.*, 1937), and in individuals with recurrent lymphangitis (Jillson and Huppert, 1949). Such reactivity has also been reported in noninfected asthmatic children (Jones *et al.*, 1973b).

Jones *et al.* (1973a, 1974b,c) found a strong correlation between immediate-type hypersensitivity and chronic infection. Naturally infected individuals with immediate-type hypersensitivity could more readily be experimentally infected with *T. mentagrophytes* then those without this type of hypersensitivity reaction.

The delayed-type reaction to "trichophy-

tin" can be suppressed by repeated intradermal injections of "trichophytin." The repeated introduction of antigen induces an immediate-type reaction which appears at the time that the delayed-type reaction disappears (Sulzberger and Wise, 1932; Jillson and Huppert, 1949).

Sulzberger and Kerr (1930) showed that the immediate reaction to "trichophytin" could be transferred with serum. Later, Marcussen (1937) showed that passive sensitization and elicitation of an immediate-type reaction in individuals who had previously had only delayed-type reactivity could suppress or diminish the delayed-type dermal reactivity to "trichophytin." Jones *et al.* (1974b) confirmed this observation and showed that the delayed-type reactivity could also be suppressed by a preceding wheal-and-flare reaction induced by a mixture of "trichophytin" and histamine.

Except for reagins (IgE) associated with immediate hypersensitivity, circulating antibodies specific for the infecting fungus have not been consistently demonstrated in dermatophytosis. Some of the differences in results may be accounted for by (1) the different methods used for serological analyses, (2) the different test antigens used, (3) the time during the course of infection at which blood was drawn, and (4) the nature of the infection, chronic vs. acute.

In general, precipitating or complement-fixing antibodies have been detected in sera of patients with (1) chronic or recurrent infections, especially due to *T. rubrum,* (2) highly inflammatory infections at the height of infection, or (3) with secondary dermatophytid eruptions (Pepys *et al.,* 1959; Grappel *et al.,* 1972; Sutter, 1917; Blumenthal and von Haupt, 1922; Kuroda, 1958; Jessner and Hoffman, 1924; Ayres and Anderson, 1934). These antibodies usually cross-reacted with antigens of other species of dermatophytes (Tomomatsu, 1962; Grappel *et al.,* 1972). Voldánová *et al.* (1967) detected precipitins in nine of 12 sera from patients with granulomatous inflammatory processes in the deep layers of the skin. As already mentioned, such antibodies could be responsible for the bizarre forms of the dermatophyte which are found in such lesions (Grappel *et al.,* 1971a,b)

Ito (1963) showed that precipitins were detectable up to 5 weeks following experimental inoculation of a subject with *T. rubrum*. They decreased at the time when type I immediate cutaneous hypersensitivity developed.

Antibodies detected by the more sensitive passive-agglutination tests or indirect fluorescent antibody techniques, using crude mycelial extracts as antigens, are generally less specific for dermatophytosis. Reyes and Friedman (1966) showed that antibodies detected by passive hemagglutination tests could be completely adsorbed with mycelia of saprophytic species of *Penicillium* and *Hormodendrum*. Passive agglutination tests using charcoal coated with mycelial extracts or polysaccharides showed higher antibody titers in sera of patients than in sera of noninfected controls (Grappel *et al.*, 1972).

With indirect fluorescent antibody tests, sera of patients were also positive with nondermatophyte fungi and sera of noninfected controls were positive with the dermatophyte antigens (Walzer and Einbinder, 1962; Miura, 1968). The use of fluorescent antibody conjugates specific for IgM and arthrospores as test antigens increased the specificity of the indirect fluorescent antibody tests (Hopfer *et al.*, 1975).

There is very little direct evidence to indicate that humoral antibodies play any role in generalized resistance to dermatophytic infections. They are more frequently associated with chronicity, deep inflammatory processes, or secondary allergic eruptions and do not persist after recovery. The experiments of Walters *et al.* (1974) suggest that circulating soluble Ag-Ab complexes could interfere with the manifestation of cell-mediated immunity or more specifically cell-mediated cutaneous hypersensitivity to dermatophyte antigens in patients with chronic infection.

Autoimmune-type antibody reactions have also been detected in dermatophytosis. Complement-fixing antibodies reactive with skin antigens were detected in sera of patients with onychomycosis due to *T. rubrum*, as well as in sera of patients with other dermatophytoses by Brusilovskaia (1970). Later, Peck *et al.* (1972) showed that one of their five patients with chronic *T. rubrum* infections produced complement-fixing antibodies to "trichophytin" which also had affinity for epithelial tissue. Hopfer *et al.* (1975) found low titers of

antibodies with an affinity for epithelial tissue in 80% of the sera of patients with chronic dermatophytoses. The antibodies, which were specific for dermatophytes, were identified as IgM and could be removed from sera by adsorption with mycelium of *T. rubrum*. Antibodies produced to the cell surface antigens, glycopeptides, of the dermatophytes may cross-react with intercellular glycoprotein of the epithelial tissue.

The fact that IgM antibodies have a shorter half-life in the circulation, and may also have an affinity for epithelial tissue, may explain some of the problems in demonstrating circulating antibodies in dermatophytosis. Such antibodies may play a role in the secondary allergic eruptions which sometimes occur.

Abraham *et al.* (1975) found that IgM levels were significantly decreased in patients who had recurrent *T. rubrum* infections. Their patients had no delayed-type cutaneous reactivity to "trichophytin."

Immediate hypersensitivity has been produced in guinea pigs, developing 40 days following experimental infection (W. Jadassohn *et al.*, 1932, 1937; Cruickshank *et al.*, 1960), and elicited in rabbits by repeated i.v. injections of *T. mentagrophytes* var. *asteroides* (K. Ito and Nishitani, 1961) and in cattle following experimental infections with *T. verrucosum* (Lepper, 1972). In cattle, the i.v. injection of 10^4 viable units of *T. verrucosum* resulted in an immediate-type reaction at the previously infected site.

Circulating antibodies have also been demonstrated in sera of animals both naturally infected and experimentally infected with dermatophytes (Verotti, 1916; Brocq-Rousseau *et al.*, 1927; Wharton *et al.*, 1950; Kuroda, 1953; K. Ito and Kashima, 1957; Cox and Moore, 1968; Kielstein, 1968). Although in most of these studies no direct relationship was found between circulating antibody titers and severity of infection or immunity, Kielstein (1968) speculated that immunity in trichophytosis in cattle is probably due to cell-bound antibodies which are responsible for recovery and the rarity of reinfection. Kielstein (1967) found that γ-globulins of infected cattle could inhibit oxygen uptake by *T. mentagrophytes in vitro*. Sera from rabbits hyperimmunized with mycelia of *T. mentagrophytes* var. *granulosum* have also been shown to inhibit growth and oxygen consumption by this dermatophyte (R. A. Calderone and S. F. Grappel, unpublished).

Lepper (1974) described an accumulation of mature plasma cells and lymphoblast cells in the dermis around capillary beds at the bases of sebaceous glands during the climax of the inflammatory response. This author postulates that such cells could be responsible for local antibody formation, which could cause Arthus-like changes or the tissue sensitization which he demonstrated at the site of previous infection. Arthrospores and hyphal fragments in the keratinized portions of the follicles and in the stratum corneum were found to be coated with γ-globulin, possibly responsible for the inhibition of the dermatophyte. γ-Globulin from immunized rabbits can completely inhibit the *in vitro* growth of *T. mentagrophytes* var. *granulosum* from infected hair (Grappel *et al.*, 1971a). Additional evidence for cell-bound antibodies at the site of previous infection was obtained in guinea pigs (Collins *et al.*, 1973). Antibodies to an antigenic keratinase isolated from *T. mentagrophytes* var. *granulosum* were detected in sections of the previously infected site but not in sections of noninfected skin. These reactions could be due to circulating antibodies with high affinity for tissue since antibodies to the keratinase do not usually persist in the circulation (Grappel, 1976), or they could be due to local antibody production, as suggested by Lepper (1974). Although generalized resistance to reinfection is not believed to be associated with circulating antibodies, cell-bound antibodies could play a role in local immunity and the relative anergy of the previously infected site.

5.2.3. Allergic Manifestations

The term "trichophytid" (= "id" or dermatophytid) was chosen by J. Jadassohn (1918) in analogy to Darrier's tuberculid. It was used to designate a generalized eruption occurring during the course of a localized trichophytosis. The "id" lesions are believed to occur primarily as a result of the reaction of circulating antigen (fungi or their allergenic products) with skin-sensitizing antibodies or possibly effector "T" lymphocytes. Williams (1927) reviewed the evidence for fungal elements in the blood of patients with dermatophytid eruptions. Although fungi were rarely demonstrable in the dermatophytid lesions, they could be demonstrated in lesions which were less than 2 days old. Such lesions usually appear at the height of infection or following a flare of the infection, probably due to a massive liberation of fungal elements. They are most often associated with suppurative type of inflammation usually caused by zoophilic species of dermatophytes, but are also found in patients infected with anthropophilic species. The "trichophytin" test for delayed-type cutaneous hypersensitivity is always positive in these patients.

X-ray treatments, "trichophytin" skin tests, and trauma inflicted at the infected site can also cause "id" lesions (Bloch, 1928; Sulzberger, 1940; Jones *et al.*, 1974c). Jadassohn (1918) observed trichophytids mainly in children suffering from tinea capitis with kerion celsi. The eruptions were located mainly on the trunk and consisted mainly of follicular nodules. More rarely, nodules resembling erythema nodosum were found on the lower extremities. Systemic symptoms, including lymphadenophathy, splenomegaly, joint involvement, and even anaphylaxis, have accompanied the acute onset of such dermatophytids (Götz, 1962).

At the present time, the "id" reaction most frequently encountered in patients occurs in adults with smooth skin infections, usually tinea pedis (Blank *et al.*, 1974; Miller, 1974). These "id" lesions occur on the fingers and palms and are usually symmetrical. The eruptions are papular, vesicular, or, rarely, bullous in appearance.

Sulzberger (1940) grouped the many varieties of eruptions into 17 forms, and Götz (1962) has classifed them as epidermal, cutaneous, subcutaneous, and vascular. The histopathological changes resemble those observed in tuberculids (Montgomery, 1967).

"Id" eruptions are not usually seen in natural infections in animals. However, "ids" have been induced following experimental infections in animals, including rabbits (Kuroda, 1959; Inaba, 1961) and guinea pigs (Henrici, 1939). Ito and Kuroda (1962) found histopathological changes in the lesions induced in rabbits to be comparable to some human dermatophytids.

6. Immunodiagnosis

Neither serological tests nor intradermal tests can be used for routine diagnosis of dermatophytosis, since they do not give reliable indications of past or present infection. However, newer *in vitro* tests for dermatophyte-specific cell-mediated hypersensitivity are providing promising tools for diagnosis.

Although delayed-type cutaneous hypersensitivity is the reaction most reliably associated with dermatophytosis, such reactions to intradermal injections of "trichophytin" have been reported in over 90% of noninfected individuals (W. Jadassohn, 1962; Jones *et al.*, 1973a). Furthermore, intradermal testing cannot establish or exclude dermatophytosis, since the "trichophytin" test may be negative in patients with chronic infections and regularly persists in patients with acute infections long after the infection is cured (Wilson, 1959).

The lack of commercially available standardized or homogeneous test antigens has also severely limited the usefulness of the "trichophytin" reaction for diagnostic purposes. There are more than ten "trichophytins" available (Seeliger, 1965). Reactivities to crude "trichophytins" have also been found in individuals with other sensitivities, including penicillin and tuberculin (Peck and Siegal, 1947; Seeliger, 1958).

So far, the most promising *in vitro* test with potential for routine immunodiagnosis comes from the investigations of Walters *et al.* (1976). These workers have recently reported that the leukocyte-adherence inhibition (LAI) test, which they used to detect cell-mediated immunity in patients with dermatophytosis, may be used for a rapid, species-specific diagnosis consistent with results of mycological cultures. The dermatophyte test antigens were powdered allergens of *T. rubrum*, *T. mentagrophytes*, and *E. flocossum* obtained from Holister Stier, Spokane, Washington. Distinction could also be made between acute and chronic infection based on the presence of blocking factors in the sera of patients. Such factors would be difficult to detect serologically, since they are likely to be antigen–antibody complexes. However, they were easily detected by their effect on the LAI test.

The specificity of the test results obtained by these investigators is surprising in light of the crude antigens used and the presence of common antigens in these species (Andrieu *et al.*, 1968; Christiansen and Svejgaard, 1976). Several workers have shown that neither acquired resistance associated with cell-mediated hypersensitivity nor delayed-cutaneous hypersensitivity to such crude antigens is species specific.

In general, tests for circulating antibodies are often positive with sera from patients with other fungus infections, as well as with sera from noninfected adults when the more sensitive tests, such as passive agglutination, are used (Grappel *et al.*, 1974). Although complement-fixing and precipitating antibodies appear to be specific for dermatophytosis, these occur less frequently and do not persist (Grappel *et al.*, 1972).

Olaru (1974) has consistently detected antidermatophyte antibodies fixed to a higher percentage of peripheral blood lymphocytes and neutrophils from patients with dermatophytoses (44–88%) than from noninfected controls (11–21%). He used fluorescein-conjugated dermatophyte extracts for detection of the cytophilic antibodies and suggested the test for diagnosis of infection.

Imamura *et al.* (1975) suggested the use of immunofluorescent staining for the detection of fungal elements in biopsy sections of kerions. They claimed that fluorescein-conjugated antibody to *T. mentagrophytes* was specific for dermatophytes and could also detect fungal antigens in the dermis which may be difficult to identify.

7. Vaccines

7.1. For Prophylaxis

There have been very few attempts at immunoprophylaxis for dermatophytosis in man. In those reported, only a local immunity of short duration has been produced by topical application of killed mycelium. However, in each case, immunity was accompanied by cutaneous sensitization.

Sutter (1917) produced a local immunity by rubbing killed mycelia of *A. quinckeanum* on the forearm. He found that resistance diminished with distance from the treatment site. Huppert and Keeney (1959) also found resistance to be greatest in the treated area. They immunized volunteers by repeated topical application of disintegrated *T. mentagrophytes* in an ointment base to one foot. On challenge, only 14% of the treated feet became infected, compared to 57% of the untreated, contralateral feet. In control subjects the infection rate averaged 86% and 71% for each foot.

Several attempts at immunoprophylaxis have been made in experimental animals. In guinea pigs parenteral inoculation of living or killed dermatophyte suspensions was capable of inducing delayed-type hypersensitivity and partial or poor protection of short duration. Subsequent cutaneous infection took an abortive course (Bloch and Massini, 1909; Saeves, 1915). Hypersensitivity and partial protection were also induced by topical application of killed mycelia (Sutter, 1917; Keeney and Huppert, 1959). Culture filtrates, even if incorporated in Freund's adjuvant, induced cutaneous hypersensitivity but no immunity to infection (Reiss and Leonard, 1956; Wharton *et al.*, 1950).

Subcutaneous injection of highly purified galactomannan peptides (Arnold *et al.*, 1976), incorporated in Freund's adjuvant, induced both delayed-type cutaneous hypersensitivity and a generalized relative resistance to *T. mentagrophytes* var. *granulosum* in guinea pigs. Subsequent experimental cutaneous infections were abortive in nature, i.e., decreased both in extent and duration (S. F. Grappel, unpublished).

Several investigators have used immunoprophylaxis successfully for the prevention of natural infection in cattle (Florian *et al.*, 1964; Kielstein and Richter, 1970; Sarkisov *et al.*, 1971). Subcutaneous inoculations of calves with extracts of killed *T. verrucosum* mycelia decreased the incidence of disease and the severity of lesions when they were exposed to infected herds. Sarkisov *et al.* (1971) reported an 85% lower incidence of infection; those lesions which occurred were small and healed spontaneously. Protection lasted up to 3–5 years.

7.2. For Treatment

At the present time, the only useful systemic antibiotic for dermatophytosis, griseofluvin, is not completely effective. At best, it has a fungistatic effect which can reduce the amount of microorganisms in the host. Complete removal of the fungus still requires activation of the body's cellular immune defenses, as well as turnover of epidermal cells.

Therapeutic vaccines have been used by several investigators in treatment trials of patients with chronic recalcitrant infections, as well as in attempts to reduce secondary dermatoallergic reactions ("ids") by desensitization. Activation of the host's defenses with killed whole mycelium or crude mycelial extracts injected intradermally or subcutaneously, the routes most useful for inducing cell-mediated hypersensitivity (Chase, 1976), has had some success in clearing resistant infections in man. However, intradermal injections of "trichophytins" prepared from culture filtrates have had little effect on the course of infection (Neisser, 1902; Truffi, 1904; Traub and Tolmach, 1935).

Repeated intradermal injections of killed mycelial suspensions were used successfully in tinea capitis by Strickler (1915) and in tinea corporis by Bazýka (1966) and more recently by Tagar *et al.* (1973). Tager *et al.* (1973) used a killed suspension of *T. rubrum* and *T. mentagrophytes* mycelia. They obtained complete cures in 22 of 39 patients and partial improvement in six with chronic superficial tinea corporis. The patients were followed for 18 months after treatment.

Various types of extracts and hydrolysates of mycelia have also been used successfully in man. Early investigations indicated that repeated injections of clasovaccines, nitric acid hydrolysates of mycelia, could cure patients with various dermatophytoses, including onychomycosis and tinea capitis (Jausion and Sohier, 1930; da Fonseca and de Área Leão, 1931). However, Lewis and Hopper (1937) found the cure rate with such vaccines disappointing and observed toxic side reactions. More recently, Longhin and Olaru (1970) used a trichloroacetic acid extract of *T. mentagrophytes* mycelia for treatment of 680 patients with profound trichophytosis. Repeated subcutaneous injections cured 530 (78%) of the patients without additional therapy. Clearing of the infection sites also cleared dermatoallergic eruptions in the patients. Such vaccine therapy in conjunction with griseofulvin cured 33 patients whose infections had recurred after griseofulvin treatment alone. The trichloroacetic acid extract consisted mainly of glycopeptides and was the same preparation later used by Arnold *et al.* (1976) for purification of galactomannan peptides which induce cellular immunity. Harada (1969) has also reported successful therapy with polysaccharide–nucleic acid antigens.

Most attempts at treatment of patients for dermatoallergic symptoms by desensitization with repeated intradermal injections of "trichophytin" have been unsuccessful. Desensitization was only temporary and usually had little effect on the "id" eruptions (Traub and Tolmach, 1935; Miller *et al.*, 1941; Sulzberger and Wise, 1932).

8. Immunotherapy

The newest form of immunotherapy for resistant dermatophytosis is the use of plasma from a donor sensitive to "trichophytin." Plasma therapy was used for a teenager who had widespread infection due to *M. audouinii* (Allen *et al.*, 1977) During the course of infection, this patient became totally anergic to all of the test antigens used for delayed-type dermal reactivity and could not be sensitized to dinitrochlorobenzene. The infection was resistant to griseofulvin, and "transfer factor" had been used without success. Plasma therapy was indicated by the results of *in vitro* lymphocyte transformation tests. Transformation was diminished in the presence of the patient's own serum, indicating blocking factors, but was normal in the presence of her mother's serum. Following intravenous transfusions with the mother's serum, which could contain unblocking factors, the patient had a minimal delayed-type dermal reaction to "trichophytin." Plasma transfusions were required repeatedly, since improvement lasted only up to 10 days following therapy. The plasma therapy was successful only in conjunction with amphotericin B.

References

Abraham, S., Pandhi, A. S., Kumar, R. K., Mohapatra, L. N., and Bhutani, L. K., 1975, A study of the immunological status of patients with dermatophytosis, *Dermatologica* 151:281–287.

Ajello, L., 1974, Natural history of the dermatophytes and related fungi, *Mycopathol. Mycol. Appl.* 53:93–110.

Allen, A. M., and Taplin, D., 1973, Epidemic *Trichophyton mentagrophytes* infections in servicemen: Source of infection, role of environment, host factors, and susceptibility, *J. Am. Med. Assoc.* 226:864–867.

Allen, D. E., Snyderman, R., Meadows, L., and Pinnell, S. R., 1977, Generalized *Microsporum audouinii* infection and depressed cellular immunity associated with a missing plasma factor required for lymphocyte blastogenesis, *Am. J. Med.* 63:991–1000.

Andrieu, S., Biguet, J., and Laloux, B., 1968, Annalyse immunoélectrophorétique comparée des structures antigéniques de 17 espèces de dermatophytes, *Mycopathol. Mycol. Appl.* 34:161–185.

Aravysky, A. N., 1959, Rare mycological findings in pathological material, *Mycopathol. Mycol. Appl.* 11:143–154.

Aravysky, A. N., 1961, Rare mycological findings in pathological material, *Mycopathol. Mycol. Appl.* 16:177–193.

Aravysky, A. N., 1964, Rare mycological findings in pathological material: Third communication of rare findings in generalized trichophytosis, *Mycopathol. Mycol. Appl.* 22:185–200.

Arnold, M. T., Grappel, S. F., Lerro, A. V., and Blank, F., 1976, Peptido polysaccharide antigens from *Trichophyton mentagrophytes* var. *granulosum, Infect. Immun.* 14:376–382.

Austwick, P. K. C., 1972, The pathogenicity of fungi, in: *Microbial Pathogenicity in Man and Animals* (H. Smith and J. H. Pearce, eds.), pp. 251–268, Cambridge University Press, Cambridge.

Ayres, S., and Anderson, N. P., 1934, Inhibition of fungi in cultures by blood serum from patients with "phytid" eruptions, *Arch. Dermatol.* 29:537–547.

Balabanoff, V. A., 1965, Dimorphism of dermatophytes with regard to the grade of parasitic adaptation and their classification, *Mycopathol. Mycol. Appl.* 25:323–350.

Barker, S. A., and Trotter, M. D., 1960, Isolation of purified trichophytin, *Nature (London)* 188:232–233.

Barker, S. A., Cruickshank, C. N. D., Morris, J. H., and Wood, S. R., 1962, The isolation of trichophytin glycopeptide and its structure in relation to the immediate and delayed reactions, *Immunology* 5:627–632.

Barker, S. A., Cruickshank, C. N. D., and Holden, J. H., 1963, Structure of a galactomannan-peptide allergen from *Trichophyton mentagrophytes, Biochim. Biophys. Acta* 74:239–246.

Barker, S. A., Basarab, O., and Cruickshank, C. N. D., 1967, Galactomannan peptides of *Trichophyton mentagrophytes, Carbohyd. Res.* 3:325–332.

Barlow, A. J. E., and Chattaway, F. W., 1958, The parasitism of ringworm group of fungi, *Arch. Dermatol.* 77:399–405.

Barlow, A. J. E., Chattaway, F. W., Brunt, R. V., and Townly, J. D., 1961, A study of susceptibility to infection by *Trichophyton rubrum, J. Invest. Dermatol.* 37:461–468.

Basarab, O., How, M. J., and Cruickshank, C. N. D.,

1968, Immunological relationships between glycopeptides of *Microsporum canis, Trichophyton mentagrophytes* and other fungi, *Sabouraudia* 6:119–126.

Bazýka, A. P., 1966, Changes in the reactivity of the organism and in the morphological structures of the affected skin in patients with mycoses of the feet under the effect of fungus immune preparations, *Vestn. Dermatol. Venerol.* 40:3–9.

Bean, S. F., and South, M. A., 1973, Cutaneous manifestations of immunogenetic disorders, *J. Invest. Dermatol.* 60:503–508.

Bibel, D. J., and LeBrun, J. R., 1975, Effect of experimental dermatophyte infection on cutaneous flora, *J. Invest. Dermatol.* 64:119–123.

Bishop, C. T., Blank, F., and Haranisavljevic-Jakovljevic, M., 1962, The water-soluble polysaccharides of dermatophytes. I. A galactomannan from *Trichophyton granulosum, Can. J. Chem.* 40:1816–1825.

Bishop, C. T., Perry, M. B., Blank, F., and Cooper, F. P., 1965, The water-soluble polysaccharides of dermatophytes. IV. Galactomannans I from *Trichophyton granulosum, Trichophyton interdigitale, Microsporum quinckeanum, Trichophyton rubrum,* and *Trichophyton schönleinii, Can. J. Chem.* 43:30–59.

Bishop, C. T., Perry, M. B., and Blank, F., 1966a, The water-soluble polysaccharides of dermatophytes. V. Galactomannans II from *Trichophyton granulosum, Trichophyton interdigitale, Microsporum quinckeanum, Trichophyton rubrum,* and *Trichophyton schönleinii, Can. J. Chem.* 44:2291–2297.

Bishop, C. T., Perry, M. B., Hulyalkar, R. K., and Blank, F., 1966b, The water-soluble polysaccharides of dermatophytes. VI. Glucans from *Trichophyton granulosum, Trichophyton interdigitale, Microsporum quinckeanum, Trichophyton rubrum,* and *Trichophyton schönleinii, Can. J. Chem.* 44:2299–2303.

Blank, F., 1955, Dermatophytes of animal origin transmissible to man, *Am. J. Med. Sci.* 299:302–316.

Blank, F., and Mann, S. J., 1975, *Trichophyton rubrum* infections according to age, anatomical distribution, and sex, *Br. J. Dermatol.* 92:171–174.

Blank, F., Mann, S. J., and Reale, R. A., 1974, Distribution of dermatophytosis according to age, ethnic group, and sex, *Sabouraudia* 12:352–361.

Blank, H., and Smith, Jr., J. G., 1960, Widespread *Trichophyton rubrum* granulomas treated with griseofulvin, *Arch. Dermatol.* 81:779–789.

Blank, H., Sagami, S., Boyd, C., and Roth, Jr., F. J., 1959, The pathogenesis of superficial fungus infections in cultured human skin, *Arch. Dermatol.* 79:524–535.

Blank, H., Taplin, D., and Zaias, N., 1969, Cutaneous *Trichophyton mentagrophytes* infections in Vietnam, *Arch. Dermatol.* 99:135–144.

Bloch, B., 1908, Zur Lehre von den Dermatomykosen, *Arch. Dermatol. Syph.* 93:157–220.

Bloch, B., 1928, Allgemeine und experimentelle Biologie der Dermatomykosen und die Trichophytide, in: *Handbuch der Haut- und Geschlechtskrankheiten,* Vol. 11

(J. Jadassohn, ed.), pp. 300–376, 564–606, J. Springer, Berlin.

Bloch, B., and Massini, R., 1909, Studien über Immunität und Überempfindlichkeit bei Hyphomycetenerkrankungen, *Z. Hyg. Infektionskr.* 63:68–89.

Bloch, B., Labouchère, A., and Schaff, F., 1925, Versuche einer chemischen Charakterisierung und Reindarstellung des Trichophytins (des aktiven, antigenen Prinzips Pathogener Hautpilze), *Arch. Dermatol. Syph.* 148:413–424.

Blumenthal, F., and von Haupt, A., 1922, Über Vorkommen von Antikörpern im Blutserum trichophytiekranker Menschen, *Dermatol. Z.* 36:313–336.

Bonk, A. F., Friedman, L., and Derbes, V. J., 1962, Experimental dermatophytosis, *J. Invest. Dermatol.* 39:281–286.

Brocq-Rousseu, D., Urbain, A., and Barotte, J., 1927, Etude des teignes du cheval et de l'immunité dans les teignes expérimentales, *Ann. Inst. Pasteur Paris* 41:513–551.

Brusilovskaia, D. A., 1970, Immunoallergic reactions of the organism in mycoses caused by *Trichophyton rubrum* and certain zoophilic fungi, *Vestn. Dermatol. Venerol.* 44:47–51.

Buckley, R. H., Wray, B. B., and Belmaker, E. Z., 1972, Extreme hyperimmunoglobulin E and undue susceptibility to infections, Pediatrics 19:59–70.

Burgoon, C. F., Blank, F., Johnson, W. C., and Grappel, S. F., 1974, Mycetoma formation in *Trichophyton rubrum* infection, *Br. J. Dermatol.* 90:155–162.

Canizares, O., Shatin, H., and Kalbert, A., 1959, Cushing's syndrome and dermatomycosis, *Arch. Dermatol.* 80:705–712.

Carlisle, D. H., Inouye, J. C., King, R. D., and Jones, H. E., 1974, Significance of serum fungal inhibitory factor in dermatophytosis, *J. Invest. Dermatol.* 63:239–241.

Caroline, L., Taschdjian, C. L., Kozinn, P. J., and Schade, A. L., 1964, Reversal of serum fungistasis by addition of iron, *J. Invest. Dermatol.* 42:415–419.

Chakraborty, A. N., Ghosh, S., and Blank, F., 1954, Isolation of *Trichophyton rubrum* fron animals, *Can. J. Comp. Med. Vet. Sci.* 18:436–438.

Chase, M. W., 1976, Developments in delayed-type hypersensitivities: 1950–1975, *J. Invest. Dermatol.* 67:136–148.

Chattaway, F. W., Ellis, D. A., and Barlow, A. J. E., 1963, Peptides of dermatophytes, *J. Invest. Dermatol.* 41:31–37.

Christiansen, A. H., and Svejgaard, E., 1976, Studies on the antigenic structure of *Trichophyton rubrum, Trichophyton mentagrophytes, Microsporum canis,* and *Epidermophyton floccosum* by crossed immuno-electrophoresis, *Acta Pathol. Microbiol. Scand.* 84:337–341.

Collins, J. P., Grappel, S. F., and Blank, F., 1973, Role of keratinases in dermatophytosis. II. Fluorescent antibody studies with keratinase II of *Trichophyton mentagrophytes, Dermatologica* 146:95–100.

Conant, N. F., Smith, D. T., Baker, R. D., and Callaway,

J. L., 1971, *Manual of Clinical Mycology,* 3rd ed., Saunders, Philadelphia.

Cox, W. A., and Moore, J. A., 1968, Experimental *Trichophyton verrucosum* infections in laboratory animals, *J. Comp Pathol.* **78:**35–41.

Cruickshank, C. N. D., 1966, Allergy, in: *Modern Trends in Dermatology,* Vol. 3 (R. M. B. MacKenna, ed.), pp. 52–83, Butterworth, Washington, D.C.

Cruickshank, C. N. D., Trotter, M. D., and Wood, S. R., 1960, Studies on trichophytin sensitivity, *J. Invest. Dermatol.* **35:**219–223.

da Fonseca, O., and de Ãrea Leão, 1931, Vaccinotherapia das epidermophyceas e dad tinhas tonsurantes: Contribuicão para o estudo das claso-vaccines, *Rev. Med. Cir. Brazil* **39:**269–277.

Dawson, C. O., 1968, Ringworm in animals, *Rev. Med. Vet. Mycol.* **6:**223–233.

Dawson, C. O., and Gentles, J. C., 1961, The perfect states of *Keratinomyces ajelloi* Vanbreuseghem, *Trichophyton terrestre* Durie and Frey, and *Microsporum nanum* Fuentes, *Sabouraudia* **1:**49–57.

DeLamater, E. D., 1941, Experimental studies with the dermatophytes. III. Development and duration of immunity and hypersensitivity in guinea pigs, *J. Invest. Dermatol.* **4:**143–158.

DeLamater, E. D., 1942, Experimental studies with the dermatophytes. IV. The influence of age upon the allergic response in experimental ringworm in the guinea pigs, *J. Invest. Dermatol.* **5:**423–429.

DeLamater, E. D., and Benham, R. W., 1938a, Experimental studies with dermatophytes. I. Primary disease in laboratory animals, *J. Invest. Dermatol.* **1:**451–467.

DeLamater, E. D., and Benham, R. W., 1938b, Experimental studies with the dermatophytes. II. Immunity and hypersensitivity produced in laboratory animals, *J. Invest. Dermatol.* **1:**469–488.

Desai, S. C., and Harvey, S. R., 1967, The study of fungistatic activity of sera from patients suffering from chronic ringworm and from healthy individuals, in: *Recent Advances of Human and Animal Mycology* (L. Chmel, ed.), pp. 313–317, Slovak Academy of Sciences, Bratislava.

Desai, S. C., Modi, P. J., and Bhat, M. L. A., 1962, Dysproteinemia in the chronic dermatomycosis due to *T. rubrum* with negative anergy to tricophytin, *J. Invest. Dermatol.* **31:**365–367.

Desai, S. C., Bhat, M. L. A., and Modi, P. J., 1963, Biology of *Trichophyton rubrum* infections, *Indian J. Med. Res.* **51:**233–243.

Desai, S. C., Khokani, A. C., and Modi, P. J., 1966, Evaluation of trichophytin reactivity in *T. rubrum* infections and its use as an exposure index, *Indian J. Med. Res.* **54:**148–156.

Eleuterio, M. K., Grappel, S. F., Caustic, C. A., and Blank, F., 1973, Role of keratinases in dermatophytosis. III. Demonstration of delayed hypersensitivity to keratinases by the capillary tube migration test, *Dermatologica* **147:**255–260.

Emmons, C. W., Binford, C. H., and Utz, J. P., 1970, *Medical Mycology,* 2nd ed., Lea and Febiger, Philadelphia.

English, M. P., 1976, Nails and fungi, *Br. J. Dermatol.* **94:**697–701.

Epstein, S., and Grünmandel, S., 1930, Untersuchungen über die spontane Abheilung von oberflächlichen Trichophytien, *Arch. Dermatol. Syph.* **161:**395–428.

Esterly, N. B., Brammer, S. R., and Crounse, R. G., 1967, The relationship of transferrin and iron to serum inhibition of *Candida albicans, J. Invest. Dermatol.* **49:**437–442.

Fielder, R. J., Grappel, S. F., Bishop, C. T., and Blank, F., 1972, The occurrence of pyruvic acid ketal in a glucan from a fungus, *Microsporum quinckeanum, Can. J. Microbiol.* **18:**701–704.

Florian, E., Nemeseri, L., and Lovas, G., 1964, Active immunization of calves against ringworm, *Magy, Allatorv. Lapja* **19:**529–530.

Fraser, R. D. B., MacRae, T. P., and Rogers, G. E., 1972, The evolution of keratins, in: *Keratins: Their Composition, Structure and Biosynthesis,* pp. 237–282, Thomas, Springfield, Ill.

Friedman, L., and Derbes, V. J., 1960, The question of immunity in ringworm infections, *Ann. N.Y. Acad. Sci.* **89:**178–183.

Fudenberg, H., Good, R. A., and Goodman, H. C., 1971, Primary immunodeficiences: Report of a World Health Organization Commitee, *Pediatrics* **47:**927–947.

Godal, T. B., Myklestad, B., Samuel, D. R., and Myrvang, B., 1971, Characterization of the cellular immune defect in lepromatous leprosy: A specific lack of circulating *Mycobacterium leprae*-reactive lymphocytes, *Clin. Exp. Immunol.* **9:**821–831.

Goodman, R. S., Temple, D. E., and Lorincz, A. L., 1961, A miniature system for extracorporeal hemodialysis with application to studies on serum antidermatophytic activity, *J. Invest. Dermatol.* **37:**535–541.

Goss, W. A., Actor, P., Jambor, W. P., and Pagano, J. F., 1963, The *Trichophyton mentagrophytes* and *Microsporum canis* infection of the guinea pig. I. The development of a chronic infection, *J. Invest. Dermatol.* **40:**299–304.

Götz, H., 1962, Die Trichophytinallergie, in: *Handbuch der Haut- und Geschlechtskrankeiten Ergänzungswerk,* Vol. 4 (3), (J. Jadassohn, ed.), pp. 123–133, Springer-Verlag, Berlin.

Graham, J. H., 1972, Superficial fungus infections, in: *Dermal Pathology* (J. H. Graham, W. C. Johnson, and E. B. Helwig, eds.), pp. 137–253, Harper and Row, Hagerstown, Md.

Grappel, S. F., 1976, Role of keratinase in dermatophytosis. IV. Reactivities of sera from guinea pigs with heat-inactivated keratinase II, *Dermatologica* **153:**157–162.

Grappel, S. F., and Blank, F., 1972, Role of keratinases in dermatophytosis. I. Immune responses of guinea pigs infected with *Trichophyton mentagrophytes* and guinea pigs immunized with keratinases, *Dermatologica* **145**:245–255.

Grappel, S. F., Blank, F., and Bishop, C. T., 1967, Immunological studies on dermatophytes. I. Serological reactivites of neutral polysaccharides with rabbit antiserum to *Microsporum quinckeanum*, *J. Bacteriol.* **93**:1001–1008.

Grappel, S. F., Blank, F., and Bishop, C. T., 1968a, Immunological studies on dermatophytes. II. Serological reactivities of mannans prepared from galactomannans I and II of *Microsporum quinckeanum*, *Trichophyton granulosum*, *Trichophyton interdigitale*, *Trichophyton rubrum*, and *Trichophyton schoenleinii*, *J. Bacteriol.* **95**:1238–1242.

Grappel, S. F., Blank, F., and Bishop, C. T., 1968b, Immunological studies on dermatophytes. III. Further analyses of the reactivites of neutral polysaccharides with rabbit antisera to *Microsporum quinckeanum*, *Trichophyton schoenleinii*, *Trichophyton rubrum*, *Trichophyton interdigitale*, and *Trichophyton granulosum*, *J. Bacteriol.* **96**:70–75.

Grappel, S. F., Blank, F., and Bishop, C. T., 1969, Immunological studies on dermatophytes. IV. Chemical structures and serological reactivities of polysaccharides from *Microsporum praecox*, *Trichophyton ferrugineum*, *Trichophyton sabouraudii*, and *Trichophyton tonsurans*, *J. Bacteriol.* **97**:23–26.

Grappel, S. F., Buscavage, C. A., Blank, F., and Bishop, C. T., 1970, Comparative serological reactivities of twenty-seven polysaccharides from nine species of dermatophytes, *Sabouraudia* **8**:116–125.

Grappel, S. F., Fethière, A., and Blank, F., 1971a, Effect of antibodies on growth and structure of *Trichophyton mentagrophytes*, *Sabouraudia* **9**:50–55.

Grappel, S. F., Fethière, A., and Blank, F., 1971b, Macroconidia of *Trichophyton schoenleinii*, *Sabouraudia* **9**:144–145.

Grappel, S. F., Blank, F., and Bishop, C. T., 1971c, Circulating antibodies in human favus, *Dermatologica* **143**:271–278.

Grappel, S. F., Blank, F., and Bishop, C. T., 1972, Circulating antibodies in dermatophytosis, *Dermatologica* **144**:1–11.

Grappel, S. F., Bishop, C. T., and Blank, F., 1974, Immunology of dermatophytes and dermatophytosis, *Bacteriol. Rev.* **38**:222–250.

Greenbaum, S. S., 1924, Immunity in ringworm infections. I. Active acquired immunity: With a note on complement fixation tests in superficial ringworm infections, *Arch. Dermatol.* **10**:279–282.

Greenberg, J. H., King, R. D., Krebs, S., and Field, R., 1976, A quantitative dermatophyte infection model in the guinea pig—A parallel to the quantitated human infection model, *J. Invest. Dermatol.* **67**:704–708.

Gregory, P. H., 1935, The dermatophytes, *Biol. Rev.* **10**:208–233.

Grin, E., and Ozegovic, L., 1963, Influence of the soil on certain dermatophytes and their evolutional trend, *My-copathol. Mycol. Appl.* **21**:23–28.

Hanifin, J. M., Ray, L. F., and Lobitz, W. C., 1974, Immunological reactivity in dermatophytosis, *Br. J. Dermatol.* **90**:1–8.

Harada, S., 1969, Vaccine therapy of mycosis, *Nippon Ika Daigaku. Zasshi.* **36**:464–465.

Hejtmánek, M., and Lenhart, K., 1970, The genetic basis of virulence in dermatophytes, *Folia Biol. (Praha)* **16**:363–366.

Hejtmánek, M., and Lenhart, K., 1971, Study of the genetic basis of resistance to dermatophytosis, in: *Comptes Rendus des Communication V Congrès de la Société Internationale de Mycologic Humáine et Animale* (H. Drouhret, ed.), pp. 113–114, Institut Pasteur, Paris.

Henrici, A. T., 1939, Experimental trichophytid in guinea pigs, *Proc. Soc. Exp. Biol. Med.* **41**:349–353.

Hildick-Smith, G., Blank, H., and Sarkany, I., 1964, *Fungus Diseases and Their Treatment*, Little, Brown, Boston.

Hill, H. R., and Quie, P. B., 1975, Defective neutrophil chemotaxis associated with hyperimmunoglobulinemia E, in: *The Phagocytic Cell in Host Resistance* (J. A. Bellanti and D. H. Dayton, eds.), pp. 249–266, Raven Press, New York.

Hopfer, R. L., Grappel, S. F., and Blank, F., 1975, Antibodies with affinity for epithelial tissue in chronic dermatophytosis, *Dermatologica* **151**:135–143.

How, M. J., Withnall, M. T., and Cruickshank, C. N. D., 1972, Allergenic glucans from dermatophytes. Part I. Isolation, purification and biological properties, *Carbohydr. Res.* **25**:341–353.

How, M. J., Withnall, M. T., and Somers, P. J., 1973, Allergenic glucans from dermatophytes. II. Enzymic degradation, *Carbohydr. Res.* **26**:21–31.

Huppert, M., 1962, Immunization against superficial fungous infection, in: *Fungi and Fungous Diseases* (G. Dalldorf, ed.), pp. 239–253, Thomas, Springfield, Ill.

Huppert, M., and Keeney, E. L., 1959, Immunization against superficial fungous infection, *J. Invest. Dermatol.* **32**:15–19.

Imamura, S., Tanaka, M., and Watanabe, S., 1975, Use of immunofluorescence staining in kerion, *Arch. Dermatol.* **111**:906–909.

Inaba, K., 1961, Experimental study on hematogenous reinfection with Trichophyton mentagrophytes, var. asteroides. VI. Experimental trichophytid (generalized) produced by hematogenous reinfection with *Trichophyton mentagr.* var. *ast.* as seen from comparative exanthematology, *Bull. Pharm. Res. Inst. Osaka* **34**:1–13.

Ito, K., 1963, Immunologic aspects of superficial fungous diseases: Trichophytin: skin and serologic reaction, in: *Proceedings of the XIIIth International Congress of Dermatology* (D. M. Pillsbury and C. S. Livingood, eds.), pp. 563–567, Excerpta Medica Foundation, New York.

Ito, K., and Kashima, R., 1957, Prolonged observation of immunobiologic follow up in *Trichophyton purpureum* rabbits receiving repeated reinoculations, and of immunobiologic relation between *T. purpureum* and *T. asteroides, Bull. Pharm. Res. Inst. Osaka* **14**:16–25.

Ito, K., and Kuroda, K., 1962, Experimental study of mycotic epidermal pathology. I. Epidermal pathology of experimental dermatophytid (produced at the ears of rabbits by dorsal cutaneous reinfection with *Trichophyton*), *Bull. Pharm. Res. Inst. Osaka* **36**:7–19.

Ito, K., and Nishitani, N., 1961, Artificial production of systemic vasculitis due to repeated sensitization by fungus antigens, *Bull. Pharm. Res. Inst. Osaka.* **35**:13–21.

Ito, Y., 1965a, On the immunologically active substances of the dermatophytes. I, *J. Invest. Dermatol.* **45**:275–284.

Ito, Y., 1965b, On the immunologically active substances of the dermatophytes. II, *J. Invest. Dermatol.* **45**:285–294.

Jadassohn, J., 1918, Über die Trichophytien, *Berliner Klin. Wochenschr.* **21**:489–494.

Jadassohn, W., 1928, Versuche über Pilzzuchtung auf Organen, *Arch. Dermatol. Syph.* **155**:203–207.

Jadassohn, W., 1962, Delayed hypersensitivity to fungal antigens, in: *Proceedings of the 4th International Congress of Allergology, New York* (E. A. Brown, ed.), pp. 220–226, Macmillan, New York.

Jadassohn, W., Schaaf, F., and Sulzberger, M. B., 1932, Der Schultz-Dalesche Versuch mit Trichophytin, *Klin. Wochenschr.* **20**:1–10.

Jadassohn, W., Schaaf, F., and Wohler, G., 1937, Analyses of composite antigens by the Schultz-Dale technic: Further experimental analyses of trichophytins, *J. Immunol.* **32**:203–227.

Jausion, H., and Sohier, R., 1930, Les claso-vaccines: Vaccinothérapie des dermatomycoses et de leurs séquelles allergiques, *Presse Med.* **30**:621–625.

Jessner, M., and Hoffman, H., 1924, Der Einflus des Serums Allergischer auf Trichophytonpilze, *Arch. Dermatol. Syph.* **145**:187–192.

Jillson, O. F., and Huppert, M., 1949, The immediate wheal and the 24–48 hour tuberculin type edematous reactions to trichophytin, *J. Invest. Dermatol.* **12**: 179–185.

Jones, H. E., Reinhardt, J. H., and Rinaldi, M. G., 1973a, A clinical, mycological, and immunological survey for dermatophytosis, *Arch. Dermatol.* **108**:61–65.

Jones, H. E., Rinaldi, M. B., Chai, H., and Kohn, G., 1973b, Apparent cross-reactivity of airborne molds and the dermatophytic fungi, *J. Allergy Clin. Immunol.* **52**:346–351.

Jones, H. E., Reinhardt, J. H., and Rinaldi, M. G., 1974a, Acquired immunity to dermatophytes, *Arch. Dermatol.* **109**:840–848.

Jones, H. E., Reinhardt, J. E., and Rinaldi, M. G., 1974b, Immunologic susceptibility to chronic dermatophytosis *Arch. Dermatol.* **110**:213–220.

Jones, H. E., Reinhardt, J. H., and Rinaldi, M. G., 1974c, Model dermatophytosis in naturally infected subjects, *Arch. Dermatol.* **110**:369–374.

Kaliciński, J., Prochacki, H., and Engelhardt-Zasada, C.,

1975, Aflatoxin-like compounds produced by dermatophytes, *Mycopathologia* **55**:23–24.

Kaplan, W., and Georg, L. K., 1957, Isolation of *Microsporum audouini* from a dog, *J. Invest. Dermatol.* **28**:313–315.

Keeney, E. L., and Huppert, M., 1959, Immunization against superficial fungous infection, *J. Invest. Dermatol.* **32**:7–13.

Kielstein, P., 1967, Zur Immunobiologie der Rindertrichophytie, *Mykosen* **10**:205.

Kielstein, P., 1968, Immunologische Untersuchungen wahrend der spontanen und experimentellen Rindertrichophytie, *Wiss. Z. Karl Marx Univ. Leipzig* **17**:177–178.

Kielstein, P., and Richter, W., 1970, Versuche zur Immunoprophylaxe der Rindertrichophytie, *Arch. Exp. Veterinaermed.* **24**:1205–1218.

King, R. D., Khan, H. A., Foye, J. C., Greenberg, J. H., and Jones, H. E., 1975, Tranferrin, iron, and dermatophyte inhibitory component definitively identified as unsaturated transferrin, *J. Lab. Clin. Med.* **86**:204–212.

Kligman, A. M., 1952, The pathogenesis of tinea capitis due to *Microsporum audouini* and *Microsporum canis*. I. Gross observations following the inoculation of humans, *J. Invest. Dermatol.* **18**:231–246.

Kligman, A. M., 1956, Pathophysiology of ringworm infections in animals with skin cycles, *J. Invest. Dermatol.* **27**:171–185.

Kligman, A. M., and Ginsberg, D., 1950, Immunity of the adult scalp to infection with *Microsporum audouini*, *J. Invest. Dermatol.* **14**:345–356.

Knight, A. G., 1972, A review of experimental human fungus infections, *J. Invest. Dermatol.* **59**:354–358.

Kogoj, F., 1926, Experimentelle Beiträge zur Lehre von den Dermatomykosen mit besonderer Berücksichtigung der Lokalisationsbestimmung hämotogener Infektionen, *Arch. Dermatol. Syph.* **150**:333–355.

Kolmer, J. A., and Strickler, A., 1915, Complement fixation in parasitic skin diseases, *J. Am. Med. Assoc.* **64**:800–804.

Kuroda, K., 1953, Serological studies of experimental trichophytosis. I. Serological reactions using a mechanically prepared antigen, *Ann. Tuberc.* **4**:15–19.

Kuroda, K., 1958, Serological studies of experimental trichophytosis. IX. Complement fixation and precipitating reactions in patients with dermatomycosis using crude polysaccharide from *T. asteroides* mechanically disintegrated as antigen, *Bull. Pharm. Res. Inst. Osaka* **15**:5–8.

Kuroda, K., 1959, Experimental study on fungus granuloma. VI. Fungus granuloma, fungus "id" reaction experimentally produced, *Bull. Pharm. Res. Inst. Osaka* **21**:7–18.

Kushida, T., and Watanabe, S., 1975, Canine ringworm caused by *Trichophyton rubrum*: Probable transmission from man to animal, *Sabouraudia* **13**:30–32.

Kwon-Chung, K. J., 1974, Genetics of fungi pathogenic to man, *CRC Crit. Rev. Microbiol.* **3**:115–133.

Lavalle, P., 1975, Effects of therapy with topical corticosteroids on dermatophytoses, in: *Mycoses: Proceedings of the 3rd International Conference, Sao Paulo 1974*, pp. 262–263, Scientific Publication No. 304, PAHO, Washington, D.C.

Lepper, A. W. D., 1969, Immunological aspects of dermatomycoses in animals and man, *Rev. Med. Vet. Mycol.* **6**:435–446.

Lepper, A. W. D., 1972, Experimental bovine *Trichophyton verrucosum* infection: Preliminary clinical, immunological, and histological observations in primary infected and reinoculated cattle, *Rev. Vet. Sci.* **13**:105–115.

Lepper, A. W. D., 1974, Experimental bovine *Trichophyton verrucosum* infection: The cellular responses in primary lesions of the skin resulting from surface or intradermal inoculation, *Res. Vet Sci.* **16**:287–298.

Levene, G. M., 1973, Chronic fungal infection (*E. floccosum*), erythroderma, immune defficiency and lymphoma, *Proc. R. Soc. Med.* **66**:745–746.

Lewis, G. M., and Hopper, M. E., 1937, Ringworm of the scalp. IV. a) Comparative reactions to cutaneous tests with trichophytin in children with and without ringworm of the scalp; b) Evaluation of therapy with stock vaccines in types of infection resistant to treatment, *Arch. Dermatol.* **36**:821–832.

Lewis, G. M., and Hopper, M. E., 1948, *An Introduction to Medical Mycology,* 3rd ed., Year Book Publishers, Chicago.

Lewis, G. M., Hopper, M. E., and Scott, M. J., 1953, Generalized *Trichophyton rubrum* infections associated with systemic lymphoblastoma, *Arch. Dermatol.* **67**:247–262.

Lewis, G. M., Hopper, M. E., Wilson, J. W., and Plunkett, O. A., 1958, *An Introduction to Medical Mycology,* 4th ed., Year Book Publishers, Chicago.

Lobitz, W. C., Jr., Honeyman, J. F., and Winkler, N. W., 1972, Suppressed cell-mediated immunity in two adults with atopic dermatitis, *Br. J. Dermatol.* **86**:317–328.

Longhin, S., and Olaru, V., 1970, The value of immunotherapy in dermatomycoses, in: *Proceedings of the 2nd International Symposium of Medical Mycology 1967* (W. Sowinski, ed.), pp. 181–183, Poznan, Poland.

Lorincz, A. L., and Sun, S. H., 1963, Dermatophyte viability at modestly raised temperatures, *Arch. Dermatol.* **88**:393–402.

Lorincz, A. L., Priestly, J. O., and Jacobs, P. A., 1958, Evidence for a humoral mechanism which prevents growth of dermatophytes, *J. Invest. Dermatol.* **31**:15–17.

McDevitt, H. O., 1976, Genetic considerations in atopic and other dermatologic conditions, *J. Invest. Dermatol.* **67**:320–326.

Mandel, E. H., 1960, Diagnosis: Tinea circinata and onychomycosis (*Trichophyton purpureum*) : Resistance to griseofulvin during uncontrolled diabetes, *Arch. Dermatol.* **82**:1027–1028.

Many, H., Derbes, V. J., and Friedman, L., 1960, *Tri-chophyton rubrum*: Exposure and infection within household groups, *Arch. Dermatol.* **82**:226–229.

Marcussen, P. V., 1937, Relationship of the urticarial to the inflammatory reaction to trichophytin, *Arch. Dermatol.* **36**:494–514.

Marks, R., and Dawber, R. P. R., 1972, In sito microbiology of the stratum corneum, *Arch. Dermatol.* **105**:216–221.

Marmor, M. F., and Barnett, E. V., 1968, Cutaneous anergy without systemic disease, *Am. J. Med.* **44**:979–989.

Marples, M. K., and Bailey, M. J., 1957, A search for the presence of pathogenic bacteria and fungi in the interdigital spaces of the foot, *Br. J. Dermatol.* **69**:379–388.

Meyer, J., Sartory, R., and Touillier, J., 1952, Sur la nature protéique des trichophytines et leur composition en amino-acides, *C. R. Acad. Sci.* **234**:2224–2226.

Miller, D. L., 1974, "Id" reactions associated with dermatophytosis, *Cutis* **13**:1019–1022.

Miller, H. E., Stewart, R. A., and Kimura, F., 1941, "Undenatured trichophytin," Preparation and clinical application, *Arch. Dermatol.* **44**:804–815.

Minocha, Y., Pastricha, J. S., Mohapatra, L. N., and Kandhari, K. C., 1972, Proteolytic activity of dermatophytes and its role in the pathogenesis of skin lesions, *Sabouraudia* **10**:79–85.

Miura, T., 1968, Clinical application of the fluorescent antibody technic to dermatomycosis, *Tohoku J. Exp. Med.* **96**:165–170.

Montgomery, H., 1967, *Dermopathology,* Vol. I, Harper and Row, New York.

Neisser, A., 1902, Plato's Versuche über die Herstellung und Verwendung von "Trichophytin," *Arch. Dermatol. Syph.* **60**:63–76.

Nelson, L. M., and McNiece, K. J., 1959, Recurrent Cushing's syndrome with *T. rubrum* infection, *Arch. Dermatol.* **80**:700–704.

Noble, W. C., and Somerville, D. A., 1974, *Microbiology of Human Skin,* W. B. Saunders, Philadelphia.

Nozawa, Y. T., Noguchi, H., Uesaka, H., and Ito, Y., 1970, Studies on the immunologically active substances of the dermatophytes: Enzymatic digestion of polysaccharide-peptide complexes isolated from *Trichophyton mentagrophytes* and their immunochemical properties, *Jpn. J. Med. Mycol.* **11**:159–165.

Nozawa, Y. T., Noguchi, T., Ito, Y., Sudo, N., and Watanabe, S., 1971, Immunochemical studies on *Trichophyton mentagrophytes, Sabouraudia* **9**:129–138.

Olaru, V., 1974, Detection of antifungal antibodies fixed to lymphocytes and polymorphonuclear neutrophils: A new immunoallergic test in dermatomycosis, in: *Dermatology: Proceedings of the XIV International Congress, Padua-Venice, 22–27, May 1972* (F. Flarer, F. Serri, and D. W. K. Cotton, eds.), pp. 744–745, Excerpta Medica, Amsterdam.

Ottaviano, P. J., Jones, H. E., Jaeger, J., King, R. D., and Bibel, D., 1974, Trichophytin extraction: Biological comparison of trichophytin extracted from Trichophyton mentagrophytes grown in a complex medium and a defined medium, *Appl. Microbiol.* **28:**271–275.

Page, W. J., and Stock, J. J., 1974, Phosphate-mediated alteration of the *Microsporum gypseum* germination protease specificity for substrate: Enhanced keratinase activity, *J. Bacteriol.* **117:**422–431.

Partridge, B. M., 1955, Multiple fungous infections with special reference to their occurrence with the *Trichophyton rubrum* syndrome, *Tr. St. John's Hosp. Dermatol. Soc.* **34:**41–46.

Peck, S. M., and Hewitt, W. L., 1945, The production of an antibiotic substance similar to penicillin by pathogenic fungi (dermatophytes), *Pub. Health Rep.* **60:** 148–163.

Peck, S. M., and Siegel, S., 1947, Immunologic relationships of the antibiotic and trichophytin: Clinical observations and animal experiments, *J. Invest. Dermatol.* **9:**165–185.

Peck, S. M., Rosenfield, H., and Glick, A. W., 1940, Fungistatic power of blood serum, *Arch. Dermatol.* **42:** 426–437.

Peck, S. M., Osserman, K. E., and Rule, A. H., 1972, Intercellular antibodies: Presence in a *Trichophyton rubrum* infection, *J. Invest. Dermatol.* **58:**133–138.

Pepys, J., Riddel, R. W., and Clayton, Y. M., 1959, Human precipitins against common pathogenic and nonpathogenic fungi, *Nature (London)* **184:**1328–1329.

Pillsbury, D. M., and Jacobson, C., 1955, Cushing's syndrome complicated by generalized *Trichophyton rubrum* infection, *Arch. Dermatol.* **67:**436.

Raubitschek, F., 1961, Mechanical versus chemical keratolysis by dermatophytes, *Sabouraudia* **1:**87–90.

Reinhardt, J. H., Allen, A. M., Gunnison, D., and Akers, W. A., 1974, Experimental human *Trichophyton mentagrophytes* infections, *J. Invest. Dermatol.* **63:**419–422.

Reiss, F., and Leonard, L., 1956, Failure of active immunization against *Trichophyton gypseum* infection in guinea pigs, *J. Invest. Dermatol.* **26:.**449–452.

Reyes, A. C., and Friedman, L., 1966, Concerning the specificity of dermatophytic reacting antibody in human and experimental animal sera, *J. Invest. Dermatol.* **47:**27–34.

Rippon, J. W., 1967, Elastase production by ringworm fungi, *Science* **157:**947.

Rippon, J. W., 1974, *Medical Mycology: The Pathogenic Fungi and the Pathogenic Actinomycetes,* W. B. Saunders, Philadelphia.

Rippon, J. W., 1975, Biochemical-genetic determinants of virulence among the dermatophytes, in: *Mycoses: Proceedings of the 3rd International Conference, Sao Paulo, 1974,* pp. 88–97, Scientific Publication No. 304, PAHO, Washington, D.C.

Rippon, J. W., and Garber, E. D., 1969, Dermatophyte pathogenicity as a function of mating type and associated enzymes, *J. Invest. Dermatol.* **53:**445–448.

Rippon, J. W., and Scherr, G. H., 1959, Induced dimorphism in dermatophytes, *Mycologia* **51:**902–914.

Rippon, J. W., and Varadi, D. P., 1968, The elastases of pathogenic fungi and actinomycetes, *J. Invest. Dermatol.* **50:**54–58.

Rivalier, E., 1960, Phénomènes d'immunité dans les dermatophyties, *Pathol. Biol.* **8:**307–317.

Roth, F. J., Boyd, C. C., Sagami, S., and Blank, H., 1959, An evaluation of the fungistatic activity of serum, *J. Invest. Dermatol.* **32:**549–556.

Rothman, S., and Lorincz, A. L., 1963, Defense mechanisms of the skin, *Annu. Rev. Med.* **14:**215–242.

Rothman, S., Smiljanic, A., Shapiro, A. L., and Weitkamp, A. W., 1947, The spontaneous cure of tinea capitis in puberty, *J. Invest. Dermatol.* **8:**81–98.

Sabouraud, R., 1910, *Maladies du Cuir Chevelu. III. Les Maladies Cryptogamiques: Les Teignes,* Masson et Cie, Paris.

Saeves, J., 1915, Experimentelle Beiträge zu Dermatomykosenlehre, *Arch. Dermatol. Syph.* **121:**161–236.

Saferstein, H. L., Strachan, A. A., Blank, F., and Bishop, C. T., 1968, Trichophytin activity and polysaccharides, *Dermatologica* **136:**151–154.

Sampei, H., 1950, On the antigenicity of trichophytin, *Jpn. J. Dermatol.* **60:**617; cited by Y. Ito (1965a).

Sarkisov, A., Petrovich, Kh. S. V., Nikiforov, L. I., Yablochnik, L. M., and Korolov, V. P., 1971, Immunization of cattle against ringworm, *Veterinarya* **47:**54–56.

Schmitt, J. A., Margard, W. L., and Meier, C. A., 1962, Variation in susceptibility to experimental dermatomycosis in genetic strains of mice. I. Preliminary studies, *Mycopathologia (Den Haag)* **18:**241–245.

Schönborn, C., 1967, Comparative studies of the geophilic *Microsporum* strains of edaphic, animal, and human origin, *Mykosen* **10:**425–440.

Schwab, J. H., 1975, Suppression of the immune response by microorganisms, *Bacteriol Rev.* **39:**121–143.

Seeliger, H. P. R., 1958, *Mykologische Serodiagnostik,* J. A. Barth, Leipzig.

Seeliger, H. P. R., 1962, Serology of fungi and deep fungus infections, in: *Fungi and Fungous Diseases* (G. Dalldorf, ed.), pp. 158–186, Thomas, Springfield, Ill.

Seeliger, H. P. R., 1965, *Progress in Immunobiological Standards,* Vol. 2, pp. 154–163, Karger, New York.

Silva, M., Kesten, B. M., and Benham, R. W., 1955, *Trichophyton rubrum* infections: A clinical, mycologic and experimental study, *J. Invest. Dermatol.* **25:**311–328.

Sorensen, G. W., and Jones, H. E., 1976, Immediate and delayed hypersensitivity in chronic dermatophytosis, *Arch. Dermatol.* **112:**40–42.

Sowinski, W., 1971, Trichophytic entrance sites into the nail in man, in: *Comptes Rendus des Communications, Vth Congrès de la Société Internationale de Mycologie Humaine et Animale* (H. Drouhet, ed.), pp. 111–112, Institut Pasteur, Paris.

Sternberg, T. H., Tarbet, J. E., Newcomer, V. D., and Winer, L. H., 1952, Deep infection of mice with *Trichophyton rubrum* (purpureum), *J. Invest. Dermatol.* **19:**373–384.

Stobo, J. D., Paul, S., Vanscoy, R. E., and Hermans, P.

E., 1976, Suppressor thymus-derived lymphocytes in fungal infection, *J. Clin. Invest.* **57**:319–328.

Stockdale, P., 1953, Nutritional requirements of the dermatophytes, *Biol. Rev.* **28**:84–104.

Stockdale, P. M., 1961, *Nannizzia incurvata* Gen. nov., sp. nov., a perfect state of *Microsporum gypseum* (Bodin) Guiart et Grigorakis, *Sabouraudia* **1**:41–48.

Strickler, A., 1915, The vaccine treatment of ringworm of the scalp, *J. Am. Med. Assoc.* **65**:224–227.

Sulzberger, M. B., 1928, The pathogenesis of trichophytids: The spontaneous passage of formed elements (spores) from the primary lesion into the circulating blood, *Arch. Dermatol.* **18**:891–901.

Sulzberger, M. B., 1929, Experimentelle Untersuchungen über die Dermatotropie der Trichophytonpilze, *Arch. Dermatol. Syph.* **157**:345–357.

Sulzberger, M. B., 1940, *Dermatologic Allergy,* Thomas, Springfield, Ill.

Sulzberger, M. B., and Kerr, P. S., 1930, *Trichophyton* hypersensitiveness of urticarial type, with circulating antibodies and passive transference, *J. Allergy* **2**:11–16.

Sulzberger, M. B., and Wise, F., 1932, Ringworm and trichophytin: Newer developments, including practical and theoretical considerations, *J. Am. Med. Assoc.* **99**:1759–1764.

Sulzberger, M. B., Rostenberg, A., and Goethe, D., 1937, Recurrent erysipelas-like manifestations of the leg, *J. Am. Med. Assoc.* **108**:2189–2193.

Sutter, E., 1917, Weitere Beiträge zur Lehre von der Immunität und Überempfindlichkeit bei Trichophytieerkrankungen, *Dermatol. Z.* **24**:65–99.

Svejgaard, E., Thomsen, M., Morling, N., and Christiansen, A. H., 1976, Lymphocyte transformation *in vitro* in dermatophytosis, *Acta Pathol. Microbiol. Scand. Sect. C* **84**:511–519.

Tagami, H., Watanabe, S., and Ofuji, S., 1973, Trichophytin contact sensitivity in guinea pigs with experimental dermatophytosis induced by a new inoculation method, *J. Invest. Dermatol.* **61**:237–241.

Tager, A., Lass, N., Avigad, J., and Beemer, A. M., 1973, Immunotherapy of superficial dermatomycoses, *Dermatologica* **147**:123–129.

Tate, P., 1929a, The dermatophytes or ringworm fungi, *Biol. Rev. Cambridge Philosophical Soc.* **4**:41–75.

Tate, P., 1929b, On the enzymes of certain dermatophytes or ringworm fungi, *Parasitology* **21**:31–54.

Tomomatsu, S., 1962, A serological study of experimental dermatomycoses using an antigen prepared from fungus mechanically disintegrated. V. Production of humoral antibody and skin hypersensitivity in test animals and man during griseofulvin therapy, *Bull. Pharm. Res. Inst. Osaka* **36**:20–35.

Tosti, A., Villardita, S., Fazzini, M. L., and Scalici, R., 1970, Contribution to the knowledge of dermatophytic invasion of hair—An investigation with the scanning electron microscope, *J. Invest. Dermatol.* **55**:123–134.

Traub, E. F., and Tolmach, J. A., 1935, Dermatophytosis:

Its treatment with trichophytin, *Arch. Dermatol.* **32**:413–421.

Truffi, M., 1904, Ricerche sulla tricofitina, *Clin. Med. Ital.* **64**:377–408.

Tschernogubow, N., and Muskatblüt, E., 1929, Klinische Beobachtungen über die Immunität bei oberflächlichen Pilzerkrankungen der behaarten Kopfhaut, *Arch. Dermatol. Syph.* **159**:46–72.

Turk, J. L., 1976, Leprosy as a model of subacute and chronic immunologic diseases, *J. Invest. Dermatol.* **67**:457–463.

Uri, J., Valu, G., and Békési, I., 1963, Production of 6-aminopenicillanic acid by dermatophytes, *Nature (London)* **200**:896–897.

Vanbreuseghem, R., 1961, Dermatophytes as saprophytes, *Recent Adv. Bot.* **4**:346–351.

Verotti, G., 1916, Un caso di micosi microsporica del cuoio capelluto da *Microsporum lanosum, G. Ital. Mal. Ven.* **57**:84–92.

Voldánová, K., Dvorsky, K., Bartak, P., Bilek, J., and Jilek, M., 1967, Serum antibodies in nodular granulomatose perifolliculitis of mycotic origin, in: *Recent Advances of Human and Animal Mycology* (L. Chmel, ed.), pp. 309–312, Slovak Academy of Science, Bratislava.

Walters, B. A. J., Chick, J. E. D., and Halliday, W. J., 1974, Cell-mediated immunity and serum blocking factors in patients with chronic dermatophytic infections, *Int. Arch. Allergy Appl. Immunol.* **46**:849–857.

Walters, B. A. J., Beardmore, G. L., and Halliday, W. J., 1976, Specific cell-mediated immunity in the laboratory diagnosis of dermatophyte infections, *Br. J. Dermatol.* **94**:55–61.

Walzer, R. A., and Einbinder, J., 1962, Immunofluorescent studies in dermatophyte infection, *J. Invest. Dermatol.* **39**:165–168.

Weary, P. E., 1968, Pityrosporum ovale: Observation on some aspects of host–parasite interrelationship, *Arch. Dermatol.* **98**:408.

Weary, P. E., and Canby, C. M., 1969, Further observations on the keratinolytic activity of *Trichophyton schoenleini* and *Trichophyton rubrum, J. Invest. Dermatol.* **53**:58–63.

Weitzman, I., 1964, Incompatibility in the *Microsporum gypseum* complex, *Mycologia* **56**:425–435.

Weitzman, I., Gordon, M. A., and Rosenthal, S. A., 1971, Determination of the perfect state, mating type, and elastase activity in clinical isolates of *Microsporum gypseum* complex, *J. Invest. Dermatol.* **57**:278–282.

Wharton, M. L., Reiss, F., and Wharton, D. R. A., 1950, Active immunization against *Trichophyton purpureum, J. Invest. Dermatol.* **14**:291–303.

Williams, C. M., 1927, The enlarging conception of dermatophytosis, *Arch. Dermatol.* **15**:451–469.

Wilson, J. W., 1959, Intradermal test in fungus disease, *Triangle,* **4**:30–35.

Wilson, J. W., Plunkett, O. A., and Gregersen, A., 1954, Nodular granulomatous perifolliculitis of the legs caused by *Trichophyton rubrum, Arch. Dermatol.* **69**:258–277.

Wood, S. R., and Cruickshank, C. N. D., 1962, The relation between trichophytin sensitivity and fungal infection, *Br. J. Dermatol.* **74**:329–336.

Yu, R. J., and Blank, F., 1973, On the mechanism of action of griseofulvin in dermatophytosis, *Sabouraudia* **11**:274–278.

Yu, R. J., Harmon, S. R., and Blank, F., 1968, Isolation and purification of an extracellular keratinase of *Trichophyton mentagrophytes, J. Bacteriol.* **96**:1435–1436.

Yu, R. J., Harmon, S. R., and Blank F., 1969a, Hair digestion by a keratinase of *Trichophyton mentagrophytes, J. Invest. Dermatol.* **53**:166–171.

Yu, R. J., Harmon, S. R., Wachter, P. E., and Blank, F.,

1969b, Amino acid composition and specificity of a keratinase of *Trichophyton mentagrophytes, Arch. Biochem. Biophys.* **135**:363–370.

Yu, R. J., Harmon, S. R., Grappel, S. F., and Blank, F., 1971, Two cell-bound keratinases of *Trichophyton mentagrophytes, J. Invest. Dermatol.* **56**:27–32.

Yu, R. J., Grappel, S. F., and Blank, F., 1972a, Inhibition of keratinases by α_2-macroglobulin, *Experientia* **28**:886.

Yu, R. J., Ragot, J., and Blank, F., 1972b, Keratinases: Hydrolysis of keratinous substrates by three enzymes of *Trichophyton mentagrophytes, Experientia* **28**:1512–1513.

Zaslow, L., and Derbes, V. J., 1969, The immunologic nature of kerion Celsi formation, *Dermatol. Int.* **8**:1–4.

21

Immunology of Candidiasis

J. M. A. WILTON and T. LEHNER

1. Introduction

The genus *Candida* contains a number of species which are associated with disease in man. *Candida albicans* is the principal organism associated with infection, but other species, such as *C. parapsilosis* and *C. kruseii,* are also pathogenic for man. Animal pathogenicity has been demonstrated for other species, such as *C. tropicalis* and *C. stellatoida.* The great majority of the literature on candida in man concerns *C. albicans* and thus most of this chapter will be concerned with the immunological aspects of infections by *C. albicans.*

C. albicans is a dimorphic fungus with two growth phases, the yeast (Y) form and the pseudohyphal (H) form. It is a commensal of the human gastrointestinal tract (Van Uden, 1960) and is found most frequently in the mouth but may also be recovered from the pharynx, small bowel, and feces (Cohen *et al.,* 1969). The organisms are found in the vagina but rarely recovered from normal skin (Winner, 1966). The carriage rate of the organism in the mouth, throat, and gut varies according to the population studied and the methods used for laboratory isolation, but is generally between 20% and 40% (Bartels and Blechman, 1962; Van Uden, 1960). The rate may increase if antibiotics are given (Smits *et al.,* 1966), although this not always found (McKendrick *et al.,* 1967). The number of organisms recovered from the mouth is affected by diurnal variation (Williamson, 1972) and in the vagina

J. M. A. WILTON and T. LEHNER ● Guy's Hospital Medical and Dental Schools, London Bridge, London SE1 9RT, England.

by endocrine influences, particularly those of pregnancy (Plass *et al.,* 1931). A comprehensive account of the biology of *C. albicans* has been given by Winner and Hurley (1964).

2. Classification of *C. albicans* Infections

2.1. Superficial Infections

The infections in man caused by *Candida* species, and *C. albicans* in particular, may be divided into two principal types. The most common are the superficial self-limiting infections of the oral and vaginal mucous membranes, which may be either acute or chronic. The oral infections with *Candida* (Table 1) have been classified by Lehner (1962), and the clinical manifestations of oral candidiasis have also been reviewed (Lehner, 1966a, 1975). Acute pseudomembraneous candidiasis (thrush) is most commonly found in neonates and very young children (Kozinn *et al.,* 1958). It also affects adults, particularly those with diabetes and malignant disease, especially leukemia and lymphoma (Lehner, 1964a). Acute atrophic candidiasis may follow thrush, and some cases of antibiotic sore tongue fall into this category (Lehner, 1966a). Acute atrophic candidiasis is associated with broad-spectrum antibiotic therapy, particularly the tetracyclines; the association of candida infections with antibiotic therapy has been reviewed (Seelig, 1966a,b). Corticosteroid therapy can also be associated with this type of candida infection, either topically (Lehner and Ward, 1970) or when inhaled for the treatment of asthma (Brompton Hospital–MRC, 1974). Vaginal thrush is commonly associated with pregnancy (Stanley *et*

**TABLE 1. Classification of Oral Infections
with *Candida albicans***

Acute	1.	Acute pseudomembraneous candidiasis (thrush)
	2.	Acute atrophic candidiasis
Chronic	1.	Chronic atrophic candidiasis (denture sore mouth)
	2.	Chronic hyperplastic candidiasis
		a. Chronic oral hyperplastic candidiasis
		b. Chronic localized mucocutaneous candidiasis with endocrine disorder
		c. Chronic localized mucocutaneous candidiasis
		d. Chronic extensive candidiasis

al., 1972) and occurs more frequently in women taking oral contraceptives (for review, see Barlow and English, 1973).

The most common form of chronic candida infection (Table 1) is chronic atrophic andidiasis (denture sore mouth) associated with the wearing of dentures (Cawson, 1966). The other form of chronic disease is chronic hyperplastic candidiasis. This has been further classified depending on the localization pattern of the lesions and possible endocrine involvement into four further subdivisions (Lehner, 1964b, 1975). These are (1) chronic oral candidiasis or candida leukoplakia (Cawson and Lehner, 1968); (2) the endocrine candidiasis syndrome (familial juvenile hypoparathyroidism, hypoadrenocorticism, and chronic candidiasis), where the lesions include the nails as well as the mouth; (3) chronic localized mucocutaneous candidiasis, where the mouth is the most common primary site, but the lesions also affect the nails, face, and scalp; and (4) chronic extensive candidiasis of the mouth, limbs, face, scalp, shoulders, and groin. Some cases of chronic mucocutaneous candidiasis have been associated with defective immunity, usually of the cell-mediated type, and these will be discussed later when the immunology of candida infections is reviewed.

Other forms of superficial candidiasis include candidal paronychia and interdigital candidiasis, and candidal folliculitis of the face. Candida has been associated with diaper rash and perineal and perianal candidiasis, in which case the organisms are believed to originate from the feces of the infant (Kozinn *et al.*,

1957). Candida gastroenteritis in infants has been distinguished from simple carriage (Kozinn and Taschdjian 1962). Allergy to candida has been associated with bowel disease in adults (Holti, 1966), although Davenport and Wilton (1971) found no allergy to *C. albicans* in patients with chronic atrophic candidiasis. The organism has been known to spread from the intestines to internal organs in cases of infantile gasteroenteritis (Wagner and Kissel, 1958). Such dissemination may occur more often than was previously thought, since ingestion of 10^{12} cells of *C. albicans* by an adult volunteer was followed by positive blood and urine cultures up to several hours later (Krause *et al.*, 1969). Heat and moisture are associated with candida infection, as evidenced by the interdigital candidiasis and chronic candidial paronychia which occur in workers whose hands are constantly immersed in water. Similarly, infections of the groin, axilla, and below the breast are common sites due to the warmth and occlusion by clothing.

In a study of experimental cutaneous candidiasis in normal skin, Maibach and Kligman (1962) found that skin infection would occur only when the organisms were occluded with an impervious dressing, and even then only 50% of the subjects developed infection with 5×10^5 organisms. In a later paper Rebora *et al.* (1973) were able to produce infections in 95% of the subjects within 24 hr using 10^5 organisms. These infections were a pustular dermatitis of rapid onset, and hyphal forms were rare in smears taken from the lesions. These workers also showed that skin stripped to the dermis could also be easily infected, thus concluding that the anticandida factors demonstrated *in vitro* (see later discussion) were not protective, at least in this type of infection. This type of experiment does not induce a typical infection, and other more relevant models of candida infection will be discussed in relation to the protective effects of the immune response. *C. albicans* was associated with chronic urticaria in 26% of a series of 100 patients, although the authors pointed out that food agents such as *Saccharomyces cerevisae* are antigenically cross-reactive with *C. albicans* (James and Warin, 1971). This urticaria was of both Type 1 and Type 3 (Gell and Coombs, 1968).

2.2. Disseminated Infections

Candida infection may also take the form of a disseminated systemic infection which is most commonly iatrogenic. It occurs in patients receiving broad-spectrum antibiotics (Seelig, 1966a,b), cytotoxic drugs, and corticosteroids (Steinberg et al., 1972). Systemic infection is also associated with indwelling venous catheters (Louria et al., 1962), heart valve grafts and prostheses (Murray et al., 1969), renal allografts (Rifkind et al., 1967), hyperalimentation (Curry and Quie, 1971), and burns (MacMillan et al., 1972). These predisposing factors have also been reviewed in particular relation to pediatric practice (Papageorgiou and Alqusus, 1976).

In some cases the generalized disease is associated with thrush or candida-infected gastric ulcers or cancer of the colon (Symmers, 1966). The source of the infection is often not known with certainty, although the patient may be a carrier of the organism. It appears that this type of infection has increased with widespread use of cytotoxic and immunosuppressive drugs, cardiac and transplantation surgery, and venous catheterization, since systemic candidiasis was rather rare before the introduction of these regimens (Winner and Hurley, 1966; Meyer et al., 1973; Taschdjian et al., 1973; Allen, 1976).

3. Antigenic Structure of C. albicans

The antigenic structure of C. albicans is extremely complex, and the relationship of any particular antigen or antigens with disease is not clear at the present time. C. albicans can be divided into two antigenic groups, groups A and B (Hasenclever and Mitchell, 1961b). The group A organisms contain at least one more antigen than the group B organisms, when assayed by agglutination using cross-adsorbed antisera to each of the two groups. Tsuchiya et al. (1961) using the agglutination method detected seven antigenic determinants on the surface of C. albicans yeast forms, and this extended to ten antigens by Murray and Buckley (1966), also using agglutination tests.

The cell wall polysaccharides of C. albicans include glucan, mannan, and chitin (Bishop et al., 1960), and the hyphal form contains more chitin but less mannose than the blastospore (Chattaway et al., 1968). A glucomannan–protein complex was isolated from Candida species by Kemp and Solotorowsky (1964) and Kessler and Nickerson (1959). The former workers showed that the antigens were located in the cell wall of C. albicans and that they are shared by not only other Candida species but also Torulopsis glabrata. In addition, some antigens were apparently present in both the cell wall and cytoplasm, although protein antigens were not found in cell walls of the yeast form. Other studies have shown that the principal antigen in the cell wall is mannan, a highly branched polymer of mannose (Summers et al., 1964; Yu et al., 1967). Mannan has been demonstrated by electron microscopy to be evenly distributed over the cell surface of C. utilis (Gerber et al., 1973) and C. albicans (Müller et al., 1975).

The findings of Kemp and Solotorowsky (1964) that there was cross-reactivity between Candida species confirm earlier work by other investigators (see review by Salvin, 1959) and further complicate the attempts to develop a specific serodiagnostic test for candida infections in general and C. albicans in particular. Although it may be advantageous to have cross-reactivity within Candida species when screening tests are performed, the extension of this cross-reactivity to other fungi, especially when clinical isolation of the organisms is lacking or ambiguous, as in deep-seated candida infection, makes definitive serological diagnosis rather difficult. The cross-reactions of Candida species have been investigated in immunized guinea pigs and the cross-reacting antibodies reside in both the early IgM and late IgG classes (Segal et al., 1975). The cross-reactions of Candida species, including some with Mycobacterium tuberculosis and Salmonella species, have been reviewed by Seeliger et al. (1975). The use of these cell wall antigens in clinical diagnosis will be discussed later.

Extensive studies have also been made of antigens from the yeast phase cytoplasm and antigens found in cell-free culture filtrates from C. albicans. When these extracts were injected into rabbits by various routes, the antiserum contained from nine to 16 precipitin arcs, depending on the route of immunization and whether an adjuvant was used (Biguet *et al.*, 1962, 1965). In these studies, there was extensive cross-reactivity with other *Candida* species, although two antigens were apparently restricted to *C. albicans*. The complexity of cytoplasmic antigens of *Candida* has also been found by Axelsen (1971), using rabbits immunized with *C. albicans* and the technique of quantitative immunoelectrophoresis. The number of precipitin arcs detected in the immunized animals ranged from 46, using phenol-treated disrupted cells to 68 when the cells were not phenol treated. This number was later increased to 78 (Axelsen, 1973). This author (Axelsen, 1976) has reviewed the current status of quantitative immunoelectrophoresis and the usefulness of this type of analysis compared to other methods of precipitin analysis, particularly in the diagnosis of human infections. Some of the antigens have been characterized in the cell wall, particularly mannan (Yu *et al.*, 1967) and a glycoprotein (Odds and Hierholzer, 1973), but none of the specific cytoplasmic antigens has been identified to date. The cell wall glycoprotein may also be found in a cytoplasmic fraction obtained by mechanical disintegration and has been used to coat latex beads, in an attempt to develop a new diagnostic test for systemic candidiasis (Stickle *et al.*, 1972).

Cell-free supernatants from *C. albicans* cultures also contain antigens (Chew and Theus, 1967), and the polysaccharide antigens are apparently identical with those mannan antigens found in the yeast cell wall (Chew and Theus 1967) and the cytoplasm (Pepys *et al.*, 1968; Taschdjian *et al.*, 1969). An interesting finding, which does not seem to have been extended, was the demonstration of an antigen apparently specific for the hyphal form of *C. albicans* (Evans *et al.*, 1973). This antigen did not, unfortunately, have any diagnostic value and has not yet been isolated and purified (Odds *et al.*, 1975).

It is evident, then, that the antigenic structure of *Candida* species is complex and that extensive cross-reaction occurs both within the genus and with other fungi and bacteria. A virulence antigen (or antigens) has not yet been isolated. Although group A is more frequently isolated from clinical material than group B, there does not appear to be any de-

tectable differences in the pathogenicity of the two groups, at least in human infection (Hasenclever and Mitchell, 1963b). There is a great need for the preparation and interlaboratory comparison of defined antigens from *C. albicans*. Until this is done, no meaningful comparison can be made between the work of different investigators who have used a variety of antigen extraction methods from a large number of strains. In this respect, the International Union of Immunology has recently set up a subcommittee of their Standardization Committee to prepare standard antigens for lymphocyte function tests. There is general agreement that the currently used tests for candida infection, particularly disseminated infection, are unsatisfactory. Since these are difficult to diagnose clinically, and either the organisms cannot be isolated or their diagnostic significance is missed (Taschdjian *et al.*, 1973), the need for a standardized antigen preparation is self-evident. Not only must the antigen be standardized but also the method for antibody detection must be carefully controlled.

4. Pathogenicity of *C. albicans*

Candida albicans is a commensal organism, and, as will be discussed, there is little evidence that infection by the organism is due to virulent strains or to the acquisition of virulence by commensal strains. It would appear that changes in the host contribute most to the susceptibility to infection with *C. albicans* (Table 2). The precise basis for the pathogenicity of *C. albicans* is still unknown, but there is general agreement that the yeast (Y) or blastospore form is not generally associated with disease and that the hyphal (H) form is the usual pathogenic feature of both animal and human infections (Gresham and Burns, 1960; Mackenzie, 1966). Both Y and H forms are found in the infected tissues of the oral and vaginal mucosa, the commonest sites for candida infection, and both forms are also found in infections of the kidneys, lung, stomach, kidney, urine, and the ear. A general review of the different organs and tissues infected with *Candida* may be found in the symposium edited by Winner and Hurley (1966). It has clearly been shown that the clinical onset of

TABLE 2. Host Factors Contributing to the Susceptibility of Infection with *Candidia albicans*

Physiological:	Neonatal period and infancy
	Pregnancy
Genetic:	Familial chronic mucocutaneous candidiasis
Immunological:	Severe combined immunodeficiency, or Swiss and Gitlin agammaglobulinemia
	DiGeorge syndrome
	Nezelof syndrome
Traumatic:	Skin maceration
	Narcotic addiction
	Venous and urinary catheterization
Atopic:	Skin allergy
	Pulmonary allergy
Endocrine:	Diabetes mellitus
	Hypoadrenalism
	Hypothyroidism
	Hypoparathyroidism
Nutritional:	Malnutrition
	Malabsorption
Malignancy:	Leukemia
	Lymphoma, especially Hodgkin's disease
	Thymoma
	Advanced cancer
Antibiotic:	Broad-spectrum antibiotics
Drugs:	Corticosteroids
	Immunosuppressive drugs
	Cytotoxic drugs
Phagocytic:	Myeloperoxidase-deficient phagocytes
	Agranulocytosis
Miscellaneous:	Post operative, especially cardiac and transplant surgery
	Aplastic anemia
	Iron deficiency
	Oral contraceptives

thrush in neonates is preceded by hyphal transformation of the blastospore (Rogers, 1957; Taschdjian and Kozinn, 1957).

4.1. Toxicity of *Candida* Species

4.1.1. Endotoxins

In an attempt to find out the means whereby *Candida* causes disease, some investigators have looked for evidence of toxic factors produced by *Candida*. Such a toxin might cause damage to the superficial tissues and could allow the fungus to penetrate more deeply, particularly the hyphal form.

Salvin (1952) showed that mice are rapidly killed after intraperitoneal inoculation with dead *C. albicans,* especially when mixed with complete Freund's adjuvant, and attributed this mortality to an endotoxin. He also showed that soluble candida cell components and other species of *Candida* were also lethal for mice. The lethal effect of *C. albicans* cells was potentiated by mucin, which is an interesting finding in view of the infection of mucous membranes by *C. albicans*. Evidence for an endotoxin was also obtained by Dobias (1957). Mice injected intravenously with a soluble extract of sonically disintegrated *C. albicans* died after 2 hr and showed toxic symptoms. Roth and Murphy (1957) found that a similar preparation from disrupted yeast cells was not lethal for mice, unless injected in combination with chlortetracycline. A lesser effect was obtained with oxytetracycline, and none was observed with chloramphenicol or streptomycin. A culture filtrate of *C. albicans* caused erythema when injected into the skin of rabbits and guinea pigs (Winner, 1958). Both the cell-free extract from *C. albicans* and the broken cell walls were lethal for mice after intravenous injection (Mourad and Friedman, 1961). In contrast, Chattaway *et al.* (1971) could not demonstrate any toxicity when *C. albicans* extracts from yeast or hyphal forms were injected into mice, although the living cells used for the extracts were lethal after intravenous injection. These workers used the same extraction methods as previous workers (Mourad and Friedman, 1961; Kobayashi and Friedman, 1964; Louria *et al.,* 1963).

It would appear that some strains of *C. albicans* may produce an endotoxin(s) which is lethal for a number of laboratory animals, but the evidence for a toxic effect of *C. albicans* in either superficial or disseminated human infections is less convincing. It was suggested that an endotoxin was responsible for the collapse and shock seen in patients with *Candida* septicemia (Braude and Rock, 1959). This was supported to some extent by Dennis and Peterson (1964), who induced shock and, in some cases, death in dogs that had been injected intravenously with a soluble extract from disrupted *C. albicans*. A human volunteer who ingested a large dose (10^{12}) of *C. albicans* became ill with shivering, pyrexia, and headache 2 hr later. Although some organisms penetrated the gut mucosa, and could be found in blood and urine cultures taken during this time, most of the fungi remained in the gut (Krause *et al.*, 1969). More direct evidence for toxins in the pathogenesis of human candida infections was obtained from the studies of Maibach and Kligman (1962). These workers showed that a cell-free extract from ruptured cells or the cell walls would induce a pustular dermatitis in occluded skin in about 75% of volunteers; the skin was not penetrated by *C. albicans*. In a later paper it was confirmed that hyphal transformation of yeast was not necessary for this type of lesion (Rebora *et al.* 1973).

In most of the animal and human experiments cited above, the dose of *Candida* organisms and the amount of toxin used were very large, and it is questionable whether these types of experiments can be extrapolated to the disease process in man. Other workers have found a similarity between the *C. albicans* endotoxin and the lipopolysaccharide (LPS) endotoxin from gram-negative bacteria by demonstrating a fever curve similar to that given by LPS (Braude *et al.*, 1960; Isenberg *et al.*, 1963; Kobayashi and Friedman, 1964). These studies used the classical hot-phenol extraction method used for LPS (Westphal and Jann, 1965) to obtain the pyrogenic fraction. In a very extensive study of the toxicity of *C. albicans* whole cells and extracellular components, Cutler *et al.* (1972) showed that there were at least two toxic components and that contamination by bacterial endotoxin was not responsible for the toxicity shown by *C. albicans*. The phenol extracts from *C. albicans* was lethal for mice in very high doses but nonpyrogenic for rabbits, the pyrogenicity remaining in the cell residue. A glycoprotein from *C. albicans* has been shown to be toxic for newborn mice (Mankowski, 1968) and to bind to mast cells, causing them to degranulate and release histamine (Nosal *et al.*, 1974). This latter property may help to explain the relationship between *C. albicans* and allergic asthma in which serum antibodies to the organism cannot be detected (Pepys *et al.*, 1968).

The injection of viable *C. albicans* intravenously into mice caused thrombocytopenia and shortened the clotting time of plasma from treated mice. Cell-free sonicated extracts from both live and dead organisms aggregated platelets *in vitro*, but although viable *C. albicans* was lethal, killed cells and culture supernatant extracts were without effect (Holder and Nathan, 1973). This work clearly demonstrated the dissociation between virulence and toxicity of *C. albicans* which has not been previously stressed in many of the papers investigating these two properties. More recently, *C. albicans* has been shown to activate complement by the alternative pathway (Ray and Wuepper, 1975). This observation could lead to a promising line of research into the mechanisms of pathogenicity of *Candida*, since complement can function both to protect and to cause damage, as will be discussed later.

At the present time, it can only be concluded that none of the toxic effects of *C. albicans* demonstrated in animal models has as yet been clearly shown to be relevant to human infections. There is also evidence that not all strains of *C. albicans* have a toxic effect (Chattaway *et al.*, 1971) and that there is no correlation between the pathogenicity of a strain and the possession of toxic activity (Holder and Nathan, 1973). More experiments are needed to resolve the findings of different workers. It is possible that the pathogenicity of *Candida* may be associated with other factors such as thrombocytopenia, complement activation, and enzyme production.

4.1.2. Proteolytic Enzymes

A variety of enzymes have been demonstrated in *C. albicans* yeast cells and hyphal forms. These include proteases (Staib, 1965), alkaline phosphatase (Chattaway *et al.*, 1971), a cell-associated leucine aminopeptidase (Kim *et al.*, 1962), an excreted peptidase (Remold *et al.*, 1968), and a plasma coagulase (Zaikaria and Elinouv, 1968). There is some evidence for the association of enzyme-producing strains and the ability of *C. albicans* strains to infect and kill mice (Staib, 1969). Acid phosphatase can be shown in extracts of both yeast and hyphal forms, and the specific activity of the enzymes was greatest from mycelial forms but this was reversed when whole cells were used (Chattaway *et al.*, 1971). It was suggested that any correlation with pathogenicity and phosphatase activity would depend on the enzyme at the cell surface and that either the yeast or hyphal form could be pathogenic.

No toxic effects have been shown *in vivo* or *in vitro* with purified enzymes. The pH optima of many of the enzymes make it unlikely that there is any significant pathogenic effect in naturally occurring candida infections. Enzymes which have been implicated in the pathogenicity of some bacteria, such as neuraminidases or phospholipases, have not been found in *C. albicans* (Chattaway *et al.*, 1971). Although other enzymes may be isolated from *C. albicans* in the future, the present evidence is against any significant pathogenicity of *C. albicans* being associated with proteolytic enzymes.

4.2. Models of Infection with *C. albicans*

4.2.1. Comparison of Y and H Forms of *C. albicans*

It is still unclear which form of organism is responsible for the tissue penetration. Taschdjian *et al.* (1960), using a mouse model of vaginal candidiasis, showed that the Y form played an essential part in tissue penetration and that the H form initiated the tissue reaction of the host which gave the characteristic lesion. The H form of *C. albicans* was found to be more virulent than the Y form in mice, but this heightened pathogenicity was also statistically related to the culture medium used for the assay (Saltarelli *et al.*, 1975). For example, blastospores were found to transform within 1 hr of instilling the organisms into the rabbit lung (Damodaran and Chakravarty, 1973). Hyphal transformation was also enhanced by a combination of factors *in vitro* studies (Barlow *et al.*, 1974). A small polypeptide from seminal fluid and a factor (or factors) associated with albumin in serum, when combined with physiological level of glucose at about 11 μmol/liter and a temperature of 37°C, sustained mycelial growth of *C. albicans*.

The Y form will induce epithelial hyperplasia in chick chorioallantoic membranes and H forms are found invading the cells (Cawson, 1973). The important role played by glucose in the growth of *C. albicans* was emphasized by Knight and Fletcher (1971), who showed that the growth of *C. albicans* in saliva from patients with diabetes mellitus and patients treated with broad-spectrum antibiotics or corticosteroids was directly proportional to the

glucose concentration in saliva. Saliva, which was inhibitory to candida, would support the growth of the organism only when glucose was added.

In experimental animals the Y form of *C. albicans* was shown to be more pathogenic as regards both mortality after intravenous or intraperitoneal injection and lesion size after intradermal inoculation (Simonetti and Strippoli, 1973). Since no histological investigation of the lesions was performed, it cannot be said which form was predominant. Increasing doses of *C. albicans* were proportionately more lethal for mice, but increasing doses of hyphal forms had little effect on survival times (Mardon *et al.*, 1975). The cell mass and the numbers of viable units in each preparation were comparable in this study. If *C. albicans* was given orally to gnotobiotic mice, the organism colonized the gut; no hyphal forms could be found over a 4-week period and the mice remained well (Wagner and Srivastava, 1975). Hyphal forms themselves produce blastospores (Chattaway *et al.*, 1973), and, if a toxic factor or factors were produced by the blastospore which allowed tissue growth of hyphae, then the decreased pathogenicity of the Y form might be due to the time taken for sufficient blastospores to be produced by hyphae. *C. albicans* pathogenicity was related to hyphal transformation in the mouse when compared with other *Candida* species, and the Y–H transformation was demonstrated in tissue sections (Hill and Gebhardt, 1956). Nickerson *et al.* (1956) using a mutant blastospore from a previously virulent hyphal form of *C. albicans* showed that the blastospore regained virulence in the mouse. Eisman *et al.* (1953) noted that Y forms were more virulent than H forms; conversely, it has also been demonstrated that isonicotinic acid hydrazide (which inhibited hyphal growth) would protect against infection with *C. albicans* (Gresham and Whittle, 1961).

It is apparent that the morphological form of *C. albicans* in relation to the transition from commensalism to parasitism is controversial. It is appreciated that the Y–H transformation can be induced biochemically (Winsten and Murray, 1956) or by heat (Chattaway *et al.*, 1973). Thus the hyphal form may not always be a prerequisite for pathogenicity, which may depend on other diverse factors, such as the type of tissue infected, antibiotic and cytotoxic drug therapy, and the defense mechanisms of the host. An excellent account of these different factors has been presented by Winner (1969). Electron microscopic investigations do not show substantial differences between the structure of the yeast and hyphal forms, although biochemical differences between the two forms have been demonstrated (Chattaway *et al.*, 1968).

The Y form has more mannan and less glucan than the H form, and this could be related to pathogenesis in the Y form since it has been shown that the yeast form mannan is toxic for mice (Kind *et al.*, 1972). Both qualitative and quantitative differences between the antigens of the two growth phases and a mycelial specific antigen have been reported (Evans *et al.*, 1973).

4.2.2. Superficial Infection with *C. albicans*

Many of the models investigating the differences in pathogenicity between the Y and H forms used injections of organisms and have not been strictly comparable to the usual superficial infection with *Candida,* and the Y form may be as important as the H form for the initiation of systemic infections. It is possible that *C. albicans* blastospores could be a pathogenic form, since electron microscopic studies have shown blastospores and hyphae penetrating epithelial cells (Montes and Wilborn, 1968; Cawson and Rajasingham, 1972). Other workers have used models of candida infection in which the organisms are applied to the oral mucosa of experimental animals. Jones and Adams (1970) induced acute oral candidiasis in 50% of rats inoculated with *C. albicans* and the lesion resembled those found in man. In a later paper Russel and Jones (1973a) found no difference between lesions induced by oral inoculation of either the blastospore or hyphal forms of the organism, although the hyphal phase was possibly more infective when the animals were fed a carbohydrate-rich diet. Tetracycline, administered before and after *C. albicans* inoculation, both prolonged the time that the organism could be recovered from the animals and increased the number of animals showing infection of the mouth (Russel and Jones, 1973b). Palatal candidiasis was induced in the monkey by inoculation of *C. albicans* under an acrylic denture

plate (Budtz-Jorgensen, 1971) and both yeast and hyphal forms were observed in the lesions; the hyphae were found to invade the epithelium but were restricted to the keratinized layer.

4.2.3. Drug Enhancement of Infection

In some cases animals have been pretreated with drugs, such as corticosteroids, which predispose to *C. albicans* infection (Louria *et al.*, 1960; Hurley, 1966). The results of this type of experiment suggest that steroids potentiate the virulence of *C. albicans* in the mouse and rabbit. It was pointed out, however, by Hurley and Fauci (1975) that these species are hypersusceptible to the effects of steroids and that the steroid-resistant guinea pig would be a more appropriate model for human studies. Using a guinea pig model of disseminated candidiasis in which the kidneys and heart were the principal organs infected (Hurley and Fauci, 1975), it was shown that only long-acting glucocorticosteroids would potentiate infection and depress established cell-mediated immunity to *C. albicans* (Hurley *et al.*, 1975). The development of cell-mediated immunity was not affected, and the authors suggested that the use of short-acting steroids was preferable in order to reduce the risk of candida infection.

4.2.4. Humoral Immunity and Infection

Candida species, particularly *C. albicans,* are pathogenic in animals when inoculated either intraperitoneally or intravenously (Fuentes *et al.*, 1952; Mankowski, 1957; Hasenclever, 1959; Winner, 1960; Hasenclever and Mitchell, 1961a). Animals immunized with *C. albicans* develop antibodies which may be detected by agglutination and precipitation reactions (Stallybrass, 1964; Matthews and Inman, 1968). Matthews and Inman (1968) also showed that both IgG and IgM antibodies were produced and that they had specificity for a mannan-rich antigen. Winner (1956, 1958) noted that rabbits would produce agglutinating antibodies but that the antibodies did not confer resistance to infection with *C. albicans.* Injection of mice and rabbits with *C. albicans* produced antibodies, but neither active immunization nor passive transfer of antibodies protected mice against subsequent infection (Hurd and Drake, 1953). In contrast, other workers have shown that active immunization of mice with *C. albicans* will protect them from rechallenge (Mourad and Friedman, 1961; Hasenclever and Mitchell, 1963a; Soles *et al.*, 1967).

4.2.5. Complement and Candida Infection

Morelli and Rosenburg (1971a) showed that *C. albicans* was more lethal for complement (C5) deficient mice than for normal mice. In a later paper they showed that fewer PMNs phagocytosed *C. albicans* in C5-deficient mouse serum than in normal mouse serum, but this was evident only in the first 10 min of incubation. There was no difference in killing by PMNs whichever serum was used (Morelli and Rosenburg, 1971b). The part played by complement in the lesions of *C. albicans* has been assessed in a guinea pig model, in which it was shown that infection under occlusive dressings produced a massive PMN infiltrate leading to sloughing of the lesion and elimination of the organisms (Sohnle *et al.*, 1976a). These results were attributed to both a direct chemotactic factor from *C. albicans* cytoplasm and alternative complement-pathway-derived chemotactic factors. When infection was produced with occlusive dressings, the organisms were also eliminated by the scaling of the keratinized layer, but this was dependent on cell-mediated immunity and the protection was transferable by peritoneal exudate cells to non-immune animals.

The suggestion that the cell wall mannan and complement were directly chemotactic for PMNs was first made by Davies and Denning (1972a). Weeks *et al.* (1976) showed that mannan was chemotactic in plasma for human PMNs, but cytoplasmic extracts had a lower activity. Using both a mucocutaneous and a systemic model of infection in young chickens, it was also shown that there was inverse relationship between virulence and the ability of either the whole organism or extracted mannan to generate chemotactic factors. Hyphal forms also generated chemotactic activity but to a lesser degree than blastospores. The most virulent strains yielded no significant chemotactic activity.

4.2.6. Cell-Mediated Immunity and Candida Infection

Cell-mediated immunity (CMI) or delayed hypersensitivity responses have also been ex-amined in experimental animals. Using a mouse thigh lesion as a model, *C. albicans* infection induced CMI to the fungus which was suppressed with azathioprine (O'Grady *et al.*, 1977). The presence of CMI to *C. albicans* did not accelerate candidal arthritis, as compared to unsensitized controls (Hollingsworth and Carr, 1973). Immunostimulation with BCG or *Corynebacterium parvum* protected mice immunosuppressed with cyclophosphamide and infected with *C. albicans* (Sher *et al.*, 1975). Monkeys with atrophic chronic candidiasis of the palatal mucosa developed cell-mediated immunity, and the infection cleared (Budtz-Jorgensen, 1973a). If the animals were treated with azathioprine, both before and during the first 2 weeks of infection, then a thrush-like lesion developed and hyphae invaded the keratinized mucosa. The infection did not clear until CMI developed to *C. albicans,* and antibodies to the organism were not apparently protective.

Salvin *et al.* (1965) showed that neonatally thymectomized mice were less resistant to a sublethal infection with *C. albicans* than normal mice, although more normal animals died when a lethal dose was used. Cutler (1976) was the first to show that congenitally thymus-deficient (nude) mice were more resistant to a lethal dose of *C. albicans* and renal clearance of the fungus was better at all times in the nude mice. Rogers *et al.* (1976) confirmed this resistance of the nude mouse to *C. albicans* infection and further showed that nude mice reconstituted with a syngeneic thymus graft became susceptible as normal mice to intravenous injection of the organisms. They suggested that CMI might actually enhance the susceptibility of the animals to systemic candidiasis and that the protective role for CMI in man might be restricted to superficial and mucocutaneous candidiasis. As will be discussed later, defects of CMI are associated with persistent chronic mucocutaneous candidiasis in man and this rarely progresses to systemic candidiasis.

4.2.7. Hormones and Candida Infection

Animals which have been treated with estrogens have increased susceptibility to *C. albicans* infections (Mankowsky, 1957). In contrast, Rifkind and Frey (1972a) showed that male mice remained infected with *C. albicans* for longer periods than females, although the number of organisms in the urine was the same for each sex. Gonadectomy increased clearance of candidae in both sexes. In further experiments agglutinin titers to killed *C. albicans* were higher in females than in males and the titers in males increased if the mice were gonadectomized. When infected with live *C. albicans,* there was no difference between males and females in antibody titer and the antibodies were not protective (Rifkind and Frey, 1972b). Although some forms of candidiasis are associated with genetic defects and endocrine disorders, such as hypoparathyroidism, there is no apparent sexual discrimination by *C. albicans,* so that the relevance of such experiments to human candida infection is not clear at present.

5. Mechanisms of Immunity to Candida Infection

Although the majority of people have antibodies to *C. albicans* in their serum both agglutinating (Winner and Hurley, 1966; Lehner, 1966b) and precipitating antibodies (Lehner, 1966b; Chew and Theus, 1967; Axelsen *et al.*, 1975), other, nonantibody factors which protect against *C. albicans* have been described.

6. Serum and Secretory Antibodies

6.1. Direct Antibody Effector Mechanisms

The literature on the direct effect of human specific antibody on *C. albicans* blastospores and hyphal forms is contentious. Antibody enhances the growth of *C. albicans* by inhibiting the clumping factor (Louria *et al.*, 1972; Smith and Louria, 1972), but other workers have shown no effect on direct killing or clumping factor (Lehrer and Cline, 1969a; Davies and Denning, 1972a). These differences could be explained by the use of hyperimmune serum by Smith and Louria (1972) and of low-titer antibodies by Davies and Denning (1972a). Occasional reports of morphological changes apparently induced by antibody have been noted (Winner and Hurley 1966), but these observations were made *in vivo* in which it is difficult to ascribe an exact role to antibody. A direct effect of γ-globulin from rabbits

immunized with *C. albicans* was shown by Grappel and Calderone (1976), using nonimmune rabbit serum with no detectable candida agglutinin as a control. The control serum both increased oxygen uptake by blastospores and induced hyphal transformation, whereas the immune serum, or a γ-globulin fraction, inhibited oxygen uptake and hyphal transformation, although agglutinating the blastospores. These data suggest that antibodies may prevent the Y-H transformation and thus inhibit the dissemination and pathogenic potential of the organism. Agglutinating antibodies to candida will, of course, clump the organism but the *in vivo* significance of this phenomenon is obscure (Winner, 1955).

IgA antibodies might interfere with fungal colonization of mucous surfaces, and both Chilgren *et al.* (1967) and Lehner *et al.* (1972b) have found salivary IgA antibodies to *C. albicans* to be deficient in some patients with mucocutaneous candidiasis. It is not known, however, whether the defect predisposes to clinical disease or follows the disease. In addition, all the patients had defects of cell-mediated immunity and this is probably more important in determining resistance to infection. Some patients also had defects of IgG antibodies to *C. albicans* (Lehner *et al.*, 1972b). It is possible that such a defect could lead to diminished phagocytosis of the organism by phagocytes, or, alternatively, in case this is due to the formation of antigen–antibody complexes, modulate lymphocyte function. In general, though, antibody titers of all classes in serum and saliva are raised in most cases of candida infection and the protective role of these will be dealt with in the next section.

6.2. Indirect Effector Mechanisms

6.2.1. Opsonization

The principal way in which antibodies mediate their protective effect against microorganisms is to opsonise them for efficient phagocytosis (Winkelstein, 1973). At the same time complement may be activated, increasing the efficiency of the system (Scribner and Fahrney, 1976). There are many reports, both in man (Louria and Brayton, 1964b; Lehrer and Cline, 1969a; Davies and Denning, 1972b; Schmid and Brune, 1974; Verhaegen *et al.*, 1976; Wilton *et al.*, 1977a) and in animals (Hill and Gebhardt, 1956; Brune *et al.*, 1972, 1973), of phagocytosis of *C. albicans* by leukocytes, demonstrating that antibody and complement are necessary for optimal phagocytosis. In some cases complement also apparently enhanced killing (Davies and Denning 1972b; Schmid and Brune, 1974), but this is probably a function of the decreased uptake of candidae by polymorphonuclear leukocytes (PMNs). Wilton *et al.* (1977b) have shown that binding of *C. albicans* to human PMNs is complement dependent. Complement operates in phagocytosis via the IgG Fc receptor present on both the macrophage and the polymorphonuclear leukocyte (Ehlenberger and Nussenzweig, 1977).

The blastospore of *C. albicans* has been used most frequently in phagocytosis studies. Live organisms have been usually employed so that killing may also be assessed. It is generally assumed that the hyphal form could escape being phagocytosed and that this contributes to its pathogenicity. Furthermore, unless the blastospores are killed, hyphal transformation can take place and rupture the cell, leaving the organism free to proliferate. This has been shown in PMNs of the mouse and rabbit (Louria and Brayten, 1964b; Damodaran and Chakravarty, 1973) and also in mouse macrophages (Young, 1968; Stanley and Hurley, 1969; Winner, 1972). Many investigators use large inocula of *Candida*, and this may overwhelm the phagocytes. However, if small inocula are used, up to 90% of *C. albicans* blastospores are ingested and killed (Davies and Denning, 1972b), even if they are forming hyphae. In addition, it was shown that hyphal forms less than 12 μm in length were phagocytosed and killed, whereas hyphal forms less than 200 μm were killed apparently by an extracellular killing mechanism, the PMNs adhering to the large hyphae only in the presence of antibody and complement. Hyphae larger than 200 μm were not killed.

In spite of the fact that *C. albicans* is apparently phagocytosed and killed by human serum containing specific antibody and complement, patients who have high levels of candida antibodies (measured by a variety of serological techniques) have poor resistance to candida infection (Brody and Finch, 1960; Drake, 1954; Winner, 1955; Lehner 1966a,

1970; Lehner *et al.*, 1972b). This could be due to a variety of factors, such as a large antigenic load, deficient leukocyte killing, and the presence of plasma inhibitors of phagocytosis (Goldman and Th'ng, 1973; Verhaegen *et al.*, 1976); some of these will be discussed in later sections, especially in relation to systemic candidiasis. Much of the available evidence suggests that cell-mediated immunity is more important for defence against *C. albicans* than humoral antibodies and this will also be discussed later. One fact which may contribute to diminished uptake of *C. albicans*, especially in superficial lesions, was the demonstration by Wilton *et al.* (1977a,b) that inflammatory polymorphs from the gingival crevice are defective in phagocytosing candida and that this is due to a defective C3b receptor. Recent work has also shown that PMNs from rheumatoid synovial fluid have the same defect (Wilton *et al.*, 1978).

6.2.2. Phagocytic Cells

Successful elimination of microorganisms depends on the phagocytes, and this process is further dependent on opsonization discussed in the previous section. Additional studies illustrating the importance of phagocytes in *C. albicans* infections, particularly where there is a defect inherent to the phagocytic cells, will now be discussed. Such defects may occur at several stages of the inflammatory process and may consist of a failure of phagocytes to respond to chemotactic stimuli, disordered locomotion of cells, or enzyme deficiencies leading to intracellular survival of the ingested organisms.

6.3. Chemotactic Defects

As might be expected, failure of phagocytic cells to migrate to sites of inflammation predisposes to severe infections. This defect has been shown in PMNs of patients who are susceptible to candida infections, e.g., newborn infants (Miller, 1969), patients with diabetes mellitus (Mowat and Baum, 1971a). patients with Chediak-Higashi syndrome (Clark and Kimball, 1971), and patients with chronic mucocutaneous candidiasis (Van Scoy *et al.*, 1975; Lawton *et al.*, 1976). Chemotactic defects have also been reported for the monocytes in a patient with chronic mucocutaneous candidiasis (Snyderman *et al.*, 1973). In contrast, defects of chemotaxis have been reported in patients with disease in which candida infections are uncommon (Mowat and Baum, 1971b; Hill *et al.*, 1974; Dahl *et al.*, 1976). Candida infections do not seem to be associated with another defect of PMN motility, the lazy leukocyte syndrome, in which random migration of PMNs is impaired (Miller, 1975). Although some of the defects described are intrinsic to the cell, others may be due to defects of serum factors, especially complement, which generate chemotactic factors (Alper and Rosen, 1975), and even to enhanced inactivation of the chemotactic factors (Ward and Berenberg, 1974).

Pyogenic infections with a variety of bacteria are most commonly associated with defects of neutrophil chemotaxis and locomotion (for reviews, see Quie, 1972; Cline, 1976; Daughaday and Douglas, 1976). Many of these patients are receiving broad-spectrum antibiotic treatment, and some antibiotics can apparently cause depression of neutrophil chemotaxis (Martin *et al.*, 1974). These chemotactic and leukotactic defects are rarely the only defects in a patient and they may be associated with other immune defects such as hypergammaglobulinemia E and defects of cell-mediated immunity (Dahl *et al.*, 1976; Lawton *et al.*, 1976). The use of cytotoxic drugs and steroids often complicates analysis in these patients, and some of the defects observed may be the result of treatment, either with steroids (Gabrielsen and Good, 1967; Humbert, 1975) or with tetracyclines, and not intrinsic to the phagocyte. Clearly however, candida infection is not particularly common in these conditions and, when present, may be related to other immunological disorders.

6.4. Phagocytic Defects

The ability of phagocytes to ingest opsonized *C. albicans* has already been discussed. Depressed phagocytic activity to a number of bacteria is found in diseases where there is an increased susceptibility to *C. albicans* infections, such as liver disease (Rankin, 1963), diabetes mellitus (Bybee and Rogers, 1964), lymphomas and leukemias (Miller, 1962), pregnancy (Mitchell and Sbarra, 1965), and severe burns (Grogan and Miller, 1973). Candida infections are associated with acute myeloblastic leukemia (AML) (Bodey, 1966; Preisler *et al.*, 1969), but the phagocytic capacity of PMNs in these patients and those with chronic granulocytic leukemia (CGL) is a subject of controversy. Rosner *et al.* (1970) showed that untreated patients with CGL, but not AML, had a low phagocytic index against *C. albicans*. In contrast, Goldman and Th'ng (1973) using a higher candida-to-PMN ratio, could find no phagocytic defect with AML or CGL leukocytes. Leukopenia does not seem to be associated with an increased frequency of candida infection (Louria, 1976). Some patients with recurrent bacterial infections have a depressed ability to phagocytose *C. albicans* (Wilton *et al.*, 1977a). In those studies where phagocytic defects have been reported in patients prone to candidiasis, the patients have almost invariably been treated with steroids, cytotoxic drugs, and broad-spectrum antibiotics, such as aureomycin, tetracycline, hydrochloride, and sulfonamides. All these agents have been associated with depressed phagocytosis of other microorganisms, particularly by PMNs (Louria *et al.*, 1960; Munoz and Geister, 1950; Lehrer, 1971; Forsgren *et al.*, 1974). Other antibiotics such as polymyxin B and rifampicin do not appear to have this effect (Hoeprich and Martin, 1970).

There is great variation in the methods used to test phagocytic functions of PMNs and monocytes, and such factors as organism-to-phagocyte ratios, the type of serum used, and the criteria of phagocytosis have not been comparable. In addition the concentration of drugs, where these have been studied *in vitro*, are higher than those usually achieved therapeutically. In the case of tetracycline it is known that the phagocytes can actually concentrate the drug, so that these particular experiments may be relevant to the clinical situation (Park and Dow, 1970). Therapeutic concentrations of sulfonamides inhibit the candidal activity of human PMNs (Lehrer, 1971).

6.5. Killing Defects

Normal human PMNs and monocytes can kill *C. albicans in vitro*, contributing to the defenses of the host against fungal infection (Lehrer, 1971). The principal mechanism of killing by both types of phagocytes is mediated by myeloperoxidase (MPO) and hydrogen peroxide, among the principal microbicidal mechanisms of these cells (Klebanoff, 1967). The absence of MPO in PMNs has been described in two patients, one male and one female, with reduced levels of the enzyme in PMNs of four male siblings. The male patient developed systemic candidiasis at the age of 49, and his PMNs could not kill *C. albicans* blastospores but would kill *C. parapsilosis* slowly (Lehrer and Cline, 1969b). The PMNs from the three siblings tested killed *C. albicans* normally. It was later shown that the monocytes from this patient also lacked candidicidal activity for *C. albicans* but killed *C. parapsilosis* and *C. pseudotropicalis* with increased efficiency (Lehrer, 1975). Myeloperoxidase deficiency has also been described in some patients with megaloblastic anemia, in which both deficient PMNs and normal PMNs are found (Lehrer *et al.*, 1972). In chronic granulomatous disease PMNs and monocytes (Oh *et al.*, 1969) were unable to kill *C. albicans* or *C. parapsilosis* (Lehrer, 1975). The importance of this mechanism in the protection against candida infections must be seen in perspective, since other nonmyeloperoxidase fungicidal mechanisms have subsequently been described both for PMNs and monocytes (Lehrer, 1972, 1975; Lehrer *et al.*, 1975).

Polymorphonuclear leukocytes from patients with CGL appear to kill *C. albicans* normally (Lehrer and Cline, 1971; Goldman and Th'ng, 1973). However, in patients with acute myeloid or myeloblastic leukemia, *C. albicans* killing by PMNs is depressed (Lehrer and Cline, 1971; Goldman and Th'ng, 1973; Wilkinson *et al.*, 1975). The defect in most cases appears to be inherent to the cell and present in untreated cases of the disease; but plasma factors from these patients also depress the normal fungicidal acitivity of normal PMNs, the defect in the leukemic cells being partly reversible in normal homologous serum. Inhibition of phagocytosis in patients with reticuloendothelial neoplasms has also been shown in an animal model (Kimball and Brody, 1963). Killing of *C. albicans* by PMNs from patients with diabetes mellitus is normal (Cline, 1976).

7. Complement

There is no evidence that complement can have a direct effect on *C. albicans* blastospores or hyphal forms (Lehrer and Cline, 1969a). The biological effects of complement, both protective and damaging, are mediated by antigen–antibody complexes (Movat, 1976) or by the alternative pathway of complement (Götze and Muller-Eberhardt, 1971) and the generation of biologically active fragments, particularly from C3 and C5. Particularly important in resistance to infection are the chemotactic factors of PMNs and macrophages and the receptor for C3b on both types of phagocytic cell (Lay and Nussenzweig, 1968). The phagocytic cells also have a receptor for the Fc portion of IgG molecules (Messner and Jelinek, 1970), and an organism coated with specific antibody and complement is efficiently opsonized for phagocytosis. No phagocytic defect was reported by Rosenfeld *et al.* (1976) in two patients with C5 deficiency, although they attributed this to high levels of candida-specific antibody, possibly obscuring any opsonic defect due to the absence of C5. One of the two patients studied had frequent episodes of oral and vaginal candidiasis and both patients had high levels of candida antibody. In a series of 12 patients with chronic mucocutaneous candidiasis, two had depressed levels of serum complement (Kirkpatrick *et al.*, 1971a). Three patients with chronic mucocutaneous candidiasis were shown to have decreased total serum hemolytic complement, while a fourth, uninfected member of the family had normal levels (Drew, 1973). *C. albicans* was shown to activate the alternative pathway of complement (Ray and Wuepper, 1975), an observation confirmed by Sohnle *et al.* (1976b) using C2-deficient human serum and either whole *C. albicans* blastospores or a soluble extract of the yeast phase. These workers also showed that both C3 and properdin were present in three of six biopsies from patients with chronic mucocutaneous candidiasis. They postulated that complement-derived chemotactic factors were responsible for the intense PMN infiltrate in the lesions and prevented the extension of *C. albicans* into the skin.

It is clear that the activation of complement by *C. albicans,* particularly by the alternative pathway, is an important defense mechanism against this pathogen. Chemotactic attraction of PMNs to sites of candida infection and phagocytosis of the organism will at least minimize the spread of organisms in superficial infections. Patients with homozygous C3 deficiency suffer repeated infections, both superficial and systemic, although infections with *Candida* were not noted (Alper *et al.,* 1972; Alper and Rosen, 1975). The activation of complement may also potentiate tissue damage (Movat, 1976; Wilton, 1977), thus leading to prolongation of the infection; this may be most pertinent to the damage found in disseminated candidiasis, particularly of the brain, heart, and kidney (Parker *et al.,* 1976), in which inflammation may lead to rapid irreversible dysfunction. Antibiotic therapy may also inhibit C3 activation by the alternative pathway, and it was shown that sulfadiazine, tetracycline, and gentamycin in therapeutic concentrations will inhibit C3 consumption (Alexander, 1975). Failure to activate C3 could lead to deficient opsonization and PMN chemotaxis, which could in turn lead to decreased resistance to *C. albicans* infection. Such observations could at least partly explain the association between broad spectrum antibiotic therapy and susceptibility to candida infection (Seelig, 1966a,b).

8. Nonantibody Mechanisms

8.1. Candida Clumping Factor

Roth and Goldstein (1961) described a factor in the serum from normal human subjects which could inhibit the growth of *C. albicans in vitro.* A candicidal factor for *C. albicans* was also found in normal human serum (Louria and Brayton, 1964a). In later studies an inhibitory antibody was found against this candicidal factor in serum from children with endocrine deficiencies (Louria *et al.,* 1967). This candicidal factor was found to clump candida organisms, leading to lower viable counts and an apparently lethal effect (Chilgren *et al.,* 1968); it was also found that interfering antibody was of the IgG class. The factor is found in leukemic patients, only after they have become infected with *C. albicans* or *Aspergillus* species (Preisler *et al.,* 1972). Louria *et al.* (1972) investigated the candida clumping fac-

tor further and found it in 98% of adults aged 21–50, 95% of children aged from 9 months to 9 years, 82% of newborns and infants, and 82% of patients over 50 years of age. It was reduced in a variety of diseases including carcinoma, leukemia, and diabetes but was absent in patients with mucocutaneous or systemic candidiasis. It was distinct from complement components and was not potentiated by transferrin. The clumping was caused by hyphal outgrowth from the yeast phase cells. The biological role of this factor is unknown, but it is of interest that patients with candidiasis lack the factor and patients with other diseases who are prone to candida infection have reduced levels. It has been suggested that since this activity is diminished by specific IgG antibodies to *C. albicans,* antibodies may actually promote the pathogenicity of the organism. This concept is difficult to accept, since both rabbit IgG antibodies to *C. albicans* and human serum will themselves promote hyphal transformation (Hendry, 1972; Smith and Louria, 1972). Although Smith and Louria (1972) suggested that antibody might preferentially bind to blastospores and thus inhibit clumping, they presented no evidence for this hypothesis. The relationship between the clumping factor and antibody which inhibits its action is complex, although it is clear that specific anticandida antibody is associated with depressed clumping factor activity. Its exact biological significance awaits further investigation.

8.2. Iron

Iron has been shown to reverse the normal growth-inhibiting activity of *C. albicans* by human serum (Caroline *et al.,* 1964). The relevance of this mechanism to the pathogenesis of candida infections was postulated by Caroline *et al.* (1969), who showed that patients with leukemia have iron-saturated transferrin in their serum and elevated serum levels of free iron. Transferrin does not itself inhibit the growth of *C. albicans in vitro* (Esterley *et al.,* 1967). This was confirmed by Hendry (1972), who also showed that iron was necessary for hyphal transformation by the yeast form and that this change was associated with an increase of catalase activity in the blastospores. She considered that since *C. albicans* in serum is catalase deficient, this could lead to enhanced killing of the organisms by the hydrogen peroxide based fungicidal mechanisms of polymorphonuclear leukocytes (Lehrer, 1969). In addition, sufficient unsaturated transferrin in normal serum would make iron unavailable for hyphal transformation and thus inhibit the pathogenicity of candidae.

Elin and Wolff (1973b) have shown that both pH and iron concentration are critical parameters, often neglected, when studying the growth of candidae in serum. They found that the growth of *C. albicans* in human serum was iron dependent and optimal when the pH was less than 6.3. At this pH, transferrin binds iron poorly, if at all, and the iron is available for candida growth. These data may explain the inconsistencies in work on the effects of serum on candida growth and hyphal transformation, both in animal and in human studies (Roth *et al.*, 1959; Roth and Goldstein, 1961; Caroline *et al.*, 1964; Landau *et al.*, 1964; Dabrowa *et al.*, 1965; Esterley *et al.*, 1967; Louria *et al.*, 1972).

In contrast to this concept of iron promoting the pathogenicity of *C. albicans,* it has been found that some patients with chronic mucocutaneous candidiasis were iron deficient, with normal iron-binding capacity and that after iron therapy some of the patients with iron deficiency showed clinical improvement (Wells *et al.*, 1972). It was considered that the iron might exert a protective function by improving the structural integrity of the oral and cutaneous epithelium (Higgs and Wells, 1973). In some cases the immunological functions of a proportion of anergic patients returned. This beneficial effect of iron has not been confirmed by many clinicians in this field.

The patients studied by Higgs and Wells (1973) were classified as having "familial chronic mucocutaneous candidiasis," and there might be an iron-related epithelial dysfunction in these patients which may either predispose to infection by or inhibit clearance of candida organisms. The lack of candida infection generally in patients with iron deficiency indicates that the relationship between iron deficiency and fungal disease is not simple. The effect of iron on the metabolism and structure of epithelial cells has been briefly reviewed by Chandra (1976). Other effects of iron which could be important in relation to candida infection, apart from the growth requirements

of the organism, are a reduction in leukocyte myeloperoxidase, deficient phagocytosis by PMNs, inadequate antibody production, and a deficiency of cell-mediated immunity. These last two phenomena could be related to defective antigen processing by monocytes and macrophages since these cells are essential for an optimal immune response (Unanue, 1972). It is also possible that the dissociation of iron binding by transferrin at low pH *in vitro* could make iron available in inflammatory sites, where the pH is low, and thus allow *C. albicans* to grow and transform into hyphae.

8.3. Bacterial Endotoxin-Induced Factor(s)

Hasenclever and Mitchell (1962, 1963c) demonstrated the protective effect of bacterial endotoxin given to mice before challenge with *C. albicans*. This protection could also be shown *in vitro,* since serum from endotoxin-treated animals inhibited the growth of *C. albicans*. This work was confirmed by Dobias (1964), and it was shown later that the protective effects of endotoxin-treated serum could be passively transferred (Wright *et al.*, 1969). The protection was bimodal, being optimal 1 and 6 days after endotoxin administration and unrelated to antibodies; the 6-day protection, however, appeared to be related to cellular proliferation in the spleen and kidney. The growth-inhibiting properties for *C. albicans* of serum from endotoxin-treated animals were also shown in human, rabbit, and guinea pig serum but not in dog serum (Elin and Wolff, 1973a). Endotoxin will also activate macrophages both *in vivo* (Nelson, 1972) and *in vitro* (Wilton *et al.*, 1975), so it is possible that the protective effect of endotoxin is mediated by an enhanced macrophage fungicidal capacity. The role of activated macrophages in protection from *C. albicans* infection will be discussed in Section 9.

The relevance of these observations to human candida infections is not at present known, since there are no published studies in man. In addition, since the broad-spectrum antibiotics which are often given for gram-negative bacterial infections may predispose to candida infection, the end result could be a potentiating rather than protective effect on *C. albicans* of gram-negative infection and endotoxin release. The relationship between endotoxin and *C. albicans* infections in disease in man must await further investigation.

9. Cell-Mediated Immunity

9.1. Genetic Defects

The best evidence for the importance of CMI in the protection from chronic candidiasis is derived from the study of patients with genetic defects of T-lymphocyte function secondary to thymic defects. These patients suffer from intractable chronic mucocutaneous candidiasis from birth and are unable to eliminate *C. albicans* from the mucosal surfaces, although systemic candidiasis is surprisingly rare. This may be an indication of the relative importance of CMI and humoral immunity in superficial and systemic candidiasis. Patients with B-lymphocyte defects alone are not susceptible to candidiasis, unless they also have a concurrent T-cell deficiency, as in the severe combined immunodeficiency syndromes. A full account of these defects and their clinical management may be found in the textbook edited by Stiehm and Fulginati (1973).

Defective generation and/or differentiation of lymphoid stem cells as seen in patients with the Swiss and Gitlin types of agammaglobulinemia (Hitzig, 1968; Fudenberg *et al.*, 1971) and thymic dysplasia (Miller and Schicken, 1967) is associated with chronic mucocutaneous candidiasis. In patients with congenital absence of the thymus gland (Nezelof, 1968; DiGeorge, 1968) and thymoma (Montes *et al.*, 1968; Schoch, 1971; Kirkpatrick and Montes, 1974), thrush, which progresses to chronic mucocutaneous candidiasis, is invariably an early sign of the underlying T-lymphocyte defect. Such profound deficiencies of the CMI system are rare, usually lethal, syndromes. Most cases of chronic mucocutaneous candidiasis cannot, however, be ascribed to them but consist of more subtle, nonlethal defects of T lymphocytes and macrophages.

9.2. Defects of Lymphocyte Function

The persistence of candida infections in patients with underlying cell-mediated immunodeficiencies was noted by Hermans *et al.* (1969). These patients are commonly anergic to skin testing with *C. albicans* and may also be anergic to other antigens and often are incapable to responding to a sensitizing dose of DNCB. In addition, many patients show single or multiple defects of *in vitro* lymphocyte function, both to *C. albicans* and to other antigens, when assayed by LT, MMI, and lymphocyte cytotoxicity tests (Chilgren *et al.*, 1967; Buckley *et al.*, 1968; Imperato *et al.*, 1968; Canales *et al.*, 1969; Folb and Trounce, 1970; Goldberg *et al.*, 1971; Kirkpatrick *et al.*, 1971a; Lehner *et al.*, 1972b; Budtz-Jorgensen, 1973b; Valdimarsson *et al.*, 1970, 1973). Patients with chronic mucocutaneous candidiasis are a very heterogeneous group and may have other abnormalities, such as endocrine dysfunction (Lehner, 1966a; Kirkpatrick *et al.*, 1971a; Montes *et al.*, 1972), ectodermal defects (Wuepper and Fudenberg, 1967; Kirkpatrick *et al.*, 1971a), malabsorption (Hermans *et al.*, 1969; Kirkpatrick *et al.*, 1971a), autoantibodies (Wuepper and Fudenberg, 1967; Kirkpatrick *et al.*, 1971a), and selective antibody deficiencies of all classes, particularly IgA (Chilgren *et al.*, 1967; Lehner *et al.*, 1972b). The exact mechanism leading to defective CMI seen in such conditions as malnutrition is obscure, but there is evidence that protein–calorie malnutrition is associated with generalized depression of CMI, defective antibody production, depressed levels of C3 (Escobar, 1976; Gross and Newberne, 1976), and defective PMN phagocytosis and bacterial killing (Douglas and Schopfer, 1974).

The association of defective CMI and autoantibodies is similarly obscure but may be associated with a lack of suppressor T lymphocytes which normally ensure homeostatic control of immune responsiveness. The presence of suppressor T cells has been demonstrated in patients with disseminated histoplasmosis and disseminated cryptococcosis but not in anergic patients with chronic mucocutaneous candidiasis (Stobo *et al.*, 1976). In a study of a patient with chronic mucocutaneous candidiasis with defective CMI, increased IgG anticandida antibodies, and no detectable IgA antibodies to *C. albicans*, transfer factor therapy was followed by a fall in titer of IgG antibodies and the appearance of IgA antibodies (DeSousa *et al.*, 1976). Since there was also an improvement in CMI *in vitro* assays to *C. albicans*, it was speculated that a population of suppressor T lymphocytes, which controlled antibody formation, had been stimulated by transfer factor to exert CMI responses and also to correct the defective antibody production.

9.3. Macrophage Activation

While it is clear that impaired cell-mediated immunity predisposes to *C. albicans* infection, the precise mechanism of protection by CMI is still unknown. Many of the lymphokines produced by antigen-activated lymphocytes affect the macrophage, and it is known that macrophages exposed to these lymphokines become activated in a number of different ways. Activated macrophages show increased glass adherence and spreading, with increased metabolic activity and enhanced phagocytic capacity (Nathan *et al.*, 1971, 1973; Simon and Sheagren, 1971, 1972a). It has also been demonstrated that biosynthesis of the cell membrane is decreased, leading to a decreased cellular motility, and that the levels of some hydrolytic and respiratory enzymes are increased (Poulter and Turk, 1975a,b). The bactericidal (Simon and Sheagren, 1972a; Fowles *et al.*, 1973) and killing (Anderson and Remington, 1974) capacities of the macrophage are enhanced when animals or humans are undergoing a cell-mediated immune reaction. The specifically sensitized lymphocyte is necessary to induce the macrophage to become activated; once activated, the increased macrophage bactericidal capacity is nonspecific and is directed against any organism tested, although recall of the activation is restricted to the eliciting antigen (Simon and Sheagren, 1972a; Fowles *et al.*, 1973; Mackaness, 1975). The antigens used to induce CMI need not themselves be microbial, and many of the model systems cited above have used protein antigens, such as γ-globulin (Simon and Sheagren, 1971; Fowles *et al.*, 1973).

The protective aspects of CMI in *C. albicans* infections must be largely extrapolated from the studies with protein and bacterial or protozoal antigens, but there is some evidence that the latter also apply to candida infections. Macrophages from mice infected with *C. albicans* and yielding *in vitro* CMI, as assessed by LTT, phagocytose *C. albicans* blastospores and prevent hyphal transformation (Winner, 1972). Macrophages from mice injected with

C. albicans showed an increased capacity to phagocytose killed blastospores (Salvin, 1974). Neither of these papers showed the data on which these assertions were based, so the precise role of the activated macrophage on *C. albicans* infections must await further investigation.

It has also been found that cell-free supernatants, containing MIF, from activated macrophages produce lymphokines that will enhance macrophage phagocytosis and bacteriostasis, provided that the supernatants are not Millipore filtered (Fowles *et al.*, 1973). The failure of Simon and Sheagren (1972b) to show this activity was probably due to the use of filtered supernatants. The leukocyte inhibitory factor (LIF), which inhibits migration of PMNs (Rocklin, 1974), does not appear to have been tested for enhancing activity of PMN phagocytosis or bactericidal capacity. Lymphokines have also been reported to have a direct fungicidal effect against *C. albicans* in the mouse (Pearsall *et al.*, 1973), but no fungicidal effect could be shown in a study using human lymphocyte culture supernatants (Weedon *et al.*, 1973). Both studies showed that supernatants contained lymphotoxin and would kill target cells. Lymphokines have been demonstrated *in vivo* in the serum of animals undergoing CMI responses (Yamamoto and Takahashi, 1971; Salvin *et al.*, 1973), and the injection of lymphokines into animals reduces circulating monocyte levels, suppresses unrelated skin reactions, and increases the accummulation of macrophages in lymph nodes of immunized animals (Kelly *et al.*, 1972; Yoshida and Cohen, 1974). Pulmonary washings from BCG-immunized rabbits were shown to contain a factor which promoted fusion of macrophages (MFF), and such fluids both increased the percentage of macrophages phagocytosing *C. albicans* and increased the number of blastospores taken up by each cell (Parks and Weiner, 1975).

Although there is no reason to believe that *C. albicans* should not be susceptible to the CMI protective mechanisms against other microorganisms, only studies using *C. albicans* will resolve this point. It must also be remembered that B lymphocytes can produce lymphokines, such as MIF, macrophage activation factor, and monocyte chemotactic factor (Yoshida *et al.*, 1973; Wilton *et al.*, 1975;

Mackler *et al.*, 1974; Rocklin *et al.*, 1974). Such lymphokines should also be tested, in addition to the T-lymphocyte-derived mediators, for their protective effect against *C. albicans*.

9.4. Classification of CMI Defects in Chronic Mucocutaneous Candidiasis

An outline of the stages necessary for an intact and fully functional cell-mediated immune response is shown in Fig. 1. This figure also includes the contribution of the B lymphocyte (especially as being under T-lymphocyte control) either enhancing or suppressing the antibody response to antigen. Using this scheme, it is possible to assign some of the defects of CMI seen in chronic mucocutaneous candidiasis to the different stages of development of the immune response to *C. albicans* antigens.

The absence of T lymphocytes (A) or their defective maturation due to the absence of a functional thymus (B), as seen in the Swiss and Gitlin types of agammaglobulinemia, DiGeorge and Nezelof syndromes, and patients with thymoma would be classified as fundamental defects. Also included here would be the lymphopenia reported in a patient with chronic mucocutaneous candidiasis due to a circulating lymphocytotoxin (Schlegel *et al.*, 1970). Under normal circumstances, the sensitized lymphocytes will produce mediators, become cytotoxic cells, and proliferate in response to specific antigenic challenge. Patients with

chronic mucocutaneous candidiasis have been reported who have defects of one or more of these functions. The macrophage is necessary for *in vitro* lymphocyte stimulation (Unanue, 1972) and mediator production (Wahl *et al.*, 1975), and candidiasis has been associated with a defect of macrophage function, leading to a failure of lymphocyte proliferation in response to *C. albicans* antigens (Twomey *et al.*, 1975). These macrophages would not support proliferation by lymphocytes normally responsive to *C. albicans*, and this defect would be classified as C. The failure of lymphocytes to respond to *C. albicans* antigens either as an isolated defect or in conjunction with the absence of responses to other antigens and depressed responses to mitogens would be assigned to D. The patients of Goldberg *et al.* (1971), Kirkpatrick *et al.* (1971a), Lehner *et al.* (1972b), and Valdimarsson *et al.* (1973) include cases which would fall into this category. The defect of proliferation may also be associated with a plasma inhibitor, classified as E. Lymphocytes of patients with such plasma inhibitors have been found to respond to *C. albicans* when cultured in allogeneic normal serum (Valdimarsson *et al.*, 1973; Canales *et al.*, 1969; Paterson *et al.*, 1971; Lehner *et al.*, 1972b; Twomey *et al.*, 1975).

Patients with chronic mucocutaneous candidiasis are also known who are unable to produce cytotoxic lymphocytes after stimulation with *C. albicans*. This defect, F, probably reflects the specific immunological unresponsiveness of lymphocytes to *C. albicans*, also

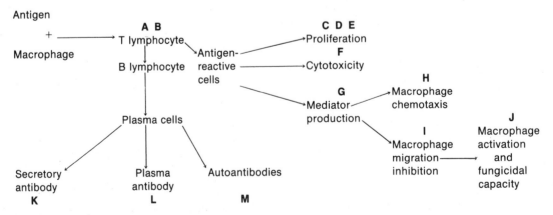

Figure 1. Successive stages in the development of cell-mediated immunity in man and a proposed classification of the defects found in patients with chronic mucocutaneous candidiasis.

manifested by failure of antigen specific pro-liferation and mediator production (Lehner *et al.*, 1972b). The failure of antigen-stimulated lymphocytes to produce MIF, although blas-togenesis is normal (Rocklin *et al.*, 1970a), leads to a defect of the efferent limb of CMI, which may be classified as G. This defect in mediator production is best correlated with the cutaneous anergy often found in these pa-tients; others have been described with cuta-neous anergy and normal *in vitro* MIF pro-duction (Valdimarsson *et al.*, 1973). Patients with defective MIF production have been de-scribed by Chilgren *et al.* (1969), Rocklin *et al.* (1970c), Kirkpatrick *et al.* (1971a), Lehner *et al.* (1972b), Schulkind *et al.* (1972), Valdi-marsson *et al.* (1973), Snyderman *et al.* (1973), Montes *et al.* (1972), and Rocklin *et al.* (1974). The failure of macrophages to respond to chemotactic stimuli (H) either lymphocyte de-rived or complement mediated has been re-ported (Snyderman *et al.*, 1973). The patients who produce MIF in response to *C. albicans* stimulation, but who have cutaneous anergy, may also have a macrophage defect of this type (Valdimarsson *et al.*, 1972b). They could also be classified in category I, since a patient with cutaneous allergy and normal MIF production has been described whose monocytes failed to respond when used as indicator cells to either autologous or homologous MIF (Goldberg *et al.*, 1971). This lack of responsiveness could also explain the failure of MIF injected *in vivo* into anergic patients to elicit a delayed hyper-sensitivity response, in contrast to the effec-tiveness of such MIF in control subjects (Val-dimarsson *et al.*, 1973). The essential fungicidal role of the macrophage (J) has been demon-strated by Lehrer and Cline (1969b). Although this defective killing was due to myeloperox-idase deficiency, the possibility also remains that monocyte or macrophage killing could be due to failure of normal macrophage activation by lymphokines. No defect of monocyte re-ceptors for immunoglobulin or complement could be found in three patients with chronic mucocutaneous candidiasis (Douglas and Goldberg, 1972).

The aberrations of antibody production are also classified in this scheme. It is likely that such abnormalities will reflect the overall T-lymphocyte control of antibody synthesis by B lymphocytes and plasma cells (Gershon, 1974). The patients with decreased titres of IgA antibodies in saliva (Chilgren *et al.*, 1967; Quie and Chilgren, 1971; Lehner *et al.*, 1972b) can be classified as K. Patients with chronic mucocutaneous candidiasis with elevated titer of serum antibody but with deficiencies of CMI (Chilgren *et al.*, 1967; Kirkpatrick *et al.*, 1971a; Lehner *et al.*, 1972b; Takeya *et al.*, 1976) are classified as L. This group possibly also includes the patients described by Cahill *et al.* (1974) who could produce only IgM an-tibodies to diphtheria toxin and who had pos-itive Schick tests even following toxoid im-munization. Finally, the frequent association of autoantibodies and chronic mucocutaneous candidiasis (Wuepper and Fudenberg, 1967; Kirkpatrick *et al.*, 1971a) is classified as M. The precise nature of the T-lymphocyte de-fects in categories K–M must await further investigation, particularly as regards whether they are due to lack of helper cells or increased suppressor cell activity. It is also possible that some of these types of defect may be due to defective macrophage function, since this cell is required for antibody production (Unanue, 1972).

The classification shown in Fig. 1 must re-main tentative at the present time, but the het-erogeneity of the defects is a prominent fea-ture. However, not all patients with chronic mucocutaneous candidiasis have demonstra-ble defect of CMI, and it may be that some of the serum factors described in previous sec-tions are responsible for the susceptibility to candida infection. The heterogeneity of CMI illustrates the delicate balance between *C. al-bicans* and host responses, such that a single defect, e.g., MIF production, can lead to a change from the commensal state to patho-genicity by the fungus.

10. Diagnosis of Candida Infections

10.1. Antibodies: Serum Antibodies to *C. albicans* in Normal Subjects

Agglutinating and immunofluorescent anti-bodies to *C. albicans* can be found in cord serum from babies at birth (Brody and Finch, 1960; Esterley, 1968; Russel and Lay, 1973), which are acquired transplacentally. There was no correlation in 50 babies between the presence of IgG antibody and neonatal colonization by *C. albicans,* or the subsequent development of thrush (Russel and Lay, 1973). Following a fall in titer during the first month of life, antibody titers rise during the infancy to the level found in adults (Brody and Finch, 1960; Esterley, 1968). Antibodies that can inhibit the growth of *Candida* (Roth *et al.,* 1959; Roth and Goldstein 1961) can also be detected which also increase in titer with age. Agglutinating antibodies are found in the serum of 20–64% of healthy adults (Drake, 1945; Winner, 1955; Salvin, 1959; Winner and Hurley, 1966; Lehner, 1966b). Immunofluorescent antibodies are also demonstrated in normal subjects (Lehner, 1966b; Esterley, 1968) in titers which correlate well with agglutinating antibody titers found in the same subjects (Lehner, 1966b). Complement-fixing antibodies have also been found in normal subjects; however, complement-fixation tests are unreliable and not in general use (Peck *et al.,* 1955; for review, see Taschdjian *et al.,* 1973). A parallel study of fluorescent agglutinating and precipitating antibodies to *C. albicans* showed that precipitating and fluorescent antibodies were of the IgG class but that agglutinating antibodies belonged to IgG, IgA, and IgM classes (Lehner *et al.,* 1972a).

10.2. Diagnosis of Candida Infections

10.2.1. Agglutinating and Immunofluorescent Antibodies to Serum and Saliva

It is evident from the many studies of antibodies to *C. albicans* in normal subjects free of clinically detectable disease that a large proportion will demonstrate agglutinating and immunofluorescent antibodies from an early age reflecting the ubiquity of the carriage of *Candida* species chiefly *C. albicans* (Lehner, 1966b). The prevalence of antibodies in the normal subject and the candida carrier makes it very difficult to diagnose candida infection with certainty.

Attempts have been made to establish the diagnosis on the basis of the titer of antibodies found. Lehner (1966b) showed that noncarriers commonly had fluorescent antibody titers of 1 : 8, carriers 1 : 16, and the majority of patients with clinical oral candidiasis had titers greater than 1 : 16. He concluded that the higher titers of fluorescent antibody, together with the clinical findings, were useful in the

diagnosis of candidiasis. Comaish *et al.* (1963) also related the titer of agglutinating antibodies to infection by using a carefully selected group of controls. In later work Lehner (1970) found significantly elevated fluorescent antibody titers in the IgG, IgA, and IgM classes in patients with candidiasis. A relationship between the severity of clinical infection and the titer of agglutinating antibodies was also found by Budtz-Jorgensen (1972), although some patients had no demonstrable antibody titer. This study also confirmed the one by Lehner (1966b) in that higher titers were found in candida carriers, as compared to normal controls. Candida antibodies have also been demonstrated in saliva from normal subjects, carriers, and patients with chronic mucocutaneous candidiasis and chronic oral hyperplastic candidiasis (Lehner, 1965). The elevated serum antibody titer was quantitatively related to the presence of antibodies in unconcentrated saliva, and it was considered that a serum titer greater than 1 : 32 and saliva titer of 1 : 1 or above indicated infection with *Candida.*

Serum agglutinating antibodies to *C. albicans* were also found to be in higher titer than the normal range in 12 patients with mucocutaneous candidiasis, but agglutinating antibodies in parotid saliva were within the normal range (Kirkpatrick *et al.,* 1970). Since there was a relationship between serum IgA and salivary secretory IgA antibodies (Lehner, 1965), it was possible to express the salivary IgA antibody levels as a ratio of the serum IgA antibodies (Chilgren *et al.,* 1967), and Lehner *et al.* (1972b) showed that normal subjects, candida carriers, and patients with candidiasis could be separated on this basis.

Although the validity of the agglutination and fluorescent antibody tests have been questioned in the diagnosis of some types of candidiasis (Winner, 1955; Taschdjian *et al.,* 1973), particularly visceral or systemic infections (Everett *et al.,* 1975), it would appear that by using a combination of carefully selected controls and estimating antibodies both in serum and in saliva, the diagnosis of oral mucocutaneous candidiasis can be made with some confidence.

10.2.2. Precipitating Antibodies

Precipitating antibodies are not detectable in so high an incidence as other types of antibodies in normal subjects; when they are found, the titers are low (Chew and Theus, 1967; Pepys *et al.*, 1968; Hellwege *et al.*, 1972). The antibodies in such studies were demonstrated with mannan-rich antigen preparations and may be a more reliable measure of the true incidence in the general population. Weiner and Yount (1976) detected mannan antibodies in nearly 100% of 234 normal subjects using a passive hemagglutination test. Other workers, however, in an attempt to find a serodiagnostic test for deep-seated or systemic candidiasis have used other candida antigens, chiefly cytoplasmic. It has been claimed that precipitating antibodies are restricted to patients with systemic candidiasis (Stallybrass, 1964; Taschdjian *et al.*, 1964, 1972; Remington *et al.*, 1972; Gaines and Remington, 1973). However, a number of normal control subjects have been found to have precipitating antibodies to cytoplasmic antigens (Stanley *et al.*, 1972; Warnock *et al.*, 1976). Although Stanley *et al.* (1972) found precipitins more frequently in patients with mycotic vulvovaginitis, Warnock *et al.* (1976) could not distinguish between patients with funguria and patients with bacteriuria and also found precipitins to *Torulopsis glabrata* mannan in the urine of patients with *C. albicans* funguria. Murray *et al.* (1969) also found precipitins in patients who had undergone cardiac surgery but who did not develop systemic candidiasis. Stanley and Hurley (1974) later considered that a positive precipitin test was useful in the diagnosis of candida vaginitis in pregnancy.

Axelsen *et al.* (1974), using an immunoelectrophoretic technique, found precipitating antibodies to a large number of *C. albicans* antigen in 15 patients with chronic mucocutaneous candidiasis but did not examine any controls. Patients with the highest precipitin titers had the highest number of individual precipitin arcs in this study. This technique is difficult to perform and requires a standardized antigen and a reference antiserum, so that it is not in general use. Until standard techniques, antigens, and antisera are available, a comparison between the results of different techniques is difficult in that the difference between studies may be methodological.

It has been suggested that in patients who are at risk of developing systemic candida infections blood should be taken before treatment starts since either a rising titer of agglutinins or the appearance of precipitating antibodies to *Candida* would be diagnostic of systemic candidiasis (Preisler *et al.*, 1969; Parsons and Nassau, 1974). Although the precipitin tests are not always positive only in infected patients, and a negative test may be due to an immunodeficiency, they are a valuable aid to diagnosis, particularly when carried out sequentially. A precipitin test, combined with the latex agglutination test, has been recommended by the American Society for Microbiology as being the best combination of tests in the present state of knowledge (Kaufman, 1976). The diagnostic serology of candida infections has been comprehensively reviewed by Taschdjian *et al.* (1973) and more recently by Axelsen (1976).

The group of patients with the endocrine candidiasis syndrome can be distinguished from other patients with chronic mucocutaneous candidiasis, even before clinical endocrine deficiency is manifest, as they possess precipitating antibodies to adrenal tissue (Heinonen *et al.*, 1976). A promising new technique, using mannan-coated erythrocytes in a hemagglutination inhibition assay has detected mannan in the blood in rising titer in 30% of cases with suspected deep-seated candida infection (Weiner and Yount, 1976). The test was negative in superficial candida infection or other invasive mycotic infections, with only three control patients being positive.

10.2.3. Secretory Antibodies in the Vagina

Antibodies to *C. albicans* mucopolysaccharide have been detected in up to 80% of vaginal secretions from healthy women using radioactive radial immunodiffusion, coprecipitation, and passive hemagglutination (Waldman *et al.*, 1971). The antibodies were shown to be of the secretory IgA class. Antibody titers in women with candida vaginitis were lower than in women not currently infected, possibly reflecting the binding of antibody to organisms *in vivo*. In contrast, Govers and Girard (1972), using a passive hemagglutination assay, found that only 48% of normal women had secretory IgA anticandida antibody and that higher titers were present in five patients with active candida infection. In a study of ten normal women secretory IgA antibodies to *C. albicans* were induced by intravaginal immunization using candida-coated pessaries; in some subjects, a rise in serum IgA antibody could also be demonstrated (Waldman *et al.*, 1972). The anticandida IgA antibodies found in oral and vaginal secretions could protect against infection by inhibiting fungal colonization.

10.3. Cell-Mediated Immunity

10.3.1. Delayed-Hypersensitivity Skin Tests

The incidence of cell-mediated immunity (CMI) to *C. albicans* reflects the widespread distribution of this organism in animal populations, as has been described for antibodies to the fungus. The commonest form of assessment for CMI is by the cutaneous delayed hypersensitivity reaction to *Candida* antigens. Using this technique, up to 95% of persons without demonstrable candidal infection will show delayed skin reactions to *C. albicans* (Salvin, 1959; Winner and Hurley, 1966; Shannon *et al.*, 1966; Davenport and Wilton, 1971). The diagnostic value of a positive skin test for candida infection is doubtful. Its value is mainly as part of a general skin test protocol to assess cell-mediated immunity, together with other bacterial antigens and contact sensitivity agents, such as dinitrochlorobenzine (DNCB), in patients with defects of CMI. The test also has some value when the results of immunotherapy in the treatment of chronic mucocutaneous candidiasis are being assessed.

10.3.2. *In Vitro* Tests of Lymphocyte Function

Recently developed *in vitro* tests of lymphocyte function have been used to investigate CMI in candida infections. These semiquantitative assays have the advantage of avoiding *in vivo* sensitization. Among the most commonly used assays is the lymphocyte transformation test (LTT). Antigen-stimulated lymphocytes, using T lymphocytes, will also produce biologically active substances which can then be assayed for their effects on other cells and provide further evidence for antigen-specific lymphocyte activation. One such test, commonly used in candida infections, is the macrophage migration inhibition test (MMI), where the normal migration of macrophages ˙ay be inhibited by supernatants containing ˙ration inhibitory factor (MIF) from anti-

gen-stimulated lymphocytes. A similar lymphocyte-dependent test in clinical use is the leukocyte migration inhibition test (LMI), using PMNs from peripheral blood. This may be carried out by incubating leukocytes from the patient together with antigen and measuring the degree of migration inhibition obtained. The LTT in general correlates well with the *in vivo* cellular hypersensitivity of the host (Mills, 1966), but the MMI and LMI appear to be the best qualitative correlates of cutaneous skin test reactivity (Rocklin *et al.*, 1970a; Budtz-Jorgensen, 1973b). There are some patients with chronic mucocutaneous candidiasis in whom the *in vitro* production of MIF is found, yet the skin test to *C. albicans* is negative (Kirkpatrick *et al.*, 1971a). These discrepancies may provide a clue to the precise nature of the underlying defect of CMI.

Antigen-stimulated lymphocytes can nonspecifically kill other target cells, such as chicken erythrocytes or tumor cells, the degree of this killing being proportional to the number of activated lymphocytes in the original population. Other tests of lymphocyte function include assays of chemotactic factors for PMNs and macrophages and activation of macrophages, detectable by their enhanced function, e.g., phagocytosis and killing of microorganisms. The clinical use of these lymphocyte function tests has been comprehensively reviewed by Rocklin (1974). When these *in vitro* tests are applied to a population without evidence of candida infection, they give essentially the same results, as skin testing for delayed hypersensitivity, although the number of positive tests is usually somewhat lower than when cutaneous testing is performed (Rocklin *et al.*, 1970a; Lehner *et al.*, 1972b, 1973; Budtz-Jorgensen, 1973b; Toh *et al.*, 1973; Valdimarsson *et al.*, 1973).

11. Immunotherapy of Candida Infections

Since deficient CMI predisposes to chronic mucocutaneous candidiasis, attempts have been made to replace the competent cells by grafting a variety of immune tissues. These techniques are particularly used when the source of cells is congenitally absent. Bone marrow grafts and thymus grafts have been used in cases of thymic aplasia and dysplasia in an attempt to provide the correct processing of the T lymphocytes. In the nonlethal candida infections, transfer factor has been used to correct the cellular immune defect (Lawrence, 1969), and this is discussed in this section.

11.1. Leukocyte Transfusion

The infusion of peripheral leukocytes from *C. albicans* sensitive donors into patients with chronic mucocutaneous candidiasis has been used in an attempt to transfer CMI (Kirkpatrick *et al.*, 1970, 1971b; Valdimarsson *et al.*, 1972a). No clinical improvement has usually been observed, and any beneficial effects have been transient. Most of the infusions have not been HLA matched, and death has invariably followed, often due to graft-vs.-host disease. The disadvantages of this technique have been reviewed by Kirkpatrick *et al.* (1971a).

11.2. Bone Marrow Transplantation

Transplantation of HLA-compatible bone marrow has been successfully used in cases of Swiss and Gitlin types of agammaglobulinemia (Gatti *et al.*, 1968). The lesions of candidiasis cleared, cutaneous delayed hypersensitivity appeared and lymphocyte function tests became normal. Two of the patients were regrafted later when the improvement showed signs of remission (Meuwissen *et al.*, 1969; Amman *et al.*, 1970). Bone marrow transplantation and intravenous amphotericin B were successful in a patient with defective CMI and chronic mucocutaneous candidiasis (Buckley *et al.*, 1968). The results in general are disappointing, and since unmatched bone marrow has usually been used (Kirkpatrick *et al.*, 1971a) most of the patients do not show clinical improvement and die.

11.3. Thymus Grafting

Early attempts to restore CMI by means of thymic grafts were uniformly unsuccessful (see review of Kirkpatrick *et al.*, 1971a). In no patient was clinical improvement noted, although some *in vitro* tests of lymphocyte function became positive. In some other patients clinical improvement with restoration of cutaneous reactivity and *in vitro* lymphocyte responses has been noted (Cleveland *et al.*,

1968; Hong *et al.*, 1968; August *et al.*, 1970; Buckley *et al.*, 1971; Levy *et al.*, 1971; Radl *et al.*, 1972). In other cases, only an improvement in lymphocyte function *in vitro* and an increase in the number of T lymphocytes has been found (Gatti *et al.*, 1972; Steele *et al.*, 1972; Kirkpatrick *et al.*, 1976). Not all the patients have survived for long periods, and the long-term effects of thymic transplantation are unknown. There are two patients who have maintained their immunological responsiveness for 6 years following transplantation (Cleveland, 1975). It is not known whether thymic grafting was appropriate for each case treated, and there is still doubt about the mechanism by which the graft exerts its restorative effect. In the patient treated by Amman *et al.* (1973) the graft acted as a source of cells since the recipient cells bore the antigens of the donor's mother. It is also possible that the thymus acts to provide humoral factors which allow the stem cells of the recipient to differentiate, as suggested by the work of Steele *et al.* (1972) and Kirkpatrick *et al.* (1976).

11.4. Transfer Factor

Transfer factor (TF) is a dialyzable, nonimmunoglobulin molecule of molecular weight 10,000, extracted from human leukocytes. It was first described by Lawrence (1955), who showed that extracts of disrupted leukocytes from donors with delayed hypersensitivity (DH) to bacterial antigens conferred specific DH to donors who were previously unresponsive to these antigens. Only DH is transferred, and there is no increase in specific antibody production following its administration (Good *et al.*, 1957; Lawrence, 1960). The identity of the cell(s) producing TF is not known at present, although the monocyte is probably not involved (Slaven and Garven, 1964).

The target cell(s) for TF is unknown. The principal target for TF is thought to be the lymphocyte, since in patients with Nezelof or Wiskot–Aldrich syndrome TF increases the number of peripheral T lymphocytes to normal levels (Wybran *et al.*, 1973; Kirkpatrick *et al.*, 1976). Restoration of DH skin reactions and the correction of some *in vitro* tests of lymphocyte function such as LT, MMI, and LMI also suggest that the lymphocyte is the principal target cell. Other cells may also be involved, however, since TF has been shown to correct defective chemotaxis and candida killing by PMNs in a patient with chronic mucocutaneous candidiasis (Lawton *et al.*, 1976) and defective monocyte chemotaxis (Snyderman *et al.*, 1973).

The therapeutic use of TF in chronic mucocutaneous candidiasis is based on an attempt to correct the defect of CMI often found in this disease. By correcting the CMI deficiency, it is hoped that the immune system will be able to eliminate the candida infection. There is no risk of graft-vs.-host reactions with TF, and, in general, the material is well tolerated with no serious side effects. The therapeutic effect is transient, and repeated injections are necessary to achieve clinical improvement and to correct the deficiencies of the *in vitro* test of lymphocyte funtion. TF is ineffective in patients with the granulomatous form of candidiasis who produce MIF but have cutaneous anergy and negative LT response to *C. albicans* (Valdimarsson *et al.*, 1973).

Clinical improvement following the administration of candida-specific TF to patients with chronic mucocutaneous candidiasis has been reported by a number of investigators (Chilgren *et al.*, 1969; Hitzig *et al.*, 1972; Pabst and Swanson. 1972: Schulkind *et al.*, 1972; Valdimarsson *et al.*, 1972b; Lawrence, 1974; Grob *et al.*, 1975; De Sousa *et al.*, 1976). In contrast, no clinical improvement was noted in some patients in whom TF was injected alone (Kirkpatrick *et al.*, 1970, 1972; Wybran *et al.*, 1973) or after the patient had received a thymus transplant (Kirkpatrick *et al.*, 1976). In most patients, DH to *C. albicans* antigens is restored; when MIF or LMIF has also been assayed, these mediators are produced *in vitro* after TF therapy. The induction of lymphocyte transformation by *C. albicans* is much more variable and reports range from no correction of negative LT (De Sousa *et al.*, 1976) to intermittent increases in LT (Kirkpatrick *et al.*, 1972; Lawton *et al.*, 1976), and there are no reported cases of permanent correction of LT. The restoration of MIF production in the absence of LT supports the findings of Rocklin *et al.* (1970) that MIF can be produced by nondividing lymphocytes.

The varied clinical and laboratory responses to TF therapy in patients with chronic muco-cutaneous candidiasis probably reflect the heterogeneity of the CMI defects in this condition (MacKie, 1975). In some cases the disappointing clinical responses may be due to the massive antigen load. Careful timing of TF therapy with antifungal therapy, such as amphotericin B, has led to successful clinical remission (Kirkpatrick and Montes, 1974). TF therapy is ineffective in patients with chronic mucocutaneous candidiasis where there is no underlying defect of CMI (Valdimarsson, 1974). Many of the reports on clinical improvement are based on studies of single patients. No double-blind trials of TF in chronic mucocutaneous candidiasis have as yet been reported. An improvement in this form of treatment must await a more precise evaluation of the cellular target(s) of TF and the identification of such cellular defects in patients with chronic mucocutaneous candidiasis.

References

Alexander, J. W., 1975, Antibiotic agents and the immune mechanisms of defense, *Bull. N.Y. Acad. Med.* **51**:1039–1045.

Allen, J. C. (ed.), 1976, *Infection and the Compromised Host*, Williams and Wilkins, Baltimore.

Alper, C. A., and Rosen, F. S., 1975, Increased susceptibility to infection in patients with defects affecting C3, *Birth Defects Orig. Art. Ser.* **11**:301–305.

Alper, C. A., Propp, R. P., Klemperer, M. R., and Rosen, F. S., 1972, Homozygous deficiency of C3 in a patient with repeated infection, *Lancet* **2**:1179–1181.

Amman, A. J., Meuwissen, H. J., Good, R. A., and Hong, R., 1970, Successful bone marrow transplantation in a patient with humoral and cell-mediated immunodeficiency, *Clin. Exp. Immunol.* **7**:343–353.

Amman, A. J., Ward, D. W., Salmon, S., and Perkins, H., 1973, Thymus transplantation: Permanent reconstitution of cellular immunity in a patient with sex linked combined immunodeficiency, *N. Engl. J. Med.* **289**:5–9.

Anderson, S. E., and Remington, J. S., 1974, Effect of normal and activated human macrophages on *Toxoplasma gondii*, *J. Exp. Med.* **139**:1154–1174.

August, C. S., Levay, R. H., Berkel, A. I., and Rosen, F. S., 1970, Establishment of immunological competence in a child with congenital thymic aplasia by a graft of fetal thymus, *Lancet* **1**:1080–1083.

Axelsen, N. H., 1971, Antigen–antibody crossed electrophoresis (Laurell) applied to the study of the antigenic structure of *Candida albicans*, *Infect. Immun.* **4**:525–527.

Axelsen, N. H., 1973, Quantitative immunoelectrophoretic methods as tools for a polyvalent approach to standardisation in the immunochemistry of *Candida albicans, Infect. Immun.* **7**:949–960.

Axelsen, N. H., 1976, Analysis of human candida precipitins by quantitative immunoelectrophoresis, *Scand. J. Immunol.* **5**:177–190.

Axelsen, N. H., Kirkpatrick, C. H., and Buckley, R. H., 1974, Precipitins to *Candida albicans* in chronic mucocutaneous candidiasis studied by crossed immunoelectrophoresis with intermediate gel, *Clin. Exp. Immunol.* **17**:385–394.

Axelsen, N. H., Buckley, H. R., Drouhet, E., Budtz-Jorgensen, E., Hattel, T., and Andersen, P. L., 1975, Crossed immunoelectrophoretic analysis of precipitins to *Candida albicans* in deep seated *Candida* infection: Possibilities for standardisation in diagnostic *Candida* serology, *Scand. J. Immunol.* **4**:217–230 (Suppl. 2).

Barlow, A. J. E., and English, M. P., 1973, Fungous diseases, in: *Recent Advances in Dermatology,* Vol. 3 (A. Rook, ed.), pp. 33–68, Churchill Livingstone, Edinburgh.

Barlow, A. J. E., Chattaway, F. W., and Aldersley, T., 1974, Factors present in serum and seminal plasma which promote germ-tube formation and mycelial growth of *Candida albicans, J. Gen. Microbiol.* **82**:261–272.

Bartels, H. A., and Blechman, H., 1962, Survey of the yeast population in saliva and an evaluation of some procedures for identification of *Candida albicans, J. Dent. Res.* **41**:1386–1390.

Biguet, J., Tran van Ky, P., Andrieu, S., and Degaey, R., 1962, Electrophoretic and immunochemical studies of the comparison of the antigen of some yeasts of the genus *Candida* (*C. albicans, C. stellatoidea, C. tropicalis, C. zeylanoides, C. krusei, C. pseudotropicalis, C. macedoniensis*), *Mycopathologica* **17**:239–254.

Biguet, J., Tran van Ky, P., Andrieu, S., and Degaey, R., 1965, Immunoelectrophoretic studies on the nature and order of appearance of precipitating antibodies as a function of the mode of immunisation with *Candida albicans, Sabouraudia* **4**:148–157.

Bishop, C. T., Blank, F., and Gardner, P. E., 1960, The cell wall polysaccharides of *Candida albicans, Can. J. Chem.* **38**:869–881.

Bodey, G. P., 1966, Fungal infection complicating acute leukaemia, *J. Chron. Dis.* **19**:667–687.

Braude, A. I., and Rock, J. A., 1959, The syndrome of acute disseminated moniliasis in adults, *Arch. Intern. Med.* **104**:91–100.

Braude, A. I., McConnell, J., and Douglas, A., 1960, Fever from pathogenic fungi, *J. Clin. Invest.* **39**:1266–1276.

Brody, J. L., and Finch, S. C., 1960, Candida-reacting antibodies in the serum of patients with lymphoma and related disorders, *Blood* **15**:830–839.

Brompton Hospital, Medical Research Council Collaberative Trial, 1974, Double-blind trial comparing two dosage schedules of beclomethasone dipropronate aerosol in the treatment of chronic bronchial asthma, *Lancet* **2**:303–307.

Brune, K., Leffel, M. S., and Spitznagel, J. K., 1972, Microbicidal activity of peroxideless chicken heterophile leucocytes, *Infect. Immun.* **5**:283–287.

Brune, K., Schmid, L., Glatt, M., and Minder, B., 1973, Correlation between antimicrobial activity and peroxidase contents of leukocytes, *Nature (London)* **245**:209–210.

Buckley, R. H., Lucas, Z. J., Hattler, B. G., Zmijewski, C. M., and Amos, D. B., 1968, Defective cellular immunity associated with chronic mucocutaneous moniliasis and recurrent staphylococcal botromycosis: Immunological reconstitution by allogeneic bone marrow, *Clin. Exp. Immunol.* **3**:153–169.

Buckely, R. H., Amos, D. B., Kremer, W. B., and Stickel, D. L., 1971, Incompatible bone marrow transplantation in lymphopenic immunologic deficiency: Circumvention of fatal graft-vs.-host disease by immunological enhancement, *N. Engl. J. Med.* **285**:1035–1042.

Budtz-Jorgensen, E., 1971, Denture stomatitis. IV. An experimental model in monkeys, *Acta. Odontol. Scand.* **29**:513–526.

Budtz-Jorgensen, E., 1972, Denture stomatitis. V. Candida agglutinins in normal sera, *Acta. Odontol. Scand.* **30**:313–325.

Budtz-Jorgensen, E., 1973a, Immune response to *C. albicans* in monkeys with experimental candidiasis of the palate, *Scand. J. Dent. Res.* **81**:360–371.

Budtz-Jorgensen, E., 1973b, Cellular immunity in acquired candidiasis of the palate, *Scand, J. Dent. Res.* **81**:372–382.

Bybee, J. D., and Rogers, D. E., 1964, The phagocytic activity of polymorphonuclear leukocytes obtained from patients with diabetes mellitus, *J. Lab. Clin. Med.* **64**:1–13.

Cahill, L. T., Ainbender, E., and Glade, P. R., 1974, Chronic mucocutaneous candidiasis; T cell deficiency associated with B cell deficiency in man, *Cell. Immunol.* **14**:215–225.

Canales, L., Middlemass, R. O., Louro, J. M., and South, M. A., 1969, Immunological observations in chronic mucocutaneous candidiasis, *Lancet* **2**:567–571.

Caroline, L., Taschdjian, C. L., Kozinn, P. J., and Schade, A. L., 1964, Reversal of serum fungistasis by addition of iron, *J. Invest. Dermatol.* **42**:415–419.

Caroline, L., Rosner, F., and Kozinn, P. J., 1969, Elevated serum iron, low unbound transferrin and candidiasis in acute leukaemia, *Blood* **34**:441–451.

Cawson, R. A., 1966, Chronic oral candidosis, denture stomatitis and chronic hyperplastic candidosis, in: *Symposium on Candida Infections* (H. I. Winner and R. Hurley, eds.), pp. 138–153, Livingstone, Edinburgh.

Cawson, R. A., 1973, Induction of epithelial hyperplasia by *Candida albicans. Br. J. Dermatol.* **89**:497–503.

Cawson, R. A., and Lehner, T., 1968, Chronic hyperplastic candidiasis—Candida leukoplakia, *Br. J. Dermatol.* **80**:9–16.

Cawson, R. A., and Rajasingham, K. C., 1972, Ultrastructural features of the invasive phase of *Candida albicans*, *Br. J. Dermatol.* **87**:435–443.

Chandra, R. K., 1976, Iron and immunocompetence, *Nutr. Rev.* **34**:129–132.

Chattaway, F. W., Holmes, M. R., and Barlow, A. J. E., 1968, Cell wall composition of mycelial and blastospore form of *Candida albicans*, *J. Gen. Microbiol.* **51**:367–376.

Chattaway, F. W., Odds, F. C., and Barlow, A. J. E., 1971, An examination of the production of hydrolytic enzymes and toxins by pathogenic strains of *Candida albicans*, *J. Gen. Microbiol.* **67**:255–263.

Chattaway, F. W., Bishop R., Holmes, M. R., Odds, F. C., and Barlow, A. J. E., 1973, Enzyme activities associated with carbohydrate synthesis and breakdown in the yeast and mycelial forms of *Candida albicans*, *J. Gen. Microbiol.* **75**:97–109.

Chew, W. H., and Theus, T. L., 1967, Candida precipitins, *J. Immunol.* **98**:220–224.

Chilgren, R. A., Quie, P. G., Meuwissen, H. J., and Hong, R., 1967, Chronic mucocutaneous candidiasis, deficiency of delayed hypersensitivity and selective antibody defect, *Lancet* **2**:688–693.

Chilgren, R. A., Hong, R., and Quie, P. G., 1968, Human serum interaction with *Candida albicans*, *J. Immunol.* **101**:128–132.

Chilgren, R. A., Quie, P. G., Meuwissen, H. J., Good, R. A., and Hong, R., 1969, The cellular immune defect in chronic mucocutaneous candidiasis, *Lancet* **1**:1286–1288.

Clark, R. A., and Kimball, H. R., 1971, Defective granulocyte chemotaxis in the Chediak–Higashi syndrome, *J. Clin. Invest.* **50**:2645–2652.

Cleveland, W. W., 1975, Immunologic reconstitution in the Di George syndrome by fetal thymic transplant, *Birth Defects Orig. Art. Ser.* **11**:352–358.

Cleveland, W. W., Fogel, B. J., Brown, W. T., and Kay, H. E. M., 1968, Foetal thymic transplant in a case of DiGeorge's syndrome, *Lancet* **2**:1211–1214.

Cline, M. J., 1976, *The White Cell*, Chap. 8, p. 139, Harvard University Press, Cambridge, Mass.

Cohen, R., Roth, F. J., Delgado, E., Ahern, D. G., and Kaiser, M. H., 1969, Fungal flora of the normal human small and large intestine, *N. Engl. J. Med.* **280**:638–641.

Comaish, J. J., Gibson, B., and Green, C. A., 1963, Candidiasis: Serology and diagnosis, *J. Invest. Dermatol.* **40**:139–142.

Curry, C. R., and Quie, P. G., 1971, Fungal septicemia in patients receiving parenteral hyperalimentation, *N. Engl. J. Med.* **285**:1221–1224.

Cutler, J. E., 1976, Acute systemic candidiasis in normal and congenitally thymic-deficient (nude) mice, *J. Reticuloendothel. Soc.* **19**:121–124.

Cutler, J. E., Friedman, L., and Milner, K. C., 1972, Biological and chemical characterisation of toxic substances from *Candida albicans*, *Infect. Immun.* **6**:616–627.

Dabrowa, N., Landau, J. W., and Newcomer, V. D., 1965, The antifungal activity of physiologic saline in serum, *J. Invest. Dermatol.* **45**:368–377.

Dahl, M. V., Greene, W. H., and Quie, P. G., 1976, Infection, dermatitis, increased IgE and impaired neutrophil chemotaxis, *Arch. Dermatol.* **112**:1387–1390.

Damodaran, V. N., and Chakravarty, S. C., 1973, Mechanisms of production of candida lesions in rabbits, *J. Med. Microbiol.* **6**:287–292.

Daughaday, C. C., and Douglas, S. D., 1976, Phagocytes: Their protective activity and their genetic and acquired defects, *Pediatr. Ann.* **25**:259–368.

Davenport, J. C., and Wilton, J. M. A., 1971, Incidence of immediate and delayed hypersensitivity to *Candida albicans* in denture stomatitis, *J. Dent. Res.* **50**:892–895.

Davies, R. R., and Denning, T. J. V., 1972a, *Candida albicans* and the fungicidal activity of blood, *Sabouraudia* **10**:301–312.

Davies, R. R., and Denning, T. J. V., 1972b, Growth and form in *Candida albicans*, *Sabouraudia* **10**:180–188.

Dennis, D. L., and Petersen, C. G., 1964, *Candida albicans* shock, *Surg. Forum* **15**:36–37.

De Sousa, M., Cochran, R., MacKie, R., Parratt, D., and Arala-Chaves, M., 1976, Chronic mucocutaneous candidiasis treated with transfer factor, *Br. J. Dermatol.* **94**:79–83.

DiGeorge, A. M., 1968, Congenital absence of the thymus and its immunologic consequences; concurrence with congential hypoparathyroidism, in: *Immunologic Deficiency Diseases in Man* (D. Bergsma and R. A. Good eds.), *Birth Defects* **4**:116–123.

Dobias, B., 1957, Moniliasis in paediatrics, *AMA J. Dis. Child.* **94**:234–251.

Dobias, B., 1964, Specific and non-specific immunity in *Candida* infections, *Acta Med. Scand.* **176**:1–79 (Suppl. 421).

Douglas, J. D., and Schopfer, K., 1974, Phagocyte function in protein calorie malnutrition, *Clin. Exp. Immunol.* **17**:121–128.

Douglas, S. D., and Goldberg, L. S., 1972, Monocyte receptors for immunoglobulin and complement in immunologic deficiency diseases, *Vox Sang.* **23**:214–217.

Drake, C. H., 1954, Natural antibodies against yeast like fungi as measured by slide agglutination, *J. Immunol.* **50**:185–189.

Drew, J. H., 1973, Chronic mucocutaneous candidiasis with abnormal function of serum complement, *Med. J. Aust.* **2**:77–79.

Ehlenberger, A., and Nussenzweig, V., 1977, The role of membrane receptors for C3b and C3d in phagocytosis, *J. Exp. Med.* **145**:357–371.

Eisman, P. C., Geftic, S. G., and Mayer, R. L., 1953, Virulence in mice of colonial variants of *Candida albicans*, *Proc. Soc. Exp. Biol. Med.* **82**:263–264.

Elin, R. J., and Wolff, S. M., 1973a, Effect of endotoxin administration on the growth of *Candida albicans* in sera from various species, *Can. J. Microbiol.* **19**:639–641.

Elin, R. J., and Wolff, S. M., 1973b, Effect of pH and

iron-concentration on the growth of *Candida albicans* in human serum, *J. Infect. Dis.* **127**:705–708.

Escobar, M. R., 1976, Immunologic aspects of nutrition, *Adv. Exp. Med. Biol.* **73**(B):444–448.

Esterley, N. B., 1968, Serum antibodies to *Candida albicans* utilising an immunofluorescent technique, *Am. J. Clin. Pathol.* **50**:291–296.

Esterley, N. B., Brammar, S. R., and Crounse, R. G., 1967, The relationship of transferrin and iron to serum inhibition of *Candida albicans, J. Invest. Dermatol.* **49**:437–442.

Evans, E. G. V., Richardson, M. D., Odds, F. C., and Holland, K. J., 1973, Relevance of antigenicity of *Candida albicans* growth phases to diagnosis of systemic candidiasis, *Br. Med. J.* **2**:86–87.

Everett, E. D., Laforce, M., and Eickhoff, T. C., 1975, Serologic studies in suspected visceral candidiasis, *Arch. Intern. Med.* **135**:1075–1078.

Folb, P. L., and Trounce, J. R., 1970, Immunological aspects of Candida infection complicating steroid and immunosuppressive therapy, *Lancet* **2**:1112–1114.

Forsgren, A., Schmelling, D., and Quie, P. G., 1974, Effect of tetracycline on the phagocytic function of human leukocytes, *J. Infect. Dis.* **130**:412–415.

Fowles, R. E., Fajardo, I. M., Leibowitz, J. L., and David, J. R., 1973, The enhancement of macrophage bacteriostatis by products of activated lymphocytes, *J. Exp. Med.* **138**:952–964.

Fudenberg, H., Good, R. A., Goodman, H. C., Hitzig, W., Kunkel, H. G., Roitt, I. M., Rosen, F. S., Rowe, D. S., Seligmann, M., and Soothill, J. R., 1971, Primary immunodeficiencies: Report of a World Health Organization Committee, *Pediatrics* **47**:927–946.

Fuentes, C. A., Schwarz, J., and Aboulafia, R., 1952, Some aspects of the pathogenicity of *Candida albicans* in laboratory animals, *Mycopathol. Mycol. Appl.* **6**:176–181.

Gabrielson, A. E., and Good, R. A., 1967, Chemical suppression of adaptive immunity. IV. Adrenal steroid hormones, *Adv. Immunol.* **6**:110–124.

Gaines, J. D., and Remington, J. S., 1973, Diagnosis of deep infection with candida: A study of candida precipitins, *Arch. Intern. Med.* **132**:699–702.

Gatti, R. A., Meuwissen, H. J., Allen, H. D., Hong, R., and Good, R. A., 1968, Immunological reconstitution of sex-linked lymphopenic immunological deficiency, *Lancet* **1**:1223–1227.

Gatti, R. A., Gershank, J. J., Levkoff, A. M., Wertelecki, W., and Good, R. A., 1972, DiGeorge syndrome associated with combined immunodeficiency, *J. Pediatr.* **81**:920–926.

Gell, P. G. H., and Coombs, R. R. A., 1968, Classification of allergic reactions responsible for clinical hypersensitivity and disease, in: *Clinical Aspects of Immunology,* 2nd ed. (P. G. H. Gell and R. R. A. Coombs, eds.), pp. 575–596, Blackwell Scientific Publications, Oxford.

Gerber, H., Horisberger, M., and Bauer, H., 1973, Immunosorbent for the isolation of specific antibodies against mannan: Localisation of antigens in yeast cell walls, *Infect. Immun.* **7**:487–492.

Gershon, R. K., 1974, T cell control of antibody production, in: *Contemporary Topics in Immunobiology,* Vol. 3 (M. D. Cooper and N. L. Warner, eds.), pp. 1–40, Plenum Press, New York.

Goldberg, L. S., Bluestone, R., Barnett, E. V., and Landau, J. W., 1971, Studies on lymphocyte and monocyte function in chronic mucocutaneous candidiasis, *Clin. Exp. Immunol.* **8**:37–43.

Goldman, J. M., and Th'ng, K. H., 1973, Phagocytic function of leucocytes from patients with acute myeloid and chronic granulocytic leukaemia, *Br. J. Haematol.* **25**:299–308.

Good, R. A., Varco, R. L., Aust, J. B., and Zak, S. J., 1957, Transplantation studies in patients with agammaglobulinaemia, *Ann. N.Y. Acad. Sci.* **64**:882–924.

Götze, O., and Muller-Eberhardt, H. J., 1971, The C3 activator system: An alternative pathway of complement activation, *J. Exp. Med.* Suppl. **134**:90–108.

Govers, J., and Girard, J. P., 1972, Some immunological properties of human cervical and vaginal secretions, *Gynecol. Invest.* **3**:184–194.

Grappel, S. F., and Calderone, R. A., 1976, Effect of antibodies on the respiration and morphology of *Candida albicans, Sabouraudia* **14**:51–60.

Gresham, G. A., and Burns, M., 1960, Tissue invasion by candida, in: *Progress in the Biological Sciences in Relation to Dermatology* (A. Rook, ed.), pp. 174–183, Cambridge University Press, London.

Gresham, G. A., and Whittle, C. H., 1961, Studies on the invasive mycelial form of *Candida albicans, Sabouraudia* **1**:30–33.

Grob, P. J., Franke, C., Reymond, J. F., and Frei-Wetenstein, M., 1975, Therapeutic use of transfer factor, *Eur. J. Clin. Invest.* **5**:33–43.

Grogan, J. B., and Miller, R. C., 1973, Impaired function of polymorphonuclear leukocytes in patients with burns and other trauma. *Surg. Gynecol. Obstet.* **137**:784–788.

Gross, R. L., and Newberne, P. M., 1976, Malnutrition, the thymolymphatic system and immunocompetence, *Adv. Exp. Med. Biol.* **73**(B):179–187.

Hasenclever, H. F., 1959, Comparative pathogenicity of *Candida albicans* for mice and rabbits, *J. Bacteriol.* **78**:105–109.

Hasenclever, H. F., and Mitchell, W. O., 1961a, Pathogenicity of *C. albicans* and *C. tropicalis, Sabouraudia* **1**:16–21.

Hasenclever, H. F., and Mitchell, W. O., 1961b, Antigenic studies of candida. I. Observation of two antigenic groups in *Candida albicans, J. Bacteriol.* **82**:570–573.

Hasenclever, H. F., and Mitchell, W. O., 1962, Production in mice of tolerance to the toxic manifestations of *Candida albicans, J. Bacteriol.* **84**:402–409.

Hasenclever, H. F., and Mitchell, W. O., 1963a, Acquired immunity to candidiasis in mice, *J. Bacteriol.* **86**:401–406.

Hasenclever, H. F., and Mitchell, W. O., 1963b, Antigenic studies of *Candida*. IV. The relationship of the antigenic groups of *Candida albicans* to their isolation from various clinical specimens, *Sabouraudia* 2:201–204.

Hasenclever, H. F., and Mitchell, W. O., 1963c, Antigenic studies of candida. I. Observation of two antigenic groups in *Candida albicans*, *J. Bacteriol.* 82:570–573.

Heinonen, E., Krohn, K., Peerheentupa, A., Aro, A., and Pelkonen, R., 1976, Association of precipitating antiadrenal antibodies with moniliasis-polyendocrinopathy syndrome, *Ann. Clin. Res.* 8:262–265.

Hellwege, H. H., Fischer, K., and Bläker, F., 1972, Diagnostic value of candida precipitins, *Lancet* 2:386.

Hendry, A. T., 1972, Inhibition of catalase activity of *Candida albicans* by serum, *Sabouraudia* 10:193–204.

Hermans, P. E., Ulrich, J. A., and Markowitz, H., 1969, Chronic mucocutaneous candidiasis as a surface expression of deep seated abnormalities, *Am. J. Med.* 47:503–519.

Higgs, J. M., and Wells, R. S., 1973, Chronic mucocutaneous candidiasis; new approaches to treatment, *Br. J. Dermatol.* 89:179–190.

Hill, D. W., and Gebhardt, J. P., 1956, Morphological transformation of *Candida albicans* in tissues of mice, *Proc. Soc. Exp. Biol. Med.* 92:640–644.

Hill, H. R., Ochs, H. D., Quie, P. G., Clark, R. A., Pabst, H. F., Klebanoff, S. S., and Wedgewood, R. J., 1974, Defect in neutrophil granulocyte chemotaxis in Job's syndrome of "cold" recurrent staphylococcal abcesses, *Lancet* 2:617–619.

Hitzig, W. H., 1968, The Swiss type of agammaglobulinaemia, in: *Immunologic Deficiency Diseases in Man* (D. Bergsma and R. A. Good, eds.), *Birth Defects* 4:82–90.

Hitzig, W. H., Fontanellaz, H. P., Müntener, U., Paul, S., Spitler, L. E., and Fudenberg, H. H., 1972, Transfer factor, *Schweiz. Med. Wochenschr.* 102:1237–1244.

Hoepvrich, P. D., and Martin, C. H., 1970, Effect of tetracyclin, polymixin B and rifampicin on phagocytosis, *Clin. Pharmacol. Ther.* 11:418–422.

Holder, I. A., and Nathan, P., 1973, Effect in mice of injection of viable *Candida albicans* and a cell-free sonic extract on circulating platelets, *Infect. Immun.* 7:468–472.

Hollingsworth, J. W., and Carr, J., 1973, Experimental candidal arthritis in the rabbit, *Sabouraudia* 11:56–58.

Holti, G., 1966, Candida allergy, in: *Symposium on Candida Infections* (H. I. Winner and R. Hurley, eds.), pp. 73–81, Livingstone, Edinburgh.

Hong, R., Kay, H. E. M., Cooper, M. D., Meuwissen, H. J., Anan, M. C. G., and Good, R. A., 1968, Immunological restitution in lymphopenic immunological deficiency syndrome, *Lancet* 1:503–506.

Humbert, J. R., 1975, *Sem. Haematol.* 12:3–5.

Hurd, R. L., and Drake, C. A., 1953, *Candida albicans* infection in actively and passively immunised animals, *Myelopathol. Mycol. App.* 6:290–297.

Hurley, D. L., and Fauci, A. S., 1975, Disseminated candidiasis. I. An experimental model in the guinea pig, *J. Infect. Dis.* 131:516–521.

Hurley, D. L., Barlow, J. E., and Fauci, A. S., 1975, Experimental disseminated candidiasis. II. Administration of glucocorticosteroids, susceptibility to infection and immunity, *J. Infect. Dis.* 132:393–398.

Hurley, R., 1966a, Experimental infection with *Candida albicans* in modified hosts, *J. Pathol. Bacteriol.* 92:57–67.

Hurley, R., 1966b, Pathogenicity of the genus *Candida*, in: *Symposium on Candida Infection* (H. I. Winner and R. Hurley, eds.), pp. 13–25, Livingstone, Edinburgh.

Imperato, P. J., Buckley, C. E., and Callaway, J. L., 1968, Candida granuloma, *Arch. Dermatol.* 97:139–146.

Isenberg, A. D., Allerhand, J., and Berkman, J. I., 1963, An endotoxin-like fraction extracted from the cells of *C. albicans*, *Nature (London)* 197:516–517.

James, J., and Warin, R. P., 1971, An assessment of the role of *Candida albicans* and food yeasts in chronic urticaria, *Br. J. Dermatol.* 84:227–237.

Jones, J. H., and Adams, D., 1970, Experimentally induced acute oral candidosis in the rat, *Br. J. Dermatol.* 83:670–673.

Kaufman, L., 1976, Serodiagnosis of fungal diseases, in: *Manual of Clinical Immunology* (N. R. Rose and H. Friedman, eds.), pp. 367–369, American Society for Microbiology, Washington D.C.

Kelly, R., Wolstencroft, R., Dumonde, D., and Balfour, F., 1972, Role of lymphocyte activation products (LAP) in cell-mediated immunity. II. Effects of lymphocyte activation products on lymph node architecture and evidence for peripheral release of LAP following antigenic stimulation, *Clin. Exp. Immunol.* 10:49–65.

Kemp, J., and Solotorowsky, M., 1964, Localisation of antigens in mechanically disrupted cells of certain species of the genera *Candida* and *Torulopsis*, *J. Immunol.* 93:305–314.

Kessler, G., and Nickerson, W. J., 1959, Glucomannan-protein complexes from the cell walls of yeasts, *J. Biol. Chem.* 234:2281–2285.

Kim, Y. P., Adachi, K., and Chow, D., 1962, Leucine aminopeptidase in *Candida* albicans, *J. Invest. Dermatol.* 38:115–116.

Kimball, S. G., and Brody, J. I., 1963, Studies of *in vivo* phagocytosis. I. Inhibition of phagocytosis by intact neoplastic body fluids, *Blood* 21:462–469.

Kind, L. S., Kaushal, P. K., and Drury, P., 1972, Fatal anaphylaxis-like reaction induced by yeast mannans in non sensitised mice, *Infect. Immun.* 5:180–182.

Kirkpatrick, C. H., and Montes, L. F., 1974, Chronic mucocutaneous candidiasis, *J. Cutaneous Path.* 1:211–229.

Kirkpatrick, C. H., Chandler, J. W., and Schimke, R. M., 1970, Chronic mucocutaneous moniliasis with impaired delayed hypersensitivity, *Clin. Exp. Immunol.* 6:373–385.

Kirkpatrick, C. H., Rich, R. R., and Bennett, J. E., 1971a, Chronic mucocutaneous candidiasis: Model building in cellular immunity, *Ann. Intern. Med.* 74:955–978.

Kirkpatrick, C. H., Rich, R. R., Graw, R. G., Smith, T. K., Mickenberg, I. D., and Rogentine, G. N., 1971b, Treatment of chronic mucocutaneous moniliasis by immunologic reconstitution, *Clin. Exp. Immunol.* **9**:733–748.

Kirkpatrick, C. H., Rich, R. R., and Smith, T. K., 1972, Effect of transfer factor on lymphocyte function in anergic patients, *J. Clin. Invest.* **51**:2948–2958.

Kirkpatrick, C. H., Ottenson, E. A., Smith, T. K., Wells, S. A., and Burdick, J. F., 1976, Reconstitution of defective cellular immunity with foetal thymus and dialsyable transfer factor: Long term studies in a patient with chronic mucocutaneous candidiasis, *Clin. Exp. Immunol.* **23**:414–428.

Klebanoff, S. J., 1967, Iodination of bacteria; a bactericidal mechanism, *J. Exp. Med.* **126**:1063–1078.

Knight, L., and Fletcher, J., 1971, Growth of *Candida albicans* in saliva: Stimulation by glucose associated with antibiotics, corticosteroids and diabetes mellitus, *J. Infect. Dis.* **123**:371–377.

Kobayashi, G. S., and Friedman, L., 1964, Characterisation of the pyrogenicity of *Candida albicans, Saccharomyces cerevisae* and *Cryptococcus neoformans, J. Bacteriol.* **88**:660–666.

Kozinn, P. J., and Taschdjian, C. L., 1962, Enteric candidiasis: Diagnosis and clinical considerations, *Pediatrics* **30**:71–85.

Kozinn, P. J., Taschdjian, C. L., Dragutsky, D., and Minsky, A., 1957, Cutaneous candidiasis in early infancy and childhood, *Pediatrics* **20**:827–834.

Kozinn, P. J., Taschdjian, C. L., Wiener, H., Dragutsky, D., and Minsky, A., 1958, Neonatal candidiasis, *Pediatr. Clin. N. Am.* **5**:803–815.

Krause, W., Matheis, H., and Wulf, K., 1969, Fungaemia and funguria after oral administration of *Candida albicans, Lancet* **1**:598–599.

Landau, J. W., Dabrowa, N., Newcomer, V. D., and Rowe, J. R., 1964, The relationship of serum transferrin and iron to the rapid formation of germ tubes by *Candida albicans, J. Invest. Dermatol.* **43**:473–482.

Lawrence, H. S., 1955, The transfer in humans of delayed skin hypersensitivity to streptococcal M substance and to tuberculin with disrupted leukocytes, *J. Clin. Invest.* **34**:219–230.

Lawrence, H. S., 1960, Delayed sensitivity and homograft sensitivity, *Ann. Rev. Med.* **11**:207–230.

Lawrence, H. S., 1969, Transfer factor, *Adv. Immunol.* **11**:195–266.

Lawrence, H. S., 1974, Selective immunotherapy with transfer factor, in: *Advances in Clinical Immunology* Vol. 4 (F. H. Baer and R. A. Good, eds.), pp. 115–152, Academic Press, New York.

Lawton, J. W. M., Costello, C., Barclay, G. R., Urbaniak, S. J., Darg, C., Raeburn, J. A., Uttley, W. S., and Kay, A. B., 1976, The effect of transfer factor on neutrophil function in chronic mucocutaneous candidiasis, *Br. J. Haematol.* **33**:137–142.

Lay, H. W., and Nussenzweig, V., 1968, Receptors for complement on leukocytes, *J. Exp. Med.* **128**:991–1007.

Lehner, T., 1962, Oral candidiasis, in: *Oral Pathology in the Child,* pp. 75–83, International Academy of Oral Pathology, London.

Lehner, T., 1964a, Oral thrush or acute pseudomembraneous candidiasis, *Oral Surg.* **18**:27–37.

Lehner, T., 1964b, Chronic candidiasis, *Tr. St. Johns Dermatol.* **50**:8–21.

Lehner, T., 1965, Immunofluorescent investigation of *Candida albicans* antibodies in human saliva, *Arch. Oral Biol.* **10**:975–980.

Lehner, T., 1966a, Classification and clinico-pathological features of candida infections in the mouth, in: *Symposium on Candida Infections* (R. I. Winner and R. Hurley, eds.), pp. 119–137, Livingstone, Edinburgh.

Lehner, T., 1966b, Immunofluorescence study of *Candida albicans* in candidiasis, carriers and controls, *J. Pathol. Bacteriol.* **91**:97–104.

Lehner, T., 1970, Serum fluorescent antibody and immunoglobulin estimation in candidosis, *J. Med. Microbiol.* **3**:475–481.

Lehner, T., 1975, Immunological aspects of oral diseases, in: *Clinical Aspects of Immunology,* 3rd ed. (P. G. H. Gell, R. R. A. Coombs, and P. J. Lachmann, eds.), pp. 1387–1427, Blackwell Scientific Publications, Oxford.

Lehner, T., and Ward, R. G., 1970, Iatrogenic oral candidosis, *Br. J. Dermatol.* **83**:161–166.

Lehner, T., Buckley, H. R., and Murray, I. G., 1972a, The relationship between fluorescent, agglutinating and precipitating antibodies to *Candida albicans* and their immunoglobulin classes, *J. Clin. Pathol.* **25**:344–348.

Lehner, T., Wilton, J. M. A., and Ivanyi, L., 1972b, Immunodeficiencies in chronic muco-cutaneous candidosis, *Immunology* **22**:775–786.

Lehner, T., Wilton, J. M. A., Shillitoe, E. J., and Ivanyi, L., 1973, Cell-mediated immunity and antibodies to *Herpesvirus hominis* type I in oral leukoplakia and carcinoma, *Br. J. Cancer* **27**:351–361.

Lehrer, R. I., 1969, Antifungal effects of peroxidase systems, *J. Bacteriol.* **99**:361–365.

Lehrer, R. I., 1971, Inhibition by sulphonamides of the candidacidal activity of human neutrophils, *J. Clin. Invest.* **50**:2498–2505.

Lehrer, R. I., 1972, Functional aspects of a second mechanism of candidicidal activity by human neutrophils, *J. Clin. Invest.* **51**:2566–2572.

Lehrer, R. I., 1975, The fungicidal mechanism of human monocytes. I. Evidence for myeloperoxidase-linked and myeloperoxidase-independent candidacidal mechanisms, *J. Clin. Invest.* **55**:338–346.

Lehrer, R. I., and Cline, M. J., 1969a, Interaction of *Candida albicans* with human leukocytes and serum, *J. Bacteriol.* **98**:996–1004.

Lehrer, R. I., and Cline, M. J., 1969b, Leukocyte myeloperoxidase deficiency and disseminated candidiasis:

The role of myeloperoxidase in resistance to *Candida* infection, *J. Clin. Invest.* **48**:1478–1488.

Lehrer, R. I., and Cline, M. J., 1971, Leukocyte candidacidal activity and resistance to systemic candidiasis in patients with cancer, *Cancer* **41**:307–337.

Lehrer, R. I., Goldberg, L. S., Rosenthal, N. P., and Apple, M. H., 1972, Refractory megaloblastic anaemia with myeloperoxidase-deficient neutrophils, *Ann. Intern. Med.* **76**:447–453.

Lehrer, R. I., Ladra, K. M., and Hake, R. B., 1975, Nonoxidative fungicidal mechanisms of mammalian granulocytes: Demonstration of components with candidacidal activity in human, rabbit and guinea pig leukocytes, *Infect. Immun.* **11**:1226–1234.

Levy, R. L., Huang, S. W., Bach, F. H., Bach, M. L., Hong, R., Amman, A. S., Borton, M., and Kay, H. E. M., 1971, Thymic transplantation in a case of chronic mucocutaneous candidiasis, *Lancet* **2**:898–900.

Louria, D. B., 1976, Defenses against Candida infections, *Int. J. Radiat. Oncol. Biol. Phys.* **1**:309–311.

Louria, D. B., and Brayton, R. G., 1964a, A substance in blood lethal for *Candida albicans, Nature (London)* **201**:309.

Louria, D. B., and Brayton, R. G., 1964b, Behaviour of Candida cells in leukocytes, *Proc. Soc. Exp. Biol. Med.* **115**:93–98.

Louria, D. B., Fallon, N., and Browne, H. G., 1960, The influence of cortisone on experimental fungus infections in mice, *J. Clin. Invest.* **39**:1435–1449.

Louria, D. B., Stiff, D. P., and Bennet, B., 1962, Disseminated moniliasis in the adult, *Medicine* **41**:307–337.

Louria, D. B., Brayton, R. G., and Funkel, G., 1963, Studies on the pathogenesis of experimental *Candida albicans* infections in mice, *Sabouraudia* **2**:271–283.

Louria, D. B., Shannon, D., Johnson, G., Caroline, L., Okai, A., and Taschdjian, C. L., 1967, The susceptibility to moniliasis in children with endocrine hypofunction, *Tr. Assoc. Am. Physicians* **80**:236–248.

Louria, D. B., Smith, J. K., Brayton, R. G., and Buse, M., 1972, Anti-candida factors in serum and their inhibition. I. Clinical and laboratory observations, *J. Infect. Dis.* **125**:102–114.

Mackaness, G., 1971, Resistance to intracellular infection, *J. Infect. Dis.* **123**:439–445.

Mackaness, G., 1975, T-cell-mediated immunity, *Arb. Paul Ehrlich Inst.* **70**:27–38.

McKendrick, A. S. W., Wilson, M. I., and Main, D. M. G., 1967, Oral candida and long term tetracyline therapy, *Arch. Oral Biol.* **12**:281–290.

Mackenzie, D. W. R., 1966, Laboratory investigation of *Candida* infections, in: *Symposium on Candida Infections* (R. I. Winner and R. Hurley, eds.), pp. 26–43, Livingstone, Edinburgh.

MacKie, R. M., 1975, Transfer factor, *Br. J. Dermatol.* **94**:107–110.

Mackler, B. F., Altman, L., Rosenstreich, D. L., and Oppenheim, J. J., 1974, Human B lymphocyte activation: Induction of lymphokine production by EAC and

of blastogenesis by soluble mitogens, *Nature (London)* **249**:834–836.

MacMillan, B. G., Law, E. J., and Holder, I. A., 1972, Experience with Candida infections in the burn patient, *Arch. Surg.* **104**:509–514.

Maibach, H. I., and Kligman, A. M., 1962, The biology of experimental human cutaneous moniliasis (*Candida albicans*), *Arch. Dermatol.* **85**:233–257.

Mankowski, Z. T., 1957, The experimental pathogenicity of various species of *Candida* in Swiss mice, *Tr. N.Y. Acad. Sci.* **19**:548–570.

Mankowski, Z. T., 1968, Production of glycoproteins by *Candida albicans* in a synthetic medium and its influence on the growth of newborn mice, *Mycopathol. Mycol. Appl.* **34**:113–118.

Mardon, D. N., Gunn, J. L., and Robinette, E., Jr., 1975, Variation in the lethal response of mice to yeast like and pseudohyphal forms of *Candida albicans, Can. J. Microbiol.* **21**:1681–1687.

Martin, R. R., Warr, G. A., Couch, R. B., Yaeger, H., and Knight, V., 1974, Effects of tetracycline on leukotaxis, *J. Infect. Dis.* **129**:110–116.

Matthews, N. M., and Inman, F. P., 1968, Identification of rabbit antibodies directed against *Candida albicans, Proc. Soc. Exp. Biol. Med.* **128**:387–392.

Messner, R. P., and Jelinek, J., 1970, Receptor for γG on human neutrophils, *J. Clin. Invest.* **49**:2165–2171.

Meuwissen, H. J., Gatti, R. A., Terasaki, P., Hong, R., and Good, R. A., 1969, Treatment of lymphopenic hypogammaglobulinaemia and bone marrow asplasia by transplantation of allogeneic marrow: Critical role of histocompatability matching, *N. Engl. J. Med.* **281**:691–697.

Meyer, R. D., Young, L. S., Armstrong, D., and Yu, B., 1973, Aspergillosis complicating neoplastic disease, *Am. J. Med.* **54**:6–15.

Miller, D. G., 1962, Patterns of immunological deficiency in lymphomas and leukemias, *Ann. Intern. Med.* **57**:703–716.

Miller, M. E., 1969, Deficiency of chemotactic function in the human noonate: A previously unrecognised defect of the inflammatory response (abstr.), *Pediatr. Res.* **3**:497.

Miller, M. E., 1975, Pathology of chemotaxis and random mobility, *Sem. Haematol.* **12**:59–81.

Miller, M. E., and Schicken, R. M., 1967, Thymic dysplasia: A separable entity from "Swiss agammaglobulinaemia," *Am. J. Med. Sci.* **253**:741–750.

Mills, J. A., 1966, The immunological significance of antigen induced lymphocyte transformation, *J. Immunol.* **97**:239–247.

Mitchell, G. W., and Sbarra, A. J., 1965, The role of the phagocyte in host parasite interactions. II. The phagocytic capabilities of leukocytes in pregnant women, *Am. J. Obstet. Gynecol.* **91**:755–762.

Montes, L. F., and Wilborn, W. H., 1968, Ultrastructural features of host–parasite relationship in oral candidiasis, *J. Bacteriol.* **96**:1349–1356.

Montes, L. F., Carter, R. E., Moreland, N., and Ceballos, R., 1968, Generalised cutaneous candidiasis associated with diffuse mycopathy and thymoma, *J. Am. Med. Assoc.* **204**:351–354.

Montes, L. F., Pittman, C. S., Moore, O. J., Taylor, C. D., and Cooper, M. D., 1972, Chronic mucocutaneous candidiasis, influence of thyroid status, *J. Am. Med. Assoc.* **221**:156–159.

Morelli, R., and Rosenberg, L. T., 1971a, Role of complement during experimental *Candida* infection in mice, *Infect. Immun.* **3**:521–523.

Morelli, R., and Rosenberg, L. T., 1971b, The role of complement in the phagocytosis of *Candida albicans* by mouse peripheral blood leukocytes, *J. Immunol.* **107**:476–480.

Mourad, S., and Friedman, L., 1961, Active immunisation of mice against *Candida albicans*, *Proc. Soc. Exp. Biol. Med.* **106**:570–572.

Movat, H. Z., 1976, Pathways to allergic inflammation: The sequelae of antigen–antibody complex formation, *Fed. Proc.* **35**:2435–2441.

Mowat, A. G., and Baum, J., 1971a, Chemotaxis of polymorphonuclear leukocytes from patients with diabetes mellitus, *N. Engl. J. Med.* **284**:621–627.

Mowat, A. G., and Baum, J., 1971b, Chemotaxis of polymorphonuclear leukocytes from patients with rheumatoid arthritis, *J. Clin. Invest.* **50**:2541–2549.

Müller, J. H., Takamiya, H., Vogt, A., and Jaeger, R., 1975, Electron-microscopic localisation of the immune reactions with *Candida* cells. I. *In vitro* incubation of *Candida albicans* with human and candida serum, *Mykosen* **19**:295–303.

Munoz, J., and Geister, R., 1950, Inhibition of phagocytosis by aureomycin, *Proc. Soc. Exp. Biol. Med.* **75**:367–370.

Murray, I. G., and Buckley, H. R., 1966, Serological study of *Candida* species, in: *Symposium on Candida infections* (R. I. Winner and R. Hurley, eds.), pp. 44–50, Livingston, Edinburgh.

Murray, I. G., Buckley, H. R., and Turner, G. C., 1969, Serological evidence of *Candida* infection after open heart surgery, *J. Med. Microbiol.* **2**:463–469.

Nathan, C. F., Karnovsky, M. L., and David, J. R., 1971, Alteration of macrophage function by mediators from lymphocytes, *J. Exp. Med.* **133**:1356–1376.

Nathan, C. F., Remold, H. G., and David, J. R., 1973, Characterisation of a lymphocyte mediator which alters macrophage functions, *J. Exp. Med.* **137**:275–290.

Nelson, D. S., 1972, Macrophages as effectors of cell-mediated immunity, in: *CRC Critical Reviews in Microbiology*, pp. 353–384, CRC Press, Cleveland.

Nezelof, C., 1968, Thymic dysplasia with normal immunoglobulins and immunologic deficiency: Pure alymphocytosis, in: *Immunologic Deficiency Diseases in Man* (D. Bergsma and R. A. Good, eds.), *Birth Defects* **4**:104–115.

Nickerson, W. J., Taber, W. A., and Falcone, G., 1956, Physiological bases of morphogenesis in fungi. V. Effect of selenite and tellurite on cellular division of yeast like fungi, *Can. J. Microbiol.* **2**:575–584.

Nosal, R., Novotny, J., and Sikl, D., 1974, The effect of glycoprotein from *Candida albicans* on isolated rat mast cells, *Toxicon* **12**:103–108.

Odds, F. C., and Hierholzer, J. C., 1973, Purification and properties of a glycoprotein acid phosphotase from *Candida albicans*, *J. Bacteriol.* **114**:257–266.

Odds, F. C., Evans, E. G., and Holland, K. T., 1975, Detection of Candida precipitins: A comparison of double diffusion and counter immunoelectrophoresis, *J. Immunol. Methods* **7**:211–218.

O'Grady, F., Pennington, J. H., and Stanfield, A. G., 1967, Delayed hypersensitivity in mouse thigh candidosis, *Br. J. Exp. Pathol.* **48**:196–203.

Oh, K. M. H., Rodey, G. E., Good, R. A., Chilgren, P. A., and Quie, P. G., 1969, Defective candidacidal activity of polymorphonuclear leukocytes: Diminished activity in chronic granulomatous disease of childhood, *J. Clin. Invest.* **46**:668–679.

Pabst, H. F., and Swanson R., 1972, Successful treatment of candidiasis with transfer factor, *Br. Med. J.* **2**:442–443.

Papageorgiou, P. S., and Alqusus, Z., 1976, Impairment of natural defenses. 1: Exogenous causes, mechanisms and opportunistic infection. *Pediatr. Ann.* **5**:439–456.

Park, J. K., and Dow, R. C., 1970, The uptake and localisation of tetracycline in human blood cells, *Br. J. Exp. Pathol.* **51**:179–182.

Parker, J. C., McCloskey, J. J., and Knauer, K. A., 1976, Pathobiologic features of human candidiasis, *Am. J. Clin. Pathol.* **65**:991–1000.

Parks, D. E., and Weiner, R. S., 1975, The role of phagocytosis and natural lymphokines in the fusion of alveolar macrophages to form Langhans giant cells, *J. Reticuloendothel. Soc.* **17**:219–228.

Parsons, E. R., and Nassau, E., 1974, Candida serology on open heart surgery, *J. Med. Microbiol.* **7**:415–423.

Paterson, P. Y., Senio, R., Blumenschein, G., and Swelstad, J., 1971, Mucocutaneous candidiasis, anergy and a plasma inhibitor of cellular immunity: Reversal after amphotericin B therapy, *Clin. Exp. Immunol.* **9**:595–602.

Pearsall, N. N., Sundsmo, J. S., and Weiser, R. S., 1973, Lymphokine toxicity for yeast cells, *J. Immunol.* **110**:1444–1446.

Peck, S. M., Bergamini, R., Kelcik, L. C., and Rein, C. R., 1955, The serodiagnosis of moniliasis, its value and limitations, *J. Invest. Dermatol.* **25**:300–310.

Pepys, J., Faux, J. A., Longbottom, J. L., McCarthy, D. S., and Hargreave, F. E., 1968, *Candida albicans* precipitins in respiratory disease in man, *J. Allergy* **41**:305–318.

Plass, E. D., Hesseltine, H. C., and Borts, I. H., 1931, Monilia vulvovaginitis, *Am. J. Obstet. Gynecol.* **21**:320–334.

Poulter, L. W., and Turk, J. L., 1975a, Studies on the effect of soluble lymphocyte products (lymphokines) on macrophage physiology. I. Early changes in enzyme activity and permeability, *Cell. Immunol.* **20**:12–24.

Poulter, L. W., and Turk, J. L., 1975b, Studies on the effect of soluble lymphocyte products (lymphokines) on macrophage physiology. II. Cytochemical changes associated with activation, *Cell. Immunol.* **20:**25–32.

Preisler, H. D., Hasenclever, H. F., Levitan, A. A., and Henderson, E. S., 1969, Serologic diagnosis of disseminated candidiasis in patients with acute leukaemia, *Ann. Intern. Med.* **70:**19–30.

Preisler, H. D., Hasenclever, H. F., Henderson, E. S., Smith, J. K., and Louria, D. B., 1972, A prospective study of anti-*Candida* interfering factor in leukemic patients, *Cancer* **30:**294–299.

Quie, P. G., 1972, Bactericidal function of polymorphonuclear leukocytes, *Pediatrics* **50:**264–270.

Quie, P. G., and Chilgren, R. A., 1971, Acute disseminated and chronic mucocutaneous candidiasis, *Sem. Haematol.* **8:**227–242.

Radl, J., Dooren, L. J., Eijsvoogel, V. P., Went, J. J., and Hijmans, W., 1972, An immunological study during post-transplantation follow up of a case of severe-combined immunodeficiency, *Clin. Exp. Immunol.* **10:**367–382.

Rankin, J. G., 1963, Phagocytosis with special reference to hepatic function and disease, *Med. Clin. N. Am.* **47:**737–752.

Ray, T. C., and Wuepper, K. D., 1975, Experimental cutaneous *Candida albicans* infections in rodents: Role of complement, *Clin. Res.* **23:**2304.

Rebora, A., Marples, R. R., and Kligman, A. M., 1973, Experimental infections with *Candida albicans, Arch. Dermatol.* **108:**69–73.

Remington, J. S., Gaines, J. D., and Gilmer, M. A., 1972, Demonstration of *Candida* precipitins in human sera by counterimmunoelectrophoresis, *Lancet* **1:**413.

Remold, H., Fasold, H., and Staib, F., 1968, Purification and characterisation of a proteolytic enzyme from *Candida albicans, Biochim. Biolphys. Acta* **167:**399–406.

Rifkind, D., and Frey, J. A., 1972a, Influence of gonadectomy on *Candida albicans* urinary tract infection in CFW mice, *Infect. Immun.* **5:**332–336.

Rifkind, D., and Frey, J. A., 1972b, Sex difference in antibody response of CFW mice to *Candida albicans, Infect. Immun.* **5:**695–698.

Rifkind, D., Marchioro, T. L., Schneck, S. A., and Hill, R. B., 1967, Systemic fungal infections complicating renal transplantation and immunosuppressive therapy, *Am. J. Med.* **43:**28–38.

Rocklin, R. E., 1974a, Products of activated lymphocytes: Leukocyte inhibitory factor (LIF) distinct from migration inhibitory factor (MIF), *J. Immunol.* **112:**1461–1466.

Rocklin, R. E., 1974b, Clinical application of *in vitro* lymphocyte tests, in: *Progress in Clinical Immunology,* Vol. 2 (R. S. Schwartz ed.), pp. 21–67, Grune and Stratton, New York.

Rocklin, R. E., Myers, D. L., and David, J., 1970a, An *in vitro* assay for cellular hypersensitivity in man, *J. Immunol.* **104:**95–102.

Rocklin, R. E., Chilgren, R. A., Hong, R., and David, J.

R., 1970b, Transfer of cellular hypersensitivity in chronic mucocutaneous candidiasis monitored *in vivo* and *in vitro, Cell. Immunol.* **1:**290–299.

Rocklin, R. E., Reardon, G., Scheffer, A., Churchill, W. H., and David, J. R., 1970c, Dissociation between two *in vitro* correlates of delayed hypersensitivity: Absence of macrophage inhibitory factor (MIF) in the presence of antigen induced incorporation of 3H thymidine, in: *Proceedings of the Fifth Leukocyte Culture Conference* (S. E. Harris, ed.), pp. 639–646, Academic Press, New York.

Rocklin, R. E., MacDermott, R. P., Chess, L., Schlossman, S. F., and David, J. R., 1974, Studies on mediator production by highly purified human T and B lymphocytes, *J. Exp. Med.* **140:**1303–1316.

Rogers, P. J., 1957, An aid to the differentiation between cases of moniliasis and monilia carriers, *J. Clin. Pathol.* **10:**406–407.

Rogers, T. J., Balish, E., and Manning, D. D. D., 1976, The role of thymus dependent cell-mediated immunity in resistance to experimental disseminated candidiasis, *J. Reticuloendothel. Soc.* **20:**291–298.

Rosenfeld, S. I., Baum, J., Steigbigel, R. T., and Leddy, J. P., 1976, Hereditary deficiency of the fifth component of complement in man. II. Biological properties of C5 deficient serum, *J. Clin. Invest.* **57:**1635–1643.

Rosner, F., Valmont, I., Kozinn, P. J., and Caroline, L., 1970, Leukocyte function in patients with leukaemia, *Cancer* **25:**835–842.

Roth, F. J., Jr., and Goldstein, M. I., 1961, Inhibition of growth of pathogenic yeasts by human serum, *J. Invest. Dermatol.* **36:**383–387.

Roth, F. J., Jr., and Murphy, W. H., Jr., 1957, Lethality of a cell free extract of *Candida albicans* for chlortetracycline treated mice, *Proc. Soc. Exp. Biol. Med.* **94:**530–532.

Roth, F. J., Jr., Boyd, C. C., Sagami, S., and Blank, H., 1959, An evaluation of the fungistatic activity of serum, *J. Invest. Dermatol.* **32:**549–556.

Russell, C., and Jones, J. H., 1973a, The effects of oral inoculation of the yeast and mycelial phases of *Candida albicans* in rats fed a normal and carbohydrate rich diets, *Arch. Oral Biol.* **18:**409–413.

Russell, C., and Jones, J. H., 1973b, Effects of oral inoculation of *Candida albicans* in tetracycline treated rats, *J. Med. Microbiol.* **6:**275–279.

Russell, C., and Lay, K. M., 1973, Natural history of *Candida* species and yeasts in the oral cavities of infants, *Arch. Oral Biol.* **18:**954–962.

Saltarelli, C. G., Gennie, K. A., and Marcuso, S. C., 1975, Lethality of Candida strains as influenced by the host, *Can. J. Microbiol.* **21:**648–654.

Salvin, S. B., 1952, Endotoxin in pathogenic fungi, *J. Immunol.* **69:**89–99.

Salvin, S. B., 1959, Current concepts of diagnostic serology and skin hypersensitivity in the mycoses, *Am. J. Med.* **27:**97–114.

Salvin, S. B., 1974, Immunity to fungal infection, in: *Prog-*

ress in Immunology II, Vol. 4 (L. Brent and J. Holborow, eds.), pp. 363–367, North-Holland, Amsterdam.

Salvin, S. B., Peterson, R. D. A., and Good, R. A., 1965, The role of the thymus in resistance to infection and endotoxin toxicity, *J. Lab. Clin. Med.* **65:**1004–1022.

Salvin, S. B., Youngner, J. S., and Lederer, W. H., 1973, Migration inhibitory factor and interferon in the circulation of mice with delayed hypersensitivity, *Infect. Immun.* **7:**68–75.

Schlegel, R. J., Bernier, G. M., Bellanti, J. A., Maybee, D. A., Osborne, G. B., Stuart, J. L., Pearlman, D. S., Ouelette, J., and Biehusen, F. C., 1970, Severe candidiasis associated with thymic dysplasia, IgA deficiency and plasma antilymphocyte effects, *Pediatrics* **45:** 926–936.

Schmid, L., and Brune, K., 1974, Assessment of phagocytic and antimicrobial activity of human granulocytes, *Infect. Immun.* **10:**1120–1126.

Schoch, E. P., 1971, Thymic conversion of *Candida albicans* from commensalism to pathogenism, *Arch. Dermatol.* **103:**311–319.

Schulkind, M. L., Adler, W. H., Altmier, W. A., and Ayoub, E. M., 1972, Transfer factor in the treatment of a case of chronic mucocutaneous candidiasis, *Cell. Immunol.* **3:**606–615.

Scribner, D. J., and Fahrney, D., 1976, Neutrophil receptors for IgG and complement: Their roles in the attachment and ingestion phases of phagocytosis, *J. Immunol.* **116:**892–897.

Seelig, M. S., 1966a, Mechanisms by which antibiotics increase the incidence and severity of candidiasis and alter the immunological defenses, *Bact. Rev.* **30:**442–459.

Seelig, M. S., 1966b, The role of antibiotics in the pathogenesis of *Candida* infections, *Am. J. Med.* **40:**887–917.

Seeliger, H. P. R., Tomsikova, A., and Torok, I., 1975, Immunological reactions among *Candida albicans, Mykosen* **18:**51–59.

Segal, E., Vardinon, N., Schwartz, J., and Eylan, E., 1975, Antigenic relationship between *Candida albicans* and various yeasts as reflected by immunoglobulin-class specificity, *Pathol. Microbiol.* **42:**49–58.

Shannon, D. L., Johnson, G., Rosen, F. S., and Austen, K. F., 1966, Cellular reactivity to *Candida albicans* antigen, *N. Engl. J. Med.* **275:**690–693.

Sher, N. A., Chaparas, S. D., Greenberg, L. E., and Bernard, S., 1975, Effects of BCG, *Corynebacterium parvum* and methanol extraction residue in the reduction of mortality from *Staphylococcus aureus* and *Candida albicans* infection in immunosuppressed mice, *Infect. Immun.* **12:**1325–1330.

Simon, H. B., and Sheagren, J. N., 1971, Cellular immunity *in vitro.* I. Immunologically mediated enhancement of macrophage bactericidal capacity, *J. Exp. Med.* **133:**137–1389.

Simon, H. B., and Sheagren, J. N., 1972a, Enhancement of macrophage bactericidal capacity by antigenically stimulated immune lymphocytes, *Cell. Immunol.* **4:**163–174.

Simon, H. B., Sheagren, J. N., 1972b, Migration inhibitory factor and macrophage bactericidal function, *Infect. Immun.* **6:**101–103.

Simonetti, N., and Strippoli, V., 1973, Pathogenicity of Y form as compared to M form in experimentally induced *Candida albicans* infections, *Mycopathol. Mycol. Appl.* **51(i):**19–28.

Slaven, R. G., and Garven, J. E., 1964, Delayed hypersensitivity in man: Transfer by lymphocyte preparations of peripheral blood, *Science* **145:**52–53.

Smith, J. K., and Louria, D. B., 1972, Anti-*Candida* factors in serum and their inhibitors. II. Identification of a *Candida*-clumping factor and the influence of the immune responses on the morphology of *Candida* and on anti-*Candida* activity of serum in rabbits, *J. Infect. Dis.* **125:**115–122.

Smits, B. J., Prior, A. P., and Arblaster, P. G., 1966, Incidence of *Candida* in hospital in-patients and the effects of antibiotic therapy, *Br. Med. J.* **1:**208–210.

Snyderman, R., Altman, L. C., Frankel, A., and Blaese, R. M., 1973, Defective mononuclear chemotaxis: a previously unrecognized immune dysfunction: Studies in a patient with chronic mucocutaneous candidiasis, *Ann. Intern. Med.* **78:**509–513.

Sohnle, P. G., Frank, M. M., and Kirkpatrick, C. H., 1976a, Mechanisms involved in elimination of organisms from experimental cutaneous *Candida albicans* infections in guinea pig, *J. Immunol.* **117:**523–530.

Sohnle, P. G., Frank, M. M., and Kirkpatrick, C. H., 1976b, Deposition of complement components in the cutaneous lesion of chronic mucocutaneous candidiasis, *Clin. Immunol. Immunopathol.* **5:**340–350.

Soles, P., Lim, L. Y., and Louria, D. B., 1967, Active immunity in experimental candidiasis in mice, *Sabouraudia* **5:**315–322.

Staib, F., 1965, Serum protein as nitrogen source for yeast like fungi, *Sabouraudia* **4:**187–193.

Staib, F., 1969, Proteolysis and pathogenicity of *Candida albicans* strains, *Mycopath, Mycol. Appl.* **37:**345–348.

Stallybrass, F. C., 1964, Candida precipitins, *J. Pathol. Bacteriol.* **87:**89–97.

Stanley, V., and Hurley, R., 1969, The growth of *Candida* species in cultures of mouse peritoneal macrophages, *J. Pathol.* **97:**357–366.

Stanley, V., and Hurley, R., 1974, Candida precipitins in pregnant women; validity of the test systems used, *J. Clin. Pathol.* **27:**66–69.

Stanley, V., Hurley, R., and Carroll, C. J., 1972, Distribution and significance of *Candida* precipitins in sera from pregnant women, *J. Med. Microbiol.* **5:**313–320.

Steele, R. W., Limas, C., Thurman, G. B., Schuelein, M., Bauer, H., and Bellanti, J. A., 1972, Familial thymic aplasia: Attempted reconstitution with fetal thymus in a millipore diffusion chamber, *N. Engl. J. Med.* **287:**787–791.

Steinberg, A. D., Plotz, P. H., Wolff, S. M., Wong, V. G., Agu, S. G., and Decker, J. L., 1972, Cytotoxic drugs in the treatment of nonmalignant disease, *Ann. Intern. Med.* 76:619–642.

Stickle, D., Kaufman, L., Blumer, S. O., and McLaughlin, D. W., 1972, Comparison of a newly developed latex agglutination test and an immunodiffusion test in the diagnosis of systemic candidiasis, *Appl. Microbiol.* 23:490–499.

Stiehm, E. R., and Fulginati, V. A., 1973, *Immunologic Disorders in Infants and Children,* Saunders, Philadelphia.

Stobo, J. D., Paul, S., Van Scoy, R. E., and Hermans, P. E., 1976, Suppressor thymus-derived lymphocytes in fungal infection, *J. Clin. Invest.* 57:319–328.

Summers, D. F., Grollman, A., and Hasenclever, H. F., 1964, Polysaccharide antigens of Candida cell wall, *J. Immunol.* 92:491–499.

Symmers, W. St. C., 1966, Septicaemic candidosis, in: *Symposium on Candida Infections* (H. I. Winner and R. Hurley, eds.), pp. 196–213, Livingstone, Edinburgh.

Takeya, K., Nomoto, T., Matsumoto, T., Mikaye, T., and Himeno, K., 1976, Chronic mucocutaneous candidiasis accompanied by enhanced antibody production, *Clin. Exp. Immunol.* 25:497–500.

Taschdjian, C. L., and Kozinn, P. J., 1957, Laboratory and clinical studies on candidiasis in the new born infant, *J. Pediatr.* 50:426–433.

Taschdjian, C. L., Reiss, F., and Kozinn, P. J., 1960, Experimental vaginal candidiasis in mice; its implication for superficial candidiasis in mice; its implication for superficial candidiasis in humans, *J. Invest. Dermatol.* 34:89–94.

Taschdjian, C. L., Kozinn, P. J., and Caroline, L., 1964, Immune studies in candidiasis III. Precipitating antibodies in systemic candidiasis, *Sabouraudia* 3:312–320.

Taschdjian, C. L., Cuesta, M. B., Kozinn, P. J., and Caroline, L., 1969, A modified antigen for the serodiagnosis of systemic candidiasis, *Am. J. Clin. Pathol.* 52:468–472.

Taschdjian, C. L., Kozinn, P. J., Cuesta, M. B., and Toni, E. F., 1972, Serodiagnosis of candidal infections, *Am. J. Clin. Pathol.* 57:195–205.

Taschdjian, C. L., Seelig, M. S., and Kozinn, P. J., 1973, Serological diagnosis of candidal infections, *CRC Crit, Rev. Clin. Lab., Sci.* 4:19–59.

Toh, B. H., Roberts-Thomson, K., Matthews, J. D., Whittingham, S., and Mackay, I. R., 1973, Depression of cell mediated immunity in old age and the immunopathic diseases, lupus erythematous, chronic hepatitis and rheumatoid arthritis, *Clin. Exp. Immunol.* 14:193–202.

Tsuchiya, T., Fukusawa, Y., and Kawakita, S., 1961, Serological classification of the genus Candida, in: *Studies on Candidiasis in Japan, Research Committee on Candidiasis,* pp. 34–46, Japanese Ministry of Education, Tokyo.

Twomey, J. J., Waddell, C. C., Krantz, S., O'Reilly, R., L'Esperance, P., and Good, R. A., 1975, Chronic mucocutaneous candidiasis with macrophage dysfunction, a plasma inhibitor and co-existent aplastic anaemia, *J. Lab. Clin. Med.* 85:968–977.

Unanue, E. R., 1972, The regulatory role of macrophages in antigenic stimulation, *Adv. Immunol.* 15:95–165.

Valdimarsson, H., 1974, Transfer factor, clinical application, in: *Progress in Immunology II,* Vol. 5 (L. Brent and J. Holborow, eds.), p. 378, North-Holland, Amsterdam.

Valdimarsson, H., Riches, H. R. C., Holt, C., and Hobbs, J. R., 1970, Lymphocyte abnormality in chronic mucocutaneous candidiasis, *Lancet* 1:1259–1261.

Valdimarsson, H., Moss, P. D., Holt, P. J. L., and Hobbs, S. R., 1972a, Treatment of chronic mucocutaneous candidiasis with leucocytes from HLA compatible sibling, *Lancet* 1:469–472.

Valdimarsson, H., Wood, C. B. S., Hobbs, J. R., and Holt, P. J. L., 1972b, Immunological features in a case of chronic granulomatous candidiasis and its treatment with transfer factor, *Clin. Exp. Immunol.* 11:151–163.

Valdimarsson, H., Higgs, J. M., Wells, R. S., Yamamura, M., Hobbs, J. R., and Holt, P. J. L., 1973, Immune abnormalities associated with chronic mucocutaneous candidiasis, *Cell. Immunol.* 6:348–361.

Van Scoy, R. E., Hill, H. R., Ritts, R. E., Jr., and Quie, P. G., 1975, Familial neutrophil chemotaxis defect, recurrent bacterial infections, mucocutaneous candidiasis and hyperimmunoglobulinaemia E, *Ann. Intern. Med.* 82:766–771.

Van Uden, N., 1960, The occurrence of Candida and other yeasts in the intestinal tracts of animals, *Ann. N.Y. Acad. Sci.* 89:59–68.

Verhaegen, H., de Cock, W., and de Cree, J., 1976, *In vitro* phagocytosis of Candida albicans by peripheral polymorphonuclear neutrophils of patients with recurrent infections: Case reports of serum-dependent abnormality, *Biomedicine* 24:164–170.

Wagner, J. M., and Kissel, I., 1958, Complications of Candida albicans infections in infancy, *Br. Med. J.* 2:362–366.

Wagner, J. M., and Srivastava, K. P., 1975, Decontamination of gnotobiotic mice experimentally monoassociated with Candida albicans, *Infect. Immun.* 12:1401–1404.

Wahl, S. M., Wilton, J. M. A., Rosenstreich, D. L., and Oppenheim, J. J., 1975, The role of macrophages in the production of lymphokines by T and B Lymphocytes, *J. Immunol.* 114:1296–1301.

Waldman, R. H., Cruz, J. M., and Rowe, D. S., 1971, Immunoglobulin levels and antibody to Candida albicans in human cervicovaginal secretions, *Clin. Exp. Immunol.* 9:427–434.

Waldman, R. H., Cruz, J. M., and Rowe, D. S., 1972, Intravaginal immunisation of humans with Candida albicans, *J. Immunol.* 109:662–664.

Ward, P. A., and Berenberg, J. L., 1974, Defective regulation of inflammatory mediators in Hodgkin's disease: Supernormal levels of chemotactic factor inactivator, *N. Engl. J. Med.* 290:76–80.

Warnock, D. W., Speller, D. C. E., Morris, J. A., and Mackie, P. H., 1976, Serological diagnosis of infection of the urinary tract by yeasts, *J. Clin. Pathol.* **29:**836–840.

Weedon, D. D., Martin, W. J., Karlson, A. G., and Shorter, R. G., 1973, *In vitro* effect of human lymphotoxin on microorganisms, *Mayo Clin. Proc.* **48:**560–564.

Weeks, B. A., Escobar, M. R., Hamilton, P. B., and Fueston, V. M., 1976, Chemotaxis of polymorphonuclear leukocytes by mannan-enriched preparations of *Candida albicans, Adv. Exp. Med. Biol.* **73**(A):161–169.

Weiner, M. H., and Yount, W. J., 1976, Mannan antigenemia in the diagnosis of invasive Candida infections, *J. Clin. Invest.* **58:**1045–1053.

Wells, R. S., Higgs, J. M., MacDonald, A., Valdimarsson, H., and Holt, P. J. L., 1972, Familial chronic mucocutaneous candidiasis, *J. Med. Genet.* **9:**302–310.

Westphal, O., and Jann, K., 1965, Bacterial lipopolysaccharides: Extraction with phenol-water and further application of the procedure, in: *Methods in Carbohydrate Chemistry* (R. L. Whistler, ed.), pp. 83–91, Academic Press, New York.

Wilkinson, P. M., Sumner, C., Delamore, I. W., Geary, C. G., and Milner, G. R., 1975, Granulocyte function in myeoblastic leukaemia, *Br. J. Cancer* **32:**574–577.

Williamson, J. J., 1972, Diurnal variation of *Candida albicans* counts in saliva, *Aust. Dent. J.* **17:**54–60.

Wilton, J. M. A., 1977, The role of complement in crevicular fluid, in: *The Borderland between Caries and Periodontal Disease* (T. Lehner, ed.), pp. 223–247, Academic Press, London.

Wilton, J. M. A., Ivanyi, L., and Lehner, T., 1972, Cell-mediated immunity in *Herpesvirus hominis* infections, *Br. Med. J.* **1:**723–726.

Wilton, J. M. A., Rosenstreich, D. L., and Oppenheim, J. J., 1975, Activation of guinea pig macrophages by bacterial lipopolysaccharide requires bone marrow derived lymphocytes, *J. Immunol.* **114:**388–393.

Wilton, J. M. A., Renggli, H. H., and Lehner, T., 1977a, A functional comparison of blood and gingival inflammatory polymorphonuclear leucocytes in man, *Clin. Exp. Immunol.* **27:**152–157.

Wilton, J. M. A., Renggli, H. H., and Lehner, T., 1977b, The role of Fc and C3b receptors in phagocytosis by inflammatory polymorphonuclear leucocytes in man, *Immunology,* **32:**955–961.

Wilton, J. M. A., Gibson, T., and Chuck, C. M., 1978, Defective phagocytosis by synovial fluid and blood polymorphonuclear leukocytes in patients with rheumatoid arthritis, *Rheumatol. Rehabil.* **17:**25–36 (Suppl.).

Winkelstein, J. A., 1973, Opsonins: Their function, identity and clinical significance, *J. Pediatr.* **82:**747–753.

Winner, H. I., 1955, Study of *Candida albicans* agglutinins in human sera, *J. Hyg.* **53:**509–512.

Winner, H. I., 1956, Immunity in experimental moniliasis, *J. Pathol. Bacteriol.* **71:**234–237.

Winner, H. I., 1958, An experimental approach to the studies of infection by yeast-like organisms, *Proc. R. Soc. Med.* **51:**496–499.

Winner, H. I., 1960, Experimental moniliasis in the guinea pig, *J. Pathol. Bacteriol.* **79:**420–421.

Winner, H. I., 1969, The transition from commensalism to parasitism, *Br. J. Dermatol.* **81:**62–68 (Suppl. 2).

Winner, H. I., 1972, Studies on *Candida, Proc. R. Soc. Med.* **65:**433–436.

Winner, R. I., 1966, General features of *Candida* infections, in: *Symposium on Candida Infection* (R. I. Winner and R. Hurley, eds.), pp. 6–12, Livingstone, Edinburgh.

Winner, R. I., and Hurley, R., 1964, *Candida albicans,* Churchill-Livingstone, London.

Winner, R. I., and Hurley, R., 1966, *Symposium on Candida Infections* (R. I. Winner and R. Hurley, eds.), Livingstone, Edinburgh.

Winsten, S., and Murray, T. J., 1956, Virulence enhancement of filamentous strain of *Candida albicans* after growth on media containing cysteine, *J. Bacteriol.* **71:**738.

Wright, L. J., Kimball, H. R., and Wolff, S. M., 1969, Alteration in host responses to experimental *Candida albicans* infections by bacterial endotoxin, *J. Immunol.* **103:**1276–1282.

Wuepper, K. D., and Fudenberg, H. H., 1967, Moniliasis "autoimmune" polyendocrinopathy and immunologic family study, *Clin. Exp. Immunol.* **2:**71–82.

Wybran, J., Levin, A. S., Spitler, L. E., and Fudenberg, H. H., 1973 Rosette forming cells, immunological deficiency diseases and transfer factor, *N. Engl. J. Med.* **288:**711–713.

Yamamoto, K., and Takahashi, Y., 1971, Macrophage migration inhibition by serum from densensitised animals previously sensitised with tubercle bacillia, *Nature (London)* **233:**261–263.

Yoshida, T., and Cohen, S., 1974, Lymphokine activity *in vivo* in relation to circulating monocyte levels and delayed skin reactivity, *J. Immunol.* **112:**1540–1547.

Yoshida, T., Sonozaki, H., and Cohen, S., 1973, The production of migration inhibition factor by B and T cells of the guinea pig, *J. Exp. Med.* **138:**784–797.

Young, G., 1968, The process of invasion and persistance of *Candida albicans* injected intraperitoneally into mice, *J. Infect. Dis.* **102:**114–121.

Yu, R. J., Bishop, C. T., Cooper, F. P., Hasenclever, H. F., and Blank, F., 1967, Structural studies of mannan from *Candida albicans* (serotypes A and B), *Candida parapsilosis, Candida stellatoidea* and *Candida tropicalis, Can. J. Chem.* **45:**2205–2211.

Zaikaria, N. A., and Elinov, N. P., 1968, Fungal plasmacoagulase, *Mycopathol. Mycol. Appl.* **35:**10–16.

22

Fungi in Pulmonary Allergic Diseases

J. PEPYS

1. General Considerations

Fungi play a variety of roles in which immunopathogenetic mechanisms are involved in the production of respiratory disease in man and other animals. They may act as primary pathogens, opportunistic pathogens, or as allergens and, as is the case with *Aspergillus fumigatus,* in more than one of these ways.

Fungal pathogens are well known and tend to have well-defined endemic areas and well-defined roles in disease. Different and formidable problems exist in trying to establish roles in disease of common commensal opportunistic fungi with or without evidence of natural infection. They are commonly present in the microflora, often regarded as simply contaminants, and are capable of inducing immunological responses in a limited number of individuals, as with *A. fumigatus,* or almost universally, as with *Candida albicans.* These responses may be epiphenomena and of no obvious clinical significance, although interpretable as evidence of the host's capacity to mount immunological responses.

The factors influencing the nature of the diseases produced are (1) the immunological reactivity of the host; (2) the nature of the fungal agent, such as its capacity to grow in the respiratory tract, invade the tissues, etc.; and (3) the circumstances of exposure.

In terms of immunological reactivity there are terminological and conceptual difficulties in assessing reactions regarded as evidence of hypersensitivity. Hypersensitivity reactions on the one hand play an important role in "immunity" and on the other are often a *sine qua non* in fungal diseases in which the end picture has characteristics pertinent to the particular infecting agent. When the fungi act as allergens, the end picture is characteristic of the type or types of allergy involved and the part or parts of the lungs affected, being similar for allergens of widely disparate nature and source. In this discussion of allergic aspects of pulmonary disease, emphasis will be laid upon the antigens, relevant antibodies, and allergic manifestations due to *A. fumigatus* and to *C. albicans.* These, in addition to their own interest, provide indications for similar studies of the pathogenic fungi, such as *Coccidioides immitis* and *Histoplasma capsulatum.*

2. Antigenic Components of Fungi

The slow growth of the organisms in fungal infections may explain the wide range and variations in immunological responsiveness, bringing into play an even larger range of antigens and their corresponding antibodies, than might be the case with more rapidly growing bacteria and viruses. The problems are complicated further by the variability of antibody responses among individuals and the capacity of fungi, termed a "mutable and

J. PEPYS • Clinical Immunology, Cardiothoracic Institute, University of London, Brompton, London SW3 6HP, England.

treacherous tribe" by Allbrech von Haller 200 years ago, to vary. The progeny of even a single spore can vary within wide biochemical limits, even though morphologically indistinguishable. These factors create problems for the preparation of antigens, the essential tools for analysis of immunological responses. The cells in any one culture are not likely to be homogeneous physiologically, and the differences are augmented by the use of different culture media and by variations in the methods of antigen preparation. These test materials are also likely to be used, in amounts in excess of those likely to be encountered at a site of infection. The responses are thus interpretable only as tests indicating previous exposure and sensitization requiring clinical correlations and not necessarily as proof of the actual allergic mechanisms involved in the particular disease.

A review of the nature and methods of preparation of antigenic components of fungi has been made by Longbottom and Pepys (1964). The main antigens to be discussed are protein, polysaccharides (often glycopeptides), and those provided by whole cells or fungal elements. Polysaccharide antigens are poor inducers of hypersensitivity, but good elicitors of reactions in sensitized subjects and, as with the mannan of *C. albicans,* can greatly enhance hypersensitivity reactions and serological responses (Pepys *et al.,* 1968a). The necessity for better knowledge of the characteristics of the antigen components in test materials is exemplified by conventional "laboratory" or commercial preparations of *C. albicans* antigens. These are commonly regarded or even titled "protein" antigens. Serological tests have shown that the usual preparations are likely to contain minimal amounts of protein antigen together with the sometimes predominant polysaccharide antigens (Fig. 1) There is also no consistency in this antigenic mixture. The different immunochemical components may elicit the same or different allergic reactions, with the same or different types of antibody response. For example, the polysaccharide cell-wall mannan of *C. albicans* can elicit immediate Type I reactions mediated by IgE and/or short-term sensitizing IgG antibodies. Together with the precipitins they may also cause Arthus Type III reactions, but not delayed Type IV reactions. The pro-

tein antigens elicit Type I, a Type III-like reaction, and in particular Type IV reactions (Pepys *et al.,* 1968a; Edge and Pepys, 1976; Edge, 1978). Under the circumstances, the proper analysis of allergic reactions which are elicited can be difficult, if not impossible. Immunological interest has been largely confined to protein antigens, but polysaccharide antigens and their effects also need to be studied more than has been the case up to now.

The use of whole organismal cells as antigens has much to be commended in that they represent the form in which the particular agent is encountered in the body.

Correlation of immunological responses with well-defined diseases and clinical manifestations can provide epidemiological, diagnostic, and prognostic information and such responses can also be a measure of immunological competence.

3.   Types of Allergic Reaction

Allergic reactions have been classified into four types by Gell *et al.* (1975). Of these, immediate, Type I; nonimmediate (late) Type III; and delayed, Type IV allergy will be discussed here. These types of allergy find their expression in responses to skin tests, which play an important part in immunological assessment. In addition to uniform use of standardized allergen preparations, it is also desirable that test methods and the ways in which the reactions are assessed be standardized and generally understood.

In Types I, III, and IV allergy, the antigen is of exogenous origin, whereas in Type II allergy the antigen is derived from an autologous cell or tissue or is produced there by combination with a hapten. The presence of Types I, III, and IV allergy to fungi can readily be shown. There is little if any evidence of fungal, Type II, allergy.

3.1.   Type I: Immediate, Skin-Test Allergic Reactions (Fig. 2)

Type I reactions are mediated mainly by the heat-labile, long-term cell sensitizing IgE antibody, reagin, demonstrable by serological tests or passive transfer tests with unheated serum. IgE antibody production is a feature

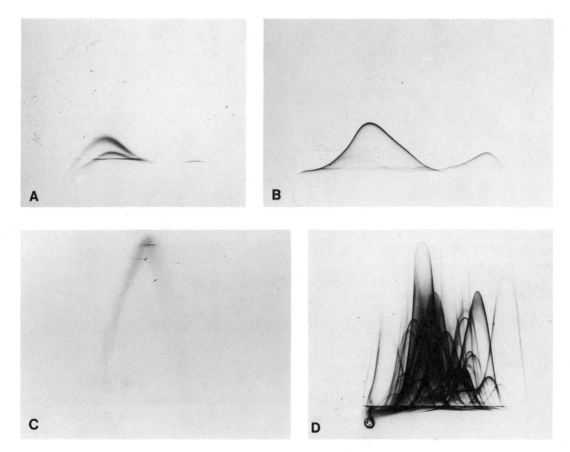

Figure 1. *C. albicans,* three commercial extracts—antigen content. Crossed immunoelectrophoresis against *C. albicans* antiserum (rabbit, Dakopatts). (A) Two mannan precipitin arcs, one small protein arc; (B) mannan precipitin arc only; (C) several protein precipitin arcs; (D) cytoplasmic protein, mannan-free, precipitin arcs.

of, but not confined to, atopic subjects (Pepys, 1975b). Atopy is of decisive importance in allergy to fungi, but little attention has been given to it in relationship to fungal infections. Type I reactions can also be mediated by heat-stable, short-term sensitizing IgG antibody as reported in man by Parish (1970). This antibody cannot be identified specifically by serological tests at present. It appears to be mainly in the IgG4 subclass and is demonstrable by passive transfer of heated serum in skin tests in man and monkey, and more recently by passive sensitization of human leukocytes (Cromwell and Pepys, 1980). STS-IgG antibody is not necessarily correlated with the presence of precipitins (see section on antibodies to *A. fumigatus*) (Pepys *et al.,* 1979). Both classes of antibody may be present to-gether against the same or different antigens in the test preparations, e.g., *C. albicans* mannan and protein antigens. Type I, IgE mediated reactions can be elicited by the precise and highly sensitive skin prick-test method (Pepys, 1975a). This method virtually eliminates the effects of nonspecific irritants and the results, from the smallest whealing reactions upward, correlate well with serological tests for specific IgE antibody (Stenius *et al.,* 1971). By contrast, for eliciting STS-IgG mediated reactions intracutaneous tests are usually necessary. Higher levels of IgG4 immunoglobulin have been reported in mold-sensitive subjects who mount positive reactions to antigen administered by the intracutaneous route but not by scratch test (Vijay *et al.,* 1978).

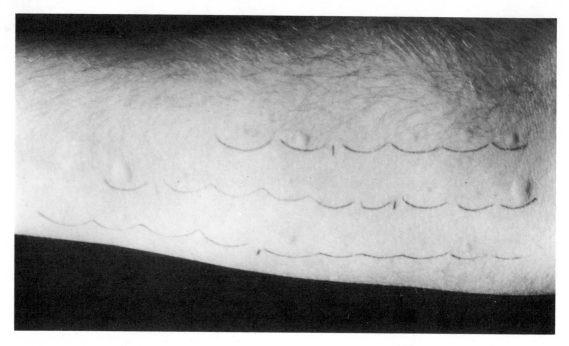

Figure 2. Type I, immediate, whealing reactions to skin prick tests with fungal and other allergens. Max. at 10–15 min and resolving in 1½–2 hr.

3.2. Type III: Nonimmediate (Late) Skin-Test Allergic Reactions (Fig. 3)

The Type III reaction appears to have two components. The immediate, Type I, reaction acts as an introductory mechanism, in experimental animals and in subjects with precipitins, for the elicitation of the more slowly appearing Type III reaction (Cochrane, 1971; Pepys, 1969). The immediate reaction is usually mediated by IgE antibody, but it can also be mediated by IgG-STS antibody (Warren et al., 1977), particularly in nonatopic subjects. There are many examples in which the presence of precipitins (e.g., the precipitins present in abundance in aspergilloma) is not accompanied by the production of Type III reactions. The usual absence of Type I reactivity may explain this. Type III reactions are sensitive to corticosteroids, which have little if any effect on Type I reactions.

In Type III reactions, soluble complexes of antigen and precipitating antibody produced in moderate excess of antigen, fix and activate the C3 component of complement by the classic pathway giving rise to the tissue damaging effects of toxic soluble-complex reactions.

Complement may also be activated by an alternative pathway without the participation of antibodies by a number of fungal or related agents such as *A. fumigatus* and *Micropolyspora faeni* (Marx and Flaherty, 1976; Edwards, 1976). The activated complement could perhaps cause tissue damage. It also activates macrophages (Schorlemmer et al., 1977), which could enhance processing of the antigen, and secondarily, the antigen-specific immunological responses. It might also play a role in the varying capacity of different fungi to produce hypersensitivity and secondary allergic disease. Macrophage activation may also contribute to resistance to infection as it does with *Mycobacterium tuberculosis* and *Listeria monocytogenes* by complement deposition (Pepys, 1976). Macrophage activation could also enhance the infection, as is the case with Histoplasma, which is modulated by the parasitisation of macrophages by *Histoplasma capsulatum*.

Another possible mode of antibody independent complement fixation is through the complement activating effect of complexes of C-reactive protein with C-substance (Kaplan and Volonakis, 1974; Siegel et al., 1975), which is present in the glycopeptides of *A. fumigatus* and other fungi.

3.3. Type IV: Delayed, Tuberculin Type, Allergic Reactions (Fig. 4)

The Type IV reaction is mediated by sensitized lymphocytes and lymphocyte-derived mediators of inflammatory tissue reactions (Pepys, 1976). This reaction is induced by protein antigens and is regarded as a classic indicator of infection. By contrast, polysaccharide antigens give rise to Types I and III, but not Type IV, reactions. More study is required to accurately assess the relevance of Type I and III reactions in infection.

Type IV reactivity to skin tests is associated with resistance to tuberculosis and also to histoplasmosis. In the latter as well as other fungal infections, depression of lymphocyte reactivity by disease or immunosuppressive drugs has an enhancing effect on infection. The *in vitro* lymphocyte responses to fungal and other antigens are used as criteria of host-defence capacity. However, lymphocyte responsiveness to antigen *in vitro* is not necessarily cor-

related with Type IV skin test reactivity and cannot be taken as equivalent to it.

As shown by tuberculin reactions, there are a number of factors capable of modifying Type IV reactivity, which can be important (Pepys, 1955a). The elicitation of Type IV reactions is strongly influenced by factors affecting the local persistence of the antigen. Increased local lymphatic absorption of the antigen from the test site will decrease reactions and vice versa. Thus immediate whealing reactions elicited by the test itself can markedly decrease or prevent subsequent Type IV reactivity from being manifest. Other factors increasing lymphatic absorption from the skin are fever; tissue edema of cachexia; pregnancy; or local reasons, such as erythema of the skin (e.g., sunburn) and inflammatory responses elicited by recent previous testing at the same site.

Some factors of this sort probably contribute to the assessment of allergy in patients with severe infections. Physiological differences in capillary distribution and thus of lymphatic absorption also have effects, so that stronger reactions are elicited on the skin of the upper

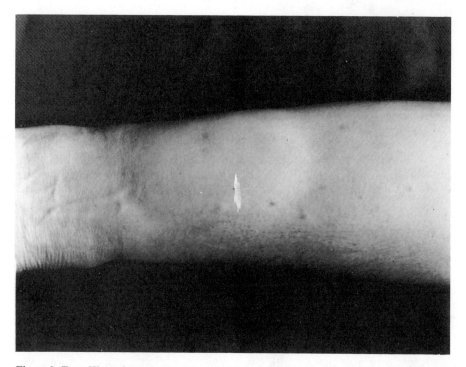

Figure 3. Type III (Arthus type) reactions to intracutaneous test with mannan of *C. albicans*. Preceded by Type I reaction and maximal at 5–8 hr resolving within about 24 hr.

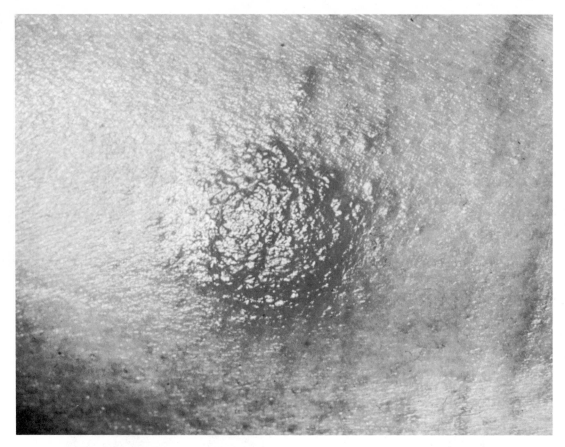

Figure 4. Type IV delayed reaction to cytoplasmic protein of *C. albicans,* maximal at 48–72 hr.

region of the back, which has a lesser capillary density than that of the lower part. Factors that decrease lymphatic absorption of the antigen enhance reactions of epicutaneous tests, such as the addition of epinephrine to the scratch or multiple puncture test for tuberculin sensitivity. Depot preparations, which are only slowly absorbed, also enhance sensitivity and reactions, such as depot tuberculin and depot lepromin. Such methods of study appear not to have been used with fungal antigens.

Repetition of skin tests can stimulate and maintain the Type IV skin test reactivity, although antigen given at frequent intervals can decrease the sensitivity, as in tuberculin desensitization.

Granulomata are usually regarded as evidence of Type IV allergy, a concept derived from their presence in association with tuberculin Type IV reactions. Evidence in sup-

port of a lymphocyte-mediated mechanism for granuloma formation is provided by the work of Boros and Warren (1973) They found that bentonite particles coated with mycobacterial or schistosomal antigen could elicit granuloma formation in sensitized subjects and that capacity for such responses could be passively transferred with lymphocytes, but not with the serum of sensitized animals. In a number of fungal respiratory diseases the spores or other fungal mycelial elements could be responsible for eliciting granuloma formation by this mechanism.

There are, however, other additional and not necessarily exclusive possibilities. Spector and Heesom (1969) showed that insoluble complexes of antigen and antibody in equivalence which do not fix and activate complement can elicit granuloma formation, whereas toxic soluble complement-activating complexes of the same antigens and antibodies cause acute inflammatory reactions. Thus the diffusible antigens of spores, in subjects with both precipitins and other elements necessary for a Type III reaction could be responsible both for this antibody-mediated acute reaction and, when insoluble complexes are formed, for the granulomatous reactions. The insoluble precipitation lines in agar–gel diffusion tests have on one side soluble complexes in antigen excess and on the other side an excess of free antibody. Gradation of antigen and antibody in tissues may also occur, leading to a variety of immunopathological responses in pulmonary fungal diseases of all sorts. Another mechanism that can contribute to the granuloma production is the activation of complement by the alternative pathway, which may lead to secondary macrophage activation.

3.4. Type II: Cytotoxic, Allergic Reactions

In this form of allergy the relevant antigen is on an autologous cell or tissue surface or is formed there by hapten conjugation. The allergic reactions that result from antibody combination are cytotoxic. It is not known whether fungal antigens cause respiratory allergic disease in this way. Polysaccharide antigens are, however, noted for their capacity to absorb to cell surfaces (Parish *et al.*, 1976), so that this possibility has to be considered.

The different types of allergy have their particular characteristic features determined by the type or types of antibody mechanism involved. They can and do exist together, and their elicitation can depend on the nature of the antigen and the test methods used. In tuberculin allergy, for example, Type I and III reactions, which are mainly directed against polysaccharide antigens, can be elicited along with Type IV reactions to proteins (Pepys, 1955). The end picture of what is regarded as a Type IV reaction may therefore show evidence of Types I and III reactions as well. The production of the Types I and III reaction can be, and has often been, overlooked where the investigators' attentions are restricted to eliciting Type IV reactions; much useful information has been lost in this way. The immunological findings in histoplasmosis and coccidioidomycosis do not make mention of this, perhaps because Type I and III reactivity

do not occur, although this is not specifically stated.

4. Aspergillus Species and Pulmonary Aspergillosis

4.1. General Considerations

Aspergillus fumigatus is the most important aspergillus species in pulmonary aspergillosis. It is ubiquitous in the environment and probably universal in distribution, although in widely different amounts. *A. fumigatus* is an allergen, a saprophyte, and an opportunistic pathogen for man and a primary pathogen for birds, cattle, and other animals. Its spores are about 3 μm in diameter and are capable of penetration to the alveolar regions. They are also present in the air in chains 8–10 μm in length, a size appropriate for being trapped in the proximal, medium-size, bronchi. The organism can grow at body temperature and at temperatures in the respiratory tract.

A. fumigatus is a model example of the influence of the immunological reactivity of the host, the nature of the causal agent, and the circumstances of exposure on the production of different forms of lung disease in atopic and nonatopic subjects.

Atopic subjects develop Type I allergy to the fungus with bronchial reactions and asthma, or peribronchial reactions with pulmonary eosinophilia termed allergic bronchopulmonary aspergillosis (ABPA), with the participation of Types I and III allergy.

In nonatopic subjects the spores can cause extrinsic allergic alveolitis, in which Type III and its introductory Type I mechanism and possibly Type IV allergy are involved; saprophytic pulmonary mycetoma or aspergilloma in damaged lung spaces; and invasive disease in patients who are immunodeficient or receiving immunosuppressive therapy.

Atopic Subjects. Type I Allergy to *A. fumigatus*. Atopic subjects can develop Type I allergy to *A. fumigatus,* just as they do to other common inhalant allergens. The reactions elicited on exposure are immediate, Type I in nature. The asthma that may develop is not complicated by pulmonary eosinophilia. Reported differences in the prevalence of Type I allergy to A. *fumigatus* in different parts of the world could be due to differences in the amounts of the fungus and its spores in the environment, to differences in the quality of the allergen test extracts, and to differences in the methods of testing and interpretation of reactions.

In the United Kingdom there may be as many as 100 times more spores of *A. fumigatus* in the air in winter than in summer (Noble and Clayton, 1963). This variation is clearly evident in our experiences with allergic bronchopulmonary aspergillosis, where the majority of the episodes of the disease occur in the winter months (McCarthy and Pepys, 1971a). A low prevalence of *A. fumigatus* in the air was found at Ann Arbor, Michigan, and there was no evidence of a winter peak (Solomon *et al.*, 1978).

The essential importance of the quality of the test extracts is shown by the fact that for many years the diagnosis of ABPA was not made in the United States. A single case was described as a "North American rarity" (Slavin *et al.*, 1969). Further investigations in Madison, Wisconsin, with more effective extracts than were previously used, elicited positive reactions to intracutaneous tests in 36% of their asthmatics. In a collaborative clinical study of patients with uncomplicated asthma, which excluded patients with allergic bronchopulmonary aspergillosis (Schwartz *et al.*, 1978), the same batch of *Aspergillus* extract, when used for prick testing, yielded a comparable frequency of Type I reactions in Cleveland (28%) and in London (23%). Similarly, serum precipitins to this antigen were detected in 7.5 and 10% of each group, respectively. This shows that for these two cities, at least, there is no difference in the incidence of allergy to *A. fumigatus*. Information on the aerobiology of two such centers would be helpful for comparison.

The method of testing is also important. The skin-prick test shows the best correlation with specific IgE antibodies to common allergens (Stenius *et al.*, 1971). The prevalence of Type I reactions reported in one series of asthmatics by Hoehne *et al.* (1971), which is higher than the incidence reported in Cleveland (Schwartz *et al.*, 1978) or in England, is probably attributable to the mode of testing. The reasons for emphasizing the skin-prick test method is that it is less likely to give doubtful or false-positive reactions (Pepys, 1975a) than the scratch and intracutaneous tests. RAST for specific IgE antibody correlates well with the skin-prick test, although IgG antibody may also play a part in ABPA (Pepys *et al.*, 1979).

Type I and III Allergy in Allergic Bronchopulmonary Aspergillosis: Clinical Aspects of ABPA. The main emphasis on pulmonary aspergillosis will be on this form of disease. ABPA was first recognized pathologically by Hinson *et al.* (1952). Immunological support for this was provided by Pepys *et al.* (1959), and it has since been the subject of many British reports (Pepys, 1969; Campbell and Clayton, 1964; Henderson *et al.*, 1968; McCarthy and Pepys, 1971a,b; Safirstein *et al.*, 1973; Malo *et al.*, 1977a–d). There are many reports of ABPA in European countries (Molina, 1976). The diagnosis was made considerably later in the United States (Rosenberg *et al.*, 1977; Wang *et al.*, 1978; Imbeau *et al.*, 1978; Bardana *et al.*, 1975) because, according to Hoehne *et al.* (1971) of the inadequacy of the *Aspergillus* antigens available.

The essential clinical features of ABPA are pulmonary eosinophilia that is transitory and often recurrent, and pulmonary shadows due to infiltration or atelectasis induced by bronchial plugging, which in many cases, are persistently associated with eosinophilia of the blood and usually the sputum. Asthma is present in almost all cases. The presence of Type I skin test reactions to *A. fumigatus* in such cases is the first diagnostic criterion of allergic bronchopulmonary aspergillosis.

In uncomplicated asthma, the immediate skin reaction is evidence only of Type I allergy comparable to that to other common inhalant allergens, and it does not in itself mean that ABPA is present. In the majority of cases of ABPA, precipitating antibodies can also be found with the elicitation on challenge of Type III as well as Type I skin, nasal, and bronchial reactions.

About 80% of British cases (McCarthy and Pepys, 1971a,b) report expectoration of tough viscid mucus plugs or gritty particles. These contain eosinophils as well as growing hyphae of *A. fumigatus*. Cylindrical and saccular bronchiectases tend to develop proximally at the sites of the plugging, so that peripheral bronchi fill normally on bronchography, unless obstructed by mucus (Scadding, 1967; McCarthy *et al.*, 1970).

4.2. Immunopathology of ABPA

The pneumonitis that develops in response to antigens from growing hyphae in sputum plugs consists of an eosinophilic reaction in which both Types I and III allergy could be involved.

The elicitation in monkeys of reactions analogous to the pulmonary eosinophilia of ABPA in man requires the participation of both IgE and precipitating antibodies (Golbert and Patterson, 1970; Slavin *et al.*, 1977).

The bronchiectasis and surrounding reaction have been included under the term bronchocentric granulomatosis (Liebow, 1973). The features of mucoid impaction, eosinophil infiltration, bronchial damage, noninvasive presence of *A. fumigatus,* and fungal allergy (Katzenstein *et al.,* 1975; Hanson *et al.,* 1977) are those of ABPA. Granulomatous changes in ABPA have also been reported by Chan-Yeung *et al.* (1971). The granulomata are usually attributed to Type IV allergy of which there is limited evidence here. Insoluble immune complexes which do not fix complement can elicit granulomata. The same immune complex in moderate antigen excess fixes complement and causes Type III reactions (Spector and Heesom, 1969). Another mechanism is suggested by the work of Boros and Warren (1973), in which antigen-coated particles elicited a granulomatous reaction that could be passively transferred with lymphocytes, but not serum.

Complement activation by the alternative pathway and associated macrophage activation could also contribute (Schorlemmer *et al.,* 1977). These various mechanisms, alone or together, are also relevant to extrinsic allergic alveolitis due to fungal spores, and have been described by Dickie and Rankin (1958) as hypersensitivity interstitial granulomatous pneumonitis.

4.3. Bronchiectasis and Type III Allergy to *A. fumigatus*

The peribronchial shadows represent a segmental eosinophilic pneumonitis, coupled with localized proximal bronchiectases developing at sites where the sputum "plugs" are formed. The first plug may be expectorated on initiation of corticosteroid treatment. With clearing of these plugs, positive sputum cultures may revert to negative. This suggests that retention of the spores in the bronchi is related to the hypersensitivity. Asthmatics in general have been found to have significantly more positive sputum cultures than other subjects with respiratory disease (Pepys *et al.,* 1959).

The antigens diffusing from the growing hyphae in the plug could be mediating Type III reactions of the sort seen in skin tests in ABPA. Limited evidence for the deposition of antigen, immunoglobulins, and activated C3 in the bronchial wall in resected lung has been reported by Katz and Kniker (1973).

Systemic evidence of immune complex formation and complement activation by the classic pathway has been reported by Geha (1977). During the acute phase, serum C3 was decreased, C1q was 60% of normal, and C4 reduced. C3 split products made up 20% of the total circulating C3. Circulating immune complexes were detected by precipitation with C1q by the method of Agnello *et al.* (1970). On retesting 10 weeks later, after cessation of corticosteroid treatment, the complement levels had returned to normal.

4.4. Prevalence of ABPA

About 80% of British patients with pulmonary eosinophilia seen at the Brompton Hospital, London, had evidence of ABPA (McCarthy and Pepys, 1971a,b).

Estimates of the prevalence of ABPA vary. According to Henderson *et al.* (1968) the prevalence was 10% in what was probably selected material. At the Brompton Hospital an estimate was made of the prevalence of ABPA in some 800 consecutive asthmatics seen for the first time, with the exclusion of those in whom ABPA had already been diagnosed. The diagnosis of ABPA was first made by us in about 1% of the cases, a value which is probably closer to its general prevalence.

4.5. Atopic Status and ABPA

Atopic status plays a role in the clinical presentation of ABPA. It can be graded (Pepys, 1975b) according to the number of Type I skin-prick test reactions to relevant common allergens, with some minor reservations, because of the possible role of IgG-STS antibody in Type I reactions.

A study of IgE and IgG-STS antibodies to *A. fumigatus* showed that in atopic patients with ABPA and with weak precipitin reactions, all have IgE antibody and one-third have IgG-STS antibody. In patients with aspergilloma, in whom very strong precipitin reactions are regularly observed, about one-quarter had IgE antibody, and none had IgG-STS antibodies (Pepys *et al.*, 1979). Thus, IgG-STS antibodies are not necessarily related to the precipitins.

ABPA patients with asthma starting before 10 years of age had the highest atopic status and comprised 57% of our material. In these patients, the first diagnosis of pulmonary eosinophilia was made after an interval of 21 years. In those patients in whom asthma developed between 11 and 30 years of age, (18%) the atopic status was lower and the interval was about 11 years. In those with asthma starting after 31 years of age (35%) the atopic status was lowest, with one-half reacting only to *A. fumigatus* and the interval before the diagnosis of ABPA was about 11/2 years (McCarthy and Pepys, 1971a,b; Malo *et al.*, 1977a–c). The clinical and immunological significance of these differences is now known. They suggest that in the more highly atopic subjects who start with asthma early in life and who are readily sensitized to produce IgE antibody, more intensive or prolonged exposure is needed to induce the production of precipitins, hence the long interval before ABPA is manifest.

In subjects with low or nonatopic status, asthma tends to appear later in life. Nonatopic subjects, i.e., those who do not readily produce IgE antibody to common allergens, tend to produce precipitins in response to inhaled organic dusts and to develop extrinsic allergic alveolitis. In the case of allergic alveolitis due to avian antigens, IgG-STS antibodies have been found (Warren *et al.*, 1977; Pepys *et al.*, 1979). These antibodies are responsible for the Type I reaction, which is necessary as an introductory mechanism for the Type III reaction. By analogy, at least one-half of the subjects with asthma starting later in life who shortly thereafter develop ABPA are of low atopic status. It seems possible that in such subjects the induction of precipitating antibodies and of IgE or IgG-STS antibodies may occur at the same time or within a short time

of each other, thus providing the immunological mechanisms for ABPA.

4.6. Corticosteroids in ABPA

Systemic corticosteroid treatment is effective in ABPA, inducing resolution of acute pulmonary shadows in most cases. As shown in a retrospective study (Safirstein *et al.*, 1973), administration of corticosteroids also reduces the incidence of episodes of pulmonary eosinophilia. There is no evidence to suggest that corticosteroid treatment in such patients who are not immunodeficient favors invasion of the tissues by the fungus or extension of disease. In patients with impairment of immunological reactivity caused by disease or immunosuppressive treatment, it is likely that corticosteroids would favor invasive infection by the fungus.

A double-blind multicenter study was made in ABPA to examine the effect of treatment with an inhaled corticosteroid, beclomethasone diproprionate, given over a period of at least 6 months, on the disease and on sputum cultures for *A. fumigatus* (BTTA, 1979). The only statistically significant finding was an association between serum antibody levels to *A. fumigatus* and episodes of pulmonary eosinophilia diagnosed radiographically. The asthma was benefited by the treatment, but there was no reduction in the episodes of pulmonary eosinophilia although these episodes usually occurred without clinical deterioration of the asthma. There were, however, more frequent, although not significantly so, positive sputum cultures for *A. fumigatus* during the period of inhalation of the corticosteroid.

4.7. Skin Test, Type I and III Reactions to *A. fumigatus*

4.7.1. Type I. Immediate Reactions

Positive Type I prick-test reactions can be elicited with both protein and polysaccharide fractions, the proteins being more potent (Longbottom, 1964); most extracts contain both in usually unknown and varying proportions.

The Type I reaction is important both in its own right and also because it provides the introductory mechanism required for the development of Type III reactions (Cochrane, 1971; Pepys, 1969).

4.7.2. Nonimmediate, Type III Reactions

Prick tests with commercial extracts give Type III reactions in about one-quarter and the protein fraction in about one-half of the ABPA patients, preceded by Type I reactions. Intracutaneous tests elicit Types I and III reactions in almost all cases. In the Type III reactions, immunofluorescence tests show the presence of IgG, IgM, IgA immunoglobulins, and activated C3 as β1C deposited in the perivascular space, in mononuclear cells, and in the endothelium of the blood vessels (Pepys et al., 1968b). Type III-like reactions without precipitins or similiar histological evidence are attributed to IgE antibody (Dolovich et al., 1973; Solley et al., 1977). Type III reactions are sensitive to corticosteroids irrespective of whether or not precipitins or other evidence for Type III allergy are concurrently demonstrable. These agents have little effect on Type I reactions.

4.8. Skin-Test Reactivity and Airway Obstruction

In ABPA there is a tendency to develop poorly reversible or "fixed" airway obstruction and significant impairment of gas transfer (Safirstein et al., 1973; Malo et al., 1977d). The Type III reactions that contribute to ABPA may be responsible for this, although a significant correlation ($p < 0.01$) was also found between skin-test reactivity to A. fumigatus and the severity of airway obstruction in asthmatics without ABPA (Schwartz et al., 1978). There is a similar tendency for the development of fixed airway obstruction in avian allergy, where there is evidence to suggest that Type III allergy is also involved.

4.9. Bronchial and Nasal Test Reactions to A. fumigatus

In ABPA patients Type I and III reactions are both elicited by bronchial and nasal tests with extracts of A. fumigatus. The two reactions can be quite distinct, with the Type I reaction lasting about $1\frac{1}{2}$ to 2 hr, several hours after which the second reaction appears. Here,

too, the Type III, but not the Type I, reaction is inhibited by corticosteroids.

4.10. Serological Tests

4.10.1. Specific and Total IgE Levels to A. fumigatus

There are many reports of raised specific IgE antibody levels and very marked increases in total IgE levels in ABPA with some relationship to the acute episodes (Patterson et al., 1973; Turner et al., 1974; Malo et al., 1977c). The specific IgE is detected by the RAST assay and assesses IgE antibody to protein antigens of A. fumigatus. Specific and total IgE levels were significantly elevated in ABPA as compared with prick-test-positive uncomplicated asthma (Malo et al., 1977c) ($p < 0.0001$). Similarly, patients with uncomplicated asthma differed from prick-test-negative subjects ($p < 0.05$), and the prick-test-negative atopic subjects differed from nonatopic subjects ($p < 0.01$). There was little overlap in the specific IgE levels in ABPA and the prick-test-positive asthmatics and even less with the others.

The total IgE levels were significantly higher ($p < 0.05$) in patients who had experienced episodes of pulmonary eosinophilia in the 3 months prior to testing, but there was no linear decline in IgE levels, suggesting the total IgE values can fall rapidly. The total IgE increases are out of proportion to the increments in specific IgE antibody (Patterson et al., 1973; Turner et al., 1974), suggesting that nonspecific increases in total IgE are due to some as yet unknown mechanism that provides a general stimulus of IgE production in response to the ongoing allergic reaction.

Raised levels of specific IgE antibody when observed between episodes can be helpful in suggesting ABPA (Malo et al., 1977c). Wang et al. (1978) found a highly significant increase ($p < 0.001$) in both IgE and IgG antibodies in ABPA and suggest that this association can be used to distinguish ABPA from uncomplicated asthma. Specific IgE levels can rise during episodes even in patients on corticosteroids and can portend a flare, although with prolonged corticosteroid therapy, levels fall toward normal (Stevens et al., 1970b; Imbeau et al., 1978).

Raised levels of specific IgE antibodies against polysaccharide antigens of *A. fumigatus* have been documented in ABPA (Baldo and Pepys, 1976; Sepulveda *et al.*, 1979) and will be discussed further under enzyme-linked immunosorbent assay (ELISA) test procedures. Occasional patients with aspergilloma have raised IgE antibodies, specific for the protein antigens of *A. fumigatus,* as shown by the ELISA test (Sepulveda *et al.*, 1979) and by the Radioallergosorbent test (RAST) and Passive Cutaneous Anaphalaxin (PCA) test in the monkey (Pepys *et al.*, 1979).

4.11. Precipitin Test Reactions to *A. fumigatus*

In the different forms of pulmonary aspergillosis, weak precipitin reactions are obtained in ABPA in contrast to very strong reactions in aspergilloma (Longbottom and Pepys, 1964; Jacoby *et al.*, 1977; Sepulveda *et al.*, 1979). Positive precipitin tests are detected in extrinsic allergic alveolitis due to *A. clavatus* and *A. fumigatus* (Vallery-Radot and Giroud, 1928; Riddle *et al.*, 1968; Yocum *et al.*, 1976). The precipitin test has not been found to be helpful in the diagnosis of invasive disease.

Positive precipitin reactions, mainly in agar-gel double-diffusion tests, can be obtained in up to about 10% of uncomplicated asthmatics (Longbottom and Pepys, 1964; Mearns *et al.*, 1967; Coleman and Kaufman, 1972; Schwartz *et al.*, 1978), and seldom in normal, healthy subjects. In ABPA about 85–90% of subjects were found to have precipitins, but in one-third of the patients concentration of the serum was needed to detect these reactions (Longbottom and Pepys, 1964; McCarthy and Pepys, 1971a,b; Safirstein *et al.*, 1973; Malo *et al.*, 1977c). Concentration of the serum increases the sensitivity of the test without loss of specificity. A significant correlation ($p < 0.02$) was found between skin-prick and precipitin test positivity (Malo *et al.*, 1977c).

In ABPA a battery of extracts is needed to establish the maximum number of positive reactions which may occur to any one or more antigens in one or more of the extracts (Longbottom, 1964; Longbottom and Pepys; Flaherty *et al.*, 1974). The precipitin reactions are stronger during acute episodes even in patients on prednisone (Imbeau *et al.*, 1978), and they correlate with the number of past episodes and the interval since the last (Malo *et al.*, 1977c).

4.12. Quantitative Measurement of IgG Antibodies to *A. fumigatus*

Agar-gel tests give only a semiquantitative measure of antibodies. The use of a solid phase coupled with anti-IgG for absorption of IgG from the test serum and the subsequent measurement of uptake of radiolabeled *A. fumigatus* protein provides an indirect quantitative measure of the amount of specific IgG, or, if so wished, of antibodies in the IgG subclasses to the particular antigen (Jacoby *et al.*, 1977). Highest concentrations of antibody are found in aspergilloma, followed by ABPA, and then asthma. The results correlate with the agar-gel test findings.

4.13. ELISA Test for IgG and IgE Antibodies to Protein and Polysaccharide Antigens of *A. fumigatus*

The ELISA, when a microplate version is used (Voller *et al.*, 1976), gives quantitative measurements of IgE and IgG antibodies to "polysaccharide" as well as protein antigens of *A. fumigatus* (Sepulveda *et al.*, 1979). In tests on ABPA, aspergilloma, and asthma sera, close correlation was found between the ELISA for IgG antibodies to *A. fumigatus* protein and the solid-phase antibody antigen uptake method. This supports the assumption that the latter test reflects antibody levels, and also correlates with the precipitin tests. There were, however, positive reactions with some precipitin-negative sera, thus showing a further value of this test.

The relative levels of IgG antibodies were higher for protein than for polysaccharide antigens in aspergilloma sera and vice versa in ABPA and asthma. This suggests that anti-polysaccharide antibodies may be relevant to the allergic phenomena in ABPA just as with the *C. albicans* mannan antigen, which is a potent allergen (Pepys *et al.*, 1968a).

4.14. Specific IgE Antibodies

The ELISA results correlated well in ABPA with the RAST for specific IgE antibody to the protein antigens. Some aspergilloma sera also gave positive and quite high IgE antibody results. Tests have not yet been made for IgE to the polysaccharide antigens, as has already been done with insolubilized polysaccharide by Baldo and Pepys (1976).

Tests methods used for antibodies to *A. fumigatus* include crossed immunoelectrophoreses, latex agglutination tests, and others. The polystyrene tube radioimmunoassay (PTRIA) and labeled antigen radioimmunoassay (LARIA) (Wang *et al.*, 1978) are similar in principle to the ELISA tests described above and give similar results. The PTRIA gave no false positive or negative results. The LARIA gave about 5% each of false positives or negatives.

4.15. Lymphocyte *in Vitro* Tests with *A. fumigatus*

Lymphocyte responses to *A. fumigatus* in ABPA (Haslam *et al.*, 1976; Rosenberg *et al.*, 1977; Forman *et al.*, 1978; Imbeau *et al.*, 1978) and in extrinsic allergic alveolitis (Yocum *et al.*, 1976) have proved to be highly variable in different series, probably due to variation in antigens, the test methods used, the small numbers of patients supplied, and the diagnostic criteria used to described them.

Lymphocyte transformation assays using unseparated whole blood have been reported to generate higher antigen-specific responses than assays that used separated lymphocytes. These differences were attributed to antigenic stimulation with immune complexes present in whole blood. (Rosenberg *et al.*, 1977). T and B cell participation in ABPA was suggested by Forman *et al.* (1978) on the basis of tests on small numbers of patients. By contrast, Haslam *et al.* (1976) found very limited evidence of lymphocyte responses, although it is suggested (Turner-Warwick, 1973) that on occasion positive results may be obtained in patients with suspected ABPA who manifest a Type IV skin test response, but negative Type I skin tests and precipitin results.

In the patient reported by Geha (1977), lymphocyte reactions of a comparable order of magnitude were obtained before and after the acute phase.

The absence of Type IV skin test reactions in infected immunocompetent individuals, could be due to the effects of Types I and III reactions on the local persistence of the allergen, as has been shown for tuberculin (Pepys, 1955). This possibility has to be explored before this apparent deficiency can be attributed to other factors, such as a histamine-induced suppressor factor (Rocklin, 1977).

4.16. Nonatopic Subjects: Extrinsic Allergic Alveolitis

The inhalation of the spores of the Aspergillus genus by nonatopic subjects can induce the production of precipitins and, on further exposure, the production of extrinsic allergic alveolitis, a severe fibrosing lung disease of which farmer's lung is the classic example.

The first report of what we would now regard as allergic alveolitis due to *A. fumigatus* was made by Vallery-Radot and Giroud (1928). The patients described had precipitins to *A. fumigatus* and gave immediate and nonimmediate skin test reactions which were probably expressions of Type I and III allergy. The authors considered the disease to be a sporomycosis.

Allergic alveolitis due to the spores of *A. clavatus* has been described in maltsters as malt-worker's lung, and is associated with the presence of precipitins (Riddle *et al.*, 1968; Yocum *et al.*, 1976). The tissue manifestations in the peripheral lung tissues are the result of allergic reactions to the inhaled spores, which have to be of an appropriate size (about 1- to 3-μm diameter) to penetrate and be retained in the alveolar regions. The acute disease responds well to corticosteroid treatment, suggesting that Type III allergy plays an important role, and that this disorder does not represent an invasive disease.

Among the many other fungal and actinomycete species listed (Pepys, 1969; Lacey *et al.*, 1972), the spores of which are causes of allergic alveolitis are the following: *Cryptostroma corticale,* causing maple bark pneumonitis; *Penicillium frequentans,* causing suberosis; *Aureobasidium pullulans* and *Graphium* sp., causing sequoiosis, and *Penicillium casei,* causing cheese-washer's lung; *Micropolyspora faeni,* causing farmer's lung in both man and cattle; *Thermoactinomyces sacchari,* causing bagassosis; and these and other thermophilic antinomycetes, causing ventilation pneumonitis.

4.17. Aspergillus Mycetoma

The development of a saprophytic *A. fumigatus* mycetoma is a pathologic process seen mainly, although not exclusively, in nonatopic subjects; it may occur together with ABPA. The aspergilloma is only locally if at all invasive, and its development is based on local damage and not on immunodeficiency. Lung cavities, predominantly those associated with or following tuberculosis, are the commonest local factor favoring the aspergilloma, and some patients may have more than one (BTA, 1968; BTTA, 1970; Villar and Cortez-Pimentel, 1970; Voisin *et al.*, 1964; Voisin and Biguet, 1970). Among other predisposing disorders are lung abscess, cavitating pneumoconiosis, sarcoidosis, bronchiectasis, and lung cavities of other unknown origin. Pleural aspergilloma may develop after surgical intervention or as a sequela to therapeutic pneumothorax. Most aspergillomata are intracavitary, in the bronchus or lung, and about 4% are pleural (Villar and Cortez-Pimentel, 1970; Voisin and Biguet 1970).

The rapid marked increase in the frequency of diagnosis of aspergilloma, e.g., in Lille, France (Voisin and Biguet, 1970) from 7 cases in 1962 to 302 in 1968, has arisen from the introduction of the precipitin test (Longbottom and Pepys, 1964). This usually gives a strong or very strong diagnostic reaction, attributable to the antigenic stimulus from the fungal mass in immune-responsive subjects.

Two British surveys were made 3–4 years apart of the prevalence of aspergilloma in patients with open-healed cavities of treated pulmonary tuberculosis (BTA, 1968; BTTA, 1970). In the first survey, positive precipitin reactions were given by 25% of cases to *A. fumigatus*, with four exceptions Radiography showed the presence of aspergilloma in 11% of the cases, all of whom gave strong precipitin reactions, and in 4% it was thought that an aspergilloma might be present. There was no radiographic evidence to suggest aspergilloma in those subjects giving weak or negative precipitin reactions.

On reexamination between 3–4 years later,

some aspergillomata had become smaller or disappeared, and the precipitin test had become negative (BTTA, 1970). Similar decreased or negative precipitin reactions were found in patients in whom the aspergilloma was removed surgically or in whom one of two aspergillomata was removed; in others the precipitin reaction increased with subsequent development of a further aspergilloma (Longbottom, 1978).

In the BTTA (1970) study, of the cases previously regarded as possible aspergillomata on radiography who also had positive precipitin tests, one-half showed the definite presence of an aspergilloma. Of those with previously weak precipitin reactions and without radiographic evidence of aspergilloma, one-sixth showed definite aspergilloma and a stronger precipitin reactions. In this survey, 25% of previously negative precipitin reactors now gave positive precipitin tests and in one-half of these a definite aspergilloma was present. Other workers (Voisin *et al.*, 1964) made similar observations and emphasized the importance of an increase in the intensity of the precipitin reaction as evidence of a latent and developing aspergilloma. In 2% of cases with a diagnosis of aspergilloma the precipitin test may be negative (Villar and Cortez-Pimentel, 1970). In one of the above surveys (Villar and Cortez-Pimentel, 1970) the aspergilloma was found to be dead in four and largely nonviable in three precipitin-negative cases. These authors found no relationship between antibiotic or corticosteroid treatment and the development of an aspergilloma.

An association of aspergilloma with ABPA in atopic subjects may occur and is associated with more severe disease. An association by hypersensitivity with aspergilloma in nonatopic subjects is reported in a small group of patients in the above BTTA survey. These patients had a raised erythrocyte sedimentation rate (ESR) and clinical signs, including malaise, fever, loss of weight, and hemoptysis, together with thickening of the cavity wall. They respond well to corticosteroid treatment (Davies and Somner, 1972). Although patients with aspergilloma are mainly nonatopic, positive and usually weak reactions are elicited by prick tests in about 20% with *A. fumigatus*, and in some the presence of specific IgE antibody has been shown by RAST and by PCA tests in the monkey. These responses, together with the presence of the precipitating antibodies, could be responsible for the hypersensitivity reactions described. Febrile, systemic reactions in response to inhalation tests with *A. fumigatus* extract in some patients with aspergilloma (Stevens *et al.,* 1970a) corresponds with the above observations, being typical of such tests in affected patients with precipitins to the particular allergen (Pepys, 1969).

The skin-prick test is not a diagnostic test for aspergilloma, whereas the strong precipitin test reaction in the presence of the appropriate clinical and radiographic findings is of high diagnostic value. By contrast in ABPA, the precipitin test is usually weak and is not diagnostic, whereas the Type I prick test reaction is diagnostic in the presence of the features of the pulmonary eosinophilia and of the bronchiectatic sequelae and cystic lung changes of ABPA.

A. fumigatus is the main cause of aspergilloma, although other species such as *A. nidulans, A. niger,* and *A. flavus* have also been identified, giving specific precipitin test reactions (Longbottom *et al.,* 1964). More than one species may be present together. In one patient, *A. versicolor* was present together with *Allescheiria boydii,* and with specific precipitins against both (McCarthy *et al.,* 1969). Pulmonary infection due to *A. boydii* affects cavity lesions, mainly from tuberculosis, with the production of a mycetoma or chronic suppurative pneumonitis (Drouhet, 1955; Creitz and Harris, 1955; Tong *et al.,* 1958, Scharyj *et al.,* 1960; Travis *et al.,* 1961; Louria *et al.,* 1966).

4.18. Invasive Aspergillosis

The spectrum of invasive aspergillosis in a group of 98 patients (Young *et al.,* 1970), of whom 90% had hematological and lymphoreticular malignant disease, showed that almost all had pulmonary involvement, consisting of pneumonia (necrotizing, hemorrhagic, or suppurative). A group of 8 subjects with noninvasive disease were termed "aspergillary bronchitis," but the limited information provided suggests that a diagnosis of ABPA would have been more appropriate.

In 15 patients with widespread invasive aspergillosis, negative tests were obtained for antibodies in the last 3 weeks of life by the double-diffusion, complement fixation, immunoelectrophoresis, and indirect fluorescent antibody methods (Young and Bennett, 1971). These findings did not confirm the report of the presence of *A. fumigatus* precipitins in patients with acute leukemia (Goldstein *et al.,* 1970).

Emphasis is laid (Young and Bennett, 1971) on the need to exclude the reaction given with C-reactive protein by polysaccharides in extracts of *A. fumigatus* capable of behaving like C-substance (Longbottom and Pepys, 1964).

Patients with leukemia and Hodgkins disease have relatively normal antibody responses to infection before receiving immunosuppressive treatment (Brown *et al.,* 1967). The negative tests for antibodies to *A. fumigatus* in such patients is in contrast to this finding, and the comment is made (Young and Bennett, 1971) that positive precipitin tests are obtained in noninvasive, and not in invasive pulmonary aspergillosis.

The problems of recognition of opportunistic invasive fungal infection by *A. fumigatus* and *C. albicans* in patients with immunodeficiency need to be resolved if early diagnosis is to be made. Serial prospective studies with the widest range of relevant antigens and of test procedures are indicated in the hope that some guidance may be obtained.

4.19. Cystic Fibrosis and *A. fumigatus*

Between one quarter to one-third of patients with cystic fibrosis had precipitins to *A. fumigatus,* with a higher incidence in severe protracted disease. Type I skin reactions were elicited in about 40% (Mearns *et al.,* 1967), and Type III reactions in many, neither showing close correlation with precipitins (Warren *et al.,* 1975), in contrast to their close relationship in ABPA. Pulmonary shadows suggestive of ABPA are seen in some cases.

4.20. Antigens, Allergens, and C-Substance in *A. fumigatus*

Antigens giving precipitin reactions appear rapidly within two days in cultures, with the highest yield in Sabouraud liquid medium after 2–6 weeks at 37°C (Longbottom and Pepys, 1964; Longbottom, 1964; Biguet *et al.,* 1964).

The culture medium is prepared further by filtration, dialysis, and freeze-drying to give a mixture of proteins and polysaccharides suitable for serological and skin and other tests *in vivo*. The cell sap of mycelium is rich in precipitating antigens, but is not suitable for intracutaneous tests, as it causes nonspecific reactions which can be confused with Type III reactions, probably because of its content of toxins.

4.21. Protein Fractions of *A. fumigatus*

These can be prepared by saturated ammonium sulfate precipitation. The protein fractions are highly potent in skin testing and should be used in very low concentrations. A small number of patients with features of ABPA, but giving negative reactions to conventional extracts, give Type I reactions to this material.

4.22. Aspergillus Antigens as Enzymes

In tests on sera giving 10 to 19 precipitin arcs, presumably from aspergilloma patients who give reactions of this intensity, antigens have been identified with activity of chymotrypsin I and II, I being the strongest; it was suggested that this could be a specific diagnostic reagent (Biguet *et al.*, 1962, 1967; Tran Van Ky *et al.*, 1966). Other enzymes so identified in the *A. fumigatus* extract include catalase (Tran Van Ky *et al.*, 1968); glucuronidase I and II and amylase (Tran Van Ky *et al.*, 1969); five carboxylic acid esterases, glucose-6 phosphate dehydrogenase, two lactic dehydrogenases, malic dehydrogenase, and alanine dehydrogenase (Tran Van Ky *et al.*, 1969, 1970). Other species of Aspergillus contain similar though not identical enzymes. In *A. flavus*, chymotryptic malic dehydrogenase enzyme was thought to be of diagnostic significance (Tran Van Ky *et al.*, 1971). It is not known whether the enzymatic activities of these many allergenic components are of immunopathogenetic importance.

4.23. Polysaccharides and C-Substance of *A. fumigatus*

The glycopeptides of *A. fumigatus* are glucogalactomannan (ratio 1 : 5 : 20) peptides (Longbottom, 1964; Longbottom and Pepys, 1964; Pepys and Longbottom, 1971).

The nitrogen content consists of a high proportion of hydroxyaminoacids, serine, and threonine together with alanine. The polysaccharides can be obtained from the supernatant after ammonium sulphate precipitation or by other methods, e.g., hot phenol extraction.

The polysaccharide and peptide moieties play different roles. The polysaccharides give fuzzy precipitin lines in agar gel. One of them also acts like pneumococcal C-substance by virtue of its calcium-dependent combination with C-reactive protein. The latter reaction can be prevented by adding a calcium chelator, e.g., sodium citrate to the agar-gel before the test. This procedure can also be used to resolve already produced precipitation reactions if added later. The precipitin reaction, but not the C-substance activity, is lost following periodic acid degradation (Longbottom, 1964). There is another polysaccharide which has identical antigenic properties but no C-substance activity.

C-substance materials which react by virtue of their phosphatidyl choline with C-reactive protein are widely distributed in nature, being found in other fungi, such as the dermatophytes, in nematode and cestode parasites and in vegetable matter, such as palm kernels. All of these can give Type I prick-test reactions in patients allergic to *A. fumigatus* (Pepys and Longbottom, 1971).

5. *Candida albicans*

5.1. General Considerations

C. albicans is an uncommon cause of pulmonary infection, being an opportunistic pathogen mainly in immunocompromised hosts. Whether it is a respiratory allergen of any importance has not been established. The fungi causing pulmonary disease, other than the usual common mould allergens range from *H. capsulatum* and *C. immitis*, which have a well-defined endemic distribution and sensitivity which constitutes evidence of infection, although not necessarily disease; and the *Aspergillus* genus, particularly *A. fumigatus*, which is widely present in the environment, which causes pulmonary disease as an allergen causing asthma or ABPA or as a saprophyte causing aspergilloma; to *C. albicans* which is universally present in the body and against which sensitization in one form or other is demonstrable in most subjects and indeed in some circumstances can be more relevant if this is shown to be absent. There is very extensive literature on serological findings in relation to *C. albicans*. Most of this work has been made with different antigens and methods and without, on the whole, sufficient knowledge of the ways in which the different antigenic components might react. The problems therefore of assessing the potential immunopathogenetic effects of *C. albicans* in respiratory disease are even more complicated than with *A. fumigatus*. No meaningful interpretation, for example, of a Type I reaction to a commercial or other extract of unknown and variable composition can be made. This reaction could be mediated by IgE or STS-IgG antibody to the polysaccharide fraction and by IgE antibody to the protein or by combinations of these. The variable characteristics of these antigens and their different immunopathogenic potential makes it essential that future studies be made with this in mind. It may not be possible to compare future work of this type with past studies for the reasons given.

5.2. Antigens of *C. albicans* and Their Immunological Reactions

The importance of a thorough characterization and standardization of allergen preparations is highlighted by the variable, different, and limited antigens in laboratory or commercial extracts of *C. albicans* (Figure 1A–D). The latter extracts are commonly regarded as protein, but they may actually contain a preponderance of polysaccharide and only limited amounts of protein. Such mixtures are hardly comparable to the multiplicity of protein antigenic components in cytoplasmic extracts which have been rendered free of polysaccharide.

5.2.1. Cell-Wall Mannan of *C. albicans*

The preparation of purified cell-wall mannose polymers, the mannan antigens (Summers *et al.*, 1964) from Group A (the more predominant in man) and from Group B, *C. albicans* (Hasenclever *et al.*, 1961) allowed

a more precise immunochemical analysis of their antigenic determinants. The mannans of Group A and B had cross-reactive as well as distinctive antigens (Hasenclever, 1965). Type A has at least three, and type B at least two fractions (Winner, 1972).

5.2.2. Protein Antigens of *C. albicans*

The main sources of protein antigens are from the culture filtrate, which contains products of cell metabolism and lysis. Polysaccharides are also present in these products. Axelsen (1973) found 78 water-soluble antigens from disrupted cells; Evans *et al.* (1973) found quantitative and qualitative differences in preparations from the two growth phases, blastospore and mycelial, and Syverson *et al.* (1975), who identified six antigens unique to each phase, suggested that antigens specific to the mycelial phase could provide a basis for a standardized antigen preparation for diagnosis in systemic candidiasis.

The various protein products also contain polysaccharide. A preparation of a polysaccharide-free cytoplasmic protein derived from disrupted cells was made by passage through an affinity chromatography column of Sepharose to which concanavalin A had been covalently bound. Concanavalin A is effective as a lectin for removal of the polysaccharide component (Longbottom *et al.*, 1976; Edge, 1978). A reference preparation of this polysaccharide-free protein is available from the National Institute for Biological Standards, Holly Hill, Hampstead, London, N.W.3.

5.3. Immunological Reactivity to Different Antigenic Preparations of *C. albicans*

In the results to be described, the yeast cells were obtained from a 48-hr continuously stirred culture at room temperature. The cells were harvested by centrifugation and were not used if mycelia were present. Such cells provide a picture of the composite antigens on their surface, in a form most likely to be encountered in the body.

Purified mannan, polysaccharide-free cytoplasmic extract, culture filtrate, and whole yeast cells were compared as antigenic preparations on the sera or skin or both of patients with a specific soft tissue *C. albicans* granuloma, termed Kimura's disease (Takenaka *et al.,* 1976) or with ABPA, asthma, or aspergilloma (Edge and Pepys, 1976; Edge, 1978).

5.4. Skin Tests

5.4.1. Reactions to Mannan

Both mannan and purified protein gave positive Type I reactions to prick tests in about 15% of atopic and nonatopic asthmatics, in contrast to ABPA where 60% or more were positive to both. This higher incidence of skin-test reactions in ABPA is paralleled by the elicitation of vigorous Types I and III reactions to intracutaneous tests with the mannan in all the ABPA subjects so tested. This suggests that allergy to *C. albicans* might play a role in ABPA and possibly, in its own right, in the occasional subjects with the features of ABPA and no evidence of allergy to *A. fumigatus.* The possibility of cross reactivity between the *C. albicans* mannan and the *A. fumigatus* glucogalactomannan was not supported by serological tests which showed specific absorption. In PCA tests in the monkey, IgE and STS-IgG antibody were demonstrable against the mannan. PCA tests showing the presence of IgE against the protein have also been made. RAST tests also showed IgE antibody to both antigens.

5.4.2. Effects of Mannan Skin Test on Degree of Sensitivity

Intracutaneous tests with the mannan had a remarkable enhancing effect on sensitivity in apparently healthy subjects. In subjects with mannan precipitins and allergic respiratory disease 77% gave Types I and III skin reactions, as compared with 14% of those without precipitins. In the subjects giving negative skin and precipitin tests (measuring about 0.25 mg antibody/ml), all gave Types I and III reactions and positive precipitin reactions on retesting within the next four weeks (Pepys *et al.,* 1968a). This has several implications. First, those using injections of this polysaccharide should take into consideration the possibility of enhancing the host's sensitivity. Second, it shows that there is a general sensitivity to the mannan in the population, which suggests the possibility of obtaining positive precipitin reactions to the mannan in all subjects tested sufficiently intensively (Chew and Theus, 1967). Third, exposure to the cell-

wall polysaccharides *in vivo* may also enhance the degree of sensitivity, which might continue to increase with increased growth of the fungus in subjects capable of responding immunologically. The mannan elicits Type I and III, but not Type IV, reactions, unlike the protein, which elicits Type IV reactions as well. Like other yeast polysaccharides the mannan could also be an activator of complement by the alternative pathway.

5.4.3. Reactions to Purified Protein

C. albicans protein is widely used in skin tests as an indication of the host's "cell-mediated" immunocompetence. It can give vigorous Type I reactions for which IgE antibody is demonstrable, followed in most cases by a Type III-like reaction for which, however, precipitins may not be demonstrable. This in turn is followed by Type IV reactions. Virtually no mention is made of the Types I and III reaction by workers using *C. albicans* antigens for such tests and their significance in terms of host defense is not known. In terms of allergic disorders, they are only the subject of unestablished speculation.

5.5. Serological Tests

5.5.1. Precipitin Tests

a. Protein Antigens. Tests for precipitins have been widely used for diagnostic purposes in deep-seated candidiasis (Taschdjian *et al.,* 1964, 1967, 1972). These precipitating antibodies are directed against protein antigens.

b. Mannan Antigens. An important feature of the precipitins to the mannan is that positive agar-gel double-diffusion reactions are obtained with low concentrations, e.g., 0.001–0.1 or 1 mg/ml, but not with higher concentrations, presumably because of the production of soluble complexes (Pepys *et al.,* 1968a). Most *C. albicans* extracts used for such tests contain amounts of polysaccharide that are probably too high for precipitation reactions, whereas this problem does not apply to the protein antigens. It may be for this reason that most attention has been focused on protein precipitation reactions in deep-seated disease.

Chew and Theus (1967) report on precipitins to the mannan in all subjects tested provided the sera are sufficiently concentrated. In contrast, precipitins to protein antigens are seldom found in uninfected subjects. Increases in amounts of antipolysaccharide precipitins might be a useful indication of systemic disease, if the subject is capable of responding immunologically. A commercial test for mannan precipitins for this purpose is prepared by F. Hoffman–LaRoche. Tests for mannan precipitins at 0.25 mg/ml level were positive in 75% of patients with ABPA, 50% with uncomplicated asthma and 20% with other disorders (Pepys *et al.*, 1968a).

5.6. Tests for Specific IgE Antibody

Polysaccharide antigens unlike proteins cannot be linked to the cyanogen bromide-activated solid-phase immunosorbents used to test for specific IgE antibodies. To overcome this, Baldo and Pepys (1977) used insolubilized mannan ground to a powder as the solid phase immunosorbent and were able to show specific IgE to the mannan and, using the same method, to *A. fumigatus* polysaccharide as well.

Positive RAST results (Edge and Pepys, 1976; Edge, 1978) for the mannan have been obtained with an epichlorohydrin-polymerized mannan prepared by Sandula and Kuniak (1974), and Edge (1978) has also used an epoxy-activated Sepharose 6B preparation, which takes up the mannan, for the same purpose.

The differences in RAST values found with mannan and cytoplasmic proteins in the different clinical groups suggest that such tests can be useful. Thus, patients with Kimura's disease (*C. albicans* soft tissue granuloma) have more mannan IgE antibody than do those with ABPA, whereas the reverse was found for antibodies to the cytoplasmic protein. RASTs using the whole yeast cells as antigen gave comparable results in these two groups, suggesting that the cell-wall antigens consist of both polysaccharide and protein. The latter tests also show that the yeast cells are a suitable solid-phase immunosorbent for these tests.

Comparison of antibodies that had combined with the cell-wall antigens in terms of their reactivity with antisera to IgG and its subclasses also showed differences (Edge, 1978). Thus, positive results were obtained with anti-IgG antisera in asthma (66%); rhinitis (46%), and ABPA (75%). With the IgG sub-class antisera, however, a different picture emerged, and for IgG1 the values were asthma 4%, rhinitis 13%, and ABPA 65%. For IgG2: asthma 0%, rhinitis 5%, and ABPA 70%. For IgG3: asthma 50%, rhinitis 25%, and ABPA 20%. For IgG4: asthma 78%, rhinitis 20%, and ABPA 85%. The ABPA group showed highly significant correlation between the total IgG antibody and that in the four subclasses. In asthma, only the total IgG and IgG3 antibodies showed a significant correlation, while in the rhinitis group total IgG correlated with IgG3 and IgG4 antibodies. The immunopathogenetic significance of these results is not known, but the fact that there are differences of this sort suggests that they may be meaningful.

The yeast cells also gave positive results in tests for IgA and IgM antibodies and titers were higher in patients with ABPA than in patients in the other groups. These findings support a possible role for *C. albicans* in ABPA. The possibility that it can cause itself a pulmonary disease similar to that caused by *Aspergillus* is suggested by the findings of Voisin *et al.* (1976). If this is so, the condition could, by analogy, be termed allergic bronchopulmonary candidiasis.

6. General Comments

Interest in fungi in allergic respiratory disease has focused largely, on the one hand, on sensitization to the common molds in the atmosphere, such as *Alternaria, Cladosporium herbarum, Aspergillus* spp., and yeasts; with the production of Type I, IgE-mediated allergy in atopic subjects; and, on the other hand, on sensitization to the pathogenic fungi with the production of delayed tuberculin-type Type IV allergy. In the course of sensitization, however, the different types of allergy can be, and often are, induced together. Emphasis in particular diseases on one or other form of immunological reactivity arises from its established or postulated relationship to a specific type of immunopathology, such as Type I allergy in immediate asthma, or from the association of a specific type of allergy, such as Type IV, and a particular type of infection, yet it can readily be shown that in allergy to the tubercle bacillus, Type I, III, and IV allergy are all demonstrable (Pepys, 1955).

J. PEPYS

Analysis of the allergic effects of fungi and of other allergens can usefully be broadened by taking these points into consideration. For example, the generally accepted Type I reaction may, as we now know, be mediated by IgE antibody or by IgG-STS antibody, or perhaps by both acting together. Furthermore, the assumption that a disease regarded as a classic example of Type I allergy, such as hay fever and asthma in the atopic, involves only immediate hypersensitivity reactions has to be questioned, because there is often evidence of reactions compatible with Type III allergy present at the same time. This may have therapeutic significance, since Type I allergy is not sensitive to corticosteroid drugs, which are very effective in Type III allergy. For example, corticosteroids can be beneficial in, hay fever, regarded as the model *par excellence* of the Type I allergy; yet evidence from skin and provocation tests shows that corticosteroids have no effect on this particular form of reactivity.

Conversely, studies of the pathogenesis of infection by the invasive fungi, have paid little attention to the participation of Type I and III allergy and, where these are present, to their significance. It would be of interest, for example, to know whether atopy, as shown by the production of IgE antibody to common allergens with or without clinical manifestations attributable to it, has any influence on such an infection.

There is clearly much to be done in analyzing the allergic state provoked by fungi. For such studies, the need for better reagents, standardized as much as possible, is evident. Differences in allergic reactivity to polysaccharide and protein antigens make it essential that these responses be assessed separately. Furthermore, the effort devoted to preparation of specific fungal extracts for clinical and research purposes needs to be matched by more comprehensive analysis of their allergenic roles.

References

Agnello, V., Winchester, R. J., and Kunkel, H. G., 1970, Precipitin reactions of the C_1q components of complement with aggregated gammaglobulin and immune-complexes in gel-diffusion, *Immunology* 19:909–919.

Axelsen, N. H., 1973, Quantitative immunoelectrophoretic methods as tools for a polyvalent approach to standardization in the immunochemistry of *Candida albicans*, *Infect. Immunol.* 7:949–960.

Baldo, B. A., and Pepys, J., 1976, Radioallergosorbent test (RAST) studies with insolubilized polysaccharides, *Clin. Allergy* 6:563–571.

Bardana, E. J., Gerber, J. D., Craig, S., and Cianculli, F. D., 1975, The general and specific humoral response to pulmonary aspergillosis, *Am. Rev. Resp. Dis.* 112:799–805.

Biguet, J., Tran Van Ky, P., Capron, A., and Fruit, J., 1962, Analyse immunochimique des fractions antigéniques solubles d'*Aspergillus fumigatus*. Orde d'apparition des anticorps expérimentaux du lapin: Comparison de ces derniers avec des anticorps naturels humains, *C. R. Acad. Sci.* 254:3768–3776.

Biguet, J., Tran Van Ky, P., and Andrieu, S., 1964, Analyse immunoélectrophoretique d'extraits cellulaires et de milieux de culture d'*Aspergillus fumigatus* par des immunserums expérimentaux et des serums de malades atteint d'aspergillome bronchopulmonaire, *Ann. Inst. Pasteur (Paris)* 107:72–97.

Biguet, J., Tran Van Ky, P., Fruit, J., and Andrieu, S., 1967, Identification d'une activité chymotrypsique au niveau de fractions remarquables de l'extrait antigénique d'*Aspergillus fumigatus*. Répercussions sur le diagnostic immunologique de l'aspergillose. *Rev. Immunol. (Paris)* 31(4–5):317–328.

Boros, D. L., and Warren, K. F., 1973, Bentonite granuloma characterisation of a model system for injection and foreign body granulomatous infiltration using soluble mycobacterial histoplasma and schistosoma antigens, *Immunology* 24:511–529.

British Thoracic and Tuberculosis Association (BTTA), 1970, Aspergilloma and residual tuberculous cavities—The results of a resurvey, *Tubercle* 51:227–245.

British Thoracic and Tuberculosis Association (BTTA), 1979, Report Inhaled beclomethasone dipropionate in allergic bronchoplumonary aspergillosis, *Br. J. Dis. Chest* 73:349–356.

British Tuberculosis Association (BTA), 1968, Aspergillus infection in persistent lung cavities after tuberculosis, *Tubercle* 49:1–11.

Brown, R. S., Haynes, H. A., Foley, H. T., Godwin, H. A., Bernard, C. W., and Carbone, P. P., 1967, Hodgkins disease: Immunologic, clinical and histologic features in 50 untreated patients, *Ann. Int. Med.* 107:291–302.

Campbell, M. D., and Clayton, Y. M., 1964, Bronchopulmonary aspergillosis, *Am. Rev. Resp. Dis.* 89:186–196.

Canetti, G., 1946, *L'allergie Tuberculeuse chez l'Homme*, Collection de l'Institut Pasteur Editions Medicales, Flammarion, Paris.

Chan-Yeung, M., Chase, W. H., and Trapp, W., 1971, Allergic broncho-pulmonary aspergillosis. Clinical and pathologic study of three cases, *Chest* 59:33–39.

Chew, W. H., and Theus, T. L., 1967, Candida precipitins, *J. Immunol.* 98:220–224.

Cochrane, C. G., 1971, Mechanism involved in the desposition of immune-complexes in tissues, *J. Exp. Med.* **134**(Suppl.):75–89.

Coleman, R. M., and Kaufman, L., 1972, Use of the immunodiffusion test in the serodiagnosis of aspergillosis, *Appl. Microbiol.* **23**:301–308.

Creitz, J., and Harris, H. W., 1955, Isolation of Allescheiria boydii from sputum. *Am. Rev. Tuberc.* **71**: 126–130.

Cromwell, O., and Pepys, J., 1980, Antigen induced histamine release mediated by heat labile IgE and heat stable STS-IgG in vitro, *Clin. Allergy* (in press).

Davies, D. G., and Somner, A. R., 1972, Pulmonary aspergillomas treated with corticosteroids, *Thorax* **27**:156–162.

Dickie, H. A., and Rankin, J., 1958, Farmer's lung: An acute granulomatous interstitial pneumonitis occurring in agricultural workers, *J. Am. Med. Assoc.* **167**:1069–1076.

Dolovich, J., Hargreave, F. E., Chalmers, R., Shier, K. J., Gouldie, J., and Bienestock, J., 1973, Late cutaneous response in isolated IgE-dependent reactions, *J. Allerg. Clin. Immunol.* **52**:38–46.

Drouhet, M., 1955, Status of fungus diseases in France, in: *Therapy of Fungus Diseases, An International Symposium* (T. H. Sternberg and V. D. Newcomer, eds.), p. 43, Little Brown, Boston.

Edge, G., and Pepys, J., 1976, RAST tests avec des antigenes proteiniques et polysaccharidiques et des cellules lavées de *Candida albicans*, *Rev. Fr. d'Allerg.* **16**:251–255.

Edge, P. G. M., 1978, Antibodies to antigens of Candida albicans in allergic respiratory disease, Ph.D. thesis, University of London.

Edwards, H. H., 1976, A quantitative study on the activation of the alternative pathway of complement by mouldy hay dust and thermophilic actinomycetes, *Clin. Allergy* **6**:19–27.

Evans, E. G. V., Richardson, M. D., Odds, F. C., and Holland, K. T., 1973, Relevance of antigenicity of C. *albicans* growth phase to diagnosis of systemic candidiasis, *Br. Med. J.* **4**:86–87.

Flaherty, D. K., Barboriak, J., Emanuel, D., Fink, J., Marx, J., Moore, J., Reed, C. E., and Roberts, R., 1974, Multilaboratory comparison of these immunodiffusion methods used for the detection of precipitating antibodies in hypersensitivity pneumonitis, *J. Lab. Clin. Med.* **84**:298–306.

Forman, S. R., Fink, J. N., Moore, U. L., Wang, J., and Patterson, R., 1978, Humoral and cellular immune responses in *Aspergillus* fumigatus pulmonary disease, *J. Allergy Clin. Immunol.* **62**:131–136.

Geha, R. S., 1977, Circulating immune-complexes and activation of the complement sequence in acute allergic bronchopulmonary apsergillosis, *J. Allergy Clin. Immunol.* **60**:357–359.

Gell, P. G. H., Coombs, R. R. A., and Lachmann, P. J.,

1975, *Clinical Aspects of Immunology,* p. 761, Blackwell Scientific Publications, Oxford.

Golbert, T. M., and Patterson, R., 1970, Pulmonary allergic aspergillosis, *Ann. Int. Med.* **73**:359–403.

Goldstein, I., Hasenclever, H., and Henderson, E., 1970, Precipitating antibodies to Aspergillus organisms in patients with acute leukaemia (abstr.), *Clin. Res.* **18**:440.

Hanson, G., Flood, N., Wells, I., Novey, H., and Galant, S., 1977, Bronchocentric granulomatosis. A complication of allergic bronchopulmonary aspergillosis, *J. Allergy Clin. Immunol.* **59**:83–90.

Hasenclever, H. F., 1965, The antigens of *Candida albicans,* *Am. Rev. Resp. Dis.* **92**(Suppl):150–158.

Hasenclever, H. F., Mitchell, W. O., and Loewi, J., 1961, Antigenic studies on Candida: 1. Observations of two antigenic groups in *C. albicans,* *J. Bacteriol.* **82**:507–573.

Haslam, R., Lukosezek, A., Longbottom, J. L., and Turner-Warwick, M., 1976, Lymphocyte sensitisation to *Aspergillus fumigatus* antigens in pulmonary diseases in man, *Clin. Allergy* **6**:277–291.

Henderson, A. H., English, M. P., and Vecht, R. J., 1968, Pulmonary aspergillosis. A survey of its occurrence in patients with chronic lung disease and a discussion of the significance of diagnostic tests, *Thorax* **23**:513–518.

Hinson, K. F. W., Moon, A. J., and Plummer, N. S., 1952, Bronchopulmonary aspergillosis, *Thorax* **7**:317–333.

Hoehne, J. H., Reed, C. E., and Dickie, H. A., 1971, Allergic aspergillosis is not rare, *J. Lab. Clin. Med.* **78**:1007–1008.

Imbeau, S. A., Nichols, D., Flaherty, D., Valdivia, E., Peters, M. E., Dickie, H., and Reed, C. E., 1978, Allergic broncho-pulmonary aspergillosis, *J. Allergy Clin. Immunol.* **62**:243–255.

Jacoby, B., Longbottom, J. L., and Pepys, J., 1977, The uptake of *Aspergillus fumigatus* protein by serum IgG antibody from patients with pulmonary aspergillosis, *Clin. Allergy* **7**:117–125.

Kaplan, M. H., and Volonakis, J. E., 1974, Interaction of C-reactive protein complexes with the complement system. I. Consumption of human complement associated with the reaction of C_3 reactive protein with pneumococcal C polysaccharide and with the choline phosphatides, lecithin and sphingomyelin, *J. Immunol.* **112**:2135–2147.

Katz, R. M., and Kniker, W. T., 1973, Infantile hypersensitivity pneumonitis as a reaction to organic antigens, *N. Engl. J. Med.* **288**:233–237.

Katzenstein, A. G., Liebow, A. A., and Friedman, P. J., 1975, Bronchocentric granulomatos, mucoid impaction and hypersensitivity reaction to fungi, *Am. Rev. Resp. Dis.* **111**:497–537.

Lacey, J., Pepys, J., and Cross, T., 1972, Actinomycete and fungus spores in air as respiratory allergens, in: *Safety in Microbiology* (D. A. Shapton and R. G. Board, eds.), p. 172, Academic Press, London.

Liebow, A. A., 1973, The J. Burns Amberson lecture—Pulmonary angiitis and granulomatosis, *Am. Rev. Resp. Dis.* **108**:2–18.

Longbottom, J. L., 1964, Immunological investigations of *Aspergillus fumigatus* in relation to disease in man, Ph. D. thesis, University of London.

Longbottom, J. L., 1978, Immunological aspects of infection and allergy due to Aspergillus species. Symposium Medical Mycology, Flims 1977, *Mykosen* I(Suppl.):207–217.

Longbottom, J. L., and Pepys, J., 1964, Pulmonary aspergillosis: Diagnostic and immunological significance of antigens and C-substance in *Aspergillus fumigatus, J. Pathol. Bacteriol.* 38:141–151.

Longbottom, J. L., Pepys, J., and Temple-Clive, F., 1964, Diagnostic precipitin test in *Aspergillus* pulmonary mycetoma, *Lancet* 1:588–589.

Longbottom, J. L., Brighton, W. D., Edge, G., and Pepys, J., 1976, Antibodies mediating Type I skin test reactions to Polysaccharide and protein antigens of *Candida albicans, Clin. Allergy* 6:41–50.

Louria, D. B., Lieberman, P. H., Collins, H. S., and Blerins, A., 1966, Pulmonary mycetoma due to *Allescheiria boyii, Arch. Int. Med.* 117:748–751.

McCarthy, D. S., Longbottom, J. L., Riddle, R. W., and Batten, J. C., 1969, Pulmonary mycetoma due to *Allescheiria boydii, Am. Rev. Resp. Dis.* 100:213–216.

McCarthy, D. S., Simon, G., and Hargreave, F. E., 1970, The radiological appearance of allergic bronchopulmonary aspergillosis, *Clin. Radiol.* 21:366–375.

McCarthy, D. S., and Pepys, J., 1971a, Allergic bronchopulmonary aspergillosis. Clinical immunology. 1. Clinical features, *Clin. Allergy* 1:261–286.

McCarthy, D. S., and Pepys, J., 1971b, Allergic bronchopulmonary aspergillosis. Clinical immunology. 2. Skin, nasal and bronchial tests, *Clin. Allergy* 1:415–532.

Malo, J. L., Hawkins, R., and Pepys, J., 1977a, Studies in chronic allergic bronchopulmonary aspergillosis. 1. Clinical and physiological findings, *Thorax* 32:254–261.

Malo, J. L., Pepys, J., and Simon, G., 1977b, Studies in chronic allergic bronchopulmonary aspergillosis. 2. Radiological findings, *Thorax* 32:262–268.

Malo, J. L., Longbottom, J. L., Mitchell, J., Hawkins, R., and Pepys, J., 1977c, Studies in chronic allergic bronchopulmonary aspergillosis. 3. Immunological findings, *Thorax* 32:269–274.

Malo, J. L., Inouye, T., Hawkins, R., Simon, G., Turner-Warwick, M., and Pepys, J., 1977d, Studies in chronic allergic bronchopulmonary aspergillosis. 4. Comparison with a group of asthmatics, *Thorax* 32:275–280.

Marx, J. J., Jr., and Flaherty, D. K., 1976, Activation of the complement sequence by extracts of bacteria and fungi associated with hypersensitivity pneumonitis, *J. Allergy Clin. Immunol.* 57:325–334.

Mearns, M., Longbottom, J. L., and Batten, J. C., 1967, Precipitating antibodies to *Aspergillus famigatus* in cystic fibrosis, *Lancet* 1:538–539.

Molina, C., 1976, *Broncho-pulmonary Immunopathology,* p. 115, Churchill Livingstone, Edinburgh.

Noble, W. C. N., and Clayton, Y. M., 1963, Fungi in the air of hospital wards, *J. Gen Microbiol.* 32:397–402.

Parish, W. E., 1970, Short-term anaphylactic antibodies in human sera, *Lancet* 2:591–592.

Parish, W. E., Welbourn, E., and Champton, R. H., 1976, Hypersensitivity to bacteria in eczema. IV. Cytotoxic effect of antibacterial antibody on skin cells acquiring bacterial antigens, *Br. J. Dermatol.* 95:493–506.

Patterson, R., Fink, J. N., Pruzansky, J. J., Read, C., Roberts, M., Slavin, R., and Zeiss, C. R., 1973, Serum immunoglobulin levels in pulmonary allergic aspergillosis and certain other lung diseases, with special reference to immunoglobulin E, *Am. J. Med.* 54:16–22.

Pepys, J., 1955, The relationship of specific and nonspecific factors in the tuberculin reaction, *Am. Rev. Tuberc.* 71:49–73.

Pepys, J., 1969, Hypersensitivity diseases of the lungs due to fungi and organic dusts, in: *Monographs in Allergy,* Vol. 4, Karger, Basel.

Pepys, J., 1974a, Skin tests in diagnosis, in: *Clinical Aspects of Immunology* (P. G. A. Gell, R. R. A. Coombs, and P. J. Lachmann, eds.), pp. 55, Blackwell, Oxford.

Pepys, J., 1975b, Atopy, in: *Clinical Aspects of Immunology* (P. G. A. Gell, R. R. A. Coombs, and P. J. Lachmann, eds.), p. 877, Blackwell, Oxford.

Pepys, J., 1976, Allergic manifestations in tuberculosis, in: *Textbook of Immunopathology* (P. A. Miescher and H. J. Muller-Eberhard, eds.), pp. 453–470, Grune & Stratton, New York.

Pepys, J., and Longbottom, J. L., 1971, Antigenic and C-substance activities of related glycopeptides from fungal, parasitic and vegetable sources, *Int. Arch. Allergy* 41:219–221.

Pepys, J., Riddell, R. W., Citron, K. M., Clayton, Y. M., and Short, E. I., 1959, Clinical and immunologic significance of *Aspergillus fumigatus* in the sputum, *Am. Rev. Resp. Dis.* 80:167–180.

Pepys, J., Faux, J. A., Longbottom, J. L., McCarthy, D. S., and Hargreave, F. E., 1968a, *Candida albicans* precipitins in respiratory disease in man, *J. Allergy* 41:305–318.

Pepys, J., Turner-Warwick, M., Dawson, P., and Hinson, K. F. W., 1968b, Arthus (Type III) skin test reactions in man: Clinical and immunopathological features, in: *Allergology* (B. Rose, M. Richter, A. Sehon, and A. W. Frankland, eds.), p. 211, Excerpta Medica International Congress Series No. 162, Amsterdam.

Pepys, J., Parish, W. E., Stenius-Aarniala, B., and Wide, L., 1979, Clinical correlations between long-term (IgE) and short-term (IgG-STS) anaphylactic antibodies in atopic and non-atopic subjects with respiratory allergic disease, *Clin. Allergy* 9:645–658.

Riddle, H. F. V., Channell, S., Blyth, W., Weir, D. M., Lloyd, M., Amos, W. M. G., and Grant, I. W. B., 1968, Allergic alveolitis in a malt worker, *Thorax* 23:271–280.

Rocklin, R. E., 1977, Histamine-induced suppressor factor (HSF) effect on migration inhibitory factor (MIF) production and proliferation, *J. Immunol.* 118:1734–1738.

Rosenberg, M., Patterson, A., Mintzer, R., Cooper, B. J., Roberts, M., and Harris, K. E., 1977, Clinical and immunologic criteria for the diagnosis of allergic broncho-pulmonary aspergillosis, *Ann. Int. Med.* **86:**405–414.

Safirstein, B., D'Souza, M. F., Simon, G., Tai, E. H. C., and Pepys, J., 1973, Five-year follow-up of allergic broncho-pulmonary aspergillosis, *Am. Rev. Resp. Dis.* **108:**450–459.

Sandula, J., and Kuniak, L., 1974, Affinity chromatography of yeast antibodies on modified mannan, *J. Chromatogr.* **91:**293–295.

Scadding, J. G., 1967, The bronchi in allergic aspergillosis, *Scand. J. Resp. Dis.* **48:**372–377.

Scharyj, M., Levene, N., and Gordon, H., 1960, Primary pulmonary infection with *Monosporium apiospermium:* Report of a case with clinical, pathologic and mycologic data, *J. Infect. Dis.* **106:**141–148.

Schorlemmer, H. V., Edwards, J. H., Davies, P., and Allison, A. C., 1977, Macrophage responses to mouldy hay dust, *Micropolyspora faeni* and zymosan activators of complement by the alternative pathway, *Clin. Exp. Immunol.* **27:**198–207.

Schwartz, H. J., Citron, K. M., Chester, E. L., Karnial, J., Barlow, P. B., Baum, G. L., and Shuyler, M. R., 1978, A comparison of the prevalence of sensitisation to *Aspergillus* antigens among asthmatics in Cleveland and London, *J. Allergy Clin. Immunol.* **62:**9–14.

Sepulveda, R., Longbottom, J. L., and Pepys, J., 1979, Enzyme linked immunosorbent assay (ELISA) for antibodies to polysaccharide and protein antigens of *A. fumigatus*, *Clin. Allergy* **9:**359–371.

Siegel, J., Osmand, A. P., Wilson, M. V., and Gewurz, H., 1975, Interactions of C-reactive proteinwith the complement system, II. C-reactive protein mediated consumption of complement by poly-1-lysine polymers and other polycations, *J. Exp. Med.* **142:**709–721.

Slavin, R. G., Stanczyk, D. J., Longigro, A. J., and Brown, S. O., Jr., 1969, Allergic bronchopulmonary aspergillosis—A North American rarity, *Am. J. Med.* **47:**306–313.

Slavin, R., Fischer, V., Levine, E., Tsai, C., and Winzerburger, P., 1977, A primate model of allergic bronchopulmonary aspergillosis, *Int. Arch. Allergy* **56:** 325–333.

Solley, G. O., Gleich, G. J., Jordan, R. E., and Schroeter, M., 1977, Late cutanious reactions due to IgE antibodies, *Monogr. Allergy* **12:**179–188.

Solomon, W. R., Burge, H. P., and Boise, J. R., 1978, Airborne *Aspergillus fumigatus* levels outside and within a large clinical center, *J. Allergy Clin. Immunol.* **62:**56–60.

Spector, W. G., and Heesom, N., 1969, The production of granulomata by antigen antibody complexes, *J. Pathol.* **98:**31–39.

Stenius, B., Wide, L., Seymour, W. M., Holford-Strevens, V., and Pepys, J., 1971, Clinical significance of specific IgE to common allergens. 1. Relationship of specific IgE against Dermatophagoides spp. and grass pollen to skin and nasal tests and history, *Clin. Allergy* **1:**37–55.

Stevens, E. A. M., Hilvering, C., and Orie, N. G. M., 1970a, Inhalation experiments with extracts of *Aspergillus fumigatus* on patients with allergic aspergillosis and aspergilloma, *Thorax* **25:**11–18.

Stevens, E. A. M., Russchen, C. J., Hilvering, C., and Orie, N. C. M., 1970b, Steroid effect on Aspergillus antibodies, *Scand. J. Resp. Dis.* **51:**55–60.

Summers, D. F., Grollman, A. O., and Hasenclever, H. F., 1964, Polysaccharide antigens of *Candida* cell wall, *J. Immunol.* **92:**491–499.

Syverson, R. E., Bucklyey, H. R., and Cambell, C. C., 1975, Cytoplasmic antigens unique to the mycelial or yeast phase of *Candida albicans, Infect. Immunol.* **12:**1184–1188.

Takenaka, T., Okude, M., Usami, A., Kawabori, S., Ogami, Y., Kubo, K., and Uda, H., 1976, Histologic and immunologic studies on eosinophilic granuloma, of soft tissues, so-called Kimura's disease, *Clin. Allergy* **6:**27–40.

Taschdjian, C. L., Kozinn, P. J., and Caroline, L., 1964, Immune studies in candidiasis. III. Precipitating antibodies in systemic candidiasis, *Sabouraudia* **3:**312–320.

Taschdjian, C. L., Kozinn, P. J., Fink, A., Cuesta, M. B., Caroline, L., and Kantrowitz, A. B., 1967, Postmortem studies of systemic candidiasis. I. Diagnostic validity of precipitin reaction and probable origin of sensitisation to cytoplasmic candidal antigens, *Sabouraudia* **7:**110–117.

Taschdjian, C. L., Kozinn, P. J., Cuesta, M. B., and Toni, E. F., 1972, Serodiagnosis of candidal infections, *Am. J. Clin. Pathol.* **57:**195–205.

Tong, J. L., Valentine, E. H., Durrance, J. R. L., Wilson, G. M., and Fischer, D. A., 1958, Pulmonary infection with Allescheiria boydii, *Am. Rev. Tuberc.* **78:**604–609.

Tran Van Ky, P., Uriel, J., and Rose, F., 1966, Caractérisation de types d'activités enzymatiques dans des extrait antigèniques d'*Aspergillus fumigatus* après eléctrophorèse et immunoléctrophorèse en agarose, *Ann. Inst. Pasteur* **111:**161–170.

Tran Van Ky, P., Biguet, J., and Vaucelle, T., 1968, Etude d'une fraction antigènique d'*Aspergillus fumigatus* support d'une activité catalasique. Consequence sur le diagnostic immunologique de l'aspergillose, *Rev. Immunol. Ther. Antimicrobiol.* **32:**37–52.

Tran Van Ky, P., Torck, C., Vaucell, T., and Floc'h, F., 1969, Etude comparée sur immunoélectrophoregramme des enzymes de l'extrait antigènique d'*Aspergillus fumigatus,* révélés par des serums expérimentaux et des serums de malades atteints d'aspergillose, *Sabouraudia* **7:**73–84.

Tran Van Ky, P., Vaucell, T., and Biguet, J., 1970, Etude comparée de la structure antigènique par analyse immunoélectrophoretique et par les réactions de caracterisation des activités enzymatiques des extraits antigèniques des champignons pathogènes du genre Aspergillus (*A. fumigatus, A. Flavus, A. terreus, A. nidulans*), *Rev. Immunol. (Paris)* **34:**357–374.

Tran Van Ky, P., Biguet, J., Vaucelle, T., and Fruit, J., 1971, Analyse immunoéléctrophoretique et caracterisation des activités enzymatiques des extraits antigèniques d'*Aspergillus flavus*. Repercussion sur la diagnostic differential des aspergilloses humaines, *Sabouraudia* **9**:210.

Travis, R. E., Ulrich, E. W., and Phillips, S., 1961, Pulmonary allescheriasis, *Ann. Int. Med.* **54**:141–152.

Turner, K. J., Elder, J. L., O'Mahoney, J., and Johansson, S. G. O., 1974, The association of lung shadowing with hypersensitivity responses in patients with allergic bronchopulmonary aspergillosis, *Clin. Allergy* **4**:149–160.

Turner-Warwick, M., 1973, Immunology of the lower respiratory tract, *Clin. Allergy* **3**(Suppl.):653–663.

Vallery-Radot, P., and Giroud, P., 1928, Sporomycose des des pelleterus de grains, *Bull. Soc. Med. Hop. Paris* **52**:1632–1645.

Vijay, J. M., Perelmutter, G., and Berstein, I. L., 1978, Possible role of IgG$_4$ in discordant correlations between intracutanious skin test and RAST, *Int. Arch. Allerg.* **56**:517–522.

Villar, T. G., and Cortez Pimental, J., 1970, Personal experience with pulmonary aspergillomas, *Bull. Int. Union Tuberc.* **43**:117–118.

Voisin, C., and Biguet, J., 1970, L'aspergillose dans les lésions pulmonaires résiduelles: Problèmes diagnostiques, prognostiques et thérapeutiques, *Bull. Int. Union Tuberc.* **43**:119–120.

Voisin, C., Biguet, J., Tran Van Ky, P., Shcouller, A., Sergeout, Y. H., and Gernez-Rieuz, C., 1964, Aspergillose latentes et tuberculose pulmonaire chronique. Interêt de la recherche systematique des précipitines seriques specifiques chez les tuberculeux cavitaires au long cours, *Rev. Tuberc. Pneum.* **28**:1311–1316.

Voisin, C., Tonnel, A. B., Jacob, M., Therol, P., Malin, P., and Lahoutte, C., 1976, Infiltrats pulmonaries avec grand eosinophilie sanguine associés à une candidose bronchique, *Rev. Franc. Allerg. Immunol. Clin.* **16**:279.

Voller, A., Bidwell, D., and Bartlett, A., 1976, Microplate enzyme immunoassays for the immunodiagnosis of virus infections, in: *Manual of Clinical Immunology*, Chapter 69, American Society for Microbiology, Washington, D.C.

Wang, J. L. F., Patterson, R., Rosenberg, M., Roberts, M., and Cooper, B. J., 1978, Serum IgE and IgG antibody activity against *Aspergillus fumigatus* as a diagnostic aid in allergic bronchopulmonary aspergillosis, *Am. Rev. Resp. Dis.* **117**:917–927.

Warren, C. P. W., Tai, E., Batten, J. C., Huthcroft, B. J., and Pepys, J., 1975, Cystic fibrosis—Immunological reactions to *A. fumigatus* and common allergens, *Clin. Allergy* **5**:1–12.

Warren, C. P., Cherniak, R. M., and Tse, K. S., 1977, Extrinsic allergic alveolitis from bird exposure. Studies on the immediate hypersensitivity reaction, *Clin. Allergy* **7**:303–314.

Winner, H. I., 1972, Studies on *Candida, Proc. R. Soc. Med.* **65**:433–436.

Yocum, M. W., Saltzman, A. R., Strong, D. Y., Donaldson, J. C., Ward, G. W., Walsh, F. M., Cobb, O. R., and Elliott, R. C., 1976, Extrinsic allergic alveilitis after *Aspergillus fumigatus* inhalation, *Am. J. Med.* **61**:939–945.

Young, R. C., and Bennett, J. E., 1971, Invasive aspergillosis. Absence of detectable antibody response, *Am. Rev. Resp. Dis.* **104**:710–716.

Young, R. C., Bennett, J. E., Voge, C. L., Cabone, P. D., and DeVita, V. T., 1970, Aspergillosis. The spectrum of the disease in 98 patients, *Medicine* **49**:146–173.

23

Immunology of Invasive Fungal Infections

RICHARD D. DIAMOND

1. Introduction

For most of the twentieth century, clinically apparent, invasive systemic mycoses have been frequently recognized and well known to physicians practicing within endemic areas. Until the last two decades the discovery of a patient with an invasive systemic mycosis outside an endemic area was a rare enough entity to incite animated conversations between interested clinicians. This relative rarity of clinical disease contrasted with the fact that potentially pathogenic fungi are widespread in nature. Human contact with these organisms must be common. In the case of some of these fungi, exposure normally leads to inapparent or mild, self-limited infections (e.g., *Histoplasma capsulatum, Coccidioides immitis*). For other pathogenic fungi there is at least circumstantial evidence that such subclinical infections occur frequently (e.g., *Paracoccidioides brasiliensis, Cryptococcus neoformans*). With some mycoses, invasive disease occurs almost exclusively in patients with specific alterations in local or systemic host defense mechanisms (e.g., *Absidia, Rhizopus,* or *Mucor* species causing mucormycosis). In recent years systemic mycoses have been recognized with greatly increased frequency. In part this is because immunosuppressive ther-

apy for other diseases has become commonplace. In addition, there have been major advances in using immunological markers for diagnosis and estimating prognosis of mycoses. In other words, the nature of the immune response that occurs in an individual patient after exposure to fungi is critical in determining the outcome and extent of infection, and also provides parameters useful in diagnosis and in following the course of therapy. This chapter will review the immune response to several agents which cause invasive mycoses in man (excluding *Candida* and *Aspergillus,* which are covered in other chapters).

2. Evolutionary Aspects

Most pathogenic fungi exist in nature as saprophytes. For several of these potential pathogens, sexual stages have been described (Kwon-Chung, 1974), which presumably help to provide genetic heterogeneity and favor survival in nature. The tissue invasive form of most pathogenic fungi differs from the saprophytic form which exists in nature (see Section 3). There is no clear evidence that host invasion and production of disease offer survival value to the fungus. In fact, fungi undoubtedly evolved long before their ecological habitats were invaded by higher animals. Features of the pathogenic forms of fungi which infect man (such as temperature dependence of the tissue invasive yeast phase of dimorphic

RICHARD D. DIAMOND ● Infectious Disease Division, Department of Medicine, University Hospital, and Boston University School of Medicine, Boston, Massachusetts 02118.

fungi) may limit known animal infections to mammals (Ajello, 1969). Invasive mycoses in man and other mammals may then represent accidental events which are "dead ends" in the evolution of fungi (Rippon, 1974). Conversely, our current knowledge of the extent of mycoses in a limited range of animal species cannot yet offer insight into the evolution of host immune responses toward invasive fungi.

3. Microbial Aspects

Several of the species of fungi which cause invasive disease in man exist in nature in mycelial phases. These forms differ from corresponding tissue invasive phases not only in morphology but also in important aspects of biochemical and antigenic composition. This group includes *Coccidioides immitis, Histoplasma capsulatum, Blastomyces dermatitidis, Paracoccidioides brasiliensis,* and *Sporothrix schenckii.* For many fungi the saprophytic mycelial phase is more easily cultivated *in vitro* than the pathogenic tissue phase. Consequently, antigens prepared from mycelial forms have been widely used in clinical and experimental studies despite their potential differences from antigens derived from tissue invasive forms. In addition, for some fungal species causing invasive disease in man there are neither well-standardized antigen preparations nor standardized antigen preparation techniques. Therefore, comparisons of studies require careful attention to the methods used for preparation and usage of immunological reagents, because differing techniques (growth phase, age of culture, temperature, pH, culture medium, etc.) may beget reagents which differ widely in sensitivity and specificity. Knowledge of the genetics of pathogenic fungi is limited, especially with respect to factors determining virulence (Kwon-Chung, 1974). Experimental animal studies have demonstrated a wide variability in virulence for different isolates of several fungal species. However, isolates from different severe human infections may also exhibit a wide range of virulence in experimental animals. In most cases, then, the host response appears to be a much more important determinant of the extent of disease in man than strain differences within fungal species.

3.1. *Coccidioides immitis*

Coccidioides immitis exists in soil and in routine laboratory cultures in a mycelial phase. Infection results when arthrospores from mycelia are inhaled. Rarely, in avascular tissue lesions (Baker and Braude, 1956) or in the center of pulmonary cavities (Puckett, 1954) *Coccidioides* may grow in mycelial phase. However, arthrospores or mycelial fragments convert in structure and grow as spherules *in vivo,* or *in vitro* when conditions permit, e.g., special media and high carbon dioxide and oxygen tension (Lubarsky and Plunkett, 1955) or addition of live neutrophils (Baker and Braude, 1956). Conversion from arthrospore to spherule is also accompanied by changes in antigens (Landay *et al.,* 1967). Spherules are complex structures approximately 30–60 µm or more in diameter. Inside spherules, hundreds of 2- to 5 µm-diameter endospores develop by progressive cleavage. Spherules mature and rupture, releasing the endospores, which then develop into spherules. Ultrastructural observations have indicated that spherule and endospore cell walls change in structure (and perhaps function and chemical composition) as they mature within lesions (Donnelly and Yunis, 1974). From experimental animal studies, it appears that spherules become more immunogenic as they mature (Levine and Kong, 1965). In addition, arthrospores, spherules, and endospores appear to have differences in chemotactic properties (Forbus and Bestebreurtje, 1946), but the specific chemical and antigenic reasons for this are unknown.

Coccidioidin is the most widely used antigenic preparation derived from this organism (Newcomer, 1974; Smith *et al.,* 1948). The commercially available material is prepared from a mycelial culture filtrate obtained from nine standard isolates of *Coccidioides immitis.* Multiple isolates are used because not all strains have identical antigenic patterns in immunodiffusion tests (Rowe *et al.,* 1963a,b). The antigen active in the delayed skin test appears to be largely mannopeptide in nature (Hassid *et al.,* 1943; Stewart and Kimura, 1940; Wheat and Chung, 1977), containing smaller amounts of 3-O-methylmannose (Wheat and Chung, 1977), glucose, and other sugars (Pappagianis *et al.,* 1961a) present in the cell wall (Ward *et al.,* 1975). The peptide or protein associated with the polysaccharide may also be active, since proteolytic enzyme treatment decreased reactivity of partially purified antigen preparations (Marcus *et al.*, 1965). The material appears to be somewhat enriched in proline, with a variety of other amino acids (Wheat and Chung, 1977). Because of batch variation, reactivity of each lot of coccidioidin must be checked against a standard preparation. Coccidioidin is also used for detection of antibodies by complement fixation (Smith *et al.*, 1956) and immunodiffusion (Huppert and Bailey, 1965). Skin testing with coccidioidin does not stimulate production of antibodies to *Coccidioides*.

Toluene extracts of mycelia have different antigenic reactivity from culture filtrates, as shown by testing of these materials using immunodiffusion (Huppert, 1970). Four separate antigen–antibody systems were noted, one of which was involved in complement fixation and immunodiffusion. Another was involved in the tube precipitation and latex particle agglutination tests (Huppert *et al.*, 1968). This latter antigen was not detected in some of the strains tested (Huppert, 1970). Toluene-induced lysates from mycelial phase cells of *C. immitis* also are effective in eliciting production of migration inhibitory factors by lymphocytes (Cox *et al.*, 1977).

Recently, spherulin, an antigen extract of lysed spherules, has been increasingly used as a sensitive, stable antigenic preparation active in skin testing and complement fixation (Levine and Scalarone, 1975). There are differences in potency of spherulins produced from different strains. There may be a wide variability in relative percentages of protein and polysaccharide in batches of spherulin produced from the same *C. immitis* strain without apparent variation in biological properties in the guinea pig. Antigen activity is associated with a large molecule (7–17 S) which contains a heat-stable sensitizing agent. This, plus the high polysaccharide content of active preparations, suggests that the major antigenic component is a polysaccharide. However, maximum activity is present only in unheated preparations, so another material (possibly protein) may be involved (Levine and Scalarone, 1975).

An alkali-soluble, water-soluble, nondialyzable antigen extracted from cell walls of *C. immitis* mycelia appears to be sensitive and specific in skin testing and eliciting production of migration inhibitory factors (Cox *et al.*, 1977).

Immunogenicity of *C. immitis* appears to reside in the cell wall (Kong *et al.*, 1963). The cell wall is composed of chitinlike material, β-glucans, and other polysaccharides, as well as the unusual sugar, 3-*O*-methylmannose (Scheer *et al.*, 1970; Wheat *et al.*, 1977). A host component may affect cell wall composition and thickness when *C. immitis* grows *in vivo* (Wheat *et al.*, 1977). Heating whole spherules for 15 min at 60–70°C markedly decreased their ability to sensitize animals, but heating for as long as 18 hr did not destroy immunogenicity completely (Levine and Kong, 1966). This work suggested the existence of two or more separate antigens or at least antigenic determinants, perhaps protein and polysaccharide in nature.

As noted above, different *C. immitis* isolates may differ in antigenic structure, as well as in virulence for laboratory animals. Thus far, however, genetic studies of *C. immitis* have been limited, partly because the organism is still known only in its asexual (imperfect) state (Kwon-Chung, 1974).

3.2. *Histoplasma capsulatum*

Histoplasma capsulatum exists in mycelial phase in nature and in cultures kept at room temperature. Human infections occur after inhalation of spores, which convert to the tissue invasive yeast phase at 37°C in tissues, as well in leukocyte cultures *in vitro* (Hempel and Goodman, 1975), or on artificial media under certain conditions. In addition, *H. capsulatum* yeasts do not grow at 40°C and grow poorly at 39°C. Environmental temperatures influence the course of experimental infections in mice (Mackinnon, 1971), although evidence that this is an important factor in human infections is slight. Genetically determined factors may prove to be important in governing infectivity of *H. capsulatum* for man. In some experimental animal studies *H. capsulatum* yeasts derived from different morphological types of the same strain appeared to have different virulence (Daniels *et al.*, 1968). The recent description of the perfect (sexual) state of *Histoplasma capsulatum* (termed *Emmon-*

siella capsulata; Kwon-Chung, 1973) now offers increased possibilities for genetic studies of virulence, as well as other factors. It was observed that the two mating types occurred with equal frequency in soil isolates (obtained from 13 states in the endemic area for histoplasmosis), but there was a 7 : 1 ratio of $(-) : (+)$ mating types in clinical isolates, and $(-)$ type mycelia tended to convert to yeast phase more readily than $(+)$ type mycelia (Kwon-Chung *et al.*, 1974).

The most commonly used reagents for immunodiagnosis of histoplasmosis are saline suspensions of whole killed yeasts and histoplasmin, a filtrate prepared from mycelial phase cultures. Histoplasmin contains a skin test active glycoprotein component (Sprouse, 1971) with three hexoses (glucose, mannose, galactose) and hexosamine, plus 18 end-group amino acid residues (Bartels, 1971). Positive histoplasmin skin tests may occur in guinea pigs after infection with a long list of pathogenic and nonpathogenic fungi, but fractionation of histoplasmin or controlled aging of cultures used for histoplasmin production may reduce cross-reactivity (Goodman, 1971; Goodman *et al.*, 1971). Antigen-specific delayed hypersensitivity to histoplasmin appears to reside in a 12,000 molecular weight glycoprotein (Sprouse, 1977). In addition to histoplasmin, polysaccharides and polysaccharide–protein complexes extracted from yeast cell walls are active skin test reagents in animals (Anderson *et al.*, 1974; Domer, 1976). A cell wall glycoprotein was found to be useful as a skin test antigen and in *in vitro* assays for migration inhibitory factors (MIFs) but not in lymphocyte transformation (Domer, 1976). Polysaccharide-rich antigens prepared from yeasts have also been used to detect antibodies in man by a passive hemagglutination technique (Hermans and Markowitz, 1969). The cell wall of the yeast phase of *H. capsulatum* consists primarily of chitin and glucan. There are two chemotypes, type I containing more chitin and less glucan than type II, with α-glucans predominating in type I, but β linkages exclusively present in type II (Davis *et al.*, 1977). Antigens extracted from the two chemotypes differ antigenically and are reactive in immunodiffusion, although are not identical to the characteristic diagnostic "H" and "M"

antigens (see Section 6.2.2) of *H. capsulatum* (Reiss *et al.*, 1977). The H and M antigens which serve to identify *H. capsulatum* in the immunodiffusion test do not appear to be located on yeast cell surfaces. In addition, complement fixation releases antigens from yeast cells which are active in the complement-fixation test (Green *et al.*, 1976).

Various *Histoplasma* yeast and mycelial cell fractions have been noted to be immunogenic (i.e., capable of inducing delayed hypersensitivity and protection against infection in experimental animal studies). These include yeast cell walls (Salvin, 1965; Domer, 1976), a protein–carbohydrate complex obtained from autolyzed yeasts (Salvin and Smith, 1959), a purified polysaccharide (Knight *et al.*, 1959), and a ribosomal preparation (RNA and protein) extracted from yeasts (Feit and Tewari, 1974; Neuhauser *et al.*, 1974). In studies using a yeast phase cell wall glycoprotein preparation, removal or alteration of protein appeared to augment induction of immediate-type hypersensitivity, while removal of carbohydrate appeared to cause a shift toward induction of strong delayed-type hypersensitivity (Domer and Ichinose, 1977).

3.3. *Blastomyces dermatitidis*

There is circumstantial evidence that *Blastomyces dermatitidis* exists in nature as a soil saprophyte. Most infections occur after inhalation of spores, which convert to yeast phase upon invading tissues (Ajello, 1969). Conversion is temperature dependent. Cultures grow on artificial media in mycelial phase at room temperature and in yeast phase at 37°C. In macrophages cultured *in vitro* at 37°C mycelia convert to yeasts within 24 hr (Hempel and Goodman, 1975). Morphological conversion is accompanied by various biochemical changes, including changes in the polysaccharide structure of the cell wall (Kanetsuna and Carbonell, 1971). Despite the frequent findings of cross-reacting antigens in *H. capsulatum* and *B. dermatitidis,* host inflammatory responses to these organisms are strikingly different (see Sections 5.2 and 5.3), yet the antigenic basis for these intriguing differences is not known. Immunodiagnostic antigens are not well characterized and, with the exception of the acetone extracts of homogenized yeasts currently used in immunodiffusion tests (Kaufman *et al.*, 1973), are nonspecific and of limited usefulness (Lancaster and Sprouse, 1976). An alkali-soluble, water-soluble cell wall fraction of yeast phase cells has been recently described and appears to be useful and specific in skin testing as well as induction of lymphocyte transformation and production of migration inhibitory factor, at least in studies in experimental animals (Deighton *et al.*, 1977). Some workers have suggested a relationship between virulence for animals and the total lipid content of *B. dermatitidis,* which is high compared with that of other fungi (Domer, 1971). In mice the granulomatous tissue response has been attributed to the presence of covalently bound phospholipids (Cox *et al.*, 1974). Genetic factors related to virulence are not well defined, but the sexual state of the organisms has been described (McDonough and Lewis, 1967), and future studies may shed light on this area.

3.4. *Paracoccidioides brasiliensis*

Paracoccidioides brasiliensis exhibits thermal dimorphism. It converts from the saprophytic mycelial phase to the yeast phase, when kept above room temperature on artificial media or in human tissues. *P. brasiliensis* grows well in the yeastlike phase at 32°C. Growth slows at 35°C, is further reduced at 37°C, is minimal at 38°C, and ceases at 39°C (Yarzabal, 1972). This temperature dependence of growth has been related to the distribution of extrapulmonary lesions. Mice kept at 37°C had rectal and paw temperatures of 38.5–39.5°C and did not develop progressive infections, but more severe disease was noted in a 14–15°C environment, and experimental infections were progressive and fatal at 9°C or less (Mackinnon *et al.*, 1960). Mucocutaneous, rectal, and testicular lesions are common in human paracoccidioidomycosis (Londero and Ramos, 1972; Sampaio, 1972; Murray *et al.*, 1974).

The conversion to the pathogenic yeastlike phase is accompanied by ultrastructural (Carbonell, 1972a) and biochemical (Kanetsuna, 1972a) changes, but factors responsible for in-

fectivity are not well defined. The cell wall (which includes the surface antigens exposed to the host) has been found to be primarily polysaccharide in nature, consisting of an inner layer of chitin and an outer layer of α-1,3-glucan (Carbonell *et al.*, 1970). The latter accounted for 90% of the cell wall polysaccharide (Kanetsuna, 1972a). It has been suggested that this cell wall structure may confer resistance to phagocytosis (San-Blas *et al.*, 1977) and to digestion by macrophage lysosomal enzymes (Kanetsuna, 1972a). Rabbits inoculated with the whole organism developed low titers of complement-fixing antibodies to the α-glucan and β-glucan (Kanetsuna, 1972a). The antigen reactive in the complement-fixation test of human sera is also a polysaccharide (Fava Netto *et al.*, 1969). The α-1,3-glucan has also been suggested to be directly involved in detection of organisms in tissue, as well as circulating antibodies by immunofluorescence (Azuma *et al.*, 1974; Carbonell, 1972b). In addition to cell wall components, some yeast antigens have enzymatic activity (Yarzabal *et al.*, 1972). However, these enzymes have not yet been directly related to infectivity of the organism, and there is no evidence that antibodies to these enzymes are protective for the host. One purified mycelial phase antigen with alkaline phosphatase activity and one with no enzymatic activity have been implicated in function of the species-specific "E" band on immunoelectrophoresis with antisera to *P. brasiliensis* (Yarzabul *et al.*, 1977). Delayed skin test reactivity has been attributed to a glycoprotein antigen (Restrepo and Schneidau, 1967).

Genetic factors contributing to pathogenicity are not well known. A sexual (perfect) state for *P. brasiliensis* is yet to be described (Kwon-Chung, 1974).

In tissues of experimental animals very small forms of the yeastlike phase have been observed early in the course of infection with *P. brasiliensis*. These minute forms have been said to be important in dissemination of organisms in the host (Fialho, 1956; Texeira *et al.*, 1969; Yarzabal, 1972). It has also been suggested that cell-wall-deficient yeastlike forms may contribute to local spreading of lesions in experimental animals (de Brito *et al.*, 1972). However, factors favoring the growth of these forms of the organism have not been clearly defined.

3.5. Sporothrix schenckii

Sporothrix schenckii exhibits thermal dimorphism. It grows in mycelial phase at room temperature, in nature, and on artificial media and converts to yeast phase at higher temperatures on artificial media, in human tissues, or in *in vitro* macrophage cultures (Hempel and Goodman, 1975). The maximum temperature for *in vitro* growth of most strains of *S. schenckii* is 38–38.5°C. As in paracoccidioidomycosis, ambient termperature has been related to the distribution of disseminated lesions in experimental animals. Disseminated infections tended to occur in animals kept in low-temperature environments, while infections were localized or absent in animals maintained at 31°C (MacKinnon and Conti-Diaz, 1963; Mackinnon *et al.*, 1964). Kwon-Chung (1979) studied 34 strains of *S. schenckii* from human cases and found that they could be grouped based on their maximum temperatures for growth *in vitro*. Conidia from 26 isolates from lymphocutaneous or disseminated lesions formed colonies at both 35°C and 37°C, while eight isolates from nonlymphocytic, fixed cutaneous lesions failed to grow at 37°C, although they grew at 35°C. Both types of isolates grew well in testes of mice after intraperitoneal infection, but only isolates which grew at 37°C developed disseminated lesions. No clinical isolates had maximum temperatures for growth below 35°C. These data correspond to the predominance of local, cutaneous disease in man, as well as the propensity of *S. schenckii* to involve peripheral joints in extracutaneous cases (Wilson *et al.*, 1967; Altner and Turner, 1970).

Antigens of *S. schenckii* responsible for immunodiagnosis and induction of the immune response are not well characterized. A wide variety of antigen preparations have been used in man, and none is standardized (McMillen, 1974). In man concentrated culture filtrates from yeast phase cells from three different strains of *S. schenckii* have been used (Schneidau *et al.*, 1964). However, in sensitized guinea pigs, skin test reactivity occurred only when whole yeast cells, cell walls, and cell wall fractions were used, and not with cyto-plasmic extracts (Nielsen, 1968). The most active preparation was produced by extracting cell walls with chloroform–methanol and sodium dodecylsulfate, followed by treatment with pronase and ribonuclease. It has been observed that blastogenic responses of human lymphocytes cultured *in vitro* with crude antigen preparations of *S. schenckii* or *Candida albicans* were closely correlated. These workers suggested that prior exposure to *C. albicans* may protect against systemic sporotrichosis (Steele *et al.*, 1976). However, this hypothesis is tenuous, in view of the small numbers of subjects tested, the nature of the antigen preparations used, the limited number of studies done using other antigens known to cross-react with *S. schenckii* (Salvin, 1963), and the lack of evidence that such *in vitro* reactivity correlates with resistance to systemic sporotrichosis.

A specific polysaccharide of *S. schenckii* and its type-specific antiserum are noted to cross-react with purified pneumococcal (types 32, 31, 23, 22, and 10) antigens and antisera (Neill *et al.*, 1955). Similarly, serological cross-reactivity has been demonstrated between *S. schenckii* and a variety of pathogenic and non-pathogenic bacteria (group B *Streptococcus*, *Ceratocystis* spp., and *Graphium* spp.). While it has been suggested that this cross-reactivity might explain low-titer agglutinins to *S. schenckii* found in normal sera (Nakamura *et al.*, 1977), the role of these relationships, if any, to host immunity is unknown.

3.6. Cryptococcus neoformans

Cryptococcus neoformans exists as a yeast in tissues, as well as in nature and on artificial media; only rare isolates have been found which produced hyphae (Shadomy and Utz, 1966). There are four serotypes, based on antigenic specificity of the capsular polysaccharide (Wilson *et al.*, 1968). Distinction between them has not been shown to be important in immunologic responses in human disease thus far (Bindschadler and Bennett, 1968). A sexual (perfect) state of *C. neoformans* (termed *Filobasidiella neoformans*) was described by Kwon-Chung (1975b).

One year later it was noted that this perfect state was produced only by serotype A or D isolates, while serotype B or C isolates produced a different perfect state on mating, termed *Filobasidiella bacillispora* (Kwon-Chung, 1976). Furthermore, compared with serotype A–D organisms, type B–C organisms have important biochemical (Bennett *et al.*, 1978), ecological, and epidemiological (Bennett *et al.*, 1977) differences. Two species have been proposed: *C. neoformans* (A–D serotypes) and *C. bacillisporus* (B–C serotypes) (Kwon-Chung *et al.*, 1978). In any case these new findings open the way for future genetic studies which deal directly with factors influencing pathogenicity in man.

Temperature tolerance appears to be related to pathogenicity of *C. neoformans*. *C. neoformans*, but usually not nonpathogenic species of *Cryptococcus*, can grow at 37°C. However, *C. neoformans* grows best at 30°C and poorly, if at all, at 39°C *in vitro*. Animals kept at 35–36°C after infection survived a lethal dose of *C. neoformans* longer than those kept at room temperature (Kuhn, 1949; Kligman *et al.*, 1961), and rabbits are resistant to experimental cryptococcosis, perhaps largely because of their 39°C body temperature (Kuhn, 1939).

The capsular polysaccharide confers unique properties on *C. neoformans* which are important in interactions with host immunological mechanisms. Excluding the capsule, most isolates of *C. neoformans* average 4–6 μm in diameter, but encapsulated yeasts vary greatly in diameter, often exceeding 30 μm in diameter in infected tissues. The capsular polysaccharide contains xylose, mannose, galactose, and glucuronic acid (Neill *et al.*, 1949; Evans and Kessel, 1951), but no amino acids or amino sugars (Einbender *et al.*, 1954). The material behaves as a polyvalent anion (Salvin, 1963). By different techniques, at least two separate fractions have been noted (Evans and Thierault, 1953; Rebers *et al.*, 1958), but they are not well characterized. After fixation for ultrastructural studies the capsule appears to be composed of intertwined microfibrils which radiate from the cell wall (Edwards *et al.*, 1967; Al-Doory, 1971). In studies using hyperimmune sera, cross-reactivity was noted between some strains of *C. neoformans* and pneumococcus types 2 (Evans *et al.*, 1953) and 14 (Rebers *et al.*, 1958), but a role for this relationship in microbe–host interactions has not been established. Anticryptococcal anti-

body activity in sera from patients with cryptococcosis could not be inhibited by as much as 1 mg/ml of type 2 or 14 pneumococcal polysaccharide (Bindschadler and Bennett, 1968). When incubated with specific antisera, a change in refractility but not size of the cryptococcal capsule has been noted (Neill *et al.*, 1949). Similar physical changes have been observed after interaction of cryptococci with complement components from fresh sera, which may be related to opsonization of the yeast for phagocytosis (Diamond *et al.*, 1974).

The capsule confers several features on the organism which affect the hose response to infection. *C. neoformans* appears to exist in soil and pigeon droppings in an unencapsulated form which is small enough to permit alveolar deposition after inhalation and initiate infections in man (Farhi *et al.*, 1970; Powell *et al.*, 1972; Neilson and Bulmer, 1975). The degree of encapsulation of different isolates observed on artificial media was not related to virulence after inoculation of mice, but capsules rapidly developed in tissues in most cases (Littman and Tsubura, 1959). In a different study unencapsulated mutants produced by ultraviolet irradiation were avirulent for mice, but some regained virulence after reverting to the encapsulated state; one strain remained unencapsulated and avirulent (Bulmer *et al.*, 1976). Cryptococcal capsular polysaccharide has a wide range of effects which might impair the immune response in human infections. These include inhibition of phagocytosis (Bulmer and Sans, 1967, 1968) and killing (Diamond *et al.*, 1972) of the yeast by human neutrophils *in vitro*, impairment of *in vitro* migration of guinea leukocytes (Drouhet and Segretain, 1951), and induction of immunological unresponsiveness in animals (Gadebusch, 1958a; Goren and Middlebrook, 1967; Murphy and Cozad, 1972). In addition, capsular polysaccharide was shown to activate the classical and alternate complement pathways in human and guinea pig sera (Diamond *et al.*, 1974). This interaction appeared to be primarily responsible for opsonization of organisms for phagocytosis. Depletion of complement components may occur in some circumstances, although only in infections severe enough to cause fungemia (Macher *et al.*, 1978). The polysaccharide has been made immunogenic for animals only after administration with adjuvants or after coupling to heterologous proteins. Even then, not all animals produced detectable levels of antibody (Goren and Middlebrook, 1967; Kozel and Cazin, 1974).

Cytoplasmic antigens appear to be most important in elicitation of delayed hypersensitivity in sensitized animals and in man. Culture filtrates containing polysaccharide, as well as proteins and other materials, have been used by some workers (Murphy *et al.*, 1974), but one active preparation prepared by urea extraction of killed cells contained only 0.2–0.3% polysaccharide (Atkinson and Bennett, 1968). Sensitization of animals with killed *C. neoformans* generally has required the use of adjuvants with injections of killed, whole yeast cells.

In addition to proteins in cytoplasm, *C. neoformans* has been said to liberate materials with acid phosphatase and proteolytic activity (Müller and Sethi, 1972; Mahvi *et al.*, 1974). A role in infection was suggested for these extracellular substances since they are capable of interaction with human proteins, but the occurrence of such reactions in infected tissues remains to be verified.

3.7. *Absidia, Mucor,* and *Rhizopus* spp.

Similar pathology results from infection by several species of the genera *Rhizopus, Mucor,* and *Absidia*. These species account for almost all cases of mucormycosis (or phycomycosis) in North America. The organisms are ubiquitous natural saprophytes which do not invade normal tissues. They grow in mycelial forms in nature, on artificial media, and in tissues of infected hosts. Only thermotolerant species (i.e., those capable of growing at or above-normal animal body temperatures) were capable of causing disease in diabetic rabbits, but not all thermotolerant species were virulent for these animals (Reinhardt *et al.*, 1970). *In vitro* growth of pathogenic isolates of *Rhizopus, Absidia,* and *Mucor* spp. occurs at 37°C or higher and is increased at acid pH levels which are commonly observed in sera of patients with diabetic ketoacidosis. Furthermore, these fungi grow well in media with high glucose content. Species of *Rhizopus*, at least, have an active ketoreductose system (Polli, 1965). These features all appear to suit it well for growth in patients with diabetic ketoacidosis. A material with endotoxinlike proper-

ties has been detected in one *Rhizopus* species (Salvin, 1952), but its role, if any, in the pathogenesis of lesions is unknown.

4. Host

For most mycoses there is either a well-documented primary, subclinical infection (e.g., histoplasmosis, coccidioidomycosis), or there is strong circumstantial evidence that such a form of infection commonly occurs (e.g., cryptococcosis, paracoccidioidomycosis). Patients who develop the unusual severe and disseminated forms of invasive mycoses often are immunosuppressed by virtue of therapy or disease (Bodey and Rodriguez, 1975; Frenkel, 1962; Hart *et al.*, 1969; Rifkind *et al.*, 1967) or have naturally occurring defects in cellular immunity. On the other hand, hypogammaglobulinemia does not appear to regularly predispose to severe forms of mycoses, although individual cases associating the two conditions have been reported.

Where available, skin test surveys suggest that males and females have an equal incidence of primary mild or subclinical fungal infections. However, the rarely occurring severe, disseminated forms of disease are far more common in males. A role for estrogens in this increased resistance in females has been suggested (Mohr *et al.*, 1972a; Muchmore *et al.*, 1972) because of direct inhibitory effects of estrogens on some fungi, as well as stimulatory effects of physiological levels of estrogens on the reticuloendothelial system (Nicol *et al.*, 1965) and on mitosis of immunocompetent cells (Kenny *et al.*, 1976). It should be noted, though, that higher levels of estrogens may have antiinflammatory effects which could conceivably impair the microbicidal function of leukocytes (Bodel *et al.*, 1972).

4.1. *Coccidioides immitis*

Although skin test surveys suggest an approximately equal sex incidence of primary pulmonary disease, disseminated (Fiese, 1958) and progressive pulmonary (Sarosi *et al.*, 1970) forms of coccidioidomycosis are much more common in males than females. The exception is late pregnancy, where the risk of dissemination is increased (Fiese, 1958; Purtilo, 1974). Over one 7-year period, coccidioidomycosis was the leading cause of maternal mortality in one general hospital located within the endemic area (Deresinski and Stevens, 1974). Postpuberal females with primary coccidioidomycosis, in contrast to the disseminated form of the disease, are at least 5 times more likely than males to develop erythema nodosum or erythema multiforme. Erythema nodosum may occur in as many as 25–40% of primary coccidioidal infections in females (Fiese, 1958; Winn, 1967) and is thought to signify a high level of immunity which reduces the liklihood of progression or dissemination of infections.

Ràcial and ethnic predispositions toward dissemination of coccidioidomycosis have been noted. In one large study, compared with whites, the risk of dissemination after primary infection was increased threefold in Mexicans, fourteenfold in blacks, and 175-fold in Filipinos (Gifford et al., 1937). More recent studies found less of a difference, although this seemed to be due to increased susceptibility in whites who have associated diseases rather than to any decrease in susceptibility among nonwhites (Drutz and Catanzaro, 1978). In addition, erythema nodosum has a much lower incidence in blacks and Filipinos than in whites (Fiese, 1958). An association of disseminated coccidioidomycosis with incidence of HLA9 has been described (Scheer et al., 1970), but this may only reflect the frequency of HLA9 in some of the ethnic groups predisposed to development of disseminated coccidioidomycosis.

Progressive pulmonary coccidioidomycosis may occur in association with diabetes mellitus (Sarosi et al., 1970). Coccidioidomycosis can also occur as an opportunistic infection associated with immunosuppressive therapy or Hodgkin's disease, but such severe infections are relatively rare, especially considering the frequency of primary infections in the endemic area (Deresinski and Stevens, 1974).

4.2. Histoplasma capsulatum

Skin test surveys and reviews of outbreaks indicate that males and females develop primáry (symptomatic and asymptomatic) pulmonary histoplasmosis with equal frequency (Sarosi et al., 1971a). However, chronic pulmonary (Baum and Schwarz, 1962) and disseminated (Reddy et al., 1970; Sarosi et al., 1971a; Smith and Utz, 1972) histoplasmosis have a strong predilection for middle-aged and elderly males. Estradiol inhibits growth of H. capsulatum in vitro (Muchmore et al., 1972) but only in concentrations higher than those circulating in normal women (Ross and Vande Wiele, 1974).

Infants are at risk for the most severe form of disseminated histoplasmosis, characterized by widespread visceral involvement with hepatosplenomegaly. Infiltration of macrophages filled with huge numbers of organisms is so prominent that blockade of the reticuloendothelial system by organisms has been postulated (Rippon, 1974). Circulating levels of IgG are usually normal or increased, histoplasmin skin tests are negative, peripheral blood leukocyte count is often decreased, and thrombocytopenia and evidence of disseminated intravascular coagulation may be found in the acute phase.

Progression of primary infection to disseminated histoplasmosis, as well as severity of disseminated disease, may be influenced by corticosteroid therapy, but healed, primary foci do not appear to reactivate (Furcolow, 1962). H. capsulatum is a rare case of opportunistic infection, considering the high incidence in endemic areas, but has been noted in association with childhood leukemia (Cox and Hughes, 1974), Hodgkin's disease, chronic lymphocytic leukemia (Israel et al., 1975), tuberculosis (Reddy et al., 1970), and immunosuppressive therapy for many different entities, including transplantation (Hood et al., 1965).

4.3. Blastomyces dermatitidis

Little is known about host factors which predispose to infection with Blastomyces dermatitidis. The existence of a common, self-limited primary pulmonary form of blastomycosis (also called North American blastomycosis) is not established, although it may occur (Sarosi et al., 1974; Tosh et al., 1974). Most infections are presumed to represent either progressive pulmonary infections or lesions disseminated from primary pulmonary infections. As in other disseminated mycoses, clinical disease is 6–15 times more common in males than in females. Most patients are between the ages of 30 and 50 (Busey et al., 1964; Witorsch and Utz, 1968). Blastomycosis is rare in children (Furcolow and Smith, 1973). Prognosis worsened with age in one series (Furcolow et al., 1968). In a review of 1476 human cases between 1885 and 1968, a three-fold increase in susceptibility of blacks was noted (Furcolow et al., 1970), although no racial predisposition was noted in other series (Kunkel et al., 1954; Leavell, 1974). While blacks appeared to fare as well as other patients after the disease was acquired in one study (Furcolow et al., 1968), other workers noted a striking increased severity of disease in blacks compared with other patients (Lockwood et al., 1968). Increased frequency and severity of blastomycosis have also been described in association with diabetes mellitus (Lockwood et al., 1968). However, there is little other evidence that blastomycosis occurs with significant increased frequency in relation to immunosuppression or underlying diseases known to compromise host defense mechanisms.

4.4. *Paracoccidioides brasiliensis*

Circumstantial evidence suggests the frequent existence of primary, self-limited mild or asymptomatic paracoccidioidomycosis (South American blastomycosis). Although there may be some lack of specificity (Schneidau, 1972), delayed skin test reactivity has been noted to be equal in both sexes (Conti-Diaz, 1972). Despite this, clinically apparent cases occur much more often in males. For example, one series noted 1344 cases in males and 110 in females (Lacaz, 1955–1956). Estradiol was shown to inhibit the growth of *P. brasiliensis in vitro* (Muchmore et al, 1972), but this occurred only in concentrations well above values observed in normal women (Ross and Vande Wiele, 1974).

Patients usually range from 30 to 75 years old, with a peak in the 40–59 age group. Disease is most common in farmers or peasants who work close to the soil, reside in subtropical or tropical forest areas, and probably have prolonged exposure to fungus (Restrepo et al., 1970). The majority of patients are white. A genetic predisposition to disease was suggested on the basis of familial cases restricted

to blood relatives (not affecting spouses) and an increased incidence in Eastern European (Polish, Ukrainian) and perhaps Japanese (Negroni, 1972) immigrants. However, others have not found such a clear association, and the importance of nutritional and socioeconomic factors has been raised (Gonzalez-Ochoa, 1975). In several studies patients with paracoccidioidomycosis have been shown to have a high frequency of defects in delayed hypersensitivity and its *in vitro* correlates (E. Mendes, 1975; Musatti, 1975; N. F. Mendes, 1975). Despite this, there is no apparent increase in incidence of opportunistic paracoccidioidomycosis in association with immunosuppression or underlying debilitating diseases. Likewise, paracoccidioidomycosis has not been associated with deficiency in immunoglobulins (Correa and Giraldo, 1972).

4.5. *Sporothrix schenckii*

The incidence of subclinical, as well as localized, primary cutaneous sporotrichosis is probably equal in both sexes (Gonzalez-Ochoa, 1965). On the other hand, most of the rare, reported cases of extracutaneous sporotrichosis have occurred in males (Wilson et al, 1967; Baum et al., 1969; Lynch et al., 1970). It has been suggested that this male predominance may be related to stronger cellular immunity to *Candida albicans*, with cross-reactivity of antigens of these two fungi providing females with additional protection (Steele et al, 1976). However, the observed correlation may reflect nonspecific increased responsiveness to antigens in females and need not imply that protective immunity is related to cross-reactivity of antigens.

In man the rare reported cases of extracutaneous sporotrichosis have sometimes been associated with concurrent predisposing factors, especially alcoholism and corticosteroid therapy (Wilson et al., 1967; Baum et al., 1969; Lynch et al., 1970; Serstock and Zinneman, 1975). Several patients with systemic sporotrichosis have had sarcoidosis or lymphoreticular malignancies but were also receiving corticosteroid therapy.

4.6. *Cryptococcus neoformans*

Delayed hypersensitivity to cryptococcal antigens, as measured by skin tests, is not rare and appears to reflect subclinical cryptococcosis (Newberry *et al.*, 1967; Atkinson and Bennett, 1968; Muchmore *et al.*, 1968). Neither pulmonary nor disseminated disease has ever been reported in laboratory workers, despite exposure sufficient to result in positive cryptococcin skin tests in 81% of those tested (Atkinson and Bennett, 1968). Therefore, strong natural resistance to this infection is presumed to be common. Despite the presumed association of cryptococcosis with defects in cellular immunity (see Section 5.6), the majority of patients have had no obvious predisposing factors (Littman and Walter, 1968; Diamond and Bennett, 1974). Nevertheless, many of these patients have defective *in vitro* cell-mediated responses to fungal antigens, which were noted in some cases years after cure (Diamond and Bennett, 1973a; Graybill and Alford, 1974; Schimpff and Bennett, 1975). It has been suggested that such defects may antedate and predispose to disseminated fungus infections, but this hypothesis remains to be established. Patients receiving corticosteroid therapy are at increased risk for cryptococcosis, and those with Hodgkin's disease, lymphosarcoma, leukemia, or sarcoidosis appear to be at increased risk even in the absence of corticosteroid or other immunosuppressive therapy (Littman and Walter, 1968; Diamond and Bennett, 1974). In one series cryptococcosis was the most common infection in patients following renal transplantation, but corticosteroid therapy appeared to be the major factor involved (Gallis *et al.*, 1975). Diabetes mellitus has also been noted in increased frequency in patients with cryptococcosis (Littman and Walter, 1968), but its position as a factor predisposing to cryptococcosis is less secure. Many of the patients termed diabetic have had abnormal glucose tolerance tests only during their active infections, while values reverted to normal after successful antifungal therapy (Diamond and Bennett, 1974).

The incidence of cryptococcosis is threefold higher in males than in females (Bennett, 1972). Concentrations of estradiol as low as 1 μg/ml were reported to inhibit growth of some isolates of *C. neoformans in vitro* (Mohr *et al.*, 1972a). In addition, leukocytes from patients with cryptococcal meningitis were found to have depressed phagocytosis of *C. neoformans* which was corrected after seven to 14 daily oral doses of 5 mg diethylstilbestrol (Mohr *et al.*, 1972b). However, these observations may not reflect a specific estrogen effect, since three of the nine patients who showed the effect were female and two were at ages likely to be premenopausal. In addition, females treated for cryptococcosis do not appear to have a better prognosis than males (Diamond and Bennett, 1974).

4.7. *Absidia, Mucor,* and *Rhizopus* spp.

Clinical forms of mucormycosis are primarily related to underlying diseases, immunosuppressive therapy, or other factors which predispose patients to infection (Baker, 1970). Diabetes, especially with ketoacidosis, underlies most cases of rhinocerebral mucormycosis. Leukemia and drug therapy (especially corticosteroids), particularly in conjunction with leukopenia, have been associated with pulmonary and disseminated forms of the disease (Baker, 1962; Meyer *et al.*, 1972). Gastrointestinal involvement has been related to nutritional deficiencies, especially kwashiorkor (Neame and Raymor, 1960). Local breakdown in tissue barriers and the presence of devitalized tissues appear to be important in some cases such as those associated with burns (Rabin *et al.*, 1961) or with injection of contaminated heroin (Hameroff *et al.*, 1970). A variety of other associated factors have been noted in individual cases (McBride *et al.*, 1960), and occasional cases have no obvious predisposing factors (Hutter, 1959).

5. Microbe–Host Interactions

Different species of fungi share many structural and antigenic features, so that similarities in microbe–host interactions are not surprising. Nevertheless, these complex agents differ in important aspects of biochemical and antigenic structure, as well as in the host responses they induce. Our knowledge of host responses to fungi is derived from three imperfect sources: clinical data and histopathology from human cases, *in vitro* studies using human leukocytes, and experimental animal studies. The normal host reaction after exposure to most of these fungi is vigorous and probably results in rapid clearing of the organisms. Most clinical and pathological materials available for study are representative of abnormal host responses which have allowed infections to become more extensive than usual. *In vitro* cellular studies and experimental animal models have obvious pitfalls in extrapolation of findings into the framework of disease in man. Nevertheless, numerous studies suggest that severe forms of invasive mycoses are often accompanied by defects in cellular immunity. Such defects have been noted even in patients who were not immunosuppressed by virtue of malignancy or drug therapy prior to the onset of mycotic infections. Defects in T-cell function, i.e., depressed skin test reactivity and *in vitro* responsiveness of cultured lymphocytes to antigens and mitogens, may predispose patients to dissemination of mycoses (Paul *et al.*, 1975). The heterogeneous defects in immunity which have been noted in association with mycoses may represent qualitative or quantitative differences in the immune responsiveness of individual patients. In some cases these immunological deficits may persist long after apparent cure of mycoses. It is not known whether these defects sometimes antedate exposure to fungi or whether immunodepression may occur as a consequence of mycotic infection. In a recent study abnormalities in T-cell function in association with disseminated mycoses were associated in some patients with suppression rather than depletion of active T cells (Stobo *et al.*, 1976). Monocytes appeared to liberate a substance which acted to generate or potentiate suppressor T cells (Stobo, 1977) to inhibit *in vitro* lymphocyte transformation in response to antigens and mitogens, although pokeweed mitogen-induced immunoglobulin synthesis was unaffected. The inhibitory substance had an approximate molecular weight of 1000, did not contain antigenic determinants detectable on human IgG, and could be readily adsorbed onto mononuclear cell surfaces.

In general, the host cellular response to fungal infections appears to be critical in determining the outcome of infection. In some cases antibodies may play a secondary role, but host antibody responses most often are important as immunological markers in diagnosis and prognosis, and may even interfere with cellular responses in some situations.

5.1. *Coccidioides immitis*

5.1.1. Primary Pulmonary Infection

After inhalation, during a 10–16 day incubation period (7–28 day extreme range), spores produce a primary bronchitis, followed by alveolar lesions with an inflammatory exudate (Fiese, 1958). This results in clinical illness in only 40% of those exposed, ranging from the more common vague respiratory symptoms to the less usual acute pneumonitis (Fiese, 1958; Winn, 1967). With heavy exposure, the percentage of symptomatic infections may be higher (Werner *et al.*, 1972).

The nature of the responding inflammatory cells in individual lesions appears to depend on stage of the fungus in tissues (Ophüls, 1905). Within lesions, arthrospores developed into mature spherules over 4–7 days (Fiese, 1958). Adult spherules were noted by Ophüls (1905) in more chronic lesions, while bursting of spherule capsules to release endospores appeared to evoke an acute inflammatory response, sometimes with abscess formation. These observations were extended in a later series based on autopsy findings (Forbus and Bestebreurtze, 1946). Different chemotactic properties were postulated for arthrospore, spherule, and endospore. When spherule capsules were intact, monocytes surrounded and partially engulfed maturing parasites, sometimes with formation of epithelioid and giant cells, but with little necrosis. With spherule capsule rupture, neutrophils invaded and attempted (usually unsuccessfully) to ingest endospores, accompanied by death of host cells, blood vessel damage, and necrosis. In man inflammatory infiltrates are usually mixed, but pulmonary lesions tend to be granulomatous, while disseminated lesions tend to be suppurative. Peripheral blood eosinophilia (4–10%) is frequent, and, if high and prolonged, may signal prolonged preliminary infection and perhaps dissemination (Fiese, 1958).

A generalized macular rash has been noted in up to 10% of patients, beginning 1–2 days after the onset of symptoms and usually subsiding within a week. This appears to differ from erythema multiforme and erythema nodosum, which may appear a few days to 3 weeks after the onset of respiratory symptoms. While dissemination of coccidioidomycosis after erythema nodosum does occur, it is much less likely. Smith *et al.* (1948) estimated a 1/200 incidence of dissemination after primary coccidioidomycosis, compared with 1/700 when primary coccidioidomycosis was accompanied by erythema nodosum. There are variable estimates of the incidence of erythema nodosum after primary coccidioidomycosis, ranging from 3% to 5% of symptomatic primary cases in males and 25% to 40% in females (Fiese, 1958; Winn, 1967). Groups with the highest incidence of erythema nodosum (e.g., postpubertal white females) are least likely to disseminate, while groups with an increased incidence of dissemination after primary infection (e.g., black males) only rarely develop erythema nodosum (Fiese, 1958). Patients with primary coccidioidomycosis and erythema nodosum typically have an extremely strong delayed skin test reaction to coccidioidin. In fact, skin testing may produce a severe local reaction, as well as exacerbation of erythema nodosum. Severe erythema nodosum or erythema multiforme has been treated with corticosteroids without apparent dissemination of primary coccidioidomycosis and without apparent depression in delayed skin reactivity to coccidioidin (Levan and Einstein, 1956; Einstein, 1967).

Delayed skin reactivity to coccidioidin is detectable 2–21 days after the onset of symptoms (Smith *et al.*, 1948). In mild cases there may be no detectable antibody rise after primary coccidioidal infection, or antibody may be noted after delayed hypersensitivity. However, more than two-thirds of patients have detectable antibodies within 1 month after the onset of symptoms, and seroconversions occur as late as 3 months after onset (Smith *et al.*, 1956). IgM antibodies appear first and are detectable in 91% of patients by the third week after onset of symptoms, then rapidly decline and disappear (Smith *et al.*, 1956). IgG antibodies may then appear in low titer, and disappear unless the primary infection fails to clear. More than 90% of primary coccioidal infections clear spontaneously, without clinically significant residual pathology. Immunity, as evidenced by positive skin test, persists for years (Smith *et al.*, 1948), as do *in vitro* correlates or delayed hypersensitivity, such as MIF and lymphocyte transformation in re-

sponse to coccidioidin (Catanzaro *et al.*, 1975). This immunity appears to depend on the presence of a functioning population of T lymphocytes (Beaman *et al.*, 1977; Deresinski *et al.*, 1977).

5.1.2. Residual and Chronic Pulmonary Infections

Several types of residual lesions may occasionally occur as sequelae of primary pulmonary coccidioidomycosis. These include nodules, cavities, and abscesses (Winn, 1967), which have been observed after 0.1–8% of symptomatic primary infections (Fiese, 1958; Hyde, 1968; Winn, 1968). Nodules, or coccidiomas, have caseous centers and fibrous capsules. Coccidioidin skin tests in patients with coccidiomas are usually positive, and complement-fixing antibodies may be present in low titer (Fiese, 1958). Lesions generally change only slowly. Central necrosis may result in abscess formation (Winn, 1968). Larger cavities, often with thin walls, also occur. In one review of 300 patients with cavitary coccidioidomycosis, 90% were under 40 years of age, 54% (106/195 tested) had positive coccidioidin skin tests (tested at 1:100 but not 1:10 dilutions), 82% had detectable antibodies (in low titers), and 64% had positive sputum cultures (Hyde, 1968). Half these cavities closed spontaneously (median time for closure of 2 years). Such cavities may cause significant local pulmonary problems. However, the risk of dissemination appears to be negligible even without systemic antifungal therapy (Fiese, 1958; Hyde, 1968; Winn, 1968), despite the apparent depression in delayed hypersensitivity observed in some of these patients.

In addition to these indolent, residual, local pulmonary lesions, a small group of patients develop chronic, progressively destructive pulmonary coccidioidomycosis (Sarosi *et al.*, 1970). Like chronic pulmonary histoplasmosis, this form of coccidioidomycosis causes worsening respiratory disease, yet is not associated with extrapulmonary dissemination. Of the 20 patients reported by Sarosi *et al.*, 16 were male, and almost all had positive sputum cultures and complement-fixing antibody in high titer. Only four of 17 skin tested with 1:100 coccidioidin were positive; an additional five of the remaining 13 were nonreactive to a 1:10 dilution of coccidioidin, although nine of 18 tested had positive intermediate or second-strength PPD skin tests. As discussed below, these skin test and serological features are similar to those in patients with disseminated coccidioidomycosis and suggest a defect in the immune response to infection.

5.1.3. Disseminated Infections

Dissemination may occur in 1/200 symptomatic primary infections and is fatal in at least 50% of untreated cases (Winn, 1967). Dissemination is generally thought to occur as a part of progression of inadequately controlled primary infection. Although viable spherules have been isolated from quiescent pulmonary lesions as late as 15 years after primary infections (Cox and Smith, 1939), reactivation or late dissemination is relatively rare, even when patients are immunosuppressed (Deresinski and Stevens, 1974).

Occasional patients with predisposing factors (lymphoma, diabetes mellitus, racial or ethnic group) develop acute, miliary disseminated coccidioidomycosis, with negative coccidioidin skin tests, low complement-fixation titers, fungemia, and rapid progression to death (Winn et al., 1967). Other disseminated lesions may have an extremely variable, chronic course. Coccidioidal lesions may localize to bone, causing chronic disease of up to 29 years' duration. Although the long-term prognosis is unfavorable, individual lesions may become quiescent spontaneously or after surgical debridement (Fiese, 1958). Coccidioidal meningitis, while almost invariably ending fatally (Sweigert et al., 1946), may have a protracted, waxing and waning clinical course, sometimes over 10 years (Fiese, 1958). Visceral lesions in some cases may persist without progression for years, or in other cases may progress steadily until the patient dies. Lesions may spontaneously exacerbate, or may remit or regress and even completely disappear, occasionally with apparent clinical and serological cure. Fiese (1958) described one patient with recurrent draining sinuses, ulcers, and abscesses occurring over a 20-year period which healed spontaneously every year or 2. Fatal spontaneous relapse has occurred more than 10 years after apparently successful antifungal therapy (Gardner and Fuller, 1969).

Dissemination of coccidioidal infection is most often heralded by a rise in complement-fixing antibodies (Smith et al., 1956), even in immunosuppressed patients (Deresinski and Stevens, 1974). In contrast, disseminated coccidioidomycosis is often accompanied by defects in delayed hypersensitivity and its in vitro correlates. In one early large study, only 30 of 100 patients with disseminated coccidioidomycosis had positive skin tests using a 1 : 100 dilution of coccidioidin, 30 of 100 remained negative even using 1 : 10 coccidioidin, and five of six who were tested with undiluted coccidioidin were negative (Smith et al., 1948). This study implied a prognostic value for the skin test: three-fourths of patients who were positive with 1 : 100 coccidioidin survived, but only one-sixth of these who were negative recovered; using the 1 : 10 coccidioidin dilution, half of those who were positive survived, while only one-tenth of those who were negative recovered. However, the relationship of coccidioidin skin test to prognosis was far from absolute. Some patients developed and died from disseminated coccidioidomycosis despite strongly positive 1 : 100 coccidioidin skin tests. Conversely, these workers cited six patients whose spontaneous recovery from disseminated coccidioidomycosis was accompanied by coccidioidin skin test conversion from negative to positive, but cited two other patients in whom recovery was not accompanied by a strongly positive skin test. These observations have been extended in several recent studies. E rosettes and total lymphocyte counts have been found to be normal (Catanzaro et al., 1975; Peterson et al., 1976). In general, comparing several studies of patients with disseminated coccidioidomycosis, results of delayed hypersensitivity to coccidioidin correlated well with in vitro determinations of MIF, but less well with lymphocyte transformation (determined by tritiated thymidine incorporation). In one study, four of eight patients with active disseminated disease had negative 1 : 100 coccidioidin skin tests, as well as depressed responses to other antigens; in addition, although 11 of 12 patients with inactive disease had positive coccidioidin skin tests, MIF and/or lymphocyte transformation in response to coccidioidin was often abnormal, and mitogen responses (phytohemagglutinin, concanavalin A) were often reduced compared with control subjects (Catanzaro *et al.,* 1975). In another study using different antigens and methodology, cellular immune defects were less obvious. Using 1 : 10 and 1 : 100 coccidioidin, 68 of 74 patients with disseminated coccidioidomycosis were skin test positive, and had positive lymphocyte transformation in response to coccidioidin as well (Opelz and Scheer, 1975). Of the six skin-test-negative patients, three had positive coccidioidin-stimulated lymphocyte transformation, although two of these three had negative responses using autologous serum, and three patients were anergic to skin test antigens other than coccidioidin. A possible role was suggested for blocking antibodies in production of anergy. Contrary to results by others (Zweiman *et al.,* 1969; Catanzaro *et al.,* 1975), there was no depression of the mitogenic response to phytohemagglutinin in subjects with negative coccidioidin skin tests.

Other workers have studied patients with disseminated disease and found unresponsiveness to skin testing and *in vitro* lymphocyte transformation restricted to coccidioidin, while most responses to unrelated antigens were positive (Peterson *et al.,* 1976). Lymphocytes from normal subjects with positive coccidioidin skin tests did not locally transfer the skin test when given intradermally to skin test negative patients. Immunogenic RNA (capable of transferring coccidioidin footpad sensitivity to normal mice) was extractable from leukocytes of normal subjects with positive coccidioidin skin tests but not from leukocytes of patients with disseminated coccidioidomycosis. Rebuck skin windows revealed an influx of neutrophils and macrophages but few lymphocytes in patients when compared with normal subjects, and active suppression of coccidioidin-committed T cells was postulated.

Disparities in results comparing different studies may be due in some cases to differences in antigen preparation and in procedures for *in vitro* studies. In some recent studies spherulin preparations were used in addition to coccidioidin (Deresinski *et al.,* 1974) and appeared to be at least as potent. The need for standardization of reagents and their usage is obvious and well recognized by workers in this area. If lymphocyte transformation is to be followed, skin-testing schedules must be carefully determined, since coccidioidin skin test may increase values for *in vitro* lymphocyte

transformation in response to coccidioidin (Kelley *et al.,* 1969). Disparate results may also occur because of differences in severity of disease in patient populations studied. For example, patients with higher complement-fixing antibody titers (signifying extensive dissemination) were more likely to have an impaired response to DNCB sensitization when compared with control subjects and with patients with less extensive coccidioidomycosis (Rea *et al.,* 1979).

In general, despite some conflicting results, it appears that patients with disseminated coccidioidomycosis often have some evidence of defects in delayed hypersensitivity or its *in vitro* correlates. In some patients with severe, active disease this may be a nonspecific depression in cellular immune responses (Catanzaro *et al.,* 1975; Rea *et al.,* 1976a). Depressed immune responses may persist after apparent cure (Catanzaro *et al.,* 1975), but there is no evidence that this represents a stable immune deficit which antedates infection.

It is apparent that the host cellular response to infection is critical in determining whether or not these infections are localized, but several questions remain. Delayed hypersensitivity is an important marker of coccidioidal immunity in man, but not a foolproof marker by any means (Smith *et al.,* 1948). Furthermore, experimental animal studies have shown that immunity to coccidioidal infection can be established in the absence of delayed hypersensitivity (Kong *et al.,* 1966; Marcus *et al.,* 1966). In dogs vaccinated with viable arthrospores or with a killed spherule preparation, phagocytosis of spores by neutrophils increased, as did coccidioidin complement-fixing antibody titers and peripheral blood leukocyte count, when compared with control animals (Wegner *et al.,* 1972). However, the specific cellular mechanisms for killing this organism in man are unknown. Soluble factors, such as circulating lysozyme, may also play a role in limiting growth of the organism (Collins and Pappagianis, 1974a,b; Rea *et al.,* 1976b). Clearly, defects in delayed hypersensitivity correlate with increased severity of coccidioidomycosis, but some of these infections remain restricted to lung and may persist or even extend locally, but do not disseminate despite documentation of the same cellular immune defects which are observed in patients with disseminated disease. The relative rarity of disseminated doccidioidomycosis as an opportunistic infection in endemic areas is also noteworthy (Deresinski and Stevens, 1974). Certainly, large numbers of immunosuppressed patients neither reactivate nor develop severe primary disease after exposure. Those who do develop opportunistic coccidioidomycosis frequently have Hodgkin's disease or other lymphoma, or have received chemotherapy for these or other diseases; but the combinations of factors which selected these patients rather than others for development of opportunistic coccidioidomycosis are not obvious at this time.

5.2. *Histoplasma capsulatum*

5.2.1. Primary Pulmonary Infection

As in coccidioidomycosis, primary, self-limited mild or asymptomatic pulmonary infections are the rule. This is indicated by a 90% incidence of positive histoplasmin skin tests in some parts of the endemic area (Ajello, 1969). Furthermore, healed histoplasmosis primary complexes have been demonstrated in lungs of 85% of consecutive autopsies performed on patients dying of other causes in a city within the endemic area (Straub and Schwarz, 1955). Unlike in tuberculosis, heavy exposure may lead to multiple primary foci, progressing to multiple healed primary complexes; these pulmonary and lymph node lesions have a strong propensity to calcify months or years after healing (Vanek and Schwarz, 1971). While development of strong cellular immunity appears to be the rule during severe acute pulmonary histoplasmosis, some patients with severe disease have been noted to have temporary depression of *in vitro* lymphocyte transformation responses to phytohemagglutinin (Cusumano *et al.*, 1974) or histoplasmin (Newberry *et al.*, 1968), followed by recovery. The majority of asymptomatic, as well as symptomatic, pulmonary infections are accompanied by asymptomatic, self-limited, hematogenous dissemination, as evidenced by autopsy demonstrations of calcified, healed foci in spleen, liver, and other tissues (Schwarz *et al.*, 1955; Okudaira *et al.*, 1961). Heavy exposure may lead to severe illness requiring prolonged hospitalization, but progressive pulmonary and disseminated dis-

ease remain rare events even under these circumstances (Vanek and Schwarz, 1971).

Where lesions were experimentally induced in mice by pulmonary infection with spores, a neutrophil response was most prominent at first, although monocytes, macrophages, and epithelioid cells appeared after several hours (Procknow *et al.*, 1960). Epithelioid cells largely replaced neutrophils in exudates by 36 hr after infection. Within 48–60 hr yeast conglomerates surrounded by epithelioid cells were noted, and monolayers containing small numbers of intracellular yeasts were more prominent. After 1 week, only few spore cell walls remained, and there were scattered granulomas with monocytes and only occasional neutrophils. Extrapulmonary dissemination occurred by day 6, but yeasts were difficult to detect within granulomas in histological sections. These and other studies suggest that neutrophils as well as monocytes and macrophages may be important in killing *Histoplasma*. *In vitro* studies have shown that neutrophils from man (Holland, 1971), guinea pig (Howard, 1973a), and mice (Howard, 1973b) can kill *H. capsulatum* yeasts. *Histoplasma* were killed by hydrogen peroxide alone (Howard, 1973a), but fungicidal effects were markedly increased in the presence of halide and myeloperoxidase (Lehrer, 1969; Howard, 1973a). In addition to the activity of this fungicidal system, studies using guinea pig neutrophil granule lysates indicated that at least three neutrophil cationic proteins could kill *H. capsulatum* (Howard, 1973a, 1975). Results of *in vitro* studies using human and animal monocytes and macrophages have been less consistent because of methodological differences, especially in view of difficulties involved in accurate, reproducible *in vitro* quantitation of viable organisms. From ultrastructural observations to determine destruction of fungi it was found that human peripheral blood monocytes ingested and killed *Histoplasma* slightly more efficiently than neutrophils (Holland, 1971). From studies employing radiolabeled organisms or uptake of radiolabeled compounds, it appeared that *H. capsulatum* yeasts survived and even multiplied within peritoneal macrophages from normal mice and guinea pigs (Howard, 1959, 1964, 1965; Howard and Otto, 1969). However, macrophages from immune animals appeared to have some increased capacity to destroy the fungus *in vivo* (Hill and Marcus, 1960) or at least limit its rate of intracellular growth *in vitro* (Howard, 1973b); macrophages from normal animals developed fungistatic properties when incubated with lymphocytes from immune animals (Howard 1975), although supernatants from "immune" lymphocytes could not increase fungistatic activity of macrophages (Howard and Otto, 1977). In one of these studies the apparent increase in ingestion and digestion of yeasts occurred independent of added or circulating antibody (Hill and Marcus, 1960). Antibodies are detectable 2–5 weeks after the onset of symptoms in man, but there is no evidence that they participate in clearing the infection, and they may interfere with some cellular immune reactions (see below).

In relation to healing of primary histoplasmosis, erythema nodosum or erythema multiforme may develop in as many as 30% of symptomatic cases, and there is a marked female preponderance (Sarosi *et al.*, 1971b). Strong immunological reactions during healing of primary foci have been related to other clinically significant sequelae of acute pulmonary histoplasmosis. Histoplasmomas are asymptomatic 1- to 3-cm diameter nodular lesions presumably resulting from healed remnants of primary lesions, which often enlarge with concentric rings of calcification and fibrosis. It has been suggested that this pattern occurs because of diffusion of antigens from the central necrotic area and precipitation in surrounding tissues (Goodwin and Snell, 1969; Vanek and Schwarz, 1971). An abnormal response to histoplasmosis involving mediastinal nodes was postulated as a cause of 26 cases of mediastinal fibrosis (Goodwin *et al.*, 1972). Similarly, in a review of 16 patients with *Histoplasma* pericarditis, it was noted that pericardial fluid was invariably culture negative, that patients recovered without antifungal therapy, and that several other features were consistent with a postinfection immunological reaction as opposed to direct extension of the infection, e.g., delayed onset after primary infection, late recurrence in six patients after complement-fixing antibodies had returned to normal, and the occurrence of sterile pleural effusions in seven patients (Picardi *et al.*, 1976). Uveitis or chro-

iditis has also been related to an immunological reaction following healed, primary histoplasmosis, but the large body of controversial, circumstantial evidence for this association will not be reviewed in this chapter (Van Metre and Maunseuee, 1964; Krill and Archer, 1970). A definite, specific relationship of this entity to histoplasmosis has not been established (Goodwin and Des Prez, 1978).

5.2.2. Chronic Pulmonary Infections

Rarely, chronic, progressive pulmonary infections develop which slowly but relentlessly destroy lung tissue unless treated, and often relapse after antifungal therapy (Baum *et al.*, 1970). In one large series 380 of 408 patients were male, and most were between 40 and 60 years of age (Parker *et al.*, 1970). On the basis of circumstantial evidence (e.g., the absence of live organisms in healed primary lesions in man and pathological data suggesting that exogenous reinfection may occur), it has been postulated that chronic pulmonary histoplasmosis represents exogenous reinfection (Baum and Schwarz, 1962). Symptomatic exogenous reinfection occurs rarely and has been followed by healing in reported cases (Powell *et al.*, 1973). Apparently, few patients fail to restrict the spread of pulmonary lesions. Most patients with chronic pulmonary histoplasmosis have had high titers of complement-fixing antibodies ($>1 : 32$) and positive histoplasmin skin tests. Histoplasmin skin tests and *in vitro* lymphocyte transformation correlated well in healthy subjects, but there was a disparity between results of skin tests and lymphocyte transformation in five patients with chronic (four pulmonary, one disseminated) histoplasmosis; in these patients, histoplasmin skin tests were positive, but lymphocyte responses to histoplasmin were depressed to ranges well below these seen in five healthy skin-test-positive subjects and close to values obtained using cells from five skin-test-negative normal subjects (Newberry *et al.*, 1968). Antibody levels did not correlate with depressed responses, but use of normal rather than autologous serum increased responses of some patients' cells, and some patients' sera could suppress responses of normal lymphocytes to histoplasmin. This was related in some cases to the presence of histoplasmin complement-fixing antibodies, although it could not be correlated directly with antibody titer (Kirkpatrick *et al.*, 1971). Of note, one patient was under treatment with amphotericin B at the time of the study, while the other four were studied 4–10 years after treatment. Differences were noted in a more recent study, which noted that lymphocyte transformation response to histoplasmin correlated with skin test results in most cases of chronic pulmonary histoplasmosis; findings in this group of patients did not differ from those in skin-test-positive normal subjects, although there was wide variation in results comparing individual patients (Alford and Goodwin, 1972). In this study six of ten patients studied with active disease had lymphocyte transformation responses to histoplasmin which exceeded those from healthy subjects with positive skin tests, while two patients with active disease had negative skin tests and depressed lymphocyte transformation response to histoplasmin, *Candida* antigen, and phytohemagglutinin. In one case this impairment was temporary. The reasons for the disparity of results in the two studies are unclear, although there were methodological differences. In addition, it may be significant that one study primarily involved patients with active disease receiving antifungal therapy. In the other most patients had been cured, and were studied years after disease. The role of defective cellular immunity in the pathogenesis of lesions in patients with chronic pulmonary histoplasmosis requires further study. It is certainly possible that subtle defects may occur (perhaps quantitative rather than qualitative, or involving parameters of cellular immunity not yet examined in this entity). Alternatively, it has been postulated that the chronic pneumonitis results from dispersion of antigen, followed by progressive infarction and necrosis in a host with a local tissue defect, i.e., centrilobular or bullous emphysema (Goodwin *et al.*, 1976). Chronically infected cavities would then form primarily because of local factors rather than a systemic immunological defect.

5.2.3. Disseminated Infections

In rare patients, organisms are not yet cleared after the dissemination which occurs in the normal course of primary infections. Progression may be rapid in infants and in patients receiving immunosuppressive therapy or debilitated from severe, underlying disease. However, the course is usually slowly progressive, with spontaneous waxing and waning of clinical manifestations. An extreme example of this is one patient recently reported with *Histoplasma* meningitis for 20 years' duration, who was clinically well after several courses of antifungal therapy but in whom the organism continued to be cultured from spinal fluid (Gelfand and Bennett, 1975). Nevertheless, most usually the disease progresses unless the organism is cleared by amphotericin B therapy. There seems to be a general relationship between prognosis and histoplasmin skin test results and antibody titers, but one not so clear as with coccidioidomycosis. Most patients have deficient delayed hypersensitivity and intact antibody responses to infection. In one series (Reddy *et al.*, 1970) 16 of 24 patients had negative histoplasmin skin tests, but only 17 of 24 had antibodies by yeast phase or histoplasmin complement-fixation tests. In another study (Sarosi *et al.*, 1971a) 27 of 52 patients had negative histoplasmin skin tests. Ten of the 27 converted to positive on retesting after clinical improvement related to antifungal chemotherapy, although 17 did not. Complement-fixing antibodies were present in 40 of 50 patients tested. Smith and Utz (1972) detected complement-fixing antibodies in 14 of 25 (46%) patients; 17 of 25 (68%) of patients had negative histoplasmin skin tests, while five of the eight patients with positive skin tests had no detectable complement-fixing antibodies. Blood cultures were done in 20 patients and were positive in ten (suggesting an active infection with many organisms); nine of these ten had negative histoplasmin skin tests, while five of ten patients with negative blood cultures had negative histoplasmin skin tests. Results of *in vitro* studies (Newberry *et al.*, 1968; Kirkpatrick *et al.*, 1971; Paul *et al.*, 1975; Stobo *et al.*, 1976) suggest that patients with disseminated histoplasmosis commonly have defects in cellular immune mechanisms, especially T-cell function. In addition, neonatally thymectomized, antithymocyte-serum-treated, or congenitally athymic ("nude") mice have significant reductions in the LD_{50} for *H. capsulatum* (Ross and Anderson, 1974; Williams *et al.*, 1978). Development of suppressor cells in spleen may be a major factor in determining the course of murine histoplasmosis (Artz and Bullock, 1979). In view of these observations it is surprising that histoplasmosis remains a rare cause of opportunistic mycoses, even in endemic areas (Furcolow, 1962; Cox and Hughes, 1974; Israel *et al.*, 1975). Local corticosteroids may be responsible for the high frequency of adrenal involvement in disseminated histoplasmosis. While corticosteroids appear to predispose to opportunistic histoplasmosis (Furcolow, 1962), inadvertent administration of high doses of corticosteroids to a patient with active (culture positive) but self-limited extrapulmonary histoplasmosis did not result in a progressive, disseminated infection after 3 years of follow-up (Lanza *et al.*, 1970). Nevertheless, disseminated histoplasmosis does occur in some immunosuppressed patients (Kauffman *et al.*, 1978). It is clear that we do not yet know the specific, critical cellular immune mechanisms which fail and thereby set the stage for progressive, disseminated histoplasmosis.

5.3. *Blastomyces dermatitidis*

It is generally accepted that almost all cases of blastomycosis (including disease which presents as isolated skin lesions) begin as a pulmonary infection which may later heal spontaneously (Schwarz and Baum, 1951). Dissemination from lungs to skin, bones, and genitourinary tract is common (Kunkel *et al.*, 1954; Witorsch and Utz, 1968). Outbreaks of mild or subclinical, self-limited primary pulmonary infections have been documented (Sarosi *et al.*, 1974; Tosh *et al.*, 1974), but the frequency of occurrence of this form of disease is not well established.

In the lungs and other tissues there is a mixed suppurative and granulomatous response to the organism. In lung the first response is accumulation of neutrophils, followed next by focal aggregates of lymphocytes, later joined by plasma cells, mast cells, histiocytes, and giant cells; healing of lesions then occurs, typically with fibrosis and scarring but not calcification (Kunkel *et al.*, 1954). Mixed with mononuclear and giant cells (which do not aggregate into well-formed granulomas), neutrophils persist, even in late lesions. Suppurative foci may develop into necrotic areas. Yeasts are found associated with leukocytes,

intracellular (usually in giant cells) or surrounded by neutrophils. *In vitro*, culture filtrates of *B. dermatitidis* were chemotactic for human neutrophils, which readily ingested *Blastomyces* yeasts but could not kill them efficiently (Sixbey *et al.*, 1979). As in coccidioidomycosis, and unlike in histoplasmosis, pulmonary lesions are not regularly associated with involvement of regional lymph nodes (Vanek *et al.*, 1970).

Cutaneous disease commonly exists as the sole, active focus. This form of the disease, when untreated, has a chronic course characterized by long spontaneous remissions, smoldering infection, and exacerbation months or years later. The disease may be disfiguring but has not appeared to greatly shorten life span in many untreated cases (Kunkel *et al.*, 1954; Tindall and Elson, 1974). Untreated systemic disease often had a prolonged course, but was almost always fatal, often after years (Kunkel *et al.*, 1954). Correlation of outcome with results of blastomycin skin test results and complement-fixation titers has been noted by some workers (Tindall and Elson, 1974), but most series have not found these tests to be helpful because of the lack of specificity of the antigens (Witorsch and Utz, 1968; Lockwood *et al.*, 1968). However, data from recent outbreaks of self-limited acute disease (Sarosi *et al.*, 1974; Tosh *et al.*, 1974) have suggested that blastomycin skin test reactivity may occur in acute, self-limited cases and may have slightly better specificity than previously thought, since several patients were blastomycin positive and histoplasmin negative. Animal studies have also associated the development of delayed hypersensitivity after sensitization of mice with protection from lethal challenge and decreased proliferation of *B. dermatitidis* in tissues (Cozad and Chang, 1975). Some human patients with blastomycosis have been noted to have defects in cellular immunity, as evidenced by cutaneous anergy or reduced *in vitro* lymphocyte mitogenic responses to phytohemagglutinin and concanavalin A (Paul *et al.*, 1975; Stobo *et al.*, 1976). Thus blastomycosis may well be associated with cellular immune defects, but more specific knowledge of cellular host defense mechanisms against this agent is limited by the quality of currently available immunologic reagents.

5.4. *Paracoccidioides brasiliensis*

Although many reports still suggest that the oral mucosa is the portal of entry in most cases of paracoccidioidomycosis, there is a large body of experimental, clinical, and pathological data indicating that pulmonary infection precedes lesions in other areas (Mackinnon, 1959; Salfelder *et al.*, 1969; Restrepo *et al.*, 1970; Gonzalez-Ochoa, 1972; Yarzabal, 1972). Existence of a self-limited, mild or asymptomatic form of the infection has been postulated (Lacaz *et al.*, 1959). Skin test surveys, as well as pathological and clinical data, suggest that such subclinical infections are common, as detailed in recent reviews (Angulo-Ortega, 1972; Furtado, 1972; Greer *et al.*, 1972; Londero, 1972; Yarzabal, 1972). The disease has a restricted geographic distribution (Mackinnon, 1972). However, clinically apparent paracoccidioidomycosis has developed in patients who had left endemic areas as long as 10 (Fountain and Sutliff, 1969), 23 (Oliveira and Baptista, 1960), and 30 (Rollier and Chenebault, 1962) years before. This suggests the possibility of prolonged latency followed by dissemination of infections.

In man a mixed inflammatory response is typical, with suppurative foci and microabscess formation, as well as granulomas with mononuclear cells and giant cells (Yarzabal, 1972). Fibrosis often occurs with healing. In many cases the tissue response to infection is minimal, and macrophages in lesions are loaded with organisms (Mendes and Raphael, 1971). In experimental animal studies, delayed hypersensitivity was apparent 7–11 days after infection (de Brito *et al.*, 1972). In man immunological reactions appear to vary according to the clinical severity of the disease (Fava Netto and Raphael, 1961; Lacaz and Fava Netto, 1969). Patients with more severe forms of disease usually have high titers of specific antibodies which decrease with clinical improvement. Conversely, impairment in delayed hypersensitivity, as well as in various *in vitro* parameters of T-cell function, has been noted in many patients with paracoccidioidomycosis and has been correlated with clinical severity of disease (Mendes and Raphael, 1971; Mendes *et al.*, 1971; E. Mendes, 1975; Musatti, 1975; N. F. Mendes, 1975). In these studies patients were noted to have an in-creased incidence of cutaneous anergy to a battery of antigens, a decreased rate of successful sensitization to dinitochlorobenzene, and prolonged survival of allografts. Conversion of tuberculin skin tests occurred in four patients after infusions of lymphocytes from normal subjects with positive tuberculin tests (Mendes and Raphael, 1971), but transfer of delayed hypersensitivity was less clear-cut in five patients who received transfer factor (E. Mendes, 1975). Compared with that in normal subjects, the percentage of E-rosette positive cells was increased, although the absolute numbers of T cells were not, considering the total peripheral blood leukocyte counts. In some cases paracortical areas of lymph nodes were depleted of lymphocytes, but this was seen only in active infected nodes, and distant nodes appeared normal (N. F. Mendes, 1975). However, other studies demonstrated a decrease in circulating T cells in some patients (Musatti *et al.*, 1976). As in coccidioidomycosis, *in vitro* MIF responses correlated well with skin results in patients, but lymphocyte transformation did not. In several cases leukocyte mitogenic responses to phytohemagglutinin and specific antigens were depressed in autologous plasma, but most of these values were significantly increased in normal plasma. Conversely, sera from seven of 17 patients depressed responses of normal cells to phytohemagglutinin. Depressed *in vitro* lymphocyte responses could not be correlated with serum antibody titers (Musatti, 1975). The mechanisms of depression of cell-mediated immunity in this disease remain unkown.

Circulating antibodies are elevated in proportion to the severity of disease but may have a useful function in host defenses beyond providing an immunological marker for activity of paracoccidioidomycosis. Peripheral blood leukocytes (approximately 70% neutrophils) were incubated *in vitro* with *P. brasiliensis* or *Rhodotorula* yeasts. Phagocytosis and intracellular killing of *P. brasiliensis* (but not *Rhodotorula*) were significantly increased in the presence of patients' sera, and an opsonic role for specific antibody was postulated. Leukocytes from 17 patients functioned as well as leukocytes from normal subjects, but there was a wide range of normal values (20–85%) comparing results in different individuals (Restrepo and Velez, 1975). Further studies of leukocyte function are needed to define the defense mechanisms which are directly involved in killing this organism within the host.

5.5. *Sporothrix schenckii*

Local disease restricted to a primary inoculation site and draining lymph nodes is the most commonly observed form of sporotrichosis (Wilson, 1963; Lynch, 1974). In a classic outbreak in over 3300 Bantu mineworkers in South Africa who were exposed to contaminated timbers, only five atypical cases were noted (including four with extracutaneous lesions), and there were no fatalities (Lurie, 1963). While a variety of skin test antigen preparations have been used, results have appeared to be universally specific and indicative of an asymptomatic, self-limited form of infection (Schneidau et al., 1964; Ingrish and Schneidau, 1967; Nielsen, 1968). Asymptomatic infections in man may occur by inhalation (Lynch, 1974). Clinically apparent pulmonary disease occurs in man in the absence of cutaneous lesions (Baum et al., 1969) and can be produced in animals by inhalation (Sethi, 1967).

In lesions there is typically a mixed pyogenic and granulomatous inflammatory response, with few organisms. Some lesions contain many plasma cells. Occasionally, a 3- to 5-μm-diameter yeastlike structure has been observed, surrounded by lines of eosinophilic material radiating outward up to 10 μm. These "asteroid bodies" have been said to represent antigen–antibody reactions (Lurie and Still, 1966).

As reviewed by Salvin (1963), a small number of studies in experimental animals have suggested a protective role in S. schenckii infections for hyperimmune serum, as well as for vaccines which were likely to have induced a cellular response. In man iodides may well exert their therapeutic effects by interaction with host defense mechanisms, since S. schenckii can grow well in media containing 10% potassium iodide (Emmons et al., 1970). It has been suggested that extracutaneous sporotrichosis, like several other disseminated responses, occurs in association with defective cellular immunity (Plouffe et al., 1979). However, studies using lymphocytes from one patient with articular sporotrichosis revealed a strong *in vitro* mitogenic response to an *S. schenckii* mycelial phase antigen (Steele et al., 1976). It is not known how the host kills this organism or whether antibodies act as opsonins or have any other protective role in host responses to sporotrichosis.

5.6. *Cryptococcus neoformans*

C. neoformans has been cultured from sputum in a number of cases in the absence of tissue invasion or clinical disease (Reiss and Szilagyi, 1965; Warr et al., 1968; Tynes et al., 1968; Howard, 1973c). The factors responsible for establishment of colonization in these patients are unknown, although many of the patients who were colonized had underlying pulmonary disease of various types. It is not known whether or not colonization may precede tissue invasion. One patient who was followed for 3½ years with C. neoformans in sputum cultures never developed clinically apparent cryptococcosis (Tynes et al., 1968).

The presumed frequent occurrence of subclinical infections was noted earlier (see Section 4.6). In addition, many symptomatic self-limited cases of cryptococcosis confined to the lungs have been observed (Warr et al., 1968; Tynes et al., 1968; Hammerman et al., 1973; Gordonson et al., 1974). It therefore appears that exposure to C. neoformans is common and that failure of immunity and development of extrapulmonary cryptococcosis is rare.

Evidence from infections in human and experimental animals suggests that cellular host defenses against C. neoformans are more important than humoral mechanisms. Resistance to local or systemic infections with cryptococci in most experimental animal models has been correlated with development of strong cellular immunity, accompanied by a vigorous cellular inflammatory response (Louria et al., 1963; Abrahams, 1966; Abrahams et al., 1970; Gentry and Remington, 1971). More severe infections with a markedly reduced cellular inflammatory reaction occurred in mice treated with corticosteroids (Song, 1971), or with antilymphocyte serum (Adamson and Cozad, 1969). In experimental animals the neutrophil has been observed to be the first line of cellular defenses against cryptococci (Bergman, 1961; Gadebusch, 1972). *In vitro* studies using human peripheral blood neutrophils showed that only cryptococci with small capsules were readily ingested by these cells (Bulmer and Sans, 1967) but that almost all intracellular fungi were killed (Diamond *et al.,* 1972). Phagocytosis was inhibited by high concentrations of soluble cryptococcal capsular polysaccharide (Bulmer and Sans, 1968; Diamond *et al.,* 1972). Intracellular killing (but not phagocytosis) of cryptococci was markedly depressed when neutrophils from three subjects with chronic granulomatous disease were used, suggesting the importance of hydrogen peroxide. Hydrogen peroxide alone (in concentrations achievable within leukocytes) killed cryptococci, but intracellular killing was significantly slowed by sodium azide treatment of leukocytes, suggesting a role for myeloperoxidase as well (Diamond *et al.,* 1972). Since killing of a fungi occurred when myeloperoxidase was completely inhibited, it appeared that an additional killing mechanism was active, such as peroxide alone, or cationic proteins (Gadebusch and Johnson, 1966). Neutrophils from 13 patients with cryptococcosis and three patients each with Hodgkin's disease, sarcoidosis, or corticosteroid therapy were found to ingest and kill cryptococci as well as those of 27 normal subjects did (Diamond *et al.,* 1972). Only three of the cryptococcosis patients had active disease at the time of study, and only one of these had a low titer of cryptococcal polysaccharide detectable in serum. Almost identical results were obtained comparing a similar number of monocytes from patients and control subjects, except that monocytes ingested large capsule yeasts as efficiently as small ones. This study therefore failed to indicate the presence of a stable defect in neutrophils, monocytes, or serum opsonins in cured cryptococcosis patients. In a later study other workers noted that sera from four patients with severe cryptococcosis depressed phagocytosis of cryptococci by autologous as well as normal neutrophils, but this defect was corrected when normal serum was used. Inhibition was attributed to high levels of polysaccharide in the sera (Tacker *et al.,* 1972). The capsular material clearly may have profound inhibitory effects on cellular responses in man, but few patients studied (in a review of 111 with cryptococcosis) had levels of cryptococcal polysaccharide in such a high range (Diamond and Bennett, 1974).

In late human as well as experimental animal lesions there may be a vigorous inflammatory response in tissue outside the brain which is usually granulomatous in nature. However, in experimental animal studies development of delayed hypersensitivity did not necessarily correlate with clearing of organisms during infections (Larsh, 1975). Despite this, most experimental studies have suggested the importance of cellular immunity in host defenses against cryptococcosis (Gentry and Remington, 1971). In man several defects in parameters of cellular immunity have been observed in patients with cryptococcosis who have no obvious predisposing factors (i.e., corticosteroid therapy or lymphoreticular malignancy). Compared with exposed normal controls (laboratory workers with positive cryptococcin skin tests), some cryptococcosis patients have been found to have depressed delayed skin responses to cryptococcin and mumps, abnormal *in vitro* MIF response to cryptococcin or killed *C. neoformans* (Schimpff and Bennett, 1975), and depressed *in vitro* lymphocyte transformation in response to killed *C. neoformans* (Diamond and Bennett, 1973a) or cryptococcin (Graybill and Alford, 1974). Some of the responses remained abnormal for several years after the patients were cured. In a different study two patients with cryptococcosis had depressed mitogenic responses *in vitro* which may have been due to production of a soluble suppressor substance (Stobo *et al.,* 1976). In experimental cryptococcosis in athymic ("nude") mice, presence of T cells appeared to be required for host immunity (Graybill and Drutz, 1978; Cauley and Murphy, 1979). Severe depression of chemotactic responses of neutrophils and monocytes may also occur in some patients with cryptococcosis, and might be one cause of cutaneous anergy (Wilson *et al.,* 1977). In addition, data from infections in guinea pigs suggest that the outcome of these experimental infections may be determined by the quantity of the inflammatory response in infectious foci, rather than the ability of individual leukocytes to kill cryptococci (Diamond, 1977). It appears that cryptococcosis may be a final common pathway for expression of several different types of defects in cellular immunity. Although this would seem to make such patients ideal candidates for immunotherapy, such therapy is difficult to evaluate because of the lack of standard antigen preparations. In additions, the disease may have a prolonged course with spontaneous remissions and exacerbations over several years in some untreated patients (Beeson, 1952; Littman and Walter, 1968).

From the above data, as well as indirect evidence from experimental animal studies (Gentry and Remington, 1971), macrophages activated by cellular immune mechanisms would be expected to be potent killers of cryptococci. Unfortunately, this expected level of activity has been difficult to document in *in vitro* studies. Peritoneal macrophages from experimental animals appeared to be able to kill only a minority of a cryptococcal inoculum. In one study glycogen-induced rat peritoneal macrophages killed only 3–49% of ingested cryptococci after 24–48 hr (Mitchell and Friedman, 1972). In another study, although visual observations suggested active killing of organisms, "activated" mouse peritoneal macrophages (stimulated by concanavalin A or endotoxin) killed only 11–29% of intracellular organisms after 5 hr. Quantitative results beyond 5 hr were not reported. Cryptococci actively grew within unstimulated macrophages or those stimulated by poly(I) · poly(C), starch, amphotericin B, or toxoplasma (Sethi and Pelster, 1973). Other investigators found that guinea pig alveolar macrophages (including cells activated by injection of animals with *Salmonella* or *Serratia*) did not kill cryptococci, and no killing was observed in one experiment using human alveolar macrophages (Bulmer and Tacker, 1975). Finally, in 144 experiments using cells from 26 different subjects, macrophages cultured from human peripheral blood monocytes not only failed to kill cryptococci but also provided a more favorable medium for growth of the fungus than serum and medium without cells. All experiments were done using at least ten macrophages for each yeast. These results were obtained even after monocytes cultured with lymphocytes were activated with streptokinase-streptodornase, in doses shown to stimulate thymidine incorporation by nonadherent lymphocytes in the culture supernatants. Similar results were observed using cells from eight normal subjects with positive cryptococcin skin tests, even if mononuclear cells were cultured with cryptococcin or infected immediately after separation with a low inoculum of cryptococci. Despite their failure to kill cryptococci, these macrophages effectively killed *Listeria* (Diamond and Bennett, 1973b). Failure to kill cryptococci may have been due to a loss of myeloperoxidase by cells in culture or its observed absence in freshly obtained "activated" alveolar macrophages (Neilsen *et al.*, 1974). Perhaps specifically activated macrophages with efficient fungicidal activity exist *in vivo,* but only at sites of active infection or stimulation by specific fungal antigens.

One feature conferred on this organism by its capsule is physical size, often large enough to preclude ingestion by phagocytic cells. There appear to be several mechanisms potentially active in killing of cryptococci by nonphagocytic effects. *In vivo* and *in vitro* experimental animal studies have indicated that phagocytic cells could surround the large, encapsulated yeasts to form "rings"; leukocytes appeared to release lysosomal enzymes into the yeasts (Kalina *et al.*, 1970). Heat-liabile opsonins were required *in vitro.* Cryptococci within monocyte rings were killed slowly (5% or less killed at 5 hr, 50% after 1–2 days), while no killing by neutrophils was noted over the 8-hr period of observation (Aronson and Kletter, 1973). In ultrastructural observations the capsules of large yeasts were penetrated by pseudopods from the leukocytes, accompanied by disintegration and phagocytosis of capsular material. It was suggested that killing occurred by release of lysosomal enzymes or other materials (Kalina *et al.,* 1974). It has also been shown that anticryptococcal antibody can induce killing of cryptococci by nonimmune peripheral blood leukocytes in the absence of serum complement components (Diamond, 1974). Studies performed since then have indicated that such killing may be mediated by monocytes, neutrophils, and perhaps lymphocytes (K cells) as well, although nonphagocytic monocytes rather than lymphocytes may be involved (Diamond and Allison, 1976).

The potential significance of these observations *in vivo* is suggested by some studies of experimental animal cryptococcosis, which demonstrated that some degree of passive protection (apparently mediated by antibody) could be induced (Gadebusch, 1958b, 1960).

In addition, in contrast to most other systemic mycoses, the presence of anticryptococcal antibody in the serum of patients with cryptococcosis has been correlated with eventual cure (Diamond and Bennett, 1974). Although specific antibody and complement do not kill cryptococci, other soluble factors may be active in the extracellular killing or at least the inhibition of growth of cryptococci within the infected host. Such factors have been noted in serum and saliva. The serum substance killed some cryptococci and inhibited growth of others *in vitro*. It was found to be nondialyzable, stable to heating at 56°C for 30 min but not 70°C for 30 min, and inactivated by trypsin and by phosphate ions. All five of Cohn serum protein fractions stimulated growth of the organism. A β-globulin-labile lipoprotein was suggested (Igel and Bolande, 1966), but later workers localized most inhibitory activity to α_2- and γ-globulin fractions. Addition of iron decreased inhibitory activity in some sera but did not eliminate it, which suggested that the inhibition of growth of yeasts by iron-binding proteins was another, separate mechanism (Reiss *et al.*, 1975). In one study serum killed 66% of a cryptococcal inoculum over a 4-hr period (Tacker *et al.*, 1972), but some *C. neoformans* isolates from patients were found to be resistant to killing by this mechanism (Diamond *et al.*, 1972). In saliva a fungicidal substance has been described which was dialyzable, stable to heating for 2 hr at 70°C, and different from amylase or lysozyme (Igel and Bolande, 1966). However, in a later study salivary antifungal activity was correlated with levels of peroxidase and was reduced, as compared to that in normal volunteers, in patients receiving irradiation or corticosteroid therapy (Dublin and Bulmer, 1974). This latter observation is consistent with the description of a three-component antimicrobial system in saliva, consisting of salivary peroxidase, thiocyanate, and hydrogen peroxide provided via microbial metabolism (Hamon and Klebanoff, 1973).

Another noteworthy feature of cryptococcosis is its predilection for localization to the central nervous system, often without evidence of lesions persisting elsewhere in the body. Spinal fluid contains thiamine and other nutrients necessary to stimulate growth of *C. neoformans* in large capsule forms (Littman,

1958) and lacks substances capable of inhibiting growth of organisms (Igel and Bolande, 1966). The interaction of cryptococci with the complement system may also provide an explanation for the tendency of cryptococcosis to localize in brain. Lesions may show a dense inflammatory response or large clusters of encapsulated yeasts with little or no surrounding inflammation. The latter response is particularly characteristic of brain lesions (Emmons *et al.*, 1970). It was observed that *C. neoformans* and its capsular polysaccharide activated the classical and alternate complement pathways in human and guinea pig sera. This interaction mediated opsonization of the organism for phagocytosis and required an intact alternate complement pathway, although the early classical complement components were necessary for optimum phagocytic kinetics. Unlike serum, spinal fluid did not opsonize cryptococci. Little or no complement was found on the surface of cryptococci obtained from spinal fluid of four patients with cryptococcosis, but it was detected on cryptococci after incubation in fresh sera from these patients (Diamond *et al.*, 1974). Studies in guinea pigs supported the hypothesis that late complement components were important in clearance of cryptococci from extraneural sites; levels of complement in the central nervous system may have been too low to aid in destruction of organisms once cryptococci disseminated to the brain (Diamond *et al.*, 1973). However, cryptococcal polysaccharide did cause an inflammatory response when injected directly into brains of rats (Hirano *et al.*, 1964, 1965). In addition, experimental animal studies suggested that the inflammatory response in brain was delayed but that organisms could be cleared from brain lesions (Staib and Mishra, 1975; Grosse *et al.*, 1975). In man it is possible that some individuals are at risk for meningeal cryptococcosis because of a decreased ability to mount a cellular response to cryptococci which reach the central nervous system.

5.7. *Absidia, Mucor,* and *Rhizopus* spp.

Absidia, Mucor, and *Rhizopus* organisms are ubiquitous, so that isolation from specimens exposed to the air is usually not significant. Because of the nature of the lesions and their rapid course, biopsies are usually needed for diagnois (Meyer *et al.*, 1972). The hallmark of lesions is invasion of blood vessels with hemorrhage, necrosis, and infarction (Hutter, 1959). There may be minimal inflammatory reaction to the hyphae, or there may be a variable reaction, although neutrophils usually predominate. Human neutrophils can damage and probably kill *Rhizopus hyphae in vitro* by a nonphagocytic mechanism (Diamond *et al.*, 1978).

Correction of acidosis appears to be critical in successful therapy of patients with diabetes, even when antifungal chemotherapy with amphotericin B is used. It has been suggested that this is related to the growth properties of the organism (see Section 3.7) as well as to the adverse effects of diabetic ketoacidosis on phagocytic cells (Abramson *et al.*, 1967). It is not surprising that the disease is difficult to produce in normal experimental animals, but a number of investigators have produced mucormycosis in alloxan-diabetic animals. Alloxan diabetes with acidosis appeared to slow and decrease the inflammatory response to *Rhizopus* (Sheldon and Bauer, 1960). Host serum factors may also be important in inhibiting the organism. The growth of *Rhizopus oryzae* was inhibited by normal human sera, but inhibitory activity was greatly reduced in sera from two of six diabetics (Gale and Welch, 1961). In one case inhibitory activity returned to normal levels when acidosis was corrected. The inhibitory activity was heat stable, dialyzable, and not attributable to antibodies. Presumably, infections occur only when normal host cutaneous or epithelial barriers are broken. It is still not known which host cellular responses are critical in helping to clear infections if metabolic disorders and leukopenia can be corrected.

6. Immunodiagnosis

Immunodiagnosis involves either detection of antigens or other products of an infectious agent or detection of the host immune response to the agent. The former method is most useful because it should correlate with active infection and may detect disease even when host immune responses are suppressed, but so far is generally available only in cryptococcosis. The latter involves a wide array of skin tests and serological tests for antibodies (circulating or fixed in tissues). Some of the procedures are well standardized and reproducible, while others are experimental (Harrell *et al.*, 1970), such as counterimmunoelectrophoresis in some mycoses, or enzyme-linked immunoadsorbant assays (ELISA). Many are available in only a few specialized laboratories. Detailed reviews of methodology have been published elsewhere (Palmer *et al.*, 1977).

6.1. *Coccidioides immitis*

6.1.1. Delayed Skin Test

Coccidioidin is the standard skin test antigen and is commercially available. Within 1 week after symptoms of primary infection, only one-eighth of patients have a negative reaction to a 1 : 100 dilution, and only 6.7% remain negative after 2 weeks (Smith *et al.*, 1948). This dilution of skin test antigen may provoke or exacerbate erythema nodosum, so testing of these subjects, if performed, is started at 1 : 1000 or 1 : 10,000 dilutions. Some patients nonreactive to a 1 : 1000 dilution of coccidioidin are positive when a 1 : 10 dilution is used, but this dilution is less specific (cross-reactivity with *Histoplasma capsulatum*). Although a small rise in *Histoplasma* yeast and mycelial phase complement-fixation titers may rarely occur after a positive coccidioidin skin test (Pappagianis *et al.*, 1967b), coccidioidal antibody titers is sensitized subjects are unaffected. The coccidioidin skin test may have some prognostic value in chronic or disseminated infections, and may also provide a useful parameter for following effects of immunotherapy. Otherwise, its clinical usefulness is limited, except as an epidemiological tool. Positive skin tests persist for years after infection, probably for life in most cases.

Spherulin, prepared from killed, cultured spherules and tested in animals (Levine *et al.*, 1969), has also been used for skin testing in man (Stevens *et al.*, 1974a, 1975a) in 2.8- and 28-μg intradermal doses. Sixteen patients were noted who had negative coccidioidin skin tests (1 : 100 dilution) but were positive when tested with 2.8 μg spherulin, while one coccidioidin-positive patient had a negative spherulin response. Patients with disseminated coccidioidomycosis also tended to react more frequently to spherulin and more often to the more dilute dosage when compared with coccidioidin responses. However, an occasional patient was coccidioidin positive and spherulin negative. In addition, data for prognostic value of skin testing in disseminated coccidioidomycosis exist for coccidioidin but not for spherulin. Nevertheless, spherulin appears to be more sensitive and perhaps more specific in concentrated form than is coccidioidin (Levine *et al.*, 1975), so it may be useful together with coccidioidin, especially in following the effects of a course of immunotherapy (Stevens *et al.*, 1975a).

6.1.2. Circulating Antibodies

After infection, IgM anticoccidioidal antibodies appear first and are detectable by a tube precipitin assay (Smith *et al.*, 1956) or by a more sensitive, but slightly less specific, latex particle agglutination technique (Huppert *et al.*, 1968). Since these antibodies are generally present in the first month after infection and disappear thereafter (even if the disease progresses), the precipitin and agglutination tests are most valuable in detecting early primary infections or exacerbations of existing disease, and have no prognostic value (Kaufman, 1975). The coccidioidin complement-fixation (Smith *et al.*, 1956) and immunodiffusion tests (Huppert and Bailey, 1965) detect IgG antibodies which appear late after primary infections. Low complement-fixation titers (>1 : 8) may represent nonspecific reactions (Smith *et al.*, 1956; Kaufman, 1975) but can be differentiated from cross-reaction with histoplasmosis and blastomycosis by the immunodiffusion test (Kaufman and Clark, 1974). Occasionally, before the coccidioidin complement-fixation test is positive, high titers are obtained using complement-fixation reagents for histoplasmosis and blastomycosis (Campbell, 1968), but the specific reaction becomes stronger with time. The coccidioidin complement-fixation titer may be negative or low in a significant percentage of primary and residual pulmonary cases but in one series was negative in only one of 722 (0.3%) cases of disseminated coccidioidomycosis (Smith *et al.*, 1956). Immunosuppression does not appear to eliminate the diagnostic value of complement-fixation titers (Deresinski and Stevens, 1974), nor does rapidly progressive miliary disease (Winn *et al.*,

1967). Complement-fixation titers $\geq 1 : 32$ are suggestive of dissemination. Similarly, titers should fall and become negative with clinical recovery; a plateau or rise in titer is a sign of continued or extending infection (Smith *et al.*, 1956). The complement-fixation test is also invaluable in diagnosis and prognosis of meningeal coccidioidomycosis, since spinal fluid cultures are frequently negative, but complement-fixing antibodies are detectable in 75% of cases (Smith *et al.*, 1956). A positive complement-fixation test is diagnostic of meningeal coccidioidomycosis, although one false-positive case (attributed to increased permeability of the meninges secondary to concomitant syphilis) has been reported. Immunodiffusion testing of concentrated spinal fluid may provide an additional aid in diagnosis of meningeal infection where complement fixation is negative, but false-positive tests may occur (probably due to penetration of serum antibodies) (Pappagianis *et al.*, 1972).

Overall, for screening sera using simple procedures, the combination of latex particle agglutination and immunodiffusion has been reported as positive in 93% of cases. However, the complement-fixation test remains invaluable because of its diagnostic specificity, as well as its critical role in determining prognosis and providing guidelines for therapy. An additional use for the immunodiffusion procedure involves use of antisera for rapid and specific identification of antigens produced by cultured isolates of *C. immitis* (Standard and Kaufman, 1977).

Spherulin has been used as a reagent for complement fixation, and is now commercially available for this purpose. Titers greater than 1 : 8 were similar, whether coccidioidin or spherulin was used as a complement fixation reagent; however, spherulin detected 31% more reactors than coccidioidin when titers were 1 : 8 or less, and appeared to be specific (Scalarone *et al.*, 1974). However, since then, others have reported that coccidioidin and spherulin were equally sensitive but that spherulin was considerably less specific (Huppert *et al.*, 1977). It has been suggested that spherulin is indeed more sensitive and that this is due to decreased potency in recent batches of coccidioidin (Drutz and Catanzaro, 1978). Spherulin has also been used as an antigen for rapid diagnosis using counterimmunoelectrophoresis, and was reported to be sensitive and specific, although only a small number of patients were tested (Aguilar-Torres *et al.,* 1976). Since then, the test has been used by others, its major advantage being speed. Spherulin (used as a complement-fixation reagent) may prove as useful as coccidioidin as a prognostic indicator and primary guideline for therapy, but this must be established by further experience.

6.1.3. Tissue Diagnosis

Fluorescent antibody (FA) techniques have been described for tissue diagnosis of *Coccidioides immitis* (Kaplan and Clifford, 1964; Kaplan and Kraft, 1969). The FA reagent will stain *C. immitis* endospores in all cases. These preparations cross-reacted with *Histoplasma, Blastomyces,* and other fungi but were specific for *Coccidioides* after adsorption with *Histoplasma capsulatum* or by dilution. The morphological distinctiveness of the organism in tissues limits the value of these FA tests to those situations where diagnostic elements of the organism are not present.

6.2. *Histoplasma capsulatum*

6.2.1. Delayed Skin Test

Up to 90% of adults within the endemic area are histoplasmin skin test positive. Skin tests probably remain positive for life after most primary infections, so that skin testing provides useful epidemiological data. However, because of these factors, skin tests are rarely useful in diagnosis of histoplasmosis, perhaps being of limited use in infancy and in the rare individual with a known recent conversion from negative to positive (Campbell, 1968; Levin, 1970; Kaufman, 1971; Buechner *et al.,* 1973). In addition, the specificity of skin test results, especially of marginal reactions, has been questioned because of data from animal studies (Goodwin *et al.,* 1972). Another disadvantage, but only in those with positive histoplasmin skin tests, is the possibility of confusion of diagnostic studies because of production of antibodies after skin testing in 12–27% of subjects (Buechner *et al.,* 1973). The mycelial phase (histoplasmin) complement-fixation test is usually affected more than the test using yeast phase antigen (see Section 6.2.2). In one study 114 healthy subjects with positive histoplasmin skin tests were bled before and 15 days after a single skin test (Kaufman, 1971). Less than 12% developed positive complement-fixation tests and most were low (in the 1 : 8–1 : 16 range), but 1.7% were 1 : 32. Precipitins developed in 17 of 114 (15%) tested.

6.2.2. Circulating Antibodies

The complement-fixation test is most widely used. It is usually but not invariably positive in acute and chronic pulmonary cases and is less reliable in disseminated infections, especially in those occurring in immunosuppressed patients (Israel *et al.,* 1975). Two antigens are used: histoplasmin (a soluble mycelial phase culture filtrate) and a suspension of merthiolate-treated intact yeasts. Sera from active cases may react with only one of the two antigen preparations, so both must be used. In one study of sera from 220 cases of active histoplasmosis, 182 (83%) were positive using mycelial phase antigen, 206 (94%) using yeast phase, and 212 (96%) using both (Kaufman, 1971). The yeast phase titer is usually higher in acute infections, but the mycelial phase is more likely to be elevated to chronic cases. This test may also be positive in other mycoses, in inactive histoplasmosis, in nonmycotic infections, and in some normal subjects as well, but usually with low titers (1 : 8–1 : 16). However, some patients with disseminated histoplasmosis have titers in this range. Conversely, while titers ≥1 : 32 are highly suggestive of active histoplasmosis, titers of 1 : 32–1 : 128 have been observed in patients with coccidioidomycosis, blastomycosis, and miscellaneous disorders (Kaufman, 1971). Titers often parallel the clinical activity of the disease, but not consistently enough to have as much usefulness as complement-fixation titers in coccidioidomycosis.

Unlike in coccidioidomycosis, no absolute titer correlates well with dissemination. Titers as high as 1 : 256–1 : 2048 have been seen in acute, self-limited pulmonary histoplasmosis (Buechner *et al.,* 1973). However, fourfold changes in titer in either direction are usually significant but infrequently observed. Plateauing of titers ≥1 : 32 for over one 1 month occasionally occurs with active disease. Titers fluctuating between negative and low levels may be seen in chronic pulmonary or extrapulmonary histoplasmosis. Patients with histoplasmosis may also respond to complement-fixation antigens for coccidioidomycosis and blastomycosis. In fact, the blastomycosis response may appear earlier and be higher than the specific antigen response in acute histoplasmosis (Kaufman, 1971). In addition, a positive coccidioidin skin test may rarely be followed by slight false elevation of the histoplasmosis yeast or mycelial phase titer (Pappagianis et al., 1967b). Rheumatoid factor or cold agglutinins in sera may interfere with the complement-fixation reaction to yeast but not mycelial antigen (Johnson and Roberts, 1976). A rapid technique for screening for antibodies by latex agglutination is available (Hill and Campbell, 1962) and correlates well with complement-fixation tests in acute cases. However, it is negative in up to 50% of chronic cases and false-positive results may result when sera contain rheumatoid factor (Oxenhandler et al., 1977) so is of limited value (Buechner et al., 1973).

Immunodiffusion, using concentrated histoplasmin preparations as antigens, has also been widely used. Sera suitable for use are prepared and evaluated at the Center for Disease Control because of recognized difficulties in antigen standardization (Gross et al., 1975). Two precipitin bands, termed H and M, have diagnostic significance (Heiner, 1958). It is necessary to use histoplasmin with a balanced H and M composition in conjunction with reference sera from human histoplasmosis cases which react with both antigens. Otherwise, no lines may form, lines may not separate or be broad and poorly defined, or the usual position of the H and M lines may reverse. The H band is most specific since it is rarely influenced by skin testing, but is found up to 2 years after recovery, as well as in active and progressive histoplasmosis. The M band has been detected in sera from patients with acute and chronic histoplasmosis but also occurs in healthy subjects after positive skin tests; it therefore may signify active infection, past infection, or a recent skin test (Kaufman, 1971). Both bands usually are present, but the H band rarely occurs alone. Sera from patients with blastomycosis, coccidioidomycosis, and aspergillosis often contain precipitating antibodies against components of histoplasmin, but these do not conform to the H and M bands and are easily separable using standard positive reference sera (Bauman and Smith, 1975). Sera from patients with paracoccidioidomycosis have been reported to produce sometimes an M band (Restrepo and Moncada, 1974), but Kaufman (1972) found the immunodiffusion test for histoplasmosis and paracoccidioidomycosis to be specific.

The immunodiffusion test appears to be highly specific for histoplasmosis (Kaufman and Clark, 1974; Bauman and Smith, 1975), at least among mycoses commonly seen in North America, and has been capable of detecting from 79% (Kaufman and Clark, 1974) to 90% (Bauman and Smith, 1975) of cases. When used together with complement-fixation tests, antibodies were detectable in all but a few cases (Kaufman, 1971; Kaufman and Clark, 1974; Bauman and Smith, 1975). In addition to detection of antibodies, standard antisera may be used in immunodiffusion tests to detect antigens produced by cultures, providing a means for rapid and specific identification of H. capsulatum organisms (Standard and Kaufman, 1976). Agar gel immunoelectrophoresis appeared to offer a rapid and still reliable method for detection of H and M precipitin lines (Kleger and Kaufman, 1973). Serum antibodies in chronic and disseminated histoplasmosis have also been quantitated by a hemagglutination technique, which demonstrated 19 S as well as 7 S antibodies late in the course of disease (Hermans and Markowitz, 1969).

6.2.3. Tissue Diagnosis

Fluorescent antibody conjugates have been prepared for use in detection of H. capsulatum yeasts in tissues (Kaplan, 1971). Such preparations are available at the Center for Disease Control and some state health laboratories. To obtain specificity, it is necessary to adsorb reagents with other fungi and to use more than one conjugate (adsorbed using different procedures).

6.3. Blastomyces dermatitidis

6.3.1. Delayed Skin Test

The role of blastomycin in diagnosis is minimal. In one series, only 56 of 136 cases (41%)

were positive (Busey *et al.*, 1964), while none of 25 was positive in another series (Witorsch and Utz, 1968). However, recent evidence from self-limited infections associated with acute outbreaks suggests some potential usefulness and perhaps specificity, since some of the patients who were blastomycin positive had negative histoplasmin skin tests. Blastomycin skin testing may cause a rise in *Histoplasma* complement-fixation titers (Levin, 1970). Because of this lack of specificity, blastomycin would not be expected to be useful in *in vitro* studies of cell-mediated mechanisms.

6.3.2. Circulating Antibodies

Complement-fixation tests in this disease are extremely unreliable. They are positive in less than half of active cases (Busey *et al.*, 1964; Witorsch and Utz, 1968; Lockwood *et al.*, 1968). Positive titers may also occur in coccidioidomycosis, histoplasmosis, and paracoccidioidomycosis (Kaufman, 1975), and blastomycosis titers may exceed the specific response. Therefore, this test can neither exclude nor establish the presence of the disease.

An immunodiffusion test (agar gel double diffusion), using a homogenized yeast antigen, has been described, which detected 80% of sera from proven cases and was 100% specific when used with appropriate reference sera (Kaufman *et al.*, 1973). Previous immunodiffusion tests for blastomycosis were sensitive but lacked specificity (Busey and Hinton, 1967). Two diagnostic precipitins (designated A and B) were described which were distinct from the H and M bands of *H. capsulatum*, as well as bands of *C. immitis* (Kaufman *et al.*, 1973). Disappearance of precipitin lines may be associated with a favorable outcome of infections, although it usually lags well behind clinical responses. Positive precipitins may persist in cured patients for 30 days or more after therapy (Kaufman, 1975).

6.3.3. Tissue Diagnosis

Fluorescent antibody conjugates have been described which are specific enough to be useful in identification of the organism in culture, as well as formalin-fixed tissue preparations (Kaplan and Kaufman, 1963; Kaplan and Kraft, 1969).

6.4. *Paracoccidioides brasiliensis*

6.4.1. Delayed Skin Test

The active material in *P. brasiliensis* appears to be a glycopeptide (Restrepo and Schneidau, 1967), but a variety of methods of preparation and materials have been used and no standardized material is commercially available. Cross-reactivity with *Histoplasma capsulatum* and *Sporothrix schenckii* antigens may be common (ContiDiaz, 1972) Therefore, while there is great potential usefulness of these antigens for skin tests and *in vitro* studies, better standardization and characterization of specificity are necessary (Schneidau, 1972).

6.4.2. Circulating Antibodies

Precipitins are the first antibodies detectable, disappear first after successful therapy, and reappear after relapse. The number of visible precipitin bands has also been correlated with clinical activity of the disease. Since various methods and antigens have been used by different workers, it is not at all surprising that variable numbers of patterns of specific and nonspecific precipitin bands have been observed (Restrepo and Drouhet, 1970; Yarzabal, 1972; Kaufman, 1972, 1975). However, results appear to be consistent, sensitive, and specific with each individual method. While Kaufman (1972) found the test to be 100% specific, Restrepo (1972) reported rare false-positive precipitin tests in histoplasmosis. It was later suggested that one characteristic precipitin band in paracoccidioidomycosis sera is identical to the M antigen in histoplasmosis (Restrepo and Moncada, 1974). Counterimmunoelectrophoresis has been used to detect precipitins and reportedly gave sensitive and specific results within hours (Negroni, 1972). Precipitins with both IgG and IgA mobilities were detected in patients' sera.

Complement-fixing antibodies appear later in the course of infections and rise proportional to the severity of clinical disease, but may persist in low titer long after cure. The different antigen preparations used may cross-react in other mycoses (especially histoplasmosis), but heterologous titers are usually lower than the specific titer (Fava Netto, 1972; Kaufman, 1975). The titer is often used as a guide in therapy; therapy is continued until titers are $\geq 1:10$. However, patients with widespread involvement in disseminated infections may have low titers, and serological relapses occasionally occur in the absence of clinical relapses (Fava Netto, 1972; Negroni, 1972). Conglutinating complement-fixing antibodies have been measured and noted to be more sensitive than direct hemolytic complement-fixation procedures for detection of sera from patients with active disease (Singer and Fava Netto, 1972); this may reflect a specific IgM response to infection.

6.4.3. Tissue Diagnosis

Fluorescent antibody conjugates have been made using hyperimmune sera from rabbits immunized with *P. brasiliensis* yeasts. Cross-reactivity occurred with *Coccidioides immitis*, *Histoplasma capsulatum* and *dubosii*, *Blastomyces dermatitidis*, and *Sporothrix schenckii*; however, specificity was obtained after absorptions (Kaplan, 1972), and the *P. brasiliensis* can be specifically identified using a single FA conjugate.

6.5. *Sporothrix schenckii*

6.5.1. Delayed Skin Test

A variety of antigen preparations have been used for *S. schenckii*. Results appear to be sensitive and highly specific using whole yeast cells, yeast cell extracts, or yeast culture filtrates (Schneidau *et al.*, 1964; Ingrish and Schneidau, 1967; Nielsen, 1968). The delayed response probably develops approximately 3–4 weeks after the onset of infection (Karlin and Nielsen, 1970) and probably persists for life (MacFarland, 1966). It is not definitely known, but has been presumed, that skin testing with these agents may raise specific antibody titers in sensitive subjects (Karlin and Nielsen, 1970).

6.5.2. Circulating Antibodies

In general, antibody responses to typical cutaneous sporotrichosis are minimal and transient, while extracutaneous infections produce strong and persistent serological responses (McMillen, 1974). In one study, using a yeast phase culture filtrate antigen, positive complement-fixation titers were usually elevated in patients with extracutaneous sporo-

trichosis but not in cutaneous disease, whereas immunodiffusion tests were not helpful (Jones *et al.*, 1969). However, in another study in which several different antigens and techniques were compared, the agglutination test using yeast or broth antigen-coated latex particles was more useful than immunodiffusion or complement-fixation tests (Karlin and Nielsen, 1970). In another study in which a mycelial culture filtrate antigen was used for the immunodiffusion test and a yeast phase culture filtrate or the complement-fixation test, the combination of these two tests was found to be most useful (McMillen, 1974).

6.5.3. Tissue Diagnosis

Fluorescent antibody reagents have been developed which can specifically identify the yeastlike form of *S. schenckii* in tissues and on artificial culture media (Kaplan and Ivens, 1960).

6.6. *Cryptococcus neoformans*

6.6.1. Delayed Skin Test

No standard preparation is available for *C. neoformans*. Several materials prepared using methods of varying complexity have been used. One antigen extracted from broken cells appeared to be specific (Salvin and Smith, 1961; Muchmore *et al.*, 1968) but was difficult to prepare. A urea extract from killed yeasts has been used in man but cross-reacted with *B. dermatitidis* and other fungal antigens in sensitized guinea pigs, and induced the development of anticryptococcal antibodies in 29% of 28 normal volunteers (Atkinson and Bennett, 1968) and 31% of 48 patients (Bindschadler and Bennett, 1968). A culture filtrate antigen has also been described which was sensitive and specific when used in guinea pigs and did not appear to stimulate antibody production (Murphy *et al.*, 1974).

6.6.2. Circulating Antibodies

The most widely used method is an indirect fluorescent antibody test using killed, whole yeast cells and a fluorescein conjugated anti-human immunoglobulin. In two large series antibodies were detectable in approximately 40% of patients with cryptococcosis (Kaufman and Blumer, 1968; Diamond and Bennett, 1974). All sera which contained antibodies reacted with an anti-IgG antiserum but none with an anti-IgM conjugate. Titers were low (1 : 1–1 : 32). Four of 75 patients tested had detectable capsular antigen as well as antibodies in serum (Bindschadler and Bennett, 1968). Because occasional normal sera are shown to have anticryptococcal antibodies, the test is not completely specific for diagnostic purposes. Tube agglutination has been used in combination with the fluorescent antibody test (Kaufman and Blumer, 1968). Passive hemagglutination using a culture filtrate antigen was reportedly specific and more sensitive than tube agglutination (Kozel and Cazin, 1972).

6.6.3. Tissue Diagnosis

Fluorescent antibody reagents have been used for specific identification of the organism in tissue sections, as well as rapid and specific identification in pure or contaminated cultures (Kaplan, 1975). However, other standard methods are available for these purposes and FA reagents are not commercially available, so they are not widely used.

6.6.4. Detection of Antigen

Using agglutination of latex particles coated with anticryptococcal globulin (Bloomfield *et al.*, 1963), cryptococcal polysaccharide can be detected in sera or spinal fluid of more than 90% of patients with culture-proven central nervous system cryptococcosis (Bennett and Bailey, 1971). Patients with localized lesions of cryptococcosis outside the central nervous system are less likely to have detectable antigen. A complement-fixation test is completely specific but somewhat less sensitive than the latex agglutination test, which can detect as little as 0.025 μg/ml polysaccharide (Gordon, 1975). The latex test is now commercially available. Controls must be performed with each latex test because rheumatoid-factor-positive sera cause false-positive reactions (Bennett and Bailey, 1971). In a recent report sera containing rheumatoid factor were successfully tested after treatment with dithiothreitol or 2-mercaptoethanol (Gordon and Lapa, 1974). The test is also useful in following the course of antifungal therapy and in estimating the likelihood of cure (Diamond and Bennett, 1974). While some patients with active cryptococcosis have no detectable poly-

saccharide in serum or spinal fluid, the test is considered to be highly specific when positive. A positive latex agglutination test has been suggested as adequate for the diagnosis of cryptococcosis in the absence of positive cultures (Goodman *et al.*, 1971). However, others have emphasized the need for verification of results with cultures due to the rare false-positive latex tests, coupled with the difficulties and hazards of prolonged antifungal therapy (Bennett, 1972).

6.7. *Absidia, Mucor,* and *Rhizopus* spp.

Because infection with *Absidia, Mucor,* or *Rhizopus* is an acute, fulminating disease, serology is of limited value. In view of the multiple agents capable of causing disease and their ubiquity in nature, development of useful serological techniques has been difficult. Gordon (1975) reported using soluble antigens derived from sonicated mycelia as antigens for immunodiffusion tests. Precipitins were not detected when the disease was treated in its early stages but were present in more advanced cases, and there was a great deal of cross-reactivity between antigens of *Absidia, Mucor,* and *Rhizopus.* It was not noted whether or not precipitins were detectable in patients with allergic diseases or asthma in the absence of mucormycosis. Jones and Kaufman (1978) obtained promising preliminary results using a homogenate antigen in immunodiffusion.

7. Immunoprevention

The prospects for immunoprevention of systemic mycoses are limited by several considerations. One of these has been the inability to produce consistently safe immunogenic materials usable in man. Another is the extremely high level of immunity to fungi present in most normal persons. For a vaccine to be effective, it would have to induce a protective response in those few hosts who are at risk for severe, progressive infections perhaps by virtue of some defect in the immune response to infection. In these individuals who are most in need of vaccination the protective response to vaccination might well be impaired.

Data on experimentally induced immunity to mycoses in animals have been reviewed elsewhere (Salvin, 1963; Kong and Levine, 1967; Chick, 1971). In man serious attempts at immunoprevention of invasive mycoses have been limited to coccidioidomycosis.

Studies in animals indicated that spherules were more active than mycelia or arthrospores in protection against experimental respiratory coccidioidal infections (Levine et al., 1960, 1961; Pappagianis et al., 1961b). Fungal growth was reduced in vaccinated animals compared with control animals (Kong and Levine, 1967). In the first studies in man, using a killed spherule vaccine, vaccination of six volunteers resulted in conversion of a negative coccidioidin skin test to positive (Levine and Smith, 1967). A recent review summarized the results of vaccination against coccidioidomycosis in man (Pappagianis and Levine, 1975). Of 97 human subjects vaccinated, 78 received a whole, killed spherule preparation and 18 received a killed mycelial vaccine. Two subjects with prior positive coccidioidin skin tests developed febrile reactions and high complement-fixing antibody titers after receiving spherule vaccine, but systemic effects in other subjects were minimal. Antibodies or delayed hypersensitivity to coccidioidin was only irregularly induced after vaccination (only 19 of 59 or 32% had positive skin tests using 1 : 10 coccidioidin). There was a 60% rate of coccidioidin skin test conversion in the 15 subjects who were followed after receiving the mycelial vaccine. However, as noted above, mycelial vaccines were less effective in animals. In addition, extrapolation of doses successfully used in experimental animal studies suggested that higher doses of the spherule preparation would be needed for immunization in man (Levine et al., 1961, 1962). This would require production of a concentrated, soluble preparation for use in future trials. It is also important to note that delayed hypersensitivity may not be needed for protection against experimental respiratory coccidioidal infections in animals (Levine et al., 1962), nor does the ability of immunization to produce strong delayed hypersensitivity in animals necessarily correlate with protection against experimental infection (Chaparas et al., 1975).

In summary, currently available vaccines do not necessarily induce antibody production, or, perhaps more important, do not necessarily convert coccidioidin skin tests. The protective value of these vaccines has not been determined, nor has their activity in patients most likely to develop severe forms of coccidioidomycosis. Furthermore, the duration of protection and strength of response to killed vaccines may be limited, but use of live, nonvirulent mutants is another possible alternative which has been tried in animals (Walch and Kalvoda, 1971).

8. Immunotherapy

As reviewed above (Section 5), disseminated mycoses often have a prolonged, unpredictable course, with spontaneous clinical remissions and exacerbations, as well as variations in cellular immune responsiveness. Before effective antifungal chemotherapeutic agents were available, many attempts at immunotherapy were made, usually by administration of either heterologous hyperimmune serum or vaccines prepared in various ways from killed organisms (Kong and Levine, 1967; Salvin, 1963). As might be expected, many of these individual reports were encouraging, if not wholly convincing. More recent efforts at immunotherapy must also be viewed with some caution because of the variability in the natural history of mycoses, the lack of standardized reagents (and or protocols for their use), and the difficulties in obtaining comparable patients for controlled studies.

Another factor which might confuse the evaluation of immunotherapeutic protocols is the possibility of direct effects of antifungal therapy on the immune response. Amphotericin B is currently the standard therapy for disseminated mycoses. Its toxicity and lack of total effectiveness have spurred the search for alternative modes of treatment, including immunotherapy. Nevertheless, amphotericin B remains the best available therapy for systemic mycoses, so that newer therapeutic modalities must generally be tested in combination with amphotericin B, or used alone late in the course of disease, after failure of amphotericin B therapy. However, experimental animals and in vitro studies have indicated that amphotericin B itself has immunoadjuvantlike properties which include (1) stimulation of resistance of mice to Listeria monocytogenes infection, accompanied by increased macrophage microbicidal activity and phagocytosis of bacteria and inert particles (Thomas *et al.*, 1973), (2) increased survival of mice with a transplantable leukemia (Medoff *et al.*, 1974), and (3) enhancement of T-cell-mediated reactions (graft-vs.-host reaction), as well as antibody responses to specific antigens (Blanke *et al.*, 1975). In addition to stimulation of mouse macrophage phagocytic and antibacterial activity, amphotericin B increased serum levels of colony-stimulating factor as well as numbers of pluripotent stem cell precursors of neutrophils and macrophages in mouse spleen. The observed increased phagocytic effect appeared to be due to direct effects of amphotericin B on macrophage membranes, while enhanced microbicidal activity required the presence of lymphocytes (Lin *et al.*, 1976). In some of these studies constant exposure to amphotericin B resulted in suppression rather than stimulation. Whether or not amphotericin B produces similar immunological effects in man remains to be determined. Immunological effects in man of newer antifungal agents such as flucytosine and the imidazoles (e.g., miconazole) also are in need of study, particularly the latter. The imidazoles stimulate *in vitro* reactivity of lymphocytes (Janssen Research Information Service, 1976), and are structurally related to levamisole, a drug with immunostimulant properties in man (Tripodi *et al.*, 1973). Levamisole itself has no antifungal activity but undoubtedly will be studied further in immunotherapy of mycoses. Use of the drug has already been reported in individual patients with paracoccidioidomycosis (Musatti *et al.*, 1976) and other systemic mycoses.

Transfer factor has been used in small numbers of cases of several types of disseminated mycoses, including several cases of paracoccidioidomycosis (Mendes, 1975) and isolated cases of cryptococcosis and histoplasmosis. However, coccidioidomycosis is the only invasive mycosis where sufficient data are available for meaningful evaluation of results. Several workers have published summaries of small series of patients with coccidioidomycosis of various stages and severity treated with transfer factor, in addition to amphotericin B (Graybill *et al.*, 1973; Stevens *et al.*, 1974b; Catanzaro *et al.*, 1974; Stevens, 1975). These and other workers have combined to form the Coccidioidomycosis Cooperative Treatment Group. Their combined results defining results of tests of cell-mediated immunity in 160 subjects were presented recently (Catanzaro and Spitler, 1976). Two groups were studied: (1) 82 healthy subjects, 66 of whom had never had clinically active coccidioidomycosis, and 16 with previously active disease; (2) 78 patients with active coccidioidomycosis, including 34 with progressive pulmonary and 44 with disseminated disease. Transfer factor was adminstered to 49 patients, but the amount, schedules of administration, and preparation used were not standardized. However, all transfer factor used was prepared from donors with strongly positive coccidioidin skin tests, as well as MIF and *in vitro* lymphocyte stimulation by coccidioidin. Techniques and antigen preparations used for evaluations of patients by different investigators also varied. In mose cases patients had received one or more courses of amphotericin B without cure prior to transfer factor therapy, and most continued to receive amphotericin B during transfer factor therapy.

In the 66 healthy subjects without prior clinical coccidioidomycosis, results of skin testing with coccidioidin correlated completely with MIF and almost as well with lymphocyte transformation responses to coccidioidin. Similar results were noted in the 16 patients with inactive coccidioidomycosis, although *in vitro* correlates deviated slightly from skin test results (13/16 skin test positive, 82% of whom had positive MIF, and 69% positive lymphocyte transformation). Parenthetically it should be noted that three of these 16 healthy patients had negative coccidioidin skin tests, as well as MIF and lymphocyte transformation. Of the 4 patients with pulmonary coccidioidomycosis, 23 had negative coccidioidin skin tests; MIF usually correlated with skin test results, but lymphocyte transformation was often negative with positive skin tests, and *vice versa*. Of the 44 patients with disseminated coccidioidomycosis, 34 had negative coccidioidin skin tests, and neither lymphocyte transformation nor MIF correlated with skin test results. As noted in other immunodeficiency states associated with infections, these patients had a variety of defects, and all possible patterns in test results were observed. Serial observations in some patients revealed changes in reactivity to coccidioidin (and to PHA) either spontaneously or in relation to amphotericin B therapy. Transfer factor converted negative coccidioidin skin tests to positive in 67% (24/36) of patients. Results with MIF and lymphocyte transformation were similar. However, responses to transfer factor were often brief. While transfer factor clearly affected delayed hypersensitivity and its *in vitro* correlates, clinical efficacy was not so clearcut. Of the 49 patients who received transfer factor, 30 were judged to have had a favorable clinical response, although improvement was often gradual, and was clearly temporally related to transfer factor therapy in only 12 of the 30. Nineteen patients failed to respond, four of whom deteriorated. In addition, clinical responses did not necessarily correlate with immunological responses to tranfer factor. Updated results on this group of patients were comparable (Graybill, 1977).

These studies must be interpreted with caution. In a controlled evaluation of transfer factor in treatment of a different infection (warts), no benefit was observed, although earlier, uncontrolled observations had suggested clinical efficacy (Stevens *et al.*, 1975a). In addition, adverse effects of transfer factor, although rare, have been reported and may include immunosuppression in some circumstances (Kirkpatrick and Gallin, 1975). Therefore, a controlled cooperative evaluation of transfer factor in coccidioidomycosis has been planned by Catanzaro and Spitler (1976), using wellclassified patients and standardized reagents and dosage schedules. These investigators plan to use transfer factor from both skin-test-positive and skin-test-negative donors to determine whether or not the effect of transfer factor is nonspecific. Nonspecific immunostimulation may contribute to clearing of lesions and return of immunoreactivity in some cases (Snyderman and Burch, 1974). The results of this amibitious cooperative study may then answer several important questions about immunity and immunotherapy of coccidioidomycosis and offer guidelines for studies of immunotherapy of other mycoses as well.

Such large-scale studies of immunotherapy would be of interest in some categories of disseminated histoplasmosis, cryptococcosis, paracoccidioidomycosis, and probably other invasive mycoses as well. However, as investigators have noted in studies of coccidioidomycosis summarized above, several conditions must be met for such studies to be meaningful: (1) antigens and *in vitro* procedures (as well as transfer factor preparations) must be better standardized than they are now, (2) patients to be studied must be carefully categorized according to stages of disease, (3) keeping in mind the variable natural histories of invasive mycoses (i.e., the occurrence of spontaneous remissions and exacerbations), control groups are always necessary, and (4) use of amphotericin B or other potentially effective modes of therapy must be carefully controlled so as to be equivalent between groups. Because of the rarity of most of these entities, these criteria will be difficult to meet unless the results of immunotherapy are unexpectedly dramatic. Alternatively, there must be a better understanding of the specific immunological mechanisms which are directly involved in killing these fungi *in vivo*, so that these parameters can be assessed in individual patients and related to clinical outcome.

In conclusion, the fungi which cause invasive mycoses in man include a diverse array of organisms with complex structural features. Although the organisms and the diseases that they cause have many features in common, important antigenic and physical differences between the organisms result in important differences in the immune responses which occur in the infected host. For example, the structural diversity between *Histoplasma capsulatum* yeasts and spherules of *Coccidioides immitis* are obvious, as are the differences in the inflammatory and immune response which they incite in the host. This is important in consideration of the factors involved in limiting the spread of systemic mycoses within the host. Whether or not a locally invasive mycosis will disseminate may, of course, be influenced by the degree of exposure or the virulence of the organism. Nevertheless, several immunologists have advanced the hypothesis that many cases of disseminated or locally invasive mycoses represent expressions of cellular immunodeficiency states. In this sense, many cases of disseminated mycoses may be "opportunistic" infections, although factors causing immunosuppression may not be obvious. On the other hand, in patients with disseminated mycoses who are not receiving immunosuppressive therapy, it is not clear whether there are preexisting defects in cellular immunity or whether these frequently observed immunological defects represent a product of infection. In either case it is possible that some form of rationally based immunotherapy could prove valuable in many if not most of such patients, but different mycoses might require different forms of therapy.

ACKNOWLEDGMENT

The author is the recipient of Career Development Award AI00055 from NIAID, NIH, DHEW.

References

Abrahams, I., 1966, Further studies on acquired resistance to murine cryptococcosis: Enhancing effect of *Bordetella pertussis, J. Immunol.* **96**:525–529.

Abrahams, I., and Gilleran, T. G., 1960, Studies on actively acquired resistance to experimental cryptococcosis in mice, *J. Immunol.* **85**:629–635.

Abrahams, I., Stoffer, H. R., Payette, K. M., and Singh, F. R., 1970, Cellular immunity in experimental murine cryptococcosis, *Fed. Proc.* **29**:503.

Abramson, E., Wilson, D., and Arky, R., 1967, Rhinocerebral phycomycosis in association with diabetic ketoacidosis: Report of two cases and a review of clinical and experimental experience with amphotericin B therapy, *Ann. Intern. Med.* **66**:735–742.

Adamson, D. M., and Cozad, G. C., 1969, Effect of antilymphocyte serum on animals experimentally infected with *Histoplasma capsulatum* or *Cryptococcus neoformans, J. Bacteriol.* **100**:1271–1276.

Aguilar-Torres, F. J., Jackson, L. J., Ferstenfeld, J. E., Pappagianis, D., and Rytel, M. W., 1976, Counterimmunoelectrophoresis in the detection of antibodies against *Coccidioides immitis, Ann. Intern. Med.* **85**:740–744.

Ajello, L., 1969, A comparative study of the pulmonary mycoses of Canada and the United States, *Public Health Rep.* **84**:869–877.

Al-Doory, Y., 1971, The ultrastructure of *Cryptococcus neoformans, Sabouraudia* **9**:113–118.

Alford, R. H., and Goodwin, R. A., 1972, Patterns of immune response in chronic pulmonary histoplasmosis, *J. Infect. Dis.* **125**:269–275.

Altner, P. C., and Turner, R. R., 1970, Sporotrichosis of bones and joints: Review of the literature and report of six cases, *Clin. Orth. Rel. Res.* **68**:138–148.

Anderson, K. L., Wheat, R. W., Conant, N. F., and Clingenpeel, W., 1974, Composition of the cell wall and

other fractions of the autolyzed yeast form of *Histoplasma capsulatum, Mycopathol. Mycol. Appl.* **54**: 439–451.

Angulo-Ortega, A., Calcification in paracoccidioidomycosis: Are they morphological manifestations of subclinical infections? in: *Paracoccidioidomycosis: Proceedings of the First Pan American Symposium,* pp. 129–133, Pan American Health Organization, Scientific Publication No. 254, Washington, D.C.

Aronson, M., and Kletter, J., 1973, Aspects of the defense against a large-sized parasite, the yeast, *Cryptococcus neoformans,* in: *Dynamic Aspects of Host–Parasite Relationships* (A. Zuckerman and D. W. Weiss, eds.), pp. 132–162, Academic Press, New York.

Artz, R. P., and Bullock, W. E., 1979, Immunoregulatory responses in experimental disseminated histoplasmosis: Depression of T-cell dependent and T-effector responses by activation of splenic suppressor cells, *Infect. Immun.* **23**:893–902.

Atkinson, A. J., and Bennett, J. E., 1968, Experience with a new skin test antigen prepared from *Cryptococcus neoformans, Am. Rev. Resp. Dis.* **63**:259–270.

Azuma, I., Kanetsuna, F., Tanaka, Y., Yamamura, Y., and Carbonell, L. M., 1974, Chemical and immunological properties of galactomannans obtained from *Histoplasma dubosii, Histoplasma capsulatum, Paracoccidioides brasiliensis,* and *Blastomyces dermatitidis, Mycopathol. Mycol. Appl.* **54**:111–125.

Baker, O., and Braude, A. I., 1956, A study of stimuli leading to the production of spherules in coccidioidomycosis, *J. Lab. Clin. Med.* **47**:169–181.

Baker, R. D., 1962, Leukopenia and therapy in leukemia as factors predisposing to fatal mycoses: Mucormycosis, aspergillosis, and cryptococcosis, *Am. J. Clin. Pathol.* **37**:358–373.

Baker, R. D., 1970, The phycomycoses, *Ann. N.Y. Acad. Sci.* **174**:592–605.

Bartels, P. A., 1971, Partial chemical characterization of histoplasmin H42, in: *Histoplasmosis: Proceedings of the Second National Conference* (L. Ajello, E. W. Chick, and M. L. Furcolow, eds.), pp. 56–63, Thomas, Springfield, Ill.

Baum, G. L., and Schwarz, J., 1962, Chronic pulmonary histoplasmosis, *Am. J. Med.* **33**:873–879.

Baum, G. L., Donnerberg, R. L., Stewart, D., Mulligan, W. J., and Putnam, L. R., 1969, Pulmonary sporotrichosis, *N. Engl. J. Med.* **280**:410–413.

Baum, G. L., Larkin, J. C., Jr., and Sutliff, W. D., 1970, Follow-up of patients with chronic histoplasmosis treated with amphotericin B, *Chest* **58**:562–565.

Bauman, D. S., 1971, Antigenic analysis of *Histoplasma capsulatum,* in: *Histoplasmosis: Proceedings of the Second National Conference* (L. Ajello, E. W. Chick, and M. L. Furcolow, eds.), pp. 45–55, Thomas, Springfield, Ill.

Bauman, D. S., and Smith, C. D., 1975, Comparison of immunodiffusion and complement fixation tests in the diagnosis of histoplasmosis, *J. Clin. Microbial.* **2**:77–80.

Beaman, L., Pappagianis, D., and Benjamini, E., 1977, Significance of T cells in resistance to experimental murine coccidioidomycosis, *Infect. Immun.* **17:**580–585.

Beeson, P. B., 1952, Cryptococcic meningitis of nearly sixteen years duration, *Arch. Intern. Med.* **89:**797–801.

Bennett, J. E., 1972, Cryptococcosis, in: *Infectious Diseases* (P. Hoeprich, ed.), pp. 945–952, Harper and Row, New York.

Bennett, J. E., and Bailey, J. W., 1971, Control for rheumatoid factor in the latex test for cryptococcosis, *Am. J. Clin. Path.* **56:**360–365.

Bennett, J. E., Kwon-Chung, K. S., and Howard, D. H., 1977, Epidemiologic differences among serotypes of *Cryptococcus neoformans, Am. J. Epidemiol.* **10:** 582–586.

Bennett, J. E., Kwon-Chung, K. J., and Theodore, T. S., 1978, Biochemical differences between serotypes of *Cryptococcus neoformans, Sabouraudia* **16:**167–174.

Bergman, F., 1961, Pathology of experimental cryptococcosis: A study of course and tissue response in subcutaneous induced infection in mice, *Acta Pathol. Microbiol. Scand. Suppl.* **147:**1–163.

Bindschadler, D. D., and Bennett, J. E., 1968, Serology of human cryptococcosis, *Ann. Intern. Med.* **69:**45–52.

Blanke, T., Little, R., Lynch, R., Lin, H., and Medoff, G., 1975, Immunostimulant properties of amphotericin B, in: *Critical Factors in Cancer Immunology*, Vol. 10 (J. Schultz and R. C. Leif, eds.), pp. 349–354, Miami Winter Symposia, Academic Press, New York.

Bloomfield, N., Gordon, M. A., and Elmondorf, D. F., Jr., 1963, Detection of *Cryptococcus neoformans* antigen in body fluids by latex particle agglutination, *Proc. Soc. Exp. Biol. Med.* **114:**64–67.

Bodel, P., Dillard, G. M., Jr., Kaplan, S. S., and Malawista, S. E., 1972, Anti-inflammatory effects of estradiol on human blood leukocytes, *J. Lab. Clin. Med.* **80:**373–384.

Bodey, G. P., and Rodriquez, V., 1975, Infections in cancer patients on a protected environment–prophylactic antibiotic program, *Am. J. Med.* **59:**497–504.

Buechner, H. A., Seabury, J. H., Campbell, C. C., Georg, L. K., Kaufman, L., and Kaplan, W., 1973, The current status of serologic, immunologic, and skin tests in the diagnosis of pulmonary mycoses: Report of the Committee on Fungus Diseases and Subcommittee on Criteria for Clinical Diagnosis—American College of Chest Physicians, *Chest* **63:**259–270.

Bulmer, G. S., and Sans, M. D., 1967, *Cryptococcus neoformans*. II. Phagocytosis by human leukocytes, *J. Bacteriol.* **94:**1480–1483.

Bulmer, G. S., and Sans, M. D., 1968, *Cryptococcus neoformans*. III. Inhibition of phagocytosis, *J. Bacteriol.* **95:**5–8.

Bulmer, G. S., and Tacker, J. R., 1975, Phagocytosis of *Cryptococcus neoformans* by alveolar macrophages, *Infect. Immun.* **11:**73–79.

Bulmer, G. S., Sans, M. D., and Gunn, C. M., 1976, *Cryp-*

tococcus neoformans. I. Non-encapsulated mutants, *J. Bacteriol.* **94:**1475–1479.

Busey, J. F., and Hinton, P. F., 1967, Precipitins in blastomycosis, *Am. Rev. Resp. Dis.* **95:**112–113.

Busey, J. F., Baker, R., Birch, L., Buechner, H., Chick, E. W., Justice, F. K., Matthews, J. H., McDerman, S., Pickar, D. N., Sutliff, W. D., Walkup, H. E., and Zimmerman, S., 1964, Blastomycosis. I. A review of 198 collected cases in Veterans Administration Hospitals. Blastomycosis cooperative study of the Veterans Administration, *Am. Rev. Resp. Dis.* **89:**659–672.

Butt, E. M., and Hoffman, A. M., 1945, Healed or arrested pulmonary coccidioidomycosis: Correlation of coccidioidin skin tests with autopsy findings, *Am. J. Pathol.* **21:**485–506.

Campbell, C. C., 1968, Use and interpretation of serologic and skin tests in the respiratory mycoses, *Dis. Chest. Suppl.* **54:**305–310.

Carbonell, L. M., 1972a, Ultrastructure of *Paracoccidioides brasiliensis* in culture, in: *Paracoccidioidomycosis: Proceedings of the First Pan American Symposium*, pp. 21–28, Pan American Health Organization, Scientific Publication No. 254, Washington, D.C.

Carbonell, L. M., 1972b, Discussion, in: *Paracoccidioidomycosis: Proceedings of the First Pan American Symposium*, p. 251, Pan American Health Organization, Scientific Publication No. 254, Washington, D.C.

Carbonell, L. M., Kanetsuna, F., and Gil, F., 1970, Chemical morphology of glucan and chitin in the cell wall of the yeast phase of *Paracoccidioides brasiliensis, J. Bacteriol.* **101:**636–642.

Catanzaro, A., and Spitler, L. (for the Coccidioidomycosis Cooperative Treatment Group), 1976, Clinical and immunologic results of transfer factor therapy in coccidioidomycosis, in: *Transfer Factor: Basic Properties and Clinical Applications* (M. S. Ascher, A. A. Gottlieb, and C. H. Kirkpatrick, eds.), pp. 477–494, Academic Press, New York.

Catanzaro, A., Spitler, L. E., and Moser, K. M., 1974, Immunotherapy of coccidioidomycosis, *J. Clin. Invest.* **54:**690–701.

Catanzaro, A., Spitler, L. E., and Moser, K. M., 1975, Cellular immune response in coccidioidomycosis, *Cell. Immunol.* **15:**360–371.

Cauley, L. K., and Murphy, J. W., 1979, Response of congenitally athymic (nude) and phenotypically normal mice to *Cryptococcus neoformans* infection, *Infect. Immun.* **23:**644–651.

Chaparas, S. D., Levine, H. B., Scalarone, G. M., and Pappagianis, D., 1975, Cellular responses, protective immunity, and virulence in experimental coccidioidomycosis, in: *Proceedings of the Third International Conference on the Mycoses*, pp. 80–87, Pan American Health Organization, Scientific Publication No. 304, Washington, D.C.

Chick, E. W., 1971, Vaccine development in histoplasmosis, in: *Histoplasmosis: Proceedings of the Second*

National Conference (L. Ajello, E. W. Chick, and M. L. Furcolow, eds.), pp. 387–391, Thomas, Springfield, Ill.

Collins, M. S., and Pappagianis, D., 1974a, Inhibition by lysozyme of growth of the spherule phase of *Coccidiodes immitis in vitro, Infect. Immun.* 10:616–623.

Collins, M. S., and Pappagianis, D., 1974b, Lysozyme-enhanced killing of *Candida albicans* and *Coccidioides immitis* by amphotericin B, *Sabouraudia* 12:329–340.

Conti-Diaz, I. A., 1972, Skin tests with paracoccidioidin and their importance, in: *Paracoccidioidomycosis: Proceedings of the First Pan American Symposium*, pp. 197–202, Pan American Health Organization, Scientific Publication No. 254, Washington, D.C.

Correa, A., and Giraldo, 1972, Study of immune mechanisms in paracoccidioidomycosis. I. Changes in immunoglobulins, in: *Paracoccidioidomycosis: Proceedings of the 1st Pan American Symposium*, pp. 197–202, Pan American Health Organization, Scientific Publication No. 254, Washington, D.C.

Cox, A. J., and Smith, C. E., 1973, Arrested pulmonary coccidioidomycosis granuloma, *Arch. Pathol.* 27:717–721.

Cox, F., and Hughes, W. T., 1974, Disseminated histoplasmosis and childhood leukemia, *Cancer* 33:1127–1133.

Cox, R. A., Mills, L. R., Best, G. K., and Denton, J. F., 1974, Histologic reactions to cell walls of an avirulent and a virulent strain of *Blastomyces* dermatitidis, *J. Infect. Dis.* 129:179–186.

Cox, R. A., Brunner, E., and Lecara, G., 1977, *In vitro* responses of coccidioidin skin test positive and negative persons to coccidioidin, spherulin and a *Coccidoides* cell wall antigen, *Infect. Immun.* 15:751–755.

Cozad, G. C., and Chang, C. T., 1975, Cell-mediated immunity in blastomycosis, in: *American Society for Microbiology—Abstracts, Annual Meeting*, p. 90, American Society for Microbiology, Washington, D.C.

Cusumano, C. L., Zellner, S. R., and Waldman, R. H., 1974, Transient reduction of phytohemagglutinin responses during acute pulmonary histoplasmosis, *Am. Rev. Resp. Dis.* 109:163–165.

Daniels, L. S., Berliner, M. D., and Campbell, C. C., 1968, Studies on rabbits infected with *Histoplasma capsulatum* yeasts from different filamentous types of the same strain, *J. Bacteriol.* 96:1535–1539.

Davis, T. E., Domer, J. E., and Li, Y., 1977, Cell wall studies of *Histoplasma capsulatum* and *Blastomyces dermatitidis* using autologous and heterologous enzymes, *Infect. Immun.* 15:978–987.

de Brito, T., Carvalho, R. P. S., Castro, R. M., and Furtado, J. S., 1972, Pathogenesis of experimental paracoccidioidomycosis, in: *Paracoccidioidomycosis: Proceedings of the First Pan American Symposium*, pp. 257–260, Pan American Health Organization, Scientific Publication No. 254, Washington, D.C.

Deighton, F., Cox, R. A., Hall, N. K., and Larsh, H. W., 1977, *In vivo* and *in vitro* cell-mediated immune responses to a cell wall antigen of *Blastomyces dermatitidis, Infect. Immun.* 15:429–435.

Deresinski, S. C., and Stevens, D. A., 1974, Coccidioidomycosis in compromised hosts: Experience at Stanford University Hospital, *Medicine* 54:377–395.

Deresinski, S. C., Levine, H. B., and Stevens, D. A., 1974, Soluble antigens of mycelia and spherules in the *in vitro* detection of immunity to *Coccidioides immitis, Infect. Immun.* 10:700–704.

Deresinski, S. C., Applegate, R. J., Levine, H. B., and Stevens, D. A., 1977, Cellular immunity to *Coccidioides immitis: In vitro* lymphocyte responses to spherules, arthrospores, and endospores, *Cell Immunol.* 32:110–119.

Diamond, R. D., 1974, Antibody-dependent killing of *Cryptococcus neoformans* by human peripheral blood mononuclear cells, *Nature (London)* 247:148–150.

Diamond, R. D., 1977, Effects of stimulation and suppression of cell-mediated immunity on experimental cryptococcosis, *Infect. Immun.* 17:187–194.

Diamond, R. D., and Allison, A. C., 1976, Nature of the effector cells responsible for antibody-dependent, cell-mediated killing of *Cryptococcus neoformans, Infect. Immun.* 14:716–720.

Diamond, R. D., and Bennett, J. E., 1973a, Disseminated cryptococcosis in man: Decreased lymphocyte transformation in response to *Cryptococcus neoformans, J. Infect. Dis.* 127:694–697.

Diamond, R. D., and Bennett, J. E., 1973b, Growth of *Cryptococcus neoformans* within human macrophages *in vitro, Infect. Immun.* 7:231–236.

Diamond, R. D., and Bennett, J. E., 1974, Prognostic factors in cryptococcal meningitis: A study of 111 cases, *Ann. Intern. Med.* 80:176–187.

Diamond, R. D., Root, R. K., and Bennett, J. E., 1972, Factors influencing killing of *Cryptococcus neoformans* by human leukocytes *in vitro, J. Infect. Dis.* 125:367–376.

Diamond, R. D., May, J. E., Kane, M., Frank, M. M., and Bennett, J. E., 1973, The role of late complement components and the alternate complement pathway in experimental cryptococcosis, *Proc. Soc. Exp. Biol. Med.* 144:312–315.

Diamond, R. D., May, J. E., Kane, M. A., Frank, M. M., and Bennett, J. E., 1974, The role of the classical and alternate complement pathways in host defense against *Cryptococcus neoformans* infection, *J. Immunol.* 112:2260–2270.

Diamond, R. D., Krzesicki, R., Epstein, B., and Jao, W., 1978, Damage to hyphal forms of fungi by human leukocytes *in vitro:* A possible host defense mechanism in aspergillosis and mucormycosis. *Am. J. Pathol.* 91:313–324.

Domer, J. E., 1971, Preliminary studies of the readily extracted lipid of cell walls and cell sap of the yeast-like form of *Histoplasma capsulatum*, in: *Histoplasmosis: Proceedings of the Second National Conference* (L. Ajello, E. W. Chick, and M. L. Furcolow, eds.), pp. 85–94, Thomas, Springfield, Ill.

Domer, J. E., 1976, *In vivo* and *in vitro* cellular responses to cytoplasmic and cell wall antigens of *Histoplasma capsulatum* in artificially immunized or infected guinea pigs, *Infect. Immun.* **13**:790–799.

Domer, J. E., and Ichinose, H., 1977, Cellular immune responses in guinea pigs immunized with cell walls of *Histoplasma capsulatum* prepared by several different procedures, *Infect. Immun.* **16**:223–301.

Donnelly, W. H., and Yunis, E. J., 1974, The ultrastructure of *Coccidioides immitis*: Study of a human infection, *Arch. Pathol.* **98**:227–232.

Drouhet, E., and Segretain, G., 1951, Inhibition de la migration leucocytaire *in vitro* par un polyoside capsulaire de torulopsis (*Cryptococcus neoformans*), *Ann. Inst. Pasteur* **81**:674–676.

Drutz, D. J., and Catanzaro, A., 1978, Coccidioidomycosis, *Am. Rev. Resp. Dis.* **117**:559–585, 727–771.

Dublin, M., and Bulmer, G. S., 1974, The anti-fungal activity of normal and host-compromised saliva, in: *American Society for Microbiology—Abstracts, Annual Meeting*, p. 135, American Society for Microbiology—Abstracts, Annual Meeting, p. 135, American Society for Microbiology, Washington, D.C.

Edwards, R. M., Gordon, M. A., Lapa, F. W., and Ghiorse, W. C., 1967, Micromorphology of *Cryptococcus neoformans*, *J. Bacteriol.* **94**:766–777.

Einbender, J. M., Benham, R. W., and Nelson, C. T., 1954, Chemical analysis of the capsular substance of *Cryptococcus neoformans*, *J. Invest. Dermatol.* **22**:279–283.

Einstein, H. E., 1967, Some aspects of coccidioidomycosis, in: *Proceedings of the Second Coccidioidomycosis Symposium, Phoenix, 1965* (L. Ajello, ed.), pp. 123–125, University of Arizona Press, Tucson.

Emmons, C. W., Binford, C. H., and Utz, J. P., 1970, *Medical Mycology*, 2nd ed., Lea and Febiger, Philadelphia.

Evans, E. E., and Kessel, J. F., 1951, The antigenic composition of *Cryptococcus neoformans*. II. Serologic studies with the capsular polysaccharide, *J. Immunol.* **67**:109–114.

Evans, E. E., and Theriault, R. J., 1953, The antigenic composition of *Cryptococcus neoformans*. IV. The use of paper chromatography for following purification of the capsular polysaccharide, *J. Bacteriol.* **65**:571–577.

Evans, E. E., Sorenson, L. J., and Walls, K. W., 1953, The antigenic composition of *Cryptococcus neoformans*, *J. Bacteriol.* **66**:287–293.

Farhi, F., Bulmer, G. S., and Tacker, J. R., 1970, *Cryptococcus neoformans* IV. The not-so-encapsulated yeast, *Infect. Immun.* **1**:526–531

Fava Netto, C., 1972, The serology of paracoccidioidomycosis: Present and future trends, in: *Paracoccidioidomycis: Proceedings of the First Pan American Symposium*, pp. 209–213, Pan American Health Organization, Scientific Publication No. 254, Washington, D.C.

Fava Netto, C., and Raphael, A., 1961, A reacao intradermica com polissacaride do *Paracoccidioides brasi-liensis* na blastomicose sul-americana, *Reve. Inst. Med. Trop. S. Paulo* **3**:161–165.

Fava Netto, C., Vegas, V. S., Sciannemea, I. M., and Guarnieri, D. B., 1969, Antígeno polissacaridico do *Paracoccidioides brasiliensis*: *Estudo do tempo de cultivo do P. brasiliensis* necessário ao preparo do antígeno, *Rev. Inst. Med. Trop. S. Paulo* **11**:177–181.

Feit, C., and Tewari, R. P., 1974, Immunogenicity of ribosomal preparations from yeast cells of *Histoplasma capsulatum*, *Infect. Immun.* **10**:1091–1097.

Fialho, A. S., 1956, Patogenia da blastomicose pulmonar, *Rev. Brasil Tuberc.* **24**:1531–1552.

Fiese, M. J., 1958, *Coccidioidomycosis*, Thomas, Springfield, Ill.

Forbus, W. D., and Bestebreurte, A. M., 1946, Coccidioidomycosis: A study of 95 cases of the disseminated type with special reference to the pathogenesis of the disease, *Milit. Surg.* **99**:653–719.

Fountain, F. F., and Sutliff, W. D., 1969, Paracoccidioidomycosis in the United States, *Am. Rev. Resp. Dis.* **99**:89–93.

Frenkel, J. K., 1962, Role of corticosteroids as predisposing factors in fungal diseases, *Lab. Invest.* **11**:1192–1208.

Furcolow, M. L., 1962, Opportunism in histoplasmosis, *Lab. Invest.* **2**:1134–1139.

Furcolow, M. L., and Smith, C. D., 1973, A new hypothesis on the epidemiology of blastomycosis and the ecology of *Blastomyces dermatitidis*, *Tr. N.Y. Acad. Sci.* **35**:421–430.

Furcolow, M. L., Watson, K. A., Tisdall, O. F., Julian, W. A., Saliba, N. A., and Balows, A., 1968, Some factors affecting survival in systemic blastomycosis, *Dis. Chest* **54**:285–291 (Suppl. 1).

Furcolow, M. L., Chick, E. W., Busey, J. F., and Menges, R. W., 1970, Prevalence and incidence studies of human and canine blastomycosis. I. Cases in the United States, 1885–1968, *Am. Rev. Resp. Dis.* **102**:60–67.

Furtado, T., 1972, Infection vs. disease in paracoccidioidomycosis, in: *Paracoccidioidomycosis: Proceedings of the First Pan American Symposium*, pp. 271–277, Pan American Health Organization, Scientific Publication No. 254, Washington, D.C.

Gadebusch, H. H., 1958a, Active immunization against *Cryptococcus neoformans*, *J. Infect. Dis.* **102**:219–226.

Gadebusch, H. H., 1958b, Passive immunization against *Cryptococcus neoformans*, *Proc. Soc. Exp. Biol.* **98**:611–614.

Gadebusch, H. H., 1960, Specific degradation of *Cryptococcus neoformans* 3723 capsular polysaccharide by a microbial enzyme. III. Antibody stimulation by partially decapsulated cells, *J. Infect. Dis.* **107**:406–409.

Gadebusch, H. H., 1972, Mechanism of native and acquired resistance to infection with *Cryptococcus neoformans*, *CRC Crit. Rev. Microbiol.* **1**:311–320.

Gadebusch, H. H., and Johnson, A. G., 1966, Natural host resistance to infection with *Cryptococcus neofor-*

mans. IV. The effect of some cationic proteins on the experimental disease, *J. Infect. Dis.* **116:**551–572.

Gale, D., Lockhart, E. A., and Kimbell, E., 1967, Studies of *Coccidioides immitis*. 1. Virulence factors of *C. immitis, Sabouraudia* **6:**29–36.

Gale, G. R., and Welch, A. M., 1961, Studies of opportunistic fungi. I. Inhibition of *Rhizopus oryzae* by human serum, *Am. J. Med. Sci.* **241:**604–612.

Gallis, H. A., Berman, R. A., Cate, T. R., Hamilton, J. D., Gunnells, J. C., and Stickel, D. L., 1975, Fungal infection following renal transplantation, *Arch. Intern. Med.* **135:**1163–1172.

Gardner, P., and Fuller, E. W., Jr., 1969, Fatal relapse of coccidioidomycosis ten years after treatment with amphotericin B, *N. Engl. J. Med.* **281:**950–952.

Gelfand, J. A., and Bennett, J. E., 1975, Active *Histoplasma* meningitis of 22 years duration, *J. Am. Med. Assoc.* **233:**1294–1295.

Gentry, L. O., and Remington, J. S., 1971, Resistance against *Cryptococcus* conferred by intracellular bacteria and protozoa, *J. Infect. Dis.* **123:**22–31.

Gifford, M. A., Buss, W. C., and Douds, R. J., 1937, Annual Report Kern County Health Department for the Fiscal Year July 1, 1936 to June 30, 1937, pp. 39–54.

Gonzalez-Ochoa, A., 1965, Contribuciones recientes al conaciemiento de la esporotrichosis, *Gac. Med. Mex.* **95:**463–474.

Gonzalez-Ochoa, A., 1972, Theories regarding the portal of entry of *Paracoccidioides brasiliensis:* A brief review, in: *Paracoccidioidomycosis: Proceedings of the First Pan American Symposium*, pp. 278–280, Pan American Health Organization, Scientific Publication No. 254, Washington, D.C.

Gonzalez-Ochoa, A., 1975, Prevalence, severity, and types of mycotic disease as reflected by patients' socioeconomic status, in: *Proceedings of the Third International Conference on the Mycoses*, pp. 227–230, Pan American Health Organization, Scientific Publication No. 304, Washington, D.C.

Goodman, J. S., Kaufman, L., and Koenig, M. G., 1971, Diagnosis of cryptococcal meningitis: Value of immunologic detection of cryptococcal antigen, *N. Engl. J. Med.* **285:**434–436.

Goodman, N. L., 1971, Cross-reactivity in histoplasmin skin testing, in: *Histoplasmosis: Proceedings of the Second National Conference* (L. Ajello, E. W. Chick, and M. L. Furcolow, eds.), pp. 313–320, Thomas, Springfield, Ill.

Goodman, N. L., Larsh, H. W., and Palmer, C. E., 1971, Cross reactivity in skin testing with histoplasmin, *Am. Rev. Resp. Dis.* **104:**258–260.

Goodwin, R. A., and Des Prez, R. M., 1978, Histoplasmosis, *Am. Rev. Resp. Dis.* **117:**929–956.

Goodwin, R. A., Jr., and Snell, J. D., Jr., 1969, The enlarging histoplasmoma: Concept of a tumor-like phenomenon encompassing the tuberculoma and coccidioma, *Am. Rev. Resp. Dis.* **100:**1–12.

Goodwin, R. A., Nickell, J. A., and Des Prez, R. M.,

1972, Mediastinal fibrosis complicating healed primary histoplasmosis and tuberculosis, *Medicine* **51:**227–246.

Goodwin, R. A., Jr., Owens, F. T., Snell, J. D., Hubbard, W. W., Buchanan, R. D., Terry, R. T., and Des Prez, R. M., 1976, Chronic pulmonary histoplasmosis, *Medicine* **55:**413–452.

Gordon, M. A., 1975, Current status of serology for diagnosis and prognostic evaluation of opportunistic fungus infections, in: *Proceedings of the Third International Conference on the Mycoses*, pp. 144–153, Pan American Health Organization, Scientific Publication No. 304, Washington, D.C.

Gordon, M. A., and Lapa, E. W., 1974, Elimination of rheumatoid factor in the latex test for cryptococcosis, *Am. J. Clin. Pathol.* **61:**488–494.

Gordonson, J., Birnbaum, W., Jacobson, G., and Sargent, E. N., 1974, Pulmonary *cryptococcosis, Radiology* **112:**557–561.

Goren, M. B., and Middlebrook, G. M., 1967, Protein conjugates of polysaccharide from *Cryptococcus neoformans, J. Immunol.* **98:**901–913.

Graybill, J. R., 1977, The clinical course of coccidioidomycosis following transfer factor therapy, in: *Coccidioidomycosis, Current Clinical and Diagnostic Status* (L. Ajello, ed.), pp. 335–345, Symposia Specialists, Miami Stratton Intercontinental, New York.

Graybill, J. R., and Alford, R. H., 1974, Cell-mediated immunity in cryptococcosis, *Cell. Immunol.* **14:**12–21.

Graybill, J. R., and Drutz, D. J., 1978, Host defense in cryptococcosis. II. Cryptococcosis in the nude mouse, *Cell. Immunol.* **40:**263–274.

Graybill, J. R., Silva, J., Jr., Alford, R. H., and Thor, D. E., 1973, Immunologic and clinical improvement of progressive coccidioidomycosis following administration of transfer factor, *Cell. Immunol.* **8:**120–135.

Green, J. H., Harrell, W. K., Gray, S. B., Johnson, J. E., Bolin, R. C., Gross, H., and Malcolm, G. B., 1976, H and M antigens of *Histoplasma capsulatum:* Preparation of antisera and location of these antigens in yeast-phase cells, *Infect. Immun.* **14:**826–831.

Greer, D. L., D'Costa de Estrada, D., and Agredo de Trejos, L., 1972, Dermal reactions to paracoccidioidin among family members of patients with paracoccidioidomycosis in: *Paracoccidioidomycosis: Proceedings of the First Pan American Symposium*, pp. 76–83, Pan American Health Organization, Scientific Publication No. 254, Washington, D.C.

Gross, H., Bradley, G., Pine, L., Gray, S., Green, J. H., and Harrell, W. K., 1975, Evaluation of histoplasmin for the preference of H and M antigens: Some difficulties encountered in the production and evaluation of a product suitable for the immunodiffusion test, *J. Clin. Microbiol.* **1:**330–334.

Grosse, G., Mishra, S. K., and Staib, F., 1975, Selective involvement of the brain in experimental murine cryptococcosis. II. Histopathological observations, *Zbl. Bakt. Hyg. I. Abt. Orig. A* **233:**106–122.

Hameroff, S. B., Eckholdt, J. W., and Lindenberg, R.,

1970, Cerebral phycomycosis in a heroin addict, *Neurology* **20**:261–265.

Hammerman, K. J., Powell, K. E., Christianson, C. S., Huggin, P. M., Larsh, H. W., Vivas, J. R., and Tosh, F. E., 1973, Pulmonary cryptococcosis: Clinical forms and treatment. A center for Disease Control Cooperative Mycoses Study, *Am. Rev. Resp. Dis.* **108**:1116–1123.

Hamon, C. B., and Klebanoff, S. J., 1973, A perioxidase-mediated, *Streptococcus mitis* dependent antimicrobial system in saliva, *J. Exp. Med.* **137**:438–450.

Harrell, W. K., Ashworth, H., Britt, L. E., George, J. R., Gray, S. B., Greer, J. H., Gross, H., and Johnson, J. G., 1970, *Procedural Manual for Production of Bacterial, Fungal, and Parasitic Reagents,* Biological Reagents Section, Center for Disease Control, Atlanta, Ga.

Hart, P. D., Russell, E., Jr., and Remington, J. S., 1969, The compromised host and infection. II. Deep fungal infection, *J. Infect. Dis.* **120**:169–191.

Hassid, W. Z., Baker, E. E., and McCready, R. M., 1943, An immunologically active polysaccharide produced by *Coccidioides immitis* Rixford and Gilchrist, *J. Biol. Chem.* **149**:303–311.

Heiner, D. C., 1958, Diagnosis of histoplasmosis using precipitin reactions in agar gel, *Pediatrics* **22**:616–627.

Hempel, H., and Goodman, N. L., 1975, Rapid conversion of *Histoplasma capsulatum, Blastomyces dermatitidis* and *Sporothrix schenckii* in tissue culture, *J. Clin. Microbiol.* **1**:420–424.

Hermans, P. E., and Markowitz, H., 1969, Serum antibody activity in patients with histoplasmosis as measured by passive hemagglutination, *J. Lab. Clin. Med.* **74**:453–463.

Hicks, H. R., and Northey, W. T., 1967, Studies on the response of thymectomized mice to infection with *Coccidioides immitis,* in: *Proceedings of the Second Coccidioidomycosis Symposium, Phoenix, Arizona, 1965* (L. Ajello, ed.), pp. 183–187, University of Arizona Press, Tucson.

Hill, G. A., and Marcus, S., 1960, Study of cellular mechanisms in resistance to systemic *Histoplasma capsulatum* infection, *J. Immunol.* **85**:6–13.

Hill, G. B., and Campbell, C. C., 1962, Commercially available histoplasmin sensitized latex particles in an agglutination test for histoplasmosis, *Mycopathologia* **18**:169–179.

Hirano, A., Zimmerman, H. M., and Levine, S., 1964, Fine structure of cerebral fluid accumulation. V. Transfer of fluid from extracellular to intracellular compartments in acute phase of cryptococcal polysaccharide lesions, *Arch. Neurol.* **11**:632–641.

Hirano, A., Zimmerman, H. M., and Levine, S., 1965, Fine structure of cerebral fluid accumulation. VI. Intracellular accumulation of fluid and cryptococcal polysaccharide in oligodendroglia, *Arch. Neurol.* **12**:189–196.

Holland, P., 1971, Circulating human phagocytes and *Histoplasma capsulatum*: Ultrastructural observations, in: *Histoplasmosis: Proceedings of the Second National*

Conference (L. Ajello, E. W. Chick, and M. L. Furcolow, eds.), pp. 580–583, Thomas, Springfield, Ill.

Hood, A. B., Inglis, F. G., Lowenstein, L., Dosseter, J. B., and Maclean, L. D., 1965, Histoplasmosis and thrombocytopenic purpura: Transmission by renal homotransplantation, *Can. Med. Assoc. J.* **93**:587–592.

Howard, D. H., 1959, Observations on tissue culture of mouse peritoneal exudates inoculated with *Histoplasma capsulatum, J. Bacteriol.* **78**:69–78.

Howard, D. H., 1964, Intracellular behavior of *Histoplasma capsulatum, J. Bacteriol.* **87**:33–38.

Howard, D. H., 1965, Intracellular growth of *Histoplasma capsulatum, J. Bacteriol.* **87**:518–523.

Howard, D. H., 1973a, Fate of *Histoplasma capsulatum* in guinea pig polymorphonuclear leukocytes, *Infect. Immun.* **8**:412–419.

Howard, D. H., 1973b, Further studies on the inhibition of *Histoplasma capsulatum* within macrophages from immunized animals, *Infect. Immun.* **8**:577–581.

Howard, D. H., 1973c, The commensalism of *Cryptococcus neoformans, Sabouraudia* **11**:171–174.

Howard, D. H., 1975, The role of phagocytic mechanisms in defense against *Histoplasma capsulatum,* in: *Proceedings of the Third International Conference on the Mycoses,* pp. 50–57, Pan American Health Organization, Scientific Publication No. 304, Washington, D.C.

Howard, D. H., and Otto, V., 1969, Protein synthesis by phagocytized yeast cells of *Histoplasma capsulatum, Sabouraudia* **7**:186–194.

Howard, D. H., and Otto, V., 1977, Experiments on lymphocyte-mediated cellular immunity in murine histoplasmosis, *Infect. Immun.* **16**:226–231.

Howard, D. H., Otto, V., and Gupta, R. K., 1971, Experiments on lymphocyte-mediated cellular immunity in histoplasmosis, *Infect. Immun.* **4**:504–610.

Huppert, M., 1970, Serology of coccidioidomycosis, *Mycopathol. Mycol. Appl.* **41**:107–113.

Huppert, M., and Bailey, J. W., 1965, The use of immunodiffusion tests in coccidioidomycosis cases, *Am. J. Clin. Pathol.* **44**:369–373.

Huppert, M., Krasnow, I., Vukovich, K. R., Sun, S. H., Rice, E. H., and Kutner, L. J., 1977, Comparison of coccidioidin and spherulin in complement fixation tests for coccidioidomycosis, *J. Clin. Microbiol.* **6**:33–41.

Huppert, M., Peterson, E. T., and Sun, S. H., 1968, Evaluation of a latex particle agglutination test for coccidioidomycosis, *Am. J. Clin. Pathol.* **49**:96–102.

Hutter, R. V. P., 1959, Phycomycetous infection (mucormycosis) in cancer patients: A complication of therapy, *Cancer* **12**:330–350.

Hyde, L., 1968, Coccidioidal pulmonary cavitation, *Dis. Chest* **54**:273–277 (Suppl. 1).

Igel, H. J., and Bolande, R. P., 1966, Humoral defense mechanisms in cryptococcosis: Substances in normal human serum, saliva, and cerebrospinal fluid affecting the growth of *Cryptococcus neoformans, J. Infect. Dis.* **116**:75–83.

Ingrish, F. M., and Schneidau, J. D., Jr., 1967, Cutaneous

hypersensitivity to sporotrichin in Maricopa County, Arizona, *J. Invest. Dermatol.* **49:**146–149.

Israel, K. L., Kauffman, C. A., Smith, J. W., White, A. C., and Brooks, G. F., 1975, Disseminated histoplasmosis in patients with compromised immune mechanisms, *Clin. Res.* **23:**532.

Jacobson, H. P., 1939, Immunotherapy for coccidioidal granuloma, *Arch. Dermatol. Syph.* **40:**521–540.

Janssen Research Information Service, 1976, Janssen, R., & D., Inc., New Brunswick, N.J., personal communication.

Johnson, J. E., and Roberts, G. D., 1976, Blocking effect of rheumatoid factor and cold agglutinins on complement fixation tests for histoplasmosis, *J. Clin. Microbiol.* **3:**157–160.

Jones, K. W., and Kaufman, L., 1978, Development and evaluation of an immunodiffusion test for diagnosis of systemic zygomycosis (mucormycosis): Preliminary report, *J. Clin. Microbiol.* **7:**97–103.

Jones, R. D., Sarosi, G. A., Parker, J. D., Weeks, R. J., and Tosh, F. E., 1969, The complement-fixation test in extracutaneous sporotrichosis, *Ann. Intern. Med.* **71:**913–918.

Kalina, M., Kletter, Y., Shahar, A., and Aronson, M., 1970, Acid phosphatase release from intact phagocytic cells surrounding a large-sized parasite, *Proc. Soc. Exp. Biol. Med.* **136:**407–410.

Kalina, M., Kletter, Y., and Aronson, M., 1974, The interaction of phagocytes and the large-sized parasite *Cryptococcus neoformans:* Cytochemical and ultrastructural study, *Cell Tiss. Res.* **152:**165–174.

Kanetsuna, F., 1972a, Biochemical characteristics of *Paracoccidioides brasiliensis,* in: *Paracoccidioidomycosis: Proceedings of the First Pan American Symposium,* pp. 31–37, Pan American Health Organization, Scientific Publication No. 254, Washington, D.C.

Kanetsuna, F., 1972b, Discussion, in: *Paracoccidioidomycosis: Proceedings of the First Pan American Symposium,* p. 39, Pan American Health Organization, Scientific Publication No. 254, Washington, D.C.

Kanetsuna, F., and Carbonell, L. M., 1971, Cell wall composition of the yeastlike and mycelial forms of *Blastomyces dermatitidis, J. Bacteriol.* **106:**946–948.

Kaplan, W., 1971, Application of fluorescent antibody techniques to the diagnosis and study of histoplasmosis, in: *Histoplasmosis: Proceedings of the Second National Conference* (L. Ajello, E. W. Chick, and M. L. Furcolow, eds.), pp. 327–340, Thomas, Springfield, Ill.

Kaplan, W., 1972, Application of immunofluorescence to the diagnosis of paracoccidioidomycosis, in: *Paracoccidioidomycosis: Proceedings of the First Pan American Symposium,* pp. 224–226, Pan American Health Organization, Scientific Publication No. 254, Washington, D.C.

Kaplan, W. M., 1975, Practical application of fluorescent antibody procedures in medical mycology, in: *Proceedings of the Third International Conference on Mycoses,* pp. 178–185, Pan American Health Organization, Scientific Publication No. 304, Washington, D.C.

Kaplan, W., and Clifford, M. K., 1964, Production of fluorescent antibody reagents specific for the tissue form of *Coccidioides immitis, Am. Rev. Resp. Dis.* **89:**651–658.

Kaplan, W., and Ivens, M. S., 1960, Fluorescent antibody staining of *Sporotrichum schenckii* in cultures and clinical materials, *J. Invest. Dermatol.* **35:**151–159.

Kaplan, W., and Kaufman, L., 1963, Specific fluorescent antiglobulins for the detection and identification of *Blastomyces dermatitidis* yeast phase cells, *Mycopathol. Mycol. Appl.* **26:**257–263.

Kaplan, W., and Kraft, D. E., 1969, Demonstration of pathogenic fungi in formalin-fixed tissues by immunofluorescence, *Am. J. Clin. Pathol.* **52:**420–432.

Karlin, J. V., and Nielsen, H. S., Jr., 1970, Serologic aspects of sporotrichosis, *J. Infect. Dis.* **121:**316–327.

Kaufman, L., 1971, Serological tests for histoplasmosis, in: *Histoplasmosis: Proceedings of the Second National Conference* (L. Ajello, E. W. Chick, and M. L. Furcolow, eds.), pp. 321–326, Thomas, Springfield, Ill.

Kaufman, L., 1972, Evaluation of serological tests for paracoccidioidomycosis: preliminary report, in: *Paracoccidioidomycosis: Proceedings of the First Pan American Symposium,* pp. 221–223, Pan American Health Organization, Scientific Publication No. 254, Washington, D.C.

Kaufman, L., 1975, Current status of immunology for diagnosis and prognostic evaluation of blastomycosis, coccidioidomycosis, and paracoccidioidomycosis, in: *Proceedings of the Third International Conference on the Mycoses,* pp. 137–143, Pan American Health Organization, Scientific Publication No. 304, Washington, D.C.

Kaufman, L., and Blumer, S., 1968, Value and interpretation of serological tests for the diagnosis of cryptococcosis, *Appl. Microbiol.* **16:**1907–1912.

Kaufman, L., and Clark, M. J., 1974, Value of the concomitant use of complement fixation and immunodiffusion tests in the diagnosis of coccidioidomycosis, *Appl. Microbiol.* **28:**641–643.

Kaufman, L., McLaughlin, D. W., Clark, M. J., and Blumer, S., 1973, Specific immunodiffusion test for blastomycosis, *Appl. Microbiol.* **26:**244–247.

Kauffman, C. A., Israel, K. S., Smith, J. W., White, A. C., Schwarz, J., and Brooks, G. F., 1978, Histoplasmosis in immunosuppressed patients, *Am. J. Med.* **64:**923–932.

Kelly, J. B., Stanfield, A. B., Dukes, C. O., and Parsons, J. L., 1969, Enhanced human lymphocyte response to coccidioidin *in vitro* following skin test, *Ann. Allergy* **27:**265–270.

Kenny, J. F., Pangburn, P. C., and Trail, G., 1976, Effect of estradiol on immune competence: *In vivo* and *in vitro* studies, *Infect. Immun.* **13:**448–456.

Kirkpatrick, C. H., and Gallin, J. I., 1975, Suppression

of cellular immune responses following transfer factor: Report of a case, *Cell. Immunol.* **15**:470–474.

Kirkpatrick, C. H., Chandler, J. W., Jr., Smith, T. K., and Newberry, M. W., Jr., 1971, Cellular immunologic studies in histoplasmosis, in: *Histoplasmosis: Proceedings of the Second National Conference* (L. Ajello, E. W. Chick, and M. L. Furcolow, eds.), pp. 371–379, Thomas, Springfield, Ill.

Kleger, B., and Kaufman, L., 1973, Detection and identification of diagnostic *Histoplasma capsulatum* precipitins by counterelectrophoresis, *Appl. Microbiol.* **26**:231–238.

Kligman, A. M., Crane, A. P., and Norris, R. F., 1961, Effect of temperature on survival of chick embryos infected intravenously with *Cryptococcus neoformans* (Torula histolytica), *Am. J. Med. Sci.* **221**:273–278.

Knight, R. A., Hill, G., and Marcus, S., 1959, Immunization of mice with polysaccharide of *Histoplasma capsulatum, Proc. Soc. Exp. Biol.* **100**:356–358.

Kong, Y. M., and Levine, H. B., 1967, Experimentally induced immunity in the mycoses, *Bacteriol. Rev.* **31**:35–53.

Kong, Y. M., Levine, H. B., and Smith, C. E., 1963, Immunogenic properties of non-disrupted and disrupted spherules of *Coccidioides immitis* in mice, *Sabouraudia* **2**:131–142.

Kong, Y. M., Savage, D. C., and Kong, L. N. L., 1966, Delayed dermal hypersensitivity in mice to spherule and mycelial extracts of *Coccidioides immitis, J. Bacteriol.* **91**:876–883.

Kozel, T. R., and Cazin, J., Jr., 1972, Immune response to *Cryptococcus neoformans* soluble polysaccharide. I. Serological assay for antigen and antibody, *Infect. Immun.* **5**:35–41.

Kozel, T. R., and Cazin, J., Jr., 1974, Induction of humoral antibody response by soluble polysaccharide of *Cryptococcus neoformans, Mycopath. Mycol. Appl.* **54**:21–30.

Krill, A. E., and Archer, D., 1970, Choroidal neovascularization in multifocal (presumed histoplasmin) choroiditis, *Arch. Ophthalmol.* **84**:595–604.

Kuhn, L. R., 1939, Growth and viability of *Cryptococcus hominis* at mouse and rabbit body temperatures, *Proc. Soc. Exp. Biol.* **41**:573–574.

Kuhn, L. R., 1949, Effect of elevated body temperatures on cryptococcosis in mice, *Proc. Soc. Exp. Biol.* **71**:341–343.

Kunkel, W. M., Weed, L. A., McDonald, J. R., and Clagett, O. T., 1954, North American blastomycosis—Gilchrists disease: A clinicopatholic study of ninety cases, *Surg. Gynecol. Obstet.* **99**:1–26.

Kwon-Chung, K. J., 1973, Studies on *Emmonsiella capsulata.* I. Heterothallism and the development of the ascocarp, *Mycologia* **65**:109–121.

Kwon-Chung, K. J., 1974, Genetics of fungi pathogenic for man, *CRC Crit. Rev. Microbiol.* **3**:115–133.

Kwon-Chung, K. J., 1975, A new genus, *Filobasidiella,*

the perfect state of *Cryptococcus neoformans, Mycologia* **67**:1997–1220.

Kwon-Chung, K. J., 1976, A new species of *Filobasidiella,* the sexual state of *Cryptococcus neoformans* B and C serotypes, *Mycologia* **69**:942–946.

Kwon-Chung, K. J., 1979, Comparison of isolates of *Sporothrix schenckii* obtained from fixed cutaneous lesions with isolates from other types of lesions, *J. Infect. Dis.* **139**:424–431.

Kwon-Chung, K. J., Weeks, R. J., and Larsh, H. W., 1974, Studies on *Emmonsiella capsulata (Histoplasma capsulatum).* II. Distribution of the two mating types in 13 endemic states of the United States, *Am. J. Epidemiol.* **99**:44–49.

Kwon-Chung, K. J., Bennett, J. E., and Theodore, T. S., 1978, *Cryptococcus bacillisporus* sp. nov.: Serotype B-C of *Cryptococcus neoformans, Infect. Immun.* **28**:616–620.

Lacaz, C. S., 1955–56, South American blastomycosis, *An. Fac. Med. S. Paulo* **29**:1–120.

Lacaz, C. S., and Fava Netto, C., 1969, Immunopatologia das micoses, in: *Immunopatologia Tropical* (C. S. Lacaz, E. Mendes, and V. Amata Neto, eds.), pp. 33–35, Livraria Ateneu, Rio De Janeiro.

Lacaz, C. S., Passos Filho, M. R. C., Fava Netto, C., and Macarron, B., 1959, Contribuição para o estudo da "blastomicose-infecao": Inquérito com a paracoccidioidina: Estudo sorológico e clínico-radiológico dos paracoccidioidina-positivos, *Rev. Inst. Med. Trop. S. Paulo* **1**:245–259.

Lancaster, M. V., and Sprouse, R. F., 1976, Preparative isotachophoretic separation of skin test antigens from blastomycin purified derivative, *Infest. Immun.* **3**:758–762.

Landay, M. E., Wheat, R. W., and Conant, N. F., 1967, Serological comparison of the three morphological phases of *Coccidioides immitis* by the agar gel diffusion method, *J. Bacteriol.* **93**:1–6.

Lanza, F. L., Nelson, R. S., Semayaji, B. N., 1970, Acute granulomatous hepatitis due to histoplasmosis, *Gastroenterology* **58**:392–396.

Larsh, H. W., 1975, Pathogenesis of experimental cryptococcosis and histoplasmosis induced by the airborne route, in: *Proceedings of the Third International Conference on the Mycoses,* pp. 63–71, Pan American Health Organization, Scientific Publication No. 304, Washington, D.C.

Leavell, U. W., Jr., 1974, North American blastomycosis, in: *The Diagnosis and Treatment of Fungal Infections* (H. M. Robinson, Jr., ed.), pp. 89–98, Thomas, Springfield, Ill.

Lehrer, R. T., 1969, Antifungal effects of peroxidase system, *J. Bacteriol.* **99**:361–365.

Levan, N. E., 1974, Coccidioidomycosis, in: *The Diagnosis and Treatment of Fungal Infections* (H. M. Robinson, Jr., ed.), pp. 241–257, Thomas, Springfield, Ill.

Levan, N. E., and Einstein, H. E., 1956, Cortisone in coccidioidomycosis, *Calif. Med.* **84**:193–197.

Levin, S., 1970, The fungal skin test as a diagnostic hindrance, *J. Infect. Dis.* **122**:343–345.

Levine, H. B., and Kong, Y. M., 1965, Immunity development in mice receiving killed *Coccidioides immitis* spherules: Effect of removing residual vaccine, *Sabouraudia* **4**:164–170.

Levine, H. B., and Kong, Y. M., 1966, Immunologic impairment in mice treated intravenously with killed *Coccidioides immitis* spherules: Suppressed response to intramuscular doses, *J. Immunol.* **97**:297–305.

Levine, H. B., and Scalarone, G. M., 1975, Properties of spherulin, a skin-test reagent in coccidioidomycosis, in: *Proceedings of the Third International Conference on the Mycoses*, pp. 101–110, Pan American Health Organization, Scientific Publication No. 304, Washington, D.C.

Levine, H. B., and Smith, C. E., 1967, The reactions of eight volunteers injected with *Coccidioides immitis* spherule vaccine: First human trials, in: *Coccidioidomycosis—Proceedings of the Second Coccidioidomycosis Symposium, Phoenix, Arizona, 1965* (L. Ajello, ed.), pp. 197–200, University of Arizona Press, Tucson.

Levine, H. B., Cobb, J. M., and Smith, C. G., 1960, Immunity to coccidioicomycosis induced in mice by purified spherule, arthrospore, and mycelial vaccines, *Tr. N.Y. Acad. Sci.* **22**:436–449.

Levine, H. B., Cobb, J. M., and Smith, C. E., 1961, Immunogenicity of spherule-endospore vaccines of *Coccidioides immitis* for mice, *J. Immunol.* **87**:218–227.

Levine, H. B., Miller, R. L., and Smith, C. E., 1962, Influence of vaccination on respiratory coccidioidal disease in cynomologus monkeys, *J. Immunol.* **89**:242–251.

Levine, H. B., Kong, Y. M., and Smith, C. E., 1965, Immunization of mice to *Coccidioides immitis:* Dose, regimen, and spherulation stage of killed spherule vaccines, *J. Immunol.* **94**:132–142.

Levine, H. B., Cobb, J. M., Scalarone, G. M., 1969, Spherule coccidioidin in delayed dermal sensitivity reactions of experimental animals, *Sabouraudia* **7**:20–32.

Levine, H. B., Restrepo-M, A., Ten Eyck, D. R., and Stevens, D. A., 1975, Spherulin and coccidioidin: Cross reactions in dermal sensitivity to histoplasmin and paracoccidioidin, *Am. J. Epidemiol.* **101**:512–516.

Lin, H., Medoff, G., and Kobayashi, G. S., 1976, Effects of amphotericin B on macrophages and their precursor cells, *Antimicrob. Agents Chemother.* **11**:154–160.

Littman, M. L., 1958, Capsule synthesis by *Cryptococcus neoformans, Tr. N.Y. Acad Sci.* **20**:623–648.

Littman, M. L., and Tsubura, E., 1959, Effect of degree of encapsulation upon virulence of *Cryptococcus neoformans, Proc. Soc. Exp. Biol.* **101**:773–777.

Littman, M. L., and Walter, J. E., 1968, Cryptococcosis: Current status, *Am. J. Med.* **45**:922–932.

Lockwood, W. R., Allison, F., Jr., Batson, B. E., and Busey, J. F., 1968, The treatment of North American blastomycosis: Ten years experience, *Am. Rev. Resp. Dis.* **100**:314–320.

Londero, A. T., 1972, The lung in paracoccidioidomy-

cosis, in: *Paracoccidioidomycosis: Proceedings of the First Pan American Symposium*, pp. 109–117, Pan American Health Organization, Scientific Publication No. 254, Washington, D.C.

Londero, A. T., and Ramos, C. D., 1972, Paracoccidioidomycosis: A clinical and mycologic study of forty-one cases observed in Santa Maria, RS, Brazil, *Am. J. Med.* **52**:771–775.

Louria, D. B., Kaminiski, T., and Finkel, G., 1963, Further studies on immunity in experimental cryptococcosis, *J. Exp. Med.* **117**:509–520.

Lubarsky, R., and Plunkett, O. A., 1955, *In vitro* production of the spherule phase *Coccidioides immitis, J. Bact.* **70**:182–186.

Lurie, H. I., 1963, Five unusual cases of sporotrichosis from South Africa showing lesions in muscles, bones, and visceria, *Br. J. Surg.* **50**:585–591.

Lurie, H. I., and Still, W. J. S., 1966, The capsule of *Sporotrichum schenckii* and the evolution of the asteroid body, *Sabouraudia* **7**:64–70.

Lynch, P. J., 1974, Systemic sporotrichosis, in: *The Diagnosis and Treatment of Fungal Infections* (H. M. Robinson, Jr., ed.), pp. 129–144, Thomas, Springfield, Ill.

Lynch, P. J., Voorhees, J. J., and Harrell, E. R., 1970, Systemic sporotrichosis, *Ann. Intern. Med.* **73**:23–30.

McBride, R. A., Corson, J. M., and Dammin, G. J., 1960, Mucormycosis: Two cases of disseminated disease with cultured identification of *Rhizopus:* Review of literature, *Am. J. Med.* **28**:832–846.

McDonough, E. S., and Lewis, A. L., 1967, *Blastomyces dermatitidis*: Production of the sexual stage, *Science* **156**:528–529.

McFarland, R. B., 1966, Sporotrichosis revisited: 65 year follow-up of the second reported case, *Ann. Intern. Med.* **65**:363–366.

Macher, A. M., Bennett, J. E., Gadek, J. E., and Frank, M. M., 1978, Complement depletion in cryptococcal sepsis, *J. Immunol.* **120**:1686–1690.

Mackinnon, J. E., 1959, Pathogenesis of South American blastomycosis, *Tr. R. Soc. Trop. Med. Hyg.* **53**:487–494.

Mackinnon, J. E., 1971, Histoplasmosis in Latin America, in: *Histoplasmosis: Proceedings of the Second National Conference* (L. Ajello, E. W. Chick, and M. L. Furcolow, eds.), pp. 129–139, Thomas, Springfield, Ill.

Mackinnon, J. E., 1972, Geographical distrubtion and prevalence of paracoccidioidomycosis, in: *Paracoccidioidomycosis: Proceedings of the First Pan American Symposium*, pp. 45–52, Pan American Health Organization, Scientific Publication No. 254, Washington, D.C.

Mackinnon, J. E., and Conti-Diaz, I. A., 1963, The effect of temperature on sporotrichosis, *Sabouraudia* **2**:56–59.

Mackinnon, J. E., Conti-Diaz, I. A., Yarzabal, L. A., and Tavella, N., 1960, Temperatura ambiental y blastomicosis Sudamericana, *An. Fac. Med. Montev.* **45**:310–318.

Mackinnon, J. E., Conti-Diaz, I. A., Yarzabal, L. A.,

1964, Experimental sporotrichosis, ambient temperature and amphotericin B, *Sabouraudia* 3:192–194.

McMillen, S., 1974, The serology of sporotrichosis, in: *The Diagnosis and Treatment of Fungal Infections* (H. M. Robinson, Jr., ed.), pp. 401–410, Thomas, Springfield, Ill.

Mahvi, T. A., Spicer, S. S., and Wright, N. J., 1974, Cytochemistry of acid mucosubstance and acid phasphatase in *Cryptococcus neoformans, Can. J. Microbiol.* 20:833–838.

Marcus, S., Aoki, Y., and Hill, G. A., 1965, Delayed skin test reactions induced by polysaccharide from coccidioidin, *Fed. Proc.* 24:182.

Marcus, S., Anderson, K. L., and Hill, G. A., 1966, Contribution of delayed hypersensitivity to resistance in coccidioidomycosis, *Bacteriol. Proc. (Abstr.),* p. 62.

Medoff, G., Valeriote, R. G., Lynch, D., Schlessinger, D., and Kobayashi, G., 1974, Synergistic effect of amphotericin B and 1,3-bis (2-chloroethyl)-1-nitrosourea against a transplantable AKR leukemia, *Cancer Res.* 34:974–978.

Mendes, E., 1975, Delayed hypersensitivity reactions in patients with paracoccidioidomycosis, in: *Proceedings of the Third International Conference on the Mycoses,* pp. 17–22, Pan American Health Organization, Scientific Publication No. 304, Washington, D.C.

Mendes, E., and Raphael, A., 1971, Impaired delayed hypersensitivity in patients with South American blastomycosis, *J. Allergol.* 47:17–22.

Mendes, N. F., 1975, Lymphocytes and lymph nodes in patients with paracoccidioidomycosis, in: *Proceedings of the Third International Conference on the Mycoses,* pp. 30–35, Pan American Health Organization, Scientific Publication No. 304, Washington, D.C.

Mendes, N. F., Musatti, C. C., Leao, R. C., Mendes, E., and Naspitz, C. K., 1971, Lymphocyte cultures and skin allograft survival in patients with South American blastomycosis, *J. Allergol.* 48:40–45.

Meyer, R. D., Rosen, P., and Armstrong, D., 1972, Phycomycosis complicating leukemia and lymphoma, *Ann. Intern. Med.* 77:871–879.

Mitchell, T. G., and Friedman, L., 1972, *In vitro* phagocytosis and intracellular fate of variously encapsulated strains of *Cryptococcus neoformans, Infect. Immun.* 5:491–498.

Mohr, J. A., Long, H., McKown, B. A., and Muchmore, H. G., 1972a, *In vitro* susceptibility of *Cryptococcus neoformans* to steroids, *Sabouraudia* 10:171–172.

Mohr, J. A., Muchmore, H. G., and Tacker, R., 1972b, Stimulation of phagocytosis of *Cryptococcus neoformans* in human cryptococcal meningitis, *J. Reticuloendothel. Soc.* 15:149–154.

Muchmore, H. G., Felton, F. G., Salvin, S. B., and Rhoades, 1968, Delayed hypersensitivity to cryptococcin in man, *Sabouraudia* 6:285–288.

Muchmore, H. G., McKown, B. A., and Mohr, J. A., 1972, Effect of steroid hormones on the growth of *Par-*

acoccidioides brasiliensis, in: *Paracoccidioidomycosis: Proceedings of the First Pan American Symposium,* pp. 300–304, Pan American Health Organization, Scientific Publication No. 254, Washington, D.C.

Müller, H. E., and Sethi, K. K., 1972, Proteolytic activity of *Cryptococcus neoformans* against human plasma proteins, *Med. Microbiol. Immunol.* 158:129–134.

Murphey, S. M., Drash, A. L., and Donnelly, W. H., 1971, Disseminated coccidioidomycosis associated with immunosuppressive therapy following renal transplantation, *Pediatrics* 48:144–145.

Murphy, J. W., and Cozad, G. C., 1972, Immunological unresponsiveness induced by cryptococcal capsular polysaccharide assayed by the hemolytic plaque technique, *Infect. Immun.* 5:896–901.

Murphy, J. W. Gregory, J. A., and Larsh, H. W., 1974, Skin testing of guinea pigs and foot pad testing of mice with a new antigen for detecting delayed hypersensitivity to *Cryptococcus neoformans, Infect. Immun.* 9:404–409.

Murray, H. W., Littman, M. L., and Roberts, R. B., 1974, Disseminated coccidioidomycosis (South American blastomycosis) in the United States, *Am. J. Med.* 56:209–220.

Musatti, C. C., 1975, Cell-mediated immunity in patients with paracoccidioidomycosis, in: *Proceedings of the Third International Conference on the Mycoses,* pp. 23–29, Pan American Health Organization, Scientific Publication No. 304, Washington, D.C.

Musatti, C. C., Reykallah, M. T., Mendes, E., and Mendes, N. F., 1976, *In vivo* and *in vitro* evaluation of cell-mediated immunity in patients with paracoccidioidomycosis, *Cell. Immunol.* 24:365–378.

Nakamura, Y., Ishizaki, H., and Wheat, R. W., 1977, Serological cross-reactivity between Group B *Streptococcus* and *Sporothrix schenckii, Ceratocystis* species, and *Graphium* species, *Infect. Immun.* 16:547–549.

Neame, P., and Raynor, D., 1960, Mucormycosis: Report of 22 cases, *Arch. Pathol. (Chicago)* 70:261–268.

Negroni, R., 1972, Serologic reactions in paracoccidioidomycosis, in: *Paracoccidioidomycosis: Proceedings of the First Pan American Symposium,* pp. 203–208, Pan American Health Organization, Scientific Publication No. 254, Washington, D.C.

Negroni, R., 1975, Discussion, in: *Proceedings of the Third International Conference on the Mycoses,* pp. 229–230, Pan American Health Organization, Scientific Publication No. 304, Washington, D.C.

Neill, J. M., Castillo, C. G., Smith, R. H., and Kapros, C. E., 1949, Capsular reactions and soluble antigens of *Torula histolytica* and *Sporotrichum schenckii, J. Exp. Med.* 89:93–106.

Neill, J. M., Abrahams, I., and Kapros, C. E., 1950, A comparison of the immunogenicity of weakly encapsulated and of strongly encapsulated strains of *Cryptococcus neoformans (Torula histolytica), J. Bacteriol.* 59:263–275.

Neill, J. M., Castillo, C. G., and Parker, A. H., 1955, Serological relationship between fungi and bacteria. I. cross reactions of *Sporotrichum schenckii* with pneumococcus, *J. Immunol.* **74:**120–125.

Neilson, J. B., and Bulmer, G. S., 1975, The infectious particle of *Cryptococcus neoformans,* in: *American Society for Microbiology–Abstracts, Annual Meeting,* pp. 93, American Society for Microbiology, Washington, D.C.

Neilson, J. B., Tacker, J. R., and Bulmer, G. S., 1974, The antifungal activity of myeloperoxidase, in: *American Society for Microbiology—Abstracts, Annual Meeting,* p. 135, American Society for Microbiology, Washington, D.C.

Neuhauser, S., Tewari, R. P., and Cino, P. M., 1974, Specificity of immunoprotection induced by immunization with ribosomal preparations from yeast cells, in: *American Society for Microbiology—Abstracts, Annual Meeting,* p. 136, American Society for Micobiology, Washington, D.C.

Newberry, W. M., Jr., Walter, J. E., Chandler, J. W. Jr., and Tosh, F. E., 1967, Epidemiologic study of *Cryptococcus neoformans, Ann. Intern. Med.* **67:**724–732.

Newberry, W. M., Jr., Chandler, J. W., Chin, T. D. Y., and Kirkpatrick, C. H., 1968, Immunology of the mycoses. I. Depressed lymphocyte transformation in chronic histoplasmosis, *J. Immunl.* **100:**436–443.

Newcomer, V. D., 1974, Coccidioidin, in: *The Diagnosis and Treatment of Fungal Infections* (H. M. Robinson, Jr., ed.), pp. 435–458, Thomas, Springfield, Ill.

Newcomer, V. D., Wright, T. W., Tarbet, J. E., Winer, L. H., and Sternberg, T. H., 1953, The effects of cortisone on experimental coccidioidomycosis, *J. Invest. Dermatol.* **20:**315–321.

Newcomer, V. D., Landau, J. W., Lehman, R., and Rowe, J. R., 1963, The local cellular response in patients with coccidioidomycosis, *Arch. Dermatol.* **88:**759–811.

Nicol, T., Vernon-Roberts, B., and Quantock, D. C., 1965, The influence of various hormones of the reticuloendothelial system: Endocrine control of body defense, *J. Endocrinol.* **33:**365–383.

Nielsen, H. S., Jr., 1968, Biologic properties of skin test antigen of yeast form *Sporotrichum schenckii, J. Infect. Dis.* **118:**173–180.

Okudaira, M., Straub, M., and Schwarz, J., 1961, Etiology of discrete splenic and hepatic calcifications in an endemic area of histoplasmosis, *Am. J. Pathol.* **39:**599–611.

Oliveira, H., and Baptista, A. P., 1960, Un caso de blastomicose sul-americana (23 anos de incubação; ação da sulfametoxipiridazina), *Coimbra Med.* **7:**661–684.

Opelz, G., and Scheer, M. I., 1975, Cutaneous sensitivity and *in vitro* responsiveness of lymphocytes in patients with disseminated coccidioidomycosis, *J. Infect. Dis.* **132:**250–255.

Ophüls, W., 1905, Further observations on a pathogenic mould formerly described as a protozoan *(Coccidioides immitis, Coccidioides pyogenes), J. Exp. Med.* **6:**443–485.

Oxenhandler, R. W., Adelstein, E. H., and Rogers, W A., 1977, Rheumatoid factor: A cause of false positive histoplasmin latex agglutination, *J. Clin. Microbiol.* **5:**31–33.

Palmer, D. F., Kaufman, L., Kaplan, W., and Cavallaro, J. J., 1977, *Serodiagnosis of Mycotic Diseases,* p. 191, Thomas, Springfield, Ill.

Pappagianis, D., and Levine, H. B., 1975, The present status of vaccination against coccidioidomycosis in man, *Am. J. Epidemiol.* **102:**30–41.

Pappagianis, D., Putman, E. W., and Kobayashi, G. S., 1961a, Polysaccharide of *Coccidioides immitis, J. Bacteriol.* **82:**714–723.

Pappagianis, D., Levine, H. B., Smith, C. E., Berman, R. J., and Kobayashi, G. S., 1961b, Immunization of mice with viable *Coccidioides immitis, J. Immunol.* **86:**28–34.

Pappagianis, D., Maibach, H., and Smith, C. E., 1967a, Microscopic characteristics of the cutaneous reaction to coccidioidin in humans, *Am. Rev. Resp. Dis.* **95:**317–319.

Pappagianis, D., Smith, C. E., and Campbell, C. C., 1967b, Serologic status after positive skin reactions, *Am. Rev. Resp. Dis.* **96:**520–523.

Pappagianis, D., Saito, M., and Van Hoosear, K. H., 1972, Antibody in cerebrospinal fluid in non-meningitic coccidioidomycosis, *Sabouraudia* **10:**173–179.

Parker, J. D., Sarosi, G. A., Doto, I. L., Bailey, R. E., and Tosh, F. E., 1970, Treatment of chronic pulmonary histoplasmosis: A National Communicable Disease Center Cooperative Mycoses Study, *N. Engl. J. Med.* **283:**225–229.

Paul, S., Stobo, J., D., Hermans, P. E., and Van Scoy, R. E., 1975, Immunologic defects in disseminated mycoses, in: *15th Interscience Conference on Antimicrobial Agents and Chemotherapy,* Abstract No. 301, American Society for Microbiology, Washington, D.C.

Peterson, E. A., Frey, J. A., Davis, J. R., Dinowitz, M., and Rifkind, D., 1976, Mechanism of anergy of disseminated coccidioidomycosis, *Clin. Res.* **24:**152.

Picardi, J. L., Kauffman, C. A., Schwarz, J., Holmes, J. C., Phair, J. P., and Fowler, N. O., 1976, Pericarditis caused by *Histoplasma capsulatum, Am. J. Cardiol.* **37:**82–88.

Plouffe, J. F., Jr., Silva, J., Jr., Fekety, R., Reinhalter, E., and Browne, R., 1979, Cell-mediated immune responses in sporotrichosis, *J. Infect. Dis.* **139:**152–157.

Polli, C., 1965, On the distribution of ketoreductase in microorganisms, *Pathol. Microbiol.* **28:**93–98.

Powell, K. E., Dahl, B. A., Weeks, R. J., and Tosh, F. E., 1972, Airborne *Cryptococcus neoformans*: Particles from pigeon excreta compatible with alveolar deposition, *J. Infect. Dis.* **125:**412–415.

Powell, K. E., Hammerman, K. J., Dahl, B. A., and Tosh, F. E., 1973, Acute reinfection pulmonary histoplasmosis: A report of six cases, *Am. Rev. Resp. Dis.* **107:**374–378.

Procknow, J. J., Page, M. I., and Loosli, C. G., 1960, Early pathogenesis of experimental histoplasmosis, *Arch. Pathol.* **69**:413–426.

Puckett, T. F., 1954, Hyphae of *Coccidioides immitis* in tissues of the human host, *Am. Rev. Tuberc.* **70**:320–327.

Purtilo, D. T., 1975, Opportunistic mycotic infections in pregnant women, *Am. J. Obstet. Gynecol.* **122**:607–610.

Rabin, E. R., Lundberg, G. D., and Mitchell, E. T., 1961, Mucormycosis in severely burned patients: Report of 2 cases with extensive destruction of the face and nasal cavity, *N. Engl. J. Med.* **264**:1286–1289.

Rea, T. H., Chandor, S. B., Hampson, R., and Levan, N. E., 1976, Serum lysozyme in coccidioidomycosis, *Clin. Res* **24**:97.

Rea, T. H., Johnson, R., Einstein, H., and Levan, N. E., 1979, Dinitrochlorobenzene responsivity: Difference between patients with severe pulmonary coccidioidomycosis and patients with disseminated coccidioidomycosis, *J. Infect. Dis.* **139**:353–356.

Rebers, P. A., Barker, S. A., Heidelberger, M., Dische, Z., and Evans, E. E., 1958, Precipitation of the specific polysaccharide of *Cryptococcus neoformans* A by types II and XIV antipneumococcal sera, *J. Am. Chem. Soc.* **80**:1135–1137.

Reddy, P., Gorelick, D. F., Brasher, C. A., and Larsh, H., 1970, Progressive disseminated histoplasmosis as seen in adults, *Am. J. Med.* **48**:629–636.

Reinhardt, D. J., Kaplan, W., and Ajello, L., 1970, Experimental cerebral zygomycosis in alloxan-diabetic rabbits. I. Relationship of temperature tolerance of selected zygomycetes to pathogenicity, *Infect. Immun.* **2**:404–413.

Reiss, E., Miller, S. E., Kaplan, W., and Kaufman, L., 1977, Antigenic, chemical and structural properties of cell walls of *Histoplasm a capsulatum* chemotypes 1 and 2 after serial enzymatic hydrolysis, *Infect. Immun.* **16**:690–700.

Reiss, F., and Szilagyi, G., 1965, Ecology of yeast-like fungi in a hospital population, *Arch. Dermatol.* **91**:611–614.

Reiss, F., Szilagyi, G., and Mayer, E., 1975, Immunological studies of the anticryptococcal factor of normal human serum, *Mycopathology* **55**:175–178.

Restrepo, A., 1972, Discussion, in: *Paracoccidioidomycosis: Proceedings of the First Pan American Symposium,* p. 251, Pan American Health Organization, Scientific Publication No. 254, Washington, D.C.

Restrepo, A., and Drouhet, E., 1970, Etude des anticorps précipitants dans le blastomycose sud-américaine par l'analyse immunoelectrophorétique des antigènes de *Paracoccidioides brasiliensis, Ann. Ist. Pasteur* **119**:338–346.

Restrepo, A., and Moncada, L. H., 1974, Characterization of the precipitin bands detected in the immunodiffusion test for paracoccidioidomycosis, *Appl. Microbiol.* **28**:138–144.

Restrepo, A., and Schneidau, J. D., Jr., 1967, Nature of the skin-reactive principle in culture filtrates prepared from *Paracoccidioides brasiliensis, J. Bacteriol.* **93**:1741–1748.

Restrepo, A., and Velez, H., 1975, Effectos de la fagocitosis *in vitro* sobre el *Paracoccidioides brasiliensis, Sabouraudia* **13**:10–21.

Restrepo, A., Robledo, M., Gutierrez, F., Sanclemente, M., Easteneda, E., and Calle, G., 1970, Paracoccidioidomycosis (South American blastomycosis): A study of 39 cases observed in Medellin, Colombia, *Am. J. Trop. Med.* **19**:68–76.

Rifkind, D., Marchioro, T. L., Schneck, S. A., and Hill, R. B., Jr., 1967, Systemic fungal infections complicating renal transplantation and immunosuppressive therapy, *Am. J. Med.* **43**:28–38.

Rippon, J. W., 1974, *Medical Mycology: The Pathogenic Fungi and the Pathogenic Actinomycetes,* Saunders, Philadelphia.

Rollier, R., and Chenebault, J., 1962, Sur un cas de paracoccidioidose brasilienne a localization pulmonaire, puis bucco-rhino-pharyngee, *Bull. Soc. Fr. Dermatol. Syph.* **69**:466–470.

Ross, G. T., and Vande Wiele, R. L., 1974, The ovaries, in: *Textbook of Endocrinology* (R. H. Williams, ed.), pp. 368–422, Saunders, Philadelphia.

Ross, W. D., and Anderson, K. L., 1974, Resistance of immunodeficient mice to challenge with *Histoplasma capsulatum,* in: *American Society for Microbiology—Abstracts, Annual Meeting,* p. 136, American Society for Microbiology, Washington, D.C.

Rowe, J. R., Newcomer, V. D., and Wright, E., T., 1963a, Studies of the soluble antigens of *Coccidioides immitis* by immunodiffusion, *J. Invest. Dermatol.* **41**:225–233.

Rowe, J. R., Newcomer, V. D., and Landau, J. W., 1963b, Effects of cultural conditions on the development of antigens by *Coccidioides immitis, J. Invest. Dermatol.* **41**:343–350.

Salfelder, K. G., Doehnert, G., and Doehnert, H. R., 1969, Paracoccidioidomycosis: Anatomic study with complete autopsies, *Virchow Arch. Pathol. Anat.* **348**:51–76.

Salvin, S. B., 1952, Endotoxin in pathogenic fungi, *J. Immunol.* **69**:89–99.

Salvin, S. B., 1963, Immunologic aspects of the mycoses, *Progr. Allergy* **7**:213–331.

Salvin, S. B., 1965, Constituents of the cell wall of the yeast phase of *Histoplasma capsulatum, Am. Rev. Resp. Dis.* **92**:119–125.

Salvin, S. B., and Smith, R. F., 1959, Antigens from the yeast phase of *Histoplasma capsulatum.* III. Isolation, properties, and activity of a protein-carbohydrate complex, *J. Infect. Dis.* **105**:45–53.

Salvin, S. B., and Smith, R. F., 1961, An antigen for detection for hypersensitivity to *Cryptococcus neoformans, Proc. Soc. Exp. Biol. Med.* **108**:498–501.

Sampaio, S. A. P., 1972, Clinical manifestations of paracoccidioidomycosis, in: *Paracoccidioidomycosis: Proceedings of the First Pan American Symposium,* pp. 101–108, Pan American Health Organization, Scientific Publication No. 254, Washington, D.C.

San-Blas, G., San Blas, F., and Serrano, L. E., 1977, Host parasite relationships in the yeast-like form of *Paracoccidioides brasiliensis* strain IVIC Pb9, *Infect. Immun.* **15**:343–346.

Sarosi, G. A., Parker, J. D., Doto, I. L., and Tosh, F. E., 1970, Chronic pulmonary coccidioidomycosis: A National Communicable Disease Center Cooperative Study, *N. Engl. J. Med.* **283**:325–329.

Sarosi, G. A., Voth, D. W., Dahl, B. A., Doto, I. L., and Tosh, F. E., 1971a, Disseminated histoplasmosis: Results of long-term follow-up, *Ann. Intern. Med.* **75**:511–516.

Sarosi, G. A., Parker, J. D., and Tosh, F. E., 1971b, Histoplasmosis outbreaks: Their patterns, in: *Histoplasmosis: Proceedings of the Second National Conference* (L. Ajello, E. W. Chick, and M. L. Furcolow, eds.), pp. 123–128, Thomas, Springfield, Ill.

Sarosi, G. A., Hammerman, K. J., Tosh, F. E., and Kronenberg, R. S., 1974, Clinical features of acute pulmonary blastomycosis, *N. Engl. J. Med.* **290**:540–543.

Saslow, S., and Schaefer, 1955, Relation of sex and age to resistance of mice to experimental *Histoplasma* infections, *Proc. Soc. Exp. Biol. Med.* **90**:400–402.

Scalarone, G. M., Levine, H. B., Pappagianis, D., and Chaparas, S. D., 1974, Spherulin as a complement-fixing antigen in human coccidioidomycosis, *Am. Rev. Resp. Dis.* **110**:324–328.

Scheer, E., Terai, T., Kulkarn, S., Conant, N. F., Wheat, R. W., and Lowe, E. P., 1970, Unusual reducing sugar from *Coccidioides immitis*, *J. Bacteriol.* **103**:325–326.

Schimpff, S. C., and Bennett, J. E., 1975, Abnormalities in cell-mediated immunity in patients with *Cryptococcus neoformans* infection, *J. Allergy Clin. Immunol.* **55**:430–441.

Schneidau, J. D., Jr., 1972, A cooperative study of cross-reactivity among fungal skin-test antigens in tropical Latin American, in: *Paracoccidioidomycosis: Proceedings of the First Pan American Symposium*, pp. 233–238, Pan American Health Organization, Scientific Publication No. 254, Washington, D.C.

Schneidau, J. D., Jr., Lamar, L. M., and Hairston, M. A., 1964, Cutaneous hypersensitivity to sporotrichin in Louisiana, *J. Am. Med. Assoc.* **188**:371–373.

Schwarz, J., and Baum, G. L., 1951, Blastomycosis, *Am. J. Clin. Pathol.* **21**:999–1029.

Schwarz, J., Silverman, F. N., Adriano, J. H., Straub, M., and Levine, S., 1955, The relation of splenic calcification to histoplasmosis, *N. Engl. J. Med.* **252**:887–891.

Serstock, D. S., and Zinneman, H. H., 1975, Pulmonary and articular sporotrichosis: Report of two cases, *J. Am. Med. Assoc.* **233**:1291–1293.

Sethi, K. K., 1967, Attempts to produce experimental intestinal cryptococcosis and sporotrichosis, *Mycopathol. Mycol. Appl.* **31**:245–250.

Sethi, K. K., and Pelster, B., 1974, Destruction of *Cryptococcus neoformans* by non-specifically activated murine macrophages, in: *Activation of Macrophages: Pro-*ceedings of the Second Workshop Conference Hoechst, Vol. 2 (W. H. Wagner and H. Holm, eds.), Excerpta Medica International Congress Series, No. 325, pp. 269–279, Excerpta Medica, Amsterdam.

Shadomy, H. J., and Utz, J. P., 1966, Preliminary studies on a hypha-forming mutant of *Cryptococcus neoformans*, *Mycologia* **58**:383–390.

Sheldon, W. H., and Bauer, H., 1960, Tissue mast cells and acute inflammation in experimental cutaneous mucormycosis of normal, 48/80-treated, and diabetic rats, *J. Exp. Med.* **112**:1069–1084.

Sieving, R. R., Kauffman, C. A., and Watanakunakorn, C., 1975, Deep fungal infection in systemic lupus erythematosis—Three cases reported, literature reviewed, *J. Rheumatol.* **2**:61–72.

Singer, L. M., and Fava Netto, C., 1972, Conglutinating complement-fixation reaction in paracoccidioidomycosis, in: *Paracoccidioidomycosis: Proceedings of the First Pan American Symposium*, pp. 227–232, Pan American Health Organization, Scientific Publication No. 254, Washington, D.C.

Sixbey, J. W., Fields, B. T., Sun, C. N., Clark, R. A., and Nolan, C. M., 1979, Interactions between human granulocytes and *Blastomyces dermatitidis*, *Infect. Immun.* **23**:41–44.

Smith, C. E., Whiting, E. G., Baker, E. E., Rosenberger, H. G., Beard, R. R., and Saito, M. T., 1948, The use of coccidioidin, *Am. Rev. Tuberc.* **57**:330–360.

Smith, C. E., Saito, M. T., and Simons, S. A., 1956, Pattern of 39,500 serologic tests in coccidioidomycosis, *J. Am. Med. Assoc.* **160**:546–552.

Smith, J. W., and Utz, J. P., 1972, Progressive disseminated histoplasmosis: A prospective study of 25 patients, *Ann. Intern. Med.* **76**:557–565.

Snyderman, R., and Burch, W., 1974, Induction of cellular immunity to *Coccidioides immitis* following sensitization to dinitrochlorobenzene, *Clin. Res.* **22**:30.

Song, M. M., 1971, Experimental cryptococcosis of the skin, *Sabouraudia* **12**:133–137.

Sprouse, R. F., 1971, Preparation and standardization of histoplasmin, in: *Histoplasmosis: Proceedings of the Second National Conference* (L. Ajello, E. W. Chick, and M. L. Furcolow, eds.), pp. 284–293, Thomas, Springfield, Ill.

Sprouse, R. F., 1977, Determination of molecular weight, isoelectric point, and glycoprotein moiety for the principal skin test-reactive component of histoplasmin, *Infect. Immun.* **15**:263–271.

Staib, F., and Mishra, S. K., 1975, Selective involvement of brain in experimental murine cryptococcosis. I. Microbiological observations, *Zbl. Bakt. Hyg. I. Abt. Orig.* **232**:355–364.

Standard, P. G., and Kaufman, L., 1976, Specific immunological test for the rapid identification of members of the genes *Histoplasma*, *J. Clin. Microbiol.* **3**:191–199.

Standard, P. G., and Kaufman, L., 1977, Immunologic procedure for the rapid and specific identification of

Coccidioides immitis cultures, *J. Clin. Microbiol.* 5:149–153.

Steele, R. W., Cannady, P. B., Jr., Moore, W. L., Jr., and Gentry, L. O., 1976, Skin test and blastogenic responses to *Sporotrichum schenckii, J. Clin. Invest.* 57:156–160.

Stevens, D. A., 1975, Transfer factor: Treatment in coccidioidomycosis, in: *Proceedings of the Third International Conference on the Mycoses,* pp. 72–79, Pan American Health Organization, Scientific Publication No. 304, Washington, D.C.

Stevens, D. A., Levine, H. B., and Ten Eyck, D. R., 1974a, Dermal sensitivity to different doses of spherulin and coccidioidin, *Chest* 65:530–533.

Stevens, D. A., Pappagianis, D., Marinkovich, V. A., and Waddell, T. F., 1974b, Immunotherapy in recurrent coccidioidomycosis, *Cell Immunol.* 12:37–48.

Stevens, D. A., Levine, H. B., Deresinski, S. C., and Blaine, L. J., 1975a, Spherulin in clinical coccidioidomycosis: Comparison with coccidioidin, *Chest* 68:697–702.

Stevens, D. A., Ferrington, R. A., Merigan, T. C., and Marinkovich, V. A., 1975b, Randomized trial to transfer factor treatment of human warts, *Clin. Exp. Immunol.* 21:520–524.

Stewart, R. A., and Kimura, F., 1940, Studies in the skin test for coccidioidal infection. I. The preparation and standardization of coccidioidin, *J. Infect. Dis.* 66:212–217.

Stobo, J. D., 1977, Immunosuppression in man: Suppression by macrophages can be mediated by interactions with regulatory T Cells, *J. Immunol.* 119:918–924.

Stobo, J. D., Paul, S., Van Scoy, R. E., and Hermans, P. E., 1976, Suppressor thymus derived lymphocytes in fungal infection. *J. Clin. Invest.* 57:319–328.

Straub, M. M., Schwarz, J., 1955, The healed primary complex in histoplasmosis, *Am. J. Clin. Pathol.* 25:727–741.

Sweigert, C. F., Turner, J. W., Gillespie, J. B., 1946, Clinical and roentgenological aspects of coccidioidomycosis, *Am. J. Med. Sci.* 212:652–673.

Tacker, J. R., Farhi, F., and Bulmer, G. S., 1972, Intracellular fate of *Cryptococcus neoformans, Infect. Immun.* 6:162–167.

Texeira, G. A., Kerr, I. B., Mirander, J. L., Machado Filho, J., and Oliveira, C. A. B., 1969, Blastomicose sul-americana experimental no nato (evolucao da doenca experimental en animals implantados com sarcoma de Yoshida), *Hospital (Rio)* 75:505–510.

Thomas, M. Z., Medoff, G., and Kobayashi, G. S., 1973, Changes in murine resistance to Listeria monocytogenes infection induced by amphotericin B, *J. Infect. Dis.* 127:373–377.

Tindall, J. P., and Elson, M. L., 1974, Cutaneous North American blastomycosis: A review of forty-eight patients, in: *The Diagnosis and Treatment of Fungal Infections* (H. M. Robinson, Jr., ed.), pp. 73–88, Thomas, Springfield, Ill.

Tosh, F. E., Hammerman, K. J., Weeks, R. J., and Sarosi,

G. A., 1974, A common source of epidemic of North American blastomycosis, *Am. Rev. Resp. Dis.* 109:525–529.

Tripodi, D., Parks, L. C., and Brugmans, J., 1973, Drug induced restoration of cutaneous delayed hypersensitivity in anergic patients with cancer, *N. Engl. J. Med.* 289:354–357.

Tynes, B., Mason, K. N., Jennings, A. E., and Bennett, J. E., 1968, Variant forms of pulmonary cryptococcosis, *Ann. Intern. Med.* 69:1117–1125.

Uzman, L. L., Rosen, H., and Foley, G. E., 1956, Studies on the biology of *Cryptococcus.* VI. Amino acid composition of the somatic proteins of *Cryptococcus neoformans, J. Infect. Dis.* 98:208–210.

Vanek, J., and Schwarz, J., 1971, The gamut of histoplasmosis, *Am. J. Med.* 50:89–104.

Vanek, J., Schwarz, J., and Hakim, S., 1970, North American blastomycosis: A study of ten cases, *Am. J. Clin. Pathol.* 54:384–400.

Van Metre, T. G., and Maunseuee, A. E., 1964, Specific ocular uveal lesions in patients with evidence of histoplasmosis, *Arch. Ophthalmol.* 71:304–324.

Walch, H. A., and Kalvoda, A., 1971, Immunization of mice with induced mutants of *Coccidioides immitis.* I. Characterization of mutants and preliminary studies of their use as viable vaccines, *Sabouraudia* 9:173–184.

Ward, E. R., Jr., Cox, R. A., Schmitt, J. A., Huppert, M., and Sun, S. H., 1975, Delayed-type hypersensitivity response to a cell wall fraction of the mycelial phase of *Coccidioides immitis, Infect. Immun.* 12:1093–1097.

Warr, W., Bates, J. H., and Stone, A., 1968, The spectrum of pulmonary cryptococcosis, *Ann. Intern. Med.* 69:1109–1116.

Wegner, T. N., Reed, R. E., Trautman, R. J., and Beavers, C. D., 1972, Some evidence for the development of a phagocytic response by polymorphonuclear leukocytes recovered from the venous blood of dogs inoculated with *Coccidioides immitis* or vaccinated with an irradiated spherule vaccine, *Am. Rev. Resp. Dis.* 105:845–849.

Werner, S. B., Pappagianis, D., Heindl, I., and Mickel, A., 1972, An epidemic of coccidioidomycosis among archeology students in Northern California, *N. Engl. J. Med.* 286:507–512.

Wheat, R. W., and Chung, K. S., 1977, Antigenic fractions of *Coccidioides immitis,* in: *Coccidioidomycosis, Current Clinical and Diagnostic Status* (L. Ajello, ed.), pp. 453–460, Symposia Specialists, Miami/Stratton Intercontinental, New York.

Wheat, R. W., Tritschler, C., Conant, N. F., and Lowe, E. P., 1977, Comparison of *Coccidioides immitis* arthrospore, mycelium, and spherule cell walls, and influence of growth medium on mycelial cell wall composition, *Infect. Immun.* 17:91–97.

Williams, D. M., Graybill, J. R., and Drutz, D. J., 1978, *Histoplasma capsulatum* in nude mice, *Infect. Immun.* 21:973–977.

Wilson, D. E., Mann, J. J., Bennett, J. E., and Utz, J. P.,

1967, Clinical features of extracutaneous sporotrichosis, *Medicine* **46**:265–279.

Wilson, D. E., Bennett, J. E., and Bailey, J. W., 1968, Serologic grouping of *Cryptococcus neoformans, Proc. Soc. Exp. Biol. Med.* **127**:820–823.

Wilson, J. W., 1963, Cutaneous (chancriform) syndrome in deep mycoses, *Arch. Dermatol.* **87**:81–85.

Wilson, W. E. C., Kirkpatrick, C. H., and Talmage, D. W., 1965, Suppression of immunologic responsiveness in uremia, *Ann. Intern. Med.* **62**:1–14.

Wilson, W. R., Ritts, R. E., Jr., and Hermans, P. E., 1977, Abnormal chemotaxis in patients with cutaneous anergy, *Mayo Clin. Proc.* **52**:196–201.

Winn, W. A., 1967, A working classification of coccidioidomycosis and its application to therapy, in: *Coccidioidomycosis: Proceedings of the Second Coccidioidomycosis Symposium,* pp. 3–9, University of Arizona Press, Phoenix.

Winn, W. A., 1968, A long term study of 300 patients with cavitary-abscess lesions of the lung of coccidioidal origin: An analytical study with special reference to treatment, *Dis. Chest* **54**:268–272 (Suppl. 1).

Winn, W. A., Finegold, S. M., and Huntington, R. W., Jr., 1967, Coccidioidomycosis with fungemia, in: *Coccidioidomycosis: Proceedings of the Second Coccidioidomycosis Symposium,* pp. 93–109, University of Arizona Press, Phoenix.

Witorsch, P., and Utz, J. P., 1968, North American blastomycosis: A study of 40 patients, *Medicine* **47**:169–200.

Yarzabal, L. A., 1972, Pathogenesis of paracoccidioidomycosis in man, in: *Paracoccidioidomycosis: Proceedings of the First Pan American Symposium,* pp. 261–270, Pan American Health Organization, Scientific Publication No. 254, Washington, D. C.

Yarzabal, L. A., Torres, J. M., Josef, M., Vigna, I., DaLus, S., and Andrieu, S., 1972, Antigenic mosaic of *Paracoccidioides brasiliensis,* in: *Paracoccidioides: Proceedings of the First Pan American Symposium,* pp. 239–244, Pan American Health Organization, Scientific Publication No. 254, Washington, D.C.

Yarzabal, L. A., Bout, D., Naquira, F., Fruit, J., and Andrieu, S., 1977, Identification and purification of the specific antigen of *Paracoccidioides brasiliensis* responsible for immunoelectrophoretic band E. *Sabouraudia* **15**:79–85.

Zweiman, B., Pappagianis, D., Maibach, A. H., and Hildreth, E. A., 1969, Coccidioidin delayed hypersensitivity: Skin test and *in vitro* lymphocyte reactivities, *J. Immunol.* **102**:1284–1289.

Index